MOSBY'S
Canadian
Comprehensive
Review of Nursing

MOSBY'S Canadian Comprehensive Review of Nursing

Canadian Editor

DONNA L. ROSENTRETER
RN, CAE, BScN, MEd

DOLORES F. SAXTON
RN, BSEd, MA, MPS, EdD

PATRICIA M. NUGENT
RN, AAS, BS, MS, EdM, EdD

PHYLLIS K. PELIKAN
RN, AAS, BS, MA

illustrated

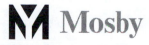 Mosby

St. Louis Baltimore Boston Carlsbad Chicago Naples New York Philadelphia Portland
London Madrid Mexico City Singapore Sydney Tokyo Toronto Wiesbaden

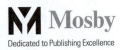
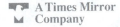

Vice President and Publisher: Nancy L. Coon
Senior Editor: Susan R. Epstein
Associate Developmental Editor: Jerry Schwartz
Project Manager: John Rogers
Production Editor: Chuck Furgason
Composition Specialist: Terri Bovay
Designer: Yael Kats
Manufacturing Manager: Theresa Fuchs

Printed in the United States of America
Composition by Mosby Electronic Production
Printing/binding by Maple-Vail Book Manufacturing Group, Binghamton

Mosby–Year Book, Inc.
11830 Westline Industrial Drive
St. Louis, Missouri 63146

Library of Congress Cataloging-in-Publication Data
Mosby's Canadian comprehensive review of nursing/Canadian editor,
Donna L. Rosentreter; [editor], Dolores F. Saxton; [associate editors], Patricia M. Nugent, Phyllis K. Pelikan.
      p.   cm.
    "Based on the fifteenth edition of Mosby's comprehensive review of nursing"—Pref.
    Includes bibliographical references and index.
    ISBN 0-8151-8673-8 (alk. paper)
    1. Nursing—Examinations, questions, etc. 2. Nursing—Outlines, syllabi, etc.   I. Rosentreter, Donna L.   II. Mosby's comprehensive review of nursing.
    [DNLM: 1. Nursing—outlines. 2. Nursing—examination questions.
3. Legislation, Nursing—Canada.   WY 18.2 M8935 1996]
RT55.M637 1996
610.73' 076—dc20
DNLM/DLC
for Library of Congress
                                       96-43174
                                          CIP

97 98 99 00 01 / 9 8 7 6 5 4 3 2 1

To my daughter, Rieva, whose enthusiasm and optimism for life and whose unremitting faith and love have been an inspiration throughout this undertaking.

Donna Rosentreter

Canadian Contributors

MELANIE BASSO, RN, BScN, MScN
Instructor, Department of Nursing
Langara College, Vancouver, British Columbia

WILLIAM FULTON, RN, BScN, MEd, CBS
Instructor, Nursing Program
Mohawk College, Chedoke Campus, Hamilton,
  Ontario

DAWN KAPLER, RN
Instructor, Health Careers Department
Alberta Vocational College, Edmonton, Alberta

JANE MIGHTON, BSN, MSN
Instructor, Department of Nursing
Langara College, Vancouver, British Columbia

DONNA ROSENTRETER, RN, CAE, BScN,
  MEd
Instructor, Department of Nursing
Langara College, Vancouver, British Columbia

ROBERTA SWANSON, RN, BSN, MSN
Instructor, Department of Nursing
Langara College, Vancouver, British Columbia

SUSAN WARD, BSc, MHA
Director of Education, Canadian Association of
  Medical Radiation Technologists
Ottawa, Ontario

Other Contributors

JANE K. BRODY, RN, BSN, MSN, PhD
Assistant Professor, Department of Nursing
Nassau Community College, Garden City, New York

JO ANN SCHMIDT FESTA, RNC, AAS, BS,
MS, PhD
Professor, Department of Nursing
Nassau Community College, Garden City, New York
President, Hygenia Registered Nursing Enterprises, P.C.

CHRISTINA ALGIERE KASPRISIN, RN, MS
Lecture in Nursing
University of Vermont School of Nursing, Burlington,
Vermont

MILDRED L. MONTAG, RN, BA, BS, MA,
EdD, LLD, LHD, DSc
Professor Emeritus
Teachers College, Columbia University, New York,
New York

THERESA A. MORAN, RN, AAS, BS, EdM, EdD
Chicago, Illinois

SELMA NEEDLEMAN, RN, BA, MA
Professor Emeritus
Nassau Community College, Garden City, New York
Adjunct Faculty, Department of Nursing
St. Petersburg Junior College, St. Petersburg, Florida

PATRICIA A. NUTZ, RN, BS, BSN, MEd, MSN
Instructor, School of Nursing
St. Francis Hospital, New Castle, Pennsylvania

TERRY F. O'DWYER, BS, PhD
Professor, Department of Engineering/Physics/
Technology
Nassau Community College, Garden City, New York

JANICE J. RUMFELT, RN, BSN, MSN, EdD
Southern Illinois University at Edwardsville School of
Nursing
Edwardsville, Illinois

LINDA CARMAN COPEL, RN, BSN, MS,
MSN, PhD
Villanova University College of Nursing
Villanova, Pennsylvania

CAROL COOKLEY GENEREUX, RN, BSN,
MSN
New England Baptist Hospital School of Nursing
Boston, Massachusetts

MARILYN M. MOHR, RN, BSN, MSN
Missouri Baptist Medical Center School of Nursing
St. Louis, Missouri

ANN T. MULLER, RN, BS, MEd, PhD
Private Practice
Dallas, Texas

MARY JANE REUMANN, RN, BSN, MSN
University of Alabama in Huntsville
Huntsville, Alabama

LINDA OWEN RIMER, RN, BSN, MSE
University of Arkansas at Little Rock
Little Rock, Arkansas

MARY ANN HELLMER SAUL, RNCS, AAS,
BS, MS, PhD
Professor, Department of Nursing
Nassau Community College, Garden City, New York

CAROL G. SCOTT, RN, AS, BSN, MSN
Lynchburg General Hospital School of Nursing
Lynchburg, Virginia

MARY SIROTNIK, Reg N, BScN, MEd
Mack Centre of Nursing Education, Niagara College
of Applied Arts and Technology
St. Catharines, Ontario, Canada

ANITA THROWE, RN, BSN, MS
Associate Professor of Nursing
Medical University of South Carolina,
College of Nursing
Satellite at Francis Marion University, Florence,
South Carolina

FRANCES A. WOLLNER, RN, BS, BSN, MN
Grand Island, New York

Canadian Reviewers

DEBBIE FRASER ASKIN, MN, RNC, CNS, NNP
St. Boniface General Hospital
Winnipeg, Manitoba

JUDITH BUCHANAN, MHSc, CPMHN (C)
Assistant Professor
University of New Brunswick
Saint John, New Brunswick

KAREN JENSEN, RN, BSN, MN
Lecturer, Faculty of Nursing
University of Manitoba
Winnipeg, Manitoba

SHARON MCMAHON, BScN, MEd, EdD, RN
Associate Professor
University of Windsor
Windsor, Ontario

MARY SIROTNIK, BScN, MEd, EdD, RN
Registered Nurse/Teacher
Mack Centre of Nursing and Education, Niagara
 College of Applied Arts and Technology
St. Catharines, Ontario

Other Reviewers

BERNADINE ADAMS, RN, BSN, MN
Associate Professor, School of Nursing
Northeast Louisiana University
Monroe, Louisiana

PATRICIA A. CASTALDI, RN, MSN
Assistant Dean, School of Nursing
Elizabeth General Medical Center
Elizabeth, New Jersey

EMILY DRAKE, RN, C, MSN
Clinical Instructor
University of Virginia
Charlottesville, Virginia

HEYWARD MICHAEL DREHER, RN, BSN, MN
Assistant Professor of Nursing
LaSalle University
Philadelphia, Pennsylvania

ELIZABETH GILBERT, RNC, MS
Associate Professor
Grand Canyon University
Phoenix, Arizona

EARL GOLDBERG, RN, MSN, CS
Associate Professor of Nursing
Bucks County Community College
Newtown, Pennsylvania

RENEE COVEY HARRISON, RN, BSN, MS
Assistant Professor
Tulsa Junior College
Tulsa, Oklahoma

MARY REUTHER HERRING, RN, BSN, MSN
Occupational Health Nurse, Motorola
Faculty, University of Phoenix
Phoenix, Arizona

DAVID C. KELLER, MS, APRN
Instructor, College of Nursing
Brigham Young University
Provo, Utah

NELLIE NELSON, RN, MSN, CARN
Nursing Faculty
Scottsdale Community College and
University of Phoenix
Phoenix, Arizona

KAREN A. PIOTROWSKI, RNC, MSN
Assistant Professor, Division of Nursing
D'Youville College
Buffalo, New York

DEBORAH SCOTT, RN, DSN
Associate Professor, School of Nursing
Acting Assistant Dean, Undergraduate Program
University of Louisville
Louisville, Kentucky

APRIL SIEH, RN, BSN, MSN
Assistant Professor of Nursing
Delta College
University Center, Michigan

DOROTHY THOMAS, RN, BSN, MSN
Associate Professor of Nursing
St. Louis Community College at Florissant Valley
St. Louis, Missouri

B. JANE THREATT, ARNP, BSN, MSN, CCRN
Assistant Professor
University of Florida
Gainesville, Florida

Preface

The material in *Mosby's Canadian Comprehensive Review of Nursing* is based on the fifteenth edition of *Mosby's Comprehensive Review of Nursing*. The progression of subject matter in each area reflects the consistent approach that has been used throughout the book. Information presented incorporates the latest knowledge, newest trends, and current practices in the profession of nursing in Canada.

In Chapter 1, direction is given on how to study and use the review to prepare for the Nurse Registration/Licensure examination. In Chapter 2, components of Canadian nursing practice are covered and include the health-illness continuum and health resources; nursing practice and the law in Canada; and the nurse's role. Highlighted in the section on the nurse's role are those topics the student of today needs to know to function as tomorrow's practitioner: communication, the nursing process, the teaching-learning environment, leadership, and the administration of medications. A list of nursing diagnoses as developed by the North American Nursing Diagnosis Association at the National Conference held in 1994 has also been included.

The medical-surgical, childbearing and women's health, pediatric, and psychiatric/mental health chapters incorporate material from the basic sciences, nutrition, pharmacology, and rehabilitation. The material is presented in the traditional clinical groupings, because when preparing for a comprehensive examination, many students refer to all the distinct parts before attempting to put them together.

Although we believe that in practice the nursing process is continuously evolving rather than remaining a clearly defined step-by-step procedure, we present the content under the headings: Data Collection, Analysis and Interpretation, Planning/Implementation, and Evaluation/Outcomes. We trust that this grouping avoids needless repetition, recognizes the abilities of our readers, and reflects current practice.

This edition contains, for every question following the individual chapters as well as for every question in the comprehensive test, the reasons why the incorrect answers are incorrect as well as why the correct answer is correct. In the comprehensive test, we have analyzed each question as to the step in the nursing process, the level of cognitive ability (or the affective domain), the area of client needs, the content area/category of concern (the specific content within the broad clinical area), and the client's age and gender.

We have added 2 steps, Collaboration and Coordination and Professional Practice to the traditional steps in the nursing process. These steps are defined by the Canadian Nurses Association (see Appendix).

The questions following each chapter are analyzed as to the step in the nursing process, area of client needs, and content area/category of concern. To further assist the user in studying/reviewing by a specific content area, questions have been grouped according to their content area/category of concern. Questions related to nutrition have been integrated into the appropriate content area/category of concern in each clinical area.

The comprehensive integrated test at the end of the text provides an opportunity to apply material from the specific clinical areas to any nursing situation. This examination consists of 250 questions and approximates the blueprint for the Nurse Registration/Licensure examination.

All the questions used in this book have been submitted by outstanding educators and practitioners of nursing. Initially the editorial panel reviewed all questions, selecting the most pertinent for inclusion in a mass field-testing project.

We would like to acknowledge and thank the following individuals for their time, support, and expertise in the preparation of this text: Marc Gluckman, Marketing Manager, for his vision; Susan Epstein,

Senior Editor, for her coordination; Jerry Schwartz, Associate Developmental Editor, for his patience and sense of humor in supervision; Ross McIvor, Marketing Representative, for his confidence, encouragement, and support; Dolores Saxton, Patricia Nugent, and Phyllis Pelikan, Editors of *Mosby's Comprehensive Review of Nursing,* for making this project a reality; and Chuck Furgason, Production Editor, for his diligence in preparing the manuscript. We would also like to recognize the numerous consultants, including Mervin Wildeman, BSP, MSc, Pharmacist, for invaluable assistance. We wish to express gratitude to the Canadian Nurses Association for sharing the Nurse Examination List of Competencies, which are appended in this text and which provide a foundation for the content area being evaluated. Also, we wish to recognize student nurses from across Canada who were a source of motivation for this project. Finally, we wish to acknowledge our families and friends for their unconditional faith in our venture.

As individuals, we are absorbed in ways to empower human beings that they might achieve and maintain health. As educators, we are equally absorbed in facilitating nursing students' education as they acquire the knowledge and confidence to meet the challenges of the Nurse Registration/Licensure examination and the requisites that are essential as they embark on a career in nursing that will take them into the new millennium.

Melanie Basso
Willian Fulton
Dawn Kapler
Jane Mighton
Donna Rosentreter
Roberta Swanson
Susan Ward

Contents

Detailed Contents

4 Psychiatric/Mental Health Nursing, *161*

CHAPTER 1

Introduction for Students Preparing for the Nurse Registration/Licensure Examination

The Nurse Registration/Licensure examinations in Canada have been integrated and comprehensive for many years. Nursing candidates are required to answer questions that necessitate a recognition and understanding of the physiologic, biologic, and social sciences, as well as the specific nursing skills and abilities involved in a given client situation.

This text contains objective multiple-choice questions. To answer the questions appropriately, a candidate needs to understand and correlate certain aspects of anatomy and physiology, the behavioral sciences, basic nursing, the effects of medications administered, the client's attitude toward illness, and other pertinent factors such as legal responsibilities. Most questions are based on nursing situations similar to those with which candidates have had experience to emphasize the nursing care of clients with representative common national health problems. Some questions, however, require candidates to apply basic principles and techniques to clinical situations with which they have had little, if any, actual experience.

To prepare adequately for an integrated comprehensive examination, it is necessary to understand the discrete parts that compose the universe under consideration. This is one of the major principles of learning on which *Mosby's Canadian Comprehensive Review of Nursing* has been developed.

Using this principle, the text first presents a review of each major clinical area. Each review is followed by questions that test the student's knowledge of principles and theories underlying nursing care in a variety of situations, in a variety of settings, and with a variety of nursing goals. Rationales for the correct answers and incorrect options follow the questions at the end of each chapter. By reviewing the rationales the student is able to verify information and reinforce knowledge.

A comprehensive examination, consisting of approximately 250 questions, is provided to approximate the Nurse Registration/Licensure Examination and Blueprint. The questions require the student to cross clinical disciplines and respond to individual and specific needs associated with given health problems. Rationales are also provided for the correct answers and the incorrect options to these questions.

Similar to those in the comprehensive registration/licensure examinations, all questions have been classified by phases of the nursing process and area of client needs. To provide a more inclusive study guide for the student, we have added the category of concern (see p. 3) to all questions and the cognitive level and client age and gender to the questions in the comprehensive test.

The following descriptions and the five sample questions on p. 4 are presented to assist you in understanding these classifications.

PHASES OF THE NURSING PROCESS (TYPES OF BEHAVIORS OF THE NURSE)

1. Data Collection (DC). The data collection (assessment) phase requires the nurse to obtain objective and subjective data from primary and secondary sources, to identify and group pertinent data, and to communicate this information to other members of the health team, which may include the client. The information necessary for making nursing decisions is obtained through a process of data collection that is founded on a nursing model or framework. Sample question 1 is a data collection question.

2. Analysis and Interpretation (AN). This phase requires the nurse to interpret data gathered during the data collection phase. A nursing diagnosis must be made, client and family needs identified, and both short-term and long-term goals set to meet the identified needs. Sample question 2 is an analysis and interpretation question.

3. Planning (PL). The planning phase requires the nurse to design a regimen with the client and family to achieve goals set during the analysis and interpretation phase. It also requires setting priorities for nursing interventions. Sample question 3 is a planning question.

4. Implementation (IM). The implementation phase requires the nurse to provide care designed during the planning phase. The client may be given total care or may be assisted and encouraged to perform activities of daily living or follow the regimen prescribed by the health professional. Implementation also includes activities such as counseling, teaching/coaching, and supervising. Sample question 4 is an implementation question.

5. Evaluation (EV). This phase requires the nurse to determine the effectiveness of nursing care. The goals of care are reviewed, the client's response to intervention identified, and a consideration made as to whether the client has achieved the predetermined outcomes and goals. Evaluation also includes appraisal of the client's response to and perception of the health plan. Sample question 5 is an evaluation question.

6. Collaboration and Coordination (CC). The collaboration and coordination activities require the nurse to liaise and work together with other members of the nursing and health care teams during the many phases of the nursing process and to ensure that the care provided is client-focused, participative, coordinated, integrated, and comprehensive. Collaboration and coordination also include activities such as communi-

cation with the health team (which may include the client), delegation, and leadership.

7. Professional Practice (PP). The professional practice activities require the nurse to practice within existing professional, legal, and ethical standards and to oversee practice according to established standards. Professional practice also includes activities such as maintaining the client's privacy and confidentiality; demonstrating respect for the client and members of the health care team; and monitoring and ensuring the quality of health care practices.

COGNITIVE LEVELS (TYPES OF INTELLECTUAL PROCESSES) AND THE AFFECTIVE DOMAIN

1. Knowledge/Comprehension (KC). The knowledge level of the intellectual process requires recollection of facts about principles, theories, terms, or procedures. Knowledge questions, which require the examinee to define, identify, or select, involve the ability to recall information (a basic cognitive skill). The comprehension level of the intellectual process requires demonstration of understanding or interpretation of the subject matter presented. The examinee is required to interpret, explain, distinguish, or predict. Sample questions 1 and 2 are knowledge/comprehension questions.

2. Application (AP). The application level of the intellectual process requires the examinee not only to know and understand information, but also to apply it to a new situation. When applying comprehended information, the examinee must show, solve, modify, change, manipulate, use, demonstrate, or teach in a specific client situation. Sample question 3 is an application question.

3. Critical Thinking (CT). The critical thinking level of the intellectual process requires the recognition of inherent structure and the relation between component parts, as well as an understanding of the underlying concepts or principles. If the examinee is required to analyze, evaluate, judge, problem-solve, select, differentiate, or interpret data from a variety of sources before responding, the question is a critical thinking question. Sample question 5 is a critical thinking question.

4. Affective Domain (AF). The affective domain reflects certain attributes which are attitudinal and do not fall strictly within the cognitive or intellectual domain. The affective domain requires the examinee to consider one's values when dealing with a client, to compare and contrast the attitudes of other care providers, and to constructively criticize conflicting values in health care. Sample question 4 is an affective domain question.

CLIENT NEEDS (REFLECT THOSE HEALTH CARE NEEDS OF THE CLIENT THAT MUST BE ADDRESSED BY THE NURSE)

1. Support and promotion of physiologic and anatomic equilibrium (PA). Meeting this need includes reducing risks that interfere with physiologic or anatomic integrity, promoting comfort and mobility, and providing basic care to assist, modify, or limit physiologic and anatomic adaptations. Sample question 1 reflects this need.

2. An environment that is safe and conducive to effective therapeutic care (TC). The nurse must provide quality, goal-directed care that is coordinated, safe, and effective. Sample questions 4 and 5 reflect this need.

3. Education and other forms of health promotion to prevent, minimize, or correct actual or potential health problems (ED). Fulfilling this need involves supporting optimal growth and development to provide for the achievement of the highest levels of functioning. This includes encouraging use of support systems and self-care directed toward promoting the prevention, recognition, and treatment of disease throughout the life cycle. Sample question 3 reflects this need.

4. Support and promotion of psychosocial and emotional equilibrium (PS). Addressing this need includes supporting individual emotional coping and adapting mechanisms to promote optimal emotional health while limiting or modifying those responses to crises that produce psychopathologic consequences. Sample question 2 reflects this need.

CATEGORY OF CONCERN (SPECIFIC CONTENT WITHIN BROAD CLINICAL AREAS)

1. The categories of concern used in medical, surgical, and pediatric nursing include emotional needs related to health problems (EH); respiratory (RE); reproductive and genitourinary (RG); neuromuscular (NM); skeletal (SK); endocrine (EN); integumentary (IT); gastrointestinal (GI); fluid and electrolyte (FE); cardiovascular (CV); blood and immunity (BI); growth and development (GD); and drug-related responses (DR). Sample question 1 reflects information related to cardiovascular content. Sample question 4

reflects information related to growth and development. Sample question 5 reflects information related to blood and immunity content.

2. The categories of concern used in childbearing and women's health nursing include emotional needs related to childbearing (EC); drug-related responses (DR); healthy childbearing (HC); high-risk neonate (HN); high-risk maternal-fetal conditions affecting childbearing (HP); normal neonate (NN); reproductive choices (RC); reproductive problems (RP); and women's health (WH). Sample question 2 reflects information related to healthy childbearing content.

3. The categories of concern used in psychiatric/mental health nursing include anxiety, somatoform, and dissociative disorders (AX); crisis situations (CS); dementia, delirium, and other cognitive disorders (DD); disorders first evident before adulthood (BA); disorders of personality (PR); disorders of mood (MO); eating disorders (EA); personality development (PD); schizophrenic disorders (SD); substance abuse (SA); emotional problems related to physical health and childbearing (EP); drug-related responses (DR); and therapeutic relationships (TR). Sample question 3 reflects information related to drug-related responses.

CLIENT AGE AND GENDER

The categories used in client age and gender include: child and adolescent (CM for males and CF for females), representing ages 0 to 18; adult (AM for males and AF for females), representing ages 19 to 64; and older adult (OM for males and OF for females), representing ages 65 years and older.

SAMPLE QUESTIONS

1. A client is admitted to the intensive care unit with a diagnosis of Adams-Stokes syndrome. What symptom should the nurse be looking for when collecting information from the client?
    1. Nausea and vertigo
    2. Flushing and slurred speech
    3. Cephalalgia and blurred vision
    4. Syncope and low ventricular rate
2. Two days after the birth of her child a client primarily focuses on her own needs. The nurse recognizes that the client is in the phase of maternal adjustment known as:
    1. Taking-in phase
    2. Letting-go phase
    3. Interdependent phase
    4. Dependent-independent phase

3. What should the nurse caution a client against when taking monoamine oxidase (MAO) inhibitors?
    1. Ingesting wine and cheeses
    2. Prolonged exposure to the sun
    3. Engaging in active physical exercise
    4. Using medications with an elixir base
4. A young boy, age 4, has been hospitalized for fever of undetermined origin (FUO). He screams and becomes uncontrollable as his mother leaves after visiting hours. What would be the best approach by the nurse?
    1. Ignore this outburst
    2. Sit quietly at his bedside
    3. Give him a favorite toy to hold
    4. Hold and pat him even though he struggles
5. After surgery, while receiving a blood transfusion, a client develops chills and headache. Based on an evaluation of the client, the nurse's best action is to:
    1. Lightly cover the client
    2. Notify the physician STAT
    3. Stop the transfusion immediately
    4. Slow the blood flow to keep the vein open

HOW TO USE THIS BOOK IN STUDYING

A. Start in one area. Study the material covered by the section. Refer to other textbooks to find additional details if you are unsure of a specific fact.
B. Answer the questions following the area. As you answer each question, write a few words about why you think that answer was correct; in other words, justify why you selected the answer. If you guess at an answer in this book you should make a special mark to identify it. This will permit you to recognize areas that need further review. It will also help you to see how correct your "guessing" can be. Remember, on the Nurse Registration/Licensure examination, you should try to answer every question, even if you guess at the option that appears best.
C. Record the answer by filling in the numbered circle next to the one you believe is correct.
D. Tear out the sheets with the answers for the area you are studying and compare your answers with those provided. If you answered the item correctly, check your reason for selecting the answer with the rationale presented. If you answered the item incorrectly, read the rationale to determine why the one you selected was incorrect. In addition, you should review the correct answer and rationale for each item answered incorrectly. If you still do not understand your mistakes, look up the theory pertaining

to these questions. You should carefully review all questions and rationales for items you identified as guesses, because you have not yet demonstrated mastery of the material being questioned.

E. Following the rationales, in the parentheses you will find a grouping of letters that classify the questions according to the following categories:

1. *Nursing process*
   - (DC) Data collection
   - (AN) Analysis and interpretation
   - (PL) Planning
   - (IM) Implementation
   - (EV) Evaluation
   - (CC) Collaboration and coordination
   - (PP) Professional practice

2. *Cognitive levels and affective domain*
   - (KC) Knowledge/Comprehension
   - (AP) Application
   - (CT) Critical thinking
   - (AF) Affective domain

3. *Area of client needs*
   - (PA) Physiologic and anatomic equilibrium
   - (TC) Therapeutic care
   - (ED) Education and health promotion
   - (PS) Psychosocial and emotional equilibrium

4. *Category of concern*

   Medical, surgical, and pediatric nursing
   - (EH) Emotional needs related to health problems
   - (RE) Respiratory
   - (RG) Reproductive and genitourinary
   - (NM) Neuromuscular
   - (SK) Skeletal
   - (EN) Endocrine
   - (IT) Integumentary
   - (GI) Gastrointestinal
   - (FE) Fluid and electrolyte
   - (CV) Cardiovascular
   - (BI) Blood and immunity
   - (GD) Growth and development
   - (DR) Drug-related responses

   Childbearing and women's health nursing
   - (EC) Emotional needs related to childbearing
   - (HC) Healthy childbearing
   - (HP) High-risk maternal-fetal conditions affecting childbearing
   - (RC) Reproductive choices
   - (RP) Reproductive problems
   - (NN) Normal neonate
   - (HN) High-risk neonate
   - (DR) Drug-related responses
   - (WH) Women's health

   Psychiatric/mental health nursing
   - (BA) Disorders first evident before adulthood
   - (EA) Eating disorders
   - (PR) Disorders of personality
   - (MO) Disorders of mood
   - (SD) Schizophrenic disorders
   - (AX) Anxiety, somatoform, and dissociative disorders
   - (SA) Substance abuse
   - (CS) Crisis situations
   - (DR) Drug-related responses
   - (TR) Therapeutic relationships
   - (DD) Dementia, delirium, and other cognitive disorders
   - (EP) Emotional problems related to physical health and childbearing
   - (PD) Personality development

5. *Client age and gender*
   - (CM) Child/adolescent male
   - (CF) Child/adolescent female
   - (AM) Adult male
   - (AF) Adult female
   - (OM) Older adult male
   - (OF) Older adult female

F. For the review questions that follow the clinical areas (e.g., Pediatric Nursing, Psychiatric/Mental Health Nursing), the series of classification letters follows the same order as for the questions in the Comprehensive Test, but is less detailed. Clinical area review questions are classified for the phase of the nursing process, area of client needs, and content area/category of concern. Comprehensive test questions are classified for the phase of the nursing process, cognitive level or affective domain, area of client needs, content area/category of concern, and client age and gender.

G. A few days later, review the area again and retake the questions following it. If you miss the same questions again, you need further study of the material.

H. To study questions for a specific content/area category of concern, refer to the list following the clinical review material in each of the clinical areas. These lists contain the content area/categories of concern for that clinical area and the numbers of the questions that deal with material related to each category. In addition the questions following the chapter are grouped by the content area/categories of concern.

I. After you have completed the clinical area questions, begin taking the comprehensive test because it will assist you in applying knowledge and principles from the specific clinical area to any nursing situation.

1. Arrange a quiet, uninterrupted time span for each part of the comprehensive test.
2. Avoid spending excessive time on any one question. Most questions can be answered in 1 to 2 minutes.
3. Make educated guesses.

4. Read carefully and answer the question asked; pay attention to specific details in the question.
5. Try putting questions and answers in your own words to test your comprehension.

J. To help analyze your mistakes on the comprehensive examination and to provide a data base for making future study plans, worksheets are included. These worksheets are designed to aid you in identifying and recording errors in the way you process information and to help you identify and record gaps in knowledge. These worksheets follow the Answers and Rationales for each part of the Comprehensive Test and are on tear-out sheets also.

K. After completing your worksheets, do the following:
1. Identify the frequency with which you made particular errors. As you review material in class notes or this review book, pay special attention to correcting your most common problems.
2. Identify the topics you want to review. It might be helpful to set priorities; review the most difficult topics first so that you will have time to review them more than once.

GENERAL CLUES FOR ANSWERING MULTIPLE-CHOICE QUESTIONS

On a multiple-choice test the question and possible answers are called a *test item*. The part of the item that asks the question or poses a problem is called the *stem*. All of the answers presented are called *options*. One of the options is the correct answer; the remainder are incorrect. The incorrect options are called *distractors* because their major purpose is to distract the test taker from the correct answer.

A. Read the question carefully before looking at the answers.
1. Attempt to determine what the question is really asking; look for key words.
2. Read each answer thoroughly and see if it completely covers the material asked by the question.
3. Narrow the choices by immediately eliminating answers you know are incorrect.

B. Because few things in life are absolute without exceptions, avoid selecting answers that include words such as always, never, all, every, and none, since answers containing these key words are rarely correct.

C. Attempt to select the answer that is most complete and includes the other answers within it. An example might be as follows:
A child's intelligence is influenced by:
1. A variety of factors

2. Heredity and environment
3. Environment and experience
4. Education and economic factors

The most correct answer is 1 because it includes all the other answers.

D. Make certain that the answer you select is reasonable and obtainable under ordinary circumstances and that the action can be carried out in the given situation.

E. Watch for grammatical inconsistencies. If one or more of the options is not grammatically consistent with the stem, the alert test taker can identify it as a probable distractor. When the stem is in the form of an incomplete sentence, each option should complete the sentence in a grammatically correct way.

F. Avoid selecting answers that state hospital rules or regulations as a reason or rationale for action.

G. Look for answers that focus on the client or are directed toward feelings.

H. If the question asks for an immediate action or response, all the answers may be correct, so base your selection on identified priorities for action.

I. Do not select answers that contain exceptions to the general rule, controversial material, or degrading responses.

J. Reread the question if the answers do not seem to make sense, because you may have missed words such as *not* or *except* in the statement.

K. Do not worry if you select the same numbered answer repeatedly, because there is usually no pattern to the answers.

L. Mark the numbered circle next to the answer you have chosen.

M. If you are not sure of an answer to a question, you can skip it and return to it later on. While answering subsequent questions on the exam, you might see something that jogs your memory on the question you skipped. Just remember that if you are skipping questions, you need to return to them later on. You should leave them blank on your computer answer sheet until such a time as you do select an answer.

PREPARING FOR THE NURSE REGISTRATION/LICENSURE EXAMINATION

A few individuals can improve their scores significantly by a highly concentrated period of study immediately before taking an examination. Most, however, profit by spreading their review over a much longer period of time, and the best time to begin studying for the Nurse Registration/Licensure examination is the first class attended.

After you have completed studying this text, you may find it beneficial and enlightening to take *Mosby's AssessTest* to evaluate your level of preparation. The *AssessTest* is a computer-scored, multiple-choice examination designed to test nursing knowledge and evaluate your ability to apply that knowledge in clinical situations. The extensive computer analysis of your performance, which is the most outstanding feature of this test, will help you design effective and efficient plans for further study and review. Identification of your own *specific* strengths and weaknesses should eliminate much of the anxiety of deciding what material to study by giving you a sense of direction and a means of setting priorities.

TAKING THE NURSE REGISTRATION/LICENSURE EXAMINATION

The two most crucial requisites for doing well on the Nurse Registration/Licensure examination are a sound understanding of the subject and a high level of reading comprehension. Determination to do well and a degree of confidence will further enhance the well-prepared individual's chances of being successful. At least three other requirements must be met if an individual's performance is to accurately reflect professional competence.

First, the candidate must follow explicitly the directions given at the beginning of the test.

Second, the candidate must read each question carefully before deciding how to answer it.

Third, the candidate must correctly transfer answers selected to the computer answer sheet.

CHAPTER 2

Components of Nursing Practice

CONCEPTUAL INTRODUCTION

THE HEALTH-WELLNESS CONTINUUM

Introduction

A. Health care is a generally accepted right; well-being is the norm toward which most governments and all health personnel direct their efforts

B. One of the primary functions of health care professions is to help individuals, families, and groups reach the highest level of wellness of which they are capable

C. A person's perception of health is based on a complex interrelationship among the physiologic, emotional, social, economic, intellectual, cultural, and developmental components of the self

D. A person's perception of health is unique and may differ from that of significant others and that of health care providers

Definition

A. The World Health Organization (WHO) states, "Health is a state of complete physical, mental, and social well-being and not just the absence of disease or infirmity"

B. This definition implies that there is:
1. Interaction between self and environment
2. Preservation of structure and function
3. Maintenance of adaptive potential

C. Significance of definition
1. Accepted right of all rather than a privilege restricted to a few; a desire to improve health is generally universal
2. Reciprocal relationships between individual health and community health
3. Need for nursing and medical practice to move toward maintenance and promotion of health and rehabilitation of the ill rather than merely to focus on provision of episodic care

D. Concerns related to the WHO definition
1. Unrealistic for underdeveloped countries and those living in poverty
2. Difficult to always determine scientifically when one is healthy and when one becomes ill
3. Many people who consider themselves healthy would not be considered healthy according to this definition
4. Presents an ideal to work toward rather than an achievable goal; health status is always changing

Basic Concepts

A. Health: a dynamic state that is continually changing
1. Moves on a continuum between optimal wellness (where potential is maximized and used with purpose) and death, rather than an absolute state

2. Change may be gradual or abrupt
3. Level attainable depends on adaptive capacity, genetic and environmental factors, and lifestyle
   a. Fluctuates throughout life cycle
   b. Varies among individuals
4. Individual may or may not be aware of change
5. Person's position on the continuum determined by:
   a. Ability to adapt
   b. Level of adaptation
   c. Culture's view of health
   d. Ability to carry out social, family, and job responsibilities
   e. Risk factors

B. Stresses affect physical, emotional, and social health
1. May be internal or external
2. Can be beneficial or detrimental to life
   a. Tension is essential to life
   b. Stress of life causes wear and tear
      (1) Produces a nonspecific response that Hans Selye identified as the general adaptation syndrome (GAS)
      (2) Three stages: alarm, resistance, and exhaustion
   c. The same stress may be detrimental to one person and beneficial to another or could be detrimental at one time during a person's life and beneficial at another
3. Elicit some response from or change in the individual
4. Vary widely for different individuals and within the same individual at different times
5. Tolerance is individual
6. Sources of stress (with examples)
   a. Physical: thermal, acoustic
   b. Chemical: gas, toxic wastes
   c. Microbiologic: viral, bacterial
   d. Physiologic: neoplasmic, hypofunctional, hyperfunctional
   e. Developmental: genetic, aging
   f. Psychologic: value conflicts, threats to self-image
7. Stress can threaten homeostasis in the physical, emotional, intellectual, social, and spiritual dimensions of the self
8. Stress can alter how a person meets basic human needs
9. That which causes a stress is a stressor
10. Stressors can be eliminated, avoided, minimized, or responded and/or adapted to
11. Illness results when one is unable to cope with stress and requires a balancing of a person's physical, social, psychological, and spiritual dimensions

C. Rehabilitation assists people in attaining their maximum level of wellness on the continuum after a negative change in health status has occurred

1. Particularly concerned with establishing function that is lost while expanding, maintaining, and supporting the limited remaining function
2. Immediate or potential needs exhibited in all health problems
3. The client is the primary rehabilitator; professional health team members assist the client and family with the process of self-rehabilitation
4. Not an isolated process; rehabilitation involves the client, family, health team, community, and society
5. Concerned with all levels of prevention: primary, secondary, and tertiary
6. Health problems that cause disabilities are socially significant because of the number of people affected, economic cost and loss, distress of personal suffering, and conditions in society that increase their incidence
7. More individuals are candidates for rehabilitation than ever before because of:
   a. Advances in technology
   b. Persons surviving birth defects and traumatic injuries that were once fatal
   c. Aging of society and more chronic illness
8. Rehabilitation focuses on interventions that improve the quality of life rather than those that are life saving; health care resources and prestige often are allocated more for critical care than rehabilitation

THE HEALTH CARE SYSTEM

SPONSORSHIP OF SERVICES

Public

A. Definition: publicly financed insurance program providing universal coverage for hospital and medical costs for all Canadians; federal-provincial funding through Canada Social Transfer Program (CST); jurisdictional authority lies within the provinces/territories

1. Canada Health Act (1984) principles: universality, comprehensiveness, accessibility, portability, public administration; user-fees and extra billing banned

B. Examples

1. National: Health Canada
2. Provincial: Ministry of Health (e.g., Ontario government administers the Ontario Health Insurance Plan [OHIP])
3. Local: regional or city departments of health

Private

A. Definition: publicly financed insurance program providing all basic health care coverage which may be supplemented by purchase of private plans to cover services beyond those covered by public insurance program (e.g., drug benefits; semi and private accomodation; dental coverage; eyeglass purchase; etc.)

B. Examples

1. Home care services: Interim Healthcare, Para-Med Health Services
2. Private Pay Care Facilities: Fraserview Intermediate Care Lodge and Courtyard Gardens in Richmond, British Columbia
3. Professional: dentists, nurses, massage therapists, chiropractors, naturopaths, psychologists, social workers

Voluntary

A. Definition: not-for-profit organizations consisting of lay and professional persons dedicated to the prevention and solution of health problems by providing educational, research, and service programs; these agencies depend on voluntary donations of funds and services as a significant component of their income, are often concerned with specific health problems

B. Examples

1. National: Heart and Stroke Foundation of Canada, Canadian Cancer Society, Multiple Sclerosis Society of Canada
2. Provincial/territorial: divisions of national organizations
3. Local: branches of provincial/territorial voluntary organizations; volunteers (e.g., hospital women's auxiliary, a Girl Guide company visiting a nursing home, a church group visiting a group home)

ENTRY INTO THE HEALTH CARE SYSTEM

A. In response to a self-identified health need
B. Emergency department of a hospital

TYPES OF SERVICES

A. Health promotion

1. Services designed to reduce risk of illness, maintain maximal function, and promote good health habits
2. Examples: prenatal nutrition classes, exercise classes, stress management classes

B. Illness prevention

1. Services designed to reduce risk factors in an effort to avoid primary, secondary, or tertiary health intervention
2. Examples: support groups to give up smoking, controlling the breeding of insects, education

programs on acquired immunodeficiency syndrome (AIDS) prevention, immunization

C. Diagnosis and treatment
   1. This has been the most commonly used service of health care; usually sought once a person feels ill or a problem is indicated
   2. Examples: teaching about breast self-examination (early diagnosis), vision-screening programs at schools, treatments provided in any health care setting

D. Rehabilitation
   1. The restoration of a person to their highest level of functioning, maximizing abilities and independence
   2. Programs have extended beyond helping those with illnesses or injuries to the nervous system; rehabilitation programs include those for cardiovascular, pulmonary, and chemical-induced impairments
   3. Involves the client, family, and the entire health team who individualize a rehabilitation program for the client
   4. Provided in various settings (e.g., hospital, home, nursing home, outpatient setting)

HEALTH CARE SERVICE SETTINGS

Institutional Care

A. Refers to all acute care hospitals, and other institutions such as homes for the elderly, institutions for the mentally and physically challenged, and treatment centers for substance abusers; special hospitals (rehabilitation, children's)
   1. Includes public and private hospitals
   2. Provides acute, chronic, and convalescent care
   3. Acute care hospitals account for most of the health care cost

B. Acute care institutions: provide short-term care for clients undergoing treatment for a health problem; intensive care to meet needs of the acutely ill client undergoing treatment for a health problem; ambulatory care for short stay surgery or medical treatment; and emergency care for acute, short-term problems

C. Rehabilitation institutions: provide multiple services and facilities that assist a client and family to make an adjustment to living; the client can obtain an optimal level of health by developing personal abilities to their fullest potential and using the following resources:
   1. Physical: total health assessment, planning, and intervention (e.g., medical, nursing, physical therapy, occupational therapy, and speech therapy)
   2. Psychosocial: personal counseling, social service, and psychiatric service

3. Vocational: work evaluation, vocational counseling, vocational training, trial employment in sheltered workshops, terminal employment in sheltered workshops, and job placement

D. Psychiatric rehabilitation institutions: provide a safe, structured environment for clients whose psychiatric illnesses and lack of personal resources do not allow for living in a less restrictive setting; comprehensive services to meet continuum of health care needs are provided

E. Extended care facilities: provide care for the elderly (levels of care provided depend on abilities of the person) and physically and mentally challenged

Continuing Care

A. Refers to all care provided outside of institutions. Terminology of care varies amongst provinces and territories

B. Consistent features include care that occurs over a long period of time which provides an integrated system of service delivery

C. Generally provides supportive, maintenance, and/or restorative interdisciplinary health intervention for individuals with chronic or long-term health problems
   1. Major components are: adult day care, group homes, homemaker services, home nursing care, community physiotherapy, and occupational therapy
      a. Adult day care: an institutional daytime program that provides all degrees of care from skilled nursing care to personal care and from rehabilitation programs to social programs, depending on whether they are based on a medical, nursing, or social model; the client is able to live at home during the evening and night, which provides an alternative to institutionalization
      b. Home care: provides comprehensive services for people who do not need to be hospitalized and yet require more care than an outpatient facility can provide; prevents or delays institutionalization; care is provided by both nonprofessional (e.g., homemakers) and professional staff (e.g., nurses)
      c. Hospice care: provides emotional, physical, and supportive care to the terminally ill client and significant others; may be provided on an inpatient or outpatient basis or in the home; provides pain control; supports quality of life; does not institute life support or other extraordinary means to prolong life
      d. Respite care: a form of short-term health care service provided in either an institution or in the home to enable the primary

caregiver to have a temporary rest; allows the primary caregiver time to pursue personal interests, enjoy time alone with other family members, be away from the home, or go on vacation

COMMUNITY HEALTH

A. Definition
   1. Provide services for people with health needs who are living at home
   2. Provide special services by organizations to meet specific client needs (e.g., Meals on Wheels and food banks)
B. Crisis intervention groups
   1. Services
      a. Provide assistance for people in crises; clients' previous methods of adaptation are inadequate to meet present needs
      b. The focus of some groups is specific (e.g., violence against women and suicide prevention) or general (e.g., walk-in mental health clinics and hospital emergency rooms)
      c. Some crisis intervention groups provide service over the phone (e.g., poison control, AIDS hot line, suicide prevention centers, and rape crisis centers), others help those who are physically present (e.g., hospital emergency rooms and walk-in mental health clinics)
   2. Success factors
      a. Help requested by the client or family
      b. Addresses the immediate need for stress reduction
      c. Immediate opportunity for exploring feelings
      d. Assists the client in perceiving the event realistically
      e. Maximizes the client's coping mechanisms
      f. Provides assistance in investigating alternative approaches to solve the problem
      g. Teaches the client methods that can be used with subsequent stressors
      h. Provides information about other health resources where the client may receive additional assistance
C. Self-help groups
   1. Services
      a. Organized by clients or their families to provide services that are not adequately supplied by previous organizations
      b. Meet the needs of clients and families with chronic problems requiring intervention over an extended period of time
      c. Focus is usually specific (e.g., Alcoholics Anonymous; Alanon; Alzheimers Society; Friends of Schizophrenics; Ileostomy Society); some deal with a range of problems (e.g., Learning Disabilities Association)
      d. Some are nonprofit (e.g., Alcoholics Anonymous); others are profit making (e.g., Weight Watchers International)
      e. Provide help to people who often are not accepted by society (e.g., a drug addict, an alcoholic, a child abuser, or one who is mentally ill, obese, or brain injured); many utilize the 12-step program developed by Alcoholics Anonymous
   2. Success factors
      a. All members are accepted as equals
      b. All members have experienced similar problems
      c. Members feel a decrease in the sense of isolation that has occurred as a result of their problems
      d. Dealing with behavior and changes in behavior rather than with underlying causes of the behavior
      e. Ready supply of human resources available
         (1) Personal resources
         (2) Assistance from peers
         (3) Finally, extension of self to others as a role model
      f. Each member has identified the problem and wants help in meeting needs—self-motivation
      g. Ritual and language specific to the group and specific to the problems
      h. Leadership remains with the membership
      i. Group interaction
         (1) Identification with peers—sense of belonging
         (2) Group expectations—discipline required of members
         (3) Small steps encouraged and, when attained, reinforced by the group
      j. As a member achieves success within the group, he or she often receives reinforcement from outside the group
      k. Participation in 12-step programs is a lifelong, continuous process; one is never "recovered" but always "recovering" a day at a time

COST OF SERVICES

A. The dramatic rise in health care costs has become a major concern of governments, professionals, and consumers; billions are being spent on a health care system that works very little in the direction of "health" and that is slowly shifting priorities from curative medicine and hospital services to community-based primary care and health promotion (e.g., Jake Epp's report "Achieving Health for All: A Framework for Health Promotion [1986])

B. Causes of increasingly high costs
  1. Increased demand for services
  2. Specialization of care
  3. High cost of new technology
  4. Inflation
  5. Increase in population
  6. Economic recession, unemployment, a large number of homeless people, and poverty
  7. Growing clients' rights groups, consumer groups, and women's movements have been instrumental in facilitating health care system changes but have also added to health care system costs
  8. Demographic trends: increase in single-parent families; increase in people living alone; increase in aging population.

C. Attempts to control costs
  1. Hospital and bed closures
  2. Restrictive lists of medications covered by provincial pharmacare plans (e.g., British Columbia's Pharmacare program: reference-based pricing; drugs on the list are less expensive and as therapeutically effective as higher-priced drugs)
  3. Restrictive coverage of some health services deemed not to be medically necessary (e.g., sterilization reversals, in vitro fertilization)
  4. Legalization of midwifery in Ontario, Alberta, and British Columbia to promote home deliveries for uncomplicated pregnancies
  5. Reorganization and amalgamation of major hospitals and revamping of hospital governance
  6. Improved efficiency of acute care hospitals (e.g., assessing admission and discharge decisions; increase in ambulatory care)
  7. Use of clinical practice guidelines focusing on outcomes related to specific clinical conditions
  8. Increase in clinical evaluation research to examine what procedures/drugs do the most for the least (e.g., Toronto's Institute for Clinical Evaluative Sciences)
  9. Shifting resources to community-based care
    a. Community health centers are used in Quebec (since 1972), Ontario, Saskatchewan, and Manitoba; physicians are paid a salary
    b. Health service organizations in Ontario provide primary care on an outpatient basis; funding is on a per capita basis
    c. Comox Valley Nursing Centre, British Columbia, practices nursing within a wellness/health promotion model

d. Regional development of health care with population needs-based assessment and delivery
e. Early discharge programs from acute care hospitals with transfer of care to the community using home care services including those provided by the Victorian Order of Nurses

PAYMENT FOR SERVICES

A. The Canadian National Health Insurance program consists of five key system components; interlocking set of provincial/territorial plans that collectively make up the national insurance program and finance hospital and medical services for Canadians; mostly autonomous personal health care system to provide hospital and medical services; provincially/territorially organized system of health services; and voluntary health care agencies organized by consumers to provide services and education for specific health problems and needs

B. Canadians receive medical care largely through the subsidization of private medical practitioners rather than through public clinics; 95% of Canadian physicians are paid on a fee-for-service basis with rates being negotiated between provincial/territorial governments and medical associations

C. Under the Canadian National Health Insurance program, individuals may consult the physician of their choice and have input into which hospital they wish treatment to be given, provided their physician has admitting privileges

PROBLEMS WITH HEALTH CARE DELIVERY

A. Overregulation: government money means government regulation and control; health care system failed to recognize this fact; impact on delivery of care is still evolving

B. Fragmentation of care: increased specialization contributes to the potential for the client to fall through the cracks regarding health care follow-up; potential for undermedication or overmedication; total health condition may not be understood

C. Some groups whose health needs may be overlooked
  1. Chronically ill
  2. Elderly
  3. Women

D. Health care costs have increased in the last decade with continuing increases predicted

TOTAL QUALITY IMPROVEMENT

A. Definition: an organized and integrated system of continuous quality improvement (CQI) aimed at meeting patients, patient's families and friends, hospital employees, physicians, outside clinical agencies expectations

B. Principles: management accountability, teamwork, continuous improvements focused on work processes, customer orientation, and statistical data analysis (Kirk, 1992)

C. Process of continuous quality improvement: problem identification, team organization, identification of causes, plan implementation, continuous monitoring

NURSING PRACTICE AND THE LAW

TYPOLOGY OF LAWS

A. Sources of law
1. English common law (custom and precedent); major source of law in Canada except in Quebec where the Napoleonic Code is used
   a. Unwritten; based on customs
   b. Precedent plays large part in judge's decisions, thus giving uniformity to decisions in like situations
   c. Nurses practice under common as well as statutory law
2. Roman civil law; has its origins in the Napoleonic Code of France; dominant influence in Quebec
3. Statutory law (legislation)
   a. Body of law enacted by federal and provincial/territorial legislation
   b. That which commands or prohibits (e.g., Nurse Practice Acts define the parameters of nursing practice)
   c. Licensing laws belong in this category
4. Municipal by-laws and ordinances: public health matters
5. Hospital by-laws: patient rights and staff responsibilities

B. The British North America (BNA) Act (1867) renamed the Constitution Act (1982); incorporates existing provisions of the BNA Act with a Canadian Charter of Rights and Freedoms; establishes the political and legal foundations, as well as fundamental rules for Canadians to govern Canada; also gives provincial/territorial governments power in health care activities

C. Public and private law: two main divisions of law; nurses exposed to liability in both public and private law
1. Public law
   a. Constitutional: includes provincial/territorial jurisdiction over health care
   b. Criminal: includes physical and sexual assault; aiding and abetting suicide
   c. Administrative: includes regulation of professionals (e.g., Nurse Practice Acts)
2. Private (civil) law
   a. Property law: wills, patents, copyrights, and trademarks
   b. Contract law: agency, conditional sales, mortgages, and bail
   c. Tort law: includes both intentional and unintentional torts, such as intentional aggression, negligence, strict liability, defamation, and invasion of privacy

TORTS AND CRIMES IMPORTANT TO NURSES

A. Torts
1. Violations of private (civil) law
2. Failure to use care or failure to prevent injury
3. Malpractice and negligence fall into this category and are unintentional torts
   a. No precise statute describes malpractice
   b. Terms often used interchangeably, but some legal experts make a distinction between them
      (1) Malpractice: professional misconduct; negligence performed in professional practice; any unreasonable lack of skill in professional duties or illegal or immoral conduct that results in injury or death to the client/consumer
      (2) Negligence: practice without a license; measurement of negligence is "reasonableness"; involves exposure of person or property of another to unreasonable risk of injury by acts of commission or omission
4. Usual standard of conduct is that which a prudent nurse would or would not do
5. Tort different from crime, but serious tort can be tried as both civil and criminal action
6. Necessary to prove negligence that may be omissive or commissive; if proven, this means that the act was performed incorrectly (commissive) or not at all (omissive) and the nurse is responsible for injury
7. Elements essential to prove negligence: four elements of a cause of action must be present for negligence; if any element is missing, one cannot proceed or succeed with a charge of negligence; negligence is not dependent on a contract
   a. Legally recognized duty of care to protect others against unreasonable risk
   b. Failure to perform according to the established standard of conduct and care, which becomes breach of duty

c. Damage to the client, which can be physical, emotional, and/or mental

d. Connection between defendant's conduct and the resulting injury referred to as "proximate cause" or "remoteness of damage"

8. Nurse responsible for own acts; if employed, employer also held responsible under the doctrine of *respondeat superior*; when responsibility is shared, nursing actions must lie within the scope of employment and legislation relating to nursing practice (such as Nurse Practice Acts)

9. Reasonableness and prudence in actions are usually determining factors in a judgment; increasing attention is being paid to the law governing the practice of nursing

10. Examples of malpractice/negligence include leaving sponges inside a client; causing burns from heating pads, hot solutions, and electric, steam, or vapor sources; medication errors; failure to prevent falls by neglecting to raise bed or crib rails; incompetent assessment of client situations, such as ignoring complaints of chest pain leading to subsequent inappropriate actions; and improper identification of clients for operative or diagnostic procedures.

11. Intentional torts occur when a person does damage to another person in a willful, intentional way and without just cause and/or excuse; includes fraud and deceit, assault and battery, false imprisonment, exposure of person or body after death, eavesdropping, libel, and slander (defamatory torts)

a. Assault: mental or physical threat
   (1) Knowingly threatening or attempting to do violence to another
   (2) Forcing a medication or treatment on a person who does not want it constitutes assault so long as touching does not occur

b. Battery: touching with or without the intent to do harm
   (1) Actually touching or wounding a person in an offensive manner
   (2) Hitting or striking a client

c. Fraud
   (1) False presentation of facts purposefully to create deception
   (2) Presenting false credentials for purposes of entering a nursing program or gaining registration, licensure, or employment

d. Invasion of privacy
   (1) Encroachment or trespass on another's body includes:
      (a) Exposure of a person: any unnecessary exposure or discussion of the client's case is actionable unless authorized by the client; after death, the client's right to be unobserved, excluded from unwarranted operations, and protected from unauthorized touching of the body persists
      (b) False imprisonment: the intentional confinement without authorization by a person who physically constricts another using force, the threat of force, or confining structures and/or clothing; even without force or malicious intent, to detain another without consent in a specified area constitutes grounds for a charge of false imprisonment; the charge is not false imprisonment if it is necessary to protect an emotionally disturbed person from harming self or others or if it is necessary to confine to defend oneself, others, or property, or to effect a lawful arrest
   (2) Defamation: concerns privileged communications and privacy; law grants the right of privacy to everyone; divulgence of privileged communication whether from charts, conversation, interview, or observation in a way that exposes the person to hatred, contempt, aversion, or a lowering of opinion; includes slander (oral) and libel (written, pictured, telecast), both of which are dependent on communication to a third party

B. Crimes
1. Criminal act: an act contrary to the Criminal Code of Canada; violates societal law; includes felonies and misdemeanors

2. Criminal Code of Canada is determined by the Parliament of Canada, is applicable to all provinces and territories, and may be amended by Parliament to reflect society's changing values

3. Law Reform Commission of Canada
   a. Has been engaged in modernizing and codifying the nation's criminal law so that it more accurately reflects twentieth-century Canadian values, the principles of the Charter of Rights and Freedoms, and the distinctive concepts and institutions of common and private (civil) law systems in Canada
   b. The Commission has succeeded in changing laws, altering legal attitudes and practices, assisting the judiciary in their decision making, stimulating research, and educating the public on matters of legal importance

c. The Commission Reports enacted, at least in part, into legislation are an Act to Amend the Criminal Code (Victims of Crime) S.C.1988 c.30; Sexual Offenses; Criteria for Determination of Death; Euthanasia; Aiding Suicide; and Cessation of Treatment

d. Additional study papers released include Sanctity of Life or Quality of Life; Consent to Medical Care; Cessation of Treatment and Suicide: A Proposal for Reform; The Right to Live and the Right to Die; Quality of Life and Treatment Decisions; Euthanasia and Homicide

4. Crimes are wrongs punishable by the crown, committed against the public, usually demonstrate that intent was present, and are tried with the crown as the complainant

5. Commission of crime requires two fundamental factors
   a. Committing a deed contrary to criminal law
   b. Omitting an act when there is a legal obligation to perform such an act (e.g., refraining from assistance with the birth of a child if such refusal results in injury to the newborn)

6. Criminal conspiracy occurs when two or more persons agree to commit a crime

7. Giving aid to another in the commission of a crime makes the person equally guilty of the offense if awareness is present that a crime is being committed

8. Ignorance of the law is usually not an adequate defense when a crime or civil wrong is committed

9. Assault may be justified in instances of self-defense if only as much force as is absolutely necessary for self-protection is used

10. Search warrants are required before property can be searched

11. Administration of narcotics by a nurse is legal only when authorized by a physician who is legally registered under the Narcotics Control Act and Regulations.
    a. If a nurse knowingly administers a drug that causes a major disability or death, a crime may be charged
    b. Illegal possession or sale of a controlled substance makes a nurse liable, as is any citizen

DEATH WITH DIGNITY, LEGAL, ETHICAL, AND EMOTIONAL ISSUES

A. Nurses' and physicians' guidelines outlining acceptable practices for making decisions in situations for which intensive treatment and resuscitative measures may not be appropriate
   1. Underlying problems are:
      a. Public concern that terminal illness is not managed appropriately by the health care team
      b. Use of aggressive treatment protocols and technologic support to unnecessarily prolong the dying process
      c. Inadequate use of the opportunity to express desires about death with dignity while competent and before becoming permanently mentally incapacitated
   2. Dignity includes two fundamental dimensions, both of which are at risk for clients in health care settings
      a. Control over one's life
      b. Respect for the worth of individuals as unique beings
   3. Must empower clients to have as much control as possible over their care and activities, recognizing that pain, increasing helplessness, and hopelessness lead to despair
   4. Living wills, "do not resuscitate" (DNR) or "no code" orders, and life-sustaining treatment protocols constitute some of the most highly debated legal/ethical issues in health care
   5. There is no need to precipitously introduce forms of legislation intended to address largely ethical/medical problems; these problems require:
      a. Assessment of public and professional attitudes toward care of the dying by institutions, organizations, and governments
      b. Education of an interested public about living wills through literature distribution and discussions
      c. Vigorous discussion and debate in scholarly journals about the medical, ethical, and legal issues involved in enactment of living will legislation
      d. Better education of all health care professionals with increased emphasis on care of dying clients and related medicolegal and ethical issues in basic curricula of health care programs
      e. Use of quality management to include assessment of the appropriate care of terminally ill clients and monitoring the use of investigations and treatments in such situations
      f. Increased availability and accessibility of palliative care services

B. Criteria of death
   1. The Law Reform Commission's (Report 15) recommendation that Parliament of Canada amend Section 28A of the Interpretation Act concerning Criteria of Death has, in part, been done using the following as guidelines for legislation review:

a. Death occurs with irreversible cessation of all brain function
b. Irreversible cessation of brain function can be determined by the prolonged absence of spontaneous circulatory and respiratory function
c. When detection of prolonged absence of spontaneous circulatory and respiratory function is made impossible by the use of artificial means of support, the irreversible cessation of brain function can be determined by any means recognized by the ordinary standards of current medical practice (Harvard criteria)

C. Do not resuscitate (DNR) or "no code" status
1. DNR status determination continues as an important issue and includes dilemmas in any health care environment including the home
    a. Documentation of DNR status includes progress notes of all DNR discussions and decisions and DNR orders in the client's cumulative medical record if the client wishes not to be resuscitated
    b. Some physicians prefer to write the DNR order as "compassionate care" once the client, family and/or substitute decision maker, and physician have agreed; "compassionate care" tends to be broader than DNR orders and includes feedings, IVs, etc.
2. Most important factors considered in determining a resuscitation order are the client's wishes, the prognosis, the client's ability to cope, and whether cardiopulmonary resuscitation (CPR) will provide benefits sufficient to make it worthwhile to endure the "burdens" of resuscitation
3. Reasons expressed by clients who choose not to be resuscitated are that the CPR will provide no benefit for them because of widespread terminal or debilitating disease; that their present quality of life is unacceptable to them; that CPR would only prolong suffering; and that the further deterioration caused by CPR would be unacceptable to them
4. The College of Nurses of Ontario (CNO) Statement on Resuscitation (1994) assists RNs and RPNs to practice competently and ethically in current health care environments by setting expectations
    a. Basic principles underlying the expectations are within three broad areas
        (1) Identifying and documenting client wishes
        (2) Respecting and following client wishes
        (3) Working within the agency's policies

b. Definitions include:
    (1) Advanced directive
    (2) Consent to treatment
    (3) Informed consent
    (4) Palliative care
5. A DNR order must be a team decision and the family and, if possible, the client must be included in the decision-making process
6. A DNR order is still not clear in implementation
7. Canadian Nurses Association, Canadian Hospital Association, and Canadian Medical Assoiciation in cooperation with the Canadian Bar Association with advice from the Law Reform Commission of Canada and the Catholic Health Association of Canada developed a Joint Statement on Terminal Illness which "is intended as a basic, national guideline for use by all those involved in the care of the terminally ill" (*Canadian Nurse* 80(6):24, 1984.)

D. Living wills and durable powers of attorney
1. Concepts
    a. Living wills gained prominence during the evolution of the patients' rights movement because these allow clients to state their wish to die in certain situations and to not be kept alive through the use of medications, artificial means, or heroic measures; the living will sets forth the client's wishes regarding health care decisions; it includes which kind of medical procedures are authorized or declined
    b. A durable power of attorney designates an agent to make health decisions according to the client's plans when the client becomes incapable of decision-making; it includes power to consent to physicians not giving or stopping treatment necessary to keep a client alive; it can be combined with a living will
2. Law
    a. Living wills are currently not recognized legal documents in Canada; at common law, the patient has the right to consent or refuse to undergo treatment, even life-saving treatment
    b. Durable power of attorney legislation enacted in Nova Scotia
3. Advantages associated with the living will are that it permits expression of the person's preferences; promotes communication between the person and caregivers, including the family; demonstrates respect for the client as a person; and supports the belief that clients have the right to self-determination as entrenched in laws and medical ethics

4. Problems related to recognition of a living will as a legal document are that there needs to be agreement and understanding of fundamental terms such as terminal illness and heroic measures, which have caused discussion of the "usefulness" or "burdensomeness" of treatments and procedures perceived by the client as inappropriate; restriction of clients' rights that ensued in provision of more rather than less care; and violation of client's autonomy when treatment is carried out despite client's expressed refusal;

E. The right to die
1. The right of clients or their designees and surrogates to refuse life-sustaining treatment is a highly debated ethical/legal issue in health care
2. Active euthanasia is a criminal offense in Canada; passive euthanasia is not illegal in Canada
3. Attempted suicide is not a crime; counseling, aiding, or abetting suicide (assisted suicide) is a criminal offense
4. The following actions are not active euthanasia or assisted suicide: respecting a person's wish to refuse or stop nonbeneficial treatment; withdrawing or withholding treatment when the burden to the dying person outweighs the benefits to the person; giving drugs to relieve pain or to promote comfort (physical and emotional) even when an unintended effect might be shortening a dying person's life
5. The Supreme Court of Canada ruled that care or treatment could be refused regardless of the consequences
6. Recent laws and court decisions have reinforced support of three basic principles: in the medical context, the presumption in favor of life is recognized; the client's autonomy and right to self-direction cannot be denied; and human life must be considered not only from the quantitative perspective, but also from the qualitative perspective, and special measures must be provided by the law to protect the incompetent client
7. The federal government is against:
   a. Legalizing or decriminalizing voluntary active euthanasia in any form and is in favor of continuing to treat it as culpable homicide
   b. Mercy killing being made an offense separate from homicide
   c. Decriminalizing assisted suicide
8. The Law Reform Commission of Canada has recommended that a physician cannot be held criminally liable merely for undertaking or continuing the administration of appropriate palliative care to eliminate or reduce the suffering of an individual only because of the effect this action might have on the latter's life expectancy, and that a physician should not incur any criminal liability if he or she decides to discontinue or not initiate treatment for an incompetent person when that treatment is no longer therapeutically useful and is not in the person's best interest

LIABILITY INSURANCE

A. Liability can be defined as a person's legal responsibility to be accountable for wrongful acts by making financial restitution to the party wronged
B. Employer's insurance protects the nurse while on duty in the course of employment (concept of vicarious liability, *respondeat superior*); a self-employed nurse can, however, be personally sued and held liable for negligent actions
C. In 1988, a professional liability protective fund operated by nurses for nurses became a reality as CNA established the Canadian Nurses' Protective Fund (CNPF) designed "to protect nurses from professional liability claims and to address inequities in the present insurance system." Included is an Adjudication Committee and nurse lawyer to provide support and help with documentation; purchased by 10 of the 12 provincial/territorial associations for their members; other associations provide liability protection as an important benefit derived from membership
D. The Canadian Nurses' Protective Society (CNPS) now offers professional liability protection to nurse members
E. In Ontario, the Registered Nurses' Association of Ontario (RNAO) has established the Legal Assistance Program (LAP) for legal assistance on a case-by-case basis; the program provides financial assistance to nurses registered with the CNO who require access to legal counsel for employment-related matters

INFORMED CONSENT

A. According to Black's Law Dictionary, consent is "an act of reason accompanied by deliberation wherein the mind weighs, as a balance, the good or evil on either side"
B. Types of consenting behaviors include inferred consenting, implied consenting, and expressed consenting
C. Purposes of informed consent
1. Makes possible a contract between two individuals with each sharing equally
2. Makes a competent decision possible for client who has the final decision

D. Consent is essential for any treatment, except in an emergency where failure to institute treatment may constitute negligence

E. In an emergency situation, two physicians may sign consent for the client when failure to intervene may cause death or the common law permits administration of health care to unconscious or mentally incompetent persons in an emergency situation as long as the client does not express non-consent while conscious or mentally competent

F. Essential elements of legally effective consents are that the consent:
   1. Is voluntary
   2. Authorizes the specific treatment or care and the person giving the treatment or care
   3. Is given by a person with the legal capacity to consent
   4. Is given by a mentally competent person
   5. Is an informed decision

G. The informed consent includes:
   1. An explanation of treatment to be done with a presentation of advantages and disadvantages
   2. Description of possible alternatives
   3. Time for decision making
   4. Absence of undue pressure
   5. Decision making that occurs before sedation is given

H. Problems arise in determining:
   1. What constitutes adequate information
   2. Who should give explanation
   3. Whether to give alternatives when one treatment is clearly preferable
   4. What constitutes mental incompetency in a client from whom consent is sought

I. The client has a right to know, agree to, or refuse, and this right is reflected in literature of the patients' rights associations and legislation

J. The nurse's responsibility is to respect the rights of the individual client, thus avoiding legal action

K. The nurse is a client/family advocate when the client cannot function in this role and when all elements of an informed consent are not in place

THE NURSE IN THE COURTS

A. Nurse may be in court either as a witness if involved personally in a case or as an expert witness because of knowledge and expertise

B. Expert witness
   1. Not an advocate
   2. If called into court, the nurse must be:
      a. Informed as to standards of care that prudent, reasonable nurses would give relative to the incident in question
      b. Knowledgeable in the field specific to the incident
      c. Without opinion unless specifically asked

   3. In some provinces and territories, the Nurse Practice Act requires that the professional nurse report a colleague's incompetence; in this way, legislation protects the public and ensures that health care providers are regulated and accountable

   4. The client's chart, to which nurses contribute, may be used in court; charting must be: accurate; complete; factual; legible; give evidence of knowledge, skill, and judgment; and reflect the plan of nursing care individualized for and with the client/family

   5. Computerization of documentation systems still requires implementation of legal principles within the evolving technology and documentation approaches

THE NURSE'S LEGAL STATUS

A. Employee
   1. Standards for nursing practice describe what actions and services the nurse performs; help the legal profession interpret the scope of nursing practice; provide a basis for job descriptions and performance appraisal systems in facilities employing nurses; and inform the patient/client/consumer of expectations of care
   2. Collective bargaining arranges contracts between employees and the employing agency
      a. Contracts are binding on both parties even though the individual nurse may not be directly involved with the deliberations
      b. Damages may be sought in court if contract is broken
      c. The grievance procedure is commonly used in the employer-employee relationship as part of the collective agreement; grievance allows either party to complain that the other has breached a term of the collective agreement; such disagreements are often sent to arbitration for a settlement

B. Independent contractor
   1. A contractor who renders direct services to clients and is in control of that service, including setting the fee for service (e.g., self-employed nurse)
   2. A private-duty nurse is an independent contractor

THE CLIENT'S RIGHTS

A. Society has become more consumer oriented and values the rights of individuals; Section 7 of the Canadian Charter of Rights and Freedoms in the

Constitution Act (1982) states that "everyone has the right to life, liberty, and security of the person and the right not to be deprived thereof except in accordance with the principles of fundamental justice"

B. The Law Reform Commission of Canada and the Manitoba Association of Rights and Liberties have recommended that clients' rights be expressly recognized; the Consumers' Association of Canada has proclaimed consumer rights in health care and has put forth a four-point statement of consumer rights (right to be informed, participate in decision-making, to be respected, and right to equal access to health care)

C. Clients have the legal right to refuse treatment (if mentally competent), to be given treatment in an emergency, to choose their own doctor, to have a proper standard of care, to execute voluntary and informed consent, to decide whether to be used for research or teaching, to be treated in confidentiality, to receive treatment free of discrimination, freedom to receive services in a hospital of one's choice, and the right to make a choice even if it is choosing to die rather than receive identified treatments

D. The federal government has set stringent rules about the use of human subjects in research

E. Clients have the right to lodge complaints to the statutory body for nursing about a nurse member and the care received when complaints are related to:
1. Professional incompetence
2. Professional misconduct
3. Physical or mental incapacity

THE NURSE'S RIGHTS AND RESPONSIBILITIES

A. Because of the close contact between clients and nurses in a variety of clinical practice settings and health care environments, it is essential for nurses to understand their rights and responsibilities

B. Consumer/patient rights movements and expansion of the scope of practice for nurses constitute reasons why nurses must develop awareness of their rights and responsibilities

C. Nurses have recently been accorded certain rights by professional groups, by contracts, and by the public; those that have been suggested are:
1. The right to be trusted by the public
2. The right to practice nursing in accordance with professionally defined standards
3. The right to participate in and to promote growth and direction of the profession
4. The right to intervene when necessary to protect clients

5. The right to be respected for one's knowledge, abilities, experience, and contributions
6. The right to be believed when speaking in the area of his or her expertise
7. The right to be trusted by colleagues
8. The right to give and receive support, guidance, and correction from colleagues
9. The right to be compensated fairly for services

D. Because of these rights nurses also have the responsibility to:
1. Practice nursing in accordance with standards of the profession
2. Fulfill professional promises made to the public
3. Intervene to protect clients from unethical and/or illegal actions by any person delivering health care
4. Participate in and promote the growth of the profession
5. Strive constantly to increase knowledge and experience
6. Speak out accurately and honestly in one's area of expertise
7. Give to and receive guidance, support, and correction from colleagues
8. Maintain continuing competence in nursing practice through professional continuing education (mandatory or voluntary)

LEGISLATION RELATED TO THE NURSING PROFESSION

A. The terms *registration* and *licensure* are used interchangeably but are not synonymous; both registration and licensure ensure a minimum level of safe practice at the time of a nurse's initial registration, thereby protecting the public's health, safety, and welfare

B. Registration: entrance of one's name on a register
1. Maintained by individual, provincial or territorial professional nurses associations (except in Ontario, where it is maintained by the College of Nurses, the statutory body for nurses in Ontario)
2. Occurs after successful completion of the registered nurses' examinations provided to provincial and territorial jurisdictions by the Canadian Nurses' Association Testing Service (CNATS)
3. In 1995 the national testing service moved from a norm-referenced to a criterion-referenced examination; the candidates' results are not influenced by the performance of others writing the examination but rather by the competencies required of nurses who are beginning to practice

4. Authorizes practice as a registered nurse
5. Protects the title of registered nurse
6. Follows automatically after licensure
7. Since 1989, CNATS has provided feedback to unsuccessful candidates in the nurse registration examinations and has evaluated this feedback process

C. Licensure: granting of a license after successful completion of the Canadian Nurses' Association Testing Service Registration Examination; in addition to licensure, practitioners are regulated by "title control," which is promoted by registration and nursing legislation that protects the use of titles such as "registered nurse," "registered practical nurse," and "nurse"

1. Mandatory licensure: all who practice nursing must be licensed; mandatory licensure protects both the title of registered nurse and the practice of nursing, the scope of which is defined in the legislation, as is the explicit delineation of nurses' functions; licensure therefore grants an exclusive right to practice nursing to only those members in good standing; practice of the profession by an unlicensed person is prohibited and punishable by law; mandatory statutes were proclaimed in Newfoundland (1953), New Brunswick (1984), Nova Scotia (1985), and Northwest Territories (1973)

2. The CNA has publicly endorsed mandatory licensure for all nurses employed by the federal government

3. Forms of regulation of nurses are different not only between provinces and territories, but also among professional groups

4. Registration and licensure may be obtained by reciprocity after initial registration is established in the province or territory where the applicant successfully completed the registration examination

5. Health Disciplines Act (Ontario) 1974 RSO 1980 has been replaced with the Regulated Health Professions Act (RHPA) 1991 as amended 1993 Chapter 37
   a. Purposes
      (a) Brings designated professions into a self-regulating framework
      (b) Protects the public
      (c) Recognizes provider autonomy, competence, and contributions
   b. 22 colleges brought under common legislation
   c. Provides for a greater public participation; established an all-public council to advise the Minister of Health on regulatory matters

6. The RHPA delineates the scope of nursing practice; the practice of nursing is the promotion of health and the assessment of the provision of care for and the treatment of health conditions by supportive, preventive, therapeutic, palliative, and rehabilitative means in order to attain or maintain optimal function

7. Nurse practice acts
   a. Nursing is recognized by provincial/territorial statutes (Nurses'/Nursing Act)
   b. Legislated definitions of scope of nursing practice are different across provinces/territories as reflected in Nursing Profession Act (Alberta 1987); Nurses (Registered) Act Rules, Part 1 (1988); and Nurses Act RSO, Chapter 1 (Quebec 1989)
   c. Purposes of registration
      (1) Protect the public from unsafe practitioners
      (2) Protect the titles of Registered Nurse or Nurse for persons who have successfully passed registration examinations
      (3) Regulate the standards of nursing education and/or nursing practice (dependent upon the province/territory)
   d. Purposes of Nurses' Acts/legislation/professional regulation
      (1) Protect public health, safety, and welfare
      (2) Regulate and monitor practice and practitioners
      (3) Credential nurses
      (4) Influence supply of qualified, competent nurses
      (5) Facilitate interprovincial registration
      (6) In some provinces, provide for the registration and licensure of nursing assistants
   e. Enactment
      (1) First in Nova Scotia (1910), followed by Manitoba (1913), New Brunswick and Alberta (1916), Saskatchewan (1917), British Columbia (1918), Prince Edward Island (1922), Ontario (1925), Quebec (1930), Newfoundland (1953), and Northwest Territories (1975)
      (2) Administered by provincial associations except in Ontario, where the College of Nurses (CNO) registers nurses, and in Quebec, where the Order of Nurses of the Province of Quebec (L'Ordre des Infirmiers et Infirmiéres du Quebec [OIIQ]) licenses nurses for nursing practice
   f. Control
      (1) In Ontario, with the Nurses' Act of 1961 amended, the College of Nurses of Ontario was established as the governing

body of nursing with provision also for governing of registered practical nurses (RPN); this is a title change from registered nursing assistants (RNA) legislated in the Regulated Health Professions Act of 1991 and amended in 1993

(2) Newfoundland was the first province to enact mandatory legislation (1953), followed by Quebec (1964), Prince Edward Island (1969), Alberta (1983), New Brunswick (1984), Nova Scotia (1985), and the Northwest Territories (1975)

(3) The Alberta Association of Registered Nurses (AARN) undertook in 1989 its legislative base and responsibilities as nurses to facilitate nursing practice as a private enterprise

(4) Yukon Nurses' Society (YNS) undertook, in 1989, the writing of a new nursing profession act; the Society realizes proclamation into law of the Yukon Health Act (1991) and worked to finalize the Yukon Nurses' Act and the renaming of the professional association to the Yukon Registered Nurses' Association; the legislation supports mandatory registration

(5) Northwest Territories Registered Nurses' Association (NWTRNA) completed a legislation review necessitated by the transfer of health to the territorial government in the Northwest Territories and requires mandatory registration

(6) Order of Nurses of Quebec (ONQ) L'Ordre des Infirmiers et Infirmiéres du Quebec (OIIQ)
  (a) February 1974: Professional Code of the Province of Quebec changed the title of Association of Nurses of the Province of Quebec (ANPQ) to Order of Nurses of Quebec (ONQ); chief purpose is protection of the public by supervising the practice of nursing and its members as legal responsibilities governed by the "Code des professions" and the "Loi sur les infirmiers et infirmiéres"
  (b) Passage of the Professional Code created 21 professional groups, of which 11 have exclusive rights to practice
  (c) Quebec Nurses' Act defines the profession of nursing as identification of persons' health needs, assisting with diagnosis, employing nursing interventions, and communication of health problems to clients
  (d) Membership in L'Ordre des Infirmiers et Infirmiéres du Quebec (OIIQ), a professional association with unique, official status, is mandatory, although OIIQ withdrew from the CNA in 1985
  (e) Because of OIIQ's withdrawal from the CNA, some Quebec nurses join other professional associations, as well as the OIIQ, to ensure membership in the CNA and ICN

(7) Northwest Territories Registered Nurses' Association (NWTRNA)
  (a) 1975: Ordinance Respecting the Nursing Profession in the Northwest Territories approved by the Territorial Council Legislation enacted 1975
  (b) Gave the NWTRNA authority to join with the Canadian Nurses' Association (1976); grant and/or revoke certificates of registration to nurses practicing in the Northwest Territories; discipline members of the nursing profession; lay claim to being the first professional group north of the sixtieth parallel to acquire registration control over its members
  (c) Is promoting development of a basic baccalaureate program

(8) Prince Edward Island (PEI) is the first province to reach the goal of accepting only a baccalaureate as education for nurse preparation (as the basis for entry to practice); the provincial government phased out diploma nursing programs on Prince Edward Island in 1988

(9) In New Brunswick, the Nurses' Association of New Brunswick (NANB) voted in favor (1989) of accepting the goal to establish a baccalaureate in nursing as the future educational requirement for entry into practice; in so doing, joined all other Canadian provinces and territories in making this a national goal

(10) The Registered Nurses' Association of British Columbia (RNABC) and the Alberta Association of Registered Nurses (AARN) have lobbied for mechanisms to directly reimburse nurses for nursing services rendered

(11) As of 1994 all provincial/territorial nurse practice acts support mandatory registration

CERTIFICATION OF SPECIALTIES

A. Certification usually refers to a nonstatutory, voluntary process that nurses may choose to achieve specialty certification
B. The noticeable trend toward specialization in the nursing profession is a result of the increasing knowledge and skill required in the judgment and decision-making processes of nursing
C. CNA has provided an interpretation of specialty: "a specifically defined area of clinical and functional nursing with a narrowed, in-depth focus, necessary for the safe delivery of the full range of services required in that area of nursing" (1982); the Canadian Nurses' Association began its certification program for specialties in 1986
D. CNA's approach to the certification processes is that the "designation process applies to an area of nursing rather than to a group or an association, and the process may be initiated by any group of nurses that is able to provide evidence that a specific nursing area meets the required criteria" (1986)
E. As of 1996, there are seven specialities certified through the CNA (occupational health nursing, neuroscience nursing, nephrology nursing, emergency nursing, critical care nursing, perioperative nursing, and psychiatric nursing)

VIOLENCE IN THE WORKPLACE

A. Violence against health workers, including nurses, is increasing
B. Restructuring in health care institutions, changes in staffing levels, improper use of staff, inadequate security, and inadequate education in preventing violence contribute to an increase in violence against nurses
C. Suggested approaches for dealing with the possibility of violence
   1. Education in recognizing signs of possible violence
   2. Proper protocols and procedures to deal with violence when it occurs
   3. Preventive measures such as:
      a. Access control
      b. Alarm systems
      c. Metal-detection systems
      d. Proper training of all personnel relative to safety measures
   4. Immediate evaluation and treatment of victims of abuse
   5. Influencing legislation that recognizes violence against nurses as a reality

THE NURSE'S ROLE

MAINTENANCE OF EFFECTIVE COMMUNICATION
Introduction

A. The need to communicate is universal
B. People communicate to satisfy needs
C. Recognition of what is communicated is basic for the establishment of a therapeutic nurse-client relationship
D. Clear and accurate communication among members of the health team, including the client, is vital to support the client's welfare
E. A person cannot avoid communicating; all behavior, even silence, has meaning, and nonverbal communication occurs even with silence

Nursing Responsibilities in Promotion of Therapeutic Communication

A. Be aware that effective communication requires skill in both sending and receiving messages
   1. Verbal: for example, words and tone of voice
   2. Written
   3. Nonverbal: for example, facial expression, eye contact, and body language
B. Recognize the high stress-anxiety potential of most health settings created in part by:
   1. Health problem itself
   2. Treatments and procedures
   3. Exclusive behavior of personnel
   4. Foreign environment
   5. Change in life-style, body image, and self-concept
   6. Inability to use normal coping skills such as exercise or talking with friends
C. Recognize the intrinsic worth of each person
   1. Listen, consider wishes when possible, and explain when necessary
   2. Avoid stereotyping, snap judgments, and unjustified comparisons
   3. Be nonjudgmental and nonpunitive in response and behavior
D. Be aware that each individual must be treated as a whole person
E. Recognize that all behavior has meaning and usually results from the attempt to cope with stress or anxiety
   1. Be aware of importance of value systems
   2. Be aware of significance of cultural differences
   3. Be sensitive to personal meaning of experiences to clients
   4. Recognize that giving information may not alter the client's behavior
   5. Recognize the defense mechanisms that the individual is using

6. Recognize own anxiety and cope with it
7. Search for patterns of adaptation on which to base action
8. Recognize that client's previous patterns of behavior may become inadequate under stress
   a. Health problems may produce a change in family or community constellations
   b. Health problems may lead to change in self-perception and role identity
9. Be aware that behavioral changes are possible only when the individual has other defenses to maintain equilibrium

F. Help the client to accept the health problem and its consequences

G. Identify the individual's needs and determine priority for care

H. Maintain a caring environment
1. Accept the client but set limits on inappropriate behavior
2. Identify and face problems honestly
3. Value the expression of feelings
4. Be nonjudgmental

I. When possible, encourage client participation in decision making

J. Recognize the client is a unique person
1. Use names rather than labels such as room numbers or diagnoses
2. Maintain the client's dignity
3. Be courteous toward the client, family, and visitors
4. Protect the client's privacy by use of curtains and avoidance of probing
5. Permit personal possessions where practical (e.g., own nightclothes, pictures, and toys)
6. Explain at the client's level of understanding and tolerance
7. Encourage expression of feelings
8. Approach the client as a person with difficulties, not as a "difficult" person

K. Support a social environment that focuses on client needs
1. Use problem-solving techniques that focus on the client (individual, family, community)
2. Be flexible in carrying out routines and policies
3. Be discreet in use of power
4. Recognize that use of medical jargon can isolate the client

RECOGNITION OF CLIENT FACTORS INFLUENCING NURSING CARE

A. Hierarchy of needs
1. Need to survive: physiologic needs for such things as air, food, and water
2. Need for safety and comfort: physical and psychologic security

3. Interpersonal needs: social needs for love, acceptance, status, and recognition
4. Intrapersonal needs: self-esteem and self-actualization

B. Developmental level
1. Infant: must adapt to a totally new environment; the stress from the transition from intrauterine to extrauterine living is compounded for the infant with a congenital defect
2. Child: maturation involves physical, functional, and emotional growth; it is an ever-changing process that produces stress; disabilities will provide additional factors that may quantitatively or qualitatively affect maturation
3. Adolescent: is experiencing a physical, psychologic, and social growth spurt; the individual is asking, "Who am I?" on the way to developing a self-image; limitations provide additional stress during identity formation
4. Adult: is expected to be independent and productive, to provide for self and family; if one cannot assume this role totally or partially, it can cause additional stress
5. Aged: our society tends to venerate youth and deplore old age; many elderly persons are experiencing multiple stresses (loss of loved ones, changes in usual life-style, loss of physical vigor, and, for many, the thought of approaching death) at a time when their ability to adapt is compromised by the anatomic, physiologic, and psychologic alterations that occur during the aging process

C. Type of condition affecting the client
1. Acute illness: caused by a health problem that produces signs and symptoms abruptly and runs a short course, from which there is usually a full recovery; an acute illness may leave an individual with a loss of a body part or function and may develop into a long-term illness
2. Chronic illness: caused by a health problem that produces signs and symptoms over time and runs a long course from which there is only partial recovery
   a. Exacerbation: period when a chronic illness becomes more active and there is a recurrence of pronounced signs and symptoms of the disease
   b. Remission: period when a chronic illness is controlled and signs and symptoms are reduced or not obvious
   c. Degenerative: continuous deterioration or increased impairment of a person's physical state
3. Terminal illness: no cure possible; death is inevitable in the near future

4. Primary health problem: original condition, developing independently of another health problem
5. Secondary health problem: direct result of another health problem

D. Personal resources
   1. Level of self-esteem: attitude that reflects the individual's perception of self-worth; it is a personal subjective judgment of oneself
   2. Experiential background: knowledge derived from one's own actions, observations, or perceptions; maturation, culture, and environment influence the individual's experiential foundation
   3. Intelligence
      a. Genetic intellectual potential
      b. Amount of formal and informal education
      c. Level of intellectual development (e.g., child versus adult)
      d. Ability to reason, conceptualize, and translate words into actions
   4. Level of motivation: internal desire or incentive to accomplish something
   5. Values: factors that are important to the individual
   6. Religion: deep personal belief in a higher force than humanity
   7. Social interaction: ability to clearly communicate needs and desires to others
   8. Stress control: development of varied effective coping skills

E. Extent of actual or perceived change in body image
   1. Obvious reminder of disability to self and others
      a. Loss of a body part or change in function
      b. Need for a prosthesis (e.g., breast, leg, or eye)
      c. Need for hardware (e.g., pacemaker, braces, hearing aid, or wheelchair)
      d. Extent of disability or limitation
      e. Need for medication
   2. Value placed on loss by self or society
      a. Image as "no longer whole" or "a cripple"
      b. Type of loss: perceptions of body part, function, or disease as being good, pleasing, repulsive, clean, or dirty
         (1) Symbols of sexuality: breast, uterus, prostate, or heart
         (2) May lack social acceptability: colostomy, mental illness, incontinence, cancer, tuberculosis, AIDS, or drug abuse
         (3) Impairment of senses and/or ability to communicate: laryngectomy, aphasia, deafness, or blindness
         (4) Altered body image resulting from anatomic changes: amputation of limb or breast, colostomy

F. Client's and family's stage of adaptation
   1. Self-protection: disbelief, denial, avoidance, and/or intellectualization; with developing awareness of implications of illness the individual defends the self further by anger, depression, and/or joking
   2. With developing realization of implications of illness the individual reorganizes self-feelings and restructures relationships with family and society
   3. As resolution occurs the individual begins to accept the consequences of the illness and acknowledges feelings about the self and further changes that must be made

G. Client's history
   1. Health history
      a. Physiologic: what physical adaptations were manifested in the past
      b. Psychologic: what psychologic methods of adaptation were exhibited in the past
   2. Sociocultural history
      a. Religion: particular denomination, specific belief (e.g., agnostic, atheist, or "energy force")
      b. Ethnic group
      c. Occupation
      d. Economic status
      e. Family members, significant others, and their personal resources
      f. Race
      g. Educational background
      h. Environment: urban versus rural, private home versus apartment
      i. Social status
      j. Life-style

USE OF THE NURSING PROCESS

Introduction

A. Basis of personalized care is planned rather than relying on intuitive intervention
B. Most efficient way to accomplish personalized care in a time of exploding knowledge and rapid social change is by the nursing process
   1. Theoretic framework used by the nurse
   2. Assists in solving or alleviating both simple and complex nursing problems
C. Changing, expanding, more responsible role demands knowledgeably planned, purposeful, and accountable action by nurses
D. Documentation of nursing care is done to:
   1. Communicate to other health care team members the nursing care provided
   2. Provide a legal document that reflects the care given to and the progress of the client
   3. Provide a data base for continuous quality improvement programs necessary for accredi-

tation; the Canadian Council on Health Services Accreditation (CCHSA) accredits health care agencies

E. Decision making that systematically selects and uses relevant information is a requisite for individualized client care

F. Cognitive, affective, and implementation nursing components can best be integrated by the nursing process

G. Process consists of assessing, diagnosing, planning, implementing, and evaluating a client's problem and its proposed solution via the nursing care plan; it is an ongoing process while the client is in the nurse's care

Steps in the Nursing Process

A. Data collection
  1. Collection of personal, social, medical, and general data
     a. Sources: primary (client and diagnostic test results) and secondary (family, colleagues, Kardex, literature)
     b. Methods
        (1) Interviewing formally (nursing health history) and informally during various nurse-client interactions
        (2) Observation
        (3) Review of records
  2. Performing a physical assessment

B. Analysis and interpretation
  1. Classification of data: screening, organizing, and grouping significant and related information
  2. Definition of client's problem: making a nursing diagnosis
     a. A nursing diagnosis is a definitive statement of the client's actual or potential difficulties, concerns, or deficits that are amenable to nursing interventions; there are two components to the statement of a nursing diagnosis joined together by the phrase "related to"
        (1) Part I: a determination of the problem (unhealthful response of client)
        (2) Part II: identification of the etiology (contributing factors)
     b. Development of diagnoses (see list of NANDA-approved Nursing Diagnoses in this chapter)
        (1) Excludes all nonnursing diagnoses; for example, medical diagnoses or diagnostic tests
        (2) Excludes medical treatments, as well as the nurse's problems with the client
        (3) Involves inductive and deductive reasoning
        (4) Includes both internal and external environmental stresses

        (5) Includes data that have been clustered (grouping of related data) during assessment

C. Planning: the nursing care plan, a blueprint for action
  1. Previously identified nursing diagnoses are written on the care plan
  2. Planned intervention may include independent and interdependent functions of the nurse; prescriptions made by physician or allied health professionals may be included
  3. New diagnoses should be noted on the nursing care plan and progress notes as they are identified
  4. Client outcomes (goals of nursing intervention) are reflected in expected changes in the client
     a. Expected client outcome is written next to each nursing diagnosis on nursing care plan
     b. These outcomes must be objective, realistic, measurable alterations in the client's behavior, activity, or physical state; a time period should be set for achievement of the outcome
     c. The outcome provides a standard of measure that can be used to determine if the goal toward which the client and nurse are working has been achieved
  5. Nursing interventions (nursing orders) are written for each nursing diagnosis and should be specific to the stated outcome or goal; each goal may have one or more applicable interventions

D. Implementation: the actual administration of the planned nursing care

E. Evaluation/outcome and revision of nursing care plan
  1. Process is ongoing throughout client's treatment/hospitalization
  2. If outcome/goal is not reached in specified time, the client is reassessed to discover the reason
  3. Reordering of priorities and new goal setting may be necessary
  4. When diagnosis/problem is resolved, the date should be noted on care plan

F. Collaboration and coordination: requires the nurse to liaise and work together with other members of the nursing and health care teams
  1. occurs during the many phases of the nursing process
  2. ensures that the care provided is client-focused, participative, coordinated, integrated, and comprehensive
  3. includes activities such as communication with the health care team (including the client), delegation, and leadership

NANDA-approved Nursing Diagnoses (1994)

Activity intolerance
Acute confusion
Altered family processes
Altered family processes: alcoholism
Altered growth and development
Altered health maintenance
Altered nutrition: less than body requirements
Altered nutrition: more than body requirements
Altered nutrition: risk for more than body requirements
Altered oral mucous membrane
Altered parenting
Altered protection
Altered role performance
Altered sexuality patterns
Altered thought processes
Altered (specify type) tissue perfusion (cerebral, cardiopulmonary, renal, gastrointestinal, peripheral)
Altered urinary elimination
Anticipatory grieving
Anxiety
Bathing/hygiene self-care deficit
Body image disturbance
Bowel incontinence
Caregiver role strain
Chronic confusion
Chronic low self-esteem
Chronic pain
Colonic constipation
Constipation
Decisional conflict (specify)
Decreased adaptive capacity: intracranial
Decreased cardiac output
Defensive coping
Diarrhea
Disorganized infant behavior
Diversional activity deficit
Dressing/grooming self-care deficit
Dysfunctional grieving
Dysfunctional ventilatory weaning response (DVWR)
Dysreflexia
Effective breastfeeding
Effective management of therapeutic regimen: individual
Energy field disturbance
Family coping: potential for growth
Fatigue
Fear
Feeding self-care deficit
Fluid volume deficit (1)
Fluid volume deficit (2)
Fluid volume excess
Functional incontinence
Health-seeking behaviors (specify) or desire for high-level wellness (specify)
Hopelessness
Hyperthermia
Hypothermia
Impaired adjustment
Impaired environmental interpretation syndrome
Impaired gas exchange
Impaired home maintenance management
Impaired memory
Impaired physical mobility
Impaired skin integrity
Impaired social interaction
Impaired swallowing
Impaired tissue integrity
Impaired verbal communication

Inability to sustain spontaneous ventilation
Ineffective airway clearance
Ineffective breastfeeding
Ineffective breathing pattern
Ineffective community coping
Ineffective denial
Ineffective family coping: compromised
Ineffective family coping: disabling
Ineffective individual coping
Ineffective infant feeding pattern
Ineffective management of therapeutic regimen (community)
Ineffective management of therapeutic regimen (families)
Ineffective management of therapeutic regimen (individual)
Ineffective thermoregulation
Interrupted breastfeeding
Knowledge deficit (specify)
Noncompliance (specify)
Pain
Parental role conflict
Perceived constipation
Personal identity disturbance
Posttrauma response
Potential for enhanced community coping
Potential for enhanced disorganized infant behavior
Potential for enhanced spiritual well-being
Powerlessness
Rape-trauma syndrome
Rape-trauma syndrome: compound reaction
Rape-trauma syndrome: silent reaction
Reflex incontinence
Relocation stress syndrome
Risk for activity intolerance
Risk for altered body temperature
Risk for altered parent/infant/child attachment
Risk for altered parenting
Risk for aspiration
Risk for caregiver role strain
Risk for disorganized infant behavior
Risk for disuse syndrome
Risk for fluid volume deficit
Risk for impaired skin integrity
Risk for infection
Risk for injury
Risk for loneliness
Risk for perioperative positioning injury
Risk for peripheral neurovascular dysfunction
Risk for poisoning
Risk for self-mutilation
Risk for suffocation
Risk for trauma
Risk for violence: self-directed or directed at others
Self-esteem disturbance
Sensory perceptual alterations (specify) (auditory, gustatory, kinesthetic, olfactory, tactile, visual)
Sexual dysfunction
Situational low self-esteem
Sleep pattern disturbance
Social isolation
Spiritual distress (distress of the human spirit)
Stress incontinence
Toileting self-care deficit
Total incontinence
Unilateral neglect
Urge incontinence
Urinary retention

G. Professional practice: requires the nurse to practice within existing professional, legal, and ethical standards and to oversee practice according to established standards
1. includes activities such as maintaining the client's privacy and confidentiality, demonstrating respect for the client and members of the health care team and
2. involves monitoring and ensuring the quality of health care practices

H. Advantages of nursing process
1. Encourages thorough individual client assessment by nurse
2. Determines priority of care
3. Provides comprehensive and systematic nursing care planning and delivery
4. Permits independent, creative, and flexible nursing intervention
5. Facilitates team cooperation by promoting:
    a. Contributions from all team members
    b. Communication among team members
    c. Coordination of care
    d. Continuity of care
6. Provides for continuous involvement and input from client
7. Facilitates nursing research
8. Provides accurate legal document of client care
9. Satisfies rules of regulatory agencies

ESTABLISHMENT OF A TEACHING-LEARNING ENVIRONMENT

Introduction

A. Teaching is communication especially structured and sequenced to produce learning
B. Learning is the activity by which knowledge, attitudes, and skills are acquired, resulting in a change in behavior
C. All problems in learning and identified knowledge deficits should be addressed when establishing the appropriate nursing diagnoses for a client
D. Goals of learning
1. Understanding or acquiring knowledge: cognitive learning (e.g., What is diabetes and how does it affect me physically?)
2. Feeling or developing attitudes: affective learning (e.g., What does this health problem mean to me?)
3. Doing or developing psychomotor skills: conative learning (e.g., How do I give myself an injection?)

Principles of Teaching-Learning Process and Related Nursing Approaches

A. Learning occurs best when there is a felt need or readiness to learn
1. Identify the client's emotional or motivational readiness: is the person ready to put forth the effort necessary to learn
2. Identify the client's experiential readiness: does the person have the necessary background of experience, skills, attitudes, and ability to learn
3. Assess the client's language abilities and reading skills
4. Determine the client's level of adaptation: different teaching strategies may be necessary during the various stages of adaptation because the client is expressing denial, anger, and/or depression; once the initial defensive compensatory reactions have passed, the individual is more receptive to teaching
5. Assess the client's level of human needs; the client whose physical and safety needs are not met will not be concerned with interpersonal and intrapersonal needs
6. Assess cognitive and motor impairment from illness or treatment, which may affect the client's ability to learn; pain, fatigue, and anxiety may impede the learning process and must be dealt with before teaching
7. Identify the client's readiness to learn
    a. Client is adapting to the initial crisis
    b. Client has a developing awareness of the health problem and its implications
    c. Client is asking direct questions
    d. Client is presenting clues that indicate indirect seeking of information
    e. Client's physical condition or behavior invites the nurse to intervene through teaching
8. Once a need has been recognized, readiness has been determined, and the time and place are appropriate, develop a plan and teach

B. The method of presentation of material influences the client's ability to learn
1. Develop a tentative teaching plan with the client and/or the client's significant others and communicate it to all members of the health team
2. Present information in an organized, accurate, and concise manner (e.g., presented in a format of simple to the complex, general to the specific)
3. Appropriate teaching methods should be instituted
    a. Teach concepts with lectures, audiovisual materials, and discussion
    b. Influence attitudes by exploring feelings, role models, discussions, and an atmosphere of acceptance
    c. Teach skills by illustrations, models, demonstration, return demonstration, and practice

4. Use teaching tools when indicated (e.g., models, filmstrips, illustrations)
5. Encourage the client and family to ask questions, which should be answered directly
6. Provide opportunities for evaluation

C. Learning is made easier when material to be learned is related to what the learner already knows
1. Find out what the client knows about the problem
2. Begin the teaching program at the client's level of understanding
3. Avoid the use of technical terminology; use simple terms or ones with which the client feels comfortable

D. Learning is purposeful; short- and long-term goals are important because they identify the behavior to be attained
1. With the client, set short- and long-term goals
2. Set goals that meet the following criteria:
   a. Client centered
   b. Specific: state exactly what is to be accomplished
   c. Measurable: set a minimum acceptable level of performance
   d. Realistic: must be potentially achievable
   e. Have a time frame

E. Learning is an active process and takes place within the learner
1. Use a teaching approach that includes the learner (e.g., programmed instruction books, discussion, questions and answers, return demonstration)
2. Provide opportunities for the client to practice motor skills
3. Encourage self-directed activities

F. Every individual has capabilities and strengths (e.g., physical strengths, emotional maturity, a supportive family) that can be used to help the client learn
1. Identify the client's personal resources
2. Build on the identified strengths
3. Use these personal resources when and where appropriate

G. Energy and endurance levels affect the client's ability to learn and perform
1. Balance teaching with sufficient rest periods
2. Provide teaching at opportune times (e.g., earlier in the day rather than at night, after periods of rest)
3. Present instruction in a manner the client can comprehend and at a pace that can be maintained
4. Be flexible and adjust the plan according to the client's rest and activity needs

H. Learning does not always progress in a straight forward-and-upward manner; the client may experience plateaus and remissions with a resulting change in adaptation and needs
1. Accept the client's feelings regarding lack of progress
2. Point out progress that has been made
3. Be patient and do not cause additional stress for the learner
4. Try alternative approaches for achieving goals
5. Identify short-term objectives for meeting goals
6. Alter long-term goals as necessary

I. Learning from previous experience can be transferred to new situations
1. Base the plan of instructions on the foundation of the client's knowledge
2. When teaching something new, relate the commonalities or similarities of previously learned experiences
3. Reinforce the known before exploring the unknown and teaching differences

Motivation

A. Definition: motivation is the process of stimulating a person to assimilate certain concepts or behavior
B. Principles of motivation and related nursing approaches
1. People are complex products of self, family, and culture; the nurse must care for the client as a unified being
   a. Respect the client as a person
   b. Accept the client's feelings without minimizing them
   c. Assist the client and family in accepting that the person's individuality and wholeness continue despite the changed physical or emotional state
   d. Involve the client in deciding what to do and how to do it
   e. Recognize the client must take precedence over the purpose of the lesson
2. Learning is fostered when the plan of instruction is designed to operate within the individual's personal attitude and value system
   a. Provide an atmosphere that allows for acceptance of differing value systems
   b. Let the client explore personal values, attitudes, and feelings concerning the health problem and its implications
   c. Explore with the family the possibilities of carrying out instruction and how to individualize it so it is acceptable and practical for the client and family
3. A motivated learner assimilates what is learned more rapidly than does one who is unmotivated
   a. Provide the client with an opportunity to explore and discover personal learning needs and feelings concerning them

b. Channel mild anxiety, which in itself is motivating

c. Avoid intense anxiety, which may reduce learning

d. Determine the client's readiness for learning

4. Intrinsic motivation (stimulated from within the learner) is preferable to extrinsic motivation (stimulated from outside the learner)

   a. Identify factors that are essential for the individual to have a feeling of meaningful achievement (e.g., being able to care for own health needs, respect and appreciation from others, acquiring new knowledge, receiving a reward)

   b. Design nursing care that will assist the client in attaining a feeling of meaningful achievement; satisfaction with learning progress promotes additional learning

   c. Encourage the client to participate as a member of the health team and to be self-directed

5. Information is learned more readily when it is relevant and meaningful to the learner

   a. Help the client interpret why the information is important and how the information gained will be useful

   b. Relate the information by building the teaching plan on the client's foundation of knowledge, experience, attitudes, and feelings

6. Learning motivated by success or rewards is preferable to learning by failure or punishment

   a. Help the client set realistic goals within the motivation zone (goals set too high may be too challenging, whereas goals set too low may lead to no action)

   b. Focus on the client's strengths and abilities rather than on failures and disabilities

   c. Select learning tasks in which the client is likely to succeed

   d. Assist the client to master or feel successful at one stage of instruction before moving on to the next

   e. Accept errors as part of the learning process

   f. Encourage tolerance for failure by providing a backlog of success that compensates for experienced failure

7. Planned reinforcement is essential for learning; operant conditioning is based on the theory that satisfaction motivates learning and that those events that occur together are associated

   a. For each client, identify and use factors that are stimulants or incentives for action (e.g., praise, smile, rewards, rest, specific privileges, being able to care for self)

b. Provide visible reinforcements (e.g., progress charts, graphs)

c. Repeat activities until they become habitual; repetition is a form of reinforcement

   (1) Provide opportunities for the client to practice old and new skills

   (2) Review information previously taught before introducing new information

d. Involve the client in groups of people who have the same health problems but are at various stages of convalescence

   (1) To be successful, it is helpful for the client to associate with successful people

   (2) Individuals can often learn more by teaching others

   (3) Seeing others who have progressed in their convalescence inspires hope and a sense that their actions will be effective

8. Evaluation of performance aids in learning

   a. Purpose

     (1) To measure and interpret results with regard to what degree the set goals are attained

     (2) To reinforce correct behavior

     (3) To help the learner realize how to change incorrect behavior

     (4) To help the teacher determine the adequacy of the teaching

   b. Together the teacher and learner should observe and evaluate the learner's response in light of the desired behavior

   c. Identify factors that may have contributed to attainment or nonattainment of goals

   d. Avoid value judgments, especially "poor" or "inadequate"; judgments must relate to the performance rather than to the individual

PROVIDING LEADERSHIP

Definition

Process of influencing the actions of an individual or group toward specific goals in a particular situation

Styles of Leadership

A. Three basic styles

1. Autocratic: leader does not seek input from the group but sets the goals, plans, makes the decisions, and evaluates the action taken

2. Democratic: leader seeks input from the group, and responsibilities for action taken are shared between the leader and the group

3. Laissez-faire: leader's input and control of the group are minimal, permitting each individual to set independent goals

B. Leadership styles influenced by the leader, the environment, and the cultural climate of the organization

C. The effective leader modifies his or her style to fit changing circumstances, problems, and people (e.g., autocratic style of leadership is appropriate in an emergency situation)

Principles of Leadership

A. Interpersonal influence depends on a knowledge of human behavior and a sensitivity to others in terms of feelings, values, and problems
   1. Explore and understand personal attitudes, feelings, and values
   2. Project self into the place of the individuals being led
   3. Know how you appear to subordinates
B. Communication is an essential component of leadership
   1. Effective communication depends on the use of the appropriate medium
      a. Communication may be verbal, written, and/or nonverbal
      b. Communication may be formal or informal
      c. Communication should have two directions: up and down the chain of command and among equals
   2. Communication style can affect the person or persons with whom the leader communicates
      a. Meanings or ideas communicated should be received or intended without distraction
      b. People react to communication differently
      c. Written communication should be in language that is understood by the person or persons intended (e.g., ancillary personnel should have a written assignment that does not require them to make judgments)
      d. Verbal communication can be influenced by facial expressions, body movement, and tone of voice
   3. Effectiveness of communication can be influenced by inappropriate timing; the information communicated may be correct, but the time may be wrong so ascertain readiness
C. Leader's success is influenced by how the leader's ability to respond to group needs effectively is perceived by those being led
   1. A role is composed of a number of expectations for the behavior of an individual in a specific position or status classification; the role a person plays may influence the dynamics of the group positively or negatively, depending on whether the role is serving the individual's or the group's needs; some roles are task oriented and help the group directly in doing the assignment; other roles are more process oriented and help the group communicate effectively
      a. Any individual's role consists of a number of expectations and relationships

b. The nurse leader, by virtue of behavior and status, can influence the perceptions of peers, clients, and colleagues
   2. Power is a leader's source of influence
   3. Power may be professional or positional
      a. Positional power: acquired through the position the leader has in the hierarchy of the organization
      b. Professional power: acquired through the knowledge or expertise displayed by the leader and/or perceived by the followers
D. Leadership moves from one person to another as changes occur in the work situation
   1. The nurse's expertise about a specific client care problem along with the availability of other resources can place the nurse in the position of providing leadership for a group
   2. A member of another discipline may assume the role of leadership in specific situations (e.g., the physician leads the cardiac arrest team; the nurse coordinates physical rehabilitation and nutrition for the client)
E. Leadership process requires the use of actions associated with problem solving: decision making, relating, influencing, and facilitating
   1. Decision making requires knowledge about and skill in solving the problem; participative decision making lends itself to the quality of the decision made, improves relationships, and influences the readiness of an individual or group to accept change (e.g., the client or the family should have the opportunity to participate in the development of the client's plan of care; unit staff may decide which primary nurse or team leader should care for a newly admitted client)
   2. Effective delegation of responsibilities is inherent in effective leadership; delegation of work requires matching the task with the appropriate position (e.g., a nursing assistant should not provide care that requires the expertise of a registered nurse; using a registered nurse for housekeeping duties is wasteful)
F. Need for change should be understood by those effecting the change, as well as those affected by the change
   1. Movement from goal setting to goal achievement involves change
   2. Resistance to change is normal and should be expected and addressed in planning
   3. Process of changing includes communication, planning, participation, and evaluation by the individual or group affected
   4. Change is more acceptable when:
      a. It has not been dictated but follows a sequence of impersonal principles

b. Individuals or groups affected have participated in its creation
c. It has been planned
d. It follows a number of successful rather than unsuccessful series of changes
e. It is initiated after other changes have been absorbed, not during the confusion of a major change
f. It does not threaten security

G. Effective use of leadership is conducive to accomplishing the goals of the group; an evaluation process is necessary if the results of efforts to attain the goals are to be interpreted accurately
   1. Goals should be identified as short term and long term
   2. Evaluation process should be ongoing
   3. Climate in which the evaluation process occurs influences its success

ADMINISTRATION OF MEDICATIONS

GENERAL INFORMATION

A. The scientific age has introduced an increasing number of pharmaceuticals appropriate for the relief of stress symptoms, for support of defense systems, and as adjuncts to other supplemental and curative therapies
B. Drug nomenclature
   1. Official name (generic, nonproprietary): designated title under which a drug is listed in official publications
   2. Chemical name: descriptive name identifying chemical composition and placement of atoms
   3. Trade name (brand, proprietary): manufacturer's registered and legally owned name for a drug
C. Sources of drugs
   1. Active constituents of plants: for example, alkaloids, glycosides, gums, resins, tannins, waxes, volatile or fixed oils
   2. Animal sources of biologic products: for example, enzymes, sera, vaccines, antitoxins, toxoids, hormones
   3. Mineral sources: for example, iron, iodine, Epsom salt
   4. Chemically and biologically engineered substances: for example human insulin
D. Types of pharmaceutical preparations
   1. Prepared by manufacturers in units for convenience of administration
   2. Forms used include capsules, extended-release capsules, tablets (enteric coated, extended release), troches, pills, suppositories, powders, ampules, vials, delayed-release (repository) suspensions, prefilled cartridges, liniments, lotions, creams, ointments, pastes, aerosols, transdermal preparations
   3. Chemical preparations: solutions (waters, true solutions, syrups), aqueous suspensions (mixtures, emulsions, magmas, gels), spirits, elixirs, tinctures, fluid extracts, extracts

BASIC CONCEPTS

A. The administration of medications requires a legally written physician's order and knowledge of the medication's cause and effect
B. Legally, morally, and ethically, independent judgment is required before prescribed medications are administered
C. Certain chemical agents alter, inactivate, or potentiate other medications when mixed either before or after administration
D. Medications may be given for local or systemic effects
E. Pharmacologic actions of drugs tend to stimulate or depress physiologic activity
F. Medications may be given in a variety of ways, depending on factors such as the effect desired, rapidity of action desired, or the effect of the chemical on the tissues

COMMONLY USED TERMINOLOGY

A. Chemotherapy: use of drugs to destroy invading organisms or abnormal tissue in the host
B. Drug: chemical agent that interacts with living systems and is employed to prevent, diagnose, or treat disease
C. Drug legislation: laws that provide the standards for drug manufacture and distribution and protect the public against fraudulent claims about drug action (e.g., Narcotics Control Act and Regulations)
D. Drug standards: criteria for drug composition established by chemical or bioassay and published in official publications (e.g., *Pharmacopoeia Internationalis*)
E. Pharmacodynamics: biochemical and physiologic effects of drugs and their mechanisms of action on living tissue
F. Pharmacology: analysis of properties of chemicals that have a biologic action
G. Pharmacotherapeutics: planned use and evaluation of the effect of drugs employed to prevent and treat disease
H. Toxicology: analysis of poisons and poisonings caused by drugs

DRUG EFFECTS

A. Desired effect: (therapeutic effect) action for which the drug is given
B. Adverse effect: action differing from the planned effect that is undesirable
C. Side effect: often predictable outcome that is unrelated to the primary action of the drug
D. Toxic effect: pathologic extension of the primary action of the drug
E. Cumulation: elevation of circulating levels of a drug consequent to slowing of metabolic pathways or excretory mechanisms
F. Drug dependence: driving need for continued use of a behavior- or mood-altering drug that leads to abuse
   1. Psychic dependence: craving requiring periodic or continued use of a drug for pleasure or relief of discomfort
   2. Physical dependence: appearance of characteristic symptoms when drug use is suspended or terminated (withdrawal or abstinence symptoms)
G. Hypersusceptibility: response to a drug action that is higher than that occurring when the same dosage is given to 90% of the population
H. Idiosyncrasy: unpredictable, highly individualized response; genetically conditioned enzymatic or receptor responsiveness that interferes with metabolic degradation of a drug
I. Paradoxical response: action of a drug producing a response that contrasts sharply with the usual therapeutic effect obtained with the same dosage of the drug
J. Receptor: cellular site where union between a drug and a cellular constituent produces a reversible action
K. Tolerance: lowering of effect obtained from an established dosage of a drug that necessitates raising the dosage to maintain the effect
L. Tachyphylaxis: rapidly developing tolerance to a drug
M. Drug allergy: response occurring when drugs are from protein sources or combine with body protein and induce an allergen-antibody reaction that releases vasoactive intermediates that cause fluid transudation into tissues
   1. Anaphylaxis: life-threatening episode of bronchial constriction and edema that obstructs the airway and causes generalized vasodilation that depletes circulating blood volume; occurs when a drug allergen is administered to an individual having antibodies produced by prior use of the drug
   2. Urticaria: generalized pruritic skin eruptions or giant hives; occurs when a drug is administered to an individual having antibodies produced by prior use of the drug
   3. Angioedema: fluid accumulation in periorbital, oral, and respiratory tissues with lengthening of the expiratory phase and wheezing as bronchial constriction gradually progresses; occurs when a drug is administered to an individual having antibodies produced by prior use of the drug
   4. Serum sickness: gradually emerging intermittent episodes of dyspnea, hypotension, generalized edema, joint pain, rash, swollen lymph glands; occurs 7 or more days after initial administration of a drug causing gradual low-level (titer) production of antibodies that interact with circulating drug to produce symptoms as long as the drug remains in the body
   5. Arthus reaction: localized area of tissue necrosis caused by disruption of blood supply; occurs when spasticity, occlusion, and degeneration of blood vessels are precipitated by injection of a drug into a site having large quantities of bivalent antibodies
   6. Delayed-reaction allergies: rash and fever occurring during drug therapy

DRUG ACTIONS

A. Local: drug acts at the site of application
B. Systemic: drug is distributed to selected internal receptor sites after being absorbed from tissues following administration; these routes include oral, sublingual, buccal, nasal, rectal, transdermal, parenteral (intradermal, subcutaneous, intramuscular, intravenous, intraspinal, intracardiac)

DRUG MECHANISMS

A. Replacement (e.g., administration of insulin required for cellular use of glucose)
B. Interruption (e.g., antimetabolic drugs tricking the cell into using an inactive component in building protein)
C. Potentiation (e.g., sulfonylurea group of oral hypoglycemic agents stimulating pancreatic beta cells to produce insulin)
D. Competition (e.g., antihistamine drugs competing with histamine for tissue-receptor sites)

FACTORS INFLUENCING DOSAGE-RESPONSE RELATIONSHIP

A. Age, weight, sex, size, physiologic status, and genetic and environmental factors affect responses and dosage required for therapeutic effect
B. The ratio between the median toxic dose and the median effective dose (TD50/ED50) of a drug provides the therapeutic index (TI), which is used as a

guide to the safe dosage range; a low TI provides a narrow margin of safety, and the client's status is monitored closely for evidence of drug-related adverse effects (e.g., antineoplastic drugs)

C. Concentration of active drug at receptors and duration of drug action are affected by:
  1. Characteristics of the drug and the rate of absorption, distribution, biotransformation, and excretion
  2. Drug affinity for particular tissues, immaturity of enzymes required for metabolism of the drug, or depressed function of tissues naturally metabolizing or excreting the drug

D. Membrane barriers (e.g., placental or blood-brain) may block or selectively pass the drug from the circulating fluids to protected areas

E. Plasma protein binding of drugs maintains tissue levels by liberating the drug when stores are lowered and by slowing renal clearance until the drug is freed from binding sites

DRUG INTERACTIONS

A. Drugs and foods may interact to affect the therapeutic plan adversely (e.g., ingestion of foods or vitamin preparations containing vitamin K may inhibit the hypothrombinemic effect of oral anticoagulants)

B. Drug antagonism: opposing effects of two drugs at receptor sites in body tissues
  1. Chemical antagonism: combining or binding of two drugs causing inactivation of the chemicals
  2. Pharmacologic antagonism: competition of two drugs for a receptor that may allow the weaker drug to block access by the more potent drug
  3. Physiologic antagonism: opposing action on physiologic systems that allows cancellation of action by either drug

C. Drug action summation: combined or concurrent action of drugs that increases therapeutic effects or incidence of adverse effects
  1. Synergism: interaction of drugs at common receptor sites that alters metabolism or excretion and enhances the effect of drugs
  2. Addition: action of two drugs at different receptors that produces an effect twice that possible when either drug is used alone
  3. Potentiation: intensified action occurring when two drugs are administered concurrently that is greater than when either drug is administered alone

NURSING RESPONSIBILITIES

A. Increasingly, as part of nursing care the nurse assumes the responsibility of administering a greater number of medications in a greater variety of forms via a greater assortment of routes; many of these substances have a narrow therapeutic index, increasing the nursing responsibilities associated with their administration

B. In the interest of client welfare and safety, it is imperative that the independent and collaborative responsibilities inherent in this function be understood and practiced

C. Ascertain the presence and correctness of a legally written order

D. Know the common symbols and equivalents in the metric/SI system

E. Know the common abbreviations denoting frequency and route of administration

F. Know the usual dosage of a drug, the usual route of administration, and the expected, unusual, untoward, or toxic effects of a drug

G. Monitor serum-drug levels for
  1. Attainment of therapeutic level
  2. Toxic level
  3. Peak and trough levels

H. Use independent judgment before administering a medication by assessing:
  1. The client's needs relative to factors such as prn medications and expected effects of the medication (e.g., diuresis or sleep)
  2. Untoward or toxic manifestations of prior doses (e.g., pruritus following an antibiotic, bradycardia and visual disturbances with digoxin)
  3. Compatibility of medications administered at the same time
    a. The presence of clouding or a precipitate when mixing injectables (e.g., phenobarbital [Luminal Sodium] and meperidine hydrochloride [Demerol])
    b. Inhibition of medication (e.g., an antacid or milk given with tetracycline interferes with absorption, resulting in decreased serum levels of the antibiotic)
    c. Potentiation of another medication (e.g., ASA given when a client is receiving anticoagulants intensifies the anticoagulant effect)
  4. Compatibility of medications with substances in the diet or environment
  5. Effects on living tissues
    a. Iron can discolor tissue and must be given through a straw in liquid form or by the Z-track method intramuscularly
    b. Abscess formation can occur when the same area is used too often for intramuscular administration; thus rotation of site is necessary
    c. Pain, irritation, or inflammation can occur during intravenous administration and may necessitate adjustments such as greater dilution or slower flow rate

I. Help the client accept ordered medications by independent actions such as:
   1. Crushing tablets that cannot be swallowed
   2. Disguising unpalatable tastes with fruit juices
   3. Reinforcing the need for medication
J. Ensure that the right medication is given to the right client at the right time, in the right dose, and by the right route
   1. Verify orders
   2. Read labels
   3. Calculate the dosage accurately when prescribed dose is not available
   4. Pour or draw up correct amounts
   5. Identify the client correctly by checking the arm band
   6. Prepare the client psychologically by providing explanations as needed
   7. Prepare the client physically by:
      a. Positioning appropriately for oral and parenteral medications
      b. Disinfecting the skin when it is to be punctured
   8. Use clean or sterile technique as indicated by route of administration; use universal precautions
   9. Use the route specified as appropriate for the ordered medication and dosage
   10. Recognize that the client has the right to refuse medication
K. For assistance with calculation of solutions and dosages, refer to a programmed text
L. Use the appropriate technique for administration
   1. Preparations such as tablets, capsules, pills, powders, or liquids may be swallowed; in addition:
      a. Tablets (e.g., nitroglycerine) may be held sublingually
      b. Powders (e.g., cromolyn sodium) may be inhaled with a Medihaler
      c. Liquids may be nebulized and inhaled or may be swabbed, sprayed, or instilled
      d. Sustained-release or enteric-coated preparations should not be crushed or broken open
      e. Suspensions should be shaken well before pouring
   2. Parenteral preparations such as ampules or vials containing the dose in solution or powder to which sterile water or saline must be added may be given in several ways
      a. Subcutaneously or intramuscularly in small volume (0.5 to 2 ml)
         (1) Subcutaneously: pinch subcutaneous tissue of anterior and lateral aspects of the thighs, lower ventral abdominal wall, lower back, or outer middle aspect of arms. Intramuscularly: spread the tissue taut on the outer surface of the upper arm (deltoid) or the anterior aspect of the thigh (vastus lateralis)
         (2) Insert a 25- to 27-gauge needle $5/8$ to 1 inch in length at a 45- to 60-degree angle or a $1/2$-inch needle (insulin or tuberculin) at a 90-degree angle, aspirate slightly, and inject the medication if there is no blood return (aspiration not indicated when heparin administered because of bruising; aspiration not recommended when insulin administered to thin adults and children who are more likely to have superficial blood vessels)
         (3) Massage to increase absorption (contraindicated when giving heparin and insulin)
      b. Intramuscularly in slightly larger volume (up to 3 ml)
         (1) Spread the tissue taut or pinch if necessary (if patient emaciated)
         (2) Use the upper outer quadrant of the buttock, ventral gluteal muscle, the vastus lateralis, or the deltoid area of the arm
         (3) When using the gluteal muscle, promote relaxation of the muscle whenever possible by placing the client in a prone position with toes pointing inward or on the side with the upper leg flexed
         (4) Insert a 20- to 22-gauge needle 1 to $1^1/2$ inches in length at a 90-degree angle quickly and smoothly
         (5) Depth of insertion depends on factors such as weight of the client and size of the muscle used
         (6) Aspirate when the needle is in place and tissue is released (unless giving a substance such as iron-dextran [Imferon], for which the Z-track method is used)
            (a) If no blood returns, continue injection
            (b) If blood is aspirated, withdraw and prepare a fresh dose
         (7) Apply pressure or massage area after injection as required (unless contraindicated, e.g., Z-track technique)
      c. Intradermally with very small volume for local effect
         (1) Use syringe with appropriate calibrations (e.g., tuberculin)
         (2) Inject at a 15-degree angle using a 26-gauge needle, $3/8$ to $1/2$ inch in length with the bevel up

d. Piggyback administration using intravenous tubing in place
   (1) If necessary, dilute medication according to directions: add 50 to 150 ml of fluid
   (2) Remove air from tubing of piggyback without losing any fluid
   (3) Cleanse diaphragm on intravenous tubing already in place with alcohol
   (4) Insert piggyback in rubber diaphragm on tubing leading from the infusion that is keeping the vein open
   (5) Stop flow of or lower the primary solution below level of the piggyback
   (6) Adjust rate of flow on piggyback medication to complete absorption in time designated—usually about 30 to 45 minutes
   (7) Remove the piggyback and readjust flow rate

3. Transdermal preparations
   a. Medication should not be touched during preparation for administration; gloves should be worn with certain medications
   b. Medication should be applied to a smooth, hairless body surface; sites should be rotated
   c. Remove old transdermal application before applying a new one

M. Clearly and accurately record and report the administration of medications and the client's response

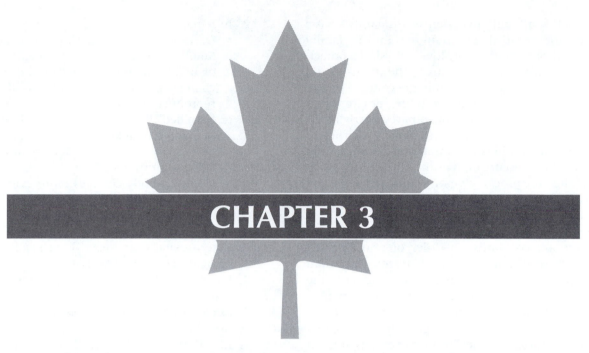

CHAPTER 3

Childbearing and Women's Health Nursing

This section, childbearing and women's health nursing, covers reproductive problems and emphasizes the pubertal changes of adolescence; the normal processes of conception, embryologic development, pregnancy, labor, birth, and postpartum developments; and family planning. In addition, the newborn and the mother are discussed in relation to prematurity, birth injuries, and complications of labor and birth. Current topics such as abortion, infant narcotic addiction, sexually transmitted diseases, sterility, and women's health issues are included.

Childbirth is a family experience. Humanity's basic needs for survival are centered in the family because without continuous love, physical contact, food, and stimulation of the senses, the infant would never survive. As each new member becomes a part of the family unit, interactions with the environment and other human beings become a part of early physical and emotional development. What is learned is determined by the kinds of stimulation received from the interactions occurring within the family. It is through this reciprocal give-and-take between the newborn and the family that each person becomes an individual, unique self.

Although childbearing patterns differ the world over, there are constants. In order of priority, they are: immediate physical contact between the infant and the parents; ability of the parents to give the infant love, food, and protection from the environment; the biologic need in men and women to reproduce; and the maturation and growth process that occurs in males and females in their changing roles as parents.

The unique and changing responsibilities in the life-cycle event of parenthood can be a real crisis. The changes occurring in society, whether social, economic, technical, or political, directly affect the patterns of childbearing and childrearing. Parenthood today is given serious thought because it concerns both the family and society, and its emphasis is on quality rather than quantity.

Women experience many gender-related health problems, such as cancer of the breast and uterus, and these problems are discussed in this chapter to reflect the current trends in health care today.

REPRODUCTIVE READINESS—PUBERTY

A period during which the organs of reproduction mature and are prepared for their reproductive function
A. Physical and physiologic changes
 1. In males
  a. Occur between 10 and 14 years of age; less dramatic than in females
  b. Heralded by deepening of voice and growth of body hair on the face, axillae, and genitalia
  c. Second year after onset: increased activity of sweat glands, spermatogenesis occurs with periodic erections and emissions of mature sperm
  d. Dramatic body growth spurt
  e. Ejaculation is beginning of fertility and end of puberty

 2. In females
  a. Occur between 9 and 13 years of age
  b. Sudden enlargement of the breasts, growth of body hair on the axillae and genitalia; changes in size and vascularity of internal reproductive organs
  c. Heralded by first menstrual flow, called menarche; unlike the male's first ejaculation, many first menstrual cycles are anovulatory (infertile)
  d. Dramatic body changes more evident than in male
B. Psychologic changes
 1. Maturational changes according to age
 2. Heterosexual interests: girls earlier than boys, girls interested in older boys
 3. Emancipation struggles with parents: independence versus dependence
 4. Need for belonging to a peer group
C. Menstrual cycle
 1. Rhythmic reproductive cycle in females extending from the onset of a period of uterine bleeding to the onset of the next period of bleeding; mean cycle length is 28 days; normal range is 20 to 45 days per cycle
 2. During each cycle, several (about 20) follicles commence maturation, but usually only one reaches full maturity and expels its contained ovum (and some surrounding granulosa cells) into the abdominal cavity
 3. The rhythmic menstrual cycles begin at puberty and cease at menopause
 4. Menstrual cycle divided into three stages based on endometrial histologic makeup and may be correlated with concentration fluctuations in hypothalamic, hypophyseal, and ovarian hormones (which cause the endometrial and other reproductive tract histologic changes)
  a. First stage—menstruation or menses: lasts 4 to 6 days; characterized by endometrial bleeding with the discharge exiting through the vagina; estrogen and progesterone blood levels are relatively low; the follicle-stimulating hormone (FSH) level is elevated and, combined with a steady low level of luteinizing hormone (LH) secretion, initiates ovarian estrogen secretion, leading to the second stage
  b. Second stage—follicular or proliferative: lasts 8 to 10 days, culminating in ovulation; endometrium regenerates and proliferates in preparation for possible implantation, and a single ovarian follicle approaches full maturation as the concentration of estradiol (the principal estrogenic hormone) in the blood rises; estradiol exerts a negative feed-

back on FSH secretion and a positive feedback on LH secretion (the latter hormone induces ovulation); estradiol's feedback effects are exerted on the hypothalamic secretion of FSH-releasing hormone (FSH-RH) and LH-releasing hormone (which control the hypophyseal secretion of FSH and LH)

   c. Third stage—luteal or secretory: final stage is 9 to 13 days and begins after ovulation; LH promotes formation of a temporary endocrine gland, the corpus luteum, from the ruptured follicle; granulosa and theca interna cells of follicle enlarge, divide into and occupy the cavity (antrum) of the follicle, and secrete progesterone and estrogen; progesterone stimulates the already proliferated endometrium to become glandular with a high glycogen-secreting potential (uterus now prepared for implantation); if fertilization does not occur, the corpus luteum functions for 7 to 8 days after ovulation and then involutes, becoming nonfunctional (corpus albicans) 10 to 12 days after ovulation; progesterone and estrogen blood levels drop, the negative feedback effect of estradiol on FSH is released, and the first stage begins again.

PREGNANCY CYCLE

▼ PRENATAL PERIOD

Development of the Embryo

A. Formation of gametes
1. The ovum and spermatozoon each have one set of 23 chromosomes; this is in contrast to other cells of the body, which have two sets, or 46 chromosomes (23 pairs)
2. The production of ova and spermatozoa requires a special type of nuclear division (meiosis) in which the chromosome number is reduced from two sets (46 chromosomes) to one set (23 chromosomes)

B. Fertilization
1. Spermatozoa are deposited in the vagina
2. Fertilization usually occurs in the fallopian tube when the ovum is about one third of the way down the tube; usually this is about 24 hours after ovulation
3. Sperm must be in the genital tract 4 to 6 hours before they are able to fertilize an ovum; during this period the enzyme hyaluronidase is activated; this enzyme is able to dissolve the cement substance (hyaluronic acid), which holds together the cells that surround the ovum
4. Male nucleus enters the cytoplasm of the ovum and several events follow
   a. Fertilization membrane forms around the ovum to prevent the entrance of other sperm
   b. Sperm tail is lost and the male nucleus (male pronucleus) moves toward the female nucleus (female pronucleus)
5. Fertilization proper occurs when the male pronucleus unites with the female pronucleus; thus the chromosome number is restored to two sets (46 chromosomes)

C. Cleavage
1. In a short time after fertilization, the zygote undergoes rapid division to produce a mass of cells (morula) that descends in the uterine tube
2. As it descends, it also divides to form a hollow ball referred to as the blastocyst

D. Implantation
1. The blastocyst implants in the uterine wall
   a. The blastocyst is differentiated into an inner cell mass, a blastocoele (internal cavity)
   b. An outer covering of cells, the trophectoderm, becomes the trophoderm and will form the fetal portion of the placenta, the vehicle for exchange of nutrients, gases, and wastes
   c. Implantation occurs 7 to 8 days after fertilization, generally in upper fundal portion
   d. Increased maternal hormonal action is necessary for continued implantation of fetus in the uterus
2. Placenta and umbilical cord development
   a. Placenta
     (1) Organ of dual origin (maternal and embryonic portions) serving interchange of food, gases, and wastes between mother and embryo (or fetus) during pregnancy
     (2) Formed from villous portion of chorion (chorion frondosum) and the portion of the uterine endometrium (called the decidua during pregnancy) directly underlying the implanted embryo (decidua basalis); chorionic villi project into placental sinuses (in decidua basalis) filled with maternal blood
     (3) Functions as the fetal digestive tract and also as fetal lungs, kidneys, and as a major endocrine gland (producing estrogens, progesterone, adrenocorticotropic hormone [ACTH], growth hormone,

gonadotropic hormones, human chorionic gonadotropin [hCG], and human placental lactogen [hPL]) (see Endocrine System in Medical-Surgical Nursing)

(4) Serves as a protective barrier against harmful effects of some drugs and microorganisms

b. Umbilical cord
(1) Inserted close to the central portion of the placenta and attached to fetus
(2) Has one vein (which transports nourishment) and two arteries (which transport wastes) between the mother and baby
(3) Wharton's jelly, a protective covering, surrounds the entire cord

E. Embryonic period
1. First 2 months is termed embryo, after this period is called a fetus
2. The inner cell mass differentiates into germ layers
a. Ectoderm: outer layer of skin and mouth cavity and nervous tissue
b. Mesoderm: connective tissue, including blood and muscle tissue
c. Endoderm: linings of the alimentary tract, respiratory system, and several glands
3. About the twelfth day after fertilization, a fetal membrane, the amnion, forms around the embryo; another membrane, the yolk sac, develops beneath embryo
a. Amnion is fluid filled (amniotic fluid) and serves as a fetal shock absorber
b. Yolk sac serves as an initial embryonic source of erythrocytes
4. Later an allantois develops that will supply the placental blood vessels
5. A chorion surrounds the embryo; this will eventually form the major part of the placenta; fingerlike projections of the chorion, called chorionic villi, grow into the decidua (formally called the endometrium); chorionic villi project into placental blood sinuses; the combination of chorionic villi, placental blood sinuses, and placental blood constitutes the placenta
6. Embryonic development—differentiation of cells occurs
a. At 14 days: heart begins to beat; brain, early spinal cord, and muscle segments present
b. At 26 days: tiny buds for arms appear
c. At 28 days: tiny buds for legs appear
d. At 30 days: embryo 0.6 to 1.2 cm in length, definite form, beginning of umbilical cord is visible
e. At 31 days: arm buds develop into hands, arms, and shoulders

f. At 33 days: finger outlines present
g. At 46 to 48 days: cartilage in upper arms replaced by first bone cells, amniotic fluid surrounds the embryo (amniotic fluid is a protective cushion, equalizes pressures, maintains temperature, and facilitates the baby's movements for adequate growth and development)
h. The first 8 weeks, known as the period of organogenesis, is a time of rapid growth and development. Any interference with maternal physiology may cause irreparable damage; no drugs should be taken during the first trimester unless absolutely necessary

7. Fetal development
a. Genitalia well developed
b. By 12 weeks: fetus moves body parts, swallows, practices inhaling and exhaling, weighs 28 g; fetal heart audible with Doptone
c. At 4 to 5 months (16 to 20 weeks): fetal movements felt by mother (known as quickening), weighs 170 g, is 20 to 25 cm in length; 200 ml of amniotic fluid present; amniocentesis is possible by 14 to 16 weeks; vernix and lanugo cover and protect the fetus
d. At 5 to 6 months (20 to 24 weeks): hair growth on head, eyelashes and brow, skeleton hardens, eyelids closed, weighs 0.45 kg, is 30.5 cm in length, fetal heart audible with fetoscope; respiratory movements become more regular
e. At 6 to 7 months (24 to 28 weeks): eyelids open, amniotic fluid increases to 1 quart with a daily exchange of 6 gallons, weighs 0.5 kg; alveolar cells of lungs produce pulmonary surfactants that minimize surface tension
f. At 7 to 8 months (28 to 32 weeks): many fat deposits, weighs 0.5 to 0.7 kg
g. At 8 to 9 months (32 to 36 weeks): stores protein for extrauterine life, gains 1.8 kg

8. Fetal circulation: contains mixed blood with less than maximal O_2 concentration; only exception is in the umbilical vein upon its immediate entrance into the liver
a. Foramen ovale is an opening between the right and left atria during fetal life, bypassing fetal lungs
b. Ductus arteriosus is a connection between pulmonary trunk and aorta, also bypassing fetal lungs
c. Ductus venosus is a connection between umbilical vein and ascending vena cava, bypassing fetal liver

Quickening
4-5 months

F. Chromosomes
1. Humans have 23 pairs of homologous chromosomes
2. In males the sex chromosomes (the X and Y) are not equal in size
3. Homologous chromosomes carry sets of matching genes (alleles) in which one may be dominant and the other recessive, or they may have blending expressions

G. Sex determination in humans
1. Genetic females have two sets of autosomes (nonsex chromosomes) and two X chromosomes, whereas genetic males have two sets of autosomes and one X chromosome and one Y chromosome
2. All ova produced by females have one set of autosomes and one X chromosome; spermatozoa produced by a male have a set of autosomes and either an X or a Y chromosome
3. If an X-bearing spermatozoon fertilizes an ovum, a female will result; if a Y-bearing spermatozoon fertilizes an ovum, a male will result

H. Genes
1. Sex-linked genes: genes carried on the X chromosome are called sex-linked genes and are always expressed in the male, even though they may be recessive; examples of such genes cause hemophilia and colorblindness
2. Multiple genes: many different genes may combine to produce cumulative effects, such as the degree of pigmentation or height
3. Multiple alleles: an example of human traits controlled by multiple alleles are the genes controlling normal blood types; the genes for type O are dominated by the genes for type A or type B; the genes for A and B are both expressed

Genes	Blood type
OO	O
AO	A
AA	A
BO	B
BB	B
AB	AB

4. Following are some other obvious human traits controlled by genes:

Dominant	Recessive
Brown eyes	Blue eyes
Normal blood clotting	Hemophilia (sex-linked)
Normal color vision	Colorblind (sex-linked)
Normal pigmentation	Albinism
Rh positive (multiple alleles)	Rh negative
Normal red blood cell development	Sickle cell trait

I. Chromosomal alterations
1. In rare cases additional sex chromosomes may appear and produce abnormal individuals
   a. X chromosome and no Y chromosome: Turner's syndrome
   b. Two or more X chromosomes and a Y chromosome: Klinefelter's syndrome
2. Translocation of chromosome: a cytogenetic abnormality such as trisomy 21 (Down syndrome)
3. Mutations
   a. Changes in DNA are mutations; there may also be chromosomal changes
   b. The frequency of mutations may be increased by certain agents such as ultraviolet radiation, x-rays, radioactive radiation, and chemical substances

Physical and Physiologic Changes in Mother During Pregnancy

Pregnancy is a normal physiologic process that affects all body systems and results in both objective and subjective changes; it is a stressful time requiring many adaptations and may lead to minor discomforts

A. Endocrine
1. During pregnancy the chorion of the placenta secretes a hormone, human chorionic gonadotropin (hCG), that maintains the corpus luteum; the continuation of progesterone and estrogen secretion from the corpus luteum maintains the pregnancy during the early weeks of development; presence of hCG hormone is an indicator of pregnancy; hCG reaches a peak in the third month and then drops; high hCG levels are found in the presence of a hydatidiform mole
2. Estrogen and progesterone increase and continue to be secreted from the placenta during the last 6 months of pregnancy; progesterone acts to inhibit uterine contractions, which might occur as the result of the uterus stretching as the fetus grows; increase in these hormones leads to sodium and water retention and muscle relaxation, which leads to fatigue
3. Thyroid activity is increased; normal pregnancy may emulate a mild hyperthyroid state
4. Human placental lactogen (hPL), sometimes called human chorionic somatomammotropin (hCS), is increased. It is a diabetogenic hormone (diminished insulin efficiency) that decreases maternal use of glucose, leaving it available for fetal use; it also affects lipid and protein metabolism
5. Estriol levels increased; sometimes used as indicator of fetal well-being
6. The posterior pituitary secretion of oxytocin, which stimulates uterine contractions, coupled

with the drop in progesterone and the increase in estrogen and prostaglandins, brings about labor; uterine contractions increase in frequency and intensity, culminating in fetal expulsion (birth); following birth oxytocin contracts the uterus which, in turn, leads to the release of prolactin to promote the let-down reflex

B. Reproductive
1. Amenorrhea occurs because the corpus luteum persists, and ovulation is inhibited by the high levels of circulating estrogen and progesterone
2. Breast changes such as fullness, tingling, soreness, and darkening of the areolae and nipples occur along with an increase in hormonal levels
3. Leukorrhea is increased as hormonal levels rise, and the increased acidity is a protection from bacterial invasion
4. Changes in the uterus are circulatory, hormonal, and related to fetal growth
    a. Softening of the cervix: Goodell's sign
    b. Softening of the lower uterine segment: Hegar's sign
    c. Purplish hue to the cervix and vaginal mucosa: Chadwick's sign
    d. Uterus enlarges in size
    e. Changes in position of the uterus: first trimester uterus is in pelvic cavity, second and third trimester uterus is in abdominal cavity before lightening occurs

C. Gastrointestinal
1. Reduction in hydrochloric acid secretion that interferes with gastric motility, causing nausea and vomiting (morning sickness) and pyrosis (heartburn)
2. Elevated estrogen levels cause excessive salivation (ptyalism)
3. Hyperemia and softening of gums with accompanying hyperacidity of oral secretions result in nonspecific gingivitis; increased vitamin C intake and regular oral hygiene are indicated
4. Decreased emptying time of gallbladder may precipitate development of gallstones
5. Food cravings may occur; only significant if substance craved is unusual (pica); for example, clay, starch, dirt
6. Heartburn (pyrosis) occurs because of delayed emptying time of stomach; client should avoid gastric irritants such as coffee, tea, and chocolate; antacids containing sodium should be avoided
7. Constipation is caused by hypoperistalsis, lack of fluids, poor dietary habits, pressure of the enlarged uterus on internal organs, effects of progesterone on muscle, and hemorrhoids

D. Excretory
1. Proximity of the uterus and bladder in early and late pregnancy causes urinary frequency
2. Bladder tone is reduced by effects of hormones on smooth muscle
3. Bladder capacity up to 1500 ml in second trimester
4. Increased urinary output results in lowered specific gravity
5. Increased excretion of sugar caused by lowered renal threshold
6. Pressure of enlarging uterus causes dilation of right ureter and kidney

E. Circulatory
1. Physiologic anemia occurs as a result of hemodilution of the blood. There is a 45% to 50% increase in blood volume expansion, of which about 75% is plasma and 25% is red blood cells (RBCs). This imbalance between the plasma and the RBCs leads to a reduced hematocrit. Blood volume is increased to meet the needs of the developing fetus
2. Cardiac output increases 25% to 50% during pregnancy, peaking at 28 to 32 weeks of gestation
3. Heart rate increases 10 to 15 beats per minute in the latter half of pregnancy: approximately 14,000 extra beats in 24 hours
4. Palpitations occur in early months from sympathetic nervous stimulation and in later months from increased thoracic pressure because of enlarged uterus
5. Blood pressure may drop slightly in second trimester
6. Supine hypotension syndrome (vena caval syndrome): in supine position weight of enlarged uterus obstructs vena cava, which decreases blood return to heart; decreased cardiac output ensues with hypotension, lightheadedness, faintness, and palpitations
7. White blood cells, fibrinogen, and other clotting factors increase
8. Varicose veins of legs, vulva, and perianal area may occur
9. Edema of extremities common in the last 6 weeks of pregnancy because of stasis of blood, hormonal changes, and possibly poor diet

F. Respiratory
1. During the third trimester, pressure of the enlarged uterus on the diaphragm and lungs may cause dyspnea that subsides when lightening occurs at about 38 weeks
2. Oxygen consumption is increased by about 15% between the sixteenth and fortieth weeks, although there may be only a slight increase in vital capacity during pregnancy

3. Hyperventilation occurs due to mother's need to blow-off increased CO_2 transferred to her from fetus

4. Nasal congestion occurs as a response to increased estrogen levels

G. Integumentary

1. Excretion of wastes through the skin causes diaphoresis

2. Skin changes: darkening of the areolae, darkening patches on the face (melasma, formally chloasma), linea alba becomes nigra on the abdomen, related to increased estrogen; striae on the abdomen and legs caused by skin stretching as pregnancy advances; erythematous changes on the palms and face in some women

H. Skeletal

1. Softening of all ligaments and joints, especially symphysis and sacroiliac joint, caused by increased hormonal action of estrogens and relaxin

2. Leg cramps may occur from an imbalance of calcium (hypocalcemia) in the body and from pressure of the gravid uterus on nerves supplying lower extremities

I. Emotional

1. Acceptance of biologic fact of pregnancy; usually occurs during first trimester

2. Acceptance of growing fetus as distinct from self; usually occurs during second trimester

3. Preparation for birth and relinquishing of child; usually occurs during third trimester

4. Ambivalence about child and parenting

5. Mood swings

6. Increase or decrease in sexual desire

7. Anxiety related to birth and adult responsibilities

J. Affirmation and confirmation of pregnancy

1. Presumptive signs: mostly subjective; may be indicative of other illnesses
   a. Amenorrhea
   b. Fatigue
   c. Nausea and vomiting
   d. Breast changes
   e. Urinary frequency
   f. Darkening of pigmentation on face, breasts, and abdomen
   g. Quickening: feeling of movement about 15 to 20 weeks

2. Probable signs: objective but still not definite confirmations of pregnancy
   a. Uterine changes
      (1) Chadwick's sign
      (2) Hegar's sign
      (3) Goodell's sign
      (4) Enlargement of the uterus
   b. Fetal outline

c. Pregnancy tests: urine and blood of pregnant woman are used to detect hCG (human chorionic gonadotropin)
   d. Ballottement
   e. Braxton Hicks contractions

3. Positive signs: confirm pregnancy
   a. Fetal heart beat
   b. Fetal outline and movement as felt by examiner
   c. Ultrasonography revealing movement of fetal heart
   d. Roentgenography of fetal skeleton (rarely used since x-ray may be damaging to fetus)

4. Estimating date of confinement (EDC) and duration of pregnancy
   a. Nägele's rule: count back 3 months from the first day of the last menstrual period and add 7 days (9 calendar months, 270 days or 10 lunar months, 280 days) and 1 year
   b. Fundal height: measurement from symphysis pubis to top of fundus; the fundus rises about 1 cm per week; at 20 weeks it should be at the umbilicus and at 36 weeks at the xiphoid process
   c. Ultrasonography: establishes fetal age from head measurements (term pregnancy: biparietal diameter is 9.8 cm or more); early in pregnancy, test is done when woman has full bladder (must be instructed to increase fluids before test)

K. Nutritional needs during pregnancy

1. Consideration of preconceptional nutritional status; obesity or underweight; age and parity of mother; biologic interactions between mother, fetus, and placenta; and individual needs, such as in times of stress

2. Weight gain should be evaluated with regard to the quality of gain (Is weight gain caused by edema or fat deposition?)

3. Severe caloric restriction during pregnancy is contraindicated, because it is a potential hazard to the mother and fetus, especially during organogenesis

4. Weight reduction should never be started as a regimen during pregnancy

5. Restriction of sodium and administration of diuretics are potentially dangerous to the mother and fetus during pregnancy; they may limit interstitial fluid reserve, which may be needed if the blood volume decreases

6. Nausea and vomiting: limited fluids with meals, small frequent feedings, restricted fat, high carbohydrate

7. Constipation: increased fluids and residue or fiber; appropriate activity level

8. Consideration of the demands of pregnancy related to growth and development of the fetus during the various trimesters; provide adequate nutrition to meet increased maternal and fetal nutrient demands
    a. Increased calories to meet increased basal metabolic needs, spare protein for growth, and promote weight gain to support pregnancy and lactation
    b. Average weight gain should be 14.4 to 16 kg but is individual according to needs; underweight women should gain even more; overweight women should gain less, about 6.8 to 11.4 kg; women carrying more than one fetus should gain more than the recommended weight
    c. Increased protein to provide for growth demands
    d. Increased vitamins, especially folic acid supplement to prevent anemia and prevent neural tube defects
    e. Increased minerals with supplement of iron to prevent anemia
    f. Iodized salt to provide needed sodium and iodine
9. Lactating mother needs additional caloric requirements
10. Dietary assessment and counseling should be an integral part of prenatal care for every pregnant woman; assess for adequate weight gain, about 1.82 kg every month after an initial 1.36 to 1.82 kg gain in the first trimester
11. Changes in dietary regimen should consider cultural, economic, and psychologic implications of food habits
12. Food guide for pregnancy is based on:
    a. Increased protein foods such as milk, eggs, and meat
    b. Additional servings from the food choices of grains, vegetables, and fruits
    c. Additional calories, protein, and fluids during lactation
    d. Daily minimum food intake during pregnancy should include: three to four dairy products; two servings of protein; eight to ten servings of bread and cereal; six to ten servings of fruits or vegetables; foods high in fiber. 1 ½ litres of fluids (6 to 8 cups) of fluid per day including water, juice, milk, and soup are recommended. A safe level of alcohol has not been established; therefore avoid alcohol completely
    e. Minerals such as iron, calcium, phosphorus, iodine, zinc, and sodium are needed in the diet

13. Adolescent nutritional needs
    a. Weight gain for normal pregnancy and expected weight gain for growth are added together
    b. Higher protein intake for young, pregnant female
    c. Iron needs higher to support enlarging muscle mass and increasing blood volume
    d. Calcium intake increased by 400 mg
L. Medical supervision during pregnancy
    1. History, including medical, surgical, gynecologic, and obstetric data; history of present pregnancy, including own and family reactions to pregnancy; history of environmental hazards and exposure to x-rays, alcohol, tobacco, and over-the-counter and prescription drugs; dietary history and nutritional status; assessment for presence of allergies; and family history of hereditary and transmittable diseases such as diabetes, tuberculosis, heart disease
    2. Physical examination of the skin, thyroid, teeth, lungs, heart, and breasts; abdominal palpation; auscultation; height of fundus; vaginal examination; and pelvic evaluation (before last 4 weeks of pregnancy)
    3. Cervical and vaginal smears for monilia, trichomonas, herpes, and chlamydia; Papanicolaou test for cancer
    4. Blood pressure; weight; and urinalysis for acetone, albumin, and glucose done at all visits
    5. Laboratory examinations for blood grouping, Rh typing and antibody screening, hematocrit and hemoglobin, serological examination for syphilis (repeated at regular intervals for high-risk clients), and blood for rubella titer
    6. Screening tests
        a. Serologic testing for hepatitis A and B, and for AIDS in high-risk clients
        b. Alpha-fetoprotein (AFP) for neural tube defects
        c. Screening for glucose intolerance by a 50 gm load followed by a 1 hour serum glucose for gestational diabetes mellitus

General Nursing Care During the Prenatal Period

A. DATA COLLECTION

1. Initial visit
    a. Date of last menstrual period
    b. Personal medical history
    c. Family history
    d. Gynecologic and obstetric history
    e. Physical examination
        (1) Baseline blood pressure, pulse, respirations
        (2) Baseline weight

f. Current nutritional status

g. Pelvic examination

  (1) Vaginal

  (2) Rectal

h. Urine examination

i. Understanding of pregnancy and related care

2. Monthly and final weekly visits

a. Blood pressure, pulse, respirations

b. Signs of supine hypotension

c. Signs of facial or digital edema

d. Weight

e. Fundal height and size

f. Fetal heart rate and fetal activity

g. Urine testing for glucose, albumin, ketones, acetone

B. ANALYSIS AND INTERPRETATION

1. Body image disturbance related to actual appearance and other physical changes of pregnancy

2. Decreased cardiac output related to pressure on vena cava by gravid uterus when in supine position

3. Constipation related to less frequent bowel movements associated with slowed peristalsis and pressure from gravid uterus

4. Family coping: potential for growth related to acceptance of pregnancy and fulfillment of parental tasks

5. Fear related to diagnosis of pregnancy, lack of knowledge about body changes, and/or impending parenthood

6. Risk for fluid volume deficit related to increasing demands of pregnancy

7. Knowledge deficit related to new experience of pregnancy

8. Altered nutrition: less than body requirements related to increased needs of pregnancy or nausea and vomiting

9. Self-esteem disturbance related to altered appearance and ambivalence about pregnancy

10. Sexual dysfunction related to altered body contour

11. Risk for trauma related to altered balance associated with increased weight of uterus and change in center of gravity

12. Altered urinary elimination related to pressure of gravid uterus

C. PLANNING/IMPLEMENTATION

1. Assist the parents in understanding the anatomy and physiology of pregnancy, labor, and birth

2. Teach mother to monitor for:

a. Visual disturbances

b. Edema of face, fingers, or feet

c. Persistent, severe headaches

d. Seizures

e. Epigastric pain

f. Persistent, severe vomiting

g. Any vaginal discharge, including blood

h. Signs of infection

i. Burning on urination

j. Abdominal pain

k. Absence of or decrease in fetal movements after initial presence

l. Signs and symptoms of premature labor

3. Teach mother about physiologic changes and related discomforts that occur during pregnancy (nausea, vomiting, backaches, varicosities, hemorrhoids, constipation, leg pain, etc.)

4. Respond to mother's questions about bathing, douching, work, sex, exercise, etc.

5. Help the parents discuss and explore feelings related to childbearing and childrearing in attempting to alleviate fears

6. Prepare the mother for the physical work of labor through the use of muscle and breathing exercises for the various phases of labor

7. Identify parents' situational support systems

8. Prepare the father or support person for a coaching and supporting role during pregnancy, labor, and birth

9. Introduce families to health facilities available for continued health care of the family

10. Teach mother to avoid alcohol, tobacco, and contact with second-hand smoke

11. Discuss various childbirth preparation techniques such as Lamaze, Read, and Bradley

12. Teach the mother to avoid over-the-counter or prescription drugs without checking with the physician because many drugs considered harmless may be teratogenic to the developing fetus

D. EVALUATION/OUTCOMES

1. Weight gain does not exceed recommended rate; total does not exceed 16 kg

2. Side-lying position used when resting

3. Childbirth technique selected; correct breathing techniques are demonstrated

4. Fetal growth and fundal enlargement within normal parameters

5. Free of signs of pregnancy-induced hypertension

6. Abstains from alcohol, drugs, and tobacco

7. Attends childbirth classes with partner

▼ INTRAPARTAL PERIOD (PERIOD OF BIRTH)

A. Labor: an involuntary physiologic process whereby the contents of the gravid uterus are expelled through the birth canal into the external environment

B. Anatomy of the bony pelvis
1. Parts: ischium, ilium, sacrum, coccyx
2. Joints: sacroiliac, sacrococcygeal, symphysis pubis (all soften during pregnancy)
3. Divisions: false pelvis supports the enlarged uterus in the abdominal cavity; true pelvis is the bony inner pelvis through which the baby must pass
4. Diameters: at inlet: true conjugate (anterior/posterior diameter), transverse (widest diameter at inlet), right and left oblique diameters; at outlet: conjugate diagonal (anterior/posterior is widest diameter), transverse (one ischial tuberosity to the other)
5. Classification of pelvis: gynecoid (normal female pelvis), android (male pelvis), anthropoid, and platypelloid
6. Normal female pelvis has an ample pubic arch, curved sacrum, curved side walls, blunt ischial spines, and a movable coccyx

C. Attitude: relationship of fetal parts to each other

D. Lie: relationship of the long axis of the fetus to the long axis of the mother

E. Presentation: fetus' body part that engages in the true pelvis
1. Cephalic (head): vertex, brow, or face
2. Breech: frank, complete, single, or double footling
3. Shoulder: cannot be delivered vaginally

F. Position: relationship of presenting parts to four quadrants of the mother's pelvis (the letters L and R are used for left or right; A and P for anterior or posterior; O for occiput; M for mentum or face; S for sacrum)
1. Vertex: occiput, LOA, LOP, ROA, ROP
2. Face: chin (mentum), LMA, LMP, RMA, RMP
3. Breech: sacrum, LSA, LSP, RSA, RSP

G. Station: relationship of presenting part to the false and true pelves
1. Floating: presenting part movable above the true pelvic inlet
2. Engaged: suboccipitobregmatic diameter fixed into the pelvic inlet
3. Station O: presenting part at level of the ischial spines: levels below spines +1, +2, +3; levels above spines −1, −2, −3

H. Amniotic fluid: about 1000 ml of fluid enclosed in membranes (amniotic sac) is present at term
1. Spontaneous rupture of membranes (SROM or SRM)): usually occurs in mid or late labor but can occur before labor begins
2. Artificial rupture of membranes (amniotomy, AROM, or ARM): expedites labor; should not be done until presenting part is at 0 or lower (+1, +2) station
3. Nitrazine paper: may be used to confirm the presence of amniotic fluid; turns dark blue because of the alkaline nature of the fluid
4. Assessment of amniotic fluid
   a. Color: normally strawlike and clear; greenish color may indicate meconium staining or breech presentation
   b. Odor: normally musky smelling but nonoffensive; foul smelling indicates infection (chorioamnionitis)
   c. Amount: 1 L of fluid at term; excessive amount is called polyhydramnios; scant amount is called oligohydramnios; scant or excessive fluid may be associated with congenital anomalies

I. Clinical findings prior to labor
1. Physiologic
   a. Lightening: fetus drops down into the true pelvis
   b. Braxton Hicks contractions: painless tryout contractions in preparation for true labor
   c. Increased vaginal secretions
   d. Softening of cervix (ripening)
   e. Rupture of membranes (ROM) may occur
   f. Bloody show; softening and effacement of cervix causes mucous plug to be expelled; this is accompanied by small blood loss
2. Psychologic: mother shows signs of nesting (increased activity) caused by sudden rise in energy level

J. Clinical findings of true labor
1. Uterine contractions that increase in frequency, strength, and duration and do not disappear when lying down or walking around
2. Effacement and progressive dilation of the cervix

K. Mechanisms of labor: rotation and descent of vertex presentation through the true pelvis
1. Engagement, descent with flexion: at onset of labor, head descends and chin flexes on the chest
2. Internal rotation: as labor contractions and uterine forces move the fetus downward, the head internally rotates to pass through the ischial spines
3. Extension: occiput emerges under the symphysis pubis and the head is delivered by extension
4. External rotation: allows for rotation of shoulders to an anterior/posterior position
5. Expulsion: rest of infant is delivered

L. Stages of labor and maternal changes
1. First stage: from the onset of true labor to complete effacement and dilation of the cervix
   a. Latent phase: mild, short contractions, cervix dilated 0 to 3 cm; mother excited and

happy that labor has started, some apprehension; follows directions readily

  b. Active phase: moderate to strong contractions 5 minutes apart, cervix dilates from 4 to 7 cm, bloody show, membranes may rupture, breathing techniques help in relaxing, medication may be necessary for discomfort, supportive measures (e.g., encouragement, praise, reassurance, keeping the mother informed of progress, providing rest between contractions, presence of a supporting person) by the partner or nurse help; has difficulty in following directions

  c. Transition phase: strong contractions 1 to 2 minutes apart (lasting 45 to 60 seconds or more with little rest in between); cervix dilates from 7 to 10 cm with a bloody show; mother becomes irritable, restless, agitated, highly emotional, belches, has leg tremors, perspires, pale white ring around mouth (circumoral pallor), flushed face, sudden nausea, and vomiting; feels need to have a bowel movement because of pressure on anus; unable to communicate or follow directions

2. Second stage: beginning with full dilation of the cervix and ending with birth of the infant; perineum bulges, pushing with contractions, grunting sounds, behavior changes from great irritability to great involvement and work, sleep and relaxation occur between contractions, leg cramps are common

3. Third stage: following birth of the infant through expulsion of the placenta; placental separation (5 to 30 minutes) after birth heralded by globular formation of uterus, lengthening of umbilical cord, and gush of blood; may have alteration in perineal structure either from episiotomy (prophylactic incision into perineum to allow for birth of head) or laceration (may be 1, 2, 3, or 4 degrees) from rapid expulsion of presenting part

4. Fourth stage: following expulsion of placenta to 1 to 2 hours after birth; fundus firm in the midline and at or slightly above the umbilicus; moderate, bloody vaginal discharge (lochia rubra); fatigue, thirst, chills, nausea; excitement and intermittent dozing

M. Oxytocics

1. Description

  a. Drugs that stimulate the uterus to contract

  b. Used in the pregnant female to initiate labor; given slowly and in small doses during labor

  c. Used to augment contractions that have already begun

  d. Capable of inducing contraction of the lacteal glands, which aids in let-down reflex for nursing

  e. Exert vasopressor and antidiuretic effects

  f. Used to control postpartum uterine atony; may be given rapidly

  g. Oxytocics are available in parenteral (IM, IV) and oral (buccal) preparations

2. Examples

  a. Ergonovine maleate (Ergot, Ergometrine)

  b. Oxytocin (syntocinon)

3. Major side effects

  a. Maternal

    (1) Hypertension (contracture of smooth muscles of blood vessels)

    (2) Tachycardia

    (3) Dysrhythmias

    (4) Uterine rupture (excessive contraction)

    (5) Water intoxication (antidiuretic effect)

    (6) Seizures (water intoxication)

    (7) Coma (water intoxication)

  b. Fetal

    (1) Anoxia, asphyxia

    (2) Dysrhythmias (premature ventricular contractions [PVBs], bradycardia)

    (3) Hyperbilirubinemia

4. Nursing needs for clients receiving oxytocics

  a. Never leave client unattended

  b. Have O_2 and emergency resuscitative equipment available

  c. Use infusion-control device for IV administration

  d. Discontinue if prolonged uterine contractions occur

  e. Monitor uterine contractions

  f. Assess blood pressure (BP) and pulse every 15 minutes

  g. Fetal monitoring is essential

  h. Instruct client on nasal administration technique

  i. Evaluate client's response to medication and understanding of teaching

N. Maternal analgesia and anaesthesia

1. Analgesia

  a. TENS (transcutaneous electronic nerve stimulation): a procedure in which two or four electrodes are placed on the mother's back or abdomen, which allows noninvasive stimulation to pass through the muscles to encourage relaxation

  b. Sedatives: such as Ativan (lorazepam) or Serax (oxazepam) may be given to help the mother to relax

  c. Entonox (laughing gas): self-administered gas given by face mask to aid in control of breathing and take the edge off the peak of the contraction pain

d. Narcotics such as Meperidine hydrochloride (Demerol) may be given via injection
e. Pudendal block: an injection which numbs the perineal area. Usually given at full dilatation to give pain relief for forceps delivery or episiotomy
f. Local anaesthetic: used for episiotomy

2. Regional analgesia and anaesthesia
a. Epidural anaesthesia: an effective pain relief method in which a local anaesthetic is administered through a small, plastic tube inserted into the epidural space, which provides pain relief from below the breasts on down; may be used for caesarean birth
b. Spinal anaesthesia: total block of all motor and pain sensations is achieved with spinal anaesthesia making it effective and efficient for planned caesarean births
c. General anaesthesia: used only for emergency caesarean section births or by specific mother's request for planned caesarean birth

3. Nursing needs for clients receiving these agents
a. Observe mother and newborn for respiratory depression if narcotic analgesic is given; monitor mother for hypotension
b. After epidural
(1) Monitor for hypotension
(2) If hypotension occurs, position client on left side, increase IV infusion, and administer oxygen
c. Evaluate client's response to medication and understanding of teaching

General Nursing Care During the Intrapartal Period

A. DATA COLLECTION (ON ADMISSION)

1. Age, weight, height
2. Parity, gravity, obstetric history
3. Allergies
4. Urine specimen
5. Time and type of last meal
6. Frequency, duration, and intensity of contractions
7. Time of onset of contractions
8. Presence of bloody show
9. Status of amniotic membrane
10. Dilation and effacement
11. Position of fetus (Leopold's maneuver)
12. Fetal heart rate and pattern
13. Vital signs and blood pressure
14. Emotional response to labor
15. Presence of support persons

B. ANALYSIS AND INTERPRETATION

MOTHER
1. Altered cardiopulmonary tissue perfusion associated with hypovolemia related to uterine relaxation following birth and/or cervical lacerations
2. Ineffective individual coping related to exhaustion
3. Fear related to lack of knowledge and unfamiliarity with labor process
4. Impaired gas exchange related to hyperventilation
5. Risk for injury related to lack of control, especially during transition phase, position during birth, and administration of anesthesia
6. Pain related to labor process and episiotomy
7. Impaired physical mobility related to need for fetal monitoring, bed rest, or positioning
8. Self-esteem disturbance related to inability to live up to behavioral expectations (self or others)
9. Altered urinary elimination related to pressure of enlarged uterus, analgesia or anesthesia, and trauma of labor and birth

INFANT
1. Ineffective airway clearance related to excessive mucus, aspiration of meconium, or inability to clear airway
2. Decreased cardiac output related to prolonged contractions, short umbilical cord, head compression, pressure on umbilical cord, or uteroplacental insufficiency
3. Risk for injury related to trauma of birth or maternal infection
4. Ineffective thermoregulation related to immature heat regulation, inability to shiver, and lack of brown fat

C. PLANNING/IMPLEMENTATION

FIRST STAGE
1. Admit mother and labor coach
a. Orient to unit
b. Obtain history
(1) Parity and gravidity
(2) Expected date of confinement (EDC)
(3) Onset of contractions
(4) Status of membranes
(5) Time and contents of last meal
(6) Allergies
(7) Intent to breastfeed or bottlefeed
(8) Prenatal care
(9) Rh, GBS, hepatitis status
c. Obtain vital signs
d. Perform Leopold's maneuvers
e. Time and assess contractions
f. Assist with vaginal examination
g. Test urine for protein, glucose, and ketones
h. Collect blood for complete blood count (CBC) and cross-match

i. Give emotional support to mother and labor coach

2. Maintain asepsis; use universal precautions
3. Monitor frequency, duration, and strength of contractions
   a. Palpate fundus
   b. Interpret data on maternal uterine monitor
4. Monitor fetal heart rate (FHR); should be done as soon as the client is admitted
   a. Fetoscope or Doppler
   b. Internal or external fetal monitor
5. Interpret data of fetal monitoring
   a. Baseline FHR: normal heart rate for a full-term infant between uterine contractions is 120 to 160 beats per minute
   b. Tachycardia: heart rate above 160 beats per minute lasting over 10 minutes
      (1) Transient tachycardia may occur with *increased* fetal activity; may be due to maternal pyrexia or dehydration; fetal infection; drugs such as Vasodilan or Ritrodrine; or increase in maternal environment temperature such as in hot shower or tub
      (2) Nursing intervention includes reducing maternal fever, increasing fluids, and monitoring for amnionitis
   c. Bradycardia: heart rate below 110 beats per minute lasting longer than 10 minutes
      (1) May be due to fetal hypoxia as a result of anesthetics used for epidural, spinal, and caudal blocks; maternal hypotension; prolonged umbilical cord compression; analgesics
      (2) Nursing intervention includes repositioning mother on side, assessing for prolapsed cord, positioning to relieve pressure on cord, elevating lower extremities, administering oxygen
   d. Variability: normal irregularity of cardiac rhythm (balance between sympathetic and parasympathetic divisions of autonomic nervous system); manifested by cyclic fluctuations and beat-to-beat changes of heart rate
      (1) Absence of these fluctuations is indicative of fetal central nervous system (CNS) depression
      (2) Associated with drugs such as narcotics and barbiturates, fetal hypoxia, acidosis, and immaturity of fetus
      (3) Nursing intervention includes administration of oxygen, repositioning of mother on side
   e. Decelerations: periodic decrease in FHR
      (1) Early decelerations
         (a) FHR decreases but not below 100 beats per minute
         (b) Occur early in contraction phase, before peak; end before uterus returns to resting tone
         (c) Indicate head compression
         (d) Assess for imminent delivery of fetus
      (2) Late decelerations
         (a) FHR rarely decreases below 100 beats per minute but, if severe, may decrease to 60 beats per minute
         (b) Begin as contraction peaks; lowest rate after peak of contraction
         (c) Long recovery time; FHR may not return to normal until well after contraction ends
         (d) Often associated with loss of variability; may be accompanied by bradycardia or tachycardia
         (e) Indicative of uteroplacental insufficiency caused by uterine tetany from oxytocin administration; maternal supine hypotension; regional anesthesia; hypertensive disorders; diabetes mellitus; and other chronic disorders
         (f) Ominous if persistent or associated with decreased variability
         (g) Nursing intervention includes discontinuing oxytocin if being administered, positioning mother on left side, administering oxygen by mask at 8 to 10 L per minute, increasing rate of intravenous fluids, assisting with fetal blood sampling; preparing for birth if there is no improvement
      (3) Variable decelerations
         (a) Abrupt transitory decrease in FHR that is variable in duration, intensity, and time in relation to contractions
         (b) FHR may decrease as low as 70 beats per minute for as long as 30 seconds with a slow return to baseline
         (c) Usually observed late in labor with fetal descent and pushing
         (d) Usually related to umbilical cord compression
         (e) Occur in about 50% of labors and are usually transient, correctable, and unrelated to low Apgar scores
         (f) Nursing intervention: in addition to nursing intervention under late decelerations, if cord is prolapsed, attempt to relieve pressure of descending part on cord

6. Prevent supine hypotension by positioning mother on side to keep gravid uterus from compressing vena cava
7. Assist the mother with breathing techniques throughout labor by teaching and encouraging appropriate breathing patterns in varying phases of labor and rebreathing techniques to correct and prevent hyperventilation
8. Use measures to promote comfort and rest by providing warmth, administering analgesics and tranquilizers as ordered, except in late phase of labor (less than 2 hours before birth) to prevent fetal depression; encourage use of relaxation techniques and positions learned in childbirth classes; support and encourage mother and coach; carefully monitor vital signs during administration of regional anesthetics
9. Observe perineum for bloody show and appearance of amniotic fluid (indicates ruptured membranes); note:
   a. Amount
   b. Color; if greenish, check for breech position and obtain fetal heart rate
   c. Odor; if foul may indicate amnionitis
   d. FHR following amniotomy to artificially rupture membranes (AROM)
10. Assess body fluids, bladder, and bowel function
11. Monitor for:
    a. Prolonged strong contractions; may indicate tetanic uterus
    b. Taut, boardlike abdomen; may indicate abruptio placentae
    c. Increase in pulse and temperature; may indicate infection
    d. Hypertension; may indicate preeclampsia
    e. Hypotension; may occur following epidural or spinal anesthesia; turn client on side
    f. Bright-red vaginal bleeding; may indicate placenta previa
    g. Meconium-stained amniotic fluid; may indicate breech position or may be a late sign of fetal distress
    h. Abnormal variations in FHR patterns; may indicate fetal distress

SECOND STAGE
1. Assist mother with pushing
2. Transfer to delivery room or prepare birthing bed
3. Monitor FHR
4. Prepare mother for birth

THIRD STAGE
1. Care of baby
   a. Clear airway of mucus
   b. Observe frequently
   c. Use Apgar scoring to determine respiratory effort and physical status
   d. Maintain body heat
   e. Assess the newborn for visible anomalies
   f. Place in parent's arms or view to begin bonding process
   g. Administer antibiotic ophthalmic medication into each eye after bonding and within 1 hour of delivery to prevent ophthalmia neonatorum
   h. Identify the mother and baby before leaving delivery room by use and application of bands and/or use of footprints
2. Assist with delivery of placenta
3. Promote attachment
4. Record birth and accompanying events

FOURTH STAGE
1. Palpate the fundus q 15 minutes for firmness and height in relation to umbilicus; if relaxed and dextroverted, check for bladder fullness
2. Check for bladder distention; determine voiding pattern; the client may hemorrhage; catheterize if necessary
3. Check the perineum for vaginal and suture line bleeding; count vaginal pads; assess for concurrent uterine relaxation; massage uterus
4. Monitor temperature, BP, and pulse; report fluctuations
5. Administer oxytocic medication as ordered; after birth an oxytocic may be administered immediately to enhance uterine contractions
6. Check episiotomy or laceration site for hematoma, bleeding, or edema; apply icebag to perineum immediately after birth to reduce edema
7. Shivering is common after birth; exact cause unknown; keeping the client warm diminishes the sensation of chilling, which is most likely caused by air-conditioned birthing room
8. Provide fluid and food as tolerated

D. EVALUATION/OUTCOMES
1. Labor progresses and culminates in safe birth; newborn and mother survive birth
2. No signs of infection present
3. No signs of hemorrhage present
4. Newborn's respiratory rate and effort sustains life without assistance
5. Newborn's Apgar is 7 or above at 5 minutes after birth

▼ POSTPARTAL PERIOD

A. Puerperium: 6-week period following birth in which the reproductive organs undergo physical and physiologic changes, a process called involution; because of the many physiologic and psychologic stresses of the postpartum period, there is a trend to increase this period to 3 months following birth and call it the fourth trimester of pregnancy

B. Systemic changes during the puerperium
1. Reproductive system
   a. Uterus: intermittent contractions bring about involution, afterpains may cause discomfort, necessitating analgesics; oxytocin release during breastfeeding speeds up involution
   b. Lochia: vaginal flow following birth changes from rubra to serosa, then becomes alba
   c. Vagina practically returns to its prepregnant state through a healing of soft tissue and cicatrization
   d. Menstruation occurs about 6 weeks after birth in nonnursing mothers and up to 24 weeks in nursing mothers
   e. Abdominal wall soft and flabby but eventually regains tone
   f. Breasts
      (1) As placenta is delivered, there is activation of luteinizing hormone in the anterior pituitary; secretion of prolactin also stimulates milk production
      (2) In breastfeeding mothers, the posterior pituitary secretes oxytocin that initiates the let-down reflex with milk ejection as the baby suckles
      (3) Absence of suckling at breast in nonnursing mothers inhibits oxytocin secretion; the let-down reflex does not occur, and milk production is inhibited
      (4) Breast engorgement occurs in both nursing and nonnursing mothers on the second or third day because of vasodilation before lactation
2. Digestive system
   a. Following birth clients are hungry and thirsty; if general anesthesia was not administered during birth, clients can be given oral nourishment
   b. Added proteins and calories to replenish those lost with the process of involution
   c. Lactating mother needs added calories and fluids
   d. Roughage, fluid, and exercise relieve constipation and distention
   e. Bowel movements usually do not occur for a few days, probably because of fear of pain from hemorrhoids and/or episiotomy and decreased food intake during labor; stool softeners may be prescribed and, if unsuccessful, suppositories or an enema may be used
3. Circulatory system
   a. Blood volume usually back to normal by the third week after birth
   b. Blood fibrinogen levels and platelets increase during the first week; this may lead to thrombus formation
   c. Increase in leukocytes; may go as high as 30,000/mm^3 if labor was lengthy
   d. Drop in hemoglobin and red blood cell count on the fourth postpartal day
4. Excretory system
   a. Increased urinary output (diuresis), second to fifth postpartal day
   b. Bladder tone altered during pregnancy; retention with overflow may occur
   c. Activation of lactogenic hormone may result in lactose in the urine
   d. Excretion of nitrogen as involution occurs
5. Integumentary system
   a. Profuse diaphoresis as wastes are being excreted
   b. Pigmentational changes such as striae, linea nigra, and darkened areolae begin to fade but do not completely return to nulliparous state
6. Vital signs
   a. Temperature elevation up to 24 hours after birth as result of exertion and dehydration
   b. Blood pressure returns to baseline; drop suggests hemorrhage; elevation suggests pregnancy-induced hypertension
   c. Pulse drops slightly because of decreased cardiac effort; blood volume is decreased
7. Emotional needs
   a. Mother may experience "blues" following "crisis" of birth; "baby blues/postpartum blues" may occur on the third day with periods of irritability, restlessness, and anxiety
   b. A mood disorder with a postpartum onset may occur within 6 months with exaggerated signs and symptoms of postpartum blues

General Nursing Care During the Postpartal Period

A. DATA COLLECTION
1. Breasts
2. Abdomen and fundus
3. Lochia
4. Perineum
   a. Episiotomy
   b. Signs of hematoma
   c. Hemorrhoids
5. Signs of thrombophlebitis
6. Vital signs
7. Hydration status
8. Voiding; bowel movements
9. Signs of interaction with or attachment to infant

B. ANALYSIS AND INTERPRETATION

1. Anxiety related to insecurities about parental role and parenting activities
2. Ineffective breastfeeding related to improper positioning, inverted nipples, or ineffective or absent infant feeding behaviors
3. Constipation related to pain upon defecation and decreased peristalsis
4. Risk for infection related to inadequate perineal care
5. Knowledge deficit about parenting activities related to lack of experience
6. Altered nutrition: less than body requirements related to increased need for protein for tissue repair and lactation
7. Pain related to episiotomy, perineal edema, breast engorgement, hemorrhoids, or afterpains
8. Altered parenting related to lack of support from significant others, interruption in bonding process, lack of knowledge, or unrealistic expectations for self, infant, or partner
9. Impaired skin integrity related to episiotomy or laceration
10. Sleep-pattern disturbance related to discomfort, parenting activities, and anxiety
11. Altered urinary elimination related to effects of anesthesia and edema of perineal area

C. PLANNING/IMPLEMENTATION

1. Use universal precautions and aseptic technique when giving perineal care
2. Teach mother and assist mother with self-care; wash perineal area from front to back
3. Teach mother breast care; inspect the breasts for tissue and nipple breakdown, palpate to rule out growths (teach breast self-examination for continued health), support breasts with well-fitted brassiere
4. Teach the importance of hand washing when caring for self and baby (important for personnel to avoid cross-contamination)
5. Observe vital signs: a temperature of 38° C or above for 2 consecutive days (excluding first 24 hours after birth) considered sign of beginning puerperal infection; bradycardia is a normal phenomenon following birth
6. Palpate the fundus for firmness and descent below the umbilical level (involution normally follows a one-fingerbreadth descent daily, by the seventh to ninth day fundus cannot be felt); a fundus that is boggy indicates poor contractile power of uterus and results in bleeding; check for full bladder
7. Administer oxytocic medication as ordered to promote involution
   a. Oxcytocin (syntocinon)
   b. Ergonovine maleate (Ergometrine)
   c. Maintains the uterus in a slightly contracted state that controls bleeding from intrauterine sites and maintains tone, rate, and amplitude of rhythmic contractions required for involution of the uterus; may cause hypertension, especially ergonovine maleate, if uterus is boggy
8. Check lochia for color, amount, clots, odor (foul odor indicates beginning infection); observe episiotomy suture line if present for redness, ecchymosis, edema, discharge, and approximation (REEDA)
9. Assess for pain; afterpains are more common in multiparas; for pain in perineal suture line, apply cold applications for the first 24 hours and then provide sitz baths
10. Promote bladder and bowel function; secure catheterization order if the client is unable to void
11. Encourage Kegel exercises to strengthen pubococcygeal muscles
12. Provide or instruct client about a diet high in proteins and calories to restore body tissues
13. Encourage early ambulation to prevent blood stasis
14. Monitor laboratory reports for hemoglobin (Hgb) and hematocrit (Hct) concentrations and white blood count (WBC)
15. Observe for "postpartal blues," which may be caused by a drop in hormonal levels; if client is discharged early, support persons should be alerted to signs and symptoms
16. Meet the mother's needs to enable her to meet the baby's needs
17. Assist the mother with care of the baby as needed
18. Provide for group discussion on breastfeeding, infant care, etc.; encourage mother
19. Discuss resumption of intercourse and family planning; include information about when to expect menses
20. If Rh-negative mother, assess need for administration of WinRho, HypRho-D
21. Give rubella vaccine if indicated
22. Provide instructions for the client who is discharged early to contact personnel when questions arise
23. Involve the family in care and teaching

D. EVALUATION/OUTCOMES

1. Involution is progressing normally
2. Free from hemorrhage
3. Free from infection
4. Free from pain
5. Bowel function has returned

6. Initiates voiding and empties bladder
7. Performs perineal care after each voiding and defecation, as taught
8. Successfully feeds and cares for infant
9. Prepared for early discharge

▼ THE NEWBORN

Family and Prenatal History

A. Chronic illness in the mother's or father's family
B. Previous medical-surgical illnesses of the mother and father
C. Age and present health status of the mother and father
D. History of previous pregnancies
E. Prenatal history
   1. Medical supervision during pregnancy
   2. Nutrition during pregnancy
   3. Course of pregnancy: illnesses, medications taken, or treatments required
   4. Duration of gestation
   5. Course and amount of sedation and anesthesia required
   6. Type of birth and significant events during the immediate period after birth
   7. Immediate response of newborn (Apgar score at 1 and 5 minutes following birth)

Parent-Child Relationships

A. Concepts basic to parent-infant relationships
   1. Early and frequent parent-infant contact is essential for survival (bonding)
   2. Parenting abilities can be fostered and developed
   3. Biologic changes that occur at puberty and during pregnancy influence the development of nurturance
   4. Interaction between mother and child begins from the moment of conception and can be shared with the father
   5. Love for the infant grows as the parents interact and care for the infant
   6. As the parent gives to the infant and the infant receives, the parent in turn receives satisfaction from parenting tasks
   7. Any disturbance in the give-and-take cycle sets up frustrations in both the parent and the infant
   8. Parental behavior is learned and frequent parent-infant contact enhances development of parenting abilities
B. Infant's basic needs
   1. Physiologic—food, clothing, bathing, and protection from environment
   2. Emotional—security, comfort, fondling, caressing, rocking, being spoken to, and contact with one person on a consistent basis
C. Mothering and fathering are:
   1. Based on a biologic inborn desire to reproduce
   2. Role concepts that begin with own childhood experiences
   3. Primitive emotional relationships
   4. Maturing processes
   5. Conceptualizations of the physiologic and psychologic processes following infant's birth
   6. Fostered by the parent-infant interaction that constantly reinforces gratification as needs are met and security develops
   7. Abilities that are learned rather than innate
D. Parent-child relationships are affected by:
   1. Readiness for pregnancy
      a Planned or unplanned
      b. Health status prior to pregnancy
      c. Financial status
      d. Determinants such as age, cultural backgrounds, number in family unit
      e. Political forces
   2. Nature of the pregnancy
      a. Health status during pregnancy
      b. Preparation for parenthood
      c. Support from family members and members of the health care team
   3. Character of the labor and birth
      a. Length and pattern of labor
      b. Type and amount of analgesia received
      c. Support from family and health team
      d. Anesthesia during birth
      e. Type of birth
E. Significant phases of maternal adjustment
   1. Taking-in phase: mother's needs have to be met before she can meet the baby's needs; talks about self rather than the baby, does not seem interested in the baby, does not touch the infant, cries easily
   2. Transition phase: characterized by the mother's starting to take hold, looking at and reaching for the baby, touching with fingertips, talking about the baby, etc.
   3. Taking-hold phase: kisses, embraces, gives care to infant, eye contact, uses whole hand to make contact, calls the baby by name, etc.
F. Supportive care to promote bonding/attachment
   1. Allow the parents to touch, fondle, and hold infant
   2. Give parents ample time to inspect and begin to identify with baby
   3. Encourage give-and-take between parents and infant: rooming-in arrangement
   4. Support these beginning relationships
   5. Identify beginning of disturbed relationships

TABLE 3-1 Apgar score chart*

Adaptation	0	1	2
Heart rate	Absent	Slow, below 100	Over 100
Respiratory effort	Absent	Weak cry	Strong cry
Muscle tone	Limp	Some flexion of extremities	Active motion
Reflex irritability	No response	Grimace	Cry
Color	Cyanotic, pale	Body pink, extremities cyanotic	Completely pink

*Scores: 7 to 10, good condition; 3 to 6, moderately depressed; 0 to 2, severely depressed.

6. Teach parents about their newborn
7. Evaluate parents' and baby's response and revise plan as necessary

Adaptation to Extrauterine Life

A. Immediate needs at the time of birth
   1. Aspiration of mucus to provide an open airway
   2. Evaluation by use of Apgar score 1 and 5 minutes following birth (Table 3-1)
   3. Maintenance of body temperature by drying infant and placing next to mother or under radiant warmer
   4. Promote interaction between parents and neonate
   5. Constant observation of physical condition
   6. Identify infant by applying an identification band to infant and mother and obtaining footprints
   7. Eye care: prophylactic instillation of ordered medicine (e.g.,erythromycin) in each eye to prevent ophthalmia neonatorum
B. Characteristics of and changes in the newborn during the first week of life
   1. Circulatory
      a. Clamping of cord at birth brings changes in fetal circulation: closure of the foramen ovale and ductus arteriosus and obliteration of the umbilical arteries produce an adultlike circulation within 1 hour after birth
      b. Heart rate regular: 120 to 160, but variable depending on the infant's activity; soft heart murmur common for first month of life
      c. Clotting mechanism poor because of low prothrombin concentration; vitamin K by injection is necessary
      d. Liver immature (although large): cannot destroy excessive red cells in the newborn, resulting in physiologic jaundice by third day
      e. Hemoglobin level high: 140 to 200 g/L of blood
      f. White blood count high: 9.0–30.0 10⁹/L
   2. Respiratory: respirations diaphragmatic, irregular, abdominal; 30 to 50 per minute, quiet with periods of apnea
   3. Temperature: axillary temperature maintained at 36.2° C or 36.6° C; environmental factors may affect temperature
   4. Excretory
      a. Kidneys immature: newborn should void during first 24 hours (at 2 weeks of age voids 20 times daily), albumin and urates (brick-red staining on diaper) common during first week because of dehydration
      b. Stools: first stool, black-green and tenacious, called meconium; by third day, becomes mixed with light yellow, called transitional
   5. Integumentary
      a. Lanugo: fine, downy hair growth over the entire body
      b. Milia: small, whitish, pinpoint spots over the nose caused by retained sebaceous secretions
      c. Mongolian spots: blue-black discolorations on back, buttocks, and sacral region that disappear by first year, usually found in oriental babies
   6. Digestive
      a. Has stores of nutrients from intrauterine existence, therefore needs very little nourishment first few days
      b. Roots and sucks when anything is brought to mouth
      c. Digests simple carbohydrates, fats, and proteins readily
      d. Cardiac sphincter of stomach not well developed, therefore regurgitates if stomach is overfull
      e. Needs to be bubbled frequently to get rid of air bubbles in stomach
   7. Metabolic
      a. All newborns normally lose 5% to 10% of their body weight by first week of life
      b. Screening for inborn errors of metabolism (IEM)
         (1) Phenylketonuria (PKU) testing done 48 hours after ingestion of nutrients; infants with absence of phenylalanine will need special diet to prevent retardation
         (2) T₄ screening; inadequate thyroxine may lead to cretinism
         (3) Lactose intolerance; eliminate milk products

8. Endocrine
   a. Enlargement of breasts in males (gynecomastia) and females is normal as a result of hormones transmitted to baby by mother
   b. Female infants may have blood in the vagina (pseudomenstruation) because of withdrawal of maternal hormones
9. Neural
   a. CNS and brain not well developed: infant needs constant supply of oxygen
   b. Breathing, sucking, and crying are early neural activities necessary for the infant's survival
10. Sleep
    a. Lowers body metabolism
    b. Helps restore energy and assimilate nutrients for growth

C. Nutrition
   1. Initial weight loss of 5% to 10% of birth weight is normal and usually regained second to third week of life
   2. Infant feeding: put to breast or bottlefeed immediately after birth
   3. Phenylalanine cannot be detected until 24 hours after first feeding; tested 48 hours after first feeding; some hospitals are testing earlier because of early discharge
   4. Newborn needs to ingest simple proteins, carbohydrates, fats, vitamins, and minerals for continued cell growth
   5. Fluid (130 to 200 ml per kilogram or 2 to 3 oz fluid per pound of body weight)
   6. Calories (110 to 130 calories per kilogram or 50 to 60 calories per pound of body weight)
   7. Protein (2.2 to 2.0 g per kilogram of body weight from birth to 6 months of age; 1.8 g per kilogram of body weight from 6 to 12 months of age)
   8. Self-regulation schedule
      a. Each infant born with different degree of maturity and rhythm of needs
      b. Superior to rigid schedule, but should be modified to meet needs of infant and parents
      c. Bottlefed infants usually fed every 4 hours
      d. Breastfeed infants on demand, usually a minimum of 8 times in 24 hours
      e. Feeding behavior and degree of satisfaction reflect psychologic development of child
      f. Close mother-infant relationship in feeding process meets basic need of trust (Erikson's stage of trust)

General Nursing Care of the Newborn

A. **DATA COLLECTION** (INCLUDING APPRAISAL OF THE NEWBORN AFTER BIRTH)
   1. Classification of gestational age/birth weight
      a. Appropriate for gestational age (AGA): weight falls between tenth and ninetieth percentile for age
      b. Large for gestational age (LGA): weight is above the ninetieth percentile for age
      c. Small for gestational age (SGA): weight is below the tenth percentile for age
      d. Low birth weight (LBW): weight of 2500 g or less at birth
      e. Intrauterine growth retardation (IUGR): fetal growth rate does not meet expected norms
      f. Preterm (premature): birth at less than 37 weeks' gestation, regardless of weight
      g. Term: birth between the thirty-eighth and forty-second week of gestation
      h. Postterm: birth after 42 weeks' gestation
      i. Postmature: birth after 42 weeks' gestation; subjected to the effects of progressive placental insufficiency
   2. Skin
      a. Body is normally pink with slight cyanosis of hands and feet (acrocyanosis); jaundice is abnormal during the first 24 hours of life
      b. Check for abrasions, rashes, crackling, and elasticity, which indicates the status of tissue hydration; at times, milia (white, pinpoint spots over the nose caused by retained sebaceous secretions), birthmarks, forceps marks, ecchymosis, or papules are present
      c. Skin turgor
   3. Respirations are abdominal and irregular, with a rate of 30 to 50 per minute (retractions—depression of the sternum—are abnormal)
   4. Head and sensory organs
      a. Head and chest circumference nearly equal to the crown-rump length; chest slightly smaller than head; if reversed the infant should be assessed for microcephaly
      b. Symmetry of face: as the baby cries, sides of the face move equally
      c. Check the head for molding, abrasions, or skin breakdowns; observe for caput succedaneum: edema of soft tissue of the scalp; cephalhematoma: edema of the scalp caused by effusion of blood between the bone and periosteum; extend the head fully in all directions for adequacy in range of motion
      d. Observe the eyes for discharge or irritation; check the pupils for reaction to light, equality of eye movements (normally there is some ocular incoordination); check the sclerae for clarity, jaundice, or hemorrhage
      e. Nose: observe for patency of both nostrils
      f. Mouth: observe the gums and hard and soft palates for any openings; mucosa of the

mouth normally clear (white patches that bleed on rubbing indicate thrush, a monilial infection)

g. Ears: auricles open; vernix covers tympanic membrane, making otoscopic examination useless (ring bell close to ear—baby should stir); both eyes should be same level as ears; upper earlobes normally curved (flatness indicative of kidney anomaly)

5. Chest and abdomen
   a. Chest auscultation: only respiratory sounds should be audible (noisy crackling sounds abnormal); heart rate: regular 120 to 160 beats per minute (rubbing or unusual sounds abnormal)
   b. Abdomen
      (1) Listen to bowel sounds over the abdomen
      (2) Palpate the spleen with fingertips under the left costal margin: tip should be palpable
      (3) Palpate liver on the right side: normally 1 cm below the costal margin
      (4) Observe umbilical cord for redness, odor, or discharge; number of vessels present (normally one vein and two arteries)
      (5) Palpate the femoral pulses gently at inner aspect of the groin: indicate intact circulation to extremities

6. Genitalia
   a. Males
      (1) Palpate the scrotum for testes: at times undescended at birth, which is normal (must descend by puberty or sperm will be destroyed by high temperature within the abdominal cavity)
      (2) Enlargement of scrotum: indicates hydrocele (diagnosis affirmed by transparent appearance of the scrotum when a flashlight is held close to the scrotal sac)
      (3) Observe tip of the penis for the urinary meatus: epispadias, meatus on upper surface of the penis; hypospadias, meatus on lower surface; voiding
   b. Females
      (1) Observe the genitalia for labia, urinary meatus, and vaginal opening
      (2) Edema of labia and bloody mucoid discharge is normal and results from transfer of maternal hormones
      (3) Check for voiding

7. Extremities
   a. Hands and arms: thumbs clenched in fist
      (1) Check for number and variation of fingers
      (2) Check the clavicles and scapulae while putting arms through normal range of motion; clicking or resistance indicates dislocation or fracture
      (3) Palpate for fractures; crepitation is indicative
   b. Feet and legs
      (1) Check toes, pattern and number
      (2) Adduct and abduct feet through range of motion; there should be no resistance or tightness
      (3) Flex both legs onto the lower abdomen; there should be no resistance or tightness; abduct knees and listen for click (Ortolani's sign, indicates hip dysplasia)
      (4) Place both feet on a flat surface and bend the knees; knees should be at the same height (when unequal, known as Allis' sign, indicates hip dislocation)

8. Back: turn the baby on the abdomen, run a finger along the vertebral column; any dimples, separations, or swellings indicative of spina bifida

9. Anus: patency confirmed with passage of meconium; inability to insert a rectal thermometer may be indicative of imperforate anus

10. Neuromuscular development: check reflexes
    a. Rooting: touch the baby's cheek; baby should search for finger
    b. Sucking: place an object close to the baby's mouth; baby should make an attempt to suck
    c. Grasp: place fingers in palm of the baby's hand and encircle palm with your hand; lift the infant off a firm surface, baby will grasp; infant's head will lag as baby is raised
    d. Babinski: run thumb up middle undersurface of infant's foot; toes will separate and flare out
    e. Plantar: run thumb up the lateral undersurface of infant's foot; toes will curl downward
    f. Moro: make a loud, sharp noise close to the baby; will result in the baby's bringing both arms and legs close to the body as if in an embrace (disappears by 4 months of age)
    g. Crawl: when the baby is on a firm surface and turned on its abdomen, crawling movements will follow
    h. Step or dance: while the infant is supported under both arms, stepping movements will occur when feet are placed on a firm surface

B. ANALYSIS AND INTERPRETATION
1. Ineffective airway clearance related to mucus obstruction
2. Risk for aspiration related to presence of meconium in amniotic fluid
3. Altered nutrition: less than body requirements related to limited fluid intake or poor sucking ability

4. Pain related to circumcision and heel sticks for glucose, hematocrit, T_4, and PKU studies, etc.
5. Altered parenting related to change in family structure
6. Ineffective thermoregulation related to immaturity of nervous system
7. Risk for trauma related to immature blood-clotting mechanisms

C. **PLANNING/IMPLEMENTATION**
1. Monitor and maintain a patent airway
   a. Suction mucus as needed to maintain an open airway
   b. Position: side-lying position to facilitate drainage of mucus
   c. Observe for signs of respiratory distress
      (1) Grunting
      (2) Flaring of nostrils
      (3) Sternal retractions
2. Provide warmth
   a. Keep in a heated crib until body temperature is stabilized to prevent chilling; baby is unable to shiver and breaks down brown fat to produce energy for warmth; premature or small-for-gestational-age infants can be compromised by chilling because they have a paucity of brown fat available for breakdown
   b. Clothing should be loose, soft
   c. Crib should be firm and provide protection
   d. Skin should be kept clean and dry to maintain integrity
3. Monitor vital signs
4. Weigh daily
5. Provide daily sponge bath
6. Provide frequent diaper changes
7. Care for cord
8. Administer Vitamin K
   a. Prevents hemorrhagic disease of the newborn; absence of bacteria in the sterile gut of the newborn prevents synthesization of clotting factors
   b. Give 0.5 mg once during the first 6 hours of life
   c. Give IM into vastus lateralis muscle via tuberculin syringe with a 25-gauge, ⅝-inch needle
9. Provide for feeding (See Breastfeeding and Bottlefeeding)
10. Teach care of infant to parents
11. Care of circumcision
    a. Observe for bleeding
    b. Observe for urination
    c. Diaper applied loosely
    d. Dressing changes
12. Provide for human contact
    a. Body contact with another human is paramount for survival
    b. Administer care with an awareness of the importance of these early, beginning relationships
    c. Talking, rocking, and singing are an essential part of body contact with the newborn

D. **EVALUATION/OUTCOMES**
1. No signs of respiratory distress present
2. Temperature is in normal range
3. Voiding commensurate with fluid intake
4. Anus is patent; passing stool
5. Initial weight loss within 10% range
6. No signs of severe jaundice, cephalic swelling, or neuromuscular impairment

▼ BREASTFEEDING

A. Advantages
   1. Psychologic value of closeness and satisfaction in beginning mother-child relationship
   2. Optimum nutritional value for infant
   3. Economic and readily accessible
   4. Greater immunity to infection
   5. Infant is less likely to be allergic to mother's milk
   6. Develops facial muscles, jaw, and nasal passages of infant because stronger sucking is necessary
   7. Assists in involution of uterus
   8. Reduces chances of infection because of maternal antibodies present in colostrum and milk

B. Prerequisites
   1. Psychologic readiness of mother is a major factor in successful breastfeeding
   2. Adequate diet must be available prenatally and postnatally to ensure high-quality milk
   3. Suitable rest, exercise, and freedom from tension for mother will provide increased satisfaction for both her and the infant
   4. Infant's sucking at the breast stimulates the maternal posterior pituitary to produce oxytocin, the properties of which, in the blood system, constrict the lactiferous sinuses to move the milk down through the nipple ducts: known as the let-down reflex; a poor sucking reflex of the child will inhibit the let-down of milk; sucking also stimulates prolactin secretion
   5. Absence of emotional stress in the mother, because anxiety inhibits the let-down reflex

C. Contraindications
   1. In mother
      a. Active tuberculosis
      b. Acute contagious disease; HIV positive
      c. Chronic disease such as cancer, advanced nephritis, cardiac disease
      d. Extensive surgery
      e. Narcotic addiction
   2. In infant: cleft lip or palate or any other condition that interferes or prevents grasp of the nipple is the only real contraindication

3. Many drugs are excreted in breast milk and have harmful effects on the developing infant; these drugs must be avoided or taken with care if they must be taken by the mother; careful monitoring of the infant is required

Nursing Care of the Mother Who Is Breastfeeding

A. DATA COLLECTION

1. Condition of nipples
2. Desire to breastfeed
3. Level of anxiety regarding breastfeeding
4. Knowledge of breastfeeding and breast care
5. Family support

B. ANALYSIS AND INTERPRETATION

1. Ineffective breastfeeding related to position, condition of nipples, and infant's sucking ability
2. Altered family processes related to the amount of time required for breastfeeding
3. Risk for infection related to cracked nipples secondary to improper positioning on nipples
4. Knowledge deficit related to feeding and maintenance of lactation

C. PLANNING/IMPLEMENTATION

1. Teach feeding schedule
   a. Self-demand schedule is desirable
   b. Length of feeding time is usually 20 minutes, with greatest quantity of milk consumed in first 5 to 10 minutes
2. Teach feeding techniques
   a. Mother and infant in comfortable position, such as semireclining or in rocking chair
   b. Entire body of infant should be turned toward mother's breast; alternate starting breast and use both breasts at each feeding
   c. Initiate feeding by stimulating rooting reflex and direct nipple straight into baby's mouth (stroking cheek toward breast, being careful not to stroke other cheek, because this will confuse infant)
   d. Burp or bubble infant during and after feeding to allow for escape of air by:
      (1) Placing infant over shoulder
      (2) Sitting infant on lap, flexed forward
      (3) Rubbing or patting back (avoid jarring infant)
   e. Breast milk intake similar to formula intake
      (1) 130 to 200 ml of milk per kilogram (2 to 3 oz of milk per pound) of body weight
      (2) From one sixth to one seventh of baby's weight per day
   f. After lactation has been established, occasional bottlefeeding can be substituted
   g. Length of time for continuing breastfeeding is variable (may be discontinued when teeth erupt, because this can be uncomfortable for mother)
3. Teach care of breasts
   a. Cleanse with plain water once daily (soap or alcohol can cause irritation and dryness)
   b. Support breasts day and night with properly fitting brassiere
   c. Nursing pads should be placed inside bra cup to absorb any milk leaking between feedings; allow nipples to air dry at intervals
   d. Plastic bra liners should be avoided because they increase heat and perspiration and decrease air circulation necessary for drying of the nipple
   e. If breasts are engorged, teach mother to take warm showers and put baby to breast more frequently

D. EVALUATION/OUTCOMES

1. Infant receiving enough milk as evidenced by six or more wet diapers daily
2. Infant sleeping between feedings
3. Mother has no signs of nipple cracking or infection

▼ BOTTLEFEEDING

A. Advantages
   1. Provides an alternative to breastfeeding
   2. Less restrictive than breastfeeding; may meet needs of working mothers
   3. Allows a more accurate assessment of intake
   4. May be indicated in the presence of a congenital anomaly such as cleft palate
   5. May be necessary for infants who require special formulas because of allergies or inborn errors of metabolism
B. Types of formulas
   1. Commercial liquid or powdered formulas
   2. Special formulas
   3. Unmodified regular cow's milk, liquid or reconstituted; not appropriate for infants before 12 months of age
C. Contraindications
   1. Inadequate intelligence to prepare formula
   2. Poor storage and refrigeration practices
   3. Contaminated water supply
   4. Cost of formula and equipment
   5. Lack of equipment to adequately prepare bottles

Nursing Care of the Mother Who Is Bottlefeeding

A. DATA COLLECTION

1. Desire to bottlefeed

2. Sucking ability of infant
3. Knowledge of formulas and formula preparation

B. ANALYSIS AND INTERPRETATION
1. Ineffective infant feeding pattern related to lack of knowledge
2. Knowledge deficit related to new experience of preparing formula and feeding infant
3. Infant's altered nutrition: less than body requirements related to sucking difficulties or formula that does not meet infant's needs

C. PLANNING/IMPLEMENTATION
1. Teach preparation of formula
   a. Calculation of formula to yield 110 to 130 calories and 130 to 200 ml of fluid per kilogram of body weight; caution regarding dangers of overdilution (water intoxication) and underdilution (excess weight gain)
   b. Proper sterilization of formula by terminal heat method and of feeding utensils by a full 25 minutes of boiling if the water supply is not purified or clear
   c. Teach about commercial formulas
   d. Proper refrigeration of formula
2. Teach feeding techniques
   a. Always hold infant during feeding to provide warm body contact (bottle propping may contribute to aspiration of formula)
   b. Hold bottle so nipple is always filled with milk to prevent excessive air ingestion
   c. Adjust size of nipple hole to needs of baby (a premature infant needs a larger hole that requires less sucking)
   d. After feeding and burping infant, place child on side to aid digestion and prevent aspiration
   e. Feeding should be offered on demand to meet the infant's needs

D. EVALUATION/OUTCOMES
1. Infant receiving enough formula as evidenced by six or more wet diapers daily
2. Infant is gaining weight
3. Infant displays no signs of discomfort related to hunger

DEVIATIONS FROM NORMAL MATERNITY CYCLE IN THE MOTHER (COMPLICATIONS OF PREGNANCY)

▼ PREGNANCY-INDUCED HYPERTENSION (PIH): GESTATIONAL

HYPERTENSION, PREECLAMPSIA, ECLAMPSIA, AND HELLP SYNDROME

Data Base
A. Characterized by a triad of symptoms: edema, hypertension, and proteinuria occurring after the twentieth to twenty-fourth week of gestation and disappearing 6 weeks after birth
B. Occurs primarily in primiparas below 17 years of age and above 35 years of age, numerous pregnancies, women with chronic hypertension, diabetes mellitus, severe nutritional deficiencies, multiple pregnancy, or trophoblastic disease are common causes
C. Clinical findings
   1. Gestational hypertension
      a. Increased blood pressure during pregnancy that resolves within 6 weeks after birth
      b. No edema or proteinuria are present
   2. Preeclampsia
      a. Mild: systolic pressure increased 30 mm Hg or more above normal; diastolic pressure increased 15 mm Hg or more above normal; proteinuria 1+; edema manifested by excessive weekly weight gain and upper-body edema
      b. Severe: BP is 160/110 or above on two readings taken 6 hours apart after bed rest; proteinuria 3+ to 4+; extensive edema (puffiness of hands and face); hyperreflexia
   3. Eclampsia: seizures and/or coma associated with hypertension, proteinuria, and edema
   4. HELLP syndrome (*H*, hemolysis; *EL*, elevated liver enzymes; *LP*, low platelet count)
      a. Occurs with little warning and often with no previous signs of PIH
      b. Right upper-quadrant pain occurs in 90% of women; proteinuria may occur
      c. Liver enzymes are elevated; platelets and RBCs are low
      d. Blood smear reveals broken red blood cells (schistocytes or burr cells)
      e. Occurs after 28 weeks' gestation or 48 to 72 hours after birth
   5. Blood chemistry: rise in hematocrit, uric acid, liver enzymes, and blood urea nitrogen concentrations and decrease in RBCs, platelets, and CO_2 combining power indicate worsening preeclampsia
   6. Qualitative urinalysis: increase in albumin output (proteinuria) and/or decreased urinary output indicates worsening preeclampsia
D. Guidelines for prevention of pregnancy-induced hypertension

1. Sound nutrition counseling during pregnancy and lactation
2. Increase protein to 60 g daily in the second and third trimesters
3. Baby aspirin or Motrin may be used daily
4. Caloric intake should be increased 10% during pregnancy; severe calorie restriction is harmful during pregnancy
5. Restriction of sodium is harmful during pregnancy and can result in electrolyte imbalance and elimination of essential nutritional components; may contribute to reduced circulatory volume
6. Diuretics are contraindicated during pregnancy because they cause hypovolemia and deplete essential nutrients for mother and fetus

E. Therapeutic interventions
1. Gestational hypertension
   a. Frequent rest periods
   b. Dietary management with increased fluid intake
   c. Treat symptoms
2. Mild preeclampsia
   a. High-protein diet
   b. Ambulatory care; frequent visits to obstetrician
   c. Frequent rest periods with feet elevated; side-lying position to enhance renal and placental perfusion
   d. Sedatives to ensure rest and sleep
3. Severe preeclampsia or eclampsia
   a. Hospitalization and complete bed rest
   b. Magnesium sulfate given IV by infusion pump to prevent or limit seizures
   c. Albumin concentrate to increase renal flow and correct the hypovolemia
   d. Antihypertensives
   e. Foley catheter
   f. Labor induction or cesarean birth once symptoms are under control
   g. Calcium gluconate for the mother and ventilations, cardiac massage, and adrenaline (epinephrine) if respiratory depression
4. HELLP syndrome
   a. Same as severe preeclampsia or eclampsia
   b. Blood or blood products may be administered if necessary

Nursing Care of Clients with Pregnancy-induced Hypertension (Preeclampsia, Eclampsia, and HELLP Syndrome)
A. DATA COLLECTION
1. Blood pressure elevation
2. Presence of edema
   a. Excessive weight gain
   b. Puffiness of hands, feet, or face
3. Albumin in urine
4. Oliguria
5. Hyperreflexia
6. Persistent headache
7. Blurred vision
8. Epigastric pain

B. ANALYSIS AND INTERPRETATION
1. Anxiety related to course of pregnancy and possible death of fetus
2. Fluid volume deficit related to fluid shift from intravascular to extravascular space secondary to vasospasm
3. Risk for injury to mother related to sedation and seizures
4. Risk for injury to fetus related to hypoxic episodes during maternal seizures
5. Risk for trauma to mother related to magnesium toxicity

C. PLANNING/IMPLEMENTATION
1. Monitor BP
   a. Every 15 minutes during critical phase
   b. Every 1 to 4 hours as condition improves
2. Monitor urine for albumin
3. Obtain daily weights
4. Assess edema
5. Maintain high-protein diet with normal salt intake
6. Monitor intake and output
7. Monitor hyperreflexia
8. Insert Foley catheter
9. Administer magnesium sulfate as ordered (check for sufficient urinary output before starting)
10. Monitor for magnesium toxicity
    a. Assess for depressed patellar reflexes
    b. Assess for depressed respirations, below 12 to 14 breaths per minute
    c. Monitor magnesium blood levels every 6 hours; therapeutic range is 0.8 to 1.2 mmol/L
    d. Have calcium gluconate available if magnesium sulfate toxicity is present
11. Maintain seizure precautions
12. Maintain on bed rest in side-lying position
13. Monitor FHR
14. Observe for labor
15. Observe for bleeding
16. Maintain quiet environment; limit visitors
17. Monitor hematologic studies to prevent HELLP syndrome
18. Assess anxieties and concerns
19. Be prepared for an induced or emergency cesarean birth
20. Continue to monitor for related complications for 48 hours after birth

D. EVALUATION/OUTCOMES
1. FHR and activity are within normal parameters

2. Absence of seizures
3. Urinary output is sufficient in relation to intake
4. Edema is reduced
5. Blood pressure is lowered

BLEEDING DURING THE FIRST TRIMESTER OF THE MATERNITY CYCLE

▼ ABORTION

Data Base
A. Definition
   1. An interruption of pregnancy in which there is complete expulsion or partial expulsion (incomplete) of the products of conception before the period of viability
   2. May be sudden, spontaneous, or induced by external mechanical force or trauma (for planned abortions, see Induced Abortion)
B. Types/clinical findings
   1. Threatened abortion: cervix is closed, but bleeding, cramping and backache are present
   2. Imminent or inevitable abortion: bleeding and cramping become more severe, cervix dilates, and products of conception are expelled
   3. Complete abortion: all products of conception are expelled within 24 to 48 hours
   4. Incomplete abortion: all the products of conception are not expelled
   5. Missed abortion: fetus dies in utero but not expelled; client must be monitored for disseminated intravascular coagulopathy (DIC)
C. Therapeutic interventions
   1. Complete bed rest
   2. Diagnostic/therapeutic blood studies: blood cell count, blood typing, Rh incompatibility, and cross-matching with availability of blood
   3. Dilation and curettage or vacuum aspiration performed if the products of conception are retained

Nursing Care of Clients Experiencing Abortion
A. DATA COLLECTION
   1. Vital signs
   2. Amount of bleeding
   3. Pain
   4. Emotional response to loss
B. ANALYSIS AND INTERPRETATION
   1. Anxiety related to impending loss of pregnancy
   2. Anticipatory grieving related to loss of expected baby
   3. Pain related to uterine contractions
   4. Situational low self-esteem related to inability to carry pregnancy to term

C. PLANNING/IMPLEMENTATION
   1. Institute measures to alleviate fear and anxiety; assist with grieving process
   2. Point out physiologic reality, but encourage client to work through feelings of guilt
   3. Encourage participation with thanatology services and bereavement groups when appropriate
   4. Monitor amount and type of bleeding
      a. Save and count number of pads
      b. Distinguish between dark clotted blood and frank bleeding, which is bright red
   5. Monitor vital signs; assess for hypovolemia and shock
   6. Monitor laboratory work; prepare for administration of blood
   7. Monitor fetal heart if pregnancy is beyond twentieth week
   8. Administer oxygen if necessary
   9. Maintain fluid and electrolyte balance
   10. Administer WinRho, HypRho-D to Rh-negative client after abortion
   11. Educate about necessity for follow-up care
D. EVALUATION/OUTCOMES
   1. No complications occur
   2. Assistance with grieving sought, if necessary

▼ ECTOPIC PREGNANCY

Data Base
A. Pregnancy in which implantation occurs outside the uterus (most frequent site is middle portion of fallopian tube, other sites are abdomen, ovaries, or cervix)
B. Early signs and symptoms are usually concealed; may be diagnosed by ultrasonography
C. Pattern in tubal pregnancy is usually one in which spotting may occur after one or two missed menstrual periods, sharp lower right or left abdominal pain radiating to shoulder develops; concealed bleeding from site of rupture leads to sudden shock
D. Clients who have had pelvic inflammatory disease (PID) or are using IUDs are predisposed to ectopic pregnancies
E. Therapeutic interventions
   1. Diagnosis confirmed by ultrasound examination, laparoscopy, or culdocentesis
   2. Immediate blood replacement if blood loss is severe
   3. Surgical repair or removal of ruptured fallopian tube may be attempted

Nursing Care of Clients with an Ectopic Pregnancy
A. DATA COLLECTION

1. Vital signs
2. Signs of shock
3. Bleeding
4. Character and location of pain
5. Level of anxiety

B. ANALYSIS AND INTERPRETATION
1. Altered cardiopulmonary tissue perfusion related to hemorrhage
2. Fear related to potential disturbance in future childbearing ability
3. Fluid volume deficit related to bleeding
4. Anticipatory grieving related to loss of expected baby
5. Pain related to tubal rupture

C. PLANNING/IMPLEMENTATION
1. Provide preoperative care
2. Assess continuously for signs of shock
3. Administer analgesics as ordered for pain
4. Administer and monitor intravenous blood therapy if ordered for excessive blood loss
5. Provide emotional support
6. Provide postoperative care
7. Give WinRho, HypRho-D immune globulin if the client is Rh negative

D. EVALUATION/OUTCOME
1. Assistance with grieving sought, if necessary
2. Able to state implications for future childbearing

BLEEDING DURING THE SECOND TRIMESTER OF THE MATERNITY CYCLE

▼ HYDATIDIFORM MOLE OR TROPHOBLASTIC DISEASE

Data Base

A. Definition
1. An abnormal pregnancy in which there is a benign growth of the chorion
2. Spontaneous expulsion usually occurs between the sixteenth and eighteenth weeks of pregnancy

B. Clinical findings
1. Uterus is generally larger for the period of gestation and fetal parts are not palpable
2. Symptoms of pregnancy-induced hypertension and hyperemesis are common
3. Potential for uterine perforation, hemorrhage, and infection

C. Therapeutic interventions
1. If spontaneous evacuation does not occur, evacuation by delicate curettage or hysterotomy is performed
2. Continued follow-up of serum gonadotropin levels is imperative for 1 year to rule out metastasis from chorionic carcinoma (increased gonadotropin levels require chemotherapy)
3. Preventing a new pregnancy is essential for 1 year

Nursing Care of Clients with Hydatidiform Mole or Trophoblastic Disease

A. DATA COLLECTION
1. Vaginal bleeding (brownish, prune juice) containing grapelike tissue
2. Uterine enlargement; fundal height is greater than that expected for length of pregnancy
3. Vomiting
4. Elevated blood pressure earlier than 24 weeks' gestation
5. Absence of fetal heart tones or activity
6. Confirmation by ultrasonography

B. ANALYSIS AND INTERPRETATION
1. Ineffective individual coping related to uncertainty of continuing a future pregnancy and frequent human chorionic gonadotropin (hCG) level monitoring
2. Fear related to the possible development of cancer
3. Risk for injury related to development of malignancy secondary to remaining remnants of mole
4. Self-esteem disturbance and/or body image disturbance related to carrying an abnormal pregnancy
5. Risk for trauma related to perforation of the uterus secondary to curettage

C. PLANNING/IMPLEMENTATION
1. See Nursing Care of Clients Experiencing Abortion
2. Teach about importance of follow-up care
3. Support through loss of expected pregnancy

D. EVALUATION/OUTCOMES
1. States intention of continuing follow-up care
2. Seeks information on preventing pregnancy for 1 year

▼ DYSFUNCTIONAL CERVIX (INCOMPETENT CERVIX)

Data Base

A. Definition
1. Cervical effacement and dilation in early second trimester resulting in expulsion of products of conception
2. Usually results from previous forceful dilation and curettage, difficult birth, or congenitally short cervix

B. Clinical findings
1. Painless contractions in midtrimester

2. Birth of dead or nonviable fetus
C. Therapeutic interventions
   1. Cerclage procedure during fourteenth to sixteenth week of gestation; suture or ribbon placed beneath cervical mucosa to close cervix
   2. At end of pregnancy cesarean birth or cutting of suture for vaginal birth

Nursing Care of Clients with a Dysfunctional Cervix
A. DATA COLLECTION
   1. Weeks of gestation
   2. Obstetric history
   3. Knowledge of the cerclage procedure
B. ANALYSIS AND INTERPRETATION
   1. Body image disturbance related to feelings of failure and feelings of guilt associated with inability to complete pregnancy
   2. Anticipatory grieving related to loss of expected baby
   3. Knowledge deficit related to cerclage procedure and effect on pregnancy
   4. Situational low self-esteem related to inability to complete pregnancy
C. PLANNING/IMPLEMENTATION
   1. Provide routine postoperative care
   2. Maintain bed rest for 24 hours
   3. Observe for rupture of membranes or bleeding
   4. Monitor FHR with Doppler ultrasound
D. EVALUATION/OUTCOMES
   1. States intention of seeking immediate medical care if labor begins
   2. Continues pregnancy to term

BLEEDING DURING THE THIRD TRIMESTER OF THE MATERNITY CYCLE

▼ PLACENTA PREVIA

Data Base
A. Definition—implantation of the placenta in the lower uterine segment
B. Types
   1. Marginal: placental edge is close to internal os
   2. Partial: placenta partially covers internal os
   3. Complete: placenta completely covers internal os
C. Clinical findings
   1. Painless, bright-red bleeding; hemorrhage
   2. Soft uterus in the latter part of pregnancy
   3. Signs of infection may be present
D. Therapeutic interventions
   1. Ultrasonography to confirm the presence of placenta previa

2. Depends on location of placenta, amount of bleeding, and status of the fetus
3. Control bleeding
4. Replace blood loss if excessive
5. Cesarean birth may be performed

Nursing Care of Clients with Placenta Previa
A. DATA COLLECTION
   1. Presence of bright-red blood with absence of pain
   2. Vital signs indicate shock (hypovolemic)
   3. Changes in or absence of FHR
   4. Level of anxiety (usually increases)
B. ANALYSIS AND INTERPRETATION
   1. Anxiety related to unknown course of pregnancy and possibility of cesarean birth
   2. Altered cardiopulmonary tissue perfusion in both mother and fetus related to hemorrhage and interruption of placental oxygen supply
   3. Fear related to acuteness of physical status and possible death of fetus and/or mother
   4. Fluid volume deficit related to hemorrhage
   5. Anticipatory grieving related to outcome of pregnancy, threat of termination of childbearing ability, and loss of body part (uterus, ovary, fallopian tube)
   6. Sleep pattern disturbance related to need for frequent assessments
C. PLANNING/IMPLEMENTATION
   1. No admission vaginal examination; if a vaginal examination is to be performed, double set-ups (vaginal and cesarean) must be provided
   2. Monitor vital signs continuously
   3. Maintain bed rest
   4. Assess color for pallor or cyanosis
   5. Administer oxygen
   6. Save all perineal pads to assess blood loss
   7. Monitor FHR continuously
   8. Prepare for cesarean birth if bleeding persists
   9. Keep mother and family informed
   10. Administer and monitor intravenous therapy and/or blood replacement
D. EVALUATION/OUTCOMES
   1. Vital signs are stable
   2. Mother and baby are in satisfactory condition
   3. Anxiety level is reduced

▼ ABRUPTIO PLACENTAE (PREMATURE SEPARATION OF PLACENTA)

Data Base
A. Definition—premature separation of a normally implanted placenta
B. Clinical findings

1. Concealed bleeding if center of the placenta separates and margins are intact
2. Dark-red blood may or may not be evident with partially detached placenta at margins
3. Moderate to agonizing abdominal pain
4. Persistent uterine contraction; normal to boardlike abdomen
5. Hyperactivity and then cessation of fetal movements
6. Frequently associated with pregnancy-induced hypertension, essential hypertension, maternal crack use, and previous history of abruptio placentae
7. Predisposes client to hemorrhage, disseminated intravascular coagulopathy (DIC), and hypofibrinogenemia

C. Therapeutic interventions
1. Replacement of blood loss
2. With fetal distress: emergency cesarean birth
3. Without fetal distress and in the presence of some cervical effacement and dilation, induction of labor may be attempted
4. Oxygen if necessary
5. Maintenance of fluid and electrolyte balance

Nursing Care of Clients with Abruptio Placentae

A. DATA COLLECTION
1. Presence of pain with or without dark-red bleeding
2. Increased tonicity of abdominal wall
3. Vital signs indicate shock
4. Changes in or absence of FHR
5. Level of anxiety usually increases

B. ANALYSIS AND INTERPRETATION
See Analysis/Nursing Diagnoses under Placenta Previa

C. PLANNING/IMPLEMENTATION
1. Monitor vital signs continuously
2. Assess color for pallor or cyanosis
3. Administer oxygen
4. Administer and monitor intravenous therapy
5. Save all perineal pads to assess blood loss
6. Monitor FHR continuously
7. Keep mother and family informed
8. Observe for signs of DIC such as seepage of blood from IV site or incisional areas

D. EVALUATION/OUTCOMES
See Evaluation/Outcomes under Placenta Previa

▼ BLEEDING DURING THE POSTPARTAL PERIOD

Data Base
A. Definition—bleeding in excess of 500 ml within the first 24 hours following birth; usually associated with uterine atony, vaginal and cervical lacerations, or retained placental fragments

B. Clinical findings
1. Large amount of frank, red bleeding
2. Boggy uterus
3. Signs of hypotension
4. Signs of disseminated intravascular coagulopathy (DIC)
   a. Profuse, uncontrollable bleeding from uterus
   b. Oozing of blood from episiotomy, laceration, or IV site
   c. Fragmented or distorted red blood cells
   d. Decreased coagulation factors (pathologic form of clotting)

C. Therapeutic interventions
1. Emptying bladder
2. Massaging of fundal portion of uterus
3. Administration of oxytocics
4. Blood replacement with severe blood loss
5. Surgical repair of vaginal and cervical lacerations
6. Manual removal of retained placental fragments
7. Cryoprecipitate, fresh frozen plasma for DIC

Nursing Care of Clients with Postpartal Bleeding

A. DATA COLLECTION
1. Identify risk factors
   a. Multiparity
   b. Prolonged labor
   c. Analgesia
   d. Multiple gestation
   e. Abruptio placentae or placenta previa
   f. PIH, especially HELLP
2. Assess for vaginal bleeding and clots
3. Palpate for boggy uterus
4. Watch for decreased urinary output
5. Monitor vital signs for signs of shock
6. Observe for pallor and fatigue
7. Monitor for increased level of anxiety

B. ANALYSIS AND INTERPRETATION
1. Altered cardiopulmonary tissue perfusion relative to hemorrhage resulting from uterine relaxation following birth and/or cervical laceration
2. Fear related to uncontrollable bleeding and possible death
3. Fluid volume deficit related to hemorrhage
4. Altered parenting related to interruption in bonding process
5. Altered cerebral or peripheral tissue perfusion related to pathologic clotting

C. PLANNING/IMPLEMENTATION

1. Check fundus for height and firmness every 15 minutes for 1 hour
2. Massage fundus if boggy
3. Keep bladder from distending so that the uterus can contract; insert Foley catheter as ordered if voiding is insufficient
4. Monitor for bleeding
   a. Save perineal pads
   b. Save all blood clots
5. Obtain vital signs every 15 minutes
6. Monitor intake and output
7. Administer oxytocin as ordered
8. Review laboratory results of blood studies
9. Reassure mother and partner about neonate

D. EVALUATION/OUTCOMES

1. Hemorrhaging has stopped
2. Vital signs are stable
3. Parent-infant attachment is maintained
4. Anxiety level is reduced

DEVIATIONS FROM NORMAL LABOR AND BIRTH PROCESS IN THE MOTHER (COMPLICATIONS OF LABOR AND BIRTH)

▼ INDUCTION OR STIMULATION OF LABOR

Data Base

A. Elective induction: initiation of labor contractions by:
1. Pharmacologic means
   a. Vaginal insertion of prostaglandin E_2 to promote cervical softening and effacement (ripening) every 6 hours up to 3 times
   b. 6 hours after prostaglandin E_2 administration pump infusion of syntocinon (Oxcytocin) to stimulate contractions
2. Mechanical means
   a. Artificial rupture of membranes (amniotomy)
   b. Insertion of *Laminaria* (dried seaweed that swells in presence of moisture) to promote cervical ripening and then induction begins
   c. Stimulation of breasts to bring about neural stimulation of posterior pituitary and secretion of oxytocin
3. May be done for medical or obstetric reasons; medical: diabetes, pyelonephritis; obstetric: PIH, Rh incompatibility, polyhydramnios, abruptio placentae, premature rupture of membranes at term without onset of labor, post-term gestation, and history of precipitate birth

B. Augmentation of labor: assisting client when labor process is not progressing normally (prolonged labor) by pharmacologic or mechanical means
C. Induction or augmentation of labor is not done with cephalopelvic disproportion, malpresentation of fetus, fetal distress, placenta previa, or active genital herpes

Nursing Care of Clients During Induction or Stimulation of Labor

A. DATA COLLECTION

1. Obstetric history, including expected date of birth
2. Maternal status
   a. Parity
   b. Contractions
   c. Status of membranes
   d. Status of cervix
   e. Ultrasonographic findings
   f. Level of anxiety
3. Fetal status
   a. Gestational age
   b. Absence of cephalopelvic disproportion
   c. Position
   d. Results of fetal monitoring

B. ANALYSIS AND INTERPRETATION

1. Anxiety related to uncertainty of the labor and birth process
2. Risk for infection related to ruptured membranes
3. Pain related to use of oxytocics
4. Risk for trauma related to possibility of sustained contractions from oxytocin or fetal cord prolapse following amniotomy

C. PLANNING/IMPLEMENTATION

1. Prepare mother and labor coach for induction
   a. Explain all procedures
   b. Obtain informed consent whenever necessary
2. Remain with mother and partner at all times
3. Obtain and record baseline information such as maternal vital signs, FHR, contractions for later comparison; continue to monitor all vital indices
4. Monitor Oxcytocin administration
   a. Gradually increase drip rate until contractions occur every 2 to 3 minutes
      (1) Slow rate if hypotension or tachycardia occurs
      (2) Keep client hydrated
   b. Discontinue Oxytocin drip if:
      (1) A sustained uterine contraction occurs
      (2) Fetal accelerations/decelerations persist
      (3) Urinary flow decreases to 30 ml per hour; (related to water intoxication)
      (4) Signs of placenta previa or abruptio placentae appear

5. Monitor effect of prostaglandin
   a. If hypertonic contractions occur, discontinue infusion
   b. If no response prepare for tocolytic therapy
6. Assist with artificial rupture of membranes (amniotomy)
   a. Maintain asepsis
   b. Immediately after rupture, monitor FHR
   c. Note color and amount of amniotic fluid
   d. Record time of rupture; prolonged rupture may predispose client to sepsis
7. Maintain hydration
8. Provide for blood typing, Rh compatibility, cross-matching
9. Have oxygen, suction, and resuscitation equipment readily available
10. Prepare for emergency cesarean birth if necessary

D. EVALUATION/OUTCOMES
1. Labor begins or increases and progresses to birth
2. Oxytocin causes no adverse effects
3. Anxiety is decreased
4. Client demonstrates no signs of infection

▼ PREMATURE RUPTURE OF MEMBRANES (PROM)

Data Base
A. Definition—spontaneous rupture of membranes before onset of labor
B. Maternal implication—ascending infection
C. Fetal implications
   1. Prolapsed cord
   2. FHR decelerations caused by cord compression from lack of amniotic fluid
   3. Sepsis from ascending infection
D. Therapeutic interventions
   1. Hospitalization with bed rest after 37 weeks of gestation
   2. Amnioinfusion of isotonic saline in some cases to allow for fetal movement and lessen danger of cord compression
   3. Prophylactic antibiotics

Nursing Care of Clients with Premature Rupture of Membranes (PROM)
A. DATA COLLECTION
1. Monitor fetal heart rate
2. Inspect perineum for prolapsed cord
3. Confirm rupture of membranes
   a. Nitrazine paper: amniotic fluid is alkaline; bluish-green result
   b. Ferning test: microscopic examination reveals fernlike crystals of sodium chloride

4. Time of rupture of membranes
5. Vital signs
6. Characteristics of leaking amniotic fluid: odor and color

B. ANALYSIS AND INTERPRETATION
1. Fear related to outcome of pregnancy
2. Impaired gas exchange to fetus related to prolapsed cord
3. Risk for infection related to premature rupture of membranes

C. PLANNING/IMPLEMENTATION
1. Monitor FHR
2. Monitor vital signs; temperature and pulse every 2 hours
3. Monitor uterine activity
4. Avoid unnecessary vaginal examinations
5. Ensure adequate hydration
6. Educate parents: amniotic fluid is still being produced
7. Provide perineal hygiene

D. EVALUATION/OUTCOMES
1. Mother shows no signs of infection
2. Cord does not prolapse
3. Fetus does not become distressed
4. Parent(s) able to verbalize implications of PROM

▼ PRETERM OR PREMATURE LABOR

Data Base
A. Labor begins after twentieth week but before thirty-eighth week of gestation
B. Contributing factors include multiple abortions, abdominal surgery, incompetent cervix, multiple pregnancies, urinary tract infections (UTI, such as nephritis and pyelitis), and use of cocaine
C. Therapeutic interventions
   1. Bed rest; side-lying position, preferably left side
   2. Tocolytic therapy directed toward postponing labor
      a. Isoxuprine (Vasodilan) to relax smooth muscle
      b. Magnesium sulfate (given in smaller doses than those that are used for PIH); affects smooth muscles by influencing the flow of calcium
      c. Ritodrine hydrochloride (Yutopar) is rarely used because of serious side effects
   3. Glucocorticoid therapy
      a. Dexamethasone
      b. Administered if birth appears inevitable 24 to 48 hours before birth
      c. Reduces incidence and severity of respiratory distress syndrome (RDS) in preterm infants; enhances formation of surfactant

Nursing Care of Clients During Preterm Labor with Tocolytic Therapy

A. DATA COLLECTION

1. Number of weeks of gestation
2. Presence of live and viable fetus
3. Presence of labor
   a. Two contractions lasting 30 seconds within a 15-minute period
   b. Cervical dilation less than 4 cm
   c. Effacement of 50% or less
4. No signs of hemorrhage or infection
5. Presence of severe pregnancy-induced hypertension
6. Prolonged rupture of membranes
7. Emotional impact on mother

B. ANALYSIS AND INTERPRETATION

1. Anxiety related to uncertainty of the labor and birth process
2. Ineffective family coping related to need for specialized care and continued hospitalization of the newborn
3. Fear related to acute status of baby and potential for death
4. Knowledge deficit related to cause and treatment of preterm labor
5. Altered parenting related to the physical condition of the baby
6. Situational low self-esteem related to failure to carry pregnancy to full term
7. Risk for trauma related to use of medications

C. PLANNING/IMPLEMENTATION

1. Monitor vital signs, FHR, contractions, and progression of labor
2. Maintain bed rest
3. Inform client about medication; obtain consent
4. Provide emotional support: reduce anxiety and prepare for possible loss of baby
5. Provide special care related to the administration of tocolytic medications
   a. Obtain baseline blood data and electrocardiographic (ECG) readings
   b. Monitor vital signs; hypotension can occur with all tocolytics; tachycardia can occur with Vasodilan and ritodrine
   c. Maintain hydration but monitor for pulmonary edema
   d. Monitor for signs of hypokalemia
   e. Monitor blood glucose levels
   f. Monitor intake and output
   g. Monitor neurologic reflexes
6. Prepare for use of glucocorticoid therapy for fetus
7. Prepare for premature birth if labor continues
8. Provide home instruction for halting preterm labor
   a. Rest periods in lateral position
   b. Increased fluid intake
   c. Avoidance of vigorous activity
   d. No sexual intercourse
   e. No nipple stimulation
   f. Avoidance of stressful events
   g. Empty bladder regularly and if contractions occur

D. EVALUATION/OUTCOMES

1. Mother's labor ceases
2. Fetus remains in utero
3. Fetal heart tones and fetal movement satisfactory
4. No ill effects from tocolytic agents
5. Anxiety decreases
6. Client and partner able to state recurring signs of preterm labor

▼ POSTTERM OR POSTDATE LABOR

Data Base

A. Extends beyond the forty-first week of gestation or 2 weeks beyond expected date of birth; 38 to 42 weeks' gestation is considered full term
B. Fetal risk
   1. Decreased amniotic fluid may lead to cord compression during labor
   2. Decreased placental function because of aging lowers oxygen and nutritional transport; fetus then becomes compromised during labor (may become asphyxic or hypoglycemic)
   3. Increasing size (mainly length) and hardening of skull may contribute to cephalopelvic disproportion
C. Maternal risk—only if infant is excessively large
D. Therapeutic intervention—induction of labor

Nursing Care of Clients During Postterm Labor

A. DATA COLLECTION

1. Fetal heart rate
2. Presence of meconium
3. Number of weeks of gestation; date of last menstrual period; EDC
4. Results of stress and nonstress tests
5. Biophysical profile, particularly amount of amniotic fluid
6. Level of anxiety related to delayed date of birth

B. ANALYSIS AND INTERPRETATION

1. Fear related to:
   a. Well-being of baby because of aging placenta and decreased amniotic fluid
   b. Traumatic birth secondary to oversized fetus
2. Risk for injury to fetus related to decreased amount of amniotic fluid
3. Knowledge deficit related to procedure for induction of labor

C. PLANNING/IMPLEMENTATION

See Planning/Implementation under Induction of Labor

D. EVALUATION/OUTCOMES
1. Labor begins and progresses to birth
2. Oxytocin causes no adverse effects
3. Anxiety is decreased
4. Neonate is stable at birth

▼ DYSFUNCTIONAL LABOR (DYSTOCIA)

Data Base

A. Mechanical factors
   1. Cephalopelvic disproportion
   2. Contracted pelvis
   3. Malpresentation or position
B. Faulty uterine contractions
   1. Hypertonic: increased frequency of contractions with decreased intensity; usually occurs in early labor; cervix does not dilate and mother becomes exhausted; increased fetal molding (caput succedaneum or cephalhematoma) may occur in older primigravidas or very anxious women
   2. Hypotonic: slowing down of rate and intensity of contractions in latter part of labor
   3. Treatment: deciding factors are length of labor, condition of mother and fetus, amount of cervical effacement and dilation, presentation, position, and station of presenting part
      a. Oxytocics to stimulate labor
      b. Cesarean birth

Nursing Care of Clients During Dysfunctional Labor (Dystocia)

A. DATA COLLECTION
1. Progress of labor
2. Status of mother
3. Status of fetus; FHR
4. Ultrasonographic results to determine fetal and pelvic size

B. ANALYSIS AND INTERPRETATION
1. Anxiety related to the uncertainty of labor process
2. Fatigue related to prolonged, difficult labor
3. Risk for fluid volume deficit related to prolonged labor
4. Pain related to prolonged unproductive contractions, administration of oxytocics, and cesarean birth if necessary
5. Risk for trauma related to failure of cervix to dilate adequately and/or mechanical problems

C. PLANNING/IMPLEMENTATION
1. Relieve back pain, caused by prolonged posterior pressure from fetus in occiput posterior position, by applying sacral pressure during contraction
2. Observe for signs of maternal exhaustion such as elevation of body temperature, dehydration, acidosis
3. Observe for signs of fetal distress
4. Have oxygen, suction, and resuscitation equipment readily available
5. Constantly monitor contractions, FHR, and vital signs when client is receiving oxytocic stimulation
6. Provide emotional support; keep client and family informed about progress
7. Administer fluids as ordered
8. Administer sedatives as ordered

D. EVALUATION/OUTCOMES
1. Labor pattern regulated
2. Safe birth occurs
3. Anxiety is reduced
4. Fluid and electrolyte status within normal limits

▼ PRECIPITATE LABOR

Data Base

A. Rapid labor and birth of less than 2-hour duration
B. Hazards to mother are perineal laceration and postpartum hemorrhage
C. Hazards to baby are anoxia and intracranial hemorrhage

Nursing Care of Clients During Precipitate Labor

A. DATA COLLECTION
1. Rapid cervical dilation
2. Accelerated fetal descent
3. History of rapid labor
4. Rapid uterine contractions with decreased uterine relaxation periods between contractions

B. ANALYSIS AND INTERPRETATION
1. Risk for maternal injury related to rapid expulsion of fetus resulting in lacerations and hemorrhage
2. Risk for fetal trauma related to cranial battering during rapid birth

C PLANNING/IMPLEMENTATION
1. Remain with mother and monitor closely
2. Keep emergency birth pack at bedside
3. Keep mother and partner informed throughout process of labor and birth
4. Guide fetal head through birth canal if birth occurs

D. EVALUATION/OUTCOMES
1. Mother is safe throughout labor and birth
2. Neonate remains injury free during birth

▼ BREECH BIRTH

Data Base
A. Position of the fetus in which the buttocks alone (frank breech), buttocks and feet (complete breech), or one or both feet (footling) descend through the birth canal first
B. Maternal implication—cesarean birth may be required, especially in primigravida
C. Fetal implications
 1. Increased mortality
 2. Occurrence of prolapsed cord leading to asphyxia
 3. Birth trauma such as brachial palsy and fracture of the upper extremities

Nursing Care of Clients During Breech Birth
A. DATA COLLECTION
 1. Recognition of breech presentation on performing Leopold's maneuvers and vaginal examination
 2. Auscultation of fetal heart tones above umbilicus
 3. Presence of meconium without signs of fetal distress
B. ANALYSIS AND INTERPRETATION
 1. Risk for injury related to difficult birth
 2. Knowledge deficit related to complications associated with breech birth
 3. Pain related to prolonged posterior pressure of fetal buttocks
 4. Risk for suffocation of fetus related to interruption in umbilical blood flow secondary to umbilical cord compression
C. PLANNING/IMPLEMENTATION
 1. Use measures to promote comfort
 2. Monitor the FHR in upper quadrants
 3. Watch for prolapsed cord; if it occurs:
  a. With a sterile gloved hand push the presenting part off the cord
  b. Place the client in the Trendelenburg position to keep presenting part away from the cord
  c. Keep prolapsed cord moist with sterile saline
 4. Observe for frank meconium; results from contraction of the uterus on lower colon of the fetus; not significant in breech birth
 5. Add Piper forceps to the delivery set-up if vaginal birth is anticipated
 6. Prepare client for cesarean birth; usually done in primigravidas
 7. Teach mother and partner about the process of breech birth
D. EVALUATION/OUTCOMES
 1. Birth is safe for mother
 2. Fetus remains free from complications

▼ CESAREAN BIRTH

Data Base
A. Birth of baby via transabdominal incision
 1. Transverse incision
 2. Lower uterine vertical incision
B. Indicated in cephalopelvic disproportion, dystocia, placenta previa and abruptio placentae, postmaturity, growths within the birth canal, multiple births, diabetes, PIH, Rh incompatibility, fetal distress, active herpes, and malpresentations such as breech birth
C. Vaginal birth after cesarean (VBAC) is being done more frequently

Nursing Care of Clients Following Cesarean Birth
A. DATA COLLECTION
 1. Vital signs
 2. Abdominal dressing: intact; presence of bleeding
 3. Fundus and lochia; lochia may be less than that with vaginal birth
 4. Urinary output
  a. Amount
  b. Specific gravity
  c. Presence of blood
 5. Numbness of extremities from spinal anesthesia
 6. Presence of pain
 7. Response to neonate
B. ANALYSIS AND INTERPRETATION
 1. Ineffective breathing pattern related to diminished respiratory exchange secondary to abdominal incision
 2. Risk for infection related to surgical incision
 3. Pain related to incision and/or flatus associated with decreased peristalsis
 4. Altered parenting related to surgical birth
 5. Situational low self-esteem related to inability to deliver vaginally
 6. Risk for trauma related to pelvic surgery
C. PLANNING/IMPLEMENTATION
 1. Assist with bonding; offer emotional support; encourage touching; include father in process
 2. Encourage early ambulation to prevent blood stasis
 3. Check vital signs, fundus, and abdominal incision
 4. Encourage eating of solids to promote peristalsis (prevents distention) when bowel sounds have returned
 5. Record intake and output
 6. Give analgesics as ordered
 7. Promote lung aeration
 8. Maintain fluid and electrolyte balance
 9. Monitor urinary output
D. EVALUATION/OUTCOMES
 1. Absence of hemorrhage

2. Absence of infection
3. Discomfort is relieved
4. Passing flatus
5. Parents and infant are bonding

▼ ASSISTED BIRTH

Data Base

A. Forceps: instrument used to shorten the second stage of labor; applied to head or presenting part to allow physician to control traction on infant's head; indicated in ineffective pushing, malposition, and large infants
B. Vacuum extraction: safer option than forceps; a cup is placed on the presenting part through which suction is applied to pull infant down; infant may develop succedaneum but is otherwise unharmed

Nursing Care During and Following Assisted Deliveries

See Nursing Care During the Intrapartal Period and Nursing Care During the Postpartal Period

MATERNAL INJURIES RESULTING FROM PREGNANCY/BIRTH

▼ EPISIOTOMY

Data Base

A. Incision into the perineum to facilitate birth and prevent lacerations and overstretching of the pelvic floor; it is usually made between the vaginal introitus and the rectum
B. Closed surgically; usually performed under regional anesthesia

Nursing Care of Clients with an Episiotomy

A. DATA COLLECTION
  1. Assess "REEDA"
     a. Redness
     b. Edema
     c. Ecchymosis
     d. Discharge or drainage
     e. Approximation of wound edges
  2. Extent of pain
  3. Signs of hematoma
B. ANALYSIS AND INTERPRETATION
  1. Risk for infection related to location of site near anal orifice
  2. Knowledge deficit related to care of episiotomy
  3. Pain related to trauma to perineum

C. PLANNING/IMPLEMENTATION
  1. Apply cold to limit edema during the first 12 to 24 hours
  2. Provide and teach perineal care
  3. Provide sitz baths
  4. Administer analgesics (as ordered) for comfort
  5. Apply local heat and spray medications (as ordered)
  6. Teach perineal exercises (Kegel)
D. EVALUATION/OUTCOMES
  1. Absence of infection
  2. Pain is relieved
  3. Perineal care performed after toileting

▼ LACERATIONS

Data Base

A. Lacerations are tears of the perineum or vulva resulting from a difficult or precipitate birth
B. Characterized as first-, second-, third-, or fourth-degree lacerations, depending on the amount of involvement; third- and fourth-degree lacerations are the most serious because the anal sphincter and rectal wall are involved
C. Therapeutic interventions
  1. Surgical repair; healing may be slower than episiotomy repair
  2. Low-residue diet if laceration is third or fourth degree

Nursing Care of Clients with Lacerations

See Nursing Care of Clients with an Episiotomy

▼ RUPTURED UTERUS

Data Base

A. Causes: perforation during attempted abortion, rupture of a previous uterine scar, spontaneous rupture of an intact uterus with the abdominal overdistention that can occur with abruptio placentae, and/or labor induction
B. During pregnancy, usually occurs after the fetus reaches a viable size
C. Therapeutic interventions
  1. Treatment for hemorrhage and shock
  2. Surgical intervention depends on extent of rupture (uterine repair or hysterectomy)

Nursing Care of Clients with a Hysterectomy for a Ruptured Uterus

A. DATA COLLECTION
  1. Vital signs
  2. Extent of bleeding
  3. Severity of pain

4. Signs of infection
5. Urinary output
6. Emotional responses

B. ANALYSIS AND INTERPRETATION
1. Knowledge deficit related to hysterectomy
2. Pain related to surgical procedure
3. Situational low self-esteem related to altered body functions or loss of childbearing ability
4. Risk for trauma related to vascularity of pelvic organs

C. PLANNING/IMPLEMENTATION
1. Maintain patency of urinary catheter
2. Assess urinary output while catheter is in place and after it is removed
3. Monitor fluid and electrolyte balance
4. Encourage coughing and deep breathing at frequent intervals
5. Assess for gas pains and administer Harris flush, if ordered
6. Institute measures, such as frequent ambulation and elevation of extremities when in a chair, to prevent thrombophlebitis
7. Provide emotional support; encourage and provide for ventilation of feelings
8. Provide postoperative teaching
   a. Explain need to avoid driving for 3 to 6 weeks
   b. Explain need to avoid sexual intercourse, dancing, jogging, and heavy lifting for 6 to 8 weeks
   c. Emphasize importance of follow-up supervision

D. EVALUATION/OUTCOMES
1. Severe pain is reduced
2. Voiding spontaneously
3. Passing flatus and stool
4. States postoperative instructions
5. Accepts loss of uterus

HEALTH PROBLEMS THAT CREATE A RISK DURING PREGNANCY

TECHNIQUES TO IDENTIFY AND/OR MONITOR HIGH-RISK PREGNANCY AND ASSOCIATED NURSING CARE

A. Alpha-fetoprotein (AFP) enzyme blood test: elevated levels may identify the pregnant woman carrying a baby with neural tube defects (spina bifida and anencephaly); may also indicate twins; if the AFP is elevated for two samples, it is followed by ultrasonography and amniocentesis for further confirmation; done at 14 to 16 weeks' gestation

B. Ultrasonography: high-frequency sound-wave testing; discerns placental location and gestational age by measurement of biparietal diameters
1. Visualization is improved if the bladder is full during the first 20 weeks of gestation; a full bladder is not necessary after 20 weeks' gestation
2. Nursing care: client is encouraged to drink and refrain from voiding before the test

C. Chorionic villi sampling (CVS): supplies same data as amniocentesis but can be done earlier and quicker results can be obtained
1. Aspiration of villi done during the eighth to twelfth week of pregnancy
2. Nursing care
   a. Obtain informed consent
   b. Instruct client to drink water so that bladder is full
   c. Place client in lithotomy position
   d. After test monitor for uterine contractions, vaginal discharge, and teach client to observe for signs of infection

D. Amniocentesis: aspiration of amniotic fluid used to detect sex, chromosomal or biochemical defects, fetal age, L/S ratio (2/1 ratio indicates lung maturity), increased bilirubin level associated with Rh disease, and phosphatidylglycerol (PG), which appears in amniotic fluid after thirty-fifth week, indicating fetal lung maturity
1. Test done after sonogram; usually after 15 to 18 weeks of gestation
2. Nursing care
   a. Obtain informed consent
   b. Explain procedure and expectations to client
   c. Have client empty bladder
   d. After test monitor for uterine contractions, vaginal discharge; teach client to observe for signs of infection and to rest

E. Serum estriol levels: confirms healthy fetal-placental functioning; used less frequently since ultrasonography
1. Results: falling levels at term may be indicative of impending fetal stress; two or more tests necessary to make diagnosis
2. Nursing care: encourage the mother to return for testing; evaluate client's response to procedure

F. Nonstress test (NST): to observe for accelerations of FHR in response to fetal movement
1. Classification of results
   a. Reactive: two or more accelerations of FHR of 15 beats per minute lasting 15 seconds throughout any fetal movement; no intervention necessary
   b. Nonreactive: no FHR acceleration or accelerations less than 15 seconds; further mon-

itoring necessary with use of the contraction stress test

    c. Unsatisfactory: recording uninterpretable; test should be repeated in 24 hours

  2. Nursing care: fasting is not necessary; observation of the fetal monitor; explain test to decrease the client's anxiety; evaluate client's response to procedure

G. Oxytocin Challenge Test (OCT): to demonstrate whether a healthy fetus can withstand a decreased oxygen supply during the stress of a contraction produced by exogenous Oxytocin (syntocinon); if late decelerations appear, the fetus may be compromised due to uteroplacental insufficiency

  1. Classification of results

    a. Negative: no late decelerations with a minimum of three contractions in 10 minutes; indicates that the fetus has good chance of surviving labor

    b. Positive: persistent and late decelerations occurring with more than half the contractions; indicates the need for considering premature intervention

    c. Suspicious: late decelerations occurring in less than half of uterine contractions; test should be repeated in 24 hours

  2. Nursing care: conscientious monitoring of the mother after the test to observe for possible initiation of labor; evaluate client's response to procedure

H. Biophysical profile (BPP): assesses breathing movements, body movements, tone, amniotic fluid volume, and FHR reactivity (NST); a score of 2 is assigned to each finding, with a score of 8 to 10 indicating a healthy fetus

  1. Used for fetus that may have intrauterine compromise

  2. Nursing care: provide emotional support

  3. Evaluate client's response to procedure

I. Maternal assessment of fetal activity: need to contact physician or midwife when there are fewer than 10 fetal movements in a 12-hour period, fewer than three fetal movements in an 8-hour period, or no fetal movements in the morning

  1. Used to determine vitality of fetus

  2. Nursing care: teach client how to record and report movements

J. Fetal scalp pH sampling: may be done during labor when fetal heart patterns begin to indicate distress; capillary blood samples are taken from the fetal scalp in utero

  1. Results: if acidosis present, immediate birth of infant is indicated

  2. Nursing care: cleanse the vaginal area to avoid contamination when the test is done

▼ HEART DISEASE

Data Base

A. Origin: 90% rheumatic (incidence expected to decrease as incidence of rheumatic fever decreases); 10% congenital lesions or syphilis

B. Normal hemodynamics of pregnancy that adversely affect the client with heart disease

  1. Oxygen consumption increased 10% to 20%; related to needs of growing fetus

  2. Plasma level and blood volume increase and RBCs remain same (physiologic anemia)

C. Functional or therapeutic classification of heart disease during pregnancy

  1. Class I: no limitation of physical activity; no symptoms of cardiac insufficiency

  2. Class II: slight limitation of physical activity; may experience excessive fatigue, palpitation, or dyspnea in last trimester

  3. Class III: moderate to marked limitation of physical activity; bed rest indicated during most of pregnancy

  4. Class IV: marked limitation of physical activity; pregnancy should be avoided; indication for termination of pregnancy

Nursing Care of Pregnant Clients with Heart Disease

A. DATA COLLECTION

  1. Prenatal period

    a. Vital signs

    b. Weight gain

    c. Stress factors such as work, household duties

    d. Signs of congestive heart failure

    e. Dietary patterns

    f. Emotional outlook

    g. Knowledge about self-care

  2. Intrapartal period

    a. Vital signs; heart rate will increase

    b. Respiratory changes; dyspnea, coughing, or crackles

    c. FHR patterns

  3. Postpartal period

    a. Signs of congestive heart failure

    b. Signs of hemorrhage

    c. Intake and output

    d. Mother and partner's response to neonate

B. ANALYSIS AND INTERPRETATION

  1. Activity intolerance related to increased cardiac workload

  2. Anxiety related to unknown course of pregnancy, possible loss of fetus, and inability to perform role responsibilities

  3. Decreased cardiac output related to stress of pregnancy and pathology associated with heart disease

4. Fear related to possible death
5. Fluid volume excess related to fluid shifts resulting from a decrease in intraabdominal pressure following birth and/or a decrease in vascular space resulting from cessation of need for fetal circulation and uterine blood flow following birth
6. Risk for altered parenting related to increased responsibility of caring for a neonate

C. PLANNING/IMPLEMENTATION
1. Prenatal period
   a. Teach importance of rest and avoidance of stress
   b. Instruct regarding use of elastic stockings
   c. Teach importance of continued medical supervision by cardiologist
   d. Teach appropriate dietary intake
      (1) Adequate calories to ensure appropriate, but not excessive, weight gain
      (2) Limited, not restricted, salt intake
   e. Administer medications as ordered; digitalis preparations, iron preparations, prophylactic antibiotics (penicillin), and anticoagulants (heparin)
   f. Monitor for signs of congestive heart failure, such as respiratory distress and tachycardia
2. Intrapartal period
   a. Encourage mother to remain in semi-Fowler's or left lateral position
   b. Provide continuous cardiac monitoring
   c. Provide electronic fetal monitoring
   d. Assist mother to cope with discomfort; minimal analgesia and anesthesia is used
   e. Assist with forceps birth in second stage of labor to avoid work of pushing
   f. Monitor for signs of congestive heart failure, such as respiratory distress and tachycardia
3. Postpartal period: most critical time because of increased circulating blood volume after birth of placenta
   a. Institute early ambulation schedule; apply elastic stockings
   b. Monitor for signs of congestive heart failure, such as respiratory distress and tachycardia
   c. Refer to various agencies for family aid, if necessary, on discharge
   d. Monitor heart rate; accelerated heart rate of mother in latter half of pregnancy puts extra workload on her heart
   e. Provide for adequate rest; the increase in oxygen consumption with contractions during labor makes length of labor a significant factor
   f. Keep under close supervision; the sudden tachycardia during birth or the sudden

bradycardia and the normal increase in cardiac output following birth may cause cardiac arrest

D. EVALUATION/OUTCOMES
1. Healthy infant is delivered
2. Maternal cardiac status maintained within acceptable limits
3. Private or community resources contacted to assist mother in home

---

▼ DIABETES MELLITUS

Data Base

A. Normal physiology of pregnancy that affects pregnant woman with diabetes
1. Vomiting during pregnancy, especially in first trimester, decreases carbohydrate intake with resulting acidosis and reduces need for insulin
2. Human placental lactogen decreases insulin response in pregnant diabetics; there is a maternal sparing of glucose, and more oxidation of fats occurs to provide fetal nourishment; this in turn leads to a greater need for insulin; although insulin production increases, resistance to insulin also increases because of the presence of placental lactogen; thus more exogenous insulin is required to maintain normal serum glucose
3. Elevated basal metabolic rate and decrease in carbon dioxide combining power increase tendency toward acidosis
4. Normal lowered renal threshold for glucose can result in glucosuria
5. Muscular activity during labor depletes glycogen; therefore carbohydrate intake must be increased
6. During puerperium insulin antagonists are removed, hypoglycemia is common as involution and lactation occur and thus insulin needs decrease

B. Hazards of diabetes during pregnancy
1. Often there is a history of anomalies, stillbirths, and fetal deaths
2. Babies are excessively large, weighing over 4000 g (macrosomia)
3. Neonatal deaths occur as a result of hypoxia, hypoglycemia, congenital anomalies, and premature labor
4. Pregnancy-induced hypertension and hydramnios are common
5. Insulin therapy instituted; oral hypoglycemics contraindicated
6. Frequent hospitalization may be necessary during prenatal period
7. Cesarean birth may be necessary

Nursing Care of Pregnant Clients with Diabetes Mellitus

A. DATA COLLECTION

1. Length of time client has had diabetes mellitus
2. Dietary patterns
3. Signs of infection
4. Blood glucose level
5. Understanding of disease in relation to pregnancy
6. Presence of support persons

B. ANALYSIS AND INTERPRETATION

1. Fear related to health of newborn
2. Fluid volume deficit related to osmotic diuresis
3. Risk for infection related to increased susceptibility
4. Knowledge deficit related to newly diagnosed diabetes mellitus or management of previously diagnosed diabetes mellitus during pregnancy
5. Altered nutrition: less than body requirements related to fetal growth and increased maternal metabolism
6. Risk for trauma related to large size of infant

C. PLANNING/IMPLEMENTATION

1. Care of mother
   a. Encourage preconception counseling and early medical and prenatal supervision
   b. Teach and encourage adherence to dietary regimen
   c. Teach signs and symptoms of hyperglycemia (acidosis) and hypoglycemia (insulin reaction)
   d. Teach hygiene and avoidance of stress
   e. Teach serum glucose testing and record keeping
   f. Teach insulin administration
   g. Reinforce need for various tests for fetal wellbeing, such as ultrasound, stress and nonstress tests, amniocentesis for phosphatidylglycerol levels and L/S ratio
   h. Prepare client for induction of labor or cesarean birth if indicated
   i. Continue monitoring for fluid and electrolyte balance and ketoacidosis during intrapartal and postpartal periods
2. Care of neonate
   a. Admit infant to neonatal intensive care unit if necessary
   b. Keep the infant warm because of poor temperature control mechanisms
   c. Observe respiration (stomach aspiration imperative at time of birth, since hydramnios inflates stomach, which pushes up and interferes with diaphragm)
   d. Observe for signs of hypoglycemia and hypocalcemia such as lethargy, poor sucking reflex, cyanosis, or muscular twitching; lowered blood glucose to 2.0 to 2.5 mmol/L
   e. Provide glucose water feeding to prevent

acidosis (with poor sucking reflex, glucose should be given parenterally)
   f. Observe for congenital anomalies; there is an increased incidence in babies of diabetic mothers
   g. Promote early mother-child interaction

D. EVALUATION/OUTCOMES

1. Serum glucose levels within normal limits
2. Dietary instructions are followed
3. Insulin regimen is followed
4. A healthy newborn is delivered

DEVIATIONS FROM NORMAL IN THE NEWBORN

▼ PRETERM (PREMATURE) OR LOW–BIRTH-WEIGHT INFANT

Data Base

A. Prevention

1. Education about nutrition and general hygiene before planning a family
2. Education about the hazards of drug use and smoking
3. Adequate and early prenatal health supervision
4. Provisions for adequate housing and financial aid to persons of lower socioeconomic means
5. Adequate community agencies to facilitate available services to persons in need
6. Higher prematurity rates, intrauterine growth retardation, and low–birth-weight babies are frequently associated with malnutrition and underweight in the mother

B. Definitions

1. Classification of newborn infants is made on the basis of gestational age as well as birth weight
2. An infant born before term (36 weeks or less) is called premature or preterm
3. A low–birth-weight infant is one who weighs 2500 g or less
4. Full-term infant may be of low birth weight; premature infant need not be

C. Management of the low–birth-weight infant (LBW) immediately after birth

1. Aspiration of mucus to maintain an open airway is vital
2. Absence of respirations necessitates direct laryngoscopy, tracheal aspiration, intubation, and mouth-to-tube resuscitation
3. Maintenance of body temperature is difficult because of heat loss by skin evaporation and limited subcutaneous fat; heated Isolette is needed

4. Aspiration of stomach contents at birth facilitates respirations and is often indicated for the low–birth-weight infant
5. Infant should be moved to the nursery in the heated unit with oxygen and resuscitation equipment available

D. Characteristics of preterm infant
1. Preterm infant has less subcutaneous fat, therefore the skin is wrinkled, blood vessels and bony structures are visible, lanugo present on face, eyebrows are absent, and ears are poorly supported by cartilage
2. Circumference of the head of the preterm infant is quite large in comparison with the chest; the fontanels are small and bones are soft
3. Skin-color changes when preterm infant is moved; upper half or one side of the body pale and lower half or one side of the body red, known as harlequin color change
4. Preterm infant's posture is one of complete relaxation with marked flexion and abduction of the thighs; random movements are common with slightest stimulus
5. Heat regulation poorly developed in the preterm infant because of poor development of CNS; heat loss caused by large skin surface area and decreased subcutaneous fat; poorly developed respiratory center with diminished oxygen consumption causing asphyxia; weak heart action, therefore slower circulation and poor oxygenation; insufficient heat production caused by inadequate metabolism
6. Respirations are not efficient in the preterm infant because of muscular weakness of lungs and rib cage and limited surfactant production; retraction at xiphoid is evidence of air hunger; infant should be stimulated if apnea occurs
7. Greater tendency toward capillary fragility and intracranial hemorrhage in the preterm infant; red and white blood cell counts are low with resulting anemia during first few months of life
8. Nutrition is difficult to maintain in the preterm infant because of weak sucking and swallowing reflexes, small capacity of stomach, low gastric acidity, and slow emptying time of the stomach; the usual caloric intake of 110 to 130 calories per kilogram of body weight may need to be increased to 200 to 220 calories per kilogram for adequate growth and development

Nursing Care of Preterm Infants
A. DATA COLLECTION
1. Respiratory rate and effort
2. Heart rate
3. Oxygen concentrations via oximeter
4. Skin color
5. Blood pressure
6. Temperature
7. Daily weight
8. Nutritional and fluid and electrolyte status
9. Ability of infant to suck
10. Parents' ability to cope with preterm birth

B. ANALYSIS AND INTERPRETATION
1. Activity intolerance related to impaired oxygenation and reduced energy reserves
2. Ineffective airway clearance related to weakness of respiratory musculature
3. Risk for aspiration related to weak or absent gag reflex and/or administration of tube feedings
4. Ineffective breathing pattern related to lung immaturity, anoxia or hypoxia, damage to the cerebral respiratory center, or cerebral immaturity
5. Impaired gas exchange related to interference with respiratory stimulation, lung immaturity, or airway obstruction
6. Hypothermia related to decreased subcutaneous fat deposits, immature thermoregulation center, inadequate shiver response, large body surface area in relation to body weight, and/or lack of flexion of extremities toward the body
7. Risk for infection related to immature/impaired immune response, stasis of respiratory secretions, and/or aspiration
8. Altered nutrition: less than body requirements related to lack of energy to suck and/or weak or absent gag and/or sucking reflex

C. PLANNING/IMPLEMENTATION
1. Maintain airway; check respirator function if employed; position to promote ventilation; suction when necessary; maintain temperature of environment
2. Observe for changes in respirations, color, and vital signs
3. Check efficacy of Isolette: maintain heat, humidity, and oxygen concentration; monitor oxygen carefully to prevent retrolental fibroplasia
4. Maintain aseptic technique to prevent infection
5. Adhere to the techniques of gavage feeding for safety of infant
6. Observe weight-gain patterns
7. Determine blood gases frequently to prevent acidosis
8. Institute phototherapy should hyperbilirubinemia occur
9. Support parents by letting them verbalize and ask questions to relieve anxiety
10. Provide flexible and liberal visiting hours for parents as soon as possible

11. Allow parents to do as much as possible for the infant after appropriate teaching
12. Arrange follow-up before and after discharge by a visiting nurse

D. EVALUATION/OUTCOMES
  1. Respiratory rate and effort within normal limits
  2. Absence of infection
  3. Body temperature within normal limits
  4. Gaining weight

NEONATAL RESPIRATORY DISTRESS

▼ ASPHYXIA NEONATORUM

Data Base

A. Asphyxia neonatorum occurs when respirations are not well established within 60 seconds after birth as a result of anoxia, cerebral damage, or narcosis
B. Therapeutic interventions
  1. Early prenatal care
  2. Prenatal education
  3. Early management of deviations from the normal pregnancy
  4. Adequate medical management during labor and birth; resuscitative measures

Nursing Care of Infants with Asphyxia Neonatorum
(See Nursing Care of Preterm Infants)

A. DATA COLLECTION
  1. Asphyxia livida: persistent generalized cyanosis and good muscle tone
  2. Asphyxia pallida: marked pallor, poor muscle tone

B. ANALYSIS AND INTERPRETATION
  1. Impaired gas exchange related to respiratory depression secondary to narcosis
  2. Inability to sustain spontaneous ventilation related to respiratory or cerebral pathology

C. PLANNING/IMPLEMENTATION
  1. Resuscitate immediately
  2. Keep infant under close observation for first 24 hours
  3. Keep equipment for intubation and oxygen administration readily available

D. EVALUATION/OUTCOMES
  1. Infant breathing on own
  2. Oxygen saturation is sufficient

▼ ATELECTASIS

Data Base

Incomplete expansion of the lung or a partial or total collapse of the lung following initial expansion; common in prematurity, oversedation, damage to the respiratory center, or results from inhalation of mucus or amniotic fluid

Nursing Care of Infants with Atelectasis
(See Nursing Care of Preterm Infants)

A. DATA COLLECTION
  1. Cyanosis
  2. Rapid, irregular respirations
  3. Flaring of nostrils
  4. Intercostal or suprasternal retractions
  5. Grunting on expiration

B. ANALYSIS AND INTERPRETATION
  Impaired gas exchange related to collapsed alveoli and/or lung

C. PLANNING/IMPLEMENTATION
  1. Maintain an open airway
  2. Administer oxygen with high humidity
  3. Stimulate respirations by frequently changing infant's position
  4. Administer antibiotics as ordered to prevent infection

D. EVALUATION/OUTCOMES
  1. Alveoli and/or lungs are expanded
  2. Breathing on own

▼ RESPIRATORY DISTRESS SYNDROME (RDS)

Data Base

A. A deficiency in surface-active (detergent-like) lipoproteins (surfactant) results in inadequate lung inflation and ventilation; commonly associated with prematurity
B. Can occur in premature infants, low–birth-weight infants, and in infants following cesarean birth
C. Therapeutic intervention: surfactant replacement given to preterm infants through endotracheal tube

Nursing Care of Infants with Respiratory Distress Syndrome (RDS)
(See Nursing Care of Preterm Infants)

A. DATA COLLECTION
  1. Cyanosis
  2. Dyspnea
  3. Sternal retractions and nasal flaring
  4. Tachypnea
  5. Grunting
  6. Respiratory acidosis
  7. Metabolic acidosis

B. ANALYSIS AND INTERPRETATION
  1. Impaired gas exchange related to inadequate lung expansion
  2. Altered nutrition: less than body requirements related to difficulty in feeding caused by RDS

C. PLANNING/IMPLEMENTATION

1. Admit to neonatal intensive care unit
2. Keep the airway patent
3. Keep the infant in an Isolette with oxygen and high humidity; prevent chilling
4. Administer surfactant by aerosol as ordered
5. Administer antibiotics as ordered
6. Maintain function of mechanical ventilation if employed
7. Correct acidosis
8. Administer feedings as ordered; prevent exhaustion

D. EVALUATION/OUTCOMES

1. Free of respiratory distress
2. Fluid and electrolytes are in balance

▼ MECONIUM ASPIRATION SYNDROME (MAS)

Data Base

A. A hypoxic insult to the fetus that causes increased intestinal peristalsis with passage of meconium into the amniotic fluid; the meconium-stained fluid is aspirated by the infant during the first few breaths after birth, causing an obstruction in the lung that results in chemical pneumonitis
B. Therapeutic interventions
   1. Suctioning after head is delivered
   2. Oxygenation and ventilation
   3. Pulmonary hygiene
   4. Prophylactic antibiotic therapy
   5. Bicarbonate for acidosis

Nursing Care for Infants with Meconium Aspiration Syndrome (MAS)
(See Nursing Care of Preterm Infants)

A. DATA COLLECTION

1. Signs of fetal hypoxia and meconium-stained amniotic fluid during intrapartum
2. Respiratory distress after birth
3. Signs of sepsis
4. Altered neurologic status (seizures)

B. ANALYSIS AND INTERPRETATION

1. Impaired gas exchange related to aspiration of meconium and amniotic fluid into lungs
2. Altered nutrition: less than body requirements related to difficulty in feeding secondary to respiratory distress

C. PLANNING/IMPLEMENTATION

1. Remove meconium and amniotic fluid from infant's nasopharynx and oropharynx immediately after birth
2. See Planning/Implementation under Respiratory Distress Syndrome (RDS)

D. EVALUATION/OUTCOMES

1. Free of respiratory distress
2. Taking feedings with no difficulty

BIRTH INJURIES

▼ CRANIAL BIRTH INJURIES

Data Base

A. Caput succedaneum: edema with extravasation of serum into scalp tissues caused by molding during the birth process; no treatment is necessary; it subsides in a few days
B. Cephalhematoma: edema of the scalp with effusion of blood between the bone and periosteum; no treatment is necessary; it disappears within a few weeks to a few months after birth; resolution of hematoma can lead to hyperbilirubinemia
C. Intracranial hemorrhage: bleeding into cerebellum, pons, and medulla oblongata caused by a tearing of the tentorium cerebelli; occurs following prolonged labor, difficult forceps birth, precipitate birth, version or breech extraction

Nursing Care of Infants with Cranial Birth Injuries

A. DATA COLLECTION

1. Abnormal respirations
2. Cyanosis
3. Shrill or weak cry
4. Flaccidity or spasticity
5. Restlessness
6. Wakefulness
7. Seizures
8. Poor sucking reflex

B. ANALYSIS AND INTERPRETATION

1. Altered cerebral tissue perfusion related to intracranial hemorrhage
2. Risk for trauma related to birth process
3. See Analysis/Nursing Diagnoses under Nursing Care of Preterm Infants

C. PLANNING/IMPLEMENTATION

1. Keep infant in Isolette with oxygen
2. Place infant in high-Fowler's position
3. Administer vitamins C and K as ordered to control and prevent further hemorrhage
4. Institute ordered gavage feedings when sucking reflex is impaired
5. Support parents because of guarded prognosis

D. EVALUATION/OUTCOMES

1. Infant is free of neurologic damage
2. Infant is taking formula and gaining weight

▼ NEUROMUSCULOSKELETAL BIRTH INJURIES

Data Base

A. Facial paralysis: asymmetry of face caused by damage to facial nerves from a difficult forceps birth

B. Erb-Duchenne paralysis (brachial palsy): caused by a difficult forceps or breech extraction birth; treatment depends on severity of paralysis

C. Dislocations and fractures are diagnosed by crepitation, immobility, and variations in range of motion; treatment depends on the site of fracture

Nursing Care of Infants with Neuromusculoskeletal Birth Injuries

A. DATA COLLECTION
1. Immobility
2. Crepitation
3. Variation in range of movement

B. ANALYSIS AND INTERPRETATION
1. Risk for disuse syndrome related to injury
2. Pain related to injury
3. Impaired physical mobility related to injured nerves, muscles, or bones; to prescribed restrictions; and/or to pain
4. Risk for impaired skin integrity related to impaired mobility and/or use of immobilizing devices
5. Risk for trauma related to birth process

C. PLANNING/IMPLEMENTATION
1. No treatment is necessary for facial paralysis because it usually is temporary and disappears in a few days
2. Erb-Duchenne paralysis
   a. Massage and exercise arm as ordered to prevent contractures
   b. Place in neutral position
   c. Apply ordered splints and braces, which are used when paralysis is severe
3. Dislocations and fractures
   a. Apply swaddling, splints, slings, or casts as ordered
   b. Position as ordered
4. Reassure parents and teach necessary care and positioning
5. Refer to public health agency to ensure continuity of care
6. Refer to other community agencies as necessary

D. EVALUATION/OUTCOMES
1. Correct alignment of limb is present
2. Movement of affected part is maintained

▼ CONGENITAL ABNORMALITIES

Data Base
A. Defects present at birth are structural or metabolic (birth injuries are not included)
B. May be genetically determined or a result of environmental interference during intrauterine life (See Pediatric Nursing, [Chapter 5] for Congenital Abnormalities)

▼ HEMOLYTIC DISEASE

Data Base
A. Rh incompatibility occurs when an Rh-negative woman is sensitized to Rh-positive blood from an Rh-positive fetus or other sources and develops antibodies against the Rh-positive blood; in subsequent pregnancies these antibodies are transferred through the placental barrier to the fetus, with a resulting agglutination and destruction of red cells (erythroblastosis fetalis); rarely a problem in first pregnancy;
Prevention: Win Rho, Hyp Rho-D, a preparation of Rh_o (D antigen) immune globulin, is now given intramuscularly to the Rh-negative mother about the twenty-eighth week of pregnancy and within 72 hours after birth or abortion to prevent the development of antibodies in this and future pregnancies; mother must be negative for Rh antibodies to receive Win Rho, Hyp Rho-D

B. ABO incompatibility occurs when the fetal blood type is A, B, or AB and the mother is type O; mother's anti-A or anti-B antibodies are transferred through the placental barrier to the fetus, causing hemolysis and resulting in fetal anemia, jaundice, and kernicterus (excessively high bilirubin levels); ABO incompatibility is more common but less severe than Rh incompatibility; previous exposures to A, B, or AB blood does not increase the formation of anti-A or anti-B antibodies, so first pregnancy can be affected

C. Therapeutic interventions
1. During pregnancy, amniotic fluid determinations are done by chemical and spectrophotometric analysis; elevated readings warrant either intrauterine transfusion or induction of labor, depending on the weeks of gestation
2. Phototherapy is used in an attempt to reduce mild to moderate kernicterus
3. Exchange transfusions are done on severely affected infants to decrease the antibody level and increase infant red blood cells and hemoglobin levels

Nursing Care of Infants with Hemolytic Disease

A. DATA COLLECTION
1. Blood incompatibility (ABO, Rh) between mother and fetus
2. Jaundice and increasing bilirubin levels during first 24 hours
3. Bilirubin, hematocrit, and hemoglobin levels
4. Lethargy or irritability
5. Poor feeding pattern
6. Vomiting
7. Signs of anemia

8. Enlargement of the liver and spleen
9. Signs of kernicterus develop without exchange transfusion
   a. Absence of Moro reflex
   b. Severe lethargy
   c. Apnea
   d. High-pitched cry
   e. Assumption of an opisthotonos position
   f. Tremors and seizures

B. ANALYSIS AND INTERPRETATION
1. Risk for injury related to:
   a. Agglutination and destruction of red blood cells secondary to maternal antibody formation
   b. Brain cell damage secondary to high bilirubin levels
2. Risk for fluid volume deficit related to phototherapy

C. PLANNING/IMPLEMENTATION
1. Monitor maternal antibody titers
2. Administer Win Rho, Hyp Rho-D within 72 hours after birth if mother is Rh negative and neonate is Rh positive
3. Teach mother why RhoGAM is necessary
4. Teach mother why an exchange transfusion for the newborn may be necessary if the bilirubin level rises over 350 μmol/L
5. Protect neonate's eyes if phototherapy is used
6. Observe for signs of dehydration

D. EVALUATION/OUTCOMES
1. Future maternal pregnancies will be free from Rh isoimmunization
2. Neonate will be free of neurologic damage

▼ INFECTIONS

Data Base
A. Usually observable during early extrauterine life
B. See disease for specific details regarding newborn infections

General Nursing Care for Infants with Infections
A. DATA COLLECTION
See Data Collection under the specific infection

B. ANALYSIS AND INTERPRETATION
1. Diarrhea related to pathogenic infection
2. Risk for fluid volume deficit related to diarrhea
3. Altered growth and development related to microbial invasion of cardiac and/or cerebral tissue
4. Hyperthermia related to microbial toxins and/or immature thermoregulatory center
5. Risk for infection related to transmission during gestation, passage through infected birth canal, and/or cross-contamination by caregiver

6. Altered nutrition: less than body requirements related to impaired sucking reflex, oral discomfort, diarrhea, and/or increased basal metabolic rate

C. PLANNING/IMPLEMENTATION
1. Collect specimens to identify causative organism
2. Institute isolation precautions
3. Use strict medical asepsis/universal precautions with meticulous hand washing
4. Use disposable feeding equipment or sterilize as necessary
5. Teach mother to wash hands before and after handling or caring for baby
6. Teach mother how to cleanse breasts or feeding equipment
7. Teach mother how to administer or apply prescribed medications
8. Support parents
9. For additional nursing care see specific infection

D. EVALUATION/OUTCOMES
Infant is free from infection

▼ THRUSH

Data Base
A. Thrush is a mouth infection caused by *Candida albicans*
B. Organism may be transmitted to the baby as the baby passes through the mother's vaginal canal, by unclean feeding utensils, or by improper handwashing techniques by staff or mother

Nursing Care of Infants with Thrush
A. DATA COLLECTION
1. White patches on tongue, palate, and inner cheeks
2. Mouth lesions bleed if touched
3. Difficulty in sucking

B. ANALYSIS AND INTERPRETATION
Altered nutrition: less than body requirements related to impaired sucking reflex, oral discomfort, diarrhea, and/or increased basal metabolic rate

C. PLANNING/IMPLEMENTATION
In addition to the items under Planning/Implementation under General Nursing Care for Infants with Infections, include:
1. Administer oral nystatin (Mycostatin)
2. Apply 1% gentian violet to oral cavity

D. EVALUATION/OUTCOMES
Infant is free from infection

▼ OPHTHALMIA NEONATORUM

Data Base

A. Ophthalmia neonatorum is an eye infection caused by *Neisseria gonorrhoeae* and *Chlamydia trachomatis*
B. Organism is transmitted from the genital tract of an infected mother during birth or by infected hands of personnel

Nursing Care of Infants with Ophthalmia Neonatorum

A. DATA COLLECTION
Purulent conjunctivitis if prophylactic treatment is not used

B. ANALYSIS AND INTERPRETATION
Risk for infection related to transmission during gestation, passage through infected birth canal, and/or cross-contamination by caregiver

C. PLANNING/IMPLEMENTATION
In addition to the items under Planning/Implementation under General Nursing Care for Infants with Infections, include:
1. Instill erythromycin or prescribed ophthalmic antibiotic after providing an opportunity for initial bonding
2. Treat infection with prescribed antibiotic

D. EVALUATION/OUTCOMES
Blindness prevented

▼ SYPHILIS

Data Base
A. A congenital systemic infection caused by *Treponema pallidum*
B. Prenatal syphilis transmitted to fetus by the mother
C. Incidence of fetal infection varies with stage of the disease in the mother at the time of pregnancy
D. Fetus seldom infected before fourth month of pregnancy; Langhans' cells in chorion are protective barrier
E. Prior to the fourth month of pregnancy, fetus not infected; after fourth month, the longer the infection goes untreated the greater the damage to the fetus; pregnant women treated immediately with penicillin

Nursing Care of Infants with Syphilis
A. DATA COLLECTION
1. Perinatal history of maternal infection
2. Maculopapular lesions of the palms of the hands and soles of the feet
3. Restlessness
4. Rhinitis
5. Hoarse cry
6. Enlargement of the spleen
7. Palpable lymph nodes
8. Enlarged ends of long bones on x-ray examination

B. ANALYSIS AND INTERPRETATION
1. Altered growth and development related to microbial invasion of cardiac and/or cerebral tissue
2. Risk for infection related to transmission during gestation, passage through infected birth canal, and/or cross-contamination by caregiver

C. PLANNING/IMPLEMENTATION
In addition to the items under Planning/Implementation under General Nursing Care for Infants with Infections, include:
1. Administer ordered antibiotics, usually penicillin
2. Teach the importance of continued medical supervision

D. EVALUATION/OUTCOMES
1. Infant will be free from infection
2. Infant will be free of sequelae from infection

▼ CHLAMYDIA INFECTION

Data Base
A. Chlamydia is a sexually transmitted disease caused by *Chlamydia trachomatis*
B. It is transferred to the infant during passage through the birth canal

Nursing Care of Infants with Chlamydia Infection

A. DATA COLLECTION
1. Perinatal history of maternal infection
2. Purulent conjunctivitis 3 to 4 days after birth, followed by pneumonia

B. ANALYSIS AND INTERPRETATION
Risk for infection related to transmission during gestation, passage through infected birth canal, and/or cross-contamination by caregiver

C. PLANNING/IMPLEMENTATION
In addition to the items under Planning/Implementation under General Nursing Care for Infants with Infections, include:
1. Instill ophthalmic antibiotics as ordered
2. Refer for ophthalmic evaluation
3. Administer medications for pneumonia
4. Monitor vital signs
5. Administer oxygen as ordered

D. EVALUATION/OUTCOMES
1. Infant will be free from infection
2. Infant will be free of sequelae from infection

▼ ACQUIRED IMMUNODEFICIENCY SYNDROME (AIDS)

Data Base
A. Generalized invasion of T cells by the human immunodeficiency virus (HIV)

B. Transmitted by mother who is HIV positive

C. Infant should be screened for HIV infection when either parent is HIV positive or at high risk for AIDS

D. Symptoms are usually not present at birth

E. If Zidovudine (AZT) was administered during the prenatal period to a woman who is HIV positive, the risk of transmission of HIV to the fetus is decreased

Nursing Care of Infants with Acquired Immunodeficiency Syndrome (AIDS)

A. DATA COLLECTION

1. Signs of prematurity or small for gestational age
2. Failure to thrive
3. Enlarged spleen and liver
4. Diarrhea
5. Weight loss
6. Neurologic deficits
7. Frequent and debilitating infections as the child ages

B. ANALYSIS AND INTERPRETATION

1. Altered growth and development related to microbial invasion of cardiac and/or cerebral tissue
2. Risk for infection related to transmission during gestation, passage through infected birth canal, and/or cross-contamination by caregiver

C. PLANNING/IMPLEMENTATION

In addition to the items under Planning/Implementation under General Nursing Care for Infants with Infections, include:

1. Obtain blood specimen for HIV testing
2. Institute and teach parents blood and body fluid precautions
3. Inform mother that the virus may be transmitted via breast milk and that infant should be bottlefed
4. Stress the importance of continued medical supervision
5. Provide human contact to meet emotional needs

D. EVALUATION/OUTCOMES

1. Universal precautions are performed
2. Medical supervision is continued
3. Infant's emotional needs are met

▼ NECROTIZING ENTEROCOLITIS (NEC)

Data Base

A. Necrotic lesions in intestines resulting from ischemia in area

B. Occurs several weeks after birth

C. More common in preterm infants

D. Therapeutic intervention—surgical excision often required, which may lead to "short bowel syndrome"

Nursing Care of Infants with Necrotizing Enterocolitis

A. DATA COLLECTION

1. Abdominal distention
2. Poor feeding
3. Vomiting
4. Loss of weight
5. Gastrointestinal bleeding
6. Disappearance of bowel sounds

B. ANALYSIS AND INTERPRETATION

1. Fluid volume deficit related to diarrhea
2. Altered nutrition: less than body requirements related to impaired sucking reflex, oral discomfort, diarrhea, and/or increased basal metabolic rate

C. PLANNING/IMPLEMENTATION

In addition to the items under Planning/Implementation under General Nursing Care for Infants with Infections, include:

1. Maintain NPO
2. Administer IV therapy as ordered, including total parenteral nutrition
3. Maintain nasogastric decompression
4. Monitor fluid and electrolyte balance
5. Provide ileostomy or colostomy care if surgery has been performed

D. EVALUATION/OUTCOMES

Infant gains weight

▼ SEPSIS

Data Base

A. Sepsis is a generalized bacterial infection

B. Sepsis is precipitated by infected amniotic fluid or break in aseptic technique

Nursing Care of Infants with Sepsis

A. DATA COLLECTION

1. Poor feeding
2. High temperature
3. Lethargy
4. Increasing irritability
5. Vomiting
6. Pallor
7. Signs of anemia
8. Increased number of stools

B. ANALYSIS AND INTERPRETATION

1. Diarrhea related to pathogenic infection
2. Risk for fluid volume deficit related to diarrhea
3. Altered growth and development related to microbial invasion of cardiac and/or cerebral tissue
4. Hyperthermia related to microbial toxins and/or immature thermoregulatory center
5. Risk for infection related to transmission dur-

ing gestation, passage through infected birth canal, and/or cross-contamination by caregiver

6. Altered nutrition: less than body requirements related to impaired sucking reflex, oral discomfort, diarrhea, and/or increased basal metabolic rate

C. PLANNING/IMPLEMENTATION

In addition to the items under Planning/Implementation under General Nursing Care for Infants with Infections, include:

1. Administer IV antibiotic therapy as ordered
2. Monitor intravenous fluid administration
3. Administer oxygen as ordered

D. EVALUATION/OUTCOMES

1. Infant will be free from infection
2. Infant will be free from sequelae of infection

▼ TORCH

Data Base

A. An acronym for the following infections:

1. *T*—Toxoplasmosis (*Toxoplasma gondii*): can be acquired by eating raw or undercooked meat or contacting cat litter; organism crosses the placenta; severity of infection related to gestational age; can cause hydrocephalus, intracranial calcifications, or chorioretinitis in the infant

2. *O*—Others (syphilis [*Treponema pallidum*], gonorrhea [*Neisseria gonorrhoeae*], varicella, beta streptococcus, and hepatitis B)

3. *R*—Rubella (rubella virus): greatest risk to the fetus when maternal infection occurs in first 12 weeks of gestation; baby may be born with encephalitis, ocular abnormalities, cardiac maldevelopment, and other defects; these infants may have active viral infection and should be isolated until pharyngeal mucus and urine are free of virus; for mothers who have not had rubella or who are serologically negative, rubella vaccine should be given in the immediate postbirth period, not during pregnancy

4. *C*—Cytomegalic inclusion disease (cytomegalovirus): pregnant women usually asymptomatic; this sexually transmitted infection may cause hemolytic anemia, hydrocephalus, microcephalus, intrauterine growth retardation, or neonatal death

5. *H*—Herpes genitalis (herpesvirus): contracted by the mother during sexual relations; characterized by periods of exacerbations and remissions; first attack most severe; during active stage the infant must be delivered by cesarean birth; if delivered vaginally, neonatal infection can be disseminated and result in death; surviving infants suffer CNS involvement

B. Therapeutic interventions: care is directed toward prevention and early treatment in the pregnant woman to eliminate or reduce risk to the fetus

▼ SUBSTANCE DEPENDENCE (NEONATAL ABSTINENCE SYNDROME)

Data Base

A. Definition: infant born with physiologic dependence on alcohol or drugs as a result of maternal drug use and/or abuse

B. Dependence: many preparations, including:

1. Alcohol
2. Methadone
3. Heroin
4. Cocaine

C. Perinatal mortality: 6 to 8 times higher than in normal control group

D. Alcohol abuse in the mother can result in fetal alcohol syndrome, producing congenital defects and retardation

E. Clinical findings

1. Infant may exhibit signs of respiratory distress, jaundice, congenital anomalies, and behavioral aberrations

2. Withdrawal symptoms appear soon after birth, severity depends on the length of maternal addiction, the type of drug used, the amount of drug taken, and the time the drug was taken before birth

Nursing Care of Infants Who Are Dependent on Alcohol or Drugs

A. DATA COLLECTION

1. Maternal intake of drug, including type, time, and amount

2. Signs of withdrawal in the infant
   a. Hyperactivity
   b. Shrill cry
   c. Tremors
   d. Sneezing, yawning
   e. Disturbed sleep
   f. Seizures
   g. Tachypnea
   h. Drooling
   i. Poor sucking reflex
   j. Vomiting
   k. Diarrhea
   l. Stuffy nose
   m. Excoriated buttocks
   n. Facial scratches

B. ANALYSIS AND INTERPRETATION

1. Ineffective breathing pattern related to mother's use of narcotic close to the time of birth

2. Altered growth and development related to addiction to narcotics, congenital anomalies, and/or mental retardation associated with fetal alcohol syndrome
3. Altered nutrition: less than body requirements related to hyperactivity or lethargy and uncoordinated sucking reflex
4. Pain related to withdrawal
5. Sleep pattern disturbance related to withdrawal and/or use of sedatives

C. PLANNING/IMPLEMENTATION
1. Monitor infant's neuromuscular status
2. Monitor vital signs; support respiratory functioning
3. Give small, frequent feedings
4. Administer supportive care to prevent injury
5. Administer sedatives or narcotics as ordered
6. Keep environmental stimuli to a minimum
7. Promote mother-infant bonding when possible; provide a constant caregiver
8. Hold and cuddle frequently but provide for periods of uninterrupted rest
9. Swaddle and rock infant when in crib
10. Use soft nipple to reduce sucking effort; administer supplemental methods of nutritional support as ordered
11. Encourage continued medical supervision
12. Refer to appropriate community-service agencies for family support and supervision

D. EVALUATION/OUTCOMES
1. Feedings are tolerated
2. Weight gain evident
3. Absence of diarrheal stools
4. Infant sleeping pattern established
5. Infant able to be held and comforted

▼ ADOLESCENT PREGNANCY

Data Base
A. High-risk pregnancy because:
1. Physical development is not yet completed
2. Developmental tasks of adolescence have not been fulfilled
3. Emotional maturity has not been achieved
B. Factors contributing to the incidence of adolescent pregnancy
1. Inadequate coping mechanisms
2. Need to enhance self-concept
3. Belief in own invulnerability
4. Lack of concern for long-term consequences; the present, not the future, becomes the focal point
5. Immature search for attention, closeness, and/or idealized or idolized love
6. Need for immediate gratification

7. Lack of knowledge about conception or contraception
8. Indulgence in risk-taking behavior
9. Sexual acting out
10. Increase in dysfunctional families
11. Change in morality and family life

Nursing Care of Adolescents Who Are Pregnant
A. DATA COLLECTION
1. Personal health
2. Family health
3. Menstrual history
4. Developmental level
5. Family or friends who constitute support system
6. Potential role of infant's father
7. Financial status
8. Understanding of responsibility of pregnancy

B. ANALYSIS AND INTERPRETATION
1. Body image disturbance related to changes associated with pregnancy
2. Ineffective family coping related to unstable family support system
3. Decisional conflict related to immature problem-solving abilities
4. Knowledge deficit related to the changes associated with pregnancy and the responsibilities of pregnancy
5. Altered nutrition: more than or less than body requirements related to food preferences, fast food, or food fads common in the adolescent
6. Risk for altered parenting related to age, lack of knowledge, or lack of support system
7. Situational low self-esteem related to the pregnancy and the individual's value system
8. Risk for trauma related to physiologic immaturity
9. Other nursing diagnoses: those associated with any pregnancy and any specific complication that may occur

C. PLANNING/IMPLEMENTATION
1. Develop trust
2. Refer to appropriate agencies and resources
3. Promote problem-solving abilities
4. Involve father, if desired by the mother
5. Provide prenatal education
6. Other nursing interventions: those associated with any pregnancy and any specific complication that may occur

D. EVALUATION/OUTCOMES
1. Able to arrive at decisions regarding the pregnancy
2. Expresses trust in nurse
3. Returns for prenatal visits
4. Attends prenatal and child-care classes
5. Father involved in planning and birth process

▼ INDUCED ABORTION

Data Base

A. Menstrual extraction or minisuction: vacuum of uterine contents with a 50-ml syringe; done 5 to 7 weeks after last menstrual period

B. Vacuum aspiration: done under local paracervical, epidural, or general anesthesia in the first 12 weeks of pregnancy; the cervix is dilated and the products of conception are suctioned by a small, hollow tube; the uterus is then curettaged to remove all fetal tissue

C. Dilation and curettage: performed during the first 12 to 14 weeks of pregnancy under local paracervical or general anesthesia; the cervix is dilated and uterus is curettaged

D. Saline injection: labor is induced when a pregnancy is 14 to 24 weeks in duration by injecting a sterile saline solution into the uterus by amniocentesis; labor usually begins within 20 to 36 hours after instillation of saline; produces a macerated fetus

E. Prostaglandin
  1. Action: used during second trimester to trigger vasoconstriction and uterine contractions that interfere with endocrine function of placenta
  2. Adverse effects: nausea, vomiting, diarrhea, pain at extrauterine sites, allergic reactions (not administered to clients with history of asthma)

F. Hysterotomy: performed after 16 weeks of pregnancy by surgically removing the fetus and placenta abdominally

Nursing Care of Clients Undergoing an Induced Abortion

A. DATA COLLECTION

  1. History and physical examination
  2. Specimens for laboratory tests
  3. Rh status
  4. Length of pregnancy
  5. Level of anxiety
  6. Understanding of procedure and postprocedure care

B. ANALYSIS AND INTERPRETATION

  1. Decisional conflict related to termination of pregnancy and the diversity of options available
  2. Risk for infection related to introduction of foreign objects or substances into the body
  3. Risk for injury related to mechanical termination of pregnancy
  4. Knowledge deficit related to self-care after the abortion and/or alternate methods of contraception
  5. Pain related to induced labor

  6. Situational low self-esteem related to possible feelings of frustration, fear, anger, or guilt

C. PLANNING/IMPLEMENTATION

  1. Obtain informed consent
  2. Be aware of own feelings about abortion (essential if the nurse is to intervene therapeutically with women having abortions)
  3. Encourage the client's expression of frustration, fear, anger, or guilt
  4. Be objective and support the client's decision about abortion
  5. Make certain that a complete history and physical examination, complete laboratory workup, pelvic examination and Papanicolaou test, and a pregnancy test are done prior to induced abortion
  6. Counsel concerning contraceptive methods if requested
  7. Administer Win Rho, Hyp Rho-D when client's blood is Rh negative and negative for antibodies

D. EVALUATION/OUTCOMES

  1. Products of conception are completely expelled
  2. Free of sequelae from procedure
  3. Returns for medical follow-up

FAMILY PLANNING

▼ CONTRACEPTIVE METHODS

Data Base

A. Oral contraceptives
  1. Description
     a. Used to prevent conception by:
        (1) Inhibiting ovulation
        (2) Causing atrophic changes in the endometrium to prevent implantation
        (3) Causing a thickening of cervical mucus to inhibit sperm travel
     b. Available in:
        (1) Combined form: inhibits hypothalamus, pituitary, and various hormone production
           (a) Monophasic: synthetic estrogen in each pill that is taken for 21 days; package usually contains 28 pills, seven of which are free of estrogen; withdrawal bleeding occurs during the 7 days when the nonmedication pills are taken
           (b) Biphasic: small amounts of estrogen are taken throughout the cycle; in a 21-day package, the first

10 pills contain small amounts of synthetic estrogen and the next 11 pills contain an increased amount of estrogen

    (c) Combined hormones: small doses of combined hormones that alter levels of estrogen and progesterone throughout the cycle

  (2) Advantages of combined oral contraceptives

    (a) 100% effective if taken correctly

    (b) Coitus independence because they are not taken during intercourse

    (c) Client can predict bleeding days

    (d) Alleviates symptoms of premenstrual syndrome (PMS), endometriosis, and dysmenorrhea

  (3) Minipills: progesterone is given alone; regimen makes uterine environment hostile to sperm

    (a) Low doses of progesterone

    (b) Can be used by lactating women

  (4) Advantages of minipills

    (a) Fewer side effects

    (b) May be taken by breastfeeding mothers

    (c) May be used by women over 35 and those with a history of headaches and mild hypertension

2. Examples

  a. Progestin products

    (1) Micronor

    (2) Norgestrol

  b. Estrogen-progestin products

    (1) Demulen

    (2) Ortho-cept

    (3) Ortho-Novum

3. Major side effects

  a. Thrombophlebitis (increased platelets and clotting factors, intimal thickening, and vein dilation)

  b. Hypertension (increased fluid retention)

  c. Libido changes (hormonal effect)

  d. Hyperglycemia (decreased carbohydrate tolerance)

  e. CNS disturbances (hormonal effects and fluid retention)

  f. Breakthrough bleeding (estrogen effect)

  g. Breast tenderness (fluid retention)

4. Contraindications for the use of oral contraceptives

  a. Hypertension

  b. Diabetes mellitus

  c. Thrombophlebitis

  d. Breast malignancy

  e. Cerebral vascular accident

  f. Breastfeeding mothers, depending on the form of drug

B. Intrauterine devices (IUD): mechanical devices inserted into isthmus of uterus; prevent pregnancy by increasing tubal motility so that ovum gets to uterus before lining is optimum for implantation; not as effective as oral contraceptives because pregnancy may occur with device in place; may cause increased menstrual bleeding

C. Diaphragm: mechanical device that fits over cervix and prevents sperm from entering cervical os; use with spermicide

D. Cervical cap: similar to a diaphragm, but smaller

E. Male condom: latex sheath that covers penis and prevents semen from entering cervical os

F. Female condom: latex vaginal sheath that is an elongated pouch with a ring at each end; one ring covers the cervix and the other covers the labia

G. Creams, jellies, foam tablets, and vaginal suppositories: spermicidal (generally low pH) preparations inserted into vaginal canal by applicator immediately prior to coitus (used in conjunction with the diaphragm and condom for added protection)

H. Coitus interruptus: withdrawal of the penis during sexual intercourse before ejaculation; least effective method

I. Fertility awareness methods: the plotting of the basal body temperature to determine fertile period so that abstinence from coitus is practiced; the basal body temperature dips slightly 24 hours before ovulation, then rises sharply; used in conjunction with cervical mucous changes (Billings method)

J. Norplant system (implantable progestin): implantation of six capsules of levonorgestrel beneath the skin of the upper arm; removal of capsules restores fertility; some difficulty is reported in removing capsules

K. Depo-Provera (injectable progestin): IM injection of medroxyprogesterone acetate that lasts from 3 to 6 months

L. Surgical sterilization

  1. Bilateral vasectomy: small incision made into the scrotum and the vas deferens is ligated, producing sterilization in the male by preventing ejaculation of sperm; usually performed on an outpatient basis

  2. Tubal ligation: interruption in the continuity of fallopian tubes by surgical transection, electric cautery, or compression with soft clamp, preventing impregnation of ovum by sperm; accomplished by laparotomy, laparoscopy, or culdoscopy; usually requires short hospitalization

Nursing Care of Clients Concerned with Family Planning

A. DATA COLLECTION
1. Medical and family history of woman
2. Clients' beliefs about sexuality, pregnancy, contraception, and abortion
3. Clients' understanding of family planning
4. Clients' readiness to learn

B. ANALYSIS AND INTERPRETATION
1. Anxiety related to potential irreversibility of some methods
2. Decisional conflict related to lack of relevant information, uncertainty about alternative contraceptive methods, lack of experience with contraceptives, and/or challenge to a personal value
3. Fear related to failure of contraceptive method resulting in pregnancy
4. Health-seeking behaviors related to desire to control future pregnancies
5. Risk for infection related to contraceptive devices
6. Risk for injury related to physiologic changes associated with oral contraceptives and/or use of contraceptive devices

C. PLANNING/IMPLEMENTATION
1. Help couples to expand their knowledge about human sexuality
2. Maintain optimum emotional and physical health of the family
3. Involve both partners in planning family size
4. Inform the couple of available methods of birth control and give them the freedom of choice
5. Assist couple in choosing the best method of birth control by providing an accepting atmosphere
6. Review specific medication/administration schedule with client and review procedure to follow if doses are missed when oral contraceptives are being used
7. Teach side effects of oral contraceptives and instruct client to inform the physician if they should occur
8. Encourage periodic physical examination for all women using any contraceptive method; should include pelvic examination, Papanicolaou test, and mammography
9. Teach couples electing surgical sterilization that in the female sterility is immediately achieved, whereas in the male sterility is not achieved until semen is free of sperm (may take up to 6 weeks); use an additional method of birth control when beginning and ending therapy

D. EVALUATION/OUTCOMES
1. Couple is successful in delaying pregnancy until desired
2. Client returns for follow-up care

▼ INFERTILITY AND STERILITY

Data Base

A. Sterility: presence of an absolute factor that makes a person unable to produce offspring
B. Infertility: inability on the part of a couple to conceive after consistent attempts for a 1-year period; woman has never conceived; man has never impregnated a woman
   1. Primary infertility occurs when the couple has never had a child
   2. Secondary infertility occurs when the couple has conceived but the woman is unable to sustain pregnancy or conceive again
C. Diagnostic measures
   1. Male: history, physical examination, semen analysis
   2. Female: history, physical examination, CBC, sedimentation rate, serologic tests, urinalysis, serum protein–bound iodine, x-ray films of the chest, basal metabolic rate determination, Sims or Huhner tests, endometrial biopsy, tubal insufflation, hysterosalpingography, culdoscopy
D. Therapeutic interventions
   1. Education about the menstrual cycle and timing of intercourse
   2. Surgery, depending on the cause
   3. Pharmacologic management
   4. In vitro fertilization and gamete transfer
   5. Therapeutic insemination
   6. Adoption
   7. Surrogate motherhood

▼ MALE INFERTILITY AND STERILITY

Data Base

A. Coital difficulties: chordee (painful, downward-curving erection) or marked obesity
B. Spermatozoal abnormalities: small ejaculatory volume, low sperm count, increased viscosity, reduced mobility of spermatozoa, and/or more than 30% abnormal sperm forms
C. Testicular abnormalities: agenesis or degenesis of testes, cryptorchidism; poor maturation of the spermatozoa; physical injury caused by trauma, irradiation, or increased temperature for prolonged periods
D. Varicocele: a swollen vein in the testicle
E. Abnormalities of the penis or urethra: hypospadias or urethral stricture
F. Prostate and seminal vesicle abnormalities: chronic prostatitis or seminal vesiculitis
G. Abnormalities of the epididymis and vas deferens: inflammation or closure
H. Severe nutritional deficiencies

I. Other factors such as radiation to testicles, excessive smoking and alcohol intake, smoking of marijuana, and in utero exposure to diethylstilbestrol (DES)

▼ FEMALE INFERTILITY AND STERILITY

Data Base

A. Endocrine disorders: pituitary, thyroid, or adrenal
B. Vaginal disorders: absence or stenosis of vagina, imperforate hymen, vaginitis, chronic infections
C. Cervical abnormalities: cervical obstruction by cervical polyps or tumors
D. Uterine abnormalities: hypoplasia, endometriosis, uterine neoplasms
E. Tubal disorders: obstruction (generally the result of infections such as chlamydia or gonorrhea), perisalpingeal adhesions
F. Ovarian abnormalities: congenital abnormalities such as ovarian dysgenesis or agenesis, infections, tumors; hormonal imbalances
G. Emotional problems: severe psychoneurosis or psychosis may cause anovulatory cycles
H. Coital factors: feminine hygiene preparations (including douches) that decrease vaginal pH may inactivate or destroy spermatozoa
I. Chronic disease states
J. Immunologic reactions to sperm
K. Nutritional factors such as a seriously faulty diet; anorexia nervosa

▼ DRUGS THAT AFFECT GONADAL FUNCTION AND FERTILITY

A. Androgens (testosterone derivatives)
   1. Used to replace deficient hormones in males after puberty and before the climacteric to improve development of secondary sex characteristics
   2. Adverse effects: adolescent males may have premature epiphyseal closure (decreased skeletal development, height stops increasing)
B. Estrogens
   1. Primarily used to replace deficient hormones to control hormonal balance in menopausal or postmenopausal women or to maintain menses and fertility in females during reproductive years
   2. Adverse effects of estrogen
      a. Anorexia (depression of appetite center)
      b. Nausea and vomiting (gastrointestinal irritation)
      c. Tissue fluid accumulation (altered tissue hydrostatic pressure)

C. Conception enhancers
   1. Ovulatory stimulants
      a. Clomiphene citrate (Clomid) is a follicle-maturing agent used during the fifth to tenth day of the menstrual cycle
      b. Bromocriptine (Parlodel) inhibits the release of prolactin, which can cause anovulation
      c. Human menopausal gonadotropin (Pergonal) acts similarly to FSH or LH to stimulate growth and maturation of ovarian follicles
      d. Gonadotropin-releasing hormone (GnRH) used when clomiphene is ineffective
   2. Hormone replacement therapy with conjugated estrogens and medroxyprogesterone
   3. For hyperplasia defects
      a. Danazol (Cyclomen) reduces endometrial hyperplasia; acts on estrogen receptors to inhibit estrogen defects
      b. Prednisone reduces adrenal hyperplasia
      c. These drugs have an androgenic effect that can cause weight gain, hirsutism, decreased breast size, and oiliness of the skin
   4. Adverse effects of conception enhancers
      a. Multiple births (increases ovulation)
      b. Visual changes (direct toxic effect)
      c. Dizziness, lightheadedness (CNS depression)
D. Alternatives to infertility
   1. Adoption
   2. Surrogate motherhood
   3. Remaining childless

Nursing Care of Clients Experiencing Infertility and Sterility

A. DATA COLLECTION

See Data Bases for Male Infertility and Sterility and Female Infertility and Sterility

B. ANALYSIS AND INTERPRETATION
   1. Impaired adjustment related to inability to achieve desired goals
   2. Anxiety related to inability to achieve a pregnancy and outcome of testing
   3. Altered family processes related to inability to achieve a pregnancy
   4. Health-seeking behaviors to obtain help related to reproduction
   5. Altered role performance related to inability to become a parent
   6. Situational low self-esteem related to inability to reproduce
   7. Sexual dysfunction related to physiologic or emotional problems preventing pregnancy

C. PLANNING/IMPLEMENTATION
   1. Apply principles of human relations and psychology

2. Listen to and discuss couple's particular problems, giving necessary support
3. Explain diagnostic procedures to alleviate anxiety and fear
4. Explain and discuss various treatment modalities
5. Encourage compliance with selected treatment modality; teach the reasons for the interventions
6. Listen to goals but point out reality
7. Help couples to support one another by:
   a. Encouraging frank discussion of feelings
   b. Avoiding blaming behaviors
   c. Adjusting to altered roles
8. Accept and work with couple's realistic frustrations and disappointments

D. **EVALUATION/OUTCOMES**
1. Conception occurs
2. Inability to conceive is accepted
3. A reproductive alternative such as adoption is selected

WOMEN'S HEALTH

STRUCTURES OF THE FEMALE REPRODUCTIVE SYSTEM

Ovaries: Female Gonads

A. Location: behind and below uterine tubes, anchored to uterus and broad ligaments
B. Size and shape of large almonds
C. Microscopic structure: each ovary of the newborn female consists of several hundred thousand graafian follicles embedded in connective tissues; follicles are epithelial sacs in which ova develop; usually, between the years of menarche and menopause, one follicle matures each month, ruptures the surface of the ovary, and expels its ovum into the pelvic cavity
D. Functions
1. Oogenesis: formation of a mature ovum in a graafian follicle
2. Ovulation: expulsion of the ovum from follicle into the pelvic cavity
3. Secretion of female hormones: maturing follicle secretes estrogens; corpus luteum secretes progesterone and estrogens (See Anatomy and Physiology of the Endocrine System in Medical-Surgical Nursing [Chapter 6])

Uterine Tubes (Fallopian Tubes, Oviducts)

A. Location: attached to upper, outer angles of uterus
B. Structure: same three coats as uterus; distal ends fimbriated and open into pelvic cavity; mucosal lining of tubes and peritoneal lining of pelvis in direct contact here (permits spread of infection from tubes to peritoneum)
C. Function: serve as ducts through which ova travel from ovaries to uterus; fertilization normally occurs in tube

Uterus

A. Location: in pelvic cavity between the bladder and rectum
B. Structure
1. Shape and size: pear-shaped organ approximately the size of a clenched fist
2. Divisions
   a. Body: upper and main part of the uterus; fundus, the bulging upper surface of the body
   b. Cervix: narrow, lower part of the uterus; projects into the vagina
3. Walls: composed of smooth muscle (myometrium) lined with mucosa (endometrium)
4. Cavities
   a. Body cavity: small and triangular with three openings into it; two from uterine tubes, one into cervical canal
   b. Cervical cavity: canal with constricted opening, internal os into body cavity and another, external os, into vagina
C. Position: flexed between body and cervix portions with the body portion lying over the bladder, pointing forward and slightly upward; cervix joins the vagina at right angles; ligaments hold the uterus in position
1. Broad ligaments (2): double fold of parietal peritoneum that forms a kind of partition across pelvic cavity, suspending uterus between its folds
2. Uterosacral ligaments (2): foldlike extensions of peritoneum from posterior surface of uterus to sacrum, one on each side of rectum
3. Posterior ligament (1): fold of peritoneum between posterior surface of uterus and rectum; forms deep pouch, cul-de-sac of Douglas (or rectouterine pouch); this pouch is the lowest point in the pelvic cavity and therefore the place where pus accumulates in pelvic inflammations; can be drained by posterior colpotomy (incision at top of the posterior vaginal wall)
4. Anterior ligament (1): fold of peritoneum between uterus and bladder; forms shallow cul-de-sac
5. Round ligaments (2): fibromuscular cords from upper, outer angles of uterus, through inguinal canals, terminating in labia majora
D. Functions
1. Menstruation
2. Pregnancy
3. Labor

Vagina

A. Location: between rectum and urethra
B. Structure: collapsible, musculomembranous tube, capable of great distention; outlet to exterior covered by fold of mucous membrane called hymen
C. Functions
   1. Receives semen from the male
   2. Constitutes lower part of birth canal
   3. Acts as excretory duct for uterine secretions and menstrual flow

Vulva

Consists of numerous structures that together constitute external genitals

A. Mons veneris: hairy, skin-covered pad of fat over the symphysis pubis
B. Labia majora: hairy, skin-covered folds
C. Labia minora: small folds covered with modified skin
D. Clitoris: small mound of erectile tissue, below junction of two labia minora
E. Urinary meatus: just below clitoris; opening into urethra
F. Vaginal orifice: below urinary meatus; opening into vagina; hymen, fold of mucosa, partially closes orifice
G. Skene's glands: small mucous glands; ducts open on each side of the urinary meatus
H. Bartholin's glands: two small, bean-shaped glands; duct from each gland opens on side of the vaginal orifice; both Bartholin's glands and Skene's glands have clinical interest because they frequently become infected (especially by gonococci)

Breasts—(Mammary Glands)

A. Location: just under skin, over the pectoralis major muscles
B. Size: depends on deposits of adipose tissue rather than on amount of glandular tissue (which is approximately same in all females)
C. Structure: divided into lobes and lobules that, in turn, are composed of racemose glands; excretory duct leads from each lobe to opening in nipple; circular pigmented area, the areola, borders nipples
D. Function: secrete milk (lactation)
   1. Shedding of placenta causes marked decrease in blood levels of estrogens and progesterone, which in turn stimulates anterior pituitary to increase prolactin secretion; high blood level of prolactin stimulates alveoli of breast to secrete milk
   2. Suckling controls lactation in two ways: by acting in some way to stimulate anterior pituitary secretion of prolactin and to stimulate posterior pituitary secretion of oxytocin, which stimulates release of milk out of alveoli into ducts from which infant can remove it by suckling (let-down reflex)

MENSTRUAL CYCLE

MENSES

A. Menarche is the first menstrual period
B. The menstrual cycle refers mainly to changes in the uterus and ovaries, which recur cyclically from the time of the menarche to the menopause
C. Length of cycle: usually 28 days, although considerable variations occur
D. Hormonal control of menstrual cycle
   1. Menses: brought on by marked decrease in blood levels of progesterone and estrogens at about cycle day 25
   2. Growth of new follicle and ovum: the low blood concentration of estrogens present for a few days before and during the menses stimulates the anterior pituitary gland to secrete follicle-stimulating hormone (FSH); the resulting high blood concentration of FSH stimulates one or more primitive graafian follicles and their ova to start growing and also stimulates the follicle cells to secrete estrogens; this leads to a high blood concentration of estrogens, which in turn has a negative feedback effect on FSH secretion by the anterior pituitary gland
   3. Endometrial thickening: in the preovulatory phase, the proliferation of endometrial cells is stimulated by the increasing concentration of estrogens in blood; the postovulatory phase is caused partly by endometrial cell proliferation and partly by fluid retention resulting from increasing progesterone concentration
   4. Ovulation: brought on by high concentrations of luteinizing hormone (LH)
   5. Postovulatory phase: increased secretion of estrogen and progesterone from corpus luteum further prepares the uterine endometrium in the event of fertilization and implantation of an ovulated egg
   6. Premenstrual phase: gradual drop in level of estrogens and progesterone, leading to menses
E. Clinical applications
   1. Contraceptive pills contain synthetic preparations of estrogen-like and/or progesterone-like compounds
   2. Most commonly used contraceptive pills prevent pregnancy by preventing ovulation: pituitary secretion of FSH inhibited

CLIMACTERIC

A. The period in a woman's life when there is gradual cessation of ovarian function and menstrual cycles is known as the climacteric
B. The last menstrual period is known as the menopause

C. Physiologic changes
1. Ovaries lose their ability to respond to gonadotropic hormones
2. Dramatic decrease in levels of circulating estrogens and progesterone because ovaries have atrophied
3. Increased FSH gonadotropin level in the blood, since production is no longer inhibited (negative feedback) by the ovaries; false-positive pregnancy test may occur

D. Clinical applications
1. Support system to deal with stress
2. Tranquilizers or phenobarbital may be necessary
3. Hormone replacement therapy (HRT): although still controversial is now being used more frequently; small doses of conjugated estrogen with progestin are thought to reduce the risk of cancer that is present with the use of estrogen alone and to prevent osteoporosis
4. Causes atrophic changes in reproductive organs resulting in dyspareunia, weight gain, facial hair growth, cardiac palpitations, hot flashes, profuse diaphoresis, constipation, pruritus, faintness; long-range changes may include osteoporosis
5. Causes emotional responses: headache, irritability; anxiety over loss of reproductive function, sexual feelings, and feelings of womanliness
6. The woman needs to understand:
   a. The changes that may occur with climacteric
   b. The need to ventilate feelings
   c. The physiologic basis for many of the temporary alterations associated with climacteric
7. Medical supervision if menopausal symptoms persist or interfere with functioning

PHARMACOLOGY RELATED TO FEMALE REPRODUCTIVE SYSTEM DISORDERS

Estrogens

(See Drugs that Affect Gonadal Function and Fertility under Infertility and Sterility)

A. Description
1. Organic compounds secreted by ovarian follicles in females; responsible for triggering the proliferative phase of the menstrual cycle
2. Used to regulate menstrual disorders, uterine bleeding, menopausal and postmenopausal problems, as well as part of a protocol to treat breast cancer and to prevent coronary artery disease; also used as a contraceptive alone or in combination with progestin
3. Available in oral, parenteral (IM, IV), intravaginal, and topical, including transdermal, preparations

B. Examples
1. Chlorotrianisene (TACE)
2. Diethylstilbestrol (DES)
3. Esterified estrogens (Neo-Estrone)
4. Estradiol preparations (Estrace, Estraderm)
5. Estrogenic substances, conjugated (Premarin)
6. Estrone (Femogen)

C. Major side effects
1. Thrombophlebitis (increased clot formation)
2. Nausea (irritation of gastric mucosa)
3. Skin disturbances (local irritation with transdermal preparations)
4. Breast tenderness (promotion of sodium and water retention)
5. Hyperglycemia (decreased carbohydrate tolerance)
6. Males: gynecomastia, loss of libido, and testicular atrophy (hormonal imbalance related to estrogen antagonism)
7. Deficiency of one or more of the B complex vitamins may be induced with prolonged use

D. Nursing care
1. Obtain client history to assess for medical problems that may contraindicate use
2. Assess client for edema formation during therapy
3. Instruct client to:
   a. Use proper procedure for application of topical or intravaginal preparations
   b. Report unusual vaginal bleeding to physician immediately
   c. Avoid smoking during therapy to decrease risk of serious cardiovascular side effects
   d. Eat foods rich in the B complex vitamins daily; B complex vitamin supplements should also be considered
4. Carefully monitor blood glucose in diabetics during therapy
5. Reassure male clients that feminizing side effects will subside when therapy is completed

Progestins

A. Description
1. Female ovarian hormones that prepare the uterus for implantation of a fertilized ovum; essential for the maintenance of pregnancy
2. Used in the treatment of endometriosis, infertility, dysmenorrhea, and threatened abortion; also used to suppress ovulation
3. Available in oral and parenteral (IM) preparations

B. Examples
1. Medroxyprogesterone acetate (Provera, Depo-Provera)
2. Megestrol acetate (Megace)
3. Norethindrone (Micronor)

5. Norethindrone acetate (Norlutate)
6. Progesterone (Progestasert, PMS progesterone, Gesterol)

C. Major side effects
1. Initial use causes profuse vaginal flow (shedding of accumulations of endometrial tissue), spotting, irregular bleeding, nausea, lethargy, jaundice
2. Edema (promotion of sodium and water retention)
3. GU disturbances (renal dysfunction aggravated by fluid retention)
4. Visual disturbances (possibility of blood clots or neuroocular lesions)
5. Scleral jaundice (hepatic alterations)
6. Thrombophlebitis (increased clot formation)
7. Depression (CNS effect)
8. Deficiency of one or more B complex vitamins may result from prolonged use

D. Nursing care
1. Obtain client history to assess for medical problems that may contraindicate drug use
2. Assess client for edema during therapy
3. Inform significant others regarding potential for development of depression
4. Instruct client to eat foods rich in the B complex vitamins daily; B complex vitamin supplements should also be considered
5. Evaluate client's response to medication and understanding of teaching

PROCEDURES RELATED TO THE FEMALE REPRODUCTIVE SYSTEM

PELVIC EXAMINATION

A. Definition
1. Examination of female reproductive structures
2. Consists of:
   a. Abdominal examination
   b. Inspection and palpation of external genitalia
   c. Vaginal examination bimanually and with a speculum
      (1) Inspect cervix and vaginal walls
      (2) As indicated or ordered, obtain specimen for:
         (a) Gonorrheal culture from endocervical canal
         (b) *Chlamydia trachomatis* smear from urethral and cervical fluorescein-monoclonal antibody test
         (c) Herpes simplex 1 and 2 viral culture of a smear from the lesion (presence of herpes may cause false positive Papanicolaou test)
         (d) Cytologic examination (Papanicolaou test) of cells from cervical junction and posterior fornix

B. Nursing care
1. Explain examination and collection of specimens to client
2. Inform client to avoid douching prior to examination
3. Request client to empty bladder prior to examination
4. Help client to relax by asking client to:
   a. Breathe slowly and deeply, exhaling with mouth open and lips in "O" shape
   b. Avoid squeezing eyes closed or clenching fists
5. Instruct client to bear down when speculum is introduced
6. If client is pregnant, observe for signs of hypotension, such as pallor, dizziness, tachycardia, nausea, and diaphoresis; if symptoms occur position client on side until symptoms subside and vital signs are within normal limits

Mammography

A. Definition
1. An x-ray study of the soft tissue of the breast
2. Technique allows detection of nonpalpable masses

B. Nursing care
1. Instruct client to avoid use of deodorants or powders prior to test
2. Maintain privacy for the client
3. Explain procedure to allay anxiety
4. Explain that stretching and compression of breast tissue may be uncomfortable
5. Stress importance of regular breast examinations for early detection; schedule examination after menstrual period when breast density and tenderness are decreased

Breast Biopsy

A. Definition
1. Excisional—removal of mass for cytologic study
2. Incisional—removal of tissue from mass for further study
3. Aspirational—removal of tissue or fluid from mass through needle for further study

B. Nursing care
1. Explain procedure to client
2. Allow ample time to express feelings
3. Instruct client to assess site for bleeding or edema
4. Stress importance of follow-up care

Infertility and Sterility Testing

Refer to Diagnostic Measures Associated with Infertility and Sterility

GENERAL NURSING DIAGNOSES FOR MAJOR DISORDERS AFFECTING WOMEN'S HEALTH

A. Body-image disturbance related to:
   1. Dependency on technology
   2. Alterations in structure
   3. Loss of function
B. Constipation related to pressure on colon
C. Altered elimination related to:
   1. Microbiologic irritants
   2. Physical obstruction
   3. Trauma
D. Anticipatory grieving related to:
   1. Loss of independence
   2. Concerns about dying
   3. Loss of body part
   4. Infertility
E. Incontinence (stress, urge) related to disease process
F. Risk for infection related to:
   1. Altered immune response
   2. Knowledge deficit
G. Knowledge deficit related to prevention/treatment protocols
H. Altered nutrition: less than body requirements related to anorexia
I. Pain related to:
   1. Inflammation
   2. Obstruction of urine
   3. Pressure
J. Impaired physical mobility related to:
   1. Pain
   2. Inflammation
   3. Limited range of motion
K. Altered role performance related to:
   1. Interference with sexual functioning
   2. Infertility
L. Sexual dysfunction related to:
   1. Altered body image
   2. Inadequate tissue perfusion
   3. Surgery
   4. Imposed restrictions
M. Altered sexuality patterns related to:
   1. Fear of transmission of infection
   2. Loss of function
N. Social isolation related to social stigma

MAJOR DISORDERS AFFECTING WOMEN'S HEALTH

▼ CYSTITIS

See Cystitis under Major Disorders of the Urinary System in Medical-Surgical Nursing (Chapter 6)

▼ CANCER OF THE CERVIX

Data Base

A. Etiology and pathophysiology
   1. Slow, malignant change in the tissue forming the neck of the uterus
   2. Multiple sexual partners and sexually transmitted diseases are considered risk factors
   3. High cure rate when diagnosed early
   4. Tends to spread by direct invasion of surrounding tissues and metastases to the lungs, bones, and liver
   5. Females exposed to diethylstilbestrol (DES) in utero have an increased risk of cervical cancer
B. Clinical findings
   1. Subjective (when invasive)
      a. Back pain
      b. Leg pain
   2. Objective
      a. Spotting between menstrual periods and after intercourse
      b. Vaginal discharge
      c. Lengthening of the menstrual period
      d. Papanicolaou cytologic finding of class V is considered conclusive of cervical cancer; Papanicolaou cytologic findings of class II, III, or IV require further studies before a conclusive diagnosis can be determined; class I is normal
C. Therapeutic interventions
   1. Type of surgical intervention depends on the extent of lesion and the physical condition of the client; staging ranges from 0 (carcinoma in situ) to IV (distant spread)
   2. Hysterosalpingo-oophorectomy (panhysterectomy) to remove the uterus, fallopian tubes, and ovaries; in advanced lesions the parametrial tissue and lymph nodes may also be removed
   3. Simple hysterectomy when preservation of ovarian function is desirable
   4. Internal or external radiation therapy alone or in conjunction with surgery may be ordered to reduce the lesion and limit metastases
   5. Laser therapy
   6. Cryosurgery
   7. Conization to remove cone-shaped area of cervix while still preserving reproductive functions

Nursing Care of Clients with Cancer of the Cervix

A. DATA COLLECTION
   1. Risk factors from history
   2. Description of onset and progression of symptoms
   3. Cervical specimen for Papanicolaou smear

B. ANALYSIS AND INTERPRETATION
   Refer to General Nursing Diagnoses for Major Dis-

orders Affecting Women's Health: A 2, D 2, D 3, and L 3

C. PLANNING/IMPLEMENTATION

1. Assist the client and family in dealing with the diagnosis of cancer
2. Allow and encourage the client to express feelings and concerns about change in self-image and sexual functioning
3. Support the client's feminine image
4. Provide care for the client receiving internal radiation
   a. Explain the side effects that may occur and the procedures involved, especially the need for isolation during treatment
   b. Instruct the client in maintaining proper positioning (supine with head of bed flat or only slightly elevated)
   c. Inspect the implant for proper position
   d. Provide low-residue diet and antidiarrheal agents to prevent bowel movements; urinary catheterization to avoid displacement of radioactive substance and irradiation of adjacent tissues
   e. Explain to the client and family that visitors and staff will be limited in the amount of time they can spend in the room to avoid their overexposure to radiation; pregnant women and children should be restricted from visiting
   f. Utilize principles of time, distance, and shielding to minimize staff exposure
   g. See Radiation in Medical-Surgical Nursing (Chapter 6)
5. Provide care following surgery
   a. Maintain patency of the urinary catheter that was inserted prior to surgery to decompress the bladder and reduce stress on the operative site
   b. Observe for reestablishment of bowel sounds
   c. Maintain accurate intake and output
   d. Following removal of the urinary catheter, note the amount of output and pattern of voiding; catheterize for residual urine if ordered and whenever necessary for urinary retention
   e. See Nursing Care for Clients with a Hysterectomy for a Ruptured Uterus and Nursing Care of Clients during the Postoperative Period in Medical-Surgical Nursing (Chapter 6)

D. EVALUATION/OUTCOMES

1. Verbalizes feelings to family and health care providers
2. Maintains satisfying sexual expression
3. Copes with effects of treatment and potential prognosis

▼ UTERINE NEOPLASMS

Data Base

A. Etiology and pathophysiology
1. Endometrial polyps
   a. Localized overgrowths of endometrial glands and stroma that occur more frequently in the fundus of the uterus
   b. Stimulated by estrogen
   c. Occur more frequently in premenopausal women who are anovulatory
2. Leiomyomas (myomas, fibromas, and fibromyomas)
   a. Benign tumors of the uterine muscle
   b. Occur more frequently in black women and women who have not been pregnant
   c. Stimulated by ovarian hormones
   d. Diminish after menopause
   e. Rarely become malignant
3. Endometrial cancer (adenocarcinoma, adenocanthoma, and adenosquamous carcinoma)
   a. Malignant overgrowth of the lining of the uterus
   b. Most common malignancy of the female reproductive system
   c. Occurs more frequently with hormone imbalance, obesity, nulliparity, late menopause, dysfunctional bleeding, anovulation, uninterrupted estrogen stimulation, diabetes mellitus, and hypertension
   d. Occurs twice as often in Caucasian women as in African American women
   e. Spreads by direct extension or metastasis
   f. Direct extension to myometrium, vagina, and paracervical tissue
   g. Metastasizes to abdominal cavity, liver, lung, brain, and bone; progression is slow and metastasis occurs late

B. Clinical findings
1. Endometrial polyps
   a. Frequently asymptomatic
   b. Intermenstrual bleeding (metrorrhagia)
2. Leiomyomas
   a. Frequently asymptomatic
   b. Excessive menstrual bleeding (menorrhagia)
   c. Signs of pressure from an enlarging mass such as low abdominal discomfort, backache, visceral displacement, and constipation
   d. Painful menstruation (dysmenorrhea)
   e. Problems with pregnancy such as preterm labor, abortion, and dystocia
3. Endometrial cancer
   a. Premenopausal recurrent metrorrhagia
   b. Postmenopausal bleeding
   c. FIGO classification system of endometrial cancer extends from stage IA G123, where

tumors are limited to the endometrium, to stage IVB, where there are distant metastases to the intraabdominal area or inguinal lymph nodes

C. Therapeutic interventions
1. Intervention depends on the type and extent of the lesion, the physical condition of the client, and the stage of the endometrial carcinoma
2. Dilation and curettage (D&C) for polyps
3. Myomectomy or hysterectomy for benign neoplasms; when surgery is not advisable, radiation therapy is employed
4. Total hysterectomy with bilateral salpingo-oophorectomy for endometrial neoplasms
5. Intracavitary radiation may be done prior to or after surgery, depending on the stage of endometrial cancer
6. Hormonal therapy with progestins for endometrial cancer
7. Combination chemotherapy with antineoplastic drugs such as cyclophosphamide (Procytox), doxorubicin (Adriamycin), and cisplatin (Platinol) for endometrial neoplasms

Nursing Care of Clients with Uterine Neoplasms

See Nursing Care for Clients with a Hysterectomy for a Ruptured Uterus and Nursing Care of Clients with Cancer of the Cervix and Nursing Care of Clients during the Postoperative Period in Medical-Surgical Nursing (Chapter 6)

▼ CANCER OF THE OVARY

Data Base

A. Etiology and pathophysiology
1. Histologic cell types influenced by age
   a. Malignant germ cell tumors more frequent between 20 to 40 years of age
   b. Epithelial cell tumors more frequent in perimenopausal women
2. More common in Caucasian women than in African American women; rare in Asian women
3. Incidence influenced by hormonal factors; environmental factors have been implicated but not proven
4. Risk factors
   a. Ovarian dysfunction
   b. Irregular menses
   c. Infertility
   d. Genetic predisposition
   e. Endometriosis
   f. Early menopause
   g. Nulliparity
   h. Use of chemicals or carcinogens in the genital area

5. Rarely diagnosed early because the abdominal cavity can accommodate an enlarging ovary without causing symptoms; poor prognosis because of the advanced stage at initial diagnosis, which is usually stage II to IV
6. Metastasizes to the peritoneum, omentum, and bowel surfaces

B. Clinical findings
1. Subjective
   a. Vague, lower abdominal discomfort
   b. Feeling of fullness
   c. Dyspepsia
   d. Rapid satiation
   e. Nausea
   f. Pelvic pressure or pain
2. Objective
   a. Increasing abdominal girth (ovarian enlargement or ascites)
   b. Constipation
   c. Anemia
   d. Increased weight
   e. Vomiting
   f. Urinary frequency
   g. Cachexia
   h. Enlarged ovary on palpation
   i. Elevated Ca 125 antigen

C. Therapeutic interventions
1. Depends on the stage of disease
2. Surgical removal of the tumor via oophorectomy, salpingo-oophorectomy, panhysterectomy, and removal of any involved structures
3. Cytoreductive surgery to debulk poorly vascularized large tumors; the smaller the remaining tumor the better the response to adjuvant therapy
4. Adjuvant therapy after tumor debulking
   a. Chemotherapy with antineoplastic drugs such as cyclophosphamide (Procytox), cisplatin (Platinol), and doxorubicin (Adriamycin) for epithelial carcinoma
   b. Intraperitoneal instillation of radioactive phosphorus (^{32}p)
   c. External radiation therapy

Nursing Care of Clients with Ovarian Cancer

See Nursing Care for Clients with a Hysterectomy for a Ruptured Uterus and Nursing Care of Clients with Cancer of the Cervix and Nursing Care of Clients during the Postoperative Period in Medical-Surgical Nursing (Chapter 6)

▼ VAGINITIS

Data Base

A. Etiology and pathophysiology
1. Trichomoniasis: overgrowth of *Trichomonas*

vaginalis, which commonly is present in the vagina

2. Candidiasis (moniliasis): caused by *Candida albicans*, a fungus; incidence is high in clients with diabetes mellitus and those receiving antibiotic therapy because of change in normal flora
3. *Gardnerella vaginalis* (bacterial vaginosis): *Gardnerella*-associated vaginitis, which is highly contagious
4. Atrophic vaginitis: common in the postmenopausal period because atrophied vaginal mucosa is prone to infection

B. Clinical findings
   1. Subjective
      a. Pruritus, burning
      b. Dyspareunia (pain with intercourse)
      c. Dysuria
   2. Objective
      a. Vaginal discharge
         (1) Malodorous, thin, yellow discharge (trichomoniasis)
         (2) White "cheesy" discharge (moniliasis)
         (3) Grayish-white discharge
      b. Vaginal smear can indicate *Trichomonas vaginalis*, *Candida albicans*, or other microorganisms

C. Therapeutic interventions
   1. Douches (acetic acid may be added)
   2. Antifungal preparations for candidiasis (see Pharmacology Related to Urinary/ Reproductive System Disorders in Medical-Surgical Nursing [Chapter 6])
      a. Nystatin (Mycostatin) vaginal suppositories or cream
      b. Miconazole nitrate (Monistat)
      c. Clotrimazole (Canesten)
   3. Antiprotozoan preparations for trichomoniasis (see Pharmacology Related to Urinary/Reproductive System Disorders)
      a. Metronidazole (Flagyl) tablets taken orally
   4. Estrogen therapy prescribed for atrophic vaginitis

Nursing Care of Clients with Vaginitis

A. DATA COLLECTION
1. History of onset and progression of symptoms
2. Presence of risk factors
   a. Improper use of tampons or douches
   b. Antibiotic use
   c. Multiple sexual partners
3. Appearance and color of vaginal discharge
4. Pelvic examination and specimen for culture

B. ANALYSIS AND INTERPRETATION
Refer to General Nursing Diagnoses for Major Disorders Affecting Women's Health: F 1, G, I 1, and M

C. PLANNING/IMPLEMENTATION

1. Advise the client to have sexual partner use a condom during coitus until vaginitis is resolved; sexual partner may also require treatment
2. Explain that frequent douching will alter the normal pH environment of the vagina, predisposing to vaginitis
3. Instruct the client to use tampons to prevent discharge from irritating vulvar area, but to change them frequently
4. Teach client the importance of wearing loose-fitting clothing and cotton underwear and to avoid wearing pantyhose and tight pants
5. Administer a douche if ordered
   a. Explain procedure to the client; provide privacy
   b. Assemble equipment, including douche can, tip, bedpan, gloves, waterproof pads, and solution at 45° C (30 ml of vinegar may be added to a liter of solution for acetic solution; alkaline solutions should never be utilized)
   c. Assist the client onto a bedpan while maintaining privacy
   d. Wearing gloves, separate the labia and insert the tip into the vagina
   e. Rotate the douche tip gently so the solution reaches all vaginal folds
   f. When all solution is used, instruct the client to bear down to expel as much remaining solution as possible; solution returns during the entire procedure
   g. Dry the perineal area gently
   h. Resterilize nondisposable equipment
6. Instruct the client who is receiving antibiotics or having recurrent vaginal infections to include yogurt or food supplements containing *Lactobacillus acidophilus* in the diet to maintain the normal vaginal flora

D. EVALUATION/OUTCOMES
1. Expresses relief of pruritis and pain
2. Cultures indicate resolution of infection
3. Discusses situation and need for precautions with sexual partner

▼ ENDOMETRIOSIS

Data Base

A. Etiology and pathophysiology
   1. Growth of endometrial cells in areas outside the uterus
   2. Generally affects young, nulliparous women
   3. Endometrial cells are stimulated by the ovarian hormones; will cause bleeding during the normal menstrual cycle (if located in ovary, a pseudocyst or chocolate cyst is formed)

4. Adhesions are common and may result in sterility
5. Adenomyosis is a similar condition affecting women 40 to 50 years old in which the endometrial cells invade the muscles of the uterus

B. Clinical findings
   1. Subjective
      a. Lower abdominal pain beginning 2 to 7 days prior to menstruation, becoming progressively worse, and then diminishing as the menstrual flow decreases
      b. Dyspareunia
      c. Pain associated with defecation
   2. Objective
      a. Abnormal uterine bleeding (metrorrhagia, menorrhagia)
      b. Infertility

C. Therapeutic interventions
   1. Hormone therapy to suppress ovulation; young married women are advised not to delay pregnancy if children are desired
   2. Surgical intervention
      a. Resection of lesions
      b. Oophorectomy, salpingectomy, and total hysterectomy if the condition is severe

Nursing Care of Clients with Endometriosis

A. DATA COLLECTION
   1. Description of onset and progression of symptoms
   2. Pelvic examination
   3. Concerns about childbearing

B. ANALYSIS AND INTERPRETATION
Refer to General Nursing Diagnoses for Major Disorders Affecting Women's Health for the following diagnoses: A 2, D 3, D 4, I 3, K 2, and L 4

C. PLANNING/IMPLEMENTATION
   1. Provide time for client to talk about feelings
   2. Administer analgesics as ordered
   3. Review contraindications, side effects, and administration of prescribed hormones (see Pharmacology Related to Reproductive System Disorders)
      a. Estrogen
      b. Progesterone
      c. Danazol (Cyclomen), a testosterone derivative
   4. Provide care following surgery (see Cancer of the Cervix and Nursing Care of Clients with a Hysterectomy for a Ruptured Uterus)
   5. Discuss alternatives if pregnancy does not occur
   6. Provide referrals to Endometriosis Society and other community-based support groups

D. EVALUATION/OUTCOMES
   1. Maintains a satisfying sexual relationship
   2. Experiences relief from pain
   3. Verbalizes concerns about altered body image and/or infertility

▼ SEXUALLY TRANSMITTED DISEASES

(See Syphilis, Gonorrhea, Chlamydia, and Acquired Immunodeficiency Syndrome [AIDS] under Sexually Transmitted Diseases in Medical-Surgical Nursing [Chapter 6])

▼ PELVIC INFLAMMATORY DISEASE (PID)

Data Base

A. Etiology and pathophysiology
   1. Occurs within female pelvic cavity; can affect the fallopian tubes (salpingitis), ovaries (oophoritis), peritoneum, surrounding connective tissue, and pelvic veins
   2. May be acute or chronic, bilateral or unilateral
   3. Caused most often by the introduction of bacteria (usually through the cervical opening), such as gonococci and chlamydia, or tubercle bacilli that are transported by the blood from the lungs
   4. If untreated, can lead to adhesions, sterility, and peritonitis

B. Clinical findings
   1. Subjective
      a. Severe cramping pain in lower abdomen
      b. Nausea
      c. Malaise
      d. Dysmenorrhea, dyspareunia
   2. Objective
      a. Temperature elevation
      b. Foul-smelling, purulent vaginal discharge
      c. Elevated WBC
      d. Cultures of vaginal discharge reveal causative organism

C. Therapeutic interventions
   1. Medication to control pain and fever
   2. Specific antibiotics, depending on the organism identified
   3. Identification and notification of sexual contacts and the state department of health if sexually transmitted disease is present

Nursing Care of Clients with Pelvic Inflammatory Disease (PID)

A. DATA COLLECTION
   1. Description of onset and progression of symptoms
   2. Potential source of infection
   3. Pelvic examination and specimens for culture
   4. Characteristics of discharge

5. Vital signs and white blood cell count for baseline data

B. ANALYSIS AND INTERPRETATION

Refer to General Nursing Diagnoses for Major Disorders Affecting Women's Health for the following diagnoses: D 4, G, I 1, K 2, L 1, L 4, M 1, and M 2

C. PLANNING/IMPLEMENTATION

1. Monitor temperature, white blood cell count, and culture reports
2. Explain the importance of completing prescribed antibiotic therapy; advise client of side effects
3. Maintain the client on bed rest in a semi-Fowler's position to localize the infection and prevent the formation of abscesses within the abdominal cavity
4. Apply heat if ordered to the abdomen or via a douche to improve circulation
5. Observe and record the amount and character of vaginal discharge
6. Change perineal pads frequently using gloves; tampons should not be used
7. Explain safety measures to prevent reinfection of the client or others; during the acute phase the client should abstain from intercourse
8. Allow time for client to verbalize feelings about illness and/or possible complication of infertility

D. EVALUATION/OUTCOMES

1. Experiences relief of pain
2. Cultures indicate resolution of infection
3. Verbalizes feelings and situation with sexual partner and health care providers
4. States importance of use of a condom to prevent transmission, if sexually active

---

▼ VAGINAL FISTULA

Data Base

A. Etiology and pathophysiology
   1. Abnormal opening between vagina and an organ
   2. May be congenital or may occur as a result of tissue trauma associated with surgery, childbirth, carcinoma, or radiation therapy
   3. Types
      a. Rectovaginal fistula: opening between the rectum and vagina
      b. Vesicovaginal fistula: opening between the bladder and vagina
      c. Ureterovaginal fistula: opening between a ureter and the vagina

B. Clinical findings
   1. Subjective
      a. Burning sensation
      b. Frequency of urination (if secondary urinary tract infection)
   2. Objective
      a. Discharge of urine, feces, or flatus from the vagina
      b. Excoriation of vaginal mucosa
      c. Odor

C. Therapeutic interventions
   1. Dietary modification including high-protein, low-residue diet with vitamin supplement
   2. Enemas, bladder irrigations, and douches
   3. Fistulas may be repaired surgically

Nursing Care of Clients with a Vaginal Fistula

A. DATA COLLECTION

1. Description of onset and progression of symptoms
2. Pelvic examination
3. Characteristics of urine, feces, and vaginal discharge
4. Condition of skin and mucous membranes in perineal area
5. Signs of urinary tract infection

B. ANALYSIS AND INTERPRETATION

Refer to General Nursing Diagnoses for Major Disorders Affecting Women's Health for the following diagnoses: C 1, E, F 1, F 2, G, I 1, I 3, K 1, L 3, and L 4

C. PLANNING/IMPLEMENTATION

1. Provide psychologic support, since the client may be embarrassed by odor and drainage and become withdrawn
2. Provide privacy during any treatments
3. Change pads frequently; sitz baths and irrigations to maintain cleanliness of area
4. Observe drainage and perineum for signs of inflammation
5. Assess urine for signs of infection; maintain patency of drainage tubes
6. Monitor for elevated temperature as an indication of secondary infection
7. Restrict diet to liquids initially and then to low residue to limit defecation and prevent strain on suture line after rectovaginal fistula repair
8. Provide care for the client who has had surgery (See Nursing Care of Clients with a Cystocele and/or Rectocele)

D. EVALUATION/OUTCOMES

1. Remains free from infection
2. Maintains skin integrity
3. Establishes satisfying sexual relationship

▼ CYSTOCELE AND/OR RECTOCELE

Data Base

A Etiology and pathophysiology

1. Cystocele: herniation of the bladder into the vagina
2. Rectocele: herniation of the rectum into the vagina
3. Both conditions may be present at the same time and are generally associated with relaxation or injury of the pelvic muscles during childbirth

B. Clinical findings
   1. Subjective
      a. Feeling of fullness in vagina
      b. Constant urge to defecate
      c. Dysuria
      d. Back pain
   2. Objective
      a. Soft, reducible mass evident during vaginal examination that increases when client is asked to bear down
      b. Stress incontinence
      c. Residual urine (60 ml or more after voiding)
      d. Constipation

C. Therapeutic interventions
   1. Anterior colporrhaphy to correct a cystocele
   2. Posterior colporrhaphy to correct a rectocele
   3. Insertion of a pessary for mild symptoms

Nursing Care of Clients with a Cystocele and/or Rectocele

A. DATA COLLECTION

1. Description of onset and progression of symptoms
2. Pelvic examination
3. Presence and extent of urinary retention
4. Impact of symptoms on client's life-style

B. ANALYSIS AND INTERPRETATION

Refer to General Nursing Diagnoses for Major Disorders Affecting Women's Health for the following diagnoses: A 3, B, C 2, E, G, I 3, L 1, and N

C. PLANNING/IMPLEMENTATION

1. Teach client care related to use of a pessary (e.g., cleaning, removing, or having it done periodically)
2. Encourage the client to perform Kegel's exercises to strengthen perineal muscles
3. Instruct client about preventing constipation (e.g., high-fiber diet, fluids, exercise, and stool softeners and laxatives as prescribed)
4. Provide postoperative care
   a. Encourage voiding every 4 hours to prevent strain on the suture line from a distended bladder (no more than 150 ml should accumulate)
   b. If the client has difficulty voiding, insert a Foley catheter if ordered
   c. After each bowel movement and voiding, cleanse perineum with warm soap and water and flush with warm water using a peri-bot-

tle; always cleanse away from the vagina and toward the anus; sitz baths can also be used
   d. Administer douches if ordered; include client instruction
   e. Apply heat lamp, anesthetic spray, or ice packs if ordered to relieve discomfort
   f. Administer ordered laxatives to limit straining at stool and pressure on the suture line
5. Encourage intake of liquids on first postoperative day and a regular diet on the second day
6. Provide time for client to verbalize fears and ask questions

D. EVALUATION/OUTCOMES

1. Maintains urinary output
2. Maintains a regular pattern of bowel elimination
3. Remains free from infection
4. Experiences less frequent episodes of stress incontinence
5. Expresses feelings about sexuality
6. Resumes satisfying sexual relationship

▼ PROLAPSED UTERUS

Data Base

A. Etiology and pathophysiology
   1. As a result of weakness of the pelvic floor, the uterus descends into the vagina; most often associated with childbirth injury or increased intraabdominal pressure
   2. If severe, the entire uterus may protrude outside the vaginal orifice; in this case, the vagina is actually inverted; referred to as procidentia
   3. Ulcerations in procidentia increase risk of cancer

B. Clinical findings
   1. Subjective
      a. Heaviness within the pelvis
      b. Low back pain
   2. Objective
      a. Mass in the lower vagina or outside the orifice
      b. Elongated cervix
      c. Urinary retention and/or incontinence

C. Therapeutic interventions
   1. Vaginal pessary to maintain the uterus in correct position
   2. Surgical intervention
      a. Suspension of the uterus and correction of retroversion
      b. Vaginal hysterectomy (if postmenopausal or if future pregnancy is not desired)

Nursing Care of Clients with a Prolapsed Uterus

A. DATA COLLECTION

1. Description of onset and progression of symptoms
2. Pelvic examination; note degree (grade) of prolapse and presence of cystocele or rectocele
3. Degree of interference with urinary and bowel elimination
4. Presence of ulcerations on skin or mucous membranes

B. ANALYSIS AND INTERPRETATION

Refer to General Nursing Diagnoses for Clients with Major Disorders Affecting Women's Health for the following diagnoses: A 2, A 3, B, C 2, D 3, E, I 3, K 1, L 1, and L 3

C. PLANNING/IMPLEMENTATION

1. Encourage the client to seek medical assistance if there is a prolapsed uterus
2. If procidentia is present, observe for ulcerations; apply warm saline compresses or protective ointment to prevent ulceration
3. Explain that if pessary is used, it must be taken out frequently by the physician and cleaned
4. Monitor the color, amount, and frequency of urination
5. Monitor the consistency, amount, and frequency of bowel movements
6. Provide postoperative care (see Nursing Care of Clients with Cancer of the Cervix)

D. EVALUATION/OUTCOMES

1. Maintains normal urine output
2. Maintains regular pattern of bowel elimination
3. Skin and mucous membranes are intact
4. Experiences a satisfying sexual relationship

▼ CANCER OF THE BREAST

Data Base

A. Etiology and pathophysiology
   1. Frequently begins as a hard, nontender, relatively fixed nodule found most often in the upper, outer quadrant of the breast
   2. Most breast cancers are adenocarcinomas originating in the ducts and lobes
   3. Incidence increases with age and is influenced by heredity and the number of menstrual cycles a woman has had (menarche before age 12, menopause after age 55, nulliparity or parity after age 35 increases the incidence because of longer exposure to estrogen); multiparas and women with early menopause have a lower incidence, as do Japanese women
   4. Familial or personal history of breast cancer greatly increases risk
   5. Recent studies have implicated a high-fat, selenium-deficient diet; oral contraceptives; estrogen-replacement therapy; and alcohol as contributing factors in the development of breast cancer

6. Most common sites of metastasis are bone, bone marrow, soft tissue, lungs, liver, and brain
7. Paget's carcinoma is a type of breast cancer that invades the nipple and milk ducts
8. Tumors may be estrogen or progesterone receptor positive
9. Extent of disease reflected by staging
   a. Stage one: localized tumor ≤2 cm; no node involvement
   b. Stage two: localized disease; tumor >2 cm but <5 cm; possible axillary node involvement
   c. Stage three: advanced localized disease in region without distant metastasis; tumor >5 cm
   d. Stage four: distant metastasis; direct extension of tumor to chest wall or skin

B. Clinical findings
   1. Subjective
      a. Lesion generally nontender
      b. Malaise in later stages
   2. Objective
      a. Asymmetry of breasts
      b. Palpable, irregularly shaped, fixed mass; most often in upper, outer quadrant
      c. Dimpling of skin by lesion
      d. Inversion and discharge from nipple
      e. Changes in color of breast over lesion; in late stages skin has orange-peel appearance
      f. Enlarged axillary lymph nodes
      g. Positive findings in following tests
         (1) Mammography: x-ray examination of the breast when there is an increased risk of developing breast cancer; baseline should be established between 35 and 40 years of age; q 1 to 2 years after 40 years of age; every year after 50 years of age
         (2) Thermography: heat-sensing device to evaluate abnormal circulatory signs
         (3) Xerography: special x-ray plate subjected to an electric charge to image all breast tissue
         (4) Biopsy for microscopic evaluation
            (a) Aspiration of specimen by syringe
            (b) Excised tissue may be sent to the laboratory for a frozen section from which thin slices are examined
            (c) Estrogen receptor assay: if positive, indicates need for alteration of the hormonal environment by surgical or chemical means
         (5) Elevated carcinoembryonic antigen (CEA) in serum, plasma, or cerebrospinal fluid: indicative of progres-

sion of cancer, particularly of the breast, ovaries, and gastrointestinal tract; also used in detecting cancer of the prostate

C. Therapeutic interventions
1. Type of surgical and medical intervention depends on the extent of the lesion and the physical condition of the client
2. Surgical intervention
   a. Partial mastectomy (lumpectomy, wide excision, segmental resection, or quadrantectomy): removal of the lump and surrounding breast tissue
   b. Simple mastectomy: removal of the breast only
   c. Radical mastectomy: removal of the breast, pectoral muscles, pectoral fascia, and nodes (pectoral, subclavicular, apical, and axillary); this procedure may be modified; rarely performed today
   d. Modified radical mastectomy: similar to a radical mastectomy but pectoral muscles are not removed
   e. Breast reconstruction
   f. Oophorectomy, adrenalectomy, and/or hypophysectomy to control metastases through alteration of the endocrine environment; most successful if normal numbers of estrogen receptor sites are maintained as determined by estrogen receptor assay
3. Radiation therapy alone or in conjunction with surgery preoperatively or postoperatively to reduce the lesion and limit metastases
4. Corticosteroids, androgens, estrogens, and antiestrogens (tamoxifen citrate) may be given to alter hormonal environment
5. Estrogen-receptor positive tumors
   a. Estrogen may be given as part of chemotherapy protocol; the increase in cell division may improve the cytotoxicity of chemotherapy
   b. Antiestrogens may be given to limit cell division
6. Chemotherapy
   a. Alkylating agents
      (1) Cyclophosphamide (Procytox)
      (2) Chlorambucil (Leukeran)
      (3) Triethylenethiophosphoramide (Thiotepa)
   b. Antimetabolites
      (1) 5-fluorouracil (5-FU, Fluorouracil)
      (2) Methotrexate (Amethopterin)
   c. Other drugs
      (1) Doxorubicin (Adriamycin)
      (2) Tamoxifen citrate (Novaldex, Tamofen)
      (3) Vincristine (Oncovin)

Nursing Care of Clients with Cancer of the Breast

A. DATA COLLECTION
1. Personal and family history of breast cancer
2. Age at menarche, menopause, and birth of first child to identify risk factors
3. Regularity of breast self-examinations and mammograms (after age 40)
4. Breast tissue, noting characteristics of lesion and skin surface
5. Enlargement of lymph nodes
6. Client's coping skills and availability of support system

B. ANALYSIS AND INTERPRETATION
Refer to General Nursing Diagnoses for Clients with Major Disorders Affecting Women's Health for the following diagnoses: A 2, D 2, D 3, F 1, F 2, G, H, I 1, J, and L 1

C. PLANNING/IMPLEMENTATION
1. Encourage and instruct the client concerning monthly breast self-examination
   a. Inspect while sitting with hands at sides and then overhead for retraction of the nipple, dimpling of skin, color change, and asymmetry
   b. Palpate the axillary and supraclavicular nodes
   c. Palpate the breast tissue using a circular pattern when lying down with the arms abducted
   d. Do after each menstrual cycle because premenstrual hormones can cause harmless nodules that will disappear after menses and the breasts will be less tender; if postmenopausal, do on the same date each month
2. Assist the client and family to cope with the diagnosis of cancer and altered body image by encouraging them to talk with staff and each other
3. Listen to and accept the client's anger and depression, and do not attempt to minimize it
4. Help the client identify feelings and encourage discussion of them
5. Support the client's feminine image
6. Care for the client following a mastectomy
   a. Observe for hemorrhage by checking all areas of the dressing underneath the client, the drainage unit, and vital signs
   b. Maintain functioning of portable vacuum drainage unit by ensuring patency of tube, emptying when necessary, and supporting to avoid tension at site of insertion; drainage should not exceed 200 ml in 8 hours
   c. Encourage correct posture and provide assistance with ambulation until the client adjusts to her altered balance
   d. Prevent or reduce lymphedema by elevat-

ing and supporting the client's hand above her elbow and the elbow above her shoulder; physician may also prescribe inflatable or elastic sleeve

e. Instruct the client who has undergone a radical mastectomy to avoid carrying heavy articles with the affected arm and to avoid cuts or bruises, having blood drawn, injections, or blood pressure readings in the affected arm because of impaired lymphatic drainage

f. Encourage active exercises of the affected arm, beginning gradually the day after surgery if approved by the physician
   (1) Wall hand climbing
   (2) Brushing hair
   (3) Turning rope

g. Instruct the client as to the types of prostheses and where to obtain them; cotton covered by gauze may be used to fill a client's bra until she is seen by a professional fitter

h. Use programs such as Reach for Recovery to help the client with physical and emotional readjustment

7. Support natural defense mechanisms of client; encourage intake of foods rich in the immune-stimulating nutrients, especially vitamins A, C, and E, and the mineral selenium; encourage low-fat diet

8. See Nursing Care of Clients with Neoplastic Disorders Receiving Either Chemotherapy or Radiation in Medical-Surgical Nursing (Chapter 6)

D. EVALUATION/OUTCOMES
1. Expresses improvement in body image
2. Participates in regular program of exercise that increases mobility and strength of affected arm
3. Identifies precautions necessary to prevent infection of the affected arm after a radical mastectomy
4. Discusses feelings with health care providers, family, and sexual partner
5. Consumes low-fat, nutritious diet
6. Utilizes community resources for additional support

▼ OSTEOPOROSIS

Data Base

A. Etiology and pathophysiology
   1. Decrease in bone substance so the bone can no longer maintain the skeletal structure
   2. Most commonly affects the vertebrae, pelvis, and femur
   3. Related factors include menopause, aging, inactivity, insufficient calcium intake or absorption, hyperparathyroidism, acromegaly,

Cushing's syndrome or long-term steroid therapy, hyperthyroidism, and consumption of caffeine and alcohol

B. Clinical findings
   1. Subjective
      a. Backache
      b. Difficulty maintaining balance
   2. Objective
      a. Decreased height resulting from compression of the vertebrae
      b. Kyphosis
      c. X-ray examination reveals a demineralization of bone and compression of the vertebrae
      d. Pathologic fractures

C. Therapeutic interventions
   1. Planned program of exercise
   2. Estrogen therapy to decrease bone reabsorption
   3. High-protein, high-calcium diet with vitamin D supplement
   4. Support for the spine (e.g., corset, Philadelphia collar, Taylor brace)
   5. Treatment of underlying disorder vital to halt the process

Nursing Care of Clients with Osteoporosis

A. DATA COLLECTION
1. Factors that may have contributed to development of osteoporosis
2. Client's usual dietary pattern and use of over-the-counter medications
3. History of fractures, loss of balance, or falls
4. Integrity of vertebral column

B. ANALYSIS AND INTERPRETATION
Refer to General Nursing Diagnoses for Clients with Neuromusculoskeletal Systems Disorders for the following diagnoses: A 3, D 1, I 1, I 3, and J 3. In addition:
1. Self-care deficit (bathing/hygiene, dressing/grooming, toileting) related to musculoskeletal impairment
2. Risk for injury related to neuromusculoskeletal impairment

C. PLANNING/IMPLEMENTATION
1. Encourage active weight-bearing exercises and assist with passive exercises
2. Instruct the client about proper body mechanics
3. Consider safety factors associated with instability; a cane or walker may be necessary for ambulation
4. Provide rest periods to prevent fatigue
5. Encourage diet rich in nutrient-dense foods such as fruits, vegetables, whole grains, and legumes to improve and maintain nutritional status; special emphasis should be placed on foods that will supply nutrients needed for mineralization of bone (vitamins A, C, and D,

and the minerals calcium, magnesium, and phosphorus)
6. Advise client to avoid caffeine, alcohol, and cigarettes
7. Encourage use of orthotic devices such as back braces for support
8. Encourage fluids in acute osteoporosis to discourage the formation of renal calculi

D. EVALUATION/OUTCOMES
1. Reports a reduction in pain
2. Complies with dietary and drug regimen
3. Participates in weight-bearing exercises
4. Remains active in family and community matters
5. Remains free from injury

CHILDBEARING AND WOMEN'S HEALTH NURSING
REVIEW QUESTIONS

Reproductive Choices

1. In a lecture on sexual functioning, the nurse plans to include the fact that ovulation occurs when the:
   1. Oxytocin level is high
   2. Blood level of LH is high
   3. Progesterone level is high
   4. Endometrial wall is sloughed off

2. After ovulation has occurred, the ovum is believed to remain viable for:
   1. 1 to 6 hours
   2. 12 to 18 hours
   3. 24 to 36 hours
   4. 48 to 72 hours

3. The time of ovulation can be determined by taking the basal temperature. During ovulation the basal temperature:
   1. Drops markedly
   2. Drops slightly and then rises
   3. Rises suddenly and then falls
   4. Rises markedly and remains high

4. The nurse explains that the efficiency of rhythm is dependent on the basal body temperature. A factor that will alter its effectiveness is:
   1. Presence of stress
   2. Length of abstinence
   3. Age of those involved
   4. Frequency of intercourse

5. A couple are desirous of using the rhythm method of contraception but do not understand how it works. The nurse's explanation to this couple about when to refrain from intercourse will be based on the fact that ovulation occurs:
   1. Fourteen days prior to the onset of menstruation
   2. Seven days before the end of the menstrual cycle
   3. Seven days after the completion of the menstrual period
   4. Fourteen days after the completion of the menstrual period

6. A biphasic antiovulatory medication of combined progestin and estrogen is prescribed for a female client. The nurse, instructing the client about the medication, should include the need to:
   1. Report any vaginal bleeding
   2. Have bimonthly Pap smears
   3. Increase her intake of calcium
   4. Temporarily restrict sexual activity

7. Following delivery a cardiac client with type II diabetes asks the nurse, "Which contraceptives will I be able to use to prevent pregnancy in the near future?" What is the nurse's best response?
   1. "You may use oral contraceptives. They are almost 100% effective in preventing a pregnancy."
   2. "You may want to use a foam and a condom to prevent pregnancy until you consult with your doctor at your postpartum visit."
   3. "The intrauterine device is best for you because it does not allow the fertilized ovum to become implanted into the uterine lining."
   4. "You do not need to worry about becoming pregnant in the near future. Clients with cardiac conditions usually become infertile."

Client Case Scenario 1: Miss Bev Campbell has recently entered into a sexual relationship with a new partner. She is seeking advice about contraception and asks the nurse about an IUD. **Items 8 to 10 refer to this client case scenario.**

8. The nurse teaches that the most frequent side effect associated with the use of IUDs is:
   1. Ectopic pregnancy
   2. Expulsion of the IUD
   3. Rupture of the uterus
   4. Excessive menstrual flow

9. The nurse should explain that a common problem that has been associated with IUDs when they are used is:
   1. Perforation of the uterus
   2. Discomfort associated with coitus
   3. Development of vaginal infections
   4. Spontaneous expulsion of the device

10. The nurse explains that the IUD provides contraception by:
    1. Blocking the cervical os
    2. Increasing the mobility of the uterus
    3. Preventing the sperm from reaching the fallopian tube
    4. Setting up a nonspecific inflammatory cell reaction in the endometrium

Client Case Scenario 2: Ms. Dena Corby is 16 to 18 weeks pregnant and requests an abortion. **Items 11 and 12 refer to this client case scenario.**

11. During the salinization method of elective abortion, the nurse should be alert for side effects such as:
    1. Edema
    2. Oliguria
    3. Headache
    4. Bradycardia

12. Following a salinization procedure for her elective abortion, Ms. Corby is told that labour will probably begin within:
    1. Two hours after the procedure
    2. Eight hours following the procedure
    3. Several minutes following the procedure
    4. Twenty-four to 72 hours after the procedure

13. In the dilation and suction evacuation method of elective abortion, *Laminarias* are used in the dilation stage of the procedure because:
    1. Dilation occurs within 2 hours
    2. They are hygroscopic and expand
    3. They are stronger in action than instruments
    4. Less anesthesia is necessary with this method

Reproductive Problems

14. In dealing with a couple who has been identified as having an infertility problem, the nurse should know that:
    1. Infertility is usually psychologic in origin
    2. Infertility and sterility are essentially the same problem
    3. The couple has been unable to have a child after trying for a year
    4. One partner has a problem that makes them unable to have children

15. A nonhemophilic woman who had a hemophilic father is married to a man with normal blood clotting. Genetically it can be predicted that:
    1. All children will be affected
    2. Female children will be unaffected
    3. All male children will be hemophiliacs
    4. Half the male children will be hemophiliacs

16. A high concentration of estrogen in the blood:
    1. Causes ovulation
    2. Stimulates lactation
    3. Inhibits secretion of FSH
    4. Is one cause of osteoporosis

17. Which test is commonly used to determine the number, motility, and activity of sperm?
    1. Rubin test
    2. Huhner test
    3. Friedman test
    4. Papanicolaou test

18. In the female, evaluation of all the pelvic organs of reproduction is accomplished by:
    1. Biopsy
    2. Cystoscopy
    3. Culdoscopy
    4. Hysterosalpingogram

19. A factor in infertility may be related to the pH of the vaginal canal. A frequent medication that is ordered to alter the vaginal pH is:
    1. Estrogen therapy
    2. Sulfur insufflations
    3. Lactic acid douches
    4. Sodium bicarbonate douches

20. A diagnostic test used to evaluate fertility is the postcoital test. It is best timed:
    1. 1 week after ovulation
    2. Immediately after menses
    3. Just prior to the next menstrual period
    4. Within 1 to 2 days of presumed ovulation

21. A tubal insufflation test is done to determine whether there is a tubal obstruction. Infertility caused by a defect in the tube is most often related to a:
    1. Past infection
    2. Fibroid tumor
    3. Congenital anomaly
    4. Previous injury to a tube

22. When assessing a client with a tentative diagnosis of hydatidiform mole, the nurse should be alert for:
    1. Hypotension
    2. Decreased FHR
    3. Unusual uterine enlargement
    4. Painless, heavy vaginal bleeding

Client Case Scenario 3: Mrs. Jennifer Hughes has had a recent confirmation of her pregnancy. She presents in the emergency room with abdominal pain not yet diagnosed. **Items 23 to 25 refer to this client case scenario.**

23. The nurse would suspect an ectopic pregnancy if Mrs. Hughes complained of:
    1. An adherent painful ovarian mass
    2. Lower abdominal cramping for a long period of time
    3. Leukorrhea and dysuria a few days after the first missed period
    4. Sharp lower right or left abdominal pain radiating to the shoulder

24. The most common type of ectopic pregnancy is tubal. Within a few weeks after conception the tube may rupture suddenly, causing:
    1. Painless vaginal bleeding
    2. Intermittent abdominal contractions
    3. Continuous dull, upper-quadrant abdominal pain
    4. Sudden knifelike, lower-quadrant abdominal pain

25. Mrs. Hughes has been complaining of vaginal bleeding and one-sided lower-quadrant pain. The nurse suspects that she has:
    1. Abruptio placentae
    2. An ectopic pregnancy
    3. An incomplete abortion
    4. A rupture of a graafian follicle

26. After a spontaneous abortion the nurse should observe the client for:
    1. Hemorrhage and infection
    2. Dehydration and hemorrhage
    3. Subinvolution and dehydration
    4. Signs of pregnancy-induced hypertension

27. Most spontaneous abortions are caused by:
    1. Physical trauma
    2. Unresolved stress
    3. Congenital defects
    4. Germ plasm defects

28. A client is admitted to the hospital with vaginal staining but no pain. The client's history reveals amenorrhea for the last 2 months and pregnancy confirmation by her physician after her first missed period. She is admitted for observation with a possible diagnosis of:
    1. Missed abortion
    2. Inevitable abortion
    3. Ectopic pregnancy
    4. Threatened abortion

29. A few hours after being admitted with a diagnosis of inevitable abortion, a client begins to experience bearing-down sensations and suddenly expels the products of conception in bed. To give safe nursing care, the nurse should first:
    1. Check the fundus for firmness
    2. Give her the sedation ordered
    3. Immediately notify the physician
    4. Take her immediately to the delivery room

30. After an incomplete abortion, a client tells the nurse that although her doctor explained what an incomplete abortion was, she did not understand. The nurse could best respond by saying:
    1. "I really don't think you should focus on what happened right now."
    2. "This is when the fetus dies but is retained in the uterus for 8 weeks or more."
    3. "I think it would be best if you asked your doctor for the answer to that question."
    4. "An incomplete abortion is when the fetus is expelled but part of the placenta and membranes are not."

31. A client is admitted to the emergency room with vaginal bleeding. When taking a history, the nurse learns that the client has had five missed periods. Later the nurse reads the chart, which states, "stillborn delivered at 8 PM. . ." The nurse understands this to mean that the fetus and other products of conception:
    1. Were previable
    2. Weighed over 500 g
    3. Were completely expelled
    4. Measured 13.4 cm in length

Healthy Childbearing

32. The outermost membrane that helps form the placenta is the:
    1. Amnion
    2. Chorion
    3. Yolk sac
    4. Allantois

33. Progesterone is normally secreted in relatively large quantities by the:
    1. Endometrium
    2. Pituitary gland
    3. Adrenal cortex
    4. Corpus luteum

34. The chief function of progesterone is the:
    1. Development of female reproductive organs
    2. Stimulation of follicles for ovulation to occur
    3. Preparation of the uterus to receive a fertilized ovum
    4. Establishment of the secondary male sex characteristics

35. The developing cells are called a fetus from the:
    1. Time the fetal heart is heard
    2. Eighth week to the time of birth
    3. Implantation of the fertilized ovum
    4. End of the second week to the onset of labour

36. During pregnancy the volume of tidal air increases because there is:
    1. An increase in total blood volume
    2. Increased expansion of the lower ribs
    3. Upward displacement of the diaphragm
    4. A relative increase in the height of the rib cage

37. The uterus rises out of the pelvis and becomes an abdominal organ at about the:
    1. Tenth week of pregnancy
    2. Eighth week of pregnancy
    3. Twelfth week of pregnancy
    4. Eighteenth week of pregnancy

38. The inner membrane that provides a fluid medium for the embryo is the:
    1. Funis
    2. Amnion
    3. Chorion
    4. Yolk sac

39. First fetal movements felt by the mother are known as:
    1. Lightening
    2. Quickening
    3. Ballottement
    4. Engagement

40. In prenatal development, when is growth most rapid?
    1. First trimester
    2. Third trimester
    3. Second trimester
    4. Implantation period

41. During the process of gametogenesis, the male and female sex cells divide, and each mature sex cell contains:
    1. Twenty-two pairs of autosomes in their nuclei
    2. Forty-six pairs of chromosomes in their nuclei
    3. A diploid number of chromosomes in their nuclei
    4. A haploid number of chromosomes in their nuclei

42. The placenta does not produce:
    1. Somatotropin
    2. Chorionic gonadotropin
    3. Follicle-stimulating hormone
    4. Progesterone precursor substances

43. After the first 3 months of pregnancy the chief source of estrogen and progesterone is the:
    1. Placenta
    2. Adrenal cortex
    3. Corpus luteum
    4. Anterior hypophysis

44. In fetal blood vessels the oxygen content is highest in the:
    1. Umbilical artery
    2. Ductus venosus
    3. Pulmonary artery
    4. Ductus arteriosus

45. A client relates that the first day of her last menstrual period was July 22. The estimated date of confinement (EDC) would be:
    1. May 5
    2. May 14
    3. April 15
    4. April 29

46. During pregnancy, a polypeptide that stimulates the melanocyte hormone is responsible for:
    1. Urinary frequency
    2. Softening of the cervix
    3. Symptoms of morning sickness
    4. Linea nigra and melasma (chloasma)

47. During pregnancy, the uterine musculature hypertrophies and is greatly stretched as the fetus grows. This stretching:
    1. By itself inhibits uterine contraction until oxytocin stimulates the birth process
    2. Is prevented from stimulating uterine contraction by high levels of estrogen during late pregnancy
    3. Inhibits uterine contraction along with the combined inhibitory effects of estrogen and progesterone
    4. Would ordinarily stimulate uterine contraction but is prevented by high levels of progesterone during pregnancy

48. When assessing a pregnant client's physical condition, the nurse is aware that a normal adaptation of pregnancy is an increased blood supply to the pelvic region that results in a purplish discoloration of the vaginal mucosa and is known as:
    1. Ladin's sign
    2. Hegar's sign
    3. Goodell's sign
    4. Chadwick's sign

49. Physiologic anemia during pregnancy is a result of:
    1. Decreased dietary intake of iron
    2. Increased blood volume of the mother

3. Decreased erythropoiesis after the first trimester
4. Increased detoxification demands on the mother's liver

50. When assessing a client, the nurse should be aware that the characteristics of the normal female pelvis include:
    1. Flat sacrum, coccyx movable, spines prominent, pubic arch wide
    2. Flat sacrum, coccyx movable, spines prominent, pubic arch narrow
    3. Well-hollowed sacrum, coccyx movable, spines not prominent, pubic arch wide
    4. Deeply hollowed sacrum, coccyx immovable, pubic arch narrow, spines not prominent

51. The anterior/posterior diameter of the birth canal is one of the important measurements of the pelvis and is known as the:
    1. Conjugate vera
    2. Diagonal conjugate
    3. Transverse diameter
    4. Transverse conjugate

52. What is a common method of locating the precise position of a fetus and placenta prior to an amniocentesis?
    1. Fetoscopy
    2. Fluoroscopy
    3. Sonography
    4. X-ray examination

53. On a first prenatal visit, a client asks the nurse, "Is it true the doctor will do an internal examination today?" The nurse should respond:
    1. "Yes, an internal is done on all mothers on the first visit."
    2. "Are you fearful of having an internal examination done?"
    3. "Yes. Have you ever had an internal examination done before?"
    4. "Yes, an internal is done on all mothers, but it is only slightly uncomfortable."

54. A normal cardiopulmonary symptom experienced by most pregnant women is:
    1. Tachycardia
    2. Dyspnea at rest
    3. Progressive dependent edema
    4. Shortness of breath on exertion

55. A primigravida in her tenth week of gestation is concerned because she has read that nutrition during pregnancy is important for proper growth and development of the baby. She wants to know something about the foods she should eat. The nurse should:
    1. Instruct her to continue eating a normal diet
    2. Assess what she eats by taking a diet history
    3. Give her a list of foods so she can better plan her meals
    4. Emphasize the importance of limiting salt and highly seasoned food

56. A client who has missed one menstrual period thinks she is pregnant. The nurse suggests a pregnancy test. This is possible because in early pregnancy the urine contains:
    1. Prolactin
    2. Estrogen
    3. Luteinizing hormone
    4. Chorionic gonadotropin

Client Case Scenario 4: Mrs. Cathy Smith is in the early first trimester of her first pregnancy. **Items 57 to 66 refer to this client case scenario.**

57. Cathy Smith visits her gynecologist to confirm a suspected pregnancy. During the nursing history she states that her last menstrual period began on April 11. Mrs. Smith states that some spotting occurred on May 8. The nurse calculates that her due date is:
    1. January 10
    2. January 18
    3. February 12
    4. February 15

58. Mrs. Smith asks the nurse why menstruation ceases once pregnancy occurs. The nurse's best response would be that this occurs because of the:
    1. "Reduction in the secretion of hormones by the ovaries."
    2. "Production of estrogen and progesterone by the ovaries."
    3. "Secretion of luteinizing hormone produced by the pituitary."
    4. "Secretion of follicle-stimulating hormone produced by the pituitary."

59. The nurse is aware that the nausea and vomiting commonly experienced by many women during the first trimester of pregnancy is an adaptation to the increased level of:
    1. Estrogen
    2. Progesterone
    3. Luteinizing hormone
    4. Chorionic gonadotropin

60. Mrs. Smith works as a keypunch operator. This would necessarily have implications for her plan of care during pregnancy. The nurse should recommend that she:
    1. Try to walk about every few hours during the workday
    2. Ask for time in the morning and afternoon to elevate her legs
    3. Tell her employer she cannot work beyond the second trimester
    4. Ask for time in the morning and afternoon to obtain nourishment

61. The nurse in the prenatal clinic should provide nutritional counseling to all newly pregnant women because:
    1. Most weight gain during pregnancy is fluid retention
    2. Dietary allowances should not increase during pregnancy
    3. Pregnant women must adhere to a specific pregnancy diet
    4. Different sources of essential nutrients are favored by different cultural groups

62. Cathy Smith is now in her eighth week of pregnancy, and complains of having to go to the bathroom often to urinate. The nurse explains to her that urinary frequency often occurs because the capacity of the bladder during pregnancy is diminished by:
    1. Atony of the detrusor muscle
    2. Compression by the ascending uterus
    3. Compromise of the autonomic reflexes
    4. Constriction of the ureteral entrance at the trigone

63. Mrs. Smith, who is now 10 weeks pregnant, calls the clinic and complains of morning sickness. To promote relief, the nurse should suggest:
    1. Eating dry crackers before arising
    2. Increasing her fat intake before bedtime
    3. Having two small meals daily and a snack at noon
    4. Drinking more high-carbohydrate fluids with her meals

64. When Mrs. Smith was 7 weeks pregnant, she confided to the nurse in the prenatal clinic that she was very sick every morning with nausea and vomiting and was sure that she was being punished for having initially thought of aborting the pregnancy. The nurse assures her that this is not punishment but a common occurrence in early pregnancy and will probably disappear by the end of the:
    1. 2nd month
    2. 3rd month
    3. 4th month
    4. 5th month

65. A nurse tells Mrs. Smith not to wear tight clothing around her abdomen because of possible damage to the fetus. What principle is responsible for the potential damage?
    1. Pascal's
    2. Newton's
    3. Einstein's
    4. Archimedes'

66. Mrs. Smith is being prepared for a pelvic examination. She complains of feeling very tired and sick to her stomach, especially in the morning. What is the best response for the nurse to make?
    1. "Perhaps you might ask the doctor about it."
    2. "This is common. There is no need to worry."
    3. "Can you tell me how you feel in the morning?"
    4. "Let's discuss some ways to deal with these common problems."

67. During a prenatal examination the nurse draws blood from a young client and explains that the determination of Rh is routinely performed on expectant mothers to predict whether the fetus is at risk for developing:
    1. Acute hemolytic anemia
    2. Protein metabolism deficiency
    3. Physiologic hyperbilirubinemia
    4. Respiratory distress syndrome

68. What is the best advice the nurse can give to a pregnant woman in her first trimester?
    1. Cut down on drugs, alcohol, and cigarettes
    2. Avoid all drugs and refrain from smoking and ingesting alcohol
    3. Avoid smoking, limit alcohol consumption, and do not take any aspirin
    4. Take only prescription drugs, especially in the second and third trimesters

Client Case Scenario 5: Mrs. Hester Jackson, 2½ months pregnant, comes through the prenatal clinic for the first time. **Items 69 to 73 refer to this client case scenario.**

69. Mrs. Jackson expresses concern about her "dark nipples" and a "dark line" from her navel to the pubis. The nurse explains that these adaptations are due to the hyperactivity of the:
    1. Ovaries
    2. Thyroid gland
    3. Adrenal gland
    4. Pituitary gland

70. The nurse can try to help Mrs. Jackson overcome first-trimester morning sickness by suggesting that she:
    1. Eat protein before sleep
    2. Take an antacid before bedtime
    3. Eat nothing until the nausea subsides
    4. Request her physician to prescribe an anti-emetic

71. Mrs. Jackson is concerned about gaining weight during pregnancy. The nurse explains that the largest part of weight gain during pregnancy is due to:
    1. The fetus
    2. Fluid retention
    3. Metabolic alterations
    4. Increased blood volume

72. Mrs. Jackson tells the nurse, "I'm worried about gaining too much weight because I have heard that it is bad for me." What is the nurse's best response?
    1. "Yes, weight gain causes complications during pregnancy."
    2. "If you gain over 7 kg, you'll have to follow a low-calorie diet."
    3. "Don't worry about gaining weight. We are more concerned if you don't gain enough weight to ensure proper growth of your baby."
    4. "An 11-kg weight gain is recommended; however, the pattern of your weight gain will be of more importance than the total amount."

73. Mrs. Jackson is concerned about regaining her figure after delivery and wishes to diet during pregnancy. The nurse should advise her that:
    1. Dieting is recommended to lessen the incidence of stillbirth
    2. Dieting is recommended to make delivery easier since she is so small
    3. Inadequate food intake during pregnancy can cause low–birth-weight infants
    4. Inadequate food intake during pregnancy can cause pregnancy-induced hypertension

74. A client is in her fourth month of pregnancy. When she comes for her monthly examination, the nurse asks if she would like to listen to the baby's heartbeat. The woman, commenting on how rapid it is, appears frightened and asks if this is normal. The nurse should respond:
    1. "The baby's heart rate is usually twice the mother's pulse rate."
    2. "The baby's heart rate is normally very rapid, so you needn't worry."

3. "The baby's heartbeat is rapid to accommodate the nutritional needs."
4. "It is far better that the heart rate is rapid; when it is slow, there is need to worry."

Client Case Scenario 6: Mrs. Kim Mann is pregnant for the first time. **Items 75 to 77 refer to this client case scenario.**

75. Kim Mann questions the nurse regarding her desire to continue working as a secretary in a large office during her pregnancy. Which of the following statements by the nurse would be the best advice to give Mrs. Mann regarding this situation?
    1. "Take hourly breaks to get up from your desk and move about."
    2. "Bring extra foodstuffs to work each day and snack at your desk."
    3. Inform your employer that it is not advisable that you continue to work after your thirtieth week of pregnancy."
    4. "Wear therapeutic elastic (antiembolic) stockings while you are on the job, removing them once you are home for the evening."

76. Kim asks the nurse if she can continue to have sexual relations. The nurse's response is based on the knowledge that coitus during pregnancy would be contraindicated only in the presence of:
    1. Leukorrhea
    2. Increased FHR
    3. Gestation of 30 weeks or more
    4. Premature rupture of membranes

77. When involved in prenatal teaching, the nurse should inform Kim that an increase in vaginal secretions during pregnancy is called leukorrhea and is caused by increased:
    1. Metabolic rates
    2. Production of estrogen
    3. Functioning of the Bartholin glands
    4. Supply of sodium chloride to the cells of the vagina

Client Case Scenario 7: Lisa Fong, a 21-year-old client who is 6 months into her second pregnancy, is experiencing increasing edema in the lower extremities. **Items 78 to 79 refer to this client case scenario.**

78. Besides advising rest with the legs elevated, the nurse discusses and gives instructions to Mrs. Fong concerning her diet. In this instance:
    1. The nutritionist should be brought in to plan a diet
    2. The foods selected should have a normal salt content
    3. Dietary preferences must influence the food that is eaten
    4. Mrs. Fong should be advised to see the physician at the prenatal clinic

79. The nurse explains the treatment for fluid retention during pregnancy, which is:
    1. Adequate fluid and a low-salt diet
    2. A low-salt diet and elevation of the lower extremities
    3. Adequate fluid and elevation of the lower extremities
    4. Judicious use of diuretics and elevation of the lower extremities

---

Client Case Scenario 8: Mrs. King and her husband Paul are attending childbirth education classes. **Items 80 to 85 refer to this client case scenario.**

80. While teaching the Kings about labour, the nurse should tell them to come to the hospital when:
    1. Contractions are 10 to 15 minutes apart
    2. Mrs. King has a bloody show and back pressure
    3. Membranes rupture or contractions are 5 to 8 minutes apart
    4. Contractions are 2 to 3 minutes apart and she cannot walk about

81. True labour can be differentiated from false labour because in true labour contractions will:
    1. Bring about progressive cervical dilation
    2. Occur immediately after membrane rupture
    3. Stop when the client is encouraged to walk around
    4. Be less uncomfortable if client is in a side-lying position

82. When teaching the prenatal class about infant feeding, the nurse is asked a question about the relationship between the size of breasts and breastfeeding. The nurse's best response would be:
    1. "Everybody can be successful at breastfeeding."
    2. "You seem to have some concern about breastfeeding."
    3. "The size of your breasts has nothing to do with the production of milk."
    4. "The amount of fat and glandular tissue in the breasts determines the amount of milk produced."

83. Mrs. King, in a class on infant feedings, asks how anyone who is breastfeeding gets anything done with a baby on demand feedings. The nurse's best response would be:
    1. "Most mothers find that feeding the baby whenever the baby cries works out fine."
    2. "Perhaps a schedule might be better because the baby is already accustomed to the hospital routine."
    3. "Most mothers find babies on breast do better on demand feeding because the amount of milk ingested varies at each feeding."
    4. "Although the baby is on demand feedings, the baby will eventually set a schedule, so there will be time for your household chores."

84. During prenatal class, the nurse should teach Mrs. King that breastfeeding is always contraindicated with:
    1. Mastitis
    2. Pregnancy
    3. Inverted nipples
    4. Herpes genitalis

85. The nurse teaches Mrs. King that the ischial spines are designated as an important landmark in labour and delivery because the distance between the spines is:
    1. The narrowest diameter of the pelvis
    2. The widest measurement of the pelvis
    3. A measurement of the floor of the pelvis
    4. A measurement of the inlet of the birth canal

Client Case Scenario 9: Mrs. Lila Jones, a 24-year-old multigravida at term is brought to the hospital in active labour. **Items 86 to 88 refer to this client case scenario.**

86. Mrs. Jones begins to tremble, becomes very tense with contractions, and is quite irritable. She frequently states, "I cannot stand this a minute longer." This kind of behavior may be indicative of the fact that she:
    1. Is entering the transition phase of labour
    2. Needs immediate administration of an analgesic or anesthetic
    3. Has been very poorly prepared for labour in the prenatal classes
    4. Is developing some abnormality in terms of uterine contractions

87. The nurse observes Lila's amniotic fluid and decides that it appears normal, since it is:
    1. Clear and dark-amber colored
    2. Milky, greenish-yellow, containing shreds of mucus

3. Clear, almost colorless, containing little white specks
4. Cloudy, greenish-yellow, containing little white specks

88. Mrs. Jones has a normal spontaneous vaginal delivery of a healthy infant. Five minutes after delivery of the infant the placenta is expressed. The nurse, upon assessing the fundus at this time, would expect the fundus to be:
1. Difficult to find
2. Just below the xiphoid process
3. At the umbilicus in the upper right quadrant
4. Halfway between the symphysis pubis and the umbilicus

89. One problem that confronts the client when an external fetal monitor is being used is the:
1. Restriction of movement
2. Inability to take sedatives
3. Interference with Lamaze techniques
4. Increased frequency of vaginal examinations

90. A primigravida, 40 weeks gestation, is admitted with q 3 to 5 min contractions, a bloody show, and intact membranes. Vaginal examination reveals that the cervix is fully effaced, 6 cm dilated, and the head is at +1 station. The nurse is aware that according to this data the client is in the:
1. Latent phase of labour
2. Active phase of labour
3. Transition phase of labour
4. Accelerated phase of labour

91. A client, 41 weeks gestation, comes to the labour suite with a bloody show and no contractions. A vaginal exam reveals that the baby's head is at +1 station. An acceptable method of inducing labor at this time is:
1. A tap-water enema
2. An IM injection of oxytocin
3. Artificial rupture of membranes
4. Administration of prostaglandins

Client Case Scenario 10: Ms. Reva Schultz, 26-year-old primigravida at term, is admitted to the labour ward. Ms Schultz is experiencing abdominal cramping and a bloody show. Her membranes are intact. **Items 92 to 94 refer to this client case scenario.**

92. A vaginal examination reveals 1 cm dilation and presenting part at +1 station. After obtaining the fetal heart rate and maternal vital signs, the nurse should:
1. Teach the client how to avoid pushing
2. Review Lamaze breathing techniques with the client

3. Provide the client with comfort measures used for women in labour
4. Prepare to type and cross-match the client's blood for a possible transfusion

93. Ms. Schultz's contractions are now q 5 to 8 minutes apart. Vaginal examination reveals 3 cm dilation and 75% effacement, +1 station with occiput anterior, and intact membranes. The client is cheerful and relaxed and asks the nurse if it is all right for her to walk around. Based on the observations of Ms. Schultz's contractions and knowledge of the physiology and mechanism of labour, the nurse could best respond:
1. "I can't make a decision on that, you will have to ask the doctor."
2. "Please stay in bed; walking may interfere with proper uterine contractions."
3. "It is quite all right for you to be up and about as long as you feel comfortable and your membranes are intact."
4. "You will have to stay in bed; otherwise your contractions cannot be timed and no one can listen to the fetal heart."

94. Ms. Schultz's labour continues and she spontaneously ruptures her membranes. The nurse should first:
1. Monitor the FHR
2. Call the physician
3. Check BP and pulse
4. Time the contractions

Client Case Scenario 11: Mrs. Lewis is a client at 36 weeks gestation. She has ruptured her membranes spontaneously. She comes to the hospital with her partner. **Items 95 to 98 refer to this client case scenario.**

95. Mrs. Lewis is examined by the nurse. Her cervix is 2 cm dilated and 75% effaced. The fetal heart rate is 136. The nurse should:
1. Place the mother in bed and attach an external fetal monitor
2. Let the mother undress while the nurse takes the history from the partner
3. Introduce the staff nurses to the couple and try to make them feel welcome
4. Have them wait in the examining room while the nurse notifies the physician that they have arrived

96. A client and her partner are working together during labour. The client is now 7 cm dilated and the presenting part is low in the midpelvis. To alleviate discomfort during contractions, the nurse should instruct the partner to encourage Mrs. Lewis to:
    1. Pant
    2. Pelvic rock
    3. Deep breathe slowly
    4. Athletic chest breathe

97. Mrs. Lewis complains of low-back pain. To increase her comfort the nurse should recommend that Mrs. Lewis' partner:
    1. Instruct her to flex her knees
    2. Place her in the supine position
    3. Apply back pressure during contractions
    4. Help her perform neuromuscular control exercises

98. The nurse withholds foods and limits fluids as Mrs. Lewis approaches the second stage of labour because:
    1. The mechanical and chemical digestive process requires energy that is needed for labor
    2. Undigested food and fluid may cause nausea and vomiting and limit the choice of anesthesia
    3. Food will further aggravate gastric peristalsis, which is already increased due to the stress of labor
    4. The gastric phase of digestion stimulates the release of hydrochloric acid and may cause dyspepsia

---

Client Case Scenario 12: Mrs. Evelyn Butler, a primigravida at 40 weeks gestation, is admitted to the birthing suite in active labour. **Items 99 to 110 refer to this client case scenario.**

99. A few hours after being admitted, Mrs. Butler becomes very restless, flushed, irritable, and perspires profusely. She states that she is going to vomit. The nurse suspects that these symptoms are indicative of:
    1. Late stage
    2. Third stage
    3. Second stage
    4. Transition stage

100. When Mrs. Butler is positioned for delivery, both legs should be positioned simultaneously to prevent:
    1. Venous stasis in the legs
    2. Pressure on the perineum
    3. Excessive pull on the fascia
    4. Trauma to the uterine ligaments

101. Mrs. Butler should be prepared for delivery when the nurse observes:
    1. Mrs. Butler becoming irritable and not following instructions
    2. That the perineum is beginning to bulge with each contraction
    3. An increase in the amount of bloody discharge from the vagina
    4. The contractions are occurring every 2 to 3 minutes and lasting 60 seconds

102. During the period of induction of labour Mrs. Butler should be observed carefully for signs of:
    1. Severe pain
    2. Uterine tetany
    3. Hypoglycemia
    4. Prolapse of the umbilical cord

103. Mrs. Butler's cervix is fully dilated, totally effaced, and the fetal head is at +2. During each contraction the nurse should encourage her to:
    1. Push with glottis open
    2. Blow so as not to grunt
    3. Relax by closing her eyes
    4. Pant to prevent cervical edema

104. During labour, station +1 indicates that the presenting part is:
    1. On the perineum
    2. High in the false pelvis
    3. Slightly below the ischial spines
    4. Slightly above the ischial spines

105. During delivery the physician performs an episiotomy. The nurse reminds Mrs. Butler that this is most commonly done to:
    1. Stretch the perineum
    2. Limit postpartal discomfort
    3. Reduce trauma to the fetus
    4. Prevent lacerations during birth

106. Four hours after a vaginal delivery Mrs. Butler still has not voided. The nurse's initial action should be to:
    1. Palpate her suprapubic area for distention
    2. Encourage voiding by placing her on a bedpan frequently
    3. Place her hands in warm water to encourage micturition
    4. Inform the physician of her inability to void and await orders

107. Mrs. Butler is at risk for postpartum complications. The two most important predisposing causes of puerperal or postpartal infection are:
    1. Hemorrhage and trauma during labour

2. Preeclampsia and retention of placenta
3. Malnutrition and anemia during pregnancy
4. Organisms present in the birth canal and trauma during labor

108. During the postpartum period it is important that Mrs. Butler voids regularly. The nurse is aware that urinary retention is unrelated to:
   1. Bladder atony
   2. Postpartum bleeding
   3. Infection of the bladder
   4. Diaphoresis following delivery

109. Eight hours after delivery the nurse notices that Mrs. Butler is voiding frequently in small amounts. Intake and output are important in the early postpartal period because small amounts of output:
   1. May indicate retention of urine with overflow
   2. Are commonly voided and should cause no alarm
   3. May be indicative of beginning glomerulonephritis
   4. Are common because less fluid is excreted following delivery

110. While checking Mrs. Butler's fundus on the second postpartum day, the nurse observes that the fundus is at the umbilicus and displaced to the right. The nurse evaluates that she probably has:
   1. A slow rate of involution
   2. A full, overdistended bladder
   3. Retained placental fragments
   4. Overstretched uterine ligaments

111. During the postpartum period following a cesarean birth, the nurse examines the client and identifies the presence of lochia serosa and feels the fundus four fingerbreadths below the umbilicus. This indicates that the time elapsed is:
   1. 1 to 3 days postpartum
   2. 4 to 5 days postpartum
   3. 6 to 7 days postpartum
   4. 8 to 9 days postpartum

112. Which pituitary hormone stimulates the secretion of milk from the mammary glands?
   1. Prolactin
   2. Oxytocin
   3. Estrogen
   4. Progesterone

113. The nurse is aware that one of the factors influencing the availability of milk in the lactating woman is the:
   1. Amount of erectile tissue in the nipples
   2. Age of the woman at the time of delivery
   3. Attitude of the woman's family toward breastfeeding
   4. Amount of milk and milk products consumed during pregnancy

114. When caring for a client with an episiotomy during the postpartum period, the nurse encourages sitz baths three times a day for 15 minutes. Sitz baths primarily aid the healing process by:
   1. Promoting vasodilation
   2. Softening the incision site
   3. Cleansing the perineal area
   4. Tightening the rectal sphincter

115. The postpartum nurse should encourage newly delivered clients to ambulate early in order to:
   1. Promote respiration
   2. Increase the tone of the bladder
   3. Maintain tone of abdominal muscles
   4. Increase peripheral vasomotor activity

Client Case Scenario 13: Mrs. Suzanne Bradshaw delivered a healthy baby boy on the previous day. She is planning on breastfeeding her baby. **Items 116 to 120 refer to this client case scenario.**

116. Mrs. Bradshaw asks about the difference between cow's milk and the milk from her breasts. The nurse should respond that cow's milk differs from human milk in that it contains:
   1. More protein, less calcium, and less carbohydrate
   2. Less protein, less calcium, and more carbohydrate
   3. More protein, more calcium, and less carbohydrate
   4. Less protein, more calcium, and more carbohydrate

117. Mrs. Bradshaw, who is now breastfeeding, is being discharged. She tells the nurse that she is worried because her neighbor's breasts dried up when she got home and she had to discontinue breastfeeding. The nurse would best reply:
   1. "This is not true; once lactation is established, this rarely happens."
   2. "You have little to worry about because you already have a good milk supply."
   3. "This commonly happens with the excitement of going home. Putting the baby to breast more frequently will reestablish lactation."
   4. "This commonly happens; however, we will give you a formula to take home so the baby won't go hungry until your milk supply returns."

118. When teaching breastfeeding the nurse should recognize Mrs. Bradshaw needs further instructions when she states, "I will:
    1. Try to empty the breast at each feeding."
    2. Use an alternate breast at each feeding."
    3. Wash breasts with water before each feeding."
    4. Wash breasts with soap and water before feeding."

119. The nurse, planning an initial home care visit following delivery of Mrs. Bradshaw's newborn, recognizes that the visit will be more productive if scheduled when:
    1. Mrs. Bradshaw is feeding the infant
    2. Mr. Bradshaw is out of the home
    3. Time is convenient for the family
    4. Nurse has time to spend with the family

120. During a postpartal visit, Mrs. Bradshaw, whose infant is now 4 weeks old, complains of leg cramps. The nurse suspects:
    1. Hypercalcemia and tells her to increase her activity
    2. Hypocalcemia and tells her to increase her intake of milk
    3. Hyperkalemia and tells her to see a physician immediately
    4. Hypokalemia and tells her to increase her intake of green, leafy vegetables

Normal Newborn

121. The blood vessels in the umbilical cord consist of:
    1. One artery and one vein
    2. One artery and two veins
    3. Two arteries and one vein
    4. Two arteries and two veins

122. Closure of the foramen ovale after birth is caused by:
    1. A decrease in the aortic blood flow
    2. A decrease in pressure in the left atrium
    3. An increase in the pulmonary blood flow
    4. An increase in the pressure in the right atrium

123. After birth, in a normal neonate, the ductus arteriosus becomes the:
    1. Venous ligament
    2. Ligamentum teres
    3. Superior vesical artery
    4. Ligamentum arteriosum

124. Immunity transferred to the fetus from an immune mother through the placenta is:
    1. Active natural immunity
    2. Active artificial immunity
    3. Passive natural immunity
    4. Passive artificial immunity

Client Case Scenario 14: Baby John, a healthy term infant, is born weighing 3690 g. **Items 125 to 139 refer to this client case scenario.**

125. Baby John is delivered precipitously in the labour room. The nurse's initial action should be to:
    1. Establish an airway for the baby
    2. Ascertain the condition of the fundus
    3. Quickly tie and cut the umbilical cord
    4. Move mother and baby to the delivery room

126. Baby John is admitted to the nursery. During the newborn assessment the nurse notes that the temperature, pulse, and respirations are within normal range. Other physical characteristics are also normal. The nurse records all observations on the baby's chart. The nurse's actions were:
    1. Correct, because the nurse met the requirements of the Nursing Process
    2. Incorrect, because making this type of medical diagnosis is not within the purview of the nurse
    3. Correct, because the assessment by the nurse is not equivalent to the physician's assessment
    4. Incorrect, because the initial assessment of the infant's physical status is the responsibility of the physician

127. The primary critical observation for Apgar scoring is the:
    1. Heart rate
    2. Respiratory rate
    3. Presence of meconium
    4. Evaluation of Moro reflex

128. When performing a newborn assessment, the nurse should measure the vital signs in the following sequence:
    1. Pulse, respirations, temperature
    2. Temperature, pulse, respirations
    3. Respirations, temperature, pulse
    4. Respirations, pulse, temperature

129. Within 3 minutes after birth the normal heart rate of the infant may range between:
    1. 100 and 180
    2. 130 and 170
    3. 120 and 160
    4. 100 and 130

130. The normal respiratory rate of an infant such as John within 3 minutes after birth may be as high as:

1. 50
2. 60
3. 80
4. 100

131. The nurse is aware that a normal newborn's respirations are:
    1. Regular, abdominal, 40 to 50 per minute, deep
    2. Irregular, abdominal, 40 to 50 per minute, shallow
    3. Irregular, initiated by chest wall, 30 to 60 per minute, deep
    4. Regular, initiated by the chest wall, 40 to 60 per minute, shallow

132. Baby John has small, whitish, pinpoint spots over the nose, which the nurse knows are caused by retained sebaceous secretions. When charting this observation, the nurse identifies it as:
    1. Milia
    2. Lanugo
    3. Whiteheads
    4. Mongolian spots

133. The nurse observes Baby John lying in a supine position with the head turned to the side, legs and arms extended on the same side and flexed on the opposite side. This is:
    1. The Moro reflex
    2. The Landau reflex
    3. A tonic neck reflex
    4. An abnormal reflex

134. The nurse may best obtain a Moro reflex by:
    1. Grasping the infant's hand
    2. Stimulating the infant's feet
    3. Creating a loud noise suddenly
    4. Changing the infant's equilibrium

135. The Moro reflex response is marked by:
    1. Extension of the arms
    2. Adduction of the arms
    3. Abduction and then adduction of the arms
    4. Extension of the legs and fanning of the toes

136. Asymmetric Moro reflexes are frequently associated with:
    1. Down syndrome
    2. Cranial nerve damage
    3. Cerebral or cerebellar injuries
    4. Brachial plexus, clavicle, or humerus injuries

137. An infant's intestines are sterile at birth, therefore lacking the bacteria necessary for the synthesis of:
    1. Bilirubin
    2. Bile salts
    3. Prothrombin
    4. Intrinsic factor

138. The nurse decides on a teaching plan for John's mother and her infant. The plan should include:
    1. Discussing the matter with her in a nonthreating manner
    2. Setting up a schedule for teaching her how to care for her baby
    3. Showing by example how to care for the infant and satisfy her own needs
    4. Supplying emotional support to her and encouraging her dependence

139. The practice of separating parents and child immediately after birth and limiting their time with the newborn in the first few days would appear to contradict studies based on:
    1. Bonding
    2. Rooming in
    3. Taking-in behaviors
    4. Taking-hold behaviors

Client Case Scenario 15: Mrs. Leslie Dowle delivers a 2811-g baby girl. **Items 140 to 145 refer to this client case scenario.**

140. After delivery, when inspecting her newborn baby girl, Mrs. Dowle notices a discharge from the nipples of both breasts of the baby. The nurse should explain that this is evidence of:
    1. Monilia contracted during birth
    2. An infection contracted in utero
    3. Congenital hormonal imbalance
    4. The influence of the mother's hormones

141. Mrs. Dowle asks the nurse why sugar was added to her baby's formula. The nurse's response would depend on the following understanding:
    1. Sugar in cow's milk is a disaccharide
    2. Sugar in cow's milk is not assimilated well
    3. Cow's milk contains fewer calories than breast milk
    4. Diluted cow's milk provides less sugar than the baby needs

142. Baby Dowle, now 2 days old, weighs 2700 g and is fed formula every 4 hours. Newborns need approximately 160.6 ml of fluid per kilo of body weight each day. Based on this information, the nurse knows that at each feeding the infant should ingest at least:
    1. 40 ml
    2. 70 ml
    3. 140 ml
    4. 420 ml

143. Mrs. Dowle notices that her infant often regurgitates after the feedings and asks the nurse if her baby is ill. The nurse explains to the mother that this is normal and due to:
    1. Intake of air while sucking
    2. A spasm at the pyloric valve
    3. An underdeveloped cardiac sphincter
    4. The position that the baby is in after feeding

144. Mrs. Dowle asks the nurse what advantage breastfeeding has over bottlefeeding. The nurse replies that one major group of substances in human milk that are of special importance to the newborn and cannot be reproduced in any bottle formula is:
    1. Amino acids
    2. Complex carbohydrates
    3. Essential ions (electrolytes)
    4. Gamma globulins (antibodies)

145. Mrs. Dowle's roommate is breastfeeding her 2-day-old infant and tells the nurse that she cannot believe her newborn wants to breastfeed again, since she just fed him 2½ hours ago. The nurse should plan to teach her that a newborn usually should be nursed:
    1. Every hour
    2. Every 2 hours
    3. Every 4 hours
    4. Every 5 hours

High-Risk Pregnancy

146. To determine if there is cephalopelvic disproportion the physician will order:
    1. Pelvimetry
    2. Fetal scalp pH
    3. Amniocentesis
    4. X-ray examination

147. When assessing the significance of estriol studies in an antenatal client, the nurse should understand that:
    1. Estriol is the hormone used in pregnancy tests
    2. Elevations in estriol levels indicate fetal demise
    3. Elevations in estriol levels indicate fetal postmaturity
    4. The fetus contributes precursors to the synthesis of estriol

148. The fetus is most likely to be damaged by the pregnant woman's ingestion of drugs during the:
    1. First trimester
    2. Second trimester
    3. Third trimester
    4. Entire pregnancy

149. A pregnant client asks the clinic nurse how smoking will affect the baby. The nurse's answer reflects the following knowledge:
    1. The placenta is permeable to specific substances
    2. Smoking relieves tension and the fetus responds accordingly
    3. Vasoconstriction will affect both fetal and maternal blood vessels
    4. Fetal and maternal circulation are separated by the placental barrier

150. A client, 12 weeks gestation, comes to the prenatal clinic complaining of severe nausea and frequent vomiting. The nurse suspects that this client has hyperemesis gravidarum and knows that this is frequently associated with:
    1. Excessive amniotic fluid
    2. A GI history of cholecystitis
    3. High levels of chorionic gonadotropin
    4. Slowed secretion of free hydrochloric acid

Client Case Scenario 16: Mrs. Miranda Allen is 2 weeks past her expected date of delivery. The physician has decided to perform an Oxytocin Challenge Test (OCT), in which IV oxytocin solution is administered, and the FHR and uterine contractions are recorded. **Items 151 to 153 refer to this client case scenario.**

151. The nurse in the prenatal clinic understands that an Oxytocin Challenge Test (OCT) is indicated for Mrs. Allen's pregnancy because of:
    1. Placenta previa
    2. Premature onset of labor
    3. A previous abruptio placentae
    4. A pregnancy of more than 40 weeks

152. Contraindications for an OCT would include:
    1. Prematurity
    2. Hypertension
    3. Drug addiction
    4. Uterine activity

153. More than half the neonatal deaths in Canada are caused by:
    1. Atelectasis
    2. Prematurity
    3. Congenital heart disease
    4. Respiratory distress syndrome

Client Case Scenario 17: Ms. Joan Tracey, 6 months pregnant, is admitted with complaints of painful urination, flank tenderness, and hematuria. **Items 154 and 155 refer to this client case scenario.**

154. A diagnosis of pyelonephritis is made. An important nursing intervention for Mrs. Tracey during the attack is:
    1. Limiting fluid intake
    2. Examining the urine for albumin
    3. Maintaining her on a low-salt diet
    4. Observing for signs of premature labor

155. The nurse encourages continued medical supervision for the pregnant woman with pyelitis because:
    1. Preeclampsia frequently occurs following pyelitis
    2. A low-protein diet is given until pregnancy is terminated
    3. Antibiotic therapy should be given until the urine is sterile
    4. Pelvic inflammatory disease occurs with untreated pyelitis

156. A client in the thirty-third week of pregnancy begins to experience contractions. She is to be treated at home with bed rest. The teaching plan for this client should include the information that the client:
    1. Needs to have the foot of the bed raised on blocks
    2. Needs to sit in bed with several large pillows supporting her back
    3. Should be placed on her side with her head raised on a small pillow
    4. Should assume the knee-chest position every 2 hours for 10 minutes while awake

157. The nurse's initial responsibility in teaching the pregnant adolescent client is:
    1. Informing her of the benefits of breastfeeding
    2. Advising her about the proper care of an infant
    3. Instructing her to watch for danger signs of preeclampsia
    4. Impressing her with the importance of consistent prenatal care

158. The major concern about pregnant, unmarried teenagers is that they are often:
    1. Diabetogenic
    2. Socially ostracized
    3. Financially dependent
    4. Prone to pregnancy-induced hypertension

159. The presence of multiple gestation should be detected as early as possible and the pregnancy managed with high risk in mind because:
    1. Postpartum hemorrhage is an expected complication
    2. Perinatal mortality is two to three times greater than in single births
    3. Maternal mortality is much higher during the prenatal period in multiple gestation
    4. The mother needs time to adjust psychologically and physiologically after delivery

160. Which is one of the most common causes of hypotonic uterine dystocia?
    1. Twin gestation
    2. Maternal anemia
    3. Pelvic contracture
    4. Pregnancy-induced hypertension

Client Case Scenario 18: Mrs. Carla Rowan is admitted to the high-risk obstetric unit. **Items 161 to 169 refer to this client case scenario.**

161. In the fifth month of pregnancy, ultrasonography is performed on Mrs. Rowan. The results indicate that the fetus is small for gestational age and there is evidence of a low-lying placenta. The nurse would use this information in the last trimester of pregnancy by assessing her for signs of possible:
    1. Placenta previa
    2. Premature labor
    3. Abruptio placentae
    4. Precipitate delivery

162. Mrs. Rowan experiences an episode of painless vaginal bleeding during the last trimester. The nurse realizes that this may be caused by:
    1. Placenta previa
    2. Abruptio placentae
    3. Frequent intercourse
    4. Excessive alcohol ingestion

163. The care of a client with placenta previa includes:
    1. Vital signs at least once per shift
    2. A tap-water enema before delivery
    3. Observation and recording of the bleeding
    4. Limited ambulation until the bleeding stops

164. Mrs. Rowan is admitted with the diagnosis of possible placenta previa. Following the physician's orders, the nurse begins IV fluids, administers oxygen, and draws blood for laboratory tests. Mrs. Rowan's apprehension is increasing and she asks the nurse what is happening. The nurse tells her not to worry, that she is going to be all right, and everything is under control. The nurse's statements are:
    1. Adequate, since all preparations are routine and need no explanation
    2. Proper, since the client's anxieties would be increased if she knew the dangers
    3. Correct, since only the physician should explain why treatments are being done
    4. Questionable, since the client has the right to know what treatment is being given and why

165. Mrs. Rowan returns to the clinic for a sonography at 36 weeks gestation. Before the test begins, she complains of severe abdominal pain. Heavy vaginal bleeding is noted and the client's BP drops while her pulse rate increases. The nurse should suspect that Mrs. Rowan has a:
    1. Hydatidiform mole
    2. Vena caval syndrome
    3. Marginal placenta previa
    4. Complete abruptio placentae

166. The nurse realizes that the abdominal pain associated with abruptio placentae initially may be caused by:
    1. Hemorrhagic shock
    2. Inflammatory reactions
    3. Concealed hemorrhage
    4. Blood in the uterine muscle

167. The nurse is aware that the bleeding following severe abruptio placentae is usually caused by:
    1. Polycythemia
    2. Hyperglobulinemia
    3. Thrombocytopenia
    4. Hypofibrinogenemia

168. Abruptio placentae is most likely to occur in a woman with:
    1. Cardiac disease
    2. Hyperthyroidism
    3. Cephalopelvic disproportion
    4. Pregnancy-induced hypertension

169. The best intervention to delay delivery of clients with vaginal bleeding in the last trimester is:
    1. Bed rest
    2. Ultrasound test
    3. Oxygen by mask
    4. Nonstress testing

170. Nursing care of women in premature labor includes:
    1. Encouraging them not to bear down
    2. Reassuring them that the situation is under control
    3. Keeping them NPO to prevent abdominal distention
    4. Explaining why pain medication is kept at a minimum

171. A predisposing factor to postpartal hemorrhage is:
    1. A short duration of labour
    2. A previous cesarean delivery
    3. The presence of a multifetal pregnancy
    4. A mother who is 40 years of age or more

172. Following a delivery of twins a client may be predisposed to experiencing a postpartum hemorrhage. The nurse understands that the reason for this is:
    1. Atony of the uterus
    2. A secondary infection
    3. A laceration of the cervix
    4. Retained placental fragments

173. When assessing clients after delivery, the nurse should be aware that postpartal hemorrhage rarely occurs as a complication of:
    1. Retained placenta
    2. Overdistended bladder
    3. Delivery of twins or hydramnios
    4. Pregnancy-induced hypotension

174. The nurse notifies the physician that a client has been admitted in her thirty-sixth week of pregnancy. The client is bleeding, has severe abdominal pain, a hard fundus, and is demonstrating signs of shock. In addition to notifying the physician, the nurse also prepares for:
    1. A high forceps delivery
    2. The insertion of a fetal monitor
    3. An immediate cesarean delivery
    4. The administration of oxytocin (Syntocinon)

175. The most common indication for cesarean delivery is:
    1. Vaginal atony
    2. Placenta previa
    3. Primary uterine inertia
    4. Cephalopelvic disproportion

176. A client undergoes a cesarean delivery because of cephalopelvic disproportion. In addition to the

routine care given to all postpartum clients during the first 24 hours, the nurse should:
1. Encourage early ambulation
2. Maintain IV infusion of oxytocin
3. Check the fundus gently but firmly
4. Check vital signs for evidence of shock

Client Case Scenario 19: Mrs. Norma Singer, a 36-year-old primigravida, has been diagnosed with pregnancy-induced hypertension at 32 weeks gestation. **Items 177 to 180 refer to this client case scenario.**

177. The first assessable objective sign of a seizure in a client with eclampsia is frequently:
    1. Epigastric pain, nausea, and vomiting
    2. Persistent headache and blurred vision
    3. Spots or flashes of light before the eyes
    4. Rolling of the eyes to one side with a fixed stare

178. The priority nursing care for a severely preeclamptic client would include:
    1. Isolating her in a dark room
    2. Maintaining her in a supine position
    3. Encouraging her to drink clear fluids
    4. Protecting her against extraneous stimuli

179. Mrs. Singer has a generalized seizure. Following the seizure, she has an elevated temperature of 39° C. The nurse suspects that the temperature may be caused by:
    1. Excessive muscular activity
    2. Development of a systemic infection
    3. Dehydration caused by rapid fluid loss
    4. Disturbance of the cerebral thermal center

180. The nurse evaluates that the danger of a seizure for Mrs. Singer ends:
    1. After labour begins
    2. After delivery occurs
    3. 24 hours postpartum
    4. 48 hours postpartum

181. A birth hazard associated with breech delivery may be:
    1. Abruptio placentae
    2. Cephalhematoma
    3. Pathologic jaundice
    4. Compression of cord

182. The safest position for a woman in labour when the nurse notes a prolapsed cord is:
    1. Prone
    2. Fowler's
    3. Lithotomy
    4. Trendelenburg

183. The normal hemodynamics of pregnancy that affect the pregnant cardiac client include the:
    1. Gradually increasing size of the uterus
    2. Decrease in the number of red blood cells
    3. Rise in cardiac output after the thirty-fourth week
    4. Cardiac acceleration in the last half of pregnancy

184. A pregnant client, with a class II cardiac condition, is concerned that her pregnancy will be an added burden on her already compromised heart. The nurse explains to this client that during pregnancy the cardiac system is most compromised during the:
    1. First trimester
    2. Third trimester
    3. Transitional phase of delivery
    4. First forty-eight hours after delivery

185. If anemia is present with a hemoglobin level of 80 g/L or lower, a mother with cardiac disease probably will develop:
    1. Heart block
    2. Cardiac failure
    3. Atrial fibrillation
    4. Cardiac compensation

Client Case Scenario 20: Mrs. Helen Reading is a Class 1 cardiac client with a history of rheumatic fever. She is admitted to the labour room in active labour. **Items 186 to 190 refer to this scenario.**

186. Proper positioning for Mrs. Reading would be:
    1. Supine; high-Fowler's
    2. Supine; semi-Fowler's
    3. Left lateral; semi-Fowler's
    4. Lying on right side; head elevated 30°

187. To prevent Mrs. Reading from developing cardiac decompensation during labor, the nurse should:
    1. Administer an IV infusion of isotonic saline
    2. Maintain an IV infusion of potassium chloride
    3. Administer oxytocin to accelerate contractions
    4. Position her on her side with shoulders elevated

188. A specific nursing intervention for labouring clients with cardiac problems is:
    1. Monitoring BP every hour
    2. Encouraging frequent voiding
    3. Auscultating for rales q 30 minutes
    4. Turning from side to side q 15 minutes

189. The nurse anticipates that after delivery Mrs. Reading will be prophylactically placed on:
    1. Lasix
    2. Heparin
    3. Digitalis
    4. Ampicillin

190. During the postpartal period it is not uncommon for a new mother to have an increased cardiac output with tachycardia. Because of this knowledge, the nurse should carefully observe Mrs. Reading for signs of:
    1. Irregular pulse
    2. Hypovolemic shock
    3. Respiratory distress
    4. Increased vaginal bleeding

191. The nurse understands that the diabetic mother's metabolism is significantly altered during pregnancy as a result of:
    1. The lower renal threshold for glucose
    2. The increased effect of insulin during pregnancy
    3. An increase in the glucose tolerance level of the blood
    4. The effect of hormones produced in pregnancy on carbohydrate and lipid metabolism

192. A pregnant client with diabetes is referred to the clinic nutritionist for nutritional assessment and counseling. The dietary program worked out for this client would be:
    1. A diet high in protein of good biologic value and decreased calories
    2. A balanced diet to meet increased dietary needs with insulin adjusted as necessary
    3. Adequate balance of carbohydrate and fat to meet energy demands and prevent ketosis
    4. A low-carbohydrate, low-calorie diet to stay within her present insulin coverage and avoid hyperglycemia

193. The nurse is aware that in the second half of pregnancy women who are diabetic require:
    1. Decreased caloric intake
    2. Increased dosage of insulin
    3. Administration of pancreatic enzymes
    4. Administration of estrogenic hormones

High-Risk Newborn

194. During labour the nurse must be aware that an early deceleration (type I dip) is evidenced by an FHR of:
    1. 80 to 100 beats per minute early in the contraction
    2. 100 to 120 beats per minute early in the contraction
    3. 120 to 140 beats per minute early in the contraction
    4. 140 to 160 beats per minute early in the contraction

195. Infants whose mothers contracted rubella in the first trimester are frequently born with:
    1. Phocomelia
    2. Otosclerosis
    3. Hydrocephalus
    4. Cardiac anomalies

196. The finding that would probably necessitate prolonged follow-up care of a newborn would be:
    1. A birth weight of 3500 g
    2. An initial Apgar score of 5
    3. An umbilical cord that contained only two vessels
    4. The aspiration of 20 ml of milky-colored fluid from the newborn's stomach

197. After a difficult delivery, a neonate is admitted to the nursery with an Apgar of 4. This would most likely indicate that this score includes the fact that the baby's:
    1. Respirations are 35
    2. Muscle tone is flaccid
    3. Heart rate is over 100
    4. Body is pink but the extremities are blue

198. An infant born in the thirty-sixth week of gestation weighs 2062 g and has an Apgar of 7/9. Upon admission to the nursery, it would be unnecessary for the nurse to:
    1. Record vital signs
    2. Administer oxygen
    3. Support body temperature
    4. Evaluate the newborn's status

199. An abandoned infant has been brought to the hospital. Ophthalmia neonatorum is diagnosed. The nurse can estimate the infant's age at:
    1. 1 day
    2. 2 days
    3. About 3 to 4 days
    4. Less than 24 hours

200. On a home visit to a known drug abuser who delivered 4 days ago, the visiting nurse assesses that the baby has a purulent discharge from the eyes. The nurse suspects that the infant has:
    1. Symptoms of *Chlamydia trachomatis* infection
    2. Retinopathy of prematurity
    3. Signs of acquired immune deficiency syndrome (AIDS)
    4. Developed a reaction to the ophthalmic antibiotic ointment instilled after birth

201. An infant develops purulent conjunctivitis on the fourth day of life and is brought to the emergency room. The nurse should:
    1. Teach the mother about hand washing
    2. Assess the infant for signs of pneumonia
    3. Secure an order for allergy testing of the infant
    4. Bathe the infant's eyes with tepid boric acid solution

202. When caring for preterm infants, the precautions that should be taken against retinopathy of prematurity (retrolental fibroplasia) include:
    1. Carefully controlling temperature and humidity
    2. Using phototherapy to prevent jaundice and retinopathy
    3. Keeping oxygen at reduced concentrations and discontinuing it as soon as feasible
    4. Maintaining a high concentration of oxygen (above 75%) together with high humidity

203. The care of a newborn infant whose mother has had untreated syphilis since the second trimester of the pregnancy would be:
    1. Assessing for a cleft palate
    2. Eliciting hypotonicity of skeletal muscles
    3. Observing for maculopapular lesions of the soles
    4. Having the baby immediately screened for syphilis

204. If a woman with an untreated chlamydial infection is allowed to deliver vaginally, the infant is in danger of being born with:
    1. Thrush
    2. Congenital syphilis
    3. Ophthalmia neonatorum
    4. Neurologic complications

205. A newborn has asymmetric gluteal folds. The nurse suspects:
    1. CNS damage
    2. A dislocated hip
    3. An inguinal hernia
    4. Peripheral nervous system damage

Client Case Scenario 21: After a long and difficult breech delivery, Baby Daniel is admitted to the neonatal nursery. **Items 206 to 208 refer to this client case scenario.**

206. Since Erb's palsy may be seen as the result of a difficult forceps or breech delivery, the nurse should assess Baby Daniel for:
    1. A flaccid arm with the elbow extended
    2. Loss of grasp reflex on the affected side

    3. Inability to turn the head to the affected side
    4. A negative Moro reflex on the unaffected side

207. Immediate nursing care for the affected arm of an infant born with Erb's palsy should include:
    1. Constant immobilization of the affected arm
    2. Teaching the parents to manipulate the muscle
    3. Immediate active ROM exercises to the affected arm
    4. Daily measurement of girth and length of the affected arm

208. After this difficult delivery, an assessment of Baby Daniel, a full-term newborn, reveals an unequal Moro reflex on one side and a flaccid arm in adduction. The nurse suspects:
    1. Brachial palsy
    2. Supratentorial tear
    3. Fracture of the clavicle
    4. Crigler-Najjar syndrome

209. A neonate admitted to the neonatal intensive care nursery has muscle twitching, convulsions, cyanosis, abnormal respirations, and a short shrill cry. The nurse suspects that this infant may have:
    1. Tetany
    2. Spina bifida
    3. Hyperkalemia
    4. Intracranial hemorrhage

210. The nurse observes a yellowish color of the skin of a baby in the newborn nursery. The immediate nursing action should be to:
    1. Ascertain the age of the infant
    2. Notify the physician of the development
    3. Take a heel blood sample and send it to the laboratory
    4. Cover the baby's eyes with a blindfold and put the baby under the ultraviolet light

211. When observing a newborn for signs of pathologic jaundice, the nurse should be alert for:
    1. Muscular irritability at birth
    2. Neurologic signs during the first 24 hours
    3. The appearance of jaundice during the first 24 hours
    4. Jaundice developing between the second and fourth day of life

Client Case Scenario 22: Baby Reisler is delivered at 29 weeks gestation. He weighs 1619 g. **Items 212 to 216 refer to this client case scenario.**

212. Based on the weight and gestational age, this neonate would be classified as:
    1. Preterm
    2. Immature
    3. Nonviable
    4. Low–birth-weight infant

213. The nurse is aware that Isolettes are used for preterm infants to maintain body temperature at a constant level, since the heat-regulation mechanism of preterm babies is one of the least developed functions. This is related to the fact that these babies:
    1. Have a smaller surface area than full-term newborns
    2. Perspire a great deal, thus losing heat almost constantly
    3. Lack subcutaneous fat, which would furnish some insulation
    4. Have a limited ability to produce antibodies against infections

214. The nurse must continuously monitor Baby Reisler's temperature and provide appropriate nursing care because the preterm infant:
    1. Has an inability to break down glycogen to glucose
    2. Has a limited ability to use shivering to produce heat
    3. Has a limited supply of brown fat available to provide heat
    4. Has an underdeveloped pituitary system to control internal heat

215. When meeting Baby Reisler's hydration needs, the nurse should know that urinary function in the premature baby:
    1. Is the same as in a full-term newborn
    2. Results in the loss of large amounts of urine
    3. Leads to urine with an elevated specific gravity
    4. Adequately maintains an acid-base and electrolyte balance

216. The nurse must continuously monitor Baby Reisler for the most common preterm complication of:
    1. Hemorrhage
    2. Brain damage
    3. Aspiration of mucus
    4. Respiratory distress

217. Twins are delivered at 30 weeks gestation and are diagnosed as having respiratory distress syndrome. The principle underlying the respiratory distress of these infants is:
    1. Surface tension
    2. Pascal's principle
    3. Archimedes' principle
    4. Second law of thermodynamics

218. When caring for preterm infants with respiratory distress, the nurse should keep:
    1. Them prone to prevent aspiration
    2. Them in a high-humidity environment
    3. Their caloric intake low to decrease metabolic rate
    4. Their oxygen concentration low to prevent eye damage

Client Case Scenario 23: Baby Barbara is delivered to a diabetic mother. **Items 219 to 221 refer to this client case scenario.**

219. In the nursery, the newborn of a mother with a history of long-standing diabetes should be provided with:
    1. Fast-acting insulin
    2. Special high-risk care
    3. Routine newborn care
    4. A decreased glucose intake

220. The nurse understands that following delivery, Baby Barbara may have tremors, periods of apnea, cyanosis, and poor sucking ability. These symptoms are associated with:
    1. Hypoglycemia
    2. Hyperglycemia
    3. Central nervous system edema
    4. Congenital depression of the islets of Langerhans

221. The nurse is aware that infants of diabetic mothers are larger than other newborns because of:
    1. Increased somatotropin and lowered glucose utilization
    2. Increased somatotropin and increased glucose utilization
    3. Decreased somatotropin and increased glucose utilization
    4. Decreased somatotropin and decreased glucose utilization

Emotional Needs Related to Childbearing and Women's Health

222. Research concerning the emotional factors of pregnancy indicates:
    1. A rejected pregnancy will result in a rejected infant

2. Ambivalence and anxiety about mothering are common
3. Maternal love is fully developed within the first week after birth
4. A good mother experiences neither ambivalence nor anxiety about mothering

223. A client enters the hospital for exploratory abdominal surgery. She is 3 months pregnant and has been informed that there are many dangers involved. The nurse has her sign a consent form for an exploratory laparotomy. Cancer of the uterus is discovered and a hysterectomy is performed. On returning from surgery the client is informed that her uterus was removed. She sues the hospital, the surgeon, and the nurse. The decision in this case will be based on the fact that:
1. General consent forms signed on admission are sufficient
2. The client received inadequate information to give consent
3. The surgeon has the legal right to do what was deemed necessary in surgery
4. Consent for exploratory surgery implies permission for removing organs if this is justified

224. When caring for a client who is having a prolonged labour, the nurse must be aware that the client is very concerned when her labour deviates from what she sees as the norm. A response conveying acceptance of the client's expressions of frustration and hostility would be:
1. "I'll rub your back; tell me if it helps."
2. "I'll leave so you can talk to your husband."
3. "All women get weary and frustrated during labour."
4. "Would you like to talk about what's bothering you?"

225. The partner of a client who is in the transitional phase of labour becomes very tense and nervous during this period and asks the nurse,"Do you think it is best for me to leave, since I don't seem to do my partner much good?" The most appropriate response by the nurse would be:
1. "This is the time your partner needs you. Don't run out on her now."
2. "This is hard for you. Let me try to help you coach her during this difficult phase."
3. "I know this is hard for you. Why don't you go have a cup of coffee and relax and come back later if you feel like it?"
4. "If you feel that way, you'd best go out and sit in the waiting room for a while because you may transmit your anxiety to your partner."

Client Case Scenario 24: After an 8-hour, uneventful labour, Mrs. Debbie Miller delivers a baby boy spontaneously. **Items 226 to 231 refer to this client case scenario.**

226. As the nurse places the baby in the mother's arms immediately following delivery, the Mrs. Miller asks, "Is he normal?" The most appropriate response by the nurse would be:
1. "Most babies are normal; of course he is."
2. "He must be all right, he has such a good strong cry."
3. "Yes, because your pregnancy and labour were so normal."
4. "Shall we unwrap him so you can look him over for yourself?"

227. Supportive nursing care in the beginning mother-infant relationship should include:
1. Requiring the mother to assist with simple aspects of her infant's care
2. Encouraging the mother to decide between breastfeeding and bottlefeeding
3. Allowing the mother ample time to undress and to carefully inspect her infant
4. Unobtrusive observation of the mother and her infant to pick up a disturbed relationship

228. While holding her baby, Mrs. Miller calls the nurse and worriedly comments that the baby seems to sneeze a lot and breathes very rapidly and irregularly. She expresses fear that her baby may be sick like her neighbor's baby was and will have to be taken back to the hospital after being home for a few days. The nurse should:
1. Pick up the baby and tell the mother that the nurses will watch the baby closely
2. Look the baby over and tell the mother that the baby is fine and nothing is wrong
3. Look the baby over and explain to the mother that sneezing is normal and helps the baby to get rid of mucus, and that a baby normally has rapid, shallow, irregular respirations
4. Assess the baby, take the baby to the nursery immediately, and return to the mother to tell her that the physician has been called, since the baby is obviously in respiratory distress

229. During the taking-hold phase, the nurse would expect Mrs. Miller to:
1. Talk about the baby
2. Call the baby by name
3. Touch the baby with her fingertips
4. Be passively involved with the baby

230. Following delivery, while considering nursing measures to help parent-child relationships, the nurse should be aware that the most important factor at this time is the:
    1. Anesthesia during labour
    2. Duration and difficulty of labour
    3. Physical condition of the infant
    4. Health status during pregnancy

231. When caring for the Millers on the postpartum unit, the nurse must be aware that all the tasks, responsibilities, and attitudes that make up child care can be called parenting, and that either parent can exhibit these qualities. A person is able to perform parenting because of:
    1. A relationship with flexible roles
    2. An inborn ability based on instinct
    3. Positive childhood roles and concepts
    4. A good education in growth and development

232. When planning care for the parents of a newborn with abnormalities, the nurse should be aware that the parents are better able to cope with this problem if informed:
    1. When bringing the baby to the mother for the first time
    2. When the parents ask if something is wrong with their baby
    3. Right after delivery while the mother is still in the delivery room
    4. After the first 24 hours, when the mother's strength has returned

233. A decision to withhold "extraordinary care" for a newborn with severe abnormalities is actually:
    1. A decision to let the newborn die
    2. The same as pediatric euthanasia
    3. Presuming that the newborn has no rights
    4. Unethical and illegal medical and nursing practice

234. It is important for the nurse to support the parents' decision to abort a fetus with a birth defect because:
    1. Supporting them will eliminate feelings of guilt
    2. It is essential for maintenance of family equilibrium
    3. The parents are legally responsible for the decision
    4. The nurse's support will relieve the pressure associated with decision making

235. Twenty-four hours after a cesarean delivery a client elects to sign herself and her baby out of the hospital because of difficulty at home with her 2-year-old son. Staff members have been unable to contact her physician. The client arrives at the nursery dressed and ready to leave and asks that her infant be given to her to dress and take home. Appropriate nursing action would be:
    1. Explain to the client that her infant must remain in the hospital until signed out by the physician and that she must leave the baby in the nursery
    2. Allow the client time with the baby to cuddle him before she leaves, but emphasize that the baby is a minor and legally must remain until orders are received
    3. Tell the client that under the circumstances hospital policy prevents the staff from releasing the infant into her care, but she will be informed when the infant is discharged
    4. Give the baby to the client to take home, making sure that she receives information regarding care and feeding of a 2-day-old infant and any potential problems which may develop

236. A newly delivered mother, with three young children at home, comments to the nursery nurse that she cannot hold the baby for feedings once she gets home. She has just too much to do, and anyhow, it spoils the baby. The best response for the nurse to make is:
    1. "You seem concerned about time. Let's talk about it."
    2. "That's entirely up to you; you have to do what works for you."
    3. "Holding the baby when feeding is important for development."
    4. "It is most unsafe to prop a bottle. The baby could aspirate the fluid."

237. After a client has a spontaneous abortion, the nurse notes that the involved couple are visibly upset. The partner has tears in his eyes and the woman has her face turned toward the wall and is sobbing quietly. The nurse's best approach would be to go over to the woman and say:
    1. "I know that you are upset now, but hopefully you will become pregnant again very soon."
    2. "I see that both of you are very upset. I brought you a cup of coffee and will be here if you want to talk."
    3. "I know how you feel, but you should not be so upset now; it will make it more difficult for you to get well quickly."
    4. "I can understand that you are upset, but be glad it happened early in your pregnancy and not after you carried the baby for the full time."

Client Case Scenario 25: Mary Flynn suspects she is pregnant, but because she is the only wage earner in her family, she is ambivalent about continuing the pregnancy. **Items 238 and 239 refer to this client case scenario.**

238. The nurse recognizes that Mary Flynn is in crisis and also remembers that pregnancy and birth are called crises because:
    1. There are mood changes during pregnancy
    2. They are periods of change and adjustment to change
    3. There are hormonal and physiologic changes in the mother
    4. Narcissism in the mother affects the male-female relationship

239. The nurse recognizes that Mary Flynn, who is seriously considering an abortion because of financial difficulties, is in crisis. The nurse should intervene to alleviate the crisis by:
    1. Understanding the family interaction
    2. Helping the mother express her feelings
    3. Involving the father in preparation classes
    4. Involving the mother in preparation classes

240. A young couple attend the prenatal clinic. The woman is 8 weeks pregnant and asks the clinic nurse for information about an abortion. The nurse expresses the opinion that abortion is immoral and that many women have long-term guilt feelings after an abortion. The couple leave the clinic in a very disturbed state. Legally, the:
    1. Client had a right to correct, unbiased information
    2. A nurse's statements need not be based on scientific knowledge
    3. Physician should have been called in, since the nurse cannot talk about it
    4. Nurse had a right to state feelings as long as they were identified as the nurse's own

241. An amniocentesis done on a client, 16 weeks gestation, reveals a Down syndrome infant. The client and her partner elect to have the pregnancy terminated. The nurse giving care to a client whose pregnancy is surgically terminated should be aware that:
    1. The risk of postoperative infection is high
    2. The client is emotionally unstable at this time
    3. Contraceptive counseling should be deferred to a later time
    4. The client needs to express her feelings of guilt, anger, and frustration

Drug-Related Responses

242. A client at 6 weeks gestation is receiving antibiotic therapy for pyelonephritis. The nurse is aware that the safest antibiotic for administration during pregnancy is:
    1. Novosoxazole
    2. Ampicillin
    3. Tetracycline
    4. Nitrofurantoin

243. A client who was admitted in active labour has only progressed from 2 cm to 3 cm in 8 hours. She is diagnosed as having hypotonic dystocia and is given oxytocin (Syntocinon) to augment her contractions. The most important aspect of nursing at this time is:
    1. Monitoring the FHR
    2. Checking perineum for bulging
    3. Timing and recording length of contractions
    4. Preparing for an emergency cesarean delivery

244. A client, 38 weeks gestation, is admitted for induction of labour. She has a history of ruptured membranes for the past 12 hours. She has no other symptoms of labour. The nurse is aware that if the proper conditions exist, the physician will prescribe:
    1. Oxytocin
    2. Progesterone
    3. Magnesium sulfate
    4. Ergometrine maleate

245. At about 5 cm, a labouring client receives medication for pain. The nurse is aware that one of the medications given to women in labour that could cause respiratory depression of the newborn is:
    1. Scopolamine
    2. Promazine (Sparine)
    3. Meperidine (Demerol)
    4. Promethazine (Phenergan)

246. A client in the midphase of labour becomes very uncomfortable and asks for medication. Meperidine (Demerol) 50 mg and Phenergan 50 mg are ordered. These medications:
    1. Act to produce amnesia
    2. Act as preliminary anesthetics
    3. Induce sleep until the time of delivery
    4. Increase the client's pain threshold, resulting in relaxation

247. A client begins preterm labour and the physician orders Ritodrine (Yutopar). After its administration, the nurse assesses the client for the therapeutic effect of:
     1. Reduction of pain in the perineal area
     2. Decrease in blood pressure from 120/80 to 90/60
     3. Decrease in frequency and duration of contractions
     4. Dilation of the cervix from 1 to 1.5 cm for every hour of labor

248. A client is on magnesium sulfate therapy for severe preeclampsia. The nurse must be alert for the first sign of an excessive blood magnesium level, which is:
     1. Disturbance in sensorium
     2. Increase in respiratory rate
     3. Development of cardiac dysrhythmia
     4. Disappearance of the knee-jerk reflex

249. Following an elective abortion via a hysterotomy, Rh_o (D) WinRho is administered intramuscularly to an Rh-negative mother to:
     1. Expand the antibody pool of the mother
     2. Prevent antibody formation in the mother
     3. Suppress the activity of Rh-negative antibodies
     4. Accelerate the mother's production of immune bodies

250. A pregnant client develops thrombophlebitis of the left leg and is admitted to the hospital for bed rest and anticoagulant therapy. The anticoagulant the nurse should expect to administer is:
     1. Heparin
     2. Dicumarol
     3. Diphenadione (Dipaxin)
     4. Warfarin (Coumadin sodium)

251. A client, undergoing treatment for infertility, is diagnosed as having endometriosis. The nurse is aware that one of the drugs that may be used to treat this condition is:
     1. Relaxin (Releasin)
     2. Danazol (Cyclomen)
     3. Ergonovine (Ergometrine)
     4. Esterified estrogen (Menrium)

Women's Health

252. The term metrorrhagia refers to:
     1. Painful intercourse
     2. Presence of blood in the vaginal discharge
     3. Severe bleeding during each menstrual period
     4. Episodes of bleeding between menstrual periods

253. Endometriosis is characterized by:
     1. Amenorrhea and insomnia
     2. Ecchymoses and petechiae
     3. Painful menstruation and backache
     4. Early osteoporosis and pelvic inflammation

254. Overstretching of perineal supporting tissues as a result of childbirth can bring about a rectocele. The most common symptom is:
     1. Crampy abdominal pain
     2. A bearing-down sensation
     3. Urinary stress incontinence
     4. Recurrent urinary tract infections

255. A client who has cervical cancer is hospitalized for internal radiation therapy. After the radiation source has been loaded, the nurse should:
     1. Check the client's voiding and catheterize if necessary
     2. Immediately place the client in a high-Fowler's position
     3. Ensure that a low-residue diet has been ordered for the client
     4. Stay with the client for half an hour and assess for symptoms of radiation sickness

Client Case Scenario 26: Mrs. Peggy Lee is scheduled to undergo an abdominal hysterectomy. **Items 256 to 258 refer to this client case scenario.**

256. To provide preoperative teaching the nurse should know that after Mrs. Lee has a hysterectomy:
     1. Menstruation ceases and ovarian hormone secretion decreases
     2. Menopause begins immediately with the cessation of ovarian hormone production
     3. The cyclical oscillation of hormones between the hypophysis and ovaries continues
     4. Ovarian hormone secretion ceases, but the hypophysis continues secretion of gonadotropic hormones

257. Mrs. Lee asks how the surgery will affect her periods. The nurse should respond:
     1. "You will no longer menstruate."
     2. "Initially your periods will increase."
     3. "Your monthly periods will be lighter."
     4. "Your monthly periods will be more regular."

258. A few days following a hysterectomy, Mrs. Lee asks for sanitary pads because she feels she is going to menstruate. The nurse should base a response on the fact that:
     1. Mrs. Lee will not menstruate because the uterus has been removed

2. It will take several weeks before Mrs. Lee reestablishes normal menstruation
3. Mrs. Lee is probably showing signs of developing an anxiety response
4. The appearance of frank vaginal bleeding is expected following this type surgery

---

259. Following a mastectomy, the nurse should position the client's arm on the affected side:
    1. In adduction supported by sandbags
    2. In abduction surrounded by sandbags
    3. With the hand higher than the arm on pillows
    4. Lower than the level of the right atrium on pillows

260. The operative procedure which would result in surgical menopause would be a:
    1. Tubal ligation
    2. Simple hysterectomy
    3. Bilateral oophorectomy
    4. Bilateral salpingectomy

261. A nurse teaches a women's group that hot flashes are caused by the:
    1. Accumulation of acetylcholine
    2. Cessation of pituitary gonadotropins
    3. Overstimulation of the adrenal medulla
    4. Hormonal stimulation of the sympathetic system

262. Menopause is the cessation of menstrual function. One of the reasons given for the cessation of menses is:
    1. A decrease in gonadotropin in the blood
    2. A decrease in the production of prostaglandins
    3. The inability of the ovary to respond to gonadotropic hormones
    4. An increase in the secretion of progesterone from the follicles in the ovary

263. When obtaining a health history the nurse would eliminate as a possible complication of endometriosis a history of:
    1. Menopause
    2. Metrorrhagia
    3. Bowel stricture
    4. Voiding difficulties

Client Case Scenario 27: Mrs. Agnes O'Brien, age 68, has been diagnosed with osteoporosis. **Items 264 to 265 refer to this client case scenario.**

264. When writing a teaching plan about osteoporosis, the nurse should recall that osteoporosis is best described as:
    1. Avascular necrosis
    2. Pathologic fractures
    3. Hyperplasia of osteoblasts
    4. A decrease in bone substance

265. The plan of care for Mrs. O'Brien includes active and passive exercises, calcium supplements, and daily vitamins. The desired effect of therapy would be noted by the nurse if Mrs. O'Brien:
    1. Increased mobility
    2. Experienced fewer muscular spasms
    3. Had fewer bruises than on admission
    4. Developed fewer cardiac irregularities

CHILDBEARING AND WOMEN'S HEALTH NURSING
ANSWERS AND RATIONALES

Reproductive Choices

1. **2** **It is the surge of LH secretion in midcycle that is responsible for ovulation. (PL; ED; RC)**
   1 This is not related; this stimulates ejection of milk into the mammary ducts.
   3 This occurs when the progesterone level is low.
   4 This occurs when the endometrial wall is built up.

2. **3** **The ovum is capable of being fertilized for only 24 to 36 hours following ovulation; after this time it travels a variable distance between the fallopian tube and uterus, disintegrates, and is phagocytized by leukocytes. (PL; PA; RC)**
   1 The ovum is viable for 24 to 36 hours.
   2 The ovum is viable a longer time.
   4 The ovum is not fertilizable after 36 hours.

3. **2** **As ovulation approaches, there may be a drop in the basal temperature because of an increased production of estrogen; when ovulation occurs, there will be a rise in the basal temperature because of an increased production of progesterone. (AN; PA; RC)**
   1 At ovulation the temperature drop is slight, not marked.
   3 At ovulation the temperature rises after a slight drop.
   4 At ovulation the temperature drops slightly and then rises.

4. **1** **Stress or infection alters the body's metabolism, causing an elevation in temperature; a rise in temperature from these causes may be misinterpreted as ovulation. (AN; PA; RC)**
   2 This may increase sperm volume but does not affect the female's basal temperature.
   3 Age is not a factor concerning efficiency of the rhythm method.
   4 Frequency of intercourse may affect the volume of sperm but does not alter the female's basal temperature.

5. **1** **Ovulation is anticipated approximately 14 days prior to menstruation; however, it is more reliable to avoid using a specific number of days and to calculate on the basis of an individual's cycle rather than an average 28-day cycle. (IM; ED; RC)**
   2 Ovulation occurs 14 days before the onset of menstruation.
   3 Same as answer 2.
   4 Ovulation is about 14 days after the start of menses.

6. **1** **Antiovulatory drugs suppress menstruation. Breakthrough bleeding is abnormal with biphasic drugs. The drug is given for only 21 days and a menstrual flow does not occur during this time. (IM; ED; RC)**
   2 There is no indication for increased Papanicolaou smears; once a year is sufficient.
   3 Increased calcium to counteract osteoporosis from menopause is not indicated for this client.
   4 No restriction of sexual activity is indicated when one is taking oral contraceptives.

7. **2** **Some type of a barrier contraceptive (condom with foam or jelly or a diaphragm) is usually recommended for the client with diabetes mellitus and a cardiac condition. (IM; ED; RC)**
   1 Oral contraceptives are not recommended because of their tendency to act as insulin antagonists.
   3 An IUD is not recommended because it may predispose the client to infection.
   4 This is untrue; clients with a cardiac condition can become pregnant again in the future.

8. **4** **Subsequent to IUD insertion, there may be an excessive menstrual flow for several cycles; this is because of an increase in the blood supply due to the inflammatory process, since the IUD is really a foreign body. (EV; ED; RC)**
   1 There is no documentation of this.
   2 This may occur but is not classified as a side effect.
   3 This may occur upon insertion but is fairly uncommon.

9. **4** **The IUD may cause irritability of the myometrium, inducing contraction of the uterus and expulsion of the device. (IM; ED; RC)**

1 This is a rare rather than a common occurrence.
2 Clients do not complain of discomfort during coitus when an IUD is in place.
3 Increased vaginal infections are not reported with the use of an IUD.

10. **4 Because of the IUD, the uterine lining is not receptive to the implantation of the fertilized egg.** (AN; PA; RC)
1 A diaphragm blocks the cervical os.
2 Mobility of the uterus is not related to contraception.
3 The sperm can reach the fallopian tube; implantation of the fertilized egg is impaired.

11. **3 A headache is a symptom of hypernatremia, which can occur with the salinization method of elective abortion.** (EV; TC; RC)
1 Edema may occur as a result of water intoxication when oxytocin is used in the saline abortion.
2 This is a serious manifestation of water intoxication occurring when oxytocin is used in the saline abortion; it is not a consequence of saline administration.
4 Bradycardia may occur with the use of spinal or regional anesthesia, not salinization.

12. **4 The saline causes puffing of the placenta, fetal death, placental separation, release of fibrin, and then labor and paradoxical hemorrhaging. This takes at least 24 hours in most cases.** (IM; ED; RC)
1 Normally labour starts 24 to 72 hours after the procedure.
2 This is too quick; it usually takes 24 to 72 hours, unless oxytocin is used to hasten labour.
3 This is too quick; it takes 24 to 72 hours for labour to begin.

13. **2 *Laminaria* is a seaweed that expands in a moist environment. It is a natural and safe method of dilating the cervix.** (AN; TC; RC)
1 It takes 24 hours for the *Laminaria* to expand.
3 This is untrue; they may not be as strong but are certainly less traumatic.
4 Anesthesia is not used in the dilation phase of abortion.

Reproductive Problems

14. **3 Infertility is the inability of a couple to conceive after at least 1 year of adequate exposure to the possibility of pregnancy.** (DC; ED; RP)

1 Infertility may be psychogenic; however, statistics show that physiologic problems are more often the cause.
2 This is untrue; infertility may be corrected, but sterility is irreversible.
4 This may or may not be true; it is possible that there is a problem with both.

15. **4 If the woman had a hemophilic father, she must have had his X chromosome, which carries the recessive gene for hemophilia (if she had had his Y chromosome, she would have been male); since her blood clots normally, her other X chromosome carries the dominant gene for normal blood clotting. With one affected chromosome, 50% of the female offspring will be carriers and 50% of the male offspring will have hemophilia.** (AN; PA; RP)
1 This could happen only if both parents were hemophiliacs.
2 Fifty percent of the offspring are affected—male hemophiliacs or female carriers.
3 Fifty percent of the male children could be normal.

16. **3 High levels of plasma estrogen inhibit pituitary secretion of FSH; this effect appears to be mediated by the hypothalamus and its releasing factors.** (AN; PA; RP)
1 LH (luteinizing hormone) causes ovulation.
2 Lactogenic hormone (prolactin) stimulates lactation.
4 Low concentrations of estrogen may precipitate demineralization of bone.

17. **2 This test determines the number and condition of sperm aspirated from the cervix within 2 hours after coitus.** (DC; PA; RP)
1 The Rubin test determines the patency of the fallopian tubes.
3 The Friedman test was a test done to establish the diagnosis of pregnancy; it has been replaced by more sophisticated tests.
4 The Papanicolaou test is used for the early diagnosis of cervical cancer.

18. **4 This test enables the examiner to visualize the uterus and fallopian tubes and the pelvic organs for reproduction.** (DC; PA; RP)
1 A biopsy is the surgical excision of tissue for diagnostic purposes.
2 A cystoscopy is used to evaluate the urinary bladder.
3 A culdoscopy is the direct examination of female pelvic viscera using an endoscope introduced through a perforation in the vagina.

19. **4 Sperm motility is increased at pH values near neutral or slightly alkaline; a sodium bicarbonate douche will reduce the acidity of fluids in the vagina and help optimize the pH. (IM; PA; RP)**
    1 Estrogen does not alter the pH.
    2 Sulfur does not change the pH in any way.
    3 This would increase the acid content and kill the sperm.

20. **4 At this time, because of increased estrogen levels, the cervical mucus is abundant, and its quality changes in such a way as to optimize sperm survival time. (PL; PA; RP)**
    1 Cervical mucus at this time is still thick and not yet receptive to spermatozoa.
    2 The cervical mucus at this time is not receptive to spermatozoa.
    3 Cervical mucus is destructive to spermatozoa at this time, and sperm penetration cannot occur.

21. **1 A past infection may cause tubal occlusions, most of which are due to postinfection adhesions. (AN; PA; RP)**
    2 This is a tumor of the uterus and does not affect the tube.
    3 This is rare; anomalies of the uterus are more common than those of a tube.
    4 This is possible, but infections in the tube are more common.

22. **3 The proliferation of trophoblastic tissue filled with fluid causes the uterus to enlarge more quickly than it would with a normally growing fetus. (DC; TC; RP)**
    1 Hypertension, not hypotension, often occurs with molar pregnancy.
    2 There is generally no living fetus with a hydatidiform mole.
    4 There may be slight vaginal bleeding without pain.

23. **4 A fallopian tube is unable to contain and sustain a pregnancy to term; as the fertilized ovum grows, there is excessive stretching or rupture of the fallopian tube, causing pain. (DC; TC; RP)**
    1 This would be difficult for the client to identify correctly.
    2 The pain is sudden, intense, knifelike, and usually located on one side.
    3 Leukorrhea and dysuria may be indicative of a vaginal or bladder infection.

24. **4 A symptom of sudden rupture of a fallopian tube is pain on the affected side, usually sudden, excruciating, and spreading over the lower abdomen; sometimes the pain is associated with nausea, vomiting, and diarrhea. (DC; TC; RP)**
    1 There may be some vaginal bleeding with ruptured tubal pregnancy; usually severe pain is present.
    2 There are no contractions since the pregnancy is not uterine.
    3 The pain is exquisite, sharp, and sudden in the lower abdomen.

25. **2 Ectopic pregnancy is one of the leading causes of first-trimester bleeding; unless an embryo and placenta happen to be located in the abdominal cavity, they cannot grow outside the uterus for more than 10 to 12 weeks without showing the classic signs of pressure and bleeding. (AN; TC; RP)**
    1 Abruptio placentae is accompanied by sharp abdominal pain with or without bleeding.
    3 Abdominal cramping pain is present with an incomplete abortion.
    4 This occurs monthly during ovulation without pain or vaginal bleeding; occasionally pain occurs when the follicle ruptures (mittelschmerz), but bleeding does not.

26. **1 Hemorrhage may be due to retained placental tissue or uterine atony; infection may occur from the introduction of contamination into the warm, moist environment, which is favorable to microbial growth. (PL; TC; RP)**
    2 There is no indication at this time that the client has been deprived of fluids or has lost large amounts of blood.
    3 Subinvolution usually occurs after a full-term delivery and may not be obvious for several days.
    4 An "abortion" would occur too early for pregnancy-induced hypertension to be present.

27. **4 About 75% of all spontaneous abortions take place between 8 and 12 weeks of gestation and show embryonic defects. (DC; PA; RP)**
    1 Though possible, physical trauma rarely causes an abortion.
    2 Unresolved stress may lead to congenital defects but is rarely associated with abortion.
    3 Congenital defects are asymptomatic during pregnancy and do not usually cause an abortion.

28. **4 Spotting in the first trimester may indi-cate that the client may be having a threat-ened abortion; any client with the possi-bility of hemorrhage should not be left alone; therefore, admitting this client for observation is safe medical practice; abor-tion is usually inevitable if accompanied by pain and cervical dilation. (AN; PA; RP)**
   1 This may not cause any outward symptoms; only the signs of pregnancy disappearing.
   2 This can be confirmed only if vaginal exami-nation reveals cervical dilation.
   3 This is usually accompanied by severe pain radiating to the shoulder on the affected side.

29. **1 After a spontaneous abortion the fundus should be checked for firmness, which would indicate effective uterine tone; if the uterus is not firm or appears to be hypotonic, hemorrhage may occur; a soft or boggy uterus may also indicate retained placental tissue. (IM; TC; RP)**
   2 The nurse would do this if necessary after checking for fundal firmness.
   3 The priority action is to check for firmness of the fundus and possible bleeding.
   4 This is unnecessary; fetal and placental con-tents are small and expelled easily in bed.

30. **4 A correct and simple definition answers the question and fulfills the client's need to know. (IM; ED; RP)**
   1 This denies the client's right to know.
   2 This is the definition of a missed abortion.
   3 The nurse can independently reinforce and clear misconceptions.

31. **2 The term stillborn is used to describe a dead fetus of more than 24 weeks gesta-tion, weighing 500 or more grams. (DC; ED; RP)**
   1 A fetus of 24 weeks gestation, which is the length of this client's pregnancy, is considered viable.
   3 Incomplete information is given for this con-clusion; only the fetus is mentioned.
   4 This length is indicative of a previable fetus, which is not classified as stillborn.

Healthy Childbearing

32. **2 The chorion is the outermost membrane that helps form the placenta. It develops villi and, through its interaction with the endometrium, becomes part of the pla-centa (AN; PA; HC)**
   1 The amnion is the innermost lining, from which amniotic fluid is secreted.
   3 The yolk sac is part of the inner structure of the blastocyst and is lined by an inner layer of cells, the endoderm; it is unrelated to placen-tal formation.
   4 The allantois is a tubular diverticulum of the posterior part of the embryo's yolk sac; it fuses with the chorion to form the placenta.

33. **4 Progesterone is secreted mainly by the corpus luteum. It helps prepare the endometrium for possible implantation of a fertilized ovum. (AN; PA; HC)**
   1 Endometrium is influenced by progesterone secretion but does not secrete it.
   2 Pituitary gland secretions stimulate the target gland (e.g., corpus luteum of the ovary) to secrete progesterone.
   3 Adrenal cortex secretions contain only minute quantities of progesterone.

34. **3 Progesterone stimulates differentiation of the endometrium into a secretory type of tissue. (AN; PA; HC)**
   1 This is influenced by estrogen.
   2 This is influenced by high levels of luteinizing hormone.
   4 Secondary male characteristics are influenced by testosterone.

35. **2 In the first 7 to 14 days the developing ovum is known as a blastocyst; it is called an embryo until the eighth week; the developing cells are then called a fetus until birth. (AN; PA; HC)**
   1 The fetal heart is heard between the twelfth and twentieth weeks; the developing cells are known as a fetus at the end of the eighth week.
   3 At the time of implantation the group of developing cells is called a blastocyst.
   4 The developing cells are known as a fetus until birth.

36. **2 To allow for the larger intake of air, the normal adaptation is to increase the size of the thoracic cavity. (AN; PA; HC)**
   1 Blood volume is not related to tidal air volume.
   3 Upward displacement would decrease tidal air volume.
   4 There is no change in the height of the rib cage.

37. **3 By this time the fetus and placenta have grown, expanding the size of the uterus. The extended uterus expands into the abdominal cavity. (AN; PA; HC)**
   1 The uterus is still within the pelvic area.
   2 The uterus is still within the pelvic area at this time.
   4 The uterus has already risen out of the pelvis and is expanding further into the abdominal area.

38. **2 The amnion encloses the embryo and the shock-protective amniotic fluid in which the embryo floats. (AN; PA; HC)**
   1 This is another name for the umbilical cord.
   3 The chorion is the outermost membrane; it does not secrete fluid.
   4 The yolk sac contains the stored nutrients of the ovum.

39. **2 The word originates from the Middle English word *quik*, which means alive. (AS; PA; HC)**
   1 Lightening is the descent of the fetus into the birth canal.
   3 Ballottement is the bouncing of the fetus in the amniotic fluid against the examiner's hand.
   4 Engagement occurs when the presenting part is at the level of the ischial spines.

40. **2 This is the period in which the fetus stores deposits of fat. (AN; PA; HC)**
   1 The first trimester is the period of organogenesis, when cells differentiate into major organ systems.
   3 Growth is occurring, but fat deposition does not occur in this period.
   4 This is the period of the blastocyst, when initial cell division takes place.

41. **4 This is the result of a reduced chromosome number, from 46 to 23, readying the sex cells for fertilization. (AN; ED; HC)**
   1 They each have one set of chromosomes (23).
   2 There are only 23 pairs of chromosomes in the nuclei.
   3 The diploid number (46 chromosomes) is reached when fertilization occurs.

42. **3 Follicle-stimulating hormone is secreted from the anterior pituitary gland. (AN; PA; HC)**
   1 This is produced by syncytiotrophoblastic tissue, a preplacental tissue.
   2 Chorionic gonadotropin is secreted by the trophoblastic tissue, which makes up part of the placenta.

4 Chorionic gonadotropin is a precursor of progesterone and is secreted by the trophoblastic tissue.

43. **1 When placental formation is complete, around the twelfth week of pregnancy, it produces progesterone and estrogen. (AN; PA; HC)**
   2 This is not the chief source of progesterone and estrogen; only small amounts are secreted.
   3 The corpus luteum supplies the estrogen and progesterone needed to sustain the pregnancy until the placenta is ready to take over.
   4 FSH is secreted by the anterior hypophysis, but it is not secreted during pregnancy.

44. **2 The umbilical vein carries blood high in oxygen from the placenta and empties it into the fetal vena cava by way of the ductus venosus. (AN; PA; HC)**
   1 The blood in the umbilical artery is more deoxygenated.
   3 The pulmonary artery carries only a small amount of oxygenated blood, since the lungs are not functioning.
   4 This contains a mixture of arterial and venous blood.

45. **4 Nägele's rule is an indirect, noninvasive method for estimating the date of confinement EDC = LMP + 7 days − 3 months + 1 year (AN; ED; HC)**
   1 This is a miscalculation.
   2 Same as answer 1
   3 Same as answer 1.

46. **4 The concentration of melanocyte-stimulating hormone rises from the end of the second month of pregnancy until term. (AN; PA; HC)**
   1 This is related to advancing growth and pressure of the uterus on the bladder.
   2 This is due to increased mucoidal secretions.
   3 High levels of chorionic gonadotropin, secreted by the chorion, are associated with nausea and vomiting.

47. **4 Progesterone acts to reduce contractility of the uterine musculature and to maintain the decidual bed. (AN; PA; HC)**
   1 Elevated progesterone levels would inhibit contractility of the uterine musculature.
   2 Progesterone, not estrogen, inhibits contractions.
   3 This would tend to stimulate contractions but is inhibited by progesterone, not estrogen.

48. **4 A purplish color results from the increased vascularity and blood vessel engorgement of the vagina.** (DC; PA; HC)
    1 This is increased vascularity and cervical softening.
    2 This is softening of the lower uterine segment.
    3 This is softening of the cervix.

49. **2 There is a 30% to 50% increase in maternal blood volume at the end of the first trimester, leading to a decrease in the concentration of hemoglobin and erythrocytes.** (DC; TC; HC)
    1 Dietary intake of iron is unrelated to the development of physiologic anemia of pregnancy.
    3 Erythropoiesis is increased after the first trimester.
    4 Detoxification demands are unchanged during pregnancy.

50. **3 Although pure types are unusual, the normal female pelvis is one most favorable for normal delivery; characteristics include well-rounded inlet, straight side walls, well-formed sacrosciatic notches, good sacral curvature and inclination, movable coccyx, moderately sized ischial spines, and well-rounded suprapubic arches.** (DC; PA; HC)
    1 The normal female pelvis is gynecoid; this describes an android pelvis.
    2 The normal female pelvis is gynecoid; this describes a platypelloid pelvis.
    4 The normal female pelvis is gynecoid; this describes an anthropoid pelvis.

51. **2 The diagonal conjugate is an estimation of the true conjugate with the lower edge of the symphysis pubis used as its anterior point and the sacral promontory posteriorly; the true conjugate uses the upper ridge of the symphysis pubis anteriorly but cannot be measured on a living woman.** (AN; PA; HC)
    1 This is the distance from the upper margin of the symphysis to the sacral promontory.
    3 This is the widest diameter at the inlet.
    4 This is the diameter between the ischial tuberosities.

52. **3 Sonography, based on sound-wave reflection and detection, locates the position of the fetus and placenta prior to insertion of the needle in amniocentesis; this minimizes the potential for fetal damage during the procedure.** (DC; TC; HC)
    1 This is visualization of the fetus through the cervix; it does not aid in placing the needle into the sac.
    2 This was formerly done; however, sonography is now the procedure of choice.
    4 X-ray examinations are contraindicated during pregnancy except at term to determine cephalopelvic disproportion.

53. **3 Before health teaching is instituted, the nurse should ascertain the client's past experiences; they will influence the teaching plan.** (DC; ED; HC)
    1 This answer does not give the client a chance to discuss her feelings about the examination.
    2 This response presupposes a "yes" or "no" answer and does not really give the client an opportunity to discuss it further.
    4 This answer does not give the client a chance to discuss her feelings about the examination; the nurse can only assume that the client's concerns are related to discomfort.

54. **4 A normal cardiopulmonary symptom in pregnancy; caused by increased ventricular rate and elevated diaphragm.** (DC; PA; HC)
    1 This is pathologic, a sign of impending cardiac decompensation.
    2 Same as answer 1.
    3 Same as answer 1.

55. **2 By taking a diet history, the nurse can assess the woman's level of nutritional knowledge and gain clues for appropriate methods of counseling.** (DC; ED; HC)
    1 Normal is too vague a term; the client will need increased protein and caloric intake.
    3 These foods may be too expensive and different from her normal choices, leading to noncompliance.
    4 Salt is no longer limited in normal pregnancy.

56. **4 Chorionic gonadotropin is present in the urine during early pregnancy and is the basis for pregnancy tests; since this hormone appears only during early pregnancy, its presence is taken as a sure sign of pregnancy.** (IM; ED; HC)
    1 Prolactin initiates milk production and is secreted after delivery.
    2 Estrogen is secreted throughout the ovulatory cycle, not just during pregnancy.
    3 This hormone is secreted into the bloodstream at the time of ovulation.

57. **2 Using Nägele's rule, subtract 3 months and add 7 days to the first day of the last menstrual period, April 11. (AN; PA; HC)**
   1 To have an EDB of January 10, the last menstrual period would have begun on April 3.
   3 To have an EDB of February 12, the last menstrual period would have begun on May 5.
   4 Even though the client had some spotting on May 8, the last normal menstrual period began April 11.

58. **1 Menstruation during pregnancy is interrupted because secretion of the ovarian hormones ceases. This response answers the client's question in understandable terms. (IM; ED; HC)**
   2 These hormones are needed to rebuild the layers of cells lining the uterus that are sloughed off during menstruation.
   3 LH stimulates the maturation of a primitive follicle into a vesicular graafian follicle; also promotes secretion of estrogen by the ovary.
   4 This brings about the development of the ova.

59. **4 Chorionic gonadotropin, secreted in large amounts by the placenta during gestation, and the metabolic changes associated with pregnancy can precipitate nausea and vomiting in early pregnancy. (AN; PA; HC)**
   1 Estrogen is elevated throughout pregnancy; symptoms of morning sickness disappear after the first trimester.
   2 Progesterone is elevated throughout pregnancy; symptoms of morning sickness disappear after the first trimester.
   3 The luteinizing hormone is present only during ovulation.

60. **1 Maintaining the sitting position for prolonged periods may constrict the vessels of the legs, particularly in the popliteal spaces, as well as diminish venous return. Walking contracts the muscles of the legs, which apply gentle pressure to the veins in the legs, and promotes venous return. (AN; PA; HC)**
   2 A better means of improving circulation would be to walk about several times each morning and afternoon; she could also keep her legs elevated while sitting at her desk.
   3 If the client is feeling well, there are no contraindications to working until her due date.
   4 Adequate nourishment can be obtained during mealtimes; the client does not require extra nutrition breaks.

61. **4 The nurse should become informed about the cultural eating patterns of clients so that foods containing the essential nutrients, which are part of these dietary patterns, will be included in the diet. (AN; PS; HC)**
   1 Fluid retention is only one component of weight gain; growth of the baby, placenta, breasts, etc., also contribute to weight gain.
   2 Calories and nutrients are increased during pregnancy.
   3 Pregnancy diets are not specific; they are merely composed of the essential nutrients.

62. **2 The uterus and bladder occupy the pelvic cavity and lie very closely together; as the uterus enlarges with the growing fetus, it impinges on the space normally occupied by the bladder and thereby diminishes bladder capacity. (IM; ED; HC)**
   1 Atony would not cause frequency; more likely it would lead to retention.
   3 This would lead to incontinence rather than frequency.
   4 This is an unlikely occurrence; the uterus would not impinge on that area.

63. **1 Nausea and vomiting in the morning occur in almost 50% of all pregnancies. Eating dry crackers before getting out of bed in the morning is a simple remedy that may provide relief. (IM; ED; HC)**
   2 Increasing fat intake does not relieve the nausea.
   3 Two small meals and a snack at noon would not meet the nutritional needs of a pregnant woman, nor would it relieve nausea. Some women find that eating five or six small meals daily instead of three large ones is helpful.
   4 This is not helpful; separating fluids from solids at mealtime is more advisable.

64. **2 Because of changes in the hormone levels, morning sickness seldom persists beyond the first trimester. (IM; ED; HC)**
   1 It is still present at this time; it is related to the high level of chorionic gonadotropin.
   3 Same as answer 1.
   4 It usually ends at the end of the third month, when the chorionic gonadotropin level falls.

65. **1 The pressure exerted anywhere in a mass of fluid in a closed container is transmitted undiminished throughout all parts of the fluid and in all directions. (IM; ED; HC)**
   2 These are laws dealing with motion, not pressure.

3 This is a theory dealing with relativity, not pressure.

4 This is a principle dealing with the displacement of fluid, not pressure.

66. **4 This is true; it allows the client to discuss her feelings and participate in her care. (IM; ED; HC)**

1 This is within the scope of the nurse's information; this also may cause the client to worry that something is seriously wrong.

2 This statement cuts off communication and denies the client's feelings.

3 The client has already told the nurse how she feels.

67. **1 When an Rh-negative mother carries an Rh-positive fetus there is a risk of maternal antibodies against Rh-positive blood; antibodies cross the placenta and destroy the fetal RBCs. (IM; PA; HC)**

2 Testing for Rh factor will not provide information about protein metabolism deficiency.

3 Physiologic bilirubinemia is a common occurrence in newborns; it is not associated with the Rh factor.

4 Determination of the lecithin-sphingomyelin ratio, not the Rh factor, may provide information about the risk of developing RDS.

68. **2 The first trimester is the period when all major organs are being laid down; drugs, alcohol, and tobacco may cause major defects. (IM; ED; HC)**

1 Cutting down is insufficient; these teratogens should be eliminated.

3 Even 30 ml of alcohol is considered harmful; baby aspirin is now given to some women who are considered at risk for pregnancy-induced hypertension.

4 Drugs, unless absolutely necessary, should be avoided throughout pregnancy; but the first trimester is most significant.

69. **4 This pigmentation is caused by the anterior pituitary hormone, melanotropin, which increases during pregnancy. (IM; ED; HC)**

1 During pregnancy, ovarian activity is very quiet because of the feedback mechanism.

2 Hyperthyroidism is manifested by increased temperature, pulse, and respirations and a fine hand tremor.

3 Hyperactivity of the adrenal glands is manifested by symptoms of Cushing's syndrome.

70. **1 Nausea and vomiting of pregnancy can be relieved with small snacks of protein before bedtime to slow digestion; presently SeaBands (used to prevent seasickness) are being used successfully on some women. (IM; TC; HC)**

2 An antacid may affect electrolyte balance; also this will not help morning sickness.

3 This is unsound advice, since both fetus and mother need nourishment.

4 Medications in the first trimester are contraindicated; this is the period of organogenesis, and congenital anomalies could result.

71. **1 The average weight gain during pregnancy is 11.9 to 15.8 kg; of this, the fetus accounts for 3.18 to 3.6 kg, the blood volume 1.4 to 2.0 kg, fluid retention 1.8 to 2.7 kg, amniotic fluid 1.0 to 1.6 kg, uterus 1.0 to 1.6 kg, placenta 0.7 to 0.9 kg, breasts 0.5 to 0.7 kg, and fat 1.8 to 3.0 kg. (IM; ED; HC)**

2 Fluid retention accounts for about 20% to 25% of weight gain.

3 Metabolic alterations do not cause a weight gain.

4 Increased blood volume accounts for about 12% to 16% of weight gain.

72. **4 A sudden, sharp increase in weight near the twentieth week of pregnancy may indicate water retention and the beginning of preeclampsia. (IM; TC; HC)**

1 This is untrue; weight gain is necessary to ensure adequate nutrition for the fetus.

2 There is no hard-and-fast number of pounds that the client should gain, and low-calorie diets may be harmful.

3 This closes off communication; it does not allow the client to ask more questions about weight gain.

73. **3 The Committee on Maternal Nutrition of the National Research Council recommends a weight gain of at least 11.3 kg during pregnancy; inadequate nutrition during pregnancy results in underweight babies. (IM; ED; HC)**

1 The cause of stillbirth is not actually known; dieting is not recommended.

2 Dieting is absolutely forbidden during pregnancy and can result in congenital anomalies.

4 There is a theory that an inadequate intake of protein is related to PIH, but it has not been totally proved.

74. 2 The FHR is usually between 120 and 160 beats per minute. This is to be expected normally, and the mother should be made aware of this fact. (IM; ED; HC)

1 This is too variable; the normal heart rate for a fetus is 120 to 160 beats per minute.

3 To accommodate the oxygen needs of the fetus, the heart rate is rapid.

4 This is unnecessary information; the mother should be informed only of that which is normal.

75. 1 Frequent changes in position are important for good circulation; moving about is a form of exercise that will promote circulation. (PL; ED; HC)

2 Added nourishment should be part of her regular mealtimes; snacking may lead to poor appetite at meals.

3 This is not true; clients may work until the day of delivery.

4 Therapeutic elastic stockings are designed to reduce the chance of the formation of thrombus in immobilized clients but are not indicated for healthy clients such as Mrs. Mann.

76. 4 Intact membranes act as a barrier against organisms that may cause an intrauterine infection. (IM; TC; HC)

1 This is common because of increased production of mucus containing exfoliated vaginal epithelial cells; intercourse is not contraindicated.

2 This may occur during sex but there is no literature indicating that it is harmful for the fetus.

3 Intercourse is not contraindicated if membranes are intact; modification of sexual positions may be needed because of an enlarged abdomen after the thirtieth week.

77. 2 The increase of estrogen during pregnancy causes hyperplasia of the vaginal mucosa, which leads to increased production of mucus by the endocervical glands. The mucus contains exfoliated epithelial cells. (IM; ED; HC)

1 Increased metabolism leads to many systemic changes but does not increase vaginal discharge.

3 Normal functioning of the glands, which lubricate the vagina during intercourse, remains unchanged during pregnancy.

4 There is no additional supply of sodium chloride to the cells during pregnancy.

78. 2 In this case the nurse has knowledge of dietary needs and their relation to the client's well-being during pregnancy. (EV; ED; HC)

1 Immediate planning based on the nurse's knowledge of proper diet is better intervention.

3 Not all preferences can be included; the diet should contain normal sodium, high protein, and sufficient calories.

4 Unless the nurse thought there was a need for medical intervention, the nurse could supervise prenatal care.

79. 3 Fluids, proteins, and salt should not be restricted, for they are necessary to the well-being of the mother and fetus; elevation of the extremities several times daily is recommended to decrease the edema. (IM; ED; HC)

1 Salt is not limited during pregnancy.

2 Same as answer 1.

4 Diuretics can be harmful and are not used during pregnancy.

80. 3 When the membranes rupture, the potential for infection is increased, and when the contractions are 5 to 8 minutes apart, they are usually of sufficient force to warrant medical supervision. Therefore, for the safety of the mother and fetus, the mother should go to the hospital. (PL; PA; HC)

1 This is too early; the client still has a great deal of time and would be better off with her family and moving about at home.

2 These may be early signs of labour or signs of posterior fetal position.

4 This is indicative of advanced labour, and the client may have difficulty getting to the hospital at this time.

81. 1 Progressive dilation of the cervix is the most accurate indication of true labour. (DC; PA; HC)

2 Contractions may not begin until 24 to 48 hours later.

3 This is untrue; contractions will increase with activity.

4 Contractions of true labour persist in any position.

82. 2 Some mothers will respond to mores and pressures by trying to nurse in spite of the fact that they would prefer to give the baby a bottle. The nurse should elicit more information before responding. (IM; PS; HC)

1 This is untrue; successful breastfeeding requires mastery, and many women are unable to do this.

3 Although this is true, the mother's statement indicates some concerns about breastfeeding and should be further explored.

4 The baby's sucking and emptying the breasts will determine the amount of milk.

83. **4 Most average-sized babies regulate themselves on an approximate 3- to 4-hour schedule. However, wide variations do exist. (IM; ED; HC)**

1 Some of the episodes of crying do not indicate that the baby is hungry; the mother will learn the difference.

2 It is best to allow the baby to set the schedule; usually close to the hospital routine.

3 Although this is true, this does not answer the mother's question concerning the time for doing things.

84. **2 During pregnancy, secretion of milk is inhibited; sucking can cause uterine contractions. (IM; ED; HC)**

1 Breastfeeding with mastitis is not always contraindicated; the baby already has the organism in the mouth, and nursing will decrease the mother's discomfort.

3 Breastfeeding is not contraindicated with inverted nipples, since a breast shield can provide mild suction to help pull out a nipple.

4 Breastfeeding is not always contraindicated with this disorder.

85. **1 This is the area through which the presenting part must enter; if it is too small it is called cephalopelvic disproportion and vaginal delivery is not possible. (AN; PA; HC)**

2 This is the narrowest measurement.

3 The measurement of the pelvic floor is not involved with the fetus' descent into the birth canal.

4 This is a measurement of the pelvic outlet.

86. **1 The contractions become stronger, last longer, and are erratic during this stage; the intervals during the contractions are shorter than the contractions themselves; much concentration and effort are needed by the mother to pace herself with each contraction. (DC; PA; HC)**

2 This is not true; administration of an analgesic or anesthetic at this point could reduce the effectiveness of labour and depress the fetus.

3 Even clients who have been adequately prepared will experience these behaviors during the transition stage.

4 There is no indication that any abnormality is developing.

87. **3 By 36 weeks gestation, normal amniotic fluid is colorless with small particles of vernix caseosa present. (DC; PA; HC)**

1 Dark-amber fluid suggests the presence of bilirubin, an ominous sign.

2 Greenish-yellow fluid may indicate the presence of meconium and suggests fetal distress.

4 Cloudy fluid suggests the presence of purulent material, and greenish-yellow may indicate the presence of meconium.

88. **4 Immediately following delivery the fundus is found midway between the symphysis pubis and the umbilicus. (DC; PA; HC)**

1 This is untrue; the fundus is easily palpable midway between the symphysis pubis and the umbilicus.

2 The fundus never gets this high.

3 The fundus is not this high until 1 hour after delivery; if the uterus is deviated to the right, it usually indicates bladder distention.

89. **1 Because the client is attached to a machine and movement may alter the tracings, movement is discouraged. (AN; PA; HC)**

2 Placement of the monitor leads does not interfere with the administration of sedatives.

3 Lamaze techniques work well with a monitor.

4 An external monitor does not necessitate more frequent vaginal examinations.

90. **2 Characteristics of the midphase of labour for the primiparous client include regular contractions 30 to 45 seconds long and 3 to 5 minutes apart, station of the presenting part at +1 to +2, and pink to bloody show in moderate amount. (AN; PA; HC)**

1 Contractions are less frequent in the early phase, and dilation is not so advanced.

3 In this phase, dilation is 8 to 10 cm, and contractions are more frequent.

4 This terminology is not appropriate for a phase of labour.

91. **3 Transcervical amniotomy (artificial rupture of the membranes) requires that the cervix be soft, partially effaced, and slightly dilated with the presenting part engaged or engaging; this client would meet these criteria, as demonstrated by the bloody show and the head at +1. (PL; PA; HC)**
  1 A tap-water enema would be ineffective for inducing labour.
  2 IM injection of oxytocin is extremely dangerous because of the physician's inability to control the effects of the drug; oxytocin by intravenous infusion is considered safe as long as maternal and fetal monitoring is continuous.
  4 Prostaglandins are used to soften and ripen the cervix. This client has a bloody show indicating that her cervical plug has already been passed and the cervix is no longer hard; in addition prostaglandins are an expensive and uncomfortable way of inducing labour.

92. **3 The client is experiencing the expected discomforts of labour; the nurse should initiate measures that will promote relaxation. (IM; PA; HC)**
  1 During the last phase of labour, pushing is unavoidable; the client is in early labour, and should not push at this time.
  2 The client is not receptive to teaching at this time; all energy is being directed inward.
  4 There is no evidence at this time that the client is losing excessive blood (hemorrhage).

93. **3 Contractions are stronger and more regular when the woman is standing; also, during walking the diameter of the pelvic inlet increases and allows for easier entrance of the head into the pelvis. (IM; PA; HC)**
  1 This denies the nurse's understanding of the physiology of labour.
  2 This is untrue; contractions of true labour are enhanced when the mother walks about.
  4 Timing can continue even if the client walks around.

94. **1 When the membranes rupture, there is always the possibility of a prolapsed cord leading to fetal distress, which would manifest itself in a slowed fetal heartbeat. (IM; TC; HC)**
  2 This is unnecessary unless there is a marked change in the FHR.
  3 This is done routinely throughout the entire labour process; at this point, fetal status takes priority.

4 This is regularly done before and after the membranes rupture; however, fetal status takes priority.

95. **3 The client is in early labour, and the first priority of care is to establish a trusting relationship with her and her husband. This will help to allay their anxiety. (IM; PS; HC)**
  1 This may be necessary later; however, it is not the first priority.
  2 The history should be taken from the client as long as she is capable of providing it.
  4 This is not an initial priority; the physician probably knows the mother is on her way.

96. **3 This slow, deep breathing expands the spaces between the ribs and raises the abdominal muscles, allowing room for the uterus to expand and preventing painful pressure of the uterus against the abdominal wall. (IM; ED; HC)**
  1 Panting is used to halt or delay the pushing out of the baby's head before complete dilation.
  2 Pelvic rocking is used during pregnancy and the puerperal period; it is not feasible during labour.
  4 Athletic chest breathing is not one of the exercises used in this stage of labour.

97. **3 The application of back pressure combined with frequent positional changes will help alleviate the discomfort. (IM; PA; HC)**
  1 Although this may be comfortable for some individuals, rubbing the back and alternating positions are more universally effective.
  2 The supine position places increased pressure on the back and often aggravates the pain.
  4 Neuromuscular control exercises are used to teach selective relaxation in childbirth classes; they will not relieve back pain.

98. **2 Gastric peristalsis often ceases during periods of stress. Abdominal contractions put pressure on the stomach and can cause nausea and vomiting, increasing the risk of aspiration. (IM; TC; HC)**
  1 Gastric activity and digestion cease during periods of stress.
  3 Same as answer 1.
  4 Although food may cause dyspepsia, the primary reason for withholding it is to prevent aspiration.

99. **4 The physiologic intensification of labour occurring during transition is caused by a**

greater energy expenditure and increased pressure on the stomach; this results in feelings of fatigue, discouragement, and nausea. (DC; PA; HC)

1 This is unclear terminology; it does not indicate the specific time of labour.

2 This stage is from delivery of the fetus to delivery of the placenta; the mother does not experience any physiologic symptoms.

3 This stage is from full dilation to expulsion; a heavy bloody show and pushing are evident at this time.

100. **4 As the uterus rises into the abdominal cavity, the uterine ligaments become elongated and hypertrophied; raising both legs at the same time limits the tension placed on these ligaments. (IM; TC; HC)**

1 Lifting the legs simultaneously does not negatively affect circulation in the legs.

2 There is already pressure on the perineum from the baby's head; this maneuver places tension on the uterine ligaments.

3 There is no effect on the fascia with this maneuver.

101. **2 The bulging perineum indicates that the fetal head is on the pelvic floor and birth is imminent. (EV; PA; HC)**

1 This is a sign that occurs during transition or the beginning of the second stage; the second stage lasts approximately 1 hour in a primipara.

3 Same as answer 1.

4 Same as answer 1.

102. **2 Uterine tetany would result from the use of oxytocin to induce labour. Since oxytocin promotes powerful uterine contractions, exogenous administration of this hormone may induce uterine tetany, which does not optimize progression of labor and may restrict fetal blood flow. (EV; TC; HC)**

1 Severe pain is associated with intense contractions.

3 This is unrelated to uterine contractions.

4 This is not likely to occur unless the baby is in the breech position.

103. **1 The contractions in this phase of labour are expulsive in nature; having the client push or bear down with the glottis open will hasten expulsion. (IM; PA; HC)**

2 Blowing is encouraged to slow down pushing; she should be encouraged to push.

3 Contractions are now frequent and intense; the client is anxious to complete the labor process; she will be unable to relax.

4 The client should be pushing; panting will prevent this.

104. **3 In reporting progress in the descent of the presenting part, the level of the tip of the ischial spines is considered to be zero, and the position of the bony prominence of the fetal head is described in centimeters—minus (above the spines) or plus (below the spines). (EV; PA; HC)**

1 This would be referred to as crowning and would be designated as +5.

2 This is designated by the term floating, meaning that the presenting part has not yet engaged.

4 Minus one (−1) would indicate that the head is above the ischial spines.

105. **4 A neat surgical incision is usually easier to repair and quicker to heal than an irregular laceration. (IM; TC; HC)**

1 Just the opposite; upon healing it will tighten up the perineum.

2 An episiotomy will contribute to rather than limit postpartal discomfort.

3 This may or may not influence birth trauma to the fetus; it usually reduces trauma to the mother.

106. **1 Physical assessment is a form of data collection. It is the first step in planning care. (DC; TC; HC)**

2 Implementation is not the initial action.

3 Same as answer 2.

4 This is too soon for medical intervention; other nursing measures should be tried first.

107. **1 Blood loss depletes the normal cellular response to infection; trauma provides an excellent medium for bacteria to grow. (DC; TC; HC)**

2 Preeclampsia is generally not a predisposing cause of postpartum infection.

3 These may create problems if hemorrhage occurs since the hemoglobin and hematocrit are already low.

4 Endogenous infection is rare; infection is usually caused by outside contamination; trauma and the denuded placental site do contribute to the development of infection.

108. **4 Diaphoresis is a normal adaptation of the postpartum period and does not relate to bladder distention; it is caused by the reduction of the antidiuretic hormone, leading to profuse perspiration. (AN; PA; HC)**
   1 This may follow anesthesia and cause retention.
   2 Postpartum bleeding may occur if the uterus is impeded from involuting because of a full bladder.
   3 Stasis of urine and infection can occur when urinary retention is present.

109. **1 Retention of urine with overflow will be manifested in small, frequent voidings. The bladder should be palpated for distention. (AN; PA; HC)**
   2 There should be large amounts of urine voided because of the increased fluid volume at this time.
   3 An elevated temperature with urinary symptoms would be indicative of impending infection.
   4 This is untrue; more circulating fluid is present, causing an increased output.

110. **2 A distended bladder will easily displace the fundus upward and laterally. (AN; PA; HC)**
   1 This would be manifested by a slow contraction and uterine descent into the pelvis.
   3 If this were true, in addition to being displaced, the uterus would be soft and boggy and vaginal bleeding would be heavy.
   4 From this assessment the nurse cannot make a judgment about over-stretched uterine ligaments.

111. **2 The fundus descends one fingerbreadth per day from the day after delivery; lochia serosa begins to flow on the fifth day. (AN; PA; HC)**
   1 The fundus would be one to three fingers below the umbilicus (one fingerbreadth per day).
   3 The fundus would be descending into the pelvis at this time.
   4 The fundus would be within the pelvis and indiscernible at this time.

112. **1 Prolactin is the hormone from the anterior pituitary that stimulates mammary gland secretion. Progesterone and estrogen are ovarian hormones that influence breast development and other female sexual characteristics. (AN; PA; HC)**
   2 Oxytocin, a posterior pituitary hormone, stimulates the uterine musculature to contract and causes the let-down reflex.
   3 Estrogen is not a pituitary hormone; it is secreted by the ovaries and placenta.
   4 Progesterone is not a pituitary hormone; it is secreted by the corpus luteum of the ovary.

113. **3 If the woman perceives a negative attitude from others, she may be tense and let-down may not occur; a positive attitude of others toward breastfeeding promotes relaxation and let-down. (AN; PA; HC)**
   1 This has no influence on lactation.
   2 Same as answer 1.
   4 Milk or milk product intake during pregnancy has little influence on lactation.

114. **1 Heat causes vasodilation and an increased blood supply to the area. (IM; TC; HC)**
   2 Sitz baths do not soften the incision site.
   3 Cleansing is done with a perineal bottle and cleansing solution immediately after voiding and defecating.
   4 Neither relaxation nor tightening of the rectal sphincter will increase healing of an episiotomy.

115. **4 There is extensive activation of the blood clotting factor after delivery; this, together with immobility, trauma, or sepsis, encourages thromboembolization, which can be limited through activity. (IM; TC; HC)**
   1 This can be accomplished by turning the client from side to side and encouraging her to deep breathe and cough.
   2 Tone would be improved by regular emptying and filling of the bladder.
   3 Abdominal muscle tone will be improved with exercise over the next 6 weeks.

116. **3 Cow's milk is diluted with water and has sugar added to make it resemble human milk. (IM; ED; HC)**
   1 Cow's milk contains more calcium.
   2 Cow's milk contains more protein and more calcium.
   4 Cow's milk contains more protein and less carbohydrate.

117. **3 Frequently the emotional excitement of going home will diminish lactation and/or the let-down reflex for a brief period. When the mother has knowledge that this may happen and how to cope with it, the problem is apt to be a minor one and easily overcome. (IM; ED; HC)**

1 Many factors (stress) inhibit lactation, and the client should be aware of this; false reassurance.

2 This supply may diminish or stop under stress factors; false reassurance.

4 This response lacks an explanation of why it happens as well as concrete instructions for remedying the situation.

118. **4 Soap irritates, cracks, and dries breasts and nipples, making it difficult for the baby to suck. (EV; ED; HC)**

1 The client should empty the breast at each feeding to keep milk flowing.

2 This is a permissible and often-used technique of breastfeeding.

3 The breasts should be washed before feeding to remove encrustations and microorganisms.

119. **3 Forcing the family to be involved at the nurse's convenience would interfere with the development of a productive relationship and affect cooperation of the family. (PL; ED; HC)**

1 This would be an inconvenient time for the mother and interfere with productivity.

2 The father should be included in the visit if at all possible.

4 This may be at a time that would be inconvenient for the family and thus interfere with productivity.

120. **2 The most likely cause is a disturbance in the ratio of calcium to phosphorus, with the amount of serum calcium reduced and the serum phosphorus increased; milk is an excellent source of calcium. (IM; PA; HC)**

1 Leg cramps are usually related to low calcium intake, not hypercalcemia.

3 Elevated potassium levels are very serious; they are not manifested by leg cramps.

4 A low potassium level is not a usual occurrence; it is not improved by ingestion of leafy vegetables.

Normal Newborn

121. **3 Two umbilical arteries arise from the fetus and go to the placenta, where waste products are exchanged for oxygen and nutrients and then returned via one umbilical vein to the baby. (DC; PA; NN)**

1 This is an anomalous number; there are two arteries and one vein.

2 Same as answer 1.

4 Same as answer 1.

122. **3 The increased pulmonary blood flow raises the pressure in the left atrium and functionally forces the septum to close the foramen ovale. (AN; PA; NN)**

1 There is an increased aortic blood flow.

2 This is caused by increased pressure in the left atrium.

4 There is decreased pressure in the right atrium.

123. **4 There is anatomic obliteration of the lumen by fibrous proliferation, leading to the term ligamentum arteriosum. (AN; PA; NN)**

1 This refers to the ductus venosus after it closes.

2 This is a descriptive term meaning a long and round ligament.

3 There is no such vessel.

124. **3 This immunity is developed from an antigen-antibody response in the mother that is passed to the fetus. (AN; PA; NN)**

1 This is acquired by an individual in response to a disease or an infection.

2 This is acquired by an individual in response to small amounts of antigenic material (e.g., vaccination).

4 This is conferred by the injection of antibodies already prepared in another host.

125. **1 Position the baby with head lower than chest and rub the infant's back to stimulate crying so he or she can oxygenate the lungs. (IM; PA; NN)**

2 This is not the priority at the present moment; the uterus still contains placenta and will not contract.

3 There is no need for haste in cutting the cord; a clear airway is the priority.

4 There is no time, and the mother will not be able to cooperate with a move to the stretcher.

126. **1 The Nursing Process requires nurses to assess and plan care. (EV; TC; NN)**

2 This is physical assessment, not medical diagnosis, and is within the nurse's role.

3 Assessment should not differ if done by the nurse.

4 Fortunately not true, since the physician may not be present; the nurse is capable of making a physical assessment.

127. **1 Heart rate is vital and is the most critical observation in Apgar scoring at birth. (DC; PA; NN)**
  2 Respiratory effort rather than rate is included in the Apgar score; the rate is very erratic.
  3 This may or may not be present at this time and is not a part of Apgar scoring.
  4 This should be assessed later, but is not a part of Apgar scoring.

128. **4 This sequence is least disturbing. Touching for pulse and inserting the thermometer increase anxiety and cause elevated vital signs. (DC; ED; NN)**
  1 Measuring the respirations should precede the pulse because the vital signs will change when the baby is touched.
  2 Temperature should be measured last.
  3 Respirations should be measured first, but temperature should be measured after the pulse.

129. **3 The heart rate varies with activity; crying will increase the rate, whereas deep sleep will lower it; a rate between 120 and 160 is within normal range. (DC; PA; NN)**
  1 Heart rates below 120 are considered bradycardia; above 180, tachycardia.
  2 The normal heart rate is between 120 and 160.
  4 A heart rate below 120 is considered bradycardia.

130. **2 The respiratory rate is associated with activity and can be as rapid as 60 breaths per minute; over 60 breaths per minute is considered tachypneic in the infant. (DC; PA; NN)**
  1 Respirations may go up to 60 with activity.
  3 Any respiratory rate above 60 is considered to be tachypneic.
  4 This respiratory rate is considered to be tachypneic in the newborn.

131. **2 Normally the newborn's breathing is abdominal and irregular in depth and rhythm; the rate ranges from 40 to 50 breaths per minute. (DC; PA; NN)**
  1 Newborns' respirations are usually irregular.
  3 Newborns' respirations are abdominal in origin.
  4 Newborns' respirations are irregular and abdominal in origin.

132. **1 Milia occur commonly, are not indicative of any illness, and eventually disappear. (AN; ED; NN)**
  2 Lanugo is fine, downy hair.
  3 This is a lay term for milia; it would not be used in charting.
  4 These are bluish-black spots on the buttocks that present on darkly pigmented infants.

133. **3 The tonic neck reflex (fencing position) is a spontaneous postural reflex of the newborn that may or may not be present during the first days of life; once apparent, it persists until the third month. (DC; PA; NN)**
  1 This is the startle reflex.
  2 This is a demonstration of muscle tone while held prone and suspended in midair.
  4 This is a normal, expected reflex in the neonate.

134. **4 Changes in equilibrium stimulate this neurologic reflex in an infant under the age of 6 months; the movements should be bilateral and symmetric; a loud noise causes the same reaction (startle reflex), but using noise as a stimulus really tests hearing. (DC; ED; NN)**
  1 This tests for the grasp reflex, not the Moro reflex.
  2 This tests for the Babinski reflex, not the Moro reflex.
  3 Although this tests the Moro reflex, it is not the best way; really tests the baby's hearing.

135. **3 The Moro reflex is a sudden extension and abduction of the arms at the shoulders and spreading of the fingers, with the index finger and thumb forming the letter "C"; this is followed by flexion and adduction; the legs may weakly flex, and the infant may cry vigorously. (EV; ED; NN)**
  1 This is only part of the normal Moro response; it should be accompanied by abduction and spreading of the fingers.
  2 The reflex is abduction.
  4 The legs generally flex weakly.

136. **4 Injury to the brachial plexus, clavicle, or humerus prevents the abductive and adductive movements of an upper extremity. (AN; ED; NN)**
  1 Children with Down syndrome exhibit a normal Moro reflex.
  2 This is not usually associated; however, if the cochlea is undeveloped or the eighth cranial (vestibulocochlear) nerve were injured, it would affect equilibrium and response to the test.

3 These injuries usually cause a symmetric loss of the Moro reflex.

137. **3 Bacteria, especially *Escherichia coli*, produce substances necessary to synthesize prothrombin. (AN; PA; NN)**
   1 This is an orange bile pigment produced by the breakdown of hemoglobin.
   2 Bile salts are manufactured in the liver, not synthesized by bacteria.
   4 This is secreted by the gastric glands, not synthesized by bacteria.

138. **3 Teaching the mother by example is a nonthreatening approach that allows her to proceed at her own pace. (PL; ED; NN)**
   1 Mothers need demonstration of appropriate mothering skills, not just a discussion.
   2 Learning does not occur by schedule; questions must be answered as they arise.
   4 Satisfying the mother's needs will allow her to develop reserves to give the child; plan should promote security in her role and facilitate more independent caregiving.

139. **1 There is a sensitive period in the first minutes or hours after birth during which it is important, for later interpersonal development to be normal, that the mother and father have close contact with their new infant. (IM; ED; NN)**
   2 Rooming-in is not usually immediate; it occurs once the mother is in the postpartal unit.
   3 Taking-in is a psychologic behavior described by Reva Rubin that occurs during the first 2 postpartal days.
   4 Taking-hold is a psychologic behavior described by Reva Rubin that occurs after the third postpartal day.

140. **4 Some maternal oxytocin crosses the placenta and induces the secretion of fluids that have accumulated in the fetal breasts (sometimes called witch's milk). (IM; ED; NN)**
   1 This is usually manifested in the oral mucosa as thrush (white, adherent patches).
   2 Evidence of infection would not appear so rapidly after birth.
   3 This is uncommon and usually undetectable in the newborn period.

141. **4 Human milk contains 42% carbohydrate, and cow's milk 30% carbohydrate; the carbohydrate in cow's milk is further diluted**
   when water is added to the formula, so additional sugar is required to supplement it. (IM; ED; NN)
   1 The sugar in cow's milk is lactose, a simple sugar.
   2 The sugar in cow's milk is assimilated well.
   3 The calorie content is about the same, 20 calories/ounce.

142. **2 Infants require approximately 160.6 ml of fluid per kilo of body weight each day. As the infant is 2.7 Kg, he would require 2.7 × 160.6 = 433.6 ml per day. Given feedings are every 4 hours this would entail 6 feedings of 433.6 ml ÷ 6 = 72 ml per feed. (PL; PA; NN)**
   1 This is too little to maintain adequate fluid intake for an infant this size.
   3 This is too much and will overhydrate an infant this size.
   4 Same as answer 3.

143. **3 The cardiac sphincter in the newborn is poorly developed; if the stomach is too full, formula backs up through the sphincter and the infant regurgitates. (IM; ED; NN)**
   1 This may cause cramping or colic; it usually does not cause regurgitation.
   2 This would be manifested by projectile vomiting, not regurgitation.
   4 This is a nondescriptive answer; the position is not described; it might happen if the baby were upside down.

144. **4 The antibodies in human milk provide the newborn infant with immunity against all or most of the pathogens that the mother has encountered. (IM; ED; NN)**
   1 This is present in commercial formulas.
   2 Complex carbohydrates are not required by the infant.
   3 Same as answer 1.

145. **2 Breast milk is digested faster than formula. Breastfed infants therefore become hungry sooner. (PL; ED; NN)**
   1 An infant may want to nurse hourly if irritable, but this is not a usual feeding pattern.
   3 A breastfed newborn must be fed more often than this.
   4 All infants must be fed more often than this.

High-Risk Pregnancy

146. **4 X-ray pelvimetry is more definitive than digital pelvimetry, but because of radiation hazards it should be limited to clients in labor in whom it is clearly essential to the outcome of pregnancy. (DC; TC; HP)**
1 This is done by external measurement; it is not an accurate assessment.
2 This is done to determine fetal acidosis.
3 This is a test of amniotic fluid; it does not reveal the actual size of the fetus or diameters of the pelvis.

147. **4 If the fetus is in a compromised state, it does not contribute to the synthesis of estriol; consequently estriol levels fall, indicating a need for intervention. (DC; TC; HP)**
1 Chorionic gonadotropin is the hormone tested for in pregnancy tests.
2 Fetal demise is generally preceded by lowered estriol levels.
3 This is untrue; elevated estriol levels indicate healthy fetal placental functioning.

148. **1 The greatest danger of drug-induced malformation is during the first trimester of pregnancy, since this is the period of organogenesis. (AN; TC; HP)**
2 This may cause problems, but organogenesis has already taken place by the second trimester.
3 The fetus is totally formed at this time, and damage from drugs would not be likely.
4 Drugs should be avoided, but the first trimester (period of organogenesis) is the most critical.

149. **3 Heavy cigarette smoking or continued exposure to a smoke-filled environment causes both maternal and fetal vasoconstriction, resulting in fetal growth retardation and increased fetal and infant mortality. (IM; ED; HP)**
1 Smoking causes vasoconstriction; permeability of the placenta to smoke is irrelevant.
2 There is no concrete evidence that smoking relieves tension; this is not a factor in the situation described.
4 The fetal and maternal circulations are separate; the answer is not related to the question.

150. **3 High levels of chorionic gonadotropin frequently are associated with severe vomiting of pregnancy, especially in the presence of hydatidiform mole and often in twin pregnancy. (AN; PA; HP)**
1 Polyhydramnios (excessive amniotic fluid) is associated with multiple gestation; maternal dehydration is generally associated with hyperemesis gravidarum.
2 Cholecystitis is unrelated to this problem; hyperemesis gravidarum is due to HCG.
4 This is associated with vomiting; undigested food remains in the stomach, which leads to a reflexive action and vomiting; this is common but not severe in early pregnancy.

151. **4 The Oxytocin Challenge Test provides data concerning the circulatory-respiratory reserve of the fetoplacental unit; a positive OCT usually indicates uteroplacental insufficiency; an OCT is contraindicated unless there is a specific indication of a problem. (PL; TC; HP)**
1 An OCT would be contraindicated in placenta previa.
2 This is contraindicated; it might accelerate the labor further.
3 This is not an indication; the OCT would be of no help in diagnosing a recurrence.

152. **1 Threatened premature labor, a history of premature births, nipple stimulation, or administration of oxytocin too early in pregnancy can cause uterine contractions and premature delivery. (AN; TC; HP)**
2 The Oxytocin Challenge Test (OCT) would be indicated because of the influence of hypertension on the placental circulation.
3 The Oxytocin Challenge Test (OCT) would be indicated to determine the fetus' response to labor.
4 Same as answer 3.

153. **2 About two thirds of neonatal deaths are caused by prematurity; there appears to be a correlation with teenage pregnancy, lack of prenatal care, nonwhite mothers, and chronic health problems. (DC; PA; HP)**
1 Atelectasis may occur from respiratory distress, which in turn is associated with prematurity, the leading cause of death.
3 Most babies who die from congenital heart disease die after the neonatal period.
4 This usually occurs as a result of prematurity, the leading cause of death.

154. **4 Pyelonephritis often causes premature labor, leading to increased neonatal morbidity and mortality. (IM; TC; HP)**

1 Fluids should be increased; the inflammatory process may lead to fever, dehydration, and an accumulation of toxins.

2 Albuminuria occurs with pregnancy-induced hypertension and is not accompanied by pain or flank tenderness; the client's symptoms are indicative of a kidney infection.

3 An inflammatory, not a degenerative, kidney process is present.

155. **3 Medical supervision requires treatment with an appropriate antibiotic for 2 to 3 weeks until two negative cultures are obtained; retreatment may be necessary if there is a recurrence; recurring pyelitis often leads to preterm birth.** (PL; PA; HP)

1 Signs of preeclampsia occur spontaneously; it is not preceded by specific infections.

2 A low-protein diet would inhibit good fetal development and is contraindicated in pregnancy.

4 Pelvic inflammatory disease is associated with infections of the genital, not the urinary, tract.

156. **3 Bed rest keeps the pressure of the fetus off the cervix, minimizing cervical dilation; the side-lying position enhances uterine perfusion.** (PL; ED; HP)

1 This position is used only when the cord is prolapsed.

2 Sitting in bed will increase pressure on the cervix; this may lead to further dilation.

4 This may aid in relieving pressure of the fetus on the cervix, but it will not enhance uterine perfusion.

157. **4 It is not uncommon for adolescents to avoid prenatal care; many do not recognize the deleterious effect that lack of prenatal care can have on them and their babies.** (IM; ED; HP)

1 This should come later in pregnancy, but not before ascertaining the client's feelings about breastfeeding.

2 This can be done in the later part of pregnancy and reinforced during the postpartal period.

3 This will have to be done, but it is not the priority intervention.

158. **4 The pregnant teenager is generally more prone to pregnancy-induced hypertension because of age, inadequate diet, and lack of prenatal care.** (AN; PA; HP)

1 This is unrelated; there is no proof that teenagers are more diabetogenic than other pregnant women.

2 This is a false assumption; societal mores vary, and the pregnancy of an unmarried female may be acceptable.

3 This may or may not be true.

159. **2 Perinatal morbidity and mortality are greatly increased in multiple pregnancy because the high metabolic demands and the possibility of malpositioning of one or both fetuses may increase the potential for medical and obstetric complications.** (DC; PA; HP)

1 Although postpartum hemorrhage does occur more frequently after multiple births, it is not a routine occurrence.

3 Maternal mortality during the prenatal period is not increased in the presence of multiple gestation.

4 Multiple gestation is usually identified prior to delivery; the mother would have this time for adjustment.

160. **1 Multiple pregnancy thins the uterine wall by over-stretching; thus the efficiency of contractions is reduced.** (AN; TC; HP)

2 Anemia may cause fatigue in the mother; it does not affect uterine contractility.

3 A pelvic contracture may lead to a difficult delivery because of cephalopelvic disproportion; it does not affect uterine contractions.

4 PIH may bring about premature labor; it does not cause hypotonic uterine dysfunction.

161. **1 Placenta previa is defined as an abnormally implanted placenta (i.e., low-lying or covering the cervical os).** (PL; PA; HP)

2 This can occur at any time; it is not specific to low-lying placentas.

3 Premature separation of the placenta can occur with normally implanted placentas.

4 This can occur without a low-lying placenta; factors such as poor muscular tone of the uterus and excessive oxytocin during induction may cause this to occur.

162. **1 As the lower uterus contracts and dilates, the edge of the low-lying placenta separates from the walls of the uterus, opening placental sinuses and allowing blood to escape.** (AN; TC; HP)

2 Abruptio placentae is usually accompanied by intense pain.

3 This is highly unlikely unless placenta previa is present.

4 Placenta previa, a low-implanted placenta, causes painless vaginal bleeding; alcohol ingestion does not.

163. **3 Observation and record keeping of bleeding are independent nursing functions and necessary for implementing safe care, since hemorrhage and shock can be life threatening.** (PL; TC; HP)
   1 Vital signs should be checked more often if bleeding persists.
   2 This is absolutely forbidden, since it may cause further separation of the placenta.
   4 The client should be restricted to complete bed rest until bleeding stops.

164. **4 The client's rights were violated. All clients have the right to a complete and accurate explanation of treatment.** (AN; PS; HP)
   1 All preparations or procedures should be explained because they are not routine to the client.
   2 The Patient's Bill of Rights states that the client should be informed.
   3 When administering treatment, the nurse is responsible for explaining to the client what the treatment is and why it is being done.

165. **4 Severe pain accompanied by bleeding at term or close to it is symptomatic of complete premature detachment of the placenta (abruptio placentae).** (DC; TC; HP)
   1 A hydatidiform mole does not usually last until 36 weeks; no severe pain accompanies it.
   2 There is no bleeding with vena caval syndrome.
   3 Bleeding caused by marginal placenta previa should not be painful.

166. **3 The blood cannot escape from behind the placenta, thus the abdomen becomes boardlike and painful because of the entrapment.** (AN; PA; HP)
   1 Symptoms of hemorrhagic shock do not include pain.
   2 This is not an immediate response; it may occur later if the client's resistance is lessened.
   4 Blood at the site of placental separation may seep into the uterine muscle (Couvelaire uterus).

167. **4 Clotting defects are common in moderate and severe abruptio placentae because of the loss of fibrinogen from severe internal bleeding.** (AN; PA; HP)
   1 An excessive amount of red blood cells is not related to the depletion of fibrinogen.
   2 Excessive globulin in the blood is unrelated to clotting.
   3 This is a decrease in the number of platelets; bleeding of abruptio placentae is caused by depletion of fibrinogen, not platelets.

168. **4 Hypertension in PIH leads to vasospasms; this in turn causes the placenta to tear away from the uterine wall (abruptio placentae).** (DC; TC; HP)
   1 Generally cardiac disease does not cause abruptio placentae.
   2 This may cause endocrine disturbance in the infant but does not affect the blood supply to the uterus.
   3 This may affect the delivery of the fetus but does not affect the placenta.

169. **1 Gravitational pull on an already-stressed placenta may cause further bleeding.** (PL; TC; HP)
   2 This provides for fetal assessment; it does not delay the delivery.
   3 Unless FHR is decelerating, this is not necessary.
   4 Same as answer 3.

170. **4 Any medication that might further depress a premature infant is given with extreme caution.** (IM; ED; HP)
   1 At the proper time the client is encouraged to bear down.
   2 This would be false reassurance; there is no absolute control of premature labor.
   3 If the client is kept NPO, it is done to lessen the risk of aspiration should anesthesia become necessary.

171. **3 Overdistention of the uterus because of a large baby, multiple gestation, or hydramnios predisposes a woman to uterine atony, which may cause postpartum hemorrhage.** (DC; TC; HP)
   1 This leads to precipitous delivery (potentially harmful to the fetus) but does not affect uterine contraction after delivery.
   2 This is not related; unless uterine atony is present, hemorrhage should not occur; a grand multipara is at risk for placenta previa.
   4 This is not a factor in involution of the uterus.

172. **1 Atony often results from an overdistended uterus; uterine contraction does not occur readily.** (AN; PA; HP)
   2 This would cause systemic responses other than hemorrhage.
   3 This is unusual and may occur with improper use of forceps; it is not indicated in this situation.

4 This can occur in any delivery (not just twins) if careful inspection of the placenta is not done.

173. 4 PIH does not interfere with uterine involution, return of uterine tone, or constriction of vessels at the placental site. (DC; TC; HP)
1 Retained placenta inhibits uterine myometrial contractions; also manual removal of placenta may cause uterine trauma.
2 This may inhibit myometrial contraction of the uterus at the placental site.
3 Overdistention of the uterus may lead to delayed or poor uterine myometrial contraction at the placental site after delivery.

174. 3 Immediate cesarean delivery is the treatment of choice for complete placental separation. The risk of fetal death is too high to delay. (IM; TC; HP)
1 This is too time consuming; a high forceps delivery is rarely used because the forceps may further complicate the situation by tearing the cervix.
2 The fetus would probably expire if this course of action were taken.
4 Same as answer 2.

175. 4 Statistically, cephalopelvic disproportion (CPD) is the most common indication for the first-time cesarean delivery. (PL; PA; HP)
1 This is a nonexistent condition.
2 This is untrue, unless the placenta covers the os or hemorrage occurs.
3 This may be improved by rest and hydration followed by an infusion of oxytocin (Syntocinon), leading to vaginal delivery.

176. 2 IV oxytocin (Syntocinon) is used to enhance postpartum uterine contractions after cesarean delivery, since massage of the fundus is difficult and painful after surgery; the drug produces effective clamping down on the vessels. (IM; PA; HP)
1 This is done for all postoperative clients.
3 This may be difficult because of the new incision.
4 This is done routinely for all postoperative clients.

177. 4 This is a sign of CNS involvement that the nurse can observe without obtaining subjective data from the client. (DC; TC; HP)
1 Pain and nausea are subjective symptoms and are not directly observable.

2 These are subjective symptoms; the client must indicate their presence.
3 This is a subjective symptom and is not obvious to the nurse.

178. 4 Absolute bed rest, a quiet room, and minimal stimulation are essential to reducing the risk of a seizure. (PL; TC; HP)
1 The client will need constant observation and should not be isolated.
2 This may cause temporary supine hypotension with resultant bradycardia in the fetus; it could also result in aspiration should a seizure occur.
3 Fluid intake depends on client's condition and physician's orders.

179. 4 Increased electric charges in the brain during a seizure may disturb the cerebral thermoregulation center. (AN; TC; HP)
1 Excessive muscular activity usually causes perspiration, leading to a drop in body temperature.
2 One elevated reading is not a conclusive sign of infection.
3 There is no rapid fluid loss during a seizure; actually this client has fluid retention.

180. 4 The danger of seizure in a woman with eclampsia ends when postpartum diuresis has occurred, usually 48 hours after delivery. (EV; TC; HP)
1 This is untrue; the danger of seizure in eclampsia ends when postpartum diuresis occurs about 48 hours after delivery.
2 Same as answer 1.
3 Same as answer 1.

181. 4 The cord may prolapse, and pressure of the baby's head on the cord may compress the cord causing fetal hypoxia. (DC; TC; HP)
1 This is associated with PIH; it is not attributable to a breech delivery.
2 In a breech delivery the head is not the presenting part bearing the brunt of pressure against the pelvic floor.
3 This is generally caused by Rh disease; it is not associated with a breech delivery.

182. 4 **A position in which the mother's head is below the level of the hips helps decrease compression of the cord and therefore maintains the blood supply to the infant.** (EV; TC; HP)

1 This does not relieve the pressure of the oncoming head on the cord.

2 This may increase the pressure of the presenting part on the cord.

3 The pressure of the presenting part on the cord is not relieved in this position.

183. 4 **The heart rate increases by about 10 beats per minute in the last half of pregnancy; this increase plus the increase in total blood volume can strain a damaged heart beyond the point at which it can efficiently compensate.** (AN; PA; HP)

1 The increased size of the uterus is related to the growth of the fetus, not to any hemodynamic change.

2 The number of RBCs does not decrease during pregnancy; plasma volume increases, simulating lowered hemoglobin.

3 Cardiac output begins to decrease by the thirty-fourth week of gestation.

184. 4 **This is the most critical period due to the rapid fluid shift as extravascular fluid returns to the bloodstream; this mobilization of fluid can place a strain on the heart and lead to cardiac decompensation.** (IM; ED; HP)

1 During the first trimester the increased amount of circulating blood volume is minimal and occurs gradually; thus it does not usually place a large burden on the heart.

2 The risk of cardiac decompensation increases as pregnancy progresses; however, the increase in blood volume occurs gradually and the mother is monitored closely.

3 There is an increased risk of stress on the heart during delivery; however, close monitoring and the use of agents to provide rest and pain relief have decreased these risks.

185. 2 **Anemia decreases the capacity of the blood to carry oxygen and thus increases the demands on the heart.** (DC; TC; HP)

1 This is due to a disturbance in the conduction of impulses, not the oxygen-carrying capacity of blood.

3 Cardiac irregularity is not associated with anemia.

4 A diseased heart is not capable of further cardiac compensation; decompensation would result.

186. 3 **The semi-Fowler's position facilitates easier oxygen exchange, and side lying promotes better venous return.** (IM; PA; HP)

1 This is too straight and uncomfortable; the gravid uterus will impede venous return from the legs.

2 The supine gravid uterus may inhibit venous return and result in placental congestion and supine hypotension.

4 At full term, clients are placed in the left side-lying position to enhance venous return.

187. 4 **The side-lying position takes the weight off large blood vessels, and blood flow to the heart is increased; elevating the shoulders relieves pressure on the diaphragm.** (IM; TC; HP)

1 Sodium leads to increased fluid retention; it is contraindicated in the cardiac client.

2 Potassium chloride is contraindicated unless lowered potassium levels indicate the need.

3 This is contraindicated unless some uterine inertia occurs.

188. 3 **Clients with cardiac problems are prone to congestive heart failure in this stage of labor.** (PL; TC; HP)

1 This is done for all laboring clients; with cardiac problems, the priority is monitoring for congestive heart failure.

2 Same as answer 1.

4 This is not necessary; clients are maintained on the side to facilitate venous return.

189. 4 **Clients who have had rheumatic fever are placed on prophylactic ampicillin therapy to minimize the development of streptococcus infections.** (PL; TC; HP)

1 This would be used only if the client was in congestive heart failure.

2 This would be used only if thrombophlebitis develops.

3 Same as answer 1.

190. 3 **A symptom of congestive heart failure is respiratory distress.** (DC; TC; HP)

1 Although pulse is important, the primary observation should be for respiratory distress, which suggests congestive heart failure.

2 Signs of congestive failure, not hypovolemic shock, might develop.

4 Increased vaginal bleeding is not caused by alterations in cardiac status.

191. 4 **The pregnant woman's increased hormones, metabolic rate, and increased**

blood volume place additional demands on the pancreas, thus altering carbohydrate and lipid metabolism. (AN; PA; HP)

1 Pregnancy lowers the renal threshold for glucose in nondiabetics as well; it does not affect metabolism.

2 The hormones of pregnancy act as antagonists to insulin, thus reducing its effect.

3 The diabetic mother's glucose tolerance does not differ from that in her prepregnant state.

192. **2 Increased metabolic demands on the body during pregnancy require an increased ingestion of glucose; appropriate levels of insulin must be provided to permit normal glucose utilization by the body. (PL; PA; HP)**

1 The caloric content is increased, not decreased, during pregnancy.

3 This diet would not be sufficient to prevent ketosis; insulin would be necessary to cover carbohydrate intake.

4 This type of diet is contraindicated; it would not meet the demands of pregnancy and the growing fetus.

193. **2 Usually, as pregnancy progresses, there are alterations in glucose tolerance and in the metabolism and utilization of insulin. The result is an increased need for exogenous insulin. (PL; PA; HP)**

1 Caloric intake is increased to meet demands of the growing fetus.

3 Pancreatic enzymes or hormones other than insulin are not taken by diabetics.

4 Estrogenic hormones are not administered during pregnancy.

High-Risk Newborn

194. **2 Early decelerations, with onset before the peak of the contraction and low point at the peak of the contraction, are due to fetal head compression; FHR rarely drops below 100 beats per minute. (DC; PA; HN)**

1 This is marked bradycardia.

3 This is not a deceleration; it is within normal limits.

4 Same as answer 3.

195. **4 Heart development occurs between the second and eighth week of gestation. (DC; ED; HN)**

1 This is associated with the intake of teratogenic drugs, not rubella.

2 This generally occurs later in life; it is not caused by rubella; rubella may cause nerve deafness from eighth cranial (vestibulocochlear) nerve or hearing-center involvement.

3 This is a neural tube defect and is not associated with rubella.

196. **3 The congenital absence of a vessel in the umbilical cord is often associated with life-threatening congenital anomalies. (EV; TC; HN)**

1 This is the average weight for a full-term newborn.

2 If the Apgar score 5 minutes later showed marked improvement, there would be no need for placing the infant in the ICU.

4 The fetus may have swallowed some amniotic fluid; this is not unusual or dangerous.

197. **2 Flaccid muscle tone is the only abnormal finding; all other choices indicate a normal newborn response and would score higher on the Apgar scale. (DC; PA; HN)**

1 This is usually much slower in an infant whose Apgar score is 4.

3 This is present with an Apgar rating of 7 to 10.

4 Apgar rating of 7 to 10 usually indicates this.

198. **2 This is unnecessary; the baby's Apgar (7/9) does not indicate a need for oxygen. (IM; PA; HN)**

1 This is an important part of record keeping on all newborns.

3 Poor thermoregulation necessitates keeping the baby warm to stabilize body temperature.

4 All newborns are evaluated immediately.

199. **3 Untreated ophthalmia neonatorum becomes apparent on the third or fourth postnatal day and is evidence that the mother may have had gonorrhea or a chlamydia infection. (DC; ED; HN)**

1 Ophthalmia neonatorum does not develop until the third day.

2 The incubation period for the organisms that cause ophthalmia neonatorum is 3 to 4 days after birth.

4 Same as answer 1.

200. 1 **This conjunctivitis occurs about 3 to 4 days after birth; if it is not treated with tetracycline, chronic follicular conjunctivitis with conjunctival scarring will occur. (AN; TC; HN)**

2 High oxygen concentrations cause vasoconstriction of retinal capillaries, which can lead to blindness.

3 AIDS in the newborn does not manifest itself in any type of conjunctivitis.

4 This chemical conjunctivitis occurs within the first 48 hours and is not purulent in nature.

201. 2 ***Chlamydia trachomatis* is associated with the development of pneumonia in the newborn infant. (DC; TC; HN)**

1 This is done at all times; the first priority here is to monitor for pneumonia, which is often associated with chlamydial infections.

3 Purulent conjunctivitis at this time suggests a chlamydial infection, not an allergic response.

4 Physician's order is required; bathing the eyes with solution will not stem the infection; the infant will be put on intensive systemic antibiotic therapy.

202. 3 **Prolonged oxygen administration at relatively high concentrations in a premature infant whose retina is incompletely differentiated and/or vascularized may result in retinopathy of prematurity (retrolental fibroplasia); when oxygen therapy is discontinued, capillary overgrowth in the retina and vitreous body may result and include capillary hemorrhage, fibrosis, and retinal detachment. (PL; TC; HN)**

1 Though true, temperature and humidity are not factors in the development of retinopathy of prematurity.

2 Phototherapy is used to decrease hyperbilirubinemia; it is unrelated to retrolental fibroplasia; however, the eyes are covered to prevent injury for all infants receiving phototherapy.

4 High oxygen concentration is dangerous and a factor in the development of retinopathy of prematurity.

203. 4 **Because congenital syphilis is difficult to detect at birth, the infant should be screened immediately to determine if treatment is necessary. (DC; TC; HN)**

1 This defect occurs in the first trimester; *Treponema pallidum* does not affect a fetus before the sixteenth week of gestation.

2 This is found in children with Down syndrome, not congenital syphilis.

3 This does not become manifest in the syphilitic infant until about 3 months of age.

204. 3 ***Chlamydia trachomatis* transmitted from the mother is usually manifested in the infant as an eye infection; it becomes apparent on the third or fourth postnatal day. (DC; PA; HN)**

1 *Monilia*, not *Chlamydia trachomatis*, causes thrush.

2 This is acquired transplacentally, not via the genital tract.

4 In newborns, opthalmic or respiratory complications, not neurologic complications, occur with exposure to this organism.

205. 2 **Asymmetry of the gluteal dorsal surface of the thighs and inguinal folds indicates congenital dislocation of the hip; folds on the affected side appear higher than those on the unaffected side. (DC; PA; HN)**

1 Impaired reflex behavior and a shrill cry, etc., would indicate CNS damage.

3 An inguinal hernia is evidenced by protrusion of the intestine into the inguinal sac.

4 Peripheral nervous system damage would be manifested by limpness or flaccidity of extremities.

206. 1 **In Erb-Duchenne paralysis there is damage to spinal nerves C5 and C6, which causes paralysis of the arm. (EV; TC; HN)**

2 The grasp reflex is intact since the fingers usually are not affected; if C8 is injured, paralysis of the hand results (Klumpke's paralysis).

3 There is no interference with turning of the head; injury usually results from excessive lateral flexion of the head during delivery of the shoulder.

4 There would be a negative Moro reflex on the affected side only.

207. 3 **Range-of-motion exercises must be done to prevent contractures. (PL; PA; HN)**

1 This would be dangerous since it would lead to permanent contractures.

2 The muscle action improves spontaneously when edema subsides.

4 The length of the arm will not change on a daily basis.

208. 1 **Brachial palsy results from excessive stretching of the nerve fibers that run from the neck, through the shoulder, and down toward the arm; the muscles of the upper arm are involved, and the infant**

holds the arm at the side with the elbow extended and the hand rotated inward. (AN; TC; HN)

2 Signs of a central nervous system disturbance would be present.

3 There would be signs of dislocation and evidence of pain with a fractured clavicle.

4 This is an inborn error of metabolism relating to the body's handling of bilirubin.

209. **4 Intracranial bleeding may occur in the subdural, subarachnoid, or intraventricular spaces of the brain, causing pressure on vital centers; clinical signs are related to the area and degree of cerebral involvement. (AN; PA; HN)**

1 This is caused by hypocalcemia; it is manifested by exaggerated muscular twitching.

2 This is an obvious defect of the spinal column; it is easily recognized.

3 Elevated potassium causes cardiac irregularities.

210. **1 Development of jaundice before 24 to 48 hours after birth may indicate a blood dyscrasia, requiring immediate medical investigation. Jaundice occurring between 48 and 72 hours after birth is a consequence of the normal physiologic breakdown of fetal red cells and immaturity of the liver. (EV; ED; HN)**

2 Unless the jaundice was pathologic (occurring in the first 24 hours of life), this is not necessary.

3 First, the age of the infant must be ascertained to see whether this is physiologic jaundice; then, the nurse can do a "heel-stick" to determine the amount of bilirubin.

4 Bilirubin studies would be done first to determine whether the amount of bilirubin present warranted phototherapy.

211. **3 Development of jaundice in the first 24 hours indicates hemolytic disease of the newborn. (DC; TC; HN)**

1 May or may not be present during first 24 hours; it usually develops later.

2 These may or may not be present in first 24 hours; they are dependent on the bilirubin level.

4 This is normal; serum bilirubin normally accumulates in the neonatal period because of the short life span of fetal erythrocytes, reaching levels of 7 mg/100 ml the second to third day, when jaundice appears.

212. **1 Preterm describes a newborn delivered at 37 weeks gestation or less, regardless of weight. (AN; ED; HN)**

2 Immature indicates an infant weighing less than 1136 g and considerably underdeveloped at birth.

3 Nonviable would be before the twenty-second week of gestation.

4 This means low birth weight for related gestational age; this infant is appropriate for gestational age.

213. **3 Much of a full-term infant's birth weight is gained during the last month of pregnancy (almost a third), and most of this final spurt is subcutaneous fat, which serves as insulation; the preterm infant has not had the time to grow in the uterus and has little of this insulating layer. (AN; ED; HN)**

1 There is a relatively larger surface area per body weight.

2 There is an extremely limited shivering and sweating response in the preterm infant.

4 This is unrelated to the maintenance of body temperature.

214. **3 Neonates are unable to shiver; they use the breakdown of brown fat to supply body heat; the preterm baby has a limited supply of brown fat available for this breakdown. (AN; ED; HN)**

1 The breakdown of glycogen into glucose does not supply body heat.

2 Newborns are unable to use shivering to supply body heat.

4 The pituitary gland does not supply body heat.

215. **2 The preterm infant has a reduced glomerular filtration rate and reduced ability to concentrate urine or conserve water. (AN; ED; HN)**

1 This is untrue; all systems of the preterm baby are less developed than in the full-term infant.

3 The opposite occurs; urine is very dilute.

4 The fluid and electrolyte balance of preterm infants is easily upset.

216. **4 Immaturity of the respiratory tract in preterm infants can be evidenced by a lack of functional alveoli, smaller lumina with increased possibility of collapse of the respiratory passages, weakness of respiratory musculature, and insufficient calcification of the bony thorax leading to respiratory distress. (PL; TC; HN)**
    1 This is not a common occurrence at the time of birth unless trauma has occurred.
    2 This is not a primary concern unless severe hypoxia occurred during labor; it is difficult to diagnose at this time.
    3 This may be a problem, but generally the air passageway is well suctioned at birth.

217. **1 The physical principle is surface tension; since the lung tissue of the infant lacks the group of detergents known as surfactant, water molecules strongly interact with each other by hydrogen bonding, and the alveolar sacs and respiratory passages do not easily expand; the result is extremely labored, if not impossible, breathing. (AN; PA; HN)**
    2 This is related to the equal distribution of external pressure throughout a fluid in a closed vessel.
    3 This has to do with a body in water being buoyed by a force equal to the weight of the fluid displaced.
    4 This has to do with the relationship between heat and mechanical energy.

218. **2 The moisture provided by the humidity liquifies the tenacious secretions, making gas exchange possible. (PL; PA; HN)**
    1 They should be side-lying rather than prone; the babies may be too immature to raise their heads from the prone position.
    3 Actually the caloric intake will be increased; the amount, number, and type of feedings will be related to the metabolic rate.
    4 This is not a routine action; oxygen concentration will depend on the babies' blood gases.

219. **2 The infant of a diabetic mother is a newborn at risk because of the interplay between the maternal disease and the developing fetus. (IM; TC; HN)**
    1 Babies of diabetic mothers are generally hypoglycemic because of oversecretion of insulin by their hypertrophied pancreas.
    3 Infants of diabetic mothers are at high risk and require intensive monitoring.
    4 The baby may be prone to hypoglycemia and will need increased glucose.

220. **1 In diabetic mothers the fetal pancreas responds to the mother's hyperglycemia by secreting more than normal amounts of insulin; this leads to infant hypoglycemia after birth. (AN; TC; HN)**
    2 Increased insulin production by the fetus diminishes the glucose content of the blood; babies are most often hypoglycemic.
    3 There may be a generalized edema, but not specific to the central nervous system.
    4 In response to the increased glucose received from the mother, the islets of Langerhans in the fetus may have become hypertrophied; they are not congenitally depressed.

221. **2 The higher-than-normal glucose level in a fetus of a diabetic mother leads to increased fat synthesis and deposition; increased glucose utilization is also promoted by the combined presence of the pituitary growth hormone and placental somatotropin. (AN; TC; HN)**
    1 This is false; glucose utilization is increased, with resultant macrosomia.
    3 This is false; somatotropin concentration is increased during pregnancy.
    4 This is false; somatotropin concentration is increased and glucose utilization is increased.

Emotional Needs Related to Childbearing and Women's Health

222. **2 Because mothering is not an inborn instinct, almost all mothers, including multiparas, report some ambivalence and anxiety about their ability to be good mothers. (DC; PS; EC)**
    1 This is untrue; very often the maternal instinct is nurtured by the sight of the infant.
    3 This is untrue; it may take a much longer time.
    4 This is untrue; ambivalent feelings are universal in response to the infant.

223. **2 Uninformed consent constitutes an artificial consent; sufficient information was not given. (EV; ED; EC)**
    1 This type of consent is not sufficient to cover invasive procedures or surgery.
    3 The surgeon may do what is necessary if an informed consent is obtained for all eventualities.
    4 Informed consent covers only that which is covered by the consent.

224. **1 This response provides the client with a comfort measure while giving her an**

opportunity to verbalize her fears about having an abnormal labour. (IM; PS; EC)

2 This closes off communication with the client.

3 This is of no help to the client; she is concerned with what is happening to her.

4 This can be answered "yes" or "no" and leaves no further avenue for discussion.

225. **2 Both partners need additional support during the transitional stage of labour. (IM; PS; EC)**

1 This statement is judgmental; this approach suggests that he will be failing his partner.

3 The partner should be present throughout labour to support the client; he should be assisted in this role.

4 This does not encourage him to fulfill his role in supporting the mother during labour.

226. **4 Mothers need to explore their infants visually and tactilely to assure themselves that the infant is normal in all respects. (DC; ED; EC)**

1 This is false reassurance; this comment closes off communication with the mother at a very opportune moment.

2 Crying is not indicative of congenital defects; a strong cry does not assure "normalcy."

3 The "normalcy" of the mother's pregnancy and labor does not always have a relationship to "normalcy" of the infant.

227. **3 Allowing the mother time to inspect the child permits viewing, touching, and holding, promoting bonding. (PL; PS; EC)**

1 The client will proceed at her own rate; requiring her to do things is not supportive.

2 The mother should have made this decision before delivery.

4 This can be done only by allowing the mother ample time to inspect and interact with her baby.

228. **3 Sneezing is the way in which the newborn clears mucus from the nose; breathing is normally rapid and irregular. (IM; PS; EC)**

1 This would discourage the mother from taking responsibility and slow the mothering process; it also implies that something could be wrong.

2 More explanation is needed, and it also shuts off communication; the mother needs to express her feelings of anxiety.

4 These are normal newborn responses and indicate no respiratory distress.

229. **2 The mother has completed the taking-in phase (the mother's needs predominate) and has moved into the taking-hold phase (active maternal involvement with self and infant) when she calls the baby by name. (DC; PS; EC)**

1 This may occur in either phase.

3 This is the initial early action of the taking-in phase.

4 This is part of the taking-in phase.

230. **3 Bonding between parent and baby is most successful when interaction is possible right after birth; if the child is ill, contact is limited. (PL; GD; EC)**

1 Though the effect of anesthesia is certainly a factor, the most important factor is the physical condition of the infant.

2 Though the duration and difficulty of labor is certainly a factor, the most important factor is the physical condition of the infant.

4 Health status during pregnancy may be a factor, but the most important factor is the physical condition of the infant.

231. **3 Parenting is not an inborn instinct but rather a learned behavior based on past experiences or current instruction. (AN; PS; EC)**

1 Partnership is not essential for good parenting.

2 This is untrue; parenting is learned, not inborn.

4 This knowledge does not assure the ability to parent.

232. **3 The parents should be informed of the birth of a child with an abnormality as early as possible, preferably in the delivery room when staff is present to support and assist them in mobilizing resources; this approach prevents fantasizing about the problem. (EV; PS; EC)**

1 This may be too much of a shock if the mother is not aware of the defect.

2 The parents may not ask and providing the information should not be delayed.

4 Crisis intervention should not be delayed; immediately informing the parents improves coping abilities.

233. **1 Based on the family's decision, extraordinary care does not have to be employed; the child's basic needs are met, and nature is allowed to take its course. (PL; PS; EC)**
2 Euthanasia is a deliberate intervention to cause death.
3 If the child's physical needs are met and comfort is provided, the child's rights are not ignored; "extraordinary," not "all," care is being withheld.
4 It is neither unethical nor illegal to withhold extraordinary treatment; once such treatment is started, it becomes a legal issue.

234. **2 Although support will help minimize guilt, it will not eliminate it; however, support will sustain family cohesion and unity. (IM; PS; EC)**
1 Support may help, but in no way does it completely alleviate guilt feelings.
3 Support does not affect the legal responsibility of the parents.
4 This may help, but cannot completely relieve pressure.

235. **4 When the client signs herself and the baby out of the hospital, she is legally responsible for her infant and must be given the baby. (IM; ED; EC)**
1 The baby belongs to the mother and can leave with the mother when she signs them out.
2 The mother is the baby's guardian and may take the baby with her when she leaves.
3 The baby is under the guardianship of the mother and may leave with the mother.

236. **1 This opens up an area of communication to get at what really is troubling the mother about feeding the baby. (IM; PS; EC)**
2 Since the nurse is aware that this is not the best method, the problem of time should be explored with the mother.
3 Holding can be accomplished at times other than feeding periods; it does not explore the client's feelings.
4 This is true, but the mother should not be frightened; a more gentle explanation should be used.

237. **2 This allows both partners to comfort each other while letting them know the nurse is available; it also allows them to recognize and accept their feelings of loss. (IM; PS; EC)**
1 This makes an assumption that another pregnancy will ensue; it also cuts off further communication.

3 Telling the client not to be upset cuts off communication and wrongly implies that it prolongs recovery.
4 Grieving for the unborn child will and should occur during any period of pregnancy.

238. **2 Normal periods of marked change and adjustment are called developmental crises and predispose the woman to a situational crisis. (AN; PS; EC)**
1 These are transient; they are similar to previous mood changes and should not affect the mother's ability to cope.
3 These occur throughout the life cycle of a mature woman and should not now be classified as a crisis.
4 It becomes a crisis only if one of the partners withdraws support.

239. **2 The ability to express one's feelings is often a first step in the recognition and resolution of a crisis. (IM; PS; EC)**
1 This is not a priority need; it may come later in the nurse-client interaction.
3 The father, as well as the mother, must indicate a readiness for learning before beginning classes.
4 Until the mother shows a readiness for learning (e.g., wants the pregnancy), she would not benefit from classes.

240. **1 Nurses with positive attitudes toward abortion should counsel women who are thinking of undergoing the procedure; they should know what services are available and the various methods that are used to induce abortion. (EV; ED; EC)**
2 Nursing practice necessitates scientific knowledge; statements must be based on fact, not personal feelings or beliefs.
3 The nurse is capable of giving information about abortion and need not defer to the physician.
4 The nurse should give the client only the information requested and should not state personal feelings.

241. **4 The client must feel comfortable enough to verbalize her feelings of guilt if she is to be able to complete the grieving process. (AN; PS; EC)**
1 This is a sterile procedure and should not predispose the client to postoperative infection.
2 This is a false assumption.
3 Studies show that contraceptive counseling at this time is most important, since the client may not return after the abortion.

Drug-related Responses

242. 2 There is no known teratogenic effect associated with penicillin. (AN; TC; DR)

1 Sulfonamides may cause hemolysis in the fetus.

3 Tetracycline causes permanent yellow staining of teeth in children whose mothers receive the drug during pregnancy.

4 This drug is contraindicated in severe renal disease.

243. 3 The oxytocic effect of Syntocinon increases the intensity and durations of contractions; prolonged contractions will jeopardize the safety of the fetus and necessitate discontinuing the drug. (IM; TC; DR)

1 This is important throughout labor.

2 Since she is only 3 to 4 cm with head floating, there will be no bulging.

4 There is no indication at this time that a cesarean delivery is necessary.

244. 1 Oxytocin is a small polypeptide hormone normally synthesized in the hypothalamus and secreted from the neurohypophysis during parturition or suckling; the synthetic form promotes powerful uterine (smooth muscle) contractions and thus is used to induce labor. (AN; PA; DR)

2 Progesterone builds up the endometrium; it does not initiate uterine contractions.

3 This drug is not for this purpose.

4 Ergometrine can lead to sustained contractions, which would be undesirable in labor.

245. 3 Respiratory depression occurs with the use of meperidine (Demerol) and produces significant depression of the infant at birth if circulating levels are high at delivery. (EV; TC; DR)

1 Scopolamine induces amnesia and forgetfulness in the mother but does not cause respiratory depression; this medication is not presently used.

2 Promazine (Sparine), an anxiolytic, augments the effects of Demerol, thereby lessening the amount of drug needed.

4 Promethazine (Phenergan), an antihistamine, does not cause respiratory depression.

246. 4 Meperidine (Demerol) is classified as a narcotic analgesic drug and is effective for the relief of pain; promethazine (Phenergan) can be classified as an analgesic potentiating drug that permits the effective use of analgesics in lower dosages. (EV; TC; DR)

1 These medications do not induce amnesia.

2 These medications act as analgesics, not anesthetics.

3 This is an undesirable effect because the mother could not participate in the delivery process.

247. 3 Ritodrine (Yutopar) is a beta receptor that acts on the smooth muscles of the uterus to reduce contractility, which in turn inhibits dilation and contractions. (EV; PA; DR)

1 Terbutaline sulfate (Brethine) has no analgesic effects.

2 Terbutaline sulfate (Brethine) does not act to decrease blood pressure.

4 Terbutaline sulfate (Brethine) acts to arrest preterm labor by relaxing the uterus; this would result in stopping cervical dilation rather than increasing it.

248. 4 Magnesium sulfate has a CNS depressant effect; therefore toxic levels will be reflected in decreased respiration and the absence of the knee-jerk reflex. (EV; TC; DR)

1 This may happen from sedation, not from magnesium sulfate.

2 There is a decrease in respirations with excessive magnesium sulfate.

3 This may be caused by increased potassium, not magnesium sulfate.

249. 2 $Rh_o(D)$ globulin attacks fetal red cells that have gained access to the maternal bloodstream at the time of delivery; it prevents antibody formation. (EV; PA; DR)

1 This is contraindicated, since antibody formation is undesirable; it sensitizes the mother and contributes to fetal red cell destruction in future pregnancies.

3 $RH_o(D)$ prevents the mother's immune system from responding to the fetal Rh-positive blood.

4 This is irrelevant; there is no production of immune bodies.

250. 1 Heparin is used because its molecular size is too large to pass the placental barrier. (PL; PA; DR)

2 This drug can pass the placental barrier and cause hemorrhage in the fetus.

3 Same as answer 2.

4 Same as answer 2.

251. 2 Danazol causes atrophy of endometrial tissue. (AN; PA; DR)

1 Relaxin is used for dysmenorrhea; it causes relaxation of the symphysis pubis.

3 Ergometrine is used to contract the uterus.

4 This is an estrogen that affects release of pituitary gonadotropins and inhibits ovulation.

Women's Health

252. 4 Metrorrhagia is uterine bleeding at any time other than during the menstrual period. (AN; PA; WH)

1 This is dyspareunia.

2 This is menstruation when it occurs in a cyclic pattern after menarche.

3 Severe menstrual bleeding is menorrhagia.

253. 3 Endometriosis is the presence of aberrant endometrial tissue outside the uterus. The tissue responds to ovarian stimulation, bleeds during menstruation, and causes severe pain. (DC; PA; WH)

1 These are not symptoms of endometriosis.

2 Ecchymoses and petechiae are not characteristic of this disorder.

4 Osteoporosis may be a complication of menopause because of decreased estrogen levels; pelvic inflammation usually results from infection.

254. 2 The posterior vaginal wall is pushed forward by the herniation of the rectum; this protrusion increases rectal pressure and causes the bearing-down sensation. (DC; PA; WH)

1 A rectocele is not accompanied by abdominal pain.

3 This is the primary symptom of a cystocele.

4 A cystocele is associated with urinary tract infections.

255. 3 Clients with internal radiation for cervical cancer are given low-residue diets and often medications to suppress peristalsis and prevent pressure from BMs. (IM; TC; WH)

1 A catheter is routinely inserted prior to loading to prevent bladder distention and possible radiation damage or alteration of implant position.

2 The head of the bed can be only slightly elevated to prevent the implant from being dislodged by gravity.

4 Since the client has the source of radiation, the nurse must limit the time spent with the client to avoid excessive exposure.

256. 3 In a hysterectomy the uterus is removed, but no other female organs. Consequently menstruation ceases but the hypophyseal and ovarian hormone cycles continue. (PL; PA; WH)

1 Removal of the uterus does not affect the secretion of ovarian hormones.

2 Normally menopause begins gradually; after an oophorectomy it begins immediately. However, an oophorectomy was not performed.

4 An oophorectomy was not performed; ovarian hormones continue to be secreted.

257. 1 An abdominal panhysterectomy in the premenopausal woman produces artificial onset of menopause. (IM; ED; WH)

2 This is untrue; because the uterus was removed, there will be no uterine endometrial proliferation and no desquamation.

3 Same as answer 2.

4 Same as answer 2.

258. 1 Menstruation is the shedding of the endometrial lining of the uterus. A woman who has undergone a hysterectomy has had her uterus removed and will no longer menstruate. (AN; PA; WH)

2 After a hysterectomy there is no endometrial lining to shed.

3 This is not an anxiety response; additional symptoms would be necessary before this diagnosis would be appropriate.

4 Frank bleeding is not expected postoperatively.

259. 3 Postoperatively the arm on the operated side is elevated on pillows with the hand higher than the arm to prevent muscle strain and edema. (IM; PA; WH)

1 Total immobilization should be avoided, and adduction may put undue pressure on the operative site.

2 Although the arm is slightly abducted, sandbags are not utilized because complete immobility should be prevented.

4 This would impair venous return and increase edema.

260. 3 The ovaries are responsible for producing the female sex hormones, estrogen and progesterone; a bilateral oophorectomy causes an abrupt cessation in the production of most of these hormones (the adrenal cortex produces small quantities of female sex hormones) and results in surgical menopause. (EV; PA; WH)

1 A tubal ligation is the surgical severing of the fallopian tubes to produce sterility, and ovarian function is unaffected.

2 A hysterectomy is the removal of the uterus, and ovarian function is unaffected.

4 A salpingectomy is the removal of the fallopian tubes, and ovarian function is unaffected.

261. **4 Alteration of ovarian hormones causes vasomotor instability; periodic systemic vasodilation is then triggered by the sympathetic nervous system, causing the feeling of warmth. (IM; ED; WH)**

1 Acetylcholine does not cause hot flashes; it is the chemical mediator of cholinergic nerve impulses.

2 Gonadotropins do not cause hot flashes; they stimulate the function of the testes and ovaries.

3 Hot flashes may be associated with understimulation of the adrenals.

262. **3 The lack of utilization of gonadotropin by the ovaries causes an elevation of gonadotropin in the blood; ovarian function is diminished; there is little or no follicular activity. (AN; PA; WH)**

1 There would be an increase in gonadotropin in the blood, for it is not used by the ovaries.

2 There would be an increase in prostaglandins.

4 There would be a decrease in secretion of progesterone.

263. **1 Menopause is a normal developmental adaptation. It is not caused by endometriosis, the abnormal bleeding of aberrant tissue outside the uterus. (DC; PA; WH)**

2 This is a possible complication; bleeding between periods is due to the bleeding of endometrial tissue outside the uterus.

3 The excessive tissue in endometriosis may impinge on the colon and cause ribbonlike stools.

4 Excessive tissue may impinge on the bladder and ureters and cause voiding difficulties.

264. **4 This defect in the bone matrix formation weakens the bones, making them unable to withstand normal stresses. (AN; ED; WH)**

1 Avascular necrosis is death of bone tissue that results from reduced circulation to bone.

2 Pathologic fractures occur during normal activity or after minimal injury in bones weakened by disease.

3 This is incorrect; hyperplasia of osteoblasts is not related to osteoporosis. This occurs during bone healing.

265. **1 This regimen limits bone demineralization. It also reduces osteoporotic pain, which promotes increased activity. (EV; PA; WH)**

2 This is unrelated to osteoporosis; it would be an expected outcome if the client were receiving calcium for hypocalcemia.

3 This is unrelated to osteoporosis; it would be expected if the client were receiving vitamin C for capillary fragility.

4 This is unrelated to osteoporosis or the rationale for therapy.

CHILDBEARING/WOMEN'S HEALTH ANSWERS

CHAPTER 4

Psychiatric/ Mental Health Nursing

S ince nursing is concerned with the basic needs of people, the nurse must be able to understand and assist the individual, being constantly aware of the many factors that influence a person's behavioral response. Individuals are constantly interacting with both the internal and the external environments and at any given moment stand as a conglomerate of their own and their forebears' experiences. The individual is continuously faced with emotional stress from the moment of birth until the moment of death. How people adapt to this stress and the problems resulting from the adaptations are the focus of psychiatric/mental health nursing. Psychiatric/mental health nursing is therefore the care of clients experiencing mental health problems and mental disorders and the promotion of mental health. But the principles used in the care of psychiatric clients are applicable to all clients regardless of their diagnosis. Nursing, which is concerned with total care, must provide for the individual's physical (soma) as well as emotional (psyche) needs.

BACKGROUND INFORMATION FROM THE BEHAVIORAL SCIENCES

BASIC CONCEPTS FROM ANTHROPOLOGY

A. All people are influenced by the culture into which they are born
B. Cultural factors include race, nationality, and religion
C. Groups that share a common race, nationality, religion, or language are known as ethnic groups
D. Society as a whole frequently develops a fixed set of expected responses for certain ethnic groups
E. When each member of an ethnic group is expected to respond in a specific manner, the expected responses are called stereotypes
F. Cultural variability occurs in all stages of the life cycle: child rearing, marriage patterns, health maintenance, etc.

Race

A. Defined as a certain combination of physical traits that are transmitted by lineage or heredity
B. Physical traits of a race include skin color; texture and/or color of hair; eye shapes and folds; shape of nose, lips, and cheekbones; contour of the head; and body build
C. Of all the factors involved in ethnic group membership, race, which is given a great deal of emphasis, appears to be a biologic phenomenon that seems to contribute few specifics to the cultural background

Nationality

A. Defined as original or acquired membership in a particular nation
B. The culture of nationalities is passed down through generations in the form of:
   1. Beliefs and superstitions
   2. Foods and national dishes
   3. Festivals and feast days
   4. Language and the meanings of certain words
   5. Mannerisms and gestures
C. Nationality and the culture that it imparts frequently become even more important when a group of people immigrate to a new country where the members tend to join together to form a subculture of the new national culture
D. The subculture provides its members with a sense of security by furnishing a collective identity and maintaining the familiar

Religion

A. Defined as the quest for values of the ideal life usually embodied in a particular set of beliefs practiced individually or within an organized system
B. Religious beliefs in some form have existed in every group during every period of history
C. Organized religions have been instrumental in developing an ethical and moral system that has frequently been based on a society's needs
D. Most of the world's religions have developed many rituals as part of their worship, and these rituals form the basis of the religious culture that is passed down from generation to generation
E. In contrast to traditional religions there exist numerous religious cults; persons seeking a sense of belonging and purpose join a religious cult that gives them a group identity through communal living and rigorous rituals

Culture and Health

A. General influences
   1. Cultural background influences the way in which people view both health and disease
   2. Cultural influences seem to be derived from the areas of nationality and religion rather than race
B. Specific influences
   1. National culture may influence an individual's:
      a. Response to illness
      b. Response to pain and even the tolerance of pain
      c. Need for superstitions and rituals
      d. Acceptance of dietary change both in type or in consistency of food
      e. Need for support and comfort from the family
      f. Ability to communicate in understandable terms
      g. Response to loss of independence
      h. Feelings about loss of privacy and exposure of parts of the body
      i. Feelings about loss of body parts
      j. Need for specific rites and rituals associated with dying
   2. Religious culture may influence an individual's:
      a. Views on conception, birth, and child care
      b. Views about the meaning of pain and suffering
      c. Feelings about the meaning of death
      d. Desire for guidance from religious leaders
      e. Acceptance of certain treatments such as immunizations and blood transfusions
      f. Concept of illness as a punishment
      g. Dietary restrictions including the types of food and their preparation
      h. Need for specific rites and rituals associated with dying

BASIC CONCEPTS FROM SOCIOLOGY

A. Every human society has institutions for the socialization of its members
  1. Process by which individuals are compelled or induced to conform to the customs of the group
     a. Group establishes rules and codes of conduct governing its members, and these become the norms, values, and mores of the group
     b. Role of members includes specified rights, duties, attitudes, and actions
  2. Controls established through a system of rewards and punishment
     a. Reward leads to acceptance as a member of the group
     b. Punishment for antisocial behavior leads to rejection and separation from the group
B. Development of society requires sanction of group members
  1. Growth takes place in social space
     a. Social boundaries separate one group from another
     b. Barriers to participation are established through mores and customs
  2. Leader's influence is always limited to conditions placed on it by the total group
  3. Behavioral roles are established by members of the group
C. A society is a reflection of all the functional relationships that occur among its individual members
  1. Products of group life are a major determinant in an individual's intellect, creativity, memory, thinking, and feeling
     a. Human beings have no memory, thought, or feeling that does not include society
     b. Intellect and creativity can be enhanced or hampered by society
  2. Members of a society have functional and rewarding social contact
     a. Members are accepted and approved and then participate in establishing rules, norms, and values
     b. The nonmembers have, at best, limited social contacts with the members; this causes a segmentation of relationships and provides few rewarding experiences for the nonmembers
D. Society or a group can change because of conflict among members
  1. This conflict is greatest when there is an absence of certain members, an introduction of new members, or a change in leadership
  2. Ensuing reorganization goes through three stages
     a. Tension: caused by conflict
     b. Integration: during which members learn about "the other's" problem
     c. Resolution: during which a reconstruction of the group's norms and values takes place
  3. Resolution of conflict and the restoring of equilibrium
     a. This takes place when people interact with one another and the group is dynamic
     b. Conflicts are not resolved when groups are rigid with fixed membership and ideas
E. Family is the primary group
  1. Helps society to establish and maintain its code of behavior
  2. Provides individual family members with:
     a. Strong emotional ties
        (1) Members experience sensory stimuli through close contacts
        (2) Members learn to care about the emotional and physical well-being of each other
        (3) Members are responsive to one another's feelings, acts, and opinions
        (4) Members learn empathy by vicariously living the experiences of others
        (5) Members view selves through the eyes of others
     b. A feeling of security by meeting dependency needs
     c. A system of communication
        (1) Overt: words
        (2) Covert: body language
     d. Role identification and intimacy that helps them to internalize the acceptable behavioral patterns of the group
     e. A spirit of cooperation and competition through sibling interaction
  3. Changes that have influenced the family's ability to indoctrinate children with the norms of society
     a. The Industrial Revolution changed an agrarian society into an industrial one
        (1) Families became nuclear rather than extended
        (2) Families depended more on secondary groups for survival
        (3) New social groups were established to replace the extended family
        (4) Labor unions replaced patriarchal management
           (a) Laws enacted to protect the rights of children and other dependent people of society
           (b) Laws enacted to establish minimum wage and hourly benefits
        (5) Increased mobility of individuals reduced contact with family

b. Altered male and female role patterns
  (1) Changing status of women
    (a) More women go outside the home to work
    (b) Women have an increased role in decision making and are better educated today
  (2) Changing status of men
    (a) More men are willing to assume homemaking responsibilities
    (b) Men share decision making with women, thus decreasing dominance
  (3) Increased partnership in home and financial management has resulted in less stereotyped sex roles
c. Factors resulting in a reduction in the size of families
  (1) Increase in financial cost involved in raising and educating children
  (2) Emphasis on limited population growth
  (3) Wide dissemination of birth control information
  (4) Legalization of abortions
  (5) Persons choosing to marry in later adulthood
  (6) Couples deciding to delay the start of a family until later years

F. Peer groups help youth to establish norms of behavior and assist in the rites of passage from the family group to society
  1. Youth learns about society through contact with the peer group
  2. Youth develops further self-concept in contact with other youths
  3. Peer group interaction can produce change in its individual members
  4. Members have a strong loyalty to the peer group because of the reciprocal relationships and other rewards the group offers
  5. Peer group norms may conflict with family or society's norms

G. Group membership helps individuals achieve goals that are not attainable through individual effort
  1. Types of groups are task oriented, therapy, self-awareness, social
  2. Group functional roles include task roles, group building or maintenance roles, individual or self-serving roles
  3. Group content refers to the subject matter or task being worked on
  4. Group process refers to what is happening among and to group members while working; it deals with morale, feeling tones, influence, competition, conflict

H. Type of leadership in a group depends on the needs of the group members as well as the personality of the leader
  1. Authoritarian leader: rigid and uses leadership role as an instrument of power; the leader makes all the decisions, which are then handed down to the membership; little communication and interrelating between leader and group
  2. Democratic leader: fair and logical, uses the leadership role to stimulate others to achieve a collective goal; the leader encourages interrelating among members by relating to all members; weaknesses as well as strengths are accepted; the contributions of all members are fostered and utilized
  3. Emotional leader: reflects the feeling tones, norms, and values of the group
  4. Laissez-faire leader: passive and unproductive; usually assumes the role of a participant-observer and exerts little control or guidance over group behavior
  5. Bureaucratic leader: rigid and assumes a role that is determined by formal criteria or rules that are inherent in the organization and frequently unrelated to the present group; the leader is not emotionally involved and avoids interrelating with the group members
  6. Charismatic leader: can assume any of the above behaviors, since the group attributes supernatural power to this person or the office and frequently follows directions without question

I. Types of roles assumed by members of the group
  1. Harmonizer: brings other group members into accord while reconciling opposing positions
  2. Questioner: asks questions, seeks information, and gives constructive criticism to other group members
  3. Deserter: talks about irrelevant material; is indifferent and usually disruptive in some manner
  4. Tension reducer: introduces levity when it is needed and appropriate
  5. Encourager: contributes to the ego of others in the group; is a warm, responsive member
  6. Monopolizer: attempts to control and assert authority over group; does not allow others to talk
  7. Clarifier: restates issues for clarification and then summarizes for rest of the group
  8. Opinion giver: uses own experience to back up opinion or belief
  9. Initiator: proposes ideas or topics for discussion and suggests possible solutions for group discussion
  10. Listener: shows interest in the group by expressions on face or by body language while making little or no comment

11. Negativist: pessimistic, argumentative, and uncooperative
12. Energizer: pushes the group into action
13. Aggressor: hostile, aggressive, seeks attention, verbally attacks other group members

J. Community is a social organization that is considered the individual's secondary group
   1. Relationships among members are usually more impersonal
   2. Individuals participate in a more delimited manner or in a specific capacity
   3. The group frequently functions as a means to an end
      a. The group enables diversified groups to communicate
      b. The group helps other groups to identify community problems and possible solutions
   4. The secondary group is usually rather large and meets on an intermittent basis; contacts are usually maintained through correspondence
   5. Leaders of the community facilitate group interaction
      a. They have a knowledge of the community and its needs
      b. They have the skill to stimulate others to act
   6. Secondary groups help establish laws that are necessary to limit antisocial behavior
      a. Laws provide diversified groups with a common base of acceptable behavior
      b. Some laws may favor and protect the vested interests of specific groups within the society

Sociology and Health

A. Role of society
   1. Traditionally societies have placed great emphasis on caring for their members when they are ill
   2. Recently society's role in health maintenance and the prevention of disease has been given an increased priority
   3. Society's provisions for health maintenance include:
      a. Protection of food, water, and drug supplies
      b. Coordination of public health agencies for the supervision, prevention, and control of disease and illness and the promotion of health
      c. Maintenance of public education programs
      d. Awarding scholarships/grants for health education and research
      e. Ongoing unemployment insurance programs
      f. Maintenance of worker's compensation insurance
      g. Maintenance of government-funded health care programs
      h. Supervision of medical and hospital insurance programs

B. Health agency as a social institution has:
   1. A bureaucratic structure
   2. Policies, rules, and regulations governing behavior of its members
   3. An impersonal viewpoint
   4. A status hierarchy
   5. An increasingly specialized subculture

C. Hospital as a subculture of society
   1. Employees develop both written and unwritten hospital policies that:
      a. Set standards of acceptable behavior for both clients and staff
      b. Regulate the hospitalized client's contact with the primary group by limiting visitors
      c. Force both clients and staff to relate to the secondary group
      d. Punish unacceptable behavior by any members of the group, including the client
   2. Folklores and folkways of the hospital serve to:
      a. Maintain the mystique of medicine by fostering the use of a unique language and system of symbols
      b. Attach stigmas to various social illnesses such as AIDS and other sexually transmitted diseases, mental illness, drug addiction, and alcoholism, which are associated with certain patterns of living and acting that are not acceptable to the group
      c. Perpetuate the roles and values of the health team members and maintain the status quo
   3. Hospital has several functions
      a. Primary: to help the client regain health and resume a role in society by providing services directed toward:
         (1) Treatment of illness
         (2) Rehabilitation
         (3) Maintenance and promotion of health
         (4) Protecting the client's legal rights
      b. Secondary: to help society by providing services directed toward:
         (1) Education of health professionals
         (2) The education of the general public
         (3) Research

D. Delivery of health services: responsibility of the community
   1. Members of society become active participants in promotion of health and prevention of illness or injury
   2. Community-health services provide care for the ill in the home rather than in the hospital
   3. Extended care facilities are established with a more community and homelike atmosphere
   4. Nonmedical community leaders take an active role in establishing health policy for society

5. Lay members of the community become involved with health agencies' policies and decisions
6. Health maintenance and treatment are no longer considered a privilege, but the right of all members of society

BASIC CONCEPTS FROM NEUROSCIENCE

Neurophysiologic Theory of Behavior

A. Studies reveal that a malfunction of certain CNS neurons, which secrete substances known as neurotransmitters, appears to inhibit or trigger impulses in other neurons and may be responsible for distortions of behavior associated with psychiatric disorders
B. Neurotransmitters
   1. Dopamine: an excess has been strongly linked with schizophrenia; a deficiency has been found in individuals with Parkinson's disease
   2. Norepinephrine: an excess has been linked to manic behavior; a deficiency has been linked to depressed behavior
   3. Serotonin: an excess has been found to result in hypersomnia (pathologically excessive sleep or drowsiness); a deficiency has been found to result in insomnia (abnormal wakefulness)

BASIC CONCEPTS FROM PSYCHOLOGY

A. Human beings must be able to perceive and interpret stimuli to interact with the environment
   1. Perception and cognitive functioning are influenced by:
      a. The nature of the stimuli
      b. Culture, beliefs, attitudes, and age
      c. Past experiences
      d. Present physical and emotional needs
   2. Individual's personality development is influenced by the ability to perceive and interpret stimuli
      a. Through these processes the external world is internalized
      b. The external world may in turn be distorted by the individual's perceptions
B. Humans must communicate to be able to interact with the environment
   1. Communication is a behavior that is learned through the process of acculturation
   2. People must communicate with others to make needs known
      a. Infant uses the cry to bring attention to needs
      b. Hearing is essential to the development of effective speech, because one learns to form words by hearing the words of others

c. Written word usually replaces the spoken word when face-to-face encounters are impractical and supplements the spoken word when further clarification is necessary
   3. Productive communication depends on the consensual validation of all involved
      a. To understand the intent of the message, each person must be aware of the meaning of the spoken word as well as the inflections in the speaker's voice (verbal and nonverbal communication)
      b. Validation can best be accomplished when participants are empathetic
      c. Language and channels of communication must be adapted to the person and the purpose for which they are intended
      d. Feedback is necessary to evaluate the effectiveness of the words and guide the communication
      e. Satisfaction is enhanced for all involved when lines of communication are kept open
   4. Barriers to effective communication include:
      a. Variations in culture, language, and education
      b. Problems in hearing, speech, or comprehension: ineffective reception or perception
      c. Refusal to listen to another point of view: inability to evaluate
      d. Use of selective inattention, which may cause an interruption or distortion of the message
   5. Nonverbal behavior communicates the inner feelings of the individual performing the behavior
      a. Facial expression, posture, and body movement may express the anxiety, pain, tension, fear, happiness, joy, or satisfaction the individual is experiencing
      b. Nonverbal communication may transmit a different message than the individual's verbal communication (covert versus overt messages)
      c. Confusion arises when there is a difference in the verbal and nonverbal message received
C. Psychologic experiences provide the energy that is transformed into behavior
   1. Anxiety frequently provides the push that moves people to action because it:
      a. Develops when two goals or needs are in conflict
      b. Is a state of apprehension or tension aroused by impulses from within
      c. Prepares one for action or completely overwhelms and inhibits action
   2. Anxiety develops in stages that progress from increased alertness to panic

3. The sympathetic nervous system prepares the body's physiologic defense for fight or flight by stimulating the adrenal medulla to secrete epinephrine and norepinephrine
   a. The heartbeat is accelerated to pump more blood to the muscles
   b. The peripheral blood vessels constrict to provide more blood to the vital organs
   c. The bronchioles dilate, and breathing becomes rapid and deep to supply more oxygen to the cells
   d. The pupils dilate to provide increased vision
   e. The liver releases glucose for quick energy
   f. The prothrombin time is shortened to protect the body from loss of blood in the event of injury
4. Selye's general adaptation syndrome (GAS) is the body's physiologic adaptation to stress (anxiety)
   a. The adrenal cortex secretes cortisone during the emergency stage
   b. When stress continues, the increased secretion of cortisone causes the body to go through a resistive stage
   c. If the process continues, the last stage is exhaustion and death
5. Defense mechanisms serve to protect the personality by controlling anxiety and reducing emotional pressures

DEVELOPMENT OF THE PERSONALITY

DEFINITION

A. Sum of all traits that differentiate one individual from another
B. Total behavior pattern of an individual through which the inner interests are expressed
C. The individual's unique and distinctive way of behaving and interacting with others
D. Constellation of defense mechanisms for dealing with inner and outer pressures
E. A functional role within a family system

FACTORS INVOLVED IN PERSONALITY DEVELOPMENT

A. Behavior is a learned response that develops as a result of past experiences
B. To protect the individual's emotional well-being, these experiences are organized in the psyche on three different levels
   1. Conscious: composed of past experiences, easily recalled, that create little if any emotional discomfort and tend to be somewhat pleasant
   2. Subconscious: composed of material that has been deliberately pushed out of the conscious but can be recalled with some effort
   3. Unconscious: contains the largest body of material; greatly influences behavior
      a. This material cannot be deliberately brought back into awareness because it is usually unacceptable and painful to the individual
      b. If recalled, it is usually disguised or distorted, as in dreams; however, it is still capable of producing a good deal of anxiety
C. According to Freud the personality consists of three parts: the id, ego, and superego
   1. Id contains the instincts, impulses, and urges; is totally self-centered and unconscious
   2. Ego is the conscious self, the "I" that deals with reality; the part of the personality that is shown to the environment
   3. Superego controls, inhibits, and regulates impulses and instincts whose uncontrolled expression would endanger the emotional well-being of the individual and the stability of the society

CRITICAL PERIODS IN THE FORMATION OF THE PERSONALITY

A. Personality of an individual develops in overlapping stages that shade and merge together
   1. Certain goals must be accomplished during each stage in the development from infancy to maturity
   2. If these goals are not accomplished at specific periods, the basic structure of the personality will be weakened
   3. Factors in each stage persist as a permanent part of the personality
   4. Each stage has particular frustrations and major traumas that must be overcome
   5. Successful resolution of the conflicts associated with each stage is essential to development
   6. Unresolved conflicts remain in the unconscious and may, at times, result in maladaptive behavior
B. Tasks related to personality development during infancy
   1. Freud: oral stage—infant obtains gratification by taking everything in; begins to develop self-concept from the responses of others
   2. Erikson: trust versus mistrust—trust develops from the inner feeling of self-worth that is transmitted through maternal care; child learns to depend on the satisfaction that is derived from this care, and when the need is met, trust develops

3. Sullivan: need for security—infant learns to rely on others to gratify needs and satisfy wishes; develops a sense of basic trust, security, and self-worth when this occurs

4. Piaget: sensorimotor stage—infant develops physically with a gradual increase in the ability to think and use language; progresses from simple reflex responses through repetitive behaviors to deliberate and imaginative activity

C. Tasks related to personality development during early childhood
1. Freud: anal stage—struggle of giving of self and breaking the symbiotic ties to mother; as the ties are broken, the child learns independence
2. Erikson: autonomy versus shame and doubt—the struggle of holding on to or letting go; an internal struggle for self-identity; love versus hate
3. Sullivan: child learns to communicate needs through the use of words and the acceptance of delayed gratification and interference with wish fulfillment
4. Piaget: preoperational thought stage—child learns to imitate and play; begins to use symbols and language although interpretation is literal

D. Tasks related to personality development during preschool period
1. Freud: oedipal stage—love for and desire to possess parent of the opposite sex creates fear and guilt feelings; desires are repressed and role identification with parent of the same sex occurs
2. Erikson: initiative versus guilt—stage of intensive activity, play, and consuming fantasies where child interjects parents' social consciousness
3. Sullivan: development of body image and self-perception—organizes and uses experiences in terms of approval and disapproval received; begins using selective inattention and disassociates those experiences that cause physical or emotional discomfort and pain
4. Piaget: preoperational thought stage continues—child begins understanding relationships and develops basic conceptual thought and intuitive reasoning

E. Tasks related to personality development during school age or preadolescence
1. Freud: latency stage—period of low sexual activity; identifies with peer groups
2. Erikson: industry versus inferiority—the child learns how to make things with others and strives to achieve success
3. Sullivan: the period of learning to form satisfying relationships with peers—uses competition, compromise, and cooperation; the preadolescent learns to relate to peers of the same sex

4. Piaget: concrete operational thought stage—thinking is more socialized and logical with increased intellectual and conceptual development; begins problem-solving by use of inductive reasoning and logical thought

F. Tasks related to personality development during adolescence
1. Freud: genital stage—sexual activity increases; sexual identity is strengthened or attacked
2. Erikson: identity versus identity diffusion—childhood identifications are integrated with the basic drives, native endowments, and opportunities offered in social roles
3. Sullivan: learns independence and how to establish satisfactory relationships with members of the opposite sex
4. Piaget: formal operational stage—develops true abstract thought by application of logical tests; achieves conceptual independence and problem-solving ability

G. Tasks related to personality development during young adulthood
1. Erikson: intimacy versus isolation—moves from the relative security of self-identity to the relative insecurity involved in establishing intimacy with another
2. Sullivan: becomes economically, intellectually, and emotionally self-sufficient

H. Tasks related to personality development during later adulthood
1. Erikson: generativity versus self-absorption—the mature person becomes interested in establishing and guiding the next generation
2. Sullivan: learns to be interdependent and assumes responsibility for others

I. Tasks related to personality development during senescence
1. Erikson: adapts to triumphs and disappointments with a certain ego integrity
2. Sullivan: develops an acceptance of responsibility for what life is and was and of its place in the flow of history

INFLUENCE OF BASIC NEEDS ON THE DEVELOPMENT OF THE PERSONALITY

A. Humanity has certain basic needs that must be satisfied
1. Need to communicate
   a. Through communication, humans maintain contact with reality
      (1) The individual needs to validate findings with others to correctly interpret reality
      (2) Validation is enhanced when communication conveys an understanding of feelings

b. Through communication, the individual develops a concept of self in relation to others
2. Need for security
   a. To feel secure an assurance of survival is fundamental
   b. Fear emerges when survival is threatened
   c. Initially the infant's security is related to the satisfaction of physical needs
   d. Security is enhanced when the same individual meets the infant's physical needs in a consistent manner
   e. The infant must also perceive love to feel secure
   f. Security is derived from the individual's perception of self in relation to others
   g. How the individual handles these perceptions influences personality development
3. Need to move from dependence to independence
   a. The infant is dependent on the parents but through learning acquires faculties for independence
   b. There is no real security or deep assurance of survival in being dependent on others, because uncertainties develop if one's security is totally derived from this source
   c. The infant must feel love and security before reaching out to struggle with the problems in the environment
   d. When the need for love and security is met, the child is sustained in the failures and hurts associated with learning and independence
   e. Denial of the opportunity to learn or frustration in the drive for independence will produce emotional problems
4. Need to develop a self-concept
   a. Self-concept begins to develop early in infancy
   b. Determination of the self-concept develops primarily through interaction with significant persons in the environment
   c. An integral part of the self-concept is the body image
   d. First and most deeply learned perception of body image develops from the attitudes of significant others, because children view themselves as others view them
   e. Concept of the self is root of security and future developmental needs
   f. Communication enhances the development of self
   g. A person's self-concept is the basis for emotional stability or instability; a secure person has strength and capacity for independence and becomes less anxious when circumstances require the help of others

5. Need to find relief from organic discomfort
   a. Through experience, one learns the most satisfying ways of relieving discomfort
   b. Adjustment to illness depends on how the individual adjusts to life
B. Needs of a specific individual at a given time will vary according to internal and external environmental factors
C. To attain psychologic equilibrium and achieve need satisfaction, the individual attempts to maintain a feeling of safety and comfort in adapting to life's situations; this is often achieved by maintaining a feeling of worth and a feeling of being needed by others

ANXIETY AND BEHAVIOR

A. Anxiety:
   1. Is a state of apprehension, tension, or uneasiness
   2. Is an internal phenomenon aroused by impulses
   3. Occurs when the ego is threatened
   4. Frequently stems from an anticipation of danger
   5. May arise from known, unknown, or unrecognized sources
B. Levels of anxiety
   1. Alertness level: automatic response of the central nervous system that:
      a. Prepares the body for danger by regulating internal processes
      b. Concentrates all energies for internal activity
   2. Apprehension level: response to anticipation of short-term danger that:
      a. Prepares the individual for efficient performance
      b. Occurs when facing new situations
      c. Creates some conscious awareness of discomfort
   3. Free-floating level: response to generalized anxiety that:
      a. Creates a feeling of impending doom
      b. Produces an acute feeling of discomfort
   4. Panic level: total response to anxiety characterized by uncontrolled, unrealistic behavior that:
      a. Lessens perception of the environment to protect the ego from awareness
      b. Increases the danger to the entire system
C. Behavioral defenses against anxiety
   1. Conscious: these are the first-line defenses against anxiety; used by all people in times of stress; comprise the individual's deliberate effort to maintain control, reduce tension, and limit anxiety (individual may be aware of behavior but is not always aware of underlying reason); the individual:

a. Removes self from the source of anxiety
b. Escapes through bodily satisfactions
c. Focuses psychic energy on other, more pleasant, activities
d. Uses substitute gratifications
e. Consciously avoids painful subjects
f. Gives socially acceptable reasons for behavior
g. Releases tensions by acting out impulsively

2. Unconscious: these include the second-, third-, and fourth-line defenses against anxiety; may be used by all people in extremely stressful situations; however, if used consistently, indicate that the individual is emotionally ill
   a. Second-line defenses are the personality traits developed to handle interpersonal relationships and protect the ego; these defenses include:
      (1) Exaggerated dependency and immaturity
      (2) Passive submission
      (3) Domination of others
      (4) Aggression toward others
      (5) Withdrawal from others
      (6) Compulsive ambition
      (7) Perfectionism and grandiosity
   b. Third-line defenses are the neurotic traits developed to handle interpersonal relationships and protect the ego; these defenses include:
      (1) Repudiation and opposition of inner drives by the use of reaction formation
      (2) Avoidance of emotional or feeling level by placing complete emphasis on intellectual reasoning
      (3) Inhibition of affective, autonomic, and visceral functions to deaden actual awareness of repressed impulses
      (4) Displacement of impulses to an external object, which is then feared and avoided
      (5) Use of compulsive rituals to magically neutralize inner impulses
   c. Fourth-line defenses are the psychotic traits developed to handle interpersonal relationships and protect the ego; these defenses include:
      (1) Regression to dependency level of development frequently accompanied by childish attitudes and behavior
      (2) Denial and withdrawal from others and reality
      (3) Internalization of hostility
      (4) Excited, uncontrolled acting out

3. As anxiety and the threat to the ego are increased or decreased, shifts in the lines of defense will occur; the individual's behavior is altered by these shifts

D. Major sources of anxiety
   1. Threat to one's biologic integrity; interference with one's basic physiologic needs
   2. Threat to one's self-system: self-esteem, self-worth, self-respect

PERSONALITY DEFENSES
Defense Mechanisms

A. Defense mechanisms provide initial protection for the personality
B. Although all individuals may, in times of severe emotional stress, use many of the behaviors listed, it is the repetitive use of these behaviors in most situations that is indicative of problems
C. Identifiable patterns of response begin to form when individuals respond to most situations they encounter with the same type of behavior
D. Commonly used normal defense mechanisms that help an individual to deal with reality are:
   1. Compensation: the individual makes up for a perceived lack in one area by emphasizing capabilities in another
   2. Compromise: reciprocal give-and-take necessary in many relationships to salvage some part of the situation or the goal
   3. Identification: the individual internalizes the characteristics of an idealized person
   4. Rationalization: the individual makes acceptable excuses for behavior and feelings; attempts to explain behavior by logical reasoning
   5. Sublimation: a socially acceptable behavior is substituted for an unacceptable instinct; this mechanism is used when the expression of these instincts would prove a threat to the self
   6. Substitution: the individual replaces one goal for another
E. In addition to the normal defenses, all individuals may use compensatory-type defenses in times of stress; these, when used in moderation, are adaptive; if used to excess, they frequently create greater emotional problems
   1. As the use of these compensatory defenses increases and encompasses more of the individual's life, contact with reality is interrupted and distortions begin
   2. These patterns of behavior are considered deviations and are usually looked on as symptoms of emotional problems
      a. Conversion: emotional conflict is unconsciously changed into a physical symptom that can be expressed openly and without anxiety
      b. Denial: emotional conflict is blocked from the conscious mind and the individual refuses to recognize its existence

c. Displacement: emotions related to an emotionally charged situation or object are shifted to a relatively safe substitute situation or object

d. Fantasy: conscious distortion of unconscious wishes and needs to obtain gratification and satisfaction

e. Intellectualization: use of thinking, ideas, or intellect to avoid emotions

f. Introjection: complete acceptance of another's opinions and values as one's own

g. Projection: unconscious denial of unacceptable feelings and emotions in oneself while attributing them to others

h. Reaction formation: the individual unconsciously reverses unacceptable feelings and behaves in the exact opposite manner

i. Regression: return to an earlier stage of behavior when stress creates problems at the present stage

j. Repression: involuntary exclusion from consciousness of those ideas, feelings, and situations that are creating conflict and causing discomfort

k. Suppression: voluntary exclusion from consciousness of those ideas, feelings, and situations that are creating conflict and causing discomfort

l. Transference: positive or negative feelings and emotions that were previously present toward important figures are applied and attributed to another person in the present

MOTIVATION, LEARNING, AND BEHAVIOR

A. All behavior is motivated
1. Motive always implies some purpose
2. Social motives are often changed through learning
3. Symbolic rewards are the major factors in learning
4. Social approval is an important form of symbolic reward

B. Behavior and emotions
1. Emotions act as motives for behavior, because they often involve a reaction to some external situation
2. Behavior is always accompanied and often controlled by the emotions
3. Emotions may facilitate or hinder the learning process
4. Emotions exert a strong influence on the thinking process

C. Automatic behavior
1. Is the predetermined or repetitive type behavior that has been used successfully in prior situations
2. Requires little effort or thought
3. Is adapted to definite situations and can be difficult to alter if the situation changes
4. Is integrated with cognition in the functioning of a mature and independent adult

D. Life is a continually changing process, and when these changes occur in areas of significance they often produce rather distinct emotional responses; these changes include:
1. Resistance to change: the individual hesitates to accept or adapt to the change and may attempt to deny its occurrence or reject its outcome
2. Regression: the individual returns to an earlier type of behavior that, at the time, provided some satisfaction and gratification and now provides an escape from the unacceptable or anxiety-producing situation
3. Acceptance and progression: the individual adapts to the change and expends energy on outside objects rather than self-centered aims

▼ DEVIANT PATTERNS OF BEHAVIOR
Withdrawn Behavior

A. Definition: pathologic retreat from or an avoidance of people and the world of reality

B. Developmental factors
1. Unhappy childhood caused by conflict, tension, and anxiety in the home
2. Inconsistent relationships with parents
   a. Lack of firm standards for reward or punishment
   b. Variations between verbal and nonverbal communications
3. Failure to develop a sense of security
4. Failure to develop a positive self-image
5. Interpersonal relationships create a continuous source of anxiety
6. Chronic anxiety results in loss of interest in interpersonal relationships and reality testing
7. Extreme sensitivity, narcissism, and introversion develop

C. Compensatory mechanisms used to reduce and avoid stress include:
1. Fixation
2. Rationalization
3. Reaction formation
4. Regression
5. Rigidity and compulsiveness
6. Sublimation

D. Effects of compensatory mechanisms on behavior
   1. Isolation and failure to test reality result in greater distortions of reality
   2. Behavior can progress until loss of contact with reality develops and the individual retreats into the condition usually identified as schizophrenia

Projective Behavior

A. Definition: pathologic denial of one's own feelings, faults, failures, and emotions while continually attributing them to others
B. Developmental factors
   1. Parents set extremely high demands and continually raise expected standards of performance
   2. Expectations of failure are fostered, creating feelings of inadequacy and feelings of inferiority
   3. Childhood experiences continue to reinforce these feelings and chronic insecurity, suspiciousness, and extreme sensitivity develop
   4. Feelings of hostility develop and cannot be expressed
   5. Inability to establish relationships with others interferes with reality testing
   6. The individual develops a rigid, structured, narcissistic personality
   7. Competitive society fosters and supports projective patterns of behavior
C. Compensatory mechanisms used to reduce and avoid stress include:
   1. Delusions
   2. Denial
   3. Displacement
   4. Ideas of reference
   5. Projection
   6. Rationalization
   7. Rigidity
D. Effects of compensatory mechanisms on behavior
   1. The individual is unable to tolerate suspense, prolonged anxiety, or tension
   2. Unacceptable impulses and wishes are denied and faults and failures are disclaimed for self and attributed to others
   3. Delusional ideas develop and begin to dominate behavior
   4. Ideas of reference result in continual misinterpretation of events
   5. Delusions become more systematized and spread out
   6. Behavior can progress until loss of contact with reality is complete and the individual retreats into the condition usually identified as paranoid-type schizophrenia or paranoid states

Aggressive Behavior

A. Definition: pathologic anger and hostility that are turned outward onto others or inward on oneself

B. Developmental factors
   1. Security chronically threatened, resulting in a continual struggle to maintain it
   2. Strong need for approval
   3. Failure to develop self-concept and self-esteem
   4. Chronic anxiety and tension, which are often increased by the real or imagined loss of a love object
   5. Demands and responsibilities are high
C. Compensatory mechanisms used to reduce and avoid stress include:
   1. Denial
   2. Displacement
   3. Hostility that can be directed on
      a. Self
      b. Environment
   4. Rationalization
   5. Repression
   6. Rigidity
D. Effects of compensatory mechanisms on behavior
   1. Need for approval results in compliance to demands
   2. Necessary compliance creates resentment
   3. Hostility develops and fosters feeling of guilt
   4. Self-doubt increases anxiety and tension
   5. Increased anxiety and tension reduce interpersonal relationships and reality testing
   6. Behavior can progress until there is a loss of contact with reality and the individual retreats into the condition usually identified as a mood disorder

Anxiety-Related Behavior

Includes anxiety reactions, conversion reactions, phobic reactions, and obsessive-compulsive reactions
A. Definition: maladjustive type of response, characterized by many fears, anxieties, and/or physical symptoms
B. Developmental factors
   1. Usually lack a stable family life and effective guidance
   2. Frequently overprotected and fail to acquire the necessary skills to cope with problems
   3. Experience chronic insecurity, anxiety, and tension
   4. Goals are set by the parents, and acceptance depends on achieving the goals
   5. Constant struggle to gain reassurance and security
   6. Gains satisfaction from behavior and substitutes this satisfaction for the satisfaction desired but not obtained through interpersonal relations
C. Compensatory mechanisms used to reduce anxiety and avoid stress include
   1. Conversion
   2. Denial
   3. Displacement

4. Rationalization
5. Regression
6. Rigidity and compulsiveness

D. Effects of compensatory mechanisms on behavior
1. Behavior is purposeful and is unconsciously resorted to when the person feels threatened
2. Continued use of behavior can:
   a. Create new problems for the individual
   b. Be out of proportion to the degree of stress, impair social effectiveness, and dominate the individual's total life
3. When impairment of functioning occurs, the individual is usually considered to be deviating from the normal and to have an anxiety disorder

Socially Aggressive Behavior

A. Definition: maladjustive response resulting from a defect in the development of the personality that is characterized by peculiar actions or misbehavior
B. Developmental factors
1. Approval and disapproval do not appear sufficiently strong in childhood to influence the behavior along accepted patterns
2. Long history of maladjustment that creates more problems as child matures and standards for acceptable behavior are increased
3. The individual may show a history of severe emotional trauma in early life that interferes with emotional development
4. Parents frequently provide a cold, emotionally sterile environment
C. Compensatory mechanisms used to reduce anxiety and avoid stress include:
1. Denial
2. Displacement
3. Hostility
4. Regression
5. Rejection
6. Repression
D. Effects of compensatory mechanisms on behavior; the individual:
1. Appears competent but is usually unreliable; lacks a sense of responsibility
2. Has the potential to succeed but shows a history of repeated failure
3. Lacks perseverance, honesty, and sincerity
4. Is completely egocentric and incapable of emotional investment in others
5. Experiences no remorse or shame
6. Is explosive under pressure
7. Is unable to tolerate criticism
8. Fails to profit from past experiences and cares little about the consequences of present acts
9. Has impaired judgment, which usually creates problems and brings the individual into conflict with society; usually classified as personality disturbances

Addictive Behavior

A. Definition: repeated or chronic use of alcohol or drugs with a resulting dependency on these substances
B. Developmental factors
1. Feelings of loneliness and isolation develop
2. Chronic anxiety, fears, and low tension tolerance develop as a result of early relationships
3. Feelings of inadequacy in interpersonal relationships serve to increase anxiety
4. Inability to delay satisfaction
5. Struggle for independence yet unconsciously desire to be dependent
6. Impulsiveness and resentment of responsibility
7. Peer pressure and drug availability
8. Sexual conflict
9. Family factors
C. Compensatory mechanisms used to reduce anxiety and avoid stress include:
1. Addiction
2. Denial
3. Displacement
4. Fantasy
5. Intellectualization
6. Rationalization
7. Regression
8. Repression
D. Effects of compensatory mechanisms on behavior
1. Drug or alcohol reduces inhibitory self-control
2. Drug or alcohol allows for expression of inner feelings but increases the guilt and requires more of the substance to relieve the guilt
3. Alcohol and drugs decrease feelings of inferiority and reduce anxiety
4. Alcohol and drugs increase social isolation and cause deterioration of personal habits
5. The individual becomes increasingly less efficient and devotes less energy to goals and ambitions
6. Dependency and tolerance develop and the substances are needed in increasing amounts to achieve the same dulling of reality
7. Securing the alcohol or drug becomes the main objective and functioning is totally impaired; they are then classified as drug addicts or alcoholics

Self-Destructive Behavior

A. Definition: chronically indulging in self-destructive behavior by noncompliance with medical regimens; habitually abusing food, drugs, alcohol, or cigarettes; or engaging in high-risk activities
B. Developmental factors:
1. Failure to develop a sense of security and/or self-worth
2. Superficial interpersonal relationships

3. Inconsistent relationship with parents
   a. Lack of firm standards for reward or punishment
   b. Variations between verbal and nonverbal communications
4. Lack of faith in the future
5. Anxiety results in difficulty in changing goals and expectations
6. Sense of failure or shame when goals are not attained
7. Sense of isolation

C. Compensatory mechanisms used to reduce and avoid stress include:
   1. Denial
   2. Fantasy
   3. Rationalization
   4. Rigidity
   5. Withdrawal

D. Effects of compensatory mechanisms on behavior
   1. Greater risk of self-destructive behavior
   2. Greater risk of suicide
      a. Talking, threatening, or planning suicide in either very vague or specific terms throughout planning
      b. Making a suicide attempt in an acute crisis state by seriously and deliberately executing a plan
      c. The suicide is completed, but there is difficulty in determining whether the act was accidental or deliberate (e.g., autoeroticism practiced by adolescents; reckless driving)
      d. Copycat suicide: suicidal acts carried out by adolescents knowing or reading about similar acts

▼ PSYCHOLOGIC FACTORS AFFECTING PHYSICAL CONDITION

A. Physical illnesses where emotional factors are the predominant causative agents

B. Anxiety stimulates the autonomic nervous system, and the nervous and endocrine impulses appear to center on one particular organ, creating actual physical illness and changes in the tissue structure

C. Reason a certain organ is involved with one client and a different organ with another is still undetermined

D. Pathology: premorbid personality appears to be one of unexpressed aggression resulting from the unresolved struggle between dependent need and independent striving; may be familial

E. Systems
   1. Skin
      a. In neurodermatitis, dermatitis factitia, pruritus, and trichotillomania, psychic factors appear to dominate
      b. There appears to be a relationship between endocrine imbalance and disturbances in the autonomic regulation of skin physiology
      c. Stress seems to lead to rash, itching, and discomfort
   2. Musculoskeletal
      a. Anxiety and fear often create a tightening of muscles
      b. This becomes an aggravating factor in arthritis, backache, tension headache, or any other musculoskeletal disorder in which increased tension and spasm are involved
   3. Respiratory
      a. Hyperventilation syndrome
         (1) Panting occurs with tension and excitement and this forced respiration can produce biochemical changes in the blood
         (2) These changes can alter the cerebral circulation and cause a reduction in consciousness and syncope
      b. Bronchial asthma
         (1) Stress and tension appear to create increased secretions and changes in the bronchi
         (2) Individuals with asthma tend to exhibit a strong desire for protection and dependency yet fear rejection or engulfment
         (3) Wheeze associated with asthma is considered by some to be a suppressed cry for this protection
   4. Cardiovascular
      a. Essential hypertension
         (1) Anxiety and other stresses are believed to play a role in releasing a pressor from the kidneys, which causes chronic vasoconstriction of the vessels
         (2) All other primary causes for hypertension must be ruled out before this cause can be diagnosed
         (3) Individuals with hypertension have difficulty handling hostile feelings, are less assertive, and have more obsessive-compulsive traits than nonhypertensive people
         (4) Hypertension may be considered a state of chronically unexpressed rage that arises from conflicts between passive/dependent longings and the struggle for independence
      b. Coronary occlusion and angina
         (1) Coronary attacks frequently occur following periods of fatigue and anxiety
         (2) These individuals place a high value on work and success; they become depressed when inactive

5. Hemolymphatic
   a. Certain blood dyscrasias and responses can be linked to emotional stress
   b. In some individuals the neutrophil count drops, the clotting time is decreased, both blood viscosity and erythrocyte sedimentation rate rise
   c. Nature of this response to stress is still controversial
6. Gastrointestinal
   a. Peptic ulcer
      (1) Anxiety and other stress appear to create a condition of hyperactivity, hypersecretion, hyperacidity, and engorgement of the mucosa
      (2) May be related to stresses in life, particularly those concerned with conflicts between passivity and aggression
      (3) Use reaction formation to cover the strong, somewhat irrational need to achieve security from others
   b. Ulcerative colitis
      (1) Parasympathetic stimulation of the lower bowel produces an enzyme that interferes with the protective coating of the bowel
      (2) May occur as a reaction to a variety of stresses but most often in situations that demand accomplishment and arouse fear of not succeeding
      (3) Many clients are immature and have not gained any feelings of independence
7. Genitourinary
   a. Disturbances in genital and urinary problems may occur under stress
   b. Enuresis, amenorrhea, frigidity, and impotence appear to be related to psychologic factors
   c. Depression and feelings of helplessness may be related to urinary retention
   d. Fear may be related to urgency and frequency
8. Endocrine
   a. Eating patterns and dependency on food for satisfaction and reduction of stress appear related to both diabetes mellitus and obesity
   b. Feelings of insecurity and an unusual sense of responsibility appear associated with onset of hyperthyroidism
9. Organs of special sense: some evidence that certain neurologic disturbances, such as atypical facial neuralgia, are related to emotional conflict
F. Therapy: must be directed toward both the physical and emotional problems

General Nursing Care of Clients with Physical Conditions Related to Psychologic Factors

A. Reduce emotional stimulation when possible
B. Explain all procedures carefully and allow client time for questions
C. Provide the client with talking time
D. Avoid material that appears to stimulate conflict for the client
E. Accept the client's behavior and encourage expression of feelings
F. Remember that the client is really physically ill and the symptoms have a physiologic basis

NURSING IN PSYCHIATRY

BASIC PRINCIPLES OF PSYCHIATRIC/MENTAL HEALTH NURSING

Psychiatric/mental health nursing in Canada is guided by the philosophy and framework of primary health care

A. These principles:
   1. Are by necessity general in nature
   2. Form the guidelines for the promotion of mental health, the prevention of mental illness, and the provision of holistic psychiatric nursing care for all clients
B. When caring for clients, the nurse should attempt to:
   1. Accept and respect people as individuals regardless of their behavior
   2. Limit or reject inappropriate behavior without rejecting the individual
   3. Recognize that all behavior has meaning and is meeting the needs of the performer regardless of how distorted or meaningless it appears to others
   4. Accept the dependency needs of individuals while supporting and encouraging moves toward independence
   5. Help individuals set appropriate limits for themselves or set limits for them when they are unable to do so
   6. Encourage individuals to express their feelings in an atmosphere free of reprisal or judgment
   7. Recognize that individuals need to use their defenses until other defenses can be substituted
   8. Recognize how feelings affect behavior and influence relationships
   9. Recognize that individuals frequently respond to the behavioral expectations of others: family, peers, authority (staff)
   10. Recognize that all individuals have a potential for movement toward higher levels of emotional health

THERAPEUTIC NURSING RELATIONSHIPS

A. Phases
1. Orientation or introductory: the nurse establishes a trust relationship that the client tests by discussing only what he or she wishes to discuss; clients are never pushed to discuss areas of concern that are upsetting to them
2. Working: the nurse and the client discuss areas of concern and the client is helped to plan, implement, and evaluate a course of action
3. Termination: end of the therapeutic relationship between the nurse and the client; the time parameters should be set early in the relationship with meetings spaced further and further apart near the end

B. Themes of communication: recurring thoughts and ideas that give insight into what an individual is feeling and tie the communication together
1. Content: conversation may appear superficial but careful attention to the underlying theme helps the nurse identify problem areas while providing insight into the client's self-concept
2. Mood: emotion or affect that the client communicates to the nurse; includes personal appearance, facial expressions, and gestures that reflect the client's mood and feelings
3. Interaction: how the client reacts or interacts with the nurse; includes how the client relates and what role he or she assumes when communicating with the nurse and others

C. Fundamental requirements of a therapeutic relationship
1. Ability to communicate therapeutically requires a basic understanding and use of verbal and nonverbal interviewing techniques in developing a trusting relationship and the ability to use "self" therapeutically through:
   a. Open-ended rather than probing questions
   b. Reflection of words and feelings and paraphrasing
   c. Acceptance of the client's behavior
   d. Nonjudgmental, objective attitude
   e. Focusing on the emotional needs of the client
   f. Having a therapeutic goal for the interview
2. Recognition that an individual has potential for growth
   a. Individuals need to learn about their own behavior in relation to others
   b. Exchanging experiences with others provides the reassurance that reactions are valid and feelings shared
   c. Participating with groups increases knowledge of interpersonal relationships and helps individuals to identify strengths and resources

d. The identification of the individual's strengths and resources helps to convey the expectation of growth
3. Recognition that an individual needs to be accepted
   a. Acceptance is an active process designed to convey respect for another through empathetic understanding
   b. Acceptance of others implies and requires acceptance of self
   c. To be nonjudgmental, one must become aware of one's own attitudes and feelings and their effect on perception
   d. Acceptance requires that individuals be permitted and even encouraged to express their feelings and attitudes even though they may be divergent from the general viewpoint
      (1) Individuals should be encouraged to express both positive and negative feelings
      (2) This encouragement must occur on both the verbal and nonverbal level
   e. Acceptance means showing interest in another person; interest requires:
      (1) Face-to-face contact and really listening to what the other person has to say
      (2) Developing an awareness of the other person's likes and dislikes
      (3) Attempting to understand another's point of view
      (4) Using nonverbal as well as verbal expressions of acceptance
   f. Acceptance requires the development of interpersonal techniques that encourage others to express problems; the listener's:
      (1) Reflection of feelings, attitudes, and words help the speaker to identify feelings
      (2) Open-ended questions permit the speaker to focus on problems
      (3) Paraphrasing assists the speaker in clarifying statements
      (4) Use of silence provides both the listener and the speaker with the necessary time for thinking over what is being discussed
   g. Acceptance requires the recognition of factors that block communication, including:
      (1) Any overt or covert response that conveys a judgmental or superior attitude
      (2) Direct questions that convey an invasive or probing attitude
      (3) Ridicule that conveys a hostile attitude
      (4) Talking about one's own problems and not listening, which conveys a self-serving attitude and loss of interest in the speaker

D. Recognition of behavioral changes that result from physical illness
1. Anxiety, fear, and depression occur whenever there is a health problem
   a. Body image and feelings of being in control of one's body have their basis in the early developmental period
   b. Anxiety develops whenever a real or imagined threat to the body image occurs
2. Signs of the anxiety, fear, and depression associated with illness are variable and include:
   a. Indifference to symptoms: usually related to failure to accept the occurrence of a health problem
   b. Denial of reality: usually related to attempts to maintain stability and integrity of the personality
   c. Reaction formation: usually related to attempts to block the reality from consciousness and acting as if nothing is wrong
   d. Failure to keep appointments and follow health care provider's directions: usually related to fear of finding additional problems or admitting there is something wrong
   e. Overconcern with body functions and symptoms: usually related to fear of death
   f. Asking many questions and offering many complaints: usually related to attempts at keeping a staff member's attention because of fears associated with illness; fear of abandonment
   g. Constantly ventilating feelings
3. Emotional needs of the ill person include:
   a. Security of continuous relationships with friends and family members
   b. Some way of achieving the feeling of self-worth and self-esteem
   c. Assistance in accepting the dependent role of the client
   d. Assistance in resolving conflicts while maintaining security
   e. Assistance in refocusing inner resources
   f. Contact with the reality of the external world
4. To help the individual maintain the self-concept during illness, the nurse must understand the normal emotional stages of illness
   a. Denial: the individual cannot believe it is happening
   b. Anger: something has happened that one cannot control
   c. Bargaining: promising to be a better person if something occurs
   d. Depression: one grieves for loss or expected loss
   e. Acceptance of the illness and learning how to adapt: this stage can only be reached when the individual has resolved the conflicts that develop during the earlier stages
5. Common reactions occur to the change in body image associated with many health problems
   a. Attitudes toward one's body and self-concept greatly influence response
   b. Fear is a universal response; individual may focus on fear of:
      (1) Pain
      (2) Incapacitation
      (3) Disfigurement
      (4) Altered self-concept
      (5) Rejection of loved ones
      (6) Death
   c. Questioning is a universal response; the individual may focus on:
      (1) This cannot be happening to me
      (2) Is this really happening to me?
      (3) What did I do to deserve this?
      (4) Why am I being punished?
   d. Grief and mourning are universal responses; the individual may focus on:
      (1) What was in the past
      (2) What could have been for the future
      (3) Loss of missed opportunities
      (4) A magnified view of the loss
      (5) Avoiding interpersonal contacts
6. Caring for the dying client involves caring for the body, the mind, and the spirit
   a. Demands an understanding and acceptance of the nurse's own feelings, beliefs, and fears about death
   b. The last stages of life should be viewed as a positive rather than negative achievement

PHARMACOLOGY RELATED TO EMOTIONAL DISORDERS

▼ ANTIANXIETY OR ANXIOLYTIC MEDICATIONS

Description
A. Used for the treatment of anxiety and also useful in the induction of sleep
B. Exert a general depressing effect on the CNS, many also exert skeletal muscle–relaxant and anticonvulsant effects
C. Anxiolytics are available in oral and parenteral (IM, IV) preparations
D. Used when the individual has difficulty in coping with environmental stresses and accomplishing daily activities

E. Although the use of sedative-hypnotics has declined in the last decade, they are still widely used to reduce anxiety

F. These drugs were formerly called minor tranquilizers

Types

A. Benzodiazepines
   1. Alprazolam (Xanax)
   2. Chlordiazepoxide (Librium)
   3. Clorazepate (Tranxene)
   4. Diazepam (Valium)
   5. Estazolam (ProSom)
   6. Flurazepam (Dalmane)
   7. Lorazepam (Ativan)
   8. Oxazepam (Serax)
   9. Temazepam (Restoril)
   10. Triazolam (Halcion)
B. Nonbenzodiazepine or azaspirodecanedione buspirone (BuSpar)
C. Anticonvulsant benzodiazepine Clonazepam (Klonopin)
D. Propanediols
E. Quinazolines

Precautions

A. Drug interactions: drugs potentiate depressant effects of alcohol or sedatives
B. Tolerance to the sedative and hypnotic effects develops eventually with all these drugs, although it develops more slowly with the benzodiazepines than with the others
C. All of these drugs, if taken in large enough doses or for extended time periods, can lead to physical and emotional dependence
D. Tolerance can contribute to self-medication and dosage escalation
E. Adverse side effects are related to diminished mental alertness; caution about driving or operating hazardous machinery until tolerance develops
F. A drop in BP of 20 mm Hg (systolic) on standing warrants withholding the drug and notifying the physician
G. Benzodiazepine use should not be abruptly discontinued to avoid a withdrawal syndrome
H. Severe withdrawal symptoms can occur if agents are taken for a long time (over 8 months) and in high doses

Nursing Care of Clients Receiving Antianxiety or Anxiolytic Medications

A. Assess the client's medication history, knowledge level and use of current medications (prescribed, over-the-counter, and illicit drugs), medication allergies, and pattern of alcohol use
B. Explore the client's perceptions and feelings about medications; clarify misinformation, fears, etc.
C. Review psychotropic drug references for current information
D. Plan for client learning about medication
E. Administer medications as prescribed
F. Teach the client about the medication, desired effect, side effects, food or activity restrictions, and lag period between onset of treatment and symptom remission
G. Supplement verbal teaching with appropriate written or audio-visual materials
H. Administer controlled substances according to schedule restrictions
I. Evaluate client's response to medications and understanding of teaching

▼ NEUROLEPTICS (ANTIPSYCHOTIC AGENTS)

Description

A. Used to treat psychotic symptoms; that is, symptoms of being out of touch with reality
B. Act by blocking dopamine receptors in the CNS and sympathetic nervous system activity; some also exert antiemetic, anticholinergic, and antihistaminic effects
C. Available in oral and parenteral (IM, IV) preparations
D. Used to relieve psychotic symptoms noted in schizophrenia, psychoses (acute, drug-induced, organic, and severe dyscontrol), agitation in acute deliria or dementia, severe anxiety that is unabated with all other treatment, Tourette's disorder, delusional disorder, pervasive developmental disorders with severe agitation or aggression, bipolar disorder (usually administered with a mood stabilizer), and psychotic depression (usually administered with an antidepressant)
E. Antipsychotics control behavior when the client's uncontrolled actions are destructive to self, others, or the environment
F. May be prescribed in conjunction with benzodiazepines (the diazepam/valium category), which is thought to minimize the use of neuroleptics and to diminish the potential for tardive dyskinesia
G. The antipsychotic agents or neuroleptics were formerly called major tranquilizers

Types

A. Phenothiazines
   1. Aliphatics
      a. Chlorpromazine (Largactil)
      b. Triflupromazine (Vesprin)

2. Piperidines
   a. Mesoridazine (Serentil)
   b. Thioridazine (Mellaril)
3. Piperazines
   a. Fluphenazine (Prolixin, Modecate, Permitil)
   b. Perphenazine (Trilafon)
   c. Trifluoperazine (Stelazine)
B. Benzisoxazole
   Risperidone (Risperdal)
C. Butyrophenones
   1. Droperidol (Inapsine)
   2. Haloperidol (Haldol)
D. Thioxanthenes
   Thiothixene (Navane)
E. Dibenzoxazepine
   Loxapine (Loxapac)
F. Dihydroindolone
G. Dibenzodiazepine
   Clozapine (Clozaril)

Precautions

A. Drug interactions: potentiate the action of alcohol, barbiturates, antihypertensives, and anticholinergics; concomitant use should be avoided when possible; antipsychotic medications should be temporarily discontinued when spinal or epidural anesthesia is necessary
B. Adverse effects: agranulocytosis (manifested by cold or sore throat), jaundice (caused by hepatotoxicity), signs of extrapyramidal tract irritation, drowsiness (highest incidence in initial days of therapy due to CNS depression), orthostatic hypotension (CNS depression), constipation and urinary retention (anticholinergic effects), anorexia (depressed appetite center), hypersensitivity reactions (tissue fluid accumulation, photoallergic reaction, impotence, cessation of menses or ovulation), cardiac toxicity (direct toxic effect)
   1. Extrapyramidal side effects (EPSEs)
      a. Dystonia: occurs early in treatment, possibly after initial dosage; involves grimacing, torticollis, intermittent muscle spasms
      b. Pseudoparkinsonism: resembles true Parkinsonism (tremor, masklike facies, drooling, restlessness, festinating gait, rigidity)
      c. Akathisia: motor agitation (restless legs, "jitters," nervous energy); most common of all EPSEs
      d. Akinesia: fatigue, weakness (hypotonia), painful muscles, anergy (lack of energy)
      e. Tardive dyskinesia: late appearing after prolonged use of antipsychotic drugs; not related to dopamine-acetylcholine imbalance; most severe effect characterized by involuntary movements of face, jaw, and tongue; lipsmacking, grinding of teeth, rolling or pro-

trusion of tongue, tics, diaphragmatic movements that may impair breathing; condition disappears during sleep; antiparkinsonian drugs ineffective and condition is usually irreversible; all antipsychotics stopped to see if symptoms subside
      f. Neuroleptic malignant syndrome: infrequent yet extreme condition occurring in severely ill clients and is believed to be the result of dopamine blockage in the hypothalamus; associated with high-potency antipsychotic drugs, especially when given in a large loading dose; symptoms are hyperthermia, muscular rigidity, tremors, impaired ventilation, muteness, altered consciousness, and autonomic hyperactivity; high body temperature is thought to be the cardinal symptom
   2. Antiparkinsonian drugs: block the extrapyramidal symptoms
      a. Anticholinergics
         (1) Benztropine (Cogentin)
         (2) Trihexyphenidyl (Artane)
         (3) Procyclidine (Kemadrin)
         (4) Biperiden (Akineton)
      b. Antihistamine
         Diphenhydramine (Benadryl)
      c. Others
         (1) Amantadine (Symmetrel)
         (2) Benzodiazepines (Lorazepam, Diazepam, and Clonazepam), useful for akinesia and akathisia
         (3) Propranolol (Inderal), useful for treatment of EPSEs
         (4) Clonidine (Catapres), useful for treatment of EPSEs
         (5) Nifedipine (Procardia), useful for treatment of tardive dyskinesia
         (6) Verapamil (Calan), useful for treatment of tardive dyskinesia
         (7) Dantrolene (Dantrium), useful for treatment of neuroleptic malignant syndrome

Nursing Care of Clients Receiving Antipsychotic Agents

A. Monitor for signs of hepatic toxicity (e.g., jaundice)
B. Monitor for signs of infection (e.g., sore throat)
C. Monitor blood pressure in standing and supine positions
   1. Assist client to get out of bed slowly (dangle feet before ambulating)
   2. Assess for hypotension and tachycardia (which is usually a reflex response to hypotension)
   3. If hypotension occurs, monitor by measuring BP before each dose is given

4. Consult physician as to safe BP systolic/diastolic margins for each client
D. Offer sugar-free chewing gum or hard candy to increase salivation and relieve dry mouth
E. Assist with ambulation as necessary; keep siderails up when nonambulatory
F. Assess for extrapyramidal symptoms (antiparkinsonism agent may be prescribed to decrease symptoms)
G. Monitor blood work during long-term therapy
H. Instruct client to:
 1. Avoid administration with other CNS depressants, including concurrent use of alcohol
 2. Avoid engaging in potentially hazardous activities
 3. Avoid exposure to direct sunlight; wear protective clothing and sunglasses outdoors
 4. Recognize extrapyramidal symptoms and report their occurrence to the physician immediately
 5. Avoid changing positions rapidly
 6. Notify physician if sore throat, fever, or weakness occurs; avoid crowded, potentially infectious places
 7. Increase water intake and eat high-fiber diet to avoid constipation
 8. Expect weight gain (diet pills should not be taken); control weight with appropriate diet
 9. Avoid mixing neuroleptics with certain juices or liquids (coffee, tea, or cola beverages may decrease effectiveness of drug)
 10. Avoid antacids or take 1 to 2 hours after antipsychotic drug is taken (antacids decrease absorption of antipsychotics)
I. Evaluate client's response to medication and understanding of teaching

---

▼ ANTIDEPRESSANTS

Description

A. Used to improve the general behavior and mood of clients experiencing melancholia; characteristic symptoms are a severely depressed mood, loss of interests, inability to respond to pleasurable events, a depression that is worst in the morning and lifts slightly as the day progresses, early morning awakening (and inability to fall asleep again), marked psychomotor retardation or agitation, anorexia, weight loss, and guilt
B. The antidepressants are most effective in treating clients who demonstrate symptoms of melancholia
C. Antidepressant drugs increase the level of norepinephrine at subcortical neuroeffector sites
D. Available in oral and parenteral (IM) preparations

E. Norepinephrine blockers provide elevated levels of the neurohormone by preventing reuptake and storage at the axon (tricyclic compounds)
F. Monoamine oxidase inhibitors (MAOIs) elevate norepinephrine levels in brain tissues by interfering with the enzyme MAO; act as psychic energizers
G. Selective serotonin reuptake inhibitors (SSRIs) are thought to alleviate depression by preventing reuptake of serotonin in the CNS

Types

A. Norepinephrine blockers or tricyclic antidepressants (TCAs)
 1. Amitriptyline (Elavil)
 2. Amoxapine (Asendin)
 3. Clomipramine (Anafranil)
 4. Desipramine (Norpramin)
 5. Doxepin (Sinequan)
 6. Imipramine (Tofranil)
 7. Maprotiline (Ludiomil)
 8. Nortriptyline (Aventyl)
 9. Protriptyline (Triptil)
 10. Trimipramine (Surmontil)
B. Monoamine oxidase inhibitors (MAOIs)
 1. Isocarboxazid (Marplan)
 2. Phenelzine sulfate (Nardil)
 3. Tranylcypromine sulfate (Parnate)
C. Selective serotonin reuptake inhibitors (SSRIs)
 1. Bupropion (Wellbutrin)
 2. Fluoxetine (Prozac)
 3. Sertraline (Zoloft)
 4. Paroxetine (Paxil)

Precautions

A. Norepinephrine blockers or tricyclic antidepressants (TCAs)
 1. Drug interactions: potentiate effects of anticholinergic drugs and CNS depressants (e.g., alcohol and sedatives)
 2. Adverse effects: orthostatic hypotension, skin rash, drowsiness, dry mouth, blurred vision, constipation, urine retention, tachycardia, CNS stimulation in elderly clients (excitement, restlessness, incoordination, fine tremor, nightmares, delusions, disorientation, insomnia)
 3. TCAs should not be given to clients with narrow-angle glaucoma
 4. TCAs are contraindicated during the recovery phase of myocardial infarction or when client's history indicates cardiac dysrhythmias and cardiac conduction defects
 5. There should be a minimum of 14 days between switching the TCA-resistant client to MAOIs to avoid hypertensive crisis

6. Abrupt discontinuation of TCAs can cause nausea, headache, and malaise
B. Monoamine oxidase inhibitors (MAOIs)
   1. Drug interactions: MAOIs potentiate the effects of alcohol, barbiturates, anesthetic agents (cocaine), antihistamines, narcotics, corticoids, anticholinergics, and sympathomimetic drugs
   2. Drug-food interactions: hypertensive crisis with vascular rupture, occipital headache, palpitations, stiffness of neck muscles, emesis, sweating, photophobia, and cardiac dysrhythmias may occur when neurohormonal levels are elevated by ingestion of foods with high tyramine content (pickled herring, beer, wine, chicken livers, aged or natural cheese, chocolate)
   3. Adverse effects: orthostatic hypotension (CNS effect); skin rash (hypersensitivity); drowsiness (CNS depression); dry mouth, blurred vision, urinary retention, tachycardia (anticholinergic effect); sexual dysfunction (autonomic effect); nightmares, delusions, disorientation, insomnia (CNS stimulation)
C. Selective serotonin reuptake inhibitors (SSRIs)
   1. Usually these drugs are administered before noon to avoid insomnia or sleep disturbances
   2. Drug interactions: may interact with tryptophan; question concomitant use of diazepam, warfarin, and digoxin; should be discontinued 4 to 6 weeks before switching to MAOIs
   3. Adverse effects: insomnia, headache, dry mouth, sexual dysfunction, anxiety, diarrhea and other gastrointestinal-tract complaints

Nursing Care of Clients Receiving Antidepressants

A. Assess for effectiveness of drug action
B. Maintain suicide precautions, especially as depression begins to lift; carefully monitor serum glucose in diabetics
C. Instruct client to:
   1. Change positions slowly
   2. Avoid engaging in hazardous activities
   3. Utilize sugar-free chewing gum or hard candy to stimulate salivation
   4. Check with physician before taking all OTC preparations or before consuming alcohol
   5. Expect therapeutic effect to be delayed; may take 3 to 4 weeks
D. MAOIs
   1. Maintain dietary restrictions; avoid foods containing tyramine (aged cheeses, beer, chianti wine, yogurt, soy sauce, chocolate)
   2. Monitor client for occurrence of hypertensive crisis (occipital headache, palpitations, and stiff neck)

E. Avoid concurrent administration of adrenergic drugs
F. Evaluate client's response to medication and understanding of teaching

▼ ANTIMANIC AND MOOD-STABILIZING AGENTS

Description
A. Used to control the manic episode of mood disorders and for maintenance in clients with a history of mania
B. Act by reducing adrenergic neurotransmitter levels in cerebral tissue through alteration of sodium transport
C. Antimanic agents are available in oral capsules and tablets, both regular and sustained-release forms, and in concentrates
D. Improves productivity by decreasing psychomotor activity or response to environmental stimuli
E. Lithium, a norepinephrine uptake accelerator alters sodium transport in nerve and muscle cells and effects a shift in intraneural metabolism of norepinephrine

Types
A. Antimanic agents and mood stabilizers
   1. Lithium carbonate (Eskalith, Lithane, Lithonate, Lithizine, Lithobid)
   2. Lithium citrate (concentrate form)
B. Alternative antimanic agents and mood stabilizers
   1. Carbamazepine (Tegretol)
   2. Clonazepam (Klonopin)
   3. Valproic acid (Depakene, Valproate sodium)

Precautions
A. Drug interactions: diuretics increase the reabsorption of lithium resulting in possible toxic effects; haloperidol and thioridazine when given with these drugs can result in encephalopathic syndrome; sodium bicarbonate or sodium chloride increase the excretion of lithium
B. Drug-food interaction: restriction of sodium intake increases drug substitution for sodium ions, which causes signs of hyponatremia (nausea, vomiting, diarrhea, muscle fasciculations, stupor, seizures); therefore salt intake must be maintained
C. Adverse effects: excess voiding and extreme thirst caused by drug suppression of antidiuretic hormone (ADH) function, which causes dehydration; slurred speech, disorientation, confusion, cogwheel rigidity, ataxia, renal failure, respiratory depression, and coma are toxic side effects; toxic effects can easily occur because the difference between the therapeutic level and toxic level is slight

Nursing Care of Clients Receiving Antimanic and Mood-Stabilizing Agents

A. Recognize that therapeutic effects will be delayed for several weeks
B. Recognize that dehydration and hyponatremia predispose the client to lithium toxicity
C. Assess therapeutic blood levels (0.6 to 1.2 mEq/L) during course of therapy
D. Recognize that lithium is the drug of choice, but other agents such as carbamazepine or valproic acid may be used to treat acute mania
E. Avoid concurrent administration of adrenergic drugs
F. Maintain normal sodium intake during course of therapy
G. Encourage increased fluid intake
H. Supervise ambulation if necessary
I. Administer with meals to reduce GI irritation
J. Teach the client that the nausea, polyuria, and thirst that occur initially will subside after several days
K. Teach client and family to observe for signs of toxicity (diarrhea, vomiting, drowsiness, muscular weakness, ataxia, confusion, and tonic-clonic seizures)
L. Evaluate client's response to medication and understanding of teaching
M. Draw complete blood count (CBC) every 2 to 4 weeks to monitor for white blood cell count (WBC) suppression and anemia noted with carbamazepine

▼ SEDATIVE AND HYPNOTIC AGENTS

Description

A. Sedative and hypnotic agents are primarily used in general medicine rather than psychiatry
B. Insomnia and hypersomnia, narcolepsy, and parasomnias, periodic leg movements (nocturnal myoclonus), and sleep apnea are among the disorders that are responsive to these agents
C. Specific psychiatric conditions do predispose clients to insomnia (mood disorders, anxiety, and dementias)
D. Central nervous system depressants have antianxiety effects in low dosages, produce sleep in high dosages, and general anesthetic-like states in very high dosages
E. All hypnotic drugs probably alter either the character or the duration of REM sleep

Types

A. Benzodiazepines
   See antianxiety agents
B. Barbiturates
   1. Amobarbital (Amytal)
   2. Butabarbital (Butisol)
   3. Pentobarbital (Nembutal)
   4. Phenobarbital (Luminal)
   5. Secobarbital (Seconal)
C. Nonbenzodiazepines, nonbarbiturate propanediols
   1. Meprobramate (Equanil, Miltown)
   2. Tybamate (Solacen)
D. Quinazoline
   Methaqualone (Quaalude)
E. Acetylinic alcohol
   Ethchlorvynol (Placidyl)
F. Piperidinedione derivatives
G. Chloral derivatives
   1. Chloral hydrate (Noctec)
   2. Chloral betaine (Beta-Chlor)
H. Azaspirodecanediones
   Buspirone (BuSpar)
I. Historical anxiolytics
   1. Ethanol (generic)
   2. Ethchlorvynol (Placidyl)
   3. Chloral hydrate (Noctec)
   4. Paraldehyde (generic)
   5. Meprobamate (Equanil, Miltown)
   6. Tybamate (Tybatran, Solacen)
   7. Secobarbital (Seconal)
   8. Methaqualone (Quaalude, Sopor)
   9. Hydroxyzine (Atarax, Vistaril)
   10. Promethazine (Phenergan)

Precautions

A. Sedative-hypnotic preparations are generally intended for either occasional or short-term use
B. Hypnotic drugs have undesirable effects (physiologic addiction, fatal overdose potential, and dangerous interactions with other drugs)
C. Barbiturate sedatives also speed up the metabolism of anticoagulants because they induce liver enzyme synthesis
D. The historical anxiolytics listed above were used to treat anxiety prior to the development of benzodiazepines; many of these historical compounds were neither safe nor effective in long-term treatment
E. Chloral hydrate and paraldehyde should be considered obsolete for treatment of alcohol withdrawal because of toxic effects
F. The sedative-hypnotics are CNS depressants
G. Tolerance develops to sedative and hypnotic agents; therefore, the client in the outpatient setting may resort to increasing doses to produce the desired effect
H. If taken in large dosages or for a long time period, physical and emotional dependence occurs
I. Once physical dependence has developed, abrupt discontinuation of sedative-hypnotics leads to withdrawal

1. Withdrawal characteristics: insomnia, weakness, muscle tremors, anxiety, irritability, sweating, anorexia, fever, nausea and vomiting, headache, incoordination, and restlessness
2. After a few more days, severe symptoms of withdrawal may develop: postural hypotension, tinnitus, incoherence, delirium, psychosis, seizures, status epilepticus, cardiovascular collapse, loss of temperature regulation, and/or death

J. To avoid withdrawal, it is important to slowly and gradually taper the dose with the same drug or one that is cross-tolerant

K. Excess ingestion
   1. Any of the sedative-hypnotics may cause unconsciousness, coma, and death
   2. Addiction to these drugs alone or in combination has increased
   3. Removal of the drug from the stomach by aspiration, resuscitative measures (assisted ventilation, cardiac massage), hemodialysis of diffusible drug, vasopressor administration to counteract vascular collapse, and correction of acidosis
   4. Follow-up drug supervision to avoid repetition of the problem
   5. Initiate psychotherapy for depressed clients

L. Refer to antianxiety agent precautions for additional information

Nursing Care of Clients Receiving Sedative-Hypnotics

A. Assess for history of drug or alcohol abuse or suicide attempts by overdose because of the increased risk of abuse
B. Assess for pregnancy and breastfeeding, as safe use has not been established
C. Explore the client's perceptions and feelings about medications; clarify any misinformation, fears, etc.
D. Review drug reference for current information about specific sedative-hypnotic
E. Plan for client teaching about specific sedative-hypnotic agent
F. Administer medication and monitor the response
G. Assess for undesired effects (respiratory depression and increased sedation, and hypotension)
H. Teach the client about the agent and its correct use
I. Supplement verbal teaching with appropriate written or audio-visual materials
J. Administer controlled substances according to schedule restrictions
K. Evaluate client's response to medication and understanding of teaching
L. Refer to nursing care of clients receiving antianxiety agents for additional information

CLASSIFICATION OF MENTAL DISORDERS*

A. Disorders usually first diagnosed in infancy, childhood, or adolescence
   1. Mental retardation
   2. Learning disorders
   3. Motor skills disorders
   4. Communication disorders
   5. Pervasive developmental disorders
   6. Attention-deficit and disruptive behavior disorders
   7. Feeding and eating disorders (infancy or early childhood)
   8. Tic disorders
   9. Elimination disorders
   10. Other disorders

B. Delirium, dementia, and amnestic and other cognitive disorders
   1. Delirium
   2. Dementia
   3. Amnestic disorders

C. Mental disorders due to a general medical condition

D. Substance-related disorders
   Types: alcohol, amphetamine, caffeine, cannabis, cocaine, hallucinogen, inhalant, nicotine, opioid, phencyclidine, sedative, hypnotic, or anxiolytics and polysubstances
   a. Substance-use disorders are concerned with substance dependence and abuse
   b. Substance-induced disorders are concerned with mental disorders resulting in intoxications; withdrawal; delirium; hallucinations; and delusional, sleep, and sexual disorders.

E. Schizophrenia and other psychotic disorders
F. Mood disorders
   1. Depressive disorders
   2. Bipolar disorders
G. Anxiety disorders
H. Somatoform disorders
I. Factitious disorders
J. Dissociative disorders
K. Sexual and gender identity disorders
L. Eating disorders
   1. Anorexia nervosa
   2. Bulimia nervosa
M. Adjustment disorders
N. Personality disorders

---

*Adapted from *Diagnostic and Statistical Manual of Mental Disorders*, ed 4, revised, Washington, DC, 1994, American Psychiatric Association.

DISORDERS USUALLY FIRST EVIDENT IN INFANCY, CHILDHOOD, OR ADOLESCENCE

GENERAL NURSING DIAGNOSES FOR CLIENTS WITH DISORDERS USUALLY FIRST EVIDENT IN INFANCY, CHILDHOOD, OR ADOLESCENCE

A. Anxiety related to:
   1. Frequent lack of success
   2. Inability to meet expectations of others
   3. Failure to develop meaningful relationships
B. Body image disturbance related to:
   1. Inability to evaluate reality
   2. Perceptual or cognitive impairment
C. Caregiver role strain related to:
   1. Inadequate support system
   2. Difficulty in maintaining child or adolescent in the home because of threats to safety
   3. Lack of or failure to use community resources
   4. Disturbed or destructive behavior of child or adolescent
D. Impaired verbal communication related to:
   1. Cerebral deficits
   2. Psychologic barriers
E. Ineffective family coping: disabling, related to:
   1. Unresolved emotions
   2. Prolonged denial of problem
   3. Ambivalent family relationships
   4. Inadequate resources
   5. Abusive or destructive behavior
F. Ineffective individual coping related to:
   1. Inadequate support system
   2. Personal vulnerability
   3. Inability to meet basic needs
   4. Inability to meet role expectations
   5. Poorly developed or inappropriate use of defense mechanisms
G. Altered family processes related to:
   1. Disturbed family interactions
   2. Disturbed behavior of infant, child, or adolescent
   3. Failure of infant, child, or adolescent to meet role expectations
H. Risk for injury related to:
   1. Sensory deficits
   2. Altered judgment
   3. Sensorimotor deficits
I. Personal identity disturbance related to:
   1. Inability to establish self boundaries
   2. Inability to interpret reality
   3. Failure to develop meaningful relationships
   4. Nonacceptance of gender

J. Altered nutrition: less or more than body requirements related to:
   1. Disturbed body image
   2. Dysfunctional emotional conditioning in relationship to altered metabolic patterns
K. Feeding, bathing/hygiene, dressing/grooming, toileting self-care deficit related to:
   1. Perceptual or cognitive impairment
   2. Emotional dysfunctioning
L. Chronic low self-esteem related to:
   1. Perceptual or cognitive impairment
   2. Emotional dysfunctioning
   3. Disturbed relationships
   4. Frequent lack of success
M. Risk for self-mutilation
   1. Inability to discharge emotions verbally
   2. Misinterpretation of stimuli
   3. Inability to control aggression
N. Sensory/perceptual alterations (visual, auditory, kinesthetic, gustatory, tactile, olfactory) related to:
   1. Perceptual or cognitive impairment
   2. Emotional dysfunction
   3. Misinterpretation of stimuli
   4. Inability to evaluate reality
O. Sleep pattern disturbance related to emotional dysfunction
P. Altered thought processes related to:
   1. Inability to evaluate reality
   2. Disturbed interpretation of environment
   3. Disturbed mental activities
   4. Altered sensory perception, reception, and transmission
   5. Inattention and impulsivity
Q. Risk for violence: self-directed or directed at others, related to:
   1. Feelings of suspicion or distrust of others
   2. Inability to discharge emotions verbally
   3. Misinterpretation of stimuli
   4. Inability to control aggression

FUNDAMENTAL PRINCIPLES WHEN CARING FOR CLIENTS WITH DISORDERS USUALLY FIRST EVIDENT IN INFANCY, CHILDHOOD, OR ADOLESCENCE

A. Recognize that all children, especially these children, require:
   1. Protection from danger
   2. Love and acceptance
   3. Basic physiologic needs to be met
   4. Meaningful relationships
   5. An opportunity to explore the environment
B. Direct care toward helping the child grow up emotionally by:

1. Establishing a favorable environment in which the child can gain or regain a favorable equilibrium
2. Establishing a constructive relationship
3. Helping the child to see self as a worthwhile person
4. Recognizing that the behavior has meaning for the child
5. Being as realistic and as truthful as possible when dealing with the child
6. Attempting to establish trust
7. Setting limits that are as realistic as possible but as firm as necessary
8. Pointing out reality, but accepting the child's views of it while pointing it out
9. Being consistent both in approach and in rules and regulations
10. Making all explanations as clear as possible and at the appropriate cognitive developmental level
11. Supporting and encouraging the child's moves toward independence but allowing dependency when necessary

▼ DEVELOPMENTAL DISABILITY

See Developmental Disability in Pediatric Nursing (Chapter 5)

▼ LEARNING DISORDERS

Data Base

A. Psychopathology
1. Theories as to the cause are being studied; however, no one definitive cause has been established
2. Learning disorders (LD) are frequently found in association with a variety of medical conditions (lead poisoning, fetal alcohol syndrome, fragile X syndrome)
3. Although genetic predisposition, perinatal injury, neurologic and general medical conditions may be associated, the presence of such conditions does not invariably predict the learning disorder
B. Behavioral/clinical findings
1. Achievement on individually administered, standardized tests in reading, mathematics, or written expression is substantially below (defined as 2 or more standard deviations between achievement and IQ) that expected for age, schooling, and level of intelligence
2. Disorders of written expression and mathematics commonly occur in combination with a reading disorder

3. Demoralization, lower self-esteem, and deficits in social skills may be associated
4. School dropout rate for children or adolescents with an LD is approximately 1.5 times the average
5. Employment difficulties and social adjustment are noted in adolescence and adulthood
6. LD must be differentiated from normal variations in academic attainment and from scholastic difficulties due to lack of opportunity, poor teaching, or cultural factors
7. Impaired vision or hearing should be investigated through visual screening and audiometric testing
8. Disorders may persist into adulthood
C. Therapeutic interventions
1. Accept child and focus on strengths to raise self-esteem
2. Identify learning deficits early
3. Minimize long-term consequences
   a. Treatment of associated problems
   b. Infant, child stimulation
   c. Parent education
4. Multi/mega vitamin and thyroid hormone replacement therapy

Nursing Care of Clients with a Learning Disorder

A. **DATA COLLECTION**
1. Determine attainment or delay of developmental milestones (motor, language, social, etc.)
2. Observe parent behavior and attitude
   a. Expectations
   b. Acceptance or rejection
   c. Encouragement or pressure
3. Social history
   a. Social activities
   b. Peer and sibling relationships
   c. Developmental history of personal and social relationships
   d. Ascertain specific and outstanding accomplishments
4. Medical history
   a. Vision
   b. Hearing
   c. General health
   d. Birth injury
   e. Past illness
B. **ANALYSIS AND INTERPRETATION**
Refer to General Nursing Diagnoses for Clients with Disorders Usually First Evident During Infancy, Childhood, or Adolescence for the following diagnoses: A 1, A 2, A 3, C 3, D 1, D 2, E 4, F 4, G 1, G 2, G 3, H 1, H 2, L 1, L 4, N 1, N 3, P 4, P 5, Q 2, and Q 4
C. **PLANNING/IMPLEMENTATION**
1. Refer to Fundamental Principles When Caring

for Clients with Disorders Usually First Evident in Infancy, Childhood, or Adolescence
2. Provide activities consistent with disorder
3. Refer for diagnostic evaluation of specific learning disorder based upon assessments
4. Provide guidance, supervision, and habilitation
5. Maintain routines based on the child's usual schedule
6. Set consistent and firm limits for behavior
7. Refer for remediation
8. Develop a trusting relationship with the child and family
9. Assist the parents to gain an accurate understanding of their child's strengths and weaknesses

D. EVALUATION/OUTCOMES
1. Participates in school and home activities
2. Follows directions
3. Carries tasks to completion
4. Benefits from remediation

▼ MOTOR SKILLS DISORDER

Data Base

A. Psychopathology
1. No definitive cause for motor impairment has been established for developmental coordination disorder
2. No specific neurologic disorders are present
3. Lack of coordination can continue through adolescence and adulthood

B. Behavioral/clinical findings
1. A marked impairment in the development of motor coordination that interferes with academic achievement or activities of daily living
2. Coordination difficulties are not related to child's medical condition
3. If mental retardation is present, the motor difficulties are in excess of those usually observed
4. First noted when child attempts motor tasks such as running, holding a knife and fork, buttoning clothes, or playing ball games
5. Performance in daily activities requiring motor coordination is substantially below that expected for chronologic age and measured IQ

C. Therapeutic interventions
1. Direct activities toward the developmental level of the child
2. Identify motor skills deficits early
3. Accept child; develop trusting relationship
4. Assist with academic achievement or activities of daily living only as required
5. Reward achievement of motor milestones (walking, crawling, sitting, improved handwriting, etc.)

Nursing Care of Clients with a Motor Skills Disorder

A. DATA COLLECTION
1. Developmental screening for delayed milestones
2. Associated illness/risk factors
3. Visual acuity
4. Play activities
5. Child's response to lack of coordination

B. ANALYSIS AND INTERPRETATION
Refer to General Nursing Diagnoses for Clients with Disorders Usually First Evident During Infancy, Childhood, or Adolescence for the following diagnoses: A 1, A 2, A 3, C 3, E 4, F 3, G 3, H 3, and L 4.

C. PLANNING/IMPLEMENTATION
1. Teach need for prevention of injury due to falls
2. Encourage exercises such as swimming
3. Foster independence by emphasizing abilities and achievements rather than limitations
4. Help parents to cope with child's lack of coordination

D. EVALUATION/OUTCOMES
1. Maintains or increases mobility
2. Participates in desired activities
3. Verbalizes positive self-image
4. Engages in activities suitable to interests, capabilities, and developmental level

▼ COMMUNICATION DISORDERS SPEECH AND LANGUAGE DISORDERS

Data Base

A. Psychopathology
1. Developmental type: inability to begin or interruption in normal patterns of speech in the absence of physiologic causes
2. Acquired type: impairment in expressive language due to a physiologic cause (brain tumor, stroke, head trauma), which may occur at any age, with sudden onset
3. Two common types
   a. Cluttering: abnormally rapid, erratic, dysrhythmic speech patterns that make communication very difficult to follow
   b. Stuttering: frequent repetition of sounds or syllables impairing speech fluency although child has normal laryngeal skills; usually occurring at the beginning of a word or phrase

B. Behavioral/clinical findings
1. Presence of faulty speech patterns that are persistent and increased by stress
2. Anxiety
3. Avoidance of social situations
4. Loss of self-esteem

C. Therapeutic interventions

1. Speech therapy
2. Counseling to reduce anxiety
3. Provision of positive environment during diagnostics and treatments

Nursing Care of Clients with Communication Disorders

A. DATA COLLECTION

1. Characteristics, pattern, and onset of speech disorder
2. Factors or situations that precipitate disturbed speech patterns
3. Level of self-esteem
4. Levels of anxiety and frustration
5. Family history of speech disorders

B. ANALYSIS AND INTERPRETATION

Refer to General Nursing Diagnoses for Clients with Disorders Usually First Evident During Infancy, Childhood, or Adolescence for the following diagnoses: A 2, D 1, D 2, F 4, F 5, G 3, I 3, L 3, and L 4.

C. PLANNING/IMPLEMENTATION

1. Refer to Fundamental Principles When Caring for Clients with Disorders Usually First Evident in Infancy, Childhood, or Adolescence
2. Encourage client to adhere to speech therapy routine
3. Allow individual time to verbalize; do not complete word or sentence
4. Avoid nonverbal behavior that implies impatience to the client

D. EVALUATION/OUTCOMES

1. Decrease in speech-pattern disturbances
2. Participates in social and public situations
3. Increase in self-esteem
4. Continues with prescribed therapy

PERVASIVE DEVELOPMENTAL DISORDERS

▼ AUTISTIC DISORDER (AFFECTIVE /COMMUNICATION DISTORTION/DISRUPTION SYNDROME)

Data Base

A. Psychopathology
   1. Many theories as to cause are being studied; however, no definitive cause has been established
   2. Failure to develop satisfactory relationships with significant adults, regardless of the cause, appears to be an underlying problem
B. Behavioral/clinical findings
   1. An alienation or withdrawal from reality, usually evident before age 3
   2. A severe disturbance in the child's feeling of self-identity
   3. Inability to differentiate between self and environment
   4. Confusion in self-boundaries frequently characterized by speaking of self only in the third person
   5. A defect in ego formation or an inadequately functioning ego system
   6. A conflict between self and reality
   7. A defect in the adaptive, inhibitory, and steering mechanisms of the personality
   8. Interference with intellect may be so profound, child appears to be mentally retarded
   9. Lack of meaningful relationships with outside world
   10. Use of autistic fantasy resulting in communication defects
   11. Turning to inanimate objects and self-centered activity for security
   12. Symptoms associated with severe autism include:
       a. Profound apathy
       b. Looseness of association
       c. Autistic thinking
       d. Ambivalence
       e. Absence of communication skills
       f. Poor grasp of reality
       g. Bizarre, unpredictable, uncontrolled behavior
       h. Inability to relate to others
       i. Total interference with intellectual functioning
       j. Stereotypic body movements (rocking, spinning) and same routines
C. Therapeutic interventions
   1. Psychotherapy directed toward the developmental level of the child: play, group, or individual therapy
   2. Medications: neuroleptics, stimulants, and lithium provide some reduction of symptoms
   3. Removal from the home situation may be necessary, although day school situations frequently provide enough relief so that hospitalization can be avoided

Nursing Care of Clients with an Autistic Disorder

A. DATA COLLECTION

1. Behavior associated with autism
2. Rejection of physical contact with others
3. Preference for inanimate, spinning, shiny objects
4. Behavior directing emotional energy inward rather than toward the external environment

B. ANALYSIS AND INTERPRETATION

Refer to General Nursing Diagnoses for Clients with Disorders Usually First Evident During Infancy, Childhood, or Adolescence for the following diagnoses: A 3, D 1, D 2, F 4, F 5, G 3, I 3, L 3, L 4, M 1, and M 2

C. PLANNING/IMPLEMENTATION
1. Refer to Fundamental Principles When Caring for Clients with Disorders Usually First Evident in Infancy, Childhood, or Adolescence
2. Accept child's need to push away but continue to make physical contact on a regular basis
3. Provide a consistent routine for activities of daily living
4. Maintain a consistent familiar environment
5. Use picture and letter boards to assist in communication
6. Set consistent and firm limits for behavior
7. Prevent acts of self-destructive behavior
8. Support family's decision for homecare or institutionalization
9. Encourage verbalization of feelings
10. Help child establish self-boundaries by using child's name and personal pronouns and identifying belongings

D. EVALUATION/OUTCOMES
1. Sits in a group
2. Decreases self-destructive behaviors
3. Limits inappropriate behavior
4. Increases use of first-person speech
5. Uses less stereotyped and repetitive motor behaviors

ATTENTION-DEFICIT AND DISRUPTIVE BEHAVIOR DISORDERS

▼ ATTENTION-DEFICIT HYPERACTIVITY DISORDER

Data Base

A. Psychopathology
1. Diagnosis difficult, because the pathology must be separated from normal disturbances that occur during this period of life
2. Evident before 7 years of age; lasting at least 6 months

B. Behavioral/clinical findings
1. Inappropriately inattentive
2. Excessive impulsiveness
3. Short attention span
4. Squirming and fidgeting
5. Hyperactivity may or may not be present

C. Therapeutic interventions
1. Psychologic counseling
2. Psychotropic medications

Nursing Care of Clients with an Attention-Deficit Hyperactivity Disorder

A. DATA COLLECTION
1. History of child's behavior from parents and teachers
2. Behavior reflecting impulsiveness and pattern of inattention
3. Difficulty in following instructions
4. Inability to sit without fidgeting or moving about
5. Easy distractibility by extraneous stimuli
6. Sensitivities (allergies to foods, etc.)
7. History of inner ear infections, vertigo
8. Change in visual acuity

B. ANALYSIS AND INTERPRETATION
Refer to General Nursing Diagnoses for Clients with Disorders Usually First Evident During Infancy, Childhood, or Adolescence for the following diagnoses: A 2, D 2, G 2, G 3, H 2, I 2, N 3, O, and P 5

C. PLANNING/IMPLEMENTATION
1. Refer to Fundamental Principles When Caring for Clients with Disorders Usually First Evident in Infancy, Childhood, or Adolescence
2. Using a team approach, plan activities that provide a balance between expenditure of energy and quiet time
3. Set realistic, attainable goals
4. Structure situations to provide less stimulation (play with only one other child rather than a group)
5. Provide firm and consistent discipline; ignore temper tantrums
6. Test hearing, visual acuity, and postural balance
7. Provide exercises in perceptual-motor coordination and balance
8. Structure learning experience to utilize the child's ability
9. Provide opportunities so the child can experience success and satisfaction
10. Administer drugs such as methylphenidate (Ritalin) or dextroamphetamine sulfate (Dexedrine)
11. Assist child to avoid allergens
12. Treat inner ear disturbances and provide glasses as necessary

D. EVALUATION/OUTCOMES
1. Participates in school and home activities
2. Carries tasks to completion
3. Follows directions

▼ UNSPECIFIED CONDUCT DISORDERS

Data Base

A. Psychopathology

1. The child may be socialized (evidence of social attachment) or undersocialized (little evidence of social attachment)
2. The child may be aggressive or nonaggressive
3. Relabeled antisocial personality disorder after age 18
4. Theories subscribe to both genetic and environmental components

B. Behavioral/clinical findings
   1. Behavior is destructive to the child's own general aims
   2. Behavior is repeated despite rational arguments to the contrary and despite punishment
   3. Behavior leads to getting caught and punished
   4. Behavior includes stealing, truancy, running away, excessive rebelliousness, and physical cruelty to others and animals
   5. Onset may occur as early as age 5 or 6, but is usually in late childhood or early adolescence

C. Therapeutic interventions
   1. Psychologic counseling
   2. Milieu therapy

Nursing Care of Clients with Conduct Disorders

A. DATA COLLECTION
1. History of behavior and onset from family's and teachers' perspective
2. Repetitive and persistent pattern of aggressive conduct toward others
3. Aggressive conduct toward animals
4. Nonaggressive conduct that causes property loss or damage
5. Deceitfulness or theft
6. Serious violations of rules
7. Inability to attain and maintain friendships
8. Parents' expectations of child
9. Family functioning

B. ANALYSIS AND INTERPRETATION
Refer to General Nursing Diagnoses for Clients with Disorders Usually First Evident During Infancy, Childhood, or Adolescence for the following diagnoses: A 1, A 2, A 3, C 4, D 2, E 5, F 4, F 5, G 1, G 2, G 3, H 2, I 3, L 3, L 4, Q 2, and Q 4

C. PLANNING/IMPLEMENTATION
1. Refer to Fundamental Principles When Caring for Clients with Disorders Usually First Evident in Infancy, Childhood, or Adolescence
2. Utilize a firm system of rewards and punishments within set limits
3. Provide for consistency and avoid manipulation
4. Prepare for milieu therapy away from home

D. EVALUATION/OUTCOMES
1. Decreases destructive acts directed at self or others

2. Demonstrates appropriate behavior
3. Parents' expectations of child are realistic

▼ FEEDING AND EATING DISORDERS OF INFANCY OR EARLY CHILDHOOD

Data Base
A. Psychopathology
   1. Persistent failure to eat adequately resulting in failure to gain weight or significant loss of weight over 1 month
   2. Refer to Failure to Thrive (FTT) in Pediatric Nursing (Chapter 5) for nonorganic causes
   3. Disturbance is not due to organic medical conditions

B. Behavioral/clinical findings
   1. Refer to Failure to Thrive in Pediatric Nursing (Chapter 5)
   2. Onset in the first year, but can also develop in children ages 2 to 3 years
   3. Irritability and difficulty in consoling, especially during feeding
   4. Developmental delays are common
   5. Inadequate caloric intake may exacerbate irritability, developmental lags, and malnutrition
   6. Parental psychopathology and child abuse or neglect

C. Therapeutic interventions
   1. Provide sufficient nutrients to achieve a rate of growth greater than expected
   2. Attempt to limit behavioral outbursts during feedings
   3. Help parents to care for child to promote bonding

Nursing Care of Clients with Feeding and Eating Disorders of Infancy or Early Childhood

A. DATA COLLECTION
1. Accurate height and weight
2. Feeding behavior
3. Developmental level
4. Parent-child behavior

B. ANALYSIS AND INTERPRETATION
1. Refer to General Nursing Diagnoses for Clients with Disorders Usually First Evident During Infancy, Childhood, or Adolescence for the following diagnoses: A 2, A 3, C 1, E 3, G 1, G 2, G 3, J 2, M 1, M 2, and O
2. Additional diagnoses to be considered are:
   a. Altered growth and development related to physical or social neglect
   b. Altered nutrition: less than body requirements related to feeding or eating disorder
   c. Altered parenting related to knowledge deficit, age-appropriate diet

C. PLANNING/IMPLEMENTATION
1. Refer to Failure to Thrive in Pediatric Nursing (Chapter 5)
2. Record daily weights and accurate caloric intake

D. EVALUATION/OUTCOMES
1. Expected growth curve and development milestones are achieved
2. Behavior during feeding times is no longer problematic
3. Parents demonstrate ability to care for child

▼ TIC DISORDERS

Data Base

A. Psychopathology
1. Classified as gross motor movement disorders
2. Types
   a. Tourette's disorder
   b. Chronic motor or vocal
   c. Transient
   d. Unspecified
3. Duration, variety of tics, and age of onset differentiate types
   a. Tourette's disorder: duration of more than 12 months, onset before age 18, and evidence of multiple motor and at least one vocal tic
   b. Chronic motor or vocal disorder: each has a duration of more than 12 months; evidence of single or multiple motor or vocal tics, but NOT both; onset before age 18
   c. Transient disorder: evidence of motor and/or vocal tics lasting for at least 1 month, but no more than 12 consecutive months; onset before age 18
   d. Unspecified disorder: does not meet criteria for other types; may last longer than 4 weeks duration or have an onset after 18 years of age

B. Behavioral/clinical findings
1. Involuntary, uncontrolled, multiple, rapid movements of muscles such as eye blinking, twitching, and head shaking that occur in bouts throughout the day
2. Involuntary production of sounds such as throat clearing, grunting, barking, or the utterance of socially unacceptable words is usually associated with Tourette's disorder
3. Can be controlled for short duration; not usually present during sleep; increased during times of stress
4. More common in males than females

C. Therapeutic interventions
1. Treat any precipitating factor such as head injury, psychoactive substance intoxication, or infection
2. Supportive individual or group counseling
3. Medications such as sedatives or Phenytoin (Dilantin) may be prescribed, although they are not shown to be effective with these disorders

Nursing Care of Clients with Tic Disorders

A. DATA COLLECTION
1. History and presence of behavior associated with tic disorders
2. Exacerbation of tics by stress
3. Decreased tic activity during sleep
4. History of psychoactive substance use to determine if tic disorder is related to intoxication
5. History of central nervous system trauma, infection, or degeneration
6. Family history of tic disorder
7. History of neuroleptic agents to determine if tics are direct physiologic consequence of medications (medication-induced movement disorder would be the appropriate label)

B. ANALYSIS AND INTERPRETATION
1. Refer to General Nursing Diagnoses for Clients with Disorders Usually First Evident During Infancy, Childhood, or Adolescence for the following diagnoses: A 2, A 3, C 1, E 3, G 1, G 2, G 3, J 2, and O

C. PLANNING/IMPLEMENTATION
1. Refer to Fundamental Principles When Caring for Clients with Disorders Usually First Evident in Infancy, Childhood, or Adolescence
2. Accept behavior, recognizing it is often uncontrollable
3. Help client to identify precipitating factors
4. Support client's attempts to control tic

D. EVALUATION/OUTCOMES
1. Decrease in tic behavior
2. Accepts presence of tic
3. Functions socially despite presence of tic
4. With Tourette's disorder family members respond positively to advice regarding genetic counseling

▼ ELIMINATION DISORDERS

Data Base

A. Psychopathology
1. Functional encopresis: involuntary or intentional defecation in inappropriate places, including clothing
2. Functional enuresis: involuntary or intentional micturition in inappropriate places, including clothing

B. Behavioral/clinical findings
1. These disorders are more common in males than females

2. No identifiable physical problems are present
3. Chronologic age is at least 4 years or equivalent developmental level
4. Can occur before bladder training has been accomplished (primary) or after a period of controlled continence (secondary)
5. Nocturnal bedwetting is most frequent; child may or may not be aware of voiding or recall a dream about the act of urinating
6. Loss of self-esteem; anxiety and rejection by peers may cause child to avoid situations (camp, school)

C. Therapeutic interventions
1. Rule out structural or organic causes
2. Psychotherapy
3. Provide a consistent routine for activities of daily living
4. Medications such as tricyclic antidepressants for children over the age of 5 to treat enuresis
5. Bowel retraining program

Nursing Care of Clients with Elimination Disorders

A. DATA COLLECTION
1. History of toileting behaviors
2. History of school or family difficulties
3. History of traumatic events (i.e., day care start, separation from parents)
4. Level of self-esteem
5. Secondary gains achieved by behavior

B. ANALYSIS AND INTERPRETATION
Refer to General Nursing Diagnoses for Clients with Disorders Usually First Evident During Infancy, Childhood, or Adolescence for the following diagnoses: A 1, A 2, E 3, F 4, G 2, G 3, K 2, L 2, L 3, L 4, and O

C. PLANNING/IMPLEMENTATION
1. Refer to Fundamental Principles When Caring for Clients with Disorders Usually First Evident in Infancy, Childhood, or Adolescence
2. Change linen and clothing in a nonjudgmental manner to avoid further embarrassment for the client
3. Recognize and accept the fact that the act is usually not motivated by hostility
4. Help parents deal with feelings such as guilt, failure, or anger

D. EVALUATION/OUTCOMES
1. Decrease in encopresis or enuresis
2. Increase in self-esteem
3. Client verbalizes understanding that behavior is neither good nor bad but solution requires outside assistance
4. Parents verbalize understanding that behavior is related to an emotional problem, not hostility

OTHER DISORDERS OF INFANCY, CHILDHOOD, AND ADOLESCENCE

▼ ANXIETY DISORDERS

Data Base

A. Psychopathology
1. Separation anxiety disorder
   a. Excessive anxiety centered on harm befalling self, family, or those to whom child has attachment
   b. Equally common in males and females
2. Selective mutism
   a. Persistent failure to speak in specific social situations
   b. Interferes with educational, social, and occupational achievement
   c. Onset usually before age 5
3. Reactive attachment disorder
   a. Disturbed or developmentally inappropriate behavior
   b. Onset before age 5
B. Behavioral/clinical findings
1. Separation anxiety disorder
   a. Problems with sleeping unless near the person to whom child has attachment
   b. Refusal to attend school in order to remain near the person to whom child has attachment
   c. Physical complaints of headaches and stomachaches when threat of separation is anticipated
2. Selective mutism
   a. Avoidance of speaking in social environments outside the home
   b. Social involvement limited to family members or people who are familiar to the child
   c. Excessive shyness and timidity when confronted with strangers
3. Reactive attachment disorder
   a. Psychosocial deprivation resulting in child's failure to initiate or respond to most social interactions
   b. Difficulty in choice of attachment figures
   c. Onset in the first several years of life; begins before age 5
C. Therapeutic interventions
1. Psychotherapy: in children, usually in the form of play therapy
2. Psychopharmacology may be helpful (stimulants and antianxiety agents)

Nursing Care of Clients with Anxiety Disorders of Infancy, Childhood, and Adolescence

A. DATA COLLECTION
1. History of child's behavior from parents and teachers
2. Presence of sleep disturbances
3. Interpersonal functioning with others
4. Physical complaints
5. History of attendance at school
6. Child's appearance and behavior

B. ANALYSIS AND INTERPRETATION
Refer to General Nursing Diagnoses for Clients with Disorders Usually First Evident During Infancy, Childhood, or Adolescence for the following diagnoses: A 2, A 3, C 4, D 2, F 4, F 5, G 2, G 3, I 3, L 2, L 3, and O

C. PLANNING/IMPLEMENTATION
1. Refer to Fundamental Principles When Caring for Clients with Disorders Usually First Evident in Infancy, Childhood, or Adolescence
2. Provide consistent caregivers
3. Introduce child to new situations gradually; permit child to bring a familiar, comforting toy
4. Allow parent to stay with child as long as possible

D. EVALUATION/OUTCOMES
1. Decrease in sleep disturbances
2. Attends school on a consistent basis
3. Decrease in physical complaints
4. Develops relationships outside of family members and the home environment
5. Decrease in episodes of anxiety and worry
6. Initiates verbal interactions

DELIRIUM, DEMENTIA, AND AMNESTIC AND OTHER COGNITIVE DISORDERS

Disorders are associated with actual temporary or permanent changes in the tissues of the brain

GENERAL NURSING DIAGNOSES FOR CLIENTS WITH DELIRIUM, DEMENTIA, AND AMNESTIC AND OTHER COGNITIVE DISORDERS

A. Anxiety related to:
1. Recognized early memory loss
2. Threat to self-concept
3. Change in environment
4. Motor and sensory loss

B. Caregiver role strain related to dealing with progressive degeneration

C. Impaired verbal communication related to:
1. Progressive cerebral impairment
2. Progressive neurologic losses
3. Aphasia
4. Apathy and/or withdrawal from others

D. Acute confusion related to:
1. Abrupt onset or global changes and disturbances in attention, cognition, and psychomotor level of consciousness
2. Changes in the wake/sleep cycle resulting from dementia, toxic substances, or delirium

E. Chronic confusion related to:
1. Changes in brain tissue resulting in impairment of intellect and personality
2. Long-standing decreased intellectual capacity resulting in disturbances in memory, orientation, and behavior

F. Ineffective individual coping related to:
1. Change in usual communication patterns
2. Inability to meet role expectations
3. Inability to meet basic needs
4. Alteration in social participation
5. High incidence of accidents

G. Impaired environmental interpretation syndrome related to:
1. Consistent disorientation
2. Chronic state of confusion

H. Altered family processes related to:
1. Change of roles within the family
2. Change in family member's ability to function
3. Difficulty in dealing with progressive degeneration of family member; resultant guilt from feelings of resentment
4. Institutionalization of family member

I. Impaired home maintenance management related to:
1. Impaired mental status
2. Progressive inability to carry out activities of daily living
3. Difficulty in maintaining self or family in the home because of threats to safety

J. Risk for injury related to cognitive deficits and psychomotor deficits

K. Ineffective management of therapeutic regimen (individual) related to progressive degeneration of mental processes

L. Impaired memory related to:
1. Neurologic disturbances and dysfunctions
2. Pathophysiologic or situational alterations

M. Altered nutrition: less than body requirements related to:
1. Confusion
2. Depression
3. Anorexia

N. Feeding, bathing/hygiene, dressing/grooming, toileting self-care deficit related to:
1. Cognitive or sensory impairment

2. Increasing inability to carry out activities of daily living
O. Situational low self-esteem related to:
   1. Inability to handle situation or events
   2. Difficulty making decisions
P. Sensory/perceptual alterations (visual, auditory, kinesthetic, gustatory, tactile, olfactory) related to progressive cerebral impairment and progressive neurologic losses
Q. Altered thought processes related to:
   1. Inability to transmit messages
   2. Destruction of cerebral tissue
R. Risk for violence: self-directed or directed at others, related to:
   1. Sensory perceptual alterations
   2. Toxic reactions in or progressive deterioration of cerebral tissue

FUNDAMENTAL PRINCIPLES WHEN CARING FOR CLIENTS WITH DELIRIUM, DEMENTIA, AND AMNESTIC AND OTHER COGNITIVE DISORDERS

A. Provide a safe environment; provide direct supervision as necessary
B. Continually orient the client to time, date, and place
C. Keep client involved in reality and in the home situation as long as possible
D. Allow client to assume as much responsibility for self-care as possible
E. Provide a quiet environment; reduce stimuli
F. Plan care so the staff approaches these clients when they appear receptive
G. Keep the schedule of activities flexible to make use of the client's lability of mood and easy distractibility
H. Encourage adequate nutritional intake; monitor intake and output
I. Provide diversional activities including exercises that the client enjoys and can handle
J. Observe for changing physiologic and neurologic symptoms
K. Support family caregivers; maintain nonjudgmental attitude
L. Help provide some relief from responsibility of total care; refer to community agencies that provide home-care helpers or respite care if appropriate
M. Support the family's decision to place client in a special care home

▼ DELIRIUM

Data Base
A. Psychopathology

1. Syndromes from which the client usually recovers, because the changes may be reversible and temporary
2. Stressors
   a. Infection
      (1) Intracranial or nervous system (e.g., meningitis or encephalitis)
      (2) Systemic or toxic (e.g., AIDS, acute or chronic respiratory disorders)
   b. Trauma to the head
   c. Circulatory disturbances resulting in impairment of blood flow to the brain
   d. Metabolic disorders: electrolyte imbalance (e.g., dehydration, diarrhea, vomiting), fever
   e. Ingestion of psychoactive substances or the accumulative CNS effect of prescribed medications
   f. Multiple etiologies (e.g., combination of medical condition and substance interaction)
B. Behavioral/clinical findings
   1. Delirium and its accompanying confusion, hallucinations, and delusions
   2. Disorientation and confusion as to time, place, identity
   3. Memory defects for both recent and remote events and facts
   4. Slurring of speech may occur along with an indistinct pronunciation or use of words
   5. Tremors, incoordination, imbalance, and incontinence may develop
   6. Physical symptoms such as depressed respiration, cardiac irregularities, and gastrointestinal changes may occur
C. Therapeutic interventions
   1. Reduction of causative agent such as fever or toxins
   2. Prevention of further damage
   3. Provision of diet high in calories, protein, and vitamins
   4. Prescription of mild sedatives if necessary
   5. Provision of a safe environment

Nursing Care of Clients with Delirium
A. **DATA COLLECTION**
   1. History of onset and progression of symptoms from family members
   2. Orientation to time, place, and person
   3. Occurrence of memory defects
   4. Behavior associated with delirium
   5. State of consciousness
B. **ANALYSIS AND INTERPRETATION**
   Refer to General Nursing Diagnoses for Clients with Delirium, Dementia, and Amnestic and Other Cognitive Disorders for the following diagnoses: A 3, A 4, B, C 1, C 2, D 1, D 2, E 1, E 2, F 1, F 3, F 4, F 5, H 2, H 3, I 1, I 2, I 3, J, K, L, M 1, N 1, N 2, Q 1, R 1, and R 2

C. PLANNING/IMPLEMENTATION
1. Refer to Fundamental Principles When Caring for Clients with Delirium, Dementia, and Amnestic and Other Cognitive Disorders
2. Implement measures as ordered to reduce causative factors
3. Reassure family members that symptoms associated with the delirium may subside

D. EVALUATION/OUTCOMES
1. Remains free from injury
2. Oriented to time, place, and person
3. Assumes increased responsibility for self-care
4. Maintains a diet high in calories, protein, and vitamins
5. Avoids intake of pharmacologic substance associated with delirium

▼ DEMENTIA

Data Base

A. Psychopathology
1. Dementia may be progressive, static, or remitting
2. Alzheimer's disease and vascular disease are two most common causes
3. Stressors
   a. Prenatal injury or malformation (e.g., hydrocephalus, microcephalus, neurosyphilis)
   b. Infections such as tertiary syphilis
   c. Trauma in which a head injury results in permanent brain damage
   d. Circulatory disturbances causing anoxia and permanent brain damage (e.g., cerebral arteriosclerosis, CVA)
   e. Nutritional deprivation of brain cells (e.g., pellagra)
   f. Damage may result from generalized diseases (e.g., multiple sclerosis, hepatolenticular disease, Huntington's chorea, Parkinson's disease, AIDS)
   g. Damage resulting from pressure of brain tumors
   h. Toxins

B. Behavioral/clinical findings
1. Memory impairment (recall or learning)
2. One or more of the following
   a. Aphasia (language disturbance)
   b. Apraxia (impaired motor activities)
   c. Agnosia (inability to recognize familiar objects)
   d. Disturbance in planning, organizing, sequencing, and abstracting

C. Therapeutic interventions
The same as those for delirium with greater emphasis on preventing further damage

Nursing Care of Clients with Dementia

A. DATA COLLECTION
1. History of onset and progression of symptoms from family
2. Physical and emotional status in relation to needs associated with nutrition, fluid and electrolyte status, and safety
3. History of premorbid personality from family
4. History of impaired memory

B. ANALYSIS AND INTERPRETATION
Refer to General Nursing Diagnoses for Clients with Delirium, Dementia, and Amnestic and Other Cognitive Disorders for the following diagnoses: A 1, A 2, A 3, B, C 1, C 2, C 4, D 1, D 2, E 1, E 2, F 1, F 3, F 4, G 1, G 2, H 1, H 2, H 3, H 4, I 1, I 2, I 3, J, K, L 1, L 2, M 1, N 1, N 2, O 2, P, Q 1, Q 2, and R 1

C. PLANNING/IMPLEMENTATION
1. Refer to Fundamental Principles When Caring for Clients with Delirium, Dementia, and Amnestic and Other Cognitive Disorders
2. Toilet client frequently
3. Feed the client who is not able to feed self
4. Protect client from self and environment
5. Support client's attempts at independence
6. Support family's decisions regarding present and future care of client

D. EVALUATION/OUTCOMES
1. Remains free from injury
2. Maintains maximal potential for as long as possible
3. Family utilizes community resources as necessary

▼ DEMENTIA OF THE ALZHEIMER'S TYPE

Data Base

A. Psychopathology
1. Primary degenerative dementia, senile onset: occurs after age 65
2. Primary degenerative dementia, presenile onset: occurs before age 65
3. Characteristics
   a. Atrophy of brain accompanied by widened cortical sulci and enlarged cerebral ventricles
   b. Microscopic brain changes include senile plaques and a granulovascular degeneration of neurons
   c. Believed to be related to the brain's inability to produce sufficient neurotransmitters that transmit messages through the brain
4. Stressors
   a. Higher than normal amounts of aluminum deposits found in the brains of clients with Alzheimer's disease

b. Immunologic defect suspected because of higher titers of antibodies in clients with Alzheimer's disease

c. Possible chromosomal defect linked to Down syndrome

d. Previous severe head injury

B. Behavioral/clinical findings

1. Memory impairment (recall or learning)

2. One or more of the following:

a. Aphasia (language disturbance)

b. Apraxia (impaired motor activities)

c. Agnosia (inability to recognize familiar objects)

d. Disturbance in planning, organizing, sequencing, and abstracting

3. More common in females than males; affects between 2% and 4% of population over age 65 but can occur as early as 35; appears to be a familial or genetic predisposition

4. Differs from normal changes associated with aging

5. Dementia has an insidious onset with symptoms following a progressively downhill course; changes are unrelated to any other specific cause

6. Progression moves from mild forgetfulness for recent events to mutism, inability to carry out any activities of daily living, and incontinence; degeneration usually ends in a vegetative state and coma; disease is 100% fatal and death usually occurs within 5 years

C. Therapeutic interventions

1. Ruling out causes such as fluid and electrolyte or vitamin deficiencies, excessive medication, exogenous poisons, or metabolic disorders

2. Provision of supportive care including adequate nutrition with supplemental vitamins

3. Admission to a total care institution when necessary

Nursing Care of Clients with Dementia of the Alzheimer's Type

A. DATA COLLECTION

1. History of progressive memory loss and regressive behaviors

2. History of progressive degeneration of mental, emotional, and physical abilities

3. Physical and emotional status in relation to needs associated with nutrition, fluid and electrolyte status, and safety

4. History of premorbid personality from family members

5. History of medications used by client

B. ANALYSIS AND INTERPRETATION

Refer to General Nursing Diagnoses for Clients with Delirium, Dementia, and Amnestic and Other Cognitive Disorders except for M 2 and M 3

C. PLANNING/IMPLEMENTATION

1. Refer to Fundamental Principles When Caring for Clients with Delirium, Dementia, and Amnestic and Other Cognitive Disorders

2. Refer to Planning/Implementation under Nursing Care of Clients with Dementia

D. EVALUATION/OUTCOMES

Refer to Evaluation/Outcomes under Nursing Care of Clients with Dementia

---

▼ AMNESTIC DISORDERS

Data Base

A. Psychopathology

1. Disturbance in memory related to medical condition (head trauma)

2. Disturbance in memory related to persistence effects of substance (drug abuse, medication, or toxin exposure)

B. Behavioral/clinical findings

1. Impaired ability to learn new information

2. Difficulty recalling previously learned information or past events

3. No evidence of anxiety related to a traumatic event

4. Impaired social and occupational functions

C. Therapeutic interventions

Same as those for dementia with emphasis on determining causative agent

Nursing Care of Clients with Amnestic Disorder

A. DATA COLLECTION

1. History of onset and progression of symptoms from family

2. Physical and emotional status

3. History of previous functioning level

B. ANALYSIS AND INTERPRETATION

Refer to General Nursing Diagnoses for Clients with Delirium, Dementia, and Amnestic and Other Cognitive Disorders except for M 2 and M 3

C. PLANNING/IMPLEMENTATION

1. Refer to Fundamental Principles When Caring for Clients with Delirium, Dementia, and Amnestic and Other Cognitive Disorders

2. Maintain the client in a safe environment

3. Support the client's attempts at independence

4. Assist with health care team's efforts to identify causative agent

5. Support client and family regarding present and future care decisions

D. EVALUATION/OUTCOMES

1. Remission of amnesia

2. Returns to previous level of functioning

3. Family utilizes community resources

OTHER COGNITIVE DISORDERS

▼ SUBSTANCE-INDUCED COGNITIVE DISORDERS

Data Base
A. Psychopathology
1. Nervous system, particularly the CNS, directly affected by substances taken nonmedically (alcohol, opiates, barbiturates, cocaine, etc.) to alter mood and behavior
2. Usually occurs in individuals with substance-abuse disorders
3. Behavioral changes may be related to a vitamin deficiency, especially in long-term alcohol abuse such as Korsakoff's syndrome
B. Behavioral/clinical findings
1. Specific neurologic and psychologic signs and maladaptive behavior such as euphoria; dysphoria; apathy; psychomotor agitation, excitement, or depression; hypervigilance; and fighting or violent behavior
2. Symptoms of dementia or delirium may be present depending upon the substance used
3. Physical symptoms such as depressed respiration, cardiac irregularities, and gastrointestinal changes may occur
C. Therapeutic interventions
Refer to Delirium

Nursing Care of Clients with Cognitive Disorders that are Substance Induced
A. DATA COLLECTION
1. History of past and present behavior from family members
2. Orientation to time, place, and person
3. Ability to have short-term and long-term recall
4. Level of consciousness and stimulation necessary to evoke a response
5. Physiologic status
B. ANALYSIS AND INTERPRETATION
Refer to General Nursing Diagnoses for Clients with Delirium, Dementia, and Amnestic and Other Cognitive Disorders for the following diagnoses: A 2, A 3, B, C 1, C 2, C 4, D 1, D 2, E 1, E 2, F 4, F 5, G 1, H 1, H 2, I 1, I 2, I 3, J, K, L 1, L 2, M 1, M 2, M 3, P, Q 2, R 1, and R 2
C. PLANNING/IMPLEMENTATION
1. Refer to Fundamental Principles When Caring for Clients with Delirium, Dementia, and Amnestic and Other Cognitive Disorders
2. Refer to Planning/Implementation under Nursing Care of Clients with Dementia and Nursing Care of Clients with Delirium

D. EVALUATION/OUTCOMES
1. Abstains from injurious substances
2. Reduces maladaptive behavior
3. Remains free from injury

MENTAL DISORDERS DUE TO A GENERAL MEDICAL CONDITION

Refer to specific conditions in Medical-Surgical Nursing (Chapter 6) as well as Delirium, Dementia, and Amnestic and Other Cognitive Disorders

SUBSTANCE-RELATED DISORDERS

DEFINITIONS*
1. Substance refers to prescription drugs, over-the-counter medications, illicit drugs, and alcohol
2. Substance abuse: maladaptive pattern of drug use leading to impairment or distress, as manifested by one or more of the following occurring within a 12-month period
   a. Failure to fulfill major roles
   b. Use in situations that are hazardous
   c. Recurring related legal problems
   d. Continued use despite social or interpersonal problems
3. Substance intoxication: a reversible substance-specific syndrome due to recent ingestion resulting in maladaptive behavioral or psychologic changes due to effects on the central nervous system
4. Substance withdrawal: development of a substance-specific syndrome due to cessation or reduction in substance use that has been heavy or prolonged
   a. Impairment in role functioning (social, school, or occupational)
   b. Symptoms are not due to another mental disorder
5. Substance tolerance: physical dependency to a drug in which the presence of the drug in increasingly higher dosages is needed to achieve the same effects; tolerance can exceed the usual lethal limits
6. Polysubstance abuse: abuse of two or more drugs or of alcohol and drugs

*Adapted from *Diagnostic and Statistical Manual of Mental Disorders*, ed 4, revised, Washington, DC, 1994, American Psychiatric Association.

7. Potentiation: two or more substances interact in the body to produce an effect greater than the sum of the effects of each substance taken alone

8. Substance dependence: the continued use of a substance despite significant related problems in cognitive, physiologic, and behavioral components; pattern of use usually results in tolerance, withdrawal, and compulsive drug-taking behavior

   a. Physiologic dependence: evidence of tolerance or withdrawal symptoms

   b. Without physiologic dependence: no evidence of tolerance or withdrawal; pattern of compulsive use

GENERAL NURSING DIAGNOSES FOR CLIENTS WITH SUBSTANCE-RELATED DISORDERS

A. Anxiety related to:
   1. Threat to self-concept
   2. Inability to deal with responsibility
   3. Feelings of inadequacy
   4. Concern regarding continued source of abused substance

B. Impaired verbal communication related to:
   1. Inability to verbalize feelings and thoughts
   2. Mental confusion or CNS depression because of substance use

C. Acute confusion related to:
   1. Abrupt onset or global changes and disturbances in attention, cognition, and psychomotor level of consciousness
   2. Changes in the wake/sleep cycle resulting from dementia, toxic substances, or delirium

D. Chronic confusion related to:
   1. Changes in brain tissue resulting in impairment of intellect and personality
   2. Long-standing decreased intellectual capacity resulting in disturbances in memory, orientation, and behavior

E. Defensive coping related to:
   1. Denial of obvious problem
   2. Projection of blame/responsibility
   3. Rationalization of failures
   4. Lack of participation in treatment or therapy

F. Ineffective family coping: compromised, related to:
   1. Individual's preoccupation with abused substance
   2. Anger, frustration, and exhaustion associated with client's negative response to attempts at assistance or support

G. Ineffective individual coping related to:
   1. Inability to meet basic needs or role expectations
   2. Inability to tolerate frustration
   3. Inappropriate use of defense mechanisms

   4. Excessive use of an abusing substance

H. Ineffective denial related to inability to admit impact of problem on pattern of life

I. Impaired environmental interpretation syndrome related to:
   1. Consistent disorientation
   2. Chronic state of confusion

J. Altered family process: alcoholism, related to:
   1. Family history of alcoholism
   2. Addictive personality
   3. Resistance to treatment

K. Risk for injury related to:
   1. Altered cerebral or perceptual function
   2. Altered judgment
   3. Altered mobility

L. Risk for loneliness related to:
   1. Social isolation from family and friends
   2. Total involvement with addicting substance

M. Impaired memory related to:
   1. Neurologic disturbances and dysfunctions
   2. Pathophysiologic or situational alterations

N. Noncompliance with abstinence and supportive therapy related to inability to stop using substance because of dependence and refusal to alter life-style

O. Altered nutrition: less than body requirements related to:
   1. A lack of interest in food
   2. Satiety of hunger by use of "empty calories" in alcohol
   3. Chemical dependence

P. Self-esteem disturbance related to:
   1. Inability to meet role expectations
   2. Feelings of inadequacy and expectation of failure
   3. Inability to accept strengths
   4. Negative feelings about self

Q. Risk for self-mutilation related to intake of mind-altering substances

R. Sensory-perceptual alterations (visual, kinesthetic, tactile) related to intake of mind-altering substances

S. Ineffective management of therapeutic regimen (individual) related to:
   1. Unhealthy life-style secondary to substance abuse
   2. Inability to take responsibility for health needs
   3. Failure to recognize that a problem exists

T. Risk for violence: self-directed or directed at others related to:
   1. Intake of mind-altering substances
   2. Misinterpretation of stimuli
   3. Feelings of suspicion or distrust of others

▼ ALCOHOL ABUSE

Data Base

A. Psychopathology

1. Alcohol intake that interferes with normal functioning or is necessary as a prerequisite to normal functioning
2. Premorbid personality utilizes the compensatory mechanisms of the addictive pattern of behavior
3. The biologic or genetic predisposition theory is continuing to be researched

B. Behavioral/clinical findings
1. Intoxication: state in which coordination or speech is impaired and behavior is altered
2. Episodic excessive drinking: becoming intoxicated as infrequently as four times a year; episodes may vary in length from hours to days or weeks
3. Habitual excessive drinking: becoming intoxicated more than 12 times a year or being recognizably under the influence of alcohol more than once a week even though not considered intoxicated
4. Alcohol addiction: direct or strong presumptive evidence of dependence on alcohol; demonstrated by withdrawal symptoms or by the inability to go for a day without drinking; when there is a history of heavy drinking for 3 or more months, the individual is considered addicted to alcohol
5. Early symptoms of alcoholism: frequent drinking sprees, increased intake, drinking alone or in the early morning, occurrence of blackouts

C. Therapeutic interventions
1. Should be multifaceted social and medical; involves psychotherapy (group, family, and individual counseling)
2. Self-help groups such as Alcoholics Anonymous
3. Negative conditioning with disulfiram (Antabuse) appears to help but never given without the client's full knowledge, understanding, and consent
4. Naltrexone hydrochloride (ReVia) to help overcome the craving for alcohol
5. Clients can be assisted only when they admit they need help
6. Relaxation therapy
7. Physical needs must be met because dietary needs have often been ignored for long periods

Nursing Care of Clients with Alcohol Abuse

A. DATA COLLECTION
1. History of alcohol use/abuse from client and family if available
2. Client's perception of the problem
3. Sleep patterns
4. Physical and emotional status in relation to needs associated with nutrition, fluid and electrolyte status, and safety

5. Why client is seeking treatment at this time

B. ANALYSIS AND INTERPRETATION
Refer to General Nursing Diagnoses for Clients with Substance-Related Disorders

C. PLANNING/IMPLEMENTATION
1. Provide a well-controlled, alcohol-free environment
2. Plan a full program of activities but provide for adequate rest
3. Support the client without criticism or judgment
4. Expect and accept lapses as client is changing a long-term habit
5. Avoid attempting to talk client out of problem or making client feel guilty
6. Accept the smooth facade that the client may present while approaching the lonely and fearful individual behind it
7. Accept failures without judgment or punishment
8. Accept hostility without criticism or retaliation
9. Recognize ambivalence and limit the need for decision making
10. Maintain the client's interest in a therapy program
11. Refer to an appropriate 12-step group such as AA, NA, or CODA

D. EVALUATION/OUTCOMES
1. Recognizes, accepts, and seeks treatment for problem
2. Accepts responsibility for problem without blaming others
3. Achieves optimal physiologic and nutritional status
4. Learns new, more self-preserving coping mechanisms
5. Verbalizes feelings and emotions
6. Enters into and continues with community-based self-help program

▼ DRUG ABUSE

Data Base

A. Psychopathology
1. Misuse of drugs, usually by self-administration, in such a way as to bring about physical, emotional, or behavioral changes
2. Stressors: premorbid personality, utilizing compensatory mechanisms of the addictive pattern of behavior

B. Behavioral/clinical findings
1. Needle marks on limbs along the path of a vein
2. Addicted individuals may tend to wear long-sleeved shirts, even in warm weather
3. Yawning, lacrimation, rhinorrhea, and perspiration appear 10 to 15 hours after the last opi-

ate injection; unrealistic high; pronounced depression
4. Severe abdominal cramps if too much time has elapsed between injections or inhalation
5. Physical examination may reveal an underweight, malnourished individual with multiple dental caries and depressed CNS functioning
6. Job or academic failure; marital conflicts; poor reality testing; personality change
7. History of violent acting out with total disregard for human life or suffering
8. History of stealing to support habit
9. Nasal discharge with possible destruction of nasal septum if cocaine snorting has been practiced
10. Inability to maintain activities of daily living or fulfill role obligations
11. Marked tolerance with a progressive need for higher doses to achieve desired effects
12. Marked letdown with progression to severe depression after cocaine use
13. Hallucinations, hypervigilance, and paranoid ideation with cocaine use
C. Therapeutic interventions
 1. Treatment for drug overdose
  a. Narcotic antagonists
   (1) Nalorphine (Nalline), a partial antagonist, or naloxone (Narcan), a pure antagonist, will improve respiratory rate, although they may not affect level of consciousness
   (2) Nalline will increase respiratory depression if barbiturates have also been used, so Narcan is the drug of choice when in doubt about the substance used
   (3) These antagonists completely or partially reverse narcotic depression and may produce an acute abstinence (withdrawal) syndrome by blocking the euphoric and physiologic effects of the narcotic
  b. Gastric lavage may be done if substance had been taken orally within the past several hours
 2. Treatment for withdrawal symptoms
  a. Antidepressants seem to block the "high" from stimulant abuse and diminish the craving for the substance
  b. Clonidine (Catapres) suppresses narcotic withdrawal symptoms and decreases adrenergic excess while opiate receptors return to normal levels
   (1) Heroin addicts who are first stabilized on methadone before detoxification do better than those who go directly from heroin to Catapres
   (2) Catapres should not be used in those addicted individuals who also abuse

alcohol or those who have unstable psychiatric or cardiovascular conditions
  c. Decreasing amounts of tranquilizers are often administered to reduce physiologic and psychologic discomfort of withdrawal
 3. Methadone maintenance for opiate addiction: programs do not treat addiction, but change the addiction from an illegal drug to a legal drug, which is administered under supervision; has proved successful only in individuals with long-standing addictions
 4. High-calorie, high-protein, high-vitamin diet because of poor eating habits
 5. Treatment in groups run by ex-addicts
 6. Therapeutic community setting
 7. Psychotherapy and family therapy on an outpatient basis
 8. Vocational counseling

Nursing Care of Clients with Drug Abuse
A. DATA COLLECTION
 1. History of drugs being used
 2. History of length and pattern of drug dependence
 3. Time since last dose was taken
 4. Physical status of the client for signs and symptoms of drug dependence
 5. Symptoms of drug overdose or withdrawal
 6. Degree of difficulty sustained by client in relation to family members, job, school, etc.
 7. Why client is seeking treatment at this time
 8. Pending criminal charges
 9. Presence of hallucinations, paranoid ideation, and depression (often associated with cocaine use)
 10. Potential for violence toward others or self
B. ANALYSIS AND INTERPRETATION
 Refer to General Nursing Diagnoses for Clients with Substance-related Disorders except for J 1, J 2, J 3, and O 2
C. PLANNING/IMPLEMENTATION
 1. Set firm controls and keep area drug free when the client is hospitalized
 2. Keep atmosphere pleasant and cheerful but not overly stimulating
 3. Contribute to the client's self-confidence, self-respect, and security in a realistic manner
 4. Walk the fine line between a relatively permissive and a firm attitude
 5. Expect and accept evasion, manipulative behavior, and negativism, but require the client to shoulder certain standards of responsibility
 6. Accept the client without approving the behavior
 7. Do not permit the client to become isolated
 8. Introduce the client to group activities as soon as possible

9. Protect clients from themselves and others
10. Refer to appropriate 12-step group such as NA, AA, or CODA

D. EVALUATION/OUTCOMES

1. Recognizes, accepts, and seeks treatment for problem
2. Accepts responsibility for problem without blaming others
3. Achieves optimal physiologic and nutritional status
4. Learns new, more self-preserving coping mechanisms
5. Verbalizes feelings and emotions
6. Enters into and continues with community-based self-help program

SCHIZOPHRENIA AND OTHER PSYCHOTIC DISORDERS

▼ SCHIZOPHRENIC DISORDERS

Data Base

A. Psychopathology
   1. Premorbid personality: individuals use the compensatory mechanisms of the withdrawn pattern of behavior; in addition, those individuals with paranoid schizophrenia use the compensatory mechanisms of the projective pattern of behavior
   2. Severe emotional problems: although unrecognized, begin early in life; however, onset of disease most commonly occurs between 18 to 34 years of age
   3. Chronic insecurity and an almost total failure in interpersonal relationships
   4. Etiology still unknown; however, some interesting findings in life sciences (psychology, sociology) and family therapy present hope for a breakthrough
   5. Recent neurobiologic investigations are most promising in the search for the etiology (neuroscience, genetics, neuropsychology, and use of computed tomography)
   6. Regardless of the ultimate etiology, a disturbed relationship with the environment and the family is an almost universal characteristic
   7. Course of the disease: either acute or chronic; although it can stop or retrogress at any point, the disorder does not appear to permit a full restoration of integrity of the personality

B. Behavioral/clinical findings
   1. Characteristic symptoms: note two or more of the following:
      a. Delusions
      b. Hallucinations
      c. Disorganized speech
      d. Grossly disorganized or catatonic behavior
      e. Negative symptoms (e.g., flat affect)
   2. Social and occupational role dysfunction
   3. Duration of at least 6 months

C. Types
   1. Although historically much time and effort were directed toward identifying types of schizophrenia, it should be recognized that the classification is not static; there is a great deal of overlapping symptomatology; individuals diagnosed as being in one classification frequently are diagnosed at a later time in another classification
   2. Paranoid type: uses prominent delusions or auditory hallucinations; does not exhibit disorganized speech, disorganized or catatonic behavior, or flat or inappropriate behavior
   3. Disorganized type: uses disorganized speech and behavior and exhibits flat or inappropriate behavior; does not exhibit catatonic behaviors (psychomotor or language mimic)
   4. Catatonic type: features marked psychomotor disturbance that may involve motor immobility (waxy flexibility), excessive motor activity, extreme negativism, mutism, posturing, echolalia, or echopraxia
   5. Undifferentiated type: demonstrates delusions, hallucinations, disorganized speech, disorganized behavior, and does not demonstrate behaviors usually observed in paranoid, disorganized, or catatonic types
   6. Residual type: continues to use many of the compensatory mechanisms common to this disorder in the absence of prominent delusions, hallucinations, incoherence, or grossly disorganized behavior

D. Therapeutic interventions
   1. Psychotherapy (individual, family, and group counseling)
   2. Motivational therapy
   3. Occupational and vocational therapy
   4. Day-care treatment programs in community settings
   5. Pharmacologic therapy: antipsychotic or neuroleptic agents are administered to treat target symptoms of schizophrenia or other psychotic disorders (see Pharmacology Related to Emotional Disorders)

Nursing Care of Clients with Schizophrenic Disorders

A. DATA COLLECTION

1. History of start of disorder from client and family if available

2. Presence of delusional ideation and/or hallucinations
3. Presence of suspiciousness and/or feelings of paranoia
4. History of work and social functioning
5. Presence of precipitating or current stress factors
6. Unclear or incomplete client and family communication patterns
7. Physiologic status

B. ANALYSIS AND INTERPRETATION
1. Anxiety related to:
   a. Disturbed thought processes
   b. Pervasive ambivalence
   c. Mistrust of others
   d. Difficulty in dealing with reality
2. Impaired verbal communication related to:
   a. Inappropriate use of words and unique patterns of speech
   b. Anxiety
   c. Disturbed and disruptive thought processes
3. Risk for caregiver role strain related to disturbed behavior
4. Acute confusion related to:
   a. Abrupt onset or global changes and disturbances in attention, cognition, and psychomotor level of consciousness
   b. Changes in the wake/sleep cycle resulting from disturbed thinking patterns
5. Chronic confusion related to:
   a. Changes in functioning resulting in impairment of intellect and personality
   b. Long-standing decreased intellectual functioning resulting in disturbances in memory, orientation, and behavior
6. Ineffective family coping: compromised or disabling, related to:
   a. Ambivalent family relationships
   b. Abusive or destructive behavior
   c. Inadequate resources
7. Ineffective individual coping related to:
   a. Inability to meet basic needs
   b. Poorly developed or inappropriate use of defense mechanisms
   c. Inability to meet role expectations
8. Decisional conflict (generalized) related to altered perceptions and ambivalence
9. Impaired environmental interpretation syndrome related to:
   a. Consistent disorientation
   b. Chronic state of confusion
10. Personal identity disturbance related to:
    a. Altered thought processes
    b. Detachment from reality
    c. Lack of boundaries between self and environment

11. Risk for injury related to:
    a. Sensory or perceptual deficits
    b. Cognitive or psychomotor deficits
    c. Altered judgment
12. Feeding, bathing/hygiene, dressing/grooming, toileting self-care deficit related to:
    a. Perceptual or cognitive impairment
    b. Emotional dysfunction
    c. Increasing inability to carry out activities of daily living
13. Sensory perceptual alterations (visual, auditory, kinesthetic, gustatory, tactile, olfactory) related to emotional misinterpretation of stimuli and inability to test reality
14. Impaired social interaction related to:
    a. Withdrawal
    b. Delusions and hallucinations
    c. Distrust of others
15. Sleep pattern disturbance related to emotional dysfunction and the side effects of psychotrophic drugs
16. Ineffective management of therapeutic regimen (individual) related to disturbed thinking process
17. Altered thought processes related to:
    a. Inability to evaluate reality
    b. Disturbed interpretation of environment
    c. Disturbed mental activities
    d. Altered sensory perception, reception, and transmission
18. Risk for violence: self-directed or directed at others, related to:
    a. Feelings of suspicion or distrust of others
    b. Inability to discharge emotions verbally
    c. Misinterpretation of stimuli
    d. Disturbed thought processes

C. PLANNING/IMPLEMENTATION
1. Observe for adverse drug reactions whenever large doses of antipsychotic medications are being administered
2. Teach client to recognize and report extrapyramidal side effects (EPSEs) to avoid physical discomforts
3. Administer antiparkinsonian agents to prevent EPSE
4. Encourage the client to follow a plan of organized activity and the prescribed drug regimen
5. Encourage the client to continue medications even after symptoms abate
6. Respect the client as a human being with both dignity and worth
7. Accept the client at his or her present level of functioning
8. Avoid trying to argue the client out of delusions or hallucinations
9. Accept that the client's hallucinations and delusions are real and frightening

10. Encourage the development of interpersonal relationships between the client and others
11. Point out reality to the client but do not impose staff's concept of reality
12. Protect client from injury because of poor judgment

D. EVALUATION/OUTCOMES
1. Remains free from adverse side effects of psychotropic drug regimen
2. Continues taking prescribed medications
3. Hallucinations decrease
4. Differentiates between hallucinations and reality
5. Remains free from injury to self and others
6. Demonstrates a reduction in anxiety through verbalizations or body language
7. Continues therapy after discharge

▼ DELUSIONAL (PARANOID) DISORDERS

Data Base
A. Psychopathology
1. Individuals who demonstrate the suspiciousness and delusions common to paranoid conditions but do not exhibit the thinking and behavioral disorganization or the personality disintegration found in the other psychoses
2. Premorbid personality: uses the compensatory mechanisms of the projective pattern of behavior
3. Paranoid defenses considered by some to be a protective mechanism against unconscious homosexuality or overt hostility
4. Exact etiology unknown
B. Behavioral/clinical findings
1. Exhibits a rather elaborate, highly organized paranoid delusional system while preserving other functions of the personality
2. Thinking is not interfered with
3. Personality function continues
4. Delusions are drawn from real life situations
5. Hallucinations are not prominent
6. Behavior is not bizarre
7. Predominant theme of delusions determines type of paranoia (e.g., grandiose, jealous, persecutory)
C. Types
1. Erotomanic: delusion that another person is in love with the client; idealized, romantic love or spiritual union rather than sexual attraction is basic to this type
2. Grandiose: theme centers around client having some great (but unrecognized) talent or insight or having made an important discovery; less commonly, the individual claims a special relationship with a prominent person or claims to be a prominent person

3. Jealous: unfaithfulness in one's spouse or lover based upon incorrect inferences is the central theme of this type
4. Persecutory: delusion that one is being conspired against, spied upon, cheated, followed, poisoned or drugged, maligned, harassed, or obstructed in the pursuit of long-term goals
5. Somatic: delusions involving bodily functions or sensations
D. Therapeutic interventions
1. Chemotherapy with neuroleptics considered most helpful (see Pharmacology Related to Emotional Disorders)
2. Individual psychotherapy may provide some relief of symptoms
3. Paranoid clients are the most challenging to reach because none of the present therapies appear to be helpful in breaking down the delusional system

Nursing Care of Clients with Delusional (Paranoid) Disorders
A. DATA COLLECTION
1. History of start of disorder from client and family if available
2. Presence of delusional ideation
3. Presence of suspiciousness; paranoid feelings are usually limited to specific areas in the client's life
4. Absence of odd or bizarre behavior and other criteria related to schizophrenia

B. ANALYSIS AND INTERPRETATION
1. Anxiety related to:
   a. Disturbed thought processes about specific areas
   b. Mistrust of others
   c. Difficulty in dealing with certain aspects of reality
   d. Threat to security
2. Ineffective individual coping related to poorly developed or inappropriate use of defense mechanisms
3. Impaired environmental interpretation syndrome related to:
   a. Consistent misinterpretation of events
   b. Chronic state of cognitive impairment
4. Risk for loneliness related to:
   a. Mistrust of others
   b. Threat to security
5. Self-esteem disturbance related to:
   a. Perceptual or cognitive impairment
   b. Feelings of grandiosity
   c. Feelings of persecution
6. Altered thought processes related to misinterpretations of events

7. Risk for violence: directed at others, related to:
   a. Feelings of suspicion or distrust of others
   b. Misinterpretation of stimuli

C. PLANNING/IMPLEMENTATION
1. Provide an environment with some intellectual challenges that do not threaten security
2. Avoid counteraggression and retaliation against the client
3. Accept and recognize the client's need for a superior attitude
4. Meet sarcasm and ridicule in a matter-of-fact manner
5. Guard the client's self-esteem from attack by other clients
6. Accept the client's misinterpretations of events
7. Point out reality but do not directly challenge the client's delusions

D. EVALUATION/OUTCOMES
1. Continues to function in society
2. Avoids factors that stimulate delusional thinking

▼ SCHIZOAFFECTIVE DISORDER

Data Base
A. Psychopathology
   1. Does not fully meet the criteria for either schizophrenia or a mood disorder
   2. Occurs in early adulthood
B. Behavioral/clinical findings
   1. Demonstrates a mixture of symptoms from both schizophrenia and mood disorders
   2. The thought processes and bizarre behavior appear schizophrenic, but there is usually marked elation or depression; often proves to be basically schizophrenic in nature
C. Therapeutic interventions
   1. Antipsychotic or antidepressant agents may be used to treat symptoms
   2. Therapy depends on the type and severity of the symptoms exhibited

Nursing Care of Clients with a Schizoaffective Disorder
See Nursing Care of Clients with Schizophrenic Disorders and Bipolar Disorders (Depressive/Manic Episode)

MOOD DISORDERS

Characterized by a disturbance of mood, encompassing two emotional extremes; individual demonstrates the vehement energy of mania, the despair and lethargy of depression, or both

GENERAL NURSING DIAGNOSES FOR CLIENTS WITH MOOD DISORDERS

A. Anxiety related to:
   1. Disturbed thought processes
   2. Difficulty in dealing with reality
   3. Feelings of failure and unworthiness
B. Impaired verbal communication related to:
   1. Pressured speech and psychomotor activity
   2. Lethargy and psychomotor depression
   3. Inability to verbalize feelings and thoughts
C. Ineffective individual coping related to:
   1. Inadequate support system
   2. Inability to meet basic needs
   3. Inability to meet role expectations
   4. Overwhelming feeling of unworthiness
D. Dysfunctional grieving related to actual or perceived object loss
E. Risk for injury related to impaired judgment
F. Risk for loneliness related to:
   1. Disturbing behavior that keeps people at a distance
   2. Feelings of depression that can become contagious, keeping others at a distance
G. Altered nutrition: less than body requirements related to:
   1. Hyperactivity and excessive expenditure of calories
   2. Inability to sit down long enough to eat
   3. Lack of interest in food
   4. Feelings of unworthiness
H. Altered role performance related to:
   1. Disturbed sensory perceptions resulting in somatic delusions
   2. Emotional dysfunction
   3. Feelings of inadequacy
   4. Feelings of grandiosity
I. Feeding, bathing/hygiene, dressing/grooming self-care deficit related to:
   1. Disinterest in activities of daily living
   2. Emotional dysfunction
J. Self-esteem disturbance related to:
   1. Disturbed sensory perceptions resulting in somatic delusions
   2. Emotional dysfunction
   3. Feelings of inadequacy
   4. Feelings of grandiosity
K. Altered sexuality patterns related to:
   1. Increased or decreased sex drive
   2. Level of energy
L. Sleep pattern disturbance related to:
   1. Emotional dysfunction
   2. A side effect of psychotrophic drugs
M. Social isolation related to:
   1. Object loss
   2. Absence of support group
   3. Alterations in mental function

N. Altered thought processes related to:
  1. Impaired judgment
  2. Impaired ability to make decisions
  3. Altered attention span
  4. Overinvolvement with or withdrawal from environment
O. Risk for violence: self-directed or directed toward others, related to:
  1. Inability to discharge emotions verbally
  2. Disturbed thought processes
  3. Feelings of unworthiness

FUNDAMENTAL PRINCIPLES WHEN CARING FOR CLIENTS WITH MOOD DISORDERS

A. Monitor nutritional intake and elimination
B. Keep the environment nonchallenging and non-stimulating
C. Avoid irritating routines as much as possible
D. Protect the client against suicide during the entire episode
E. Keep activities simple, uncomplicated, and repetitive in nature; they should be of short duration and should require little concentration
F. Observe for adverse effects of drugs; assist in monitoring lithium blood levels weekly and white cell count less often
G. Encourage the client to continue medications even after symptoms abate
H. Caution and teach the client regarding special dietary precautions with lithium and the MAO inhibitors

▼ BIPOLAR DISORDER

Data Base

A. Presence of one or more manic or hypomanic episodes in a client with a history of depressive episodes
  1. Hypomanic episode: a distinct period of elevated or irritable mood that is clearly different from the nondepressive mood; duration at least 4 days
  2. Three or four of these symptoms are noted: grandiosity, insomnia, verbosity, flight of ideas, distractibility, goal-directed pursuits or psychomotor agitation, and engagement in pleasurable activities without regard for consequences
  3. Although the functioning level is altered, there is no marked impairment
B. Biologic, psychosocial, and family theories are offered; at present, research supports the psychobiologic theories

C. Generally occurs between 20 and 40 years of age, although it has been reported in clients over 50 years of age
D. Usually a response to a loss, change in life events, or role change
E. Biochemical changes in the body, specifically a disturbance in biogenic amines
F. Cyclic, periodic episodes of acute self-limiting mood swings; can be all manic, all depressed, or mixed manic and depressed
G. Resumption of customary activities between episodes
H. Obesity a frequent precursor of an attack; onset can be slowed or modified by dieting

▼ DEPRESSIVE EPISODE OF A BIPOLAR DISORDER

Data Base

A. Psychopathology
  See Data Base under Bipolar Disorder
B. Behavioral/clinical findings
  1. Prime symptoms are either a depressed mood or loss of interest or pleasure, occurring during a 2-week period, with a change in level of functioning, plus five or more of the following: change in weight, insomnia, psychomotor agitation or retardation, fatigue, worthless feelings or inappropriate guilt, concentration difficulties, death thoughts, suicidal ideation, or suicidal attempt
  2. Orientation and logic unaffected
  3. Sex drive decreased
  4. Constipation and urinary retention may occur
C. Therapeutic interventions
  1. Dexamethasone suppression test (DST): used to identify depressed clients who may be responsive to antidepressant drug therapy or electroconvulsant therapy (ECT)
  2. Electroconvulsive therapy to reduce depression; drugs such as succinylcholine chloride (Anectine), a depolarizing muscle relaxant causing paralysis, are used to reduce the intensity of muscle contractions during the convulsive stage; used most often for clients with recurrent depressions, delusions, suicidal ideation, and those who are resistant to drug therapy
  3. High-protein, high-carbohydrate diet is provided for energy
  4. Psychotherapy
  5. Pharmacologic approach in depressive phase: antidepressant drugs that increase the level of norepinephrine at subcortical neuroeffector sites (see Pharmacology Related to Emotional Disorders)

Nursing Care of Clients During the Depressive Episode of a Bipolar Disorder

A. DATA COLLECTION

1. Presence of feelings of worthlessness, guilt, and suicidal ideation or acting out
2. Presence of depressed mood, loss of interest or pleasure, and slowing of psychomotor activity
3. Weigh for recent changes and to establish a baseline
4. Changes in sleep patterns
5. Changes in the ability to concentrate

B. ANALYSIS AND INTERPRETATION

Refer to General Nursing Diagnoses for Clients with Mood Disorders except for B 1, G 1, G 2, H 1, and J 4

C. PLANNING/IMPLEMENTATION

1. See Fundamental Principles When Caring for Clients with Mood Disorders
2. Accept client's inability to carry out daily routines
3. Set expectations that can be achieved by the client
4. Help client express hostility and accept client's responses without rejection
5. Provide realistic praise whenever possible
6. Involve client in simple repetitious tasks and activities
7. Accept client's feelings of worthlessness as real; client's feelings should be accepted but not denied, condoned, or approved
8. Protect client against suicidal acting out, especially when the depression begins to lift; suicide is a real and ever-present danger throughout the entire illness

D. EVALUATION/OUTCOMES

1. Avoids acting out suicidal ideation
2. Verbalizes feelings
3. Verbalizes increased feelings of self-worth
4. Continues prescribed treatment regimen

▼ MANIC EPISODE OF A BIPOLAR DISORDER

Data Base

A. Psychopathology

See Data Base under Bipolar Disorder

B. Behavioral/clinical findings

1. Abnormally and persistently elevated, expansive, or irritable mood for a duration of 1 week
2. Three or more of the following symptoms are noted: grandiosity, insomnia, verbosity, flight of ideas, distractibility, increase in goal-directed behavior or psychomotor agitation, excessive involvement in pleasurable activities without regard for consequences

3. Marked impairment in occupational and social activities and in relationships
4. Extreme overactive behavior requires hospitalization to prevent harm to self or others
5. Marked impairment in functioning
6. Symptoms are unrelated to a general medical condition or physiologic effects of a substance

C. Therapeutic interventions

1. High-protein, high-carbohydrate diet is provided for energy
2. Psychotherapy
3. Pharmacologic approach: improves productivity by decreasing psychomotor activity or response to environmental stimuli (see Pharmacology Related to Emotional Disorders)

Nursing Care of Clients During the Manic Episode of a Bipolar Disorder

A. DATA COLLECTION

1. Rapid increase in manic behavior
2. Presence of elevated mood
3. Increased psychomotor agitation
4. Impairment in functioning
5. Feelings of grandiosity and euphoria
6. Adequate nutrition, hygiene, and rest patterns

B. ANALYSIS AND INTERPRETATION

Refer to General Nursing Diagnoses for Clients with Mood Disorders for the following diagnoses: A 1, A 2, B 1, C 1, C 2, C 3, E, G 1, G 2, G 3, H 2, H 4, I 2, J 2, J 4, K 1, K 2, L 1, M 3, N 1, N 2, N 3, N 4, O 1, and O 2

C. PLANNING/IMPLEMENTATION

1. See Fundamental Principles When Caring for Clients with Mood Disorders
2. Accept client while rejecting objectionable behavior
3. Permit expression of hostility and ambivalence without reinforcement of guilt feelings
4. Approach in a calm, collected manner and maintain self-control
5. Set limits for behavior
6. Communicate in a nonargumentative manner
7. Use client's easy distractibility to interrupt hyperactive behavior to avoid injury and exhaustion
8. Advise all caregivers to approach client in a consistent manner
9. Prevent physical exhaustion and maintain physical health
10. Maintain environmental safety for client, other clients, and staff
11. Monitor medications and side effects
12. Educate family as to early symptoms of hypomanic episode

D. EVALUATION/OUTCOMES

1. Decrease in manic behavior

2. Verbalizes feelings of increased self-worth
3. Improvement in judgment
4. Decrease in caustic humor
5. Increase in ability to relax
6. Adequate nutrition
7. Adheres to medication regimen

▼ MAJOR DEPRESSION

Data Base
A. Psychopathology
   1. See Data Base under Depressive Episode of a Bipolar Disorder
   2. No organic factors identified; psychosocial stresses play a role
   3. Usually occurs in late twenties but may occur at any age, including infancy
B. Behavioral/clinical findings
   1. Diminished interest or pleasure in all activities
   2. Decreased appetite with weight loss
   3. Psychomotor retardation
   4. Anxiety and tearfulness
   5. Insomnia or hypersomnia
   6. Feelings of worthlessness
   7. Inappropriate guilt
   8. Interruption in thinking and concentration that may interfere with occupational and social functioning
   9. Recurrent thoughts of death; suicidal ideation with or without a specific plan to carry it out
C. Therapeutic interventions
   Same as Depressive Episode of Bipolar Disorder

Nursing Care of Clients with a Major Depression
A. See Fundamental Principles When Caring for Clients with Mood Disorders
B. See Nursing Care of Clients During the Depressive Episode of a Bipolar Disorder

▼ MAJOR DEPRESSION— MELANCHOLIC TYPE

Data Base
A. Psychopathology
   1. Frequently there is a history of a previous major depressive episode
   2. Depression is agitated rather than retarded
   3. Depression occurs after 40 years of age and before 60 years of age
   4. Precipitating factors such as the marriage of children, loss of a job, breakup of a marriage, or death of a partner frequently are identified
   5. Depression often closely related to the

menopause or climacteric; hormonal and endocrine changes are considered by many to play an important role, although current thinking does not make a distinction between this depression and depressions occurring at other periods of life
   6. Usually rigid, inflexible, overassertive, overly meticulous, and worrisome
B. Behavioral/clinical findings
   Loss of interest or lack of reactivity to usually pleasurable stimuli, plus three or more of the following: distinct quality of the depressed mood, morning depression that is worse than other times, early morning awakening, psychomotor agitation or retardation, significant anorexia or weight loss, excessive or inappropriate guilt
C. Therapeutic interventions
   See Depressive Episode of Bipolar Disorder

Nursing Care of Clients with a Major Depression—Melancholic Type
A. See Fundamental Principles When Caring for Clients with Mood Disorders
B. See Nursing Care of Clients During the Depressive Episode of a Bipolar Disorder

▼ CYCLOTHYMIC DISORDER

Data Base
A. Psychopathology
   1. There are numerous hypomanic episodes dispersed with periods of depressed mood and lack of interest in pleasurable activities
   2. No evidence of true manic or major depressive episodes
   3. Although behavior affects life-style, it does not interfere with it
B. Behavioral/clinical findings
   1. Alternating mood swings between elation and sadness; apparently unrelated to external environment
   2. The individual is usually warm and friendly; approaches life with an obvious enthusiasm
   3. Mood swings do not demonstrate great emotional intensity
   4. Refer to Data Base under Bipolar Disorder for hypomanic symptoms
C. Therapeutic interventions
   1. Often unnecessary; if required, same as for Depressive or Manic Episode of Bipolar Disorder
   2. Medication often unnecessary; if required, same as for Depressive or Manic Episode of Bipolar Disorder

Nursing Care of Clients with a Cyclothymic Disorder

A. See Fundamental Principles When Caring for Clients with Mood Disorders
B. See Nursing Care of Clients During the Depressive Episode of a Bipolar Disorder
C. See Nursing Care of Clients During the Manic Episode of a Bipolar Disorder

▼ DYSTHYMIC DISORDER

Data Base

A. Psychopathology
   1. Guilt and depression used unconsciously to relieve anxiety
   2. Closely resembles bipolar disorder but differs in depth and awareness of reality
   3. Depression is real and suicide can occur
B. Behavioral/clinical findings
   1. Depressed mood for most of day
   2. Duration: at least 2 years in adults; in children and adolescents, mood can be irritable for at least 1 year
   3. Two or more of the following: poor appetite or overeating, insomnia, low energy or fatigue, low self-esteem, concentration/problem-solving difficulties, feelings of hopelessness
   4. Impairment in social, occupational, and other roles
   5. No evidence of manic episodes (present or past history)
C. Therapeutic interventions
   1. Often unnecessary; if required, same as for Depressive Episode of Bipolar Disorder
   2. Medication often unnecessary; if required, same as for Depressive Episode of Bipolar Disorder

Nursing Care of Clients with a Dysthymic Disorder

A. See Fundamental Principles in Caring for Clients with Mood Disorders
B. See Nursing Care of Clients During the Depressive Episode of a Bipolar Disorder

ANXIETY DISORDERS

Common responses to emotional problems that are rarely treated in psychiatric settings; disturbances in personality, but there is no great defect in reality testing or severe antisocial behavior

GENERAL NURSING DIAGNOSES FOR CLIENTS WITH ANXIETY DISORDERS

A. Anxiety related to:
   1. Threat to security
   2. Threat to self-concept
   3. Feelings of inadequacy
   4. Recall of traumatic experiences
B. Ineffective individual coping related to:
   1. Inability to meet role expectations
   2. Inadequate support system
   3. Difficulty in meeting basic needs
   4. Pervasive anxiety and fear
C. Decisional conflict related to pervasive anxiety
D. Fear related to:
   1. Feelings of panic
   2. Altered judgment
   3. Pervasive anxiety
E. Risk for injury related to:
   1. Flight from the stress-producing object or situation
   2. Feelings of panic
   3. Altered judgment
F. Powerlessness related to overwhelming, pervasive anxiety
G. Altered role performance related to:
   1. Feelings of inadequacy and hostility
   2. Disturbed relationships
   3. Pervasive anxiety
   4. Inability to meet role expectations
H. Chronic or situational low self-esteem related to:
   1. Feelings of inadequacy and hostility
   2. Disturbed relationships
   3. Pervasive anxiety
   4. Inability to meet role expectations
I. Impaired social interaction related to:
   1. Pervasive anxiety
   2. Irrational fear
J. Post-trauma response related to experiencing an event that is outside of usual human experience
K. Risk for violence: self-directed or directed toward others, related to:
   1. Altered judgment
   2. Pervasive anxiety and fear

FUNDAMENTAL PRINCIPLES WHEN CARING FOR CLIENTS WITH ANXIETY DISORDERS

A. Establish a trusting relationship
B. Accept symptoms as real to the individual
C. Attempt to limit the use of defenses, but do not stop them until the individual is ready to give them up
D. Encourage the individual to develop a balance between work and play so anxiety is lessened
E. Help the individual develop better ways of handling anxiety-producing situations through problem solving

F. Accept physical symptoms but do not emphasize or call attention to them

G. Reduce demands on the individual as much as possible

H. Recognize when anxiety is interrupting ability to think clearly

I. Intervene to protect client from acting out on impulses that may harm self or others

▼ PANIC DISORDER

Data Base

A. Psychopathology
1. Psychologic, behavioral, and biologic theories are useful to study anxiety disorders; psychobiologic investigations are promising
2. Recurrent attacks of severe anxiety may not be associated with a stimulus but can occur spontaneously
3. Development of the symptoms usually permits some measure of social adjustment
4. Commonly begins in early 20s as a result of environmental factors in childhood
5. Early life rigid and orderly
6. Pressures of decision making regarding lifestyle that occur in the early adult years seem to act as precipitating factors
7. Discrete periods of intense discomfort or fear

B. Behavioral/clinical findings
Period of intense fear or discomfort resulting in four or more of the following symptoms: palpitations or accelerated heart rate, sweating, trembling or shaking, shortness of breath, feelings of choking, chest pain or discomfort, nausea or abdominal distress, depersonalization, fear of losing control, fear of dying, paresthesias, and chills or hot flashes

C. Therapeutic interventions
1. Complete medical workup to reassure the individual and rule out medical problems
2. Psychotherapy, family therapy, group therapy
3. Sedatives and antianxiety agents useful when client is unable to cope or accomplish daily activities

Nursing Care of Clients with a Panic Disorder

A. DATA COLLECTION
1. Increase in somatic symptoms and complaints
2. Interference in activities of daily living and social and occupational functioning
3. Situational triggers may or may not precipitate the onset of an attack

B. ANALYSIS AND INTERPRETATION
Refer to General Nursing Diagnoses for Clients with Anxiety Disorders for the following diagnoses: A 1, A 2, A 4, B 1, B 4, C, D 1, D 2, D 3, E 1, E 2, E 3, F, G 3, G 4, H 3, H 4, I 1, I 2, K 1, and K 2

C. PLANNING/IMPLEMENTATION
1. See Fundamental Principles When Caring for Clients with Anxiety Disorders
2. Remain with client during an attack
3. Do not get caught up in client's panic; remain calm and in control of the situation

D. EVALUATION/OUTCOMES
1. Recognizes situations that increase anxiety
2. Demonstrates increased use of anxiety-reducing behaviors
3. Follows prescribed treatment regimen
4. Reports a decreased number of panic attacks

▼ PHOBIC DISORDERS

Data Base

A. Psychopathology
1. Multiple theories as to the cause (genetic, psychologic, developmental, and environmental) are being studied; etiology remains unverified
2. Development of the phobia usually permits some measure of social adjustment
3. Commonly begins in early 20s as a result of environmental factors in childhood
4. Early life rigid and orderly
5. Pressures of decision making regarding lifestyle that occur in the early adult years seem to act as precipitating factors
6. Anxiety unconsciously transferred to an inanimate object or situation, which then symbolically represents the conflict and can be avoided

B. Behavioral/clinical findings
1. Anxiety appears when clients find themselves in places that threaten their sense of security
2. Attempts are made to avoid these distressing situations
3. Depending on the phobic object, the individual's life-style is often greatly limited
4. Fear of being trapped, embarrassed, or humiliated in social situations
5. Adults recognize that the fear is excessive or unreasonable

C. Types
1. Agoraphobia: fear of being alone or in public places where help would not be immediately available if necessary; includes tunnels, bridges, crowds, buses, and trains
2. Social phobia: fear of public speaking or situations in which public scrutiny may occur
3. Specific phobia: fear of a specific object, animal, or situation

D. Therapeutic interventions
1. Same as Panic Disorders
2. Behavior modification: a counter-conditioning technique to overcome fears by gradually

increasing exposure to the feared object, situation, or animal (desensitization)

Nursing Care of Clients with Phobic Disorders
A. DATA COLLECTION
1. Behaviors associated with anxiety disorders
2. Presence and type of phobic symptoms
3. Interference in activities of daily living and social and occupational functioning
4. Behaviors used to avoid phobic object or stress-producing situations

B. ANALYSIS AND INTERPRETATION
Refer to General Nursing Diagnoses for Clients with Anxiety Disorders for the following diagnoses: A 1, A 2, A 3, B 1, B 3, B 4, D 3, E 1, F, G 3, G 4, H 3, H 4, I 1, I 2, and K 2

C. PLANNING/IMPLEMENTATION
1. See Fundamental Principles When Caring for Clients with Anxiety Disorders
2. Recognize client's feelings about phobic object or situation
3. Provide constant support if exposure to phobic object or situation cannot be avoided
4. Assist with relaxation techniques to control or diminish anxiety levels

D. EVALUATION/OUTCOMES
1. Tolerates desensitization process
2. Recognizes and effectively deals with anxiety-producing object or situation
3. Follows prescribed treatment regimen
4. Utilizes relaxation techniques to diminish anxiety

▼ OBSESSIVE-COMPULSIVE DISORDER

Data Base
A. Psychopathology
1. Major defensive mechanisms utilized are isolation, undoing, and reaction formation
2. Development of the ritual usually permits some measure of social adjustment
3. Commonly begins in early 20s as a result of environmental factors in childhood
4. Early life rigid and orderly
5. Pressures of decision making regarding lifestyle that occur in the early adult years seem to act as precipitating factors
6. Unconscious control of anxiety by the use of rituals and thoughts

B. Behavioral/clinical findings
1. Thoughts persist and become repetitive and obsessive
2. Thoughts may be turned into compulsions that are repetitive acts of irrational behavior that the individual is emotionally forced to carry out although they serve no rational purpose

3. Client is indecisive and demonstrates a striving for perfection and superiority
4. Intellectual and verbal defenses are used
5. Anxiety and depression may be present in various degrees, particularly if rituals are prevented
6. Adults experiencing this disorder usually recognize that obsessions or compulsions are excessive or unreasonable
7. Obsessions or compulsions interfere with activities of daily living, occupation, social activities, or relationships

C. Therapeutic interventions
1. Same as Panic Disorders
2. Behavior modification to attempt to limit the length and/or frequency of the ritual
3. Pharmacologic treatment: fluvoxamine, Prozac, or Zoloft to control obsessive-compulsive behavior

Nursing Care of Clients with an Obsessive-Compulsive Disorder
A. DATA COLLECTION
1. Behavior associated with anxiety disorders
2. Type and use of ritual or obsession
3. Level of interference in life-style
4. Degree of anxiety experienced by the client
5. Extent of danger inherent in the ritual or obsession

B. ANALYSIS AND INTERPRETATION
Refer to General Nursing Diagnoses for Clients with Anxiety Disorders for the following diagnoses: A 1, A 2, B 1, B 3, B 4, C, E 3, F, G 3, G 4, H 3, H 4, I 1, I 2, and K 2

C. PLANNING/IMPLEMENTATION
1. See Fundamental Principles When Caring for Clients with Anxiety Disorders
2. Recognize that the client understands that the ritual has no rational basis but cannot control it
3. Allow the client to continue the ritual but attempt to limit the length and frequency of the ritual
4. Support clients in their attempt to reduce dependency on the ritual

D. EVALUATION/OUTCOMES
1. Demonstrates decrease in need to perform ritual or continue obsession
2. Controls anxiety without ritual or obsession
3. Follows prescribed treatment regimen

▼ POSTTRAUMATIC STRESS DISORDER

Data Base
A. Psychopathology
1. Follows a devastating event that is outside the

range of usual human experience (e.g., rape, assault, military combat, hostage situations)

2. The traumatic event is persistently re-experienced as flashbacks, distressing dreams, sense of reliving the experience, or exposure to situations that foster recall of the event (including anniversaries)

B. Behavioral/clinical findings
1. Exposure to a traumatic event resulting in actual death, threatened death, or serious injury to others or self and/or responding to the event with intense fear, helplessness, or horror
2. Feeling of isolation
3. Difficulty sleeping
4. Violent outbursts of anger
5. Depression
6. Interrupted concentration
7. Hypervigilance

C. Therapeutic interventions
1. Same as Panic Disorders
2. Behavior modification to provide controlled exposure to recall of the event

Nursing Care of Clients with a Posttraumatic Stress Disorder

A. DATA COLLECTION
1. Behavior associated with anxiety disorders
2. History of traumatic experience
3. Sleep-pattern disturbances
4. Behavioral symptoms during recall of experience
5. Presence of depression, outbursts of anger, and/or decreased concentration

B. ANALYSIS AND INTERPRETATION
Refer to General Nursing Diagnoses for Clients with Anxiety Disorders for the following diagnoses: A 1, A 2, A 4, B 1, B 4, D 1, D 2, D 3, E 1, E 2, E 3, F, G 2, G 3, G 4, H 3, H 4, I 1, J, and K 2

C. PLANNING/IMPLEMENTATION
1. See Fundamental Principles When Caring for Clients with Anxiety Disorders
2. Stay with client when memory of the event returns to the conscious level
3. Protect client from acting out violently with disregard for the safety of self or others

D. EVALUATION/OUTCOMES
1. Develops coping mechanisms to more realistically deal with traumatic event
2. Verbalizes decrease in dreams or flashbacks regarding traumatic event
3. Follows prescribed treatment regimen

▼ GENERALIZED ANXIETY DISORDER

Data Base
A. Psychopathology
1. Psychologic, behavioral, and psychobiologic theories are all offered; the latter theory is most promising
2. Development of the anxiety usually permits some measure of social adjustment
3. Commonly begins in early 20s as a result of environmental factors in childhood
4. Early life rigid and orderly
5. Pressures of decision making regarding lifestyle that occur in the early adult years seem to act as precipitating factors
6. Excessive anxiety and worry about at least two of life situations

B. Behavioral/clinical findings
1. Excessive anxiety and worry about a number of events or activities for a 6-month duration
2. Unable to control the worry
3. Anxiety and worry associated with three or more of the following symptoms: restlessness or feeling on edge, easily fatigued, difficulty concentrating, irritability, muscle tension, and sleep disturbance
4. Impairment in social or occupational relationships caused by anxiety, worry, and physical symptoms

C. Therapeutic interventions
Same as Panic Disorder

Nursing Care of Clients with a Generalized Anxiety Disorder

A. See Fundamental Principles When Caring for Clients with Anxiety Disorders
B. See Nursing Care of Clients with a Panic Disorder

SOMATOFORM DISORDERS

GENERAL NURSING DIAGNOSES FOR CLIENTS WITH SOMATOFORM DISORDERS

A. Anxiety related to:
1. Threat to security
2. Threat to self-concept
3. Inability to meet role expectations

B. Ineffective individual coping related to:
1. Development of physical problems to escape stressful situations and control anxiety
2. Inability to verbalize feelings
3. Inability to accept that the symptoms lack a physiologic basis

C. Body image disturbance related to:
1. Passive acceptance of disabling symptoms that would alter body image
2. Inability to meet idealized role expectations and performance

D. Risk for injury related to:
1. Feeling that the physiologic problem is real
2. Inability to overcome perceived physiologic problem
E. Altered role performance related to:
1. Passive acceptance of disabling symptoms that would alter body image
2. Inability to meet idealized role expectations and performance
3. Preoccupation with physical symptoms

FUNDAMENTAL PRINCIPLES WHEN CARING FOR CLIENTS WITH SOMATOFORM DISORDERS

A. Establish a trusting relationship
B. Accept symptoms as real to the individual
C. Attempt to limit the use of defenses, but do not stop them until the individual is ready to give them up
D. Encourage the individual to develop a balance between work and play so anxiety is lessened
E. Help the individual develop better ways of handling anxiety-producing situations through problem solving
F. Accept physical symptoms but do not emphasize or call attention to them
G. Minimize sick-role behavior
H. Help client identify and label needs met by symptoms

▼ CONVERSION DISORDER

Data Base

A. Psychopathology
1. Anxiety unconsciously converted to physical symptoms that are not under voluntary control; these symptoms permit the individual to avoid some unacceptable activity
2. Development of symptoms usually permits some measure of social adjustment
3. Generally begins before 30 years of age
4. Early life often rigid and orderly; physical illness frequently used by the family as an excuse for problems
5. Pressures of decision making regarding lifestyle in the early adult years seem to be precipitating factors
B. Behavioral/clinical findings
1. Presence of symptoms or deficits affecting voluntary motor or sensory function
2. Conflicts or stressors precede the initiation or exacerbation of symptoms or deficits (paralysis, blindness, deafness)
3. Noticeable lack of concern about the problem; this lack of concern has been labeled "la belle indifférence"

4. Impairment may vary over different episodes and does not follow anatomic structure; paralysis or numbness may circle the foot or arm instead of beginning at the joint and is known as stocking-and-glove anesthesia
5. The individual appears relieved by symptoms and demonstrates little anxiety when observed
C. Therapeutic interventions
1. Complete medical workup to rule out medical problems
2. Psychotherapy, family therapy, group therapy
3. Pharmacologic approach: antianxiety agents may be used when individual has coping difficulties with environmental stress and accomplishing daily activities of living

Nursing Care of Clients with a Conversion Disorder

A. **DATA COLLECTION**
1. Presence of physical symptoms with no physiologic basis
2. Level of concern regarding physical symptoms
3. Degree of impairment
4. Level of anxiety
B. **ANALYSIS AND INTERPRETATION**
Refer to General Nursing Diagnoses for Clients with Somatoform Disorders for the following diagnoses: A 1, A 2, A 3, B 1, B 3, C 1, C 2, D 1, D 2, E 1, and E 2
C. **PLANNING/IMPLEMENTATION**
See Fundamental Principles When Caring for Clients with Somatoform Disorders
D. **EVALUATION/OUTCOMES**
1. Reduces need to develop physical symptoms to decrease anxiety
2. Develops a balance between work and play
3. Uses problem solving rather than physical symptoms to handle anxiety-producing situations

▼ BODY DYSMORPHIC DISORDER

Data Base

A. Psychopathology
1. Preoccupation with imagined defect in a normal-appearing person (not of delusional intensity)
2. Generally begins in early adolescence and lasts several years
3. No predisposing factor in early life or family patterns has been identified
4. A minor defect is grossly exaggerated
B. Behavioral/clinical findings
1. History of multiple visits to plastic surgeons to correct imagined defects
2. Preoccupation with imagined deficit causes avoidance or impairment in social and occupational relationships

3. Often exhibits symptoms of depression or obsessive-compulsive personality traits

C. Therapeutic interventions
Same as Conversion Disorder

Nursing Care of Clients with a Body Dysmorphic Disorder

A. DATA COLLECTION
1. Preoccupation with imagined physical defects
2. History of medical and surgical therapies to correct imagined defects
3. Ability to handle stressful situations
4. Level of anxiety

B. ANALYSIS AND INTERPRETATION
Refer to General Nursing Diagnoses for Clients with Somatoform Disorders for the following diagnoses: A 1, A 2, A 3, B 1, B 2, C 2, D 1, D 2, E 2, and E 3

C. PLANNING/IMPLEMENTATION
See Fundamental Principles When Caring for Clients with Somatoform Disorders

D. EVALUATION/OUTCOMES
1. Recognizes that emphasis on physical defect is exaggerated
2. Uses problem solving rather than physical defect to handle anxiety-producing situations
3. Accepts and is comfortable with self

▼ HYPOCHONDRIASIS

Data Base

A. Psychopathology
1. Preoccupation with the belief that one has a serious illness because of how physical symptoms are interpreted
2. A positive medical evaluation does not allay fears
3. Knowledge of symptoms associated with a given disease aids in the client's developing a similar set of symptoms, leading them to conclude that they have the disease
4. Psychosocial stresses are believed to lead to development of this disorder
5. Usually begins between 20 and 30 years of age

B. Behavioral/clinical findings
1. Misinterpretation and exaggeration of physical symptoms
2. Inability to accept reassurance even after exhaustive testing and therapy; leads to "doctor-shopping"
3. History of repeated absences from work
4. Duration of disturbance is at least 6 months
5. Adoption of sick role and invalid life-style

C. Therapeutic interventions
Same as Conversion Disorder

Nursing Care of Clients with Hypochondriasis

A. DATA COLLECTION
1. Level of preoccupation with symptoms
2. Past and present degree of interference with functioning related to symptoms
3. Duration and degree of disability associated with symptoms

B. ANALYSIS AND INTERPRETATION
Refer to General Nursing Diagnoses for Clients with Somatoform Disorders for the following diagnoses: A 1, A 2, A 3, B 1, B 3, C 2, E 1, E 2, and E 3

C. PLANNING/IMPLEMENTATION
See Fundamental Principles When Caring for Clients with Somatoform Disorders

D. EVALUATION/OUTCOMES
1. Accepts that there is no physical basis for the symptoms
2. Develops more effective coping mechanisms to deal with anxiety
3. Accepts need to continue therapy even after condition has improved

FACTITIOUS DISORDERS

These disorders are characterized by physical or psychologic symptoms that are intentionally produced or feigned to enable one to assume the sick role. Therefore, the client with a factitious disorder will "doctor shop," present for treatment in multiple emergency departments, and generally not be admitted to a psychiatric facility.

A factitious disorder must be distinguished from a true medical condition through a medical workup; the nurse's role is to assist with this process. Medical/Surgical Nursing (Chapter 6) and the Somatoform Disorders discussed in this chapter may be useful to help distinguish physiologic from intentional conditions.

▼ DISSOCIATIVE DISORDERS

These disorders are characterized by either a sudden or gradual disruption in the usual integrated functions of consciousness, memory, identity, or perception of the environment

GENERAL NURSING DIAGNOSES FOR CLIENTS WITH DISSOCIATIVE DISORDERS

Refer to General Nursing Diagnoses for Clients with Anxiety Disorders

FUNDAMENTAL PRINCIPLES WHEN CARING FOR CLIENTS WITH DISSOCIATIVE DISORDERS

Refer to Fundamental Principles When Caring for Clients with Anxiety Disorders

Database

A. Psychopathology
   1. Inability to recall important personal information usually of a traumatic or stressful nature
   2. Gaps are reported in recalling aspects of an individual's life history
   3. Gaps are usually related to traumatic episodes
B. Behavioral/clinical findings
   1. The disruption may be transient or may become a well-established pattern
   2. Development of these disorders is often associated with exposure to a traumatic event
   3. Sexual abuse during childhood is a frequent contributing factor
   4. Types
      a. Dissociative amnesia: characterized by an inability to recall important personal information, usually of a traumatic or stressful nature as distinguished from ordinary forgetfulness
      b. Dissociative fugue: characterized by sudden, unexpected travel accompanied by an inability to recall one's past and identity confusion or the assumption of a new identity
      c. Dissociative identity disorder: characterized by coexistence of two or more distinct personalities within an individual
      d. Depersonalization disorder: characterized by a persistent or recurrent feeling of being detached from one's mental processes or body that is accompanied by intact reality testing
C. Therapeutic interventions
   1. Complete medical workup to rule out possibility of organic causes (e.g., brain tumor versus dissociative disorder)
   2. Psychotherapy, individual and family
   3. Offer more effective and satisfying ways to handle anxiety

Nursing Care of Clients with Dissociative Disorders

A. **DATA COLLECTION**
   1. Identity
   2. Memory
   3. Consciousness
   4. Physical condition
   5. Psychosocial component to discover fundamental anxiety source

B. **ANALYSIS AND INTERPRETATION**
   Refer to General Nursing Diagnoses for Clients with Anxiety Disorders for the following diagnoses: A1, A2, B1, B2, B4, E3, G1, G2, G4, H1, H2, H3, H4, J, adding Sensory/perceptual alterations and altered thought process related to:
   1. Sudden memory loss
   2. Disorientation
   3. Loss of personal identity
   4. Alteration in state of consciousness
C. **PLANNING/IMPLEMENTATION**
   1. See Fundamental Principles When Caring for Clients with Anxiety Disorders
   2. Assist with treatment plan to alleviate the troublesome symptoms
   3. Reinforce usual coping styles
   4. Provide for family therapy
   5. Assist with problem solving
   6. Encourage involvement in long-term therapy
D. **EVALUATION/OUTCOMES**
   1. Correctly recalls and identifies past experiences
   2. Verbalizes increased satisfaction with family and work relationships
   3. Ceases incidents of being absent without explanation
   4. Develops more effective coping mechanisms to deal with anxiety

SEXUAL AND GENDER IDENTITY DISORDERS

Changing social and cultural mores have caused many of the sexual behaviors that were once considered deviations to be removed from the list of "abnormal practices." Today sexual activities are considered abnormal only if they are directed toward anything other than consenting adults or are performed under unusual circumstances.

GENERAL NURSING DIAGNOSES FOR CLIENTS WITH SEXUAL AND GENDER IDENTITY DISORDERS

A. Anxiety related to:
   1. Threat to security and fear of discovery
   2. Conflict between sexual desires and societal norms
B. Body image disturbance related to:
   1. Feelings about size and functioning of genitalia
   2. Ineffective past sexual functioning
C. Ineffective individual coping related to:
   1. Inability to meet basic sexual needs
   2. Inability to meet sexual role expectations
   3. Poor self-esteem

D. Risk for infection related to:
  1. Frequent changes in sexual partners
  2. Sadistic or masochistic acts
E. Risk for injury related to:
  1. Retaliation for sexual behavior
  2. Sadistic or masochistic acts
F. Knowledge deficit related to:
  1. Lack of sex education
  2. Lack of communication with partner regarding individual responses
  3. Ineffective sexual techniques
  4. Addiction, illness, injury, surgery, medication, or substance abuse contributing to sexual dysfunction
G. Sexual dysfunction related to:
  1. Actual or perceived sexual limitations
  2. Feelings of vulnerability
  3. Values conflict
  4. Inability to achieve sexual satisfaction without the use of paraphiliac behaviors
H. Risk for violence: directed toward others or self, related to:
  1. Choice of sex objects
  2. Obtaining sexual gratification by inflicting or receiving physical abuse

FUNDAMENTAL PRINCIPLES WHEN CARING FOR CLIENTS WITH SEXUAL AND GENDER IDENTITY DISORDERS

A. Accept the individual as a person in emotional pain
B. Avoid punitive remarks or responses
C. Protect the individual from others
D. Set limits on the individual's sexual acting out
E. Provide diversional activities

▼ PARAPHILIAS

Data Base

A. Psychopathology
  1. Sexual urges or fantasies that are directed toward nonhuman objects, the pain to self or partner, or children and other nonconsenting individuals
  2. Diagnosis is made when the individual has acted on urges or is extremely distressed by the urges
  3. Sexual arousal accompanies paraphiliac fantasies or stimuli
  4. Person may or may not be able to function sexually without the paraphiliac fantasy or stimuli
  5. May be symptomatic of other personality or psychiatric disorders
  6. May occur as a behavior aberration or a disordered personality
B. Types and behavioral/clinical findings
  1. Fetishism: substitution of an inanimate object for the genitals

2. Transvestism: wearing clothes of the opposite sex to achieve sexual pleasure
3. Exhibitionism: sexual pleasure obtained by exposing the genitals
4. Pedophilia: attraction to children as sex objects
5. Voyeurism: sexual gratification obtained by watching the sexual play of others
6. Sadism: sexual gratification obtained from cruelty to others; used as a substitute for or an accompaniment to the sex act
7. Masochism: sexual gratification obtained from self-suffering; used as a substitute for or an accompaniment to the sex act
8. Frotteurism: sexual pleasure obtained by touching or rubbing against a nonconsenting person; usually occurs in crowds or on public transportation
9. Necrophilia: sexual gratification obtained from sexual relations with a corpse
10. Telephone scatologia: sexual gratification from or during lewdness on the telephone
C. Therapeutic interventions
  1. Rather unsuccessful with these individuals unless they really want to change
  2. If change is desired, psychotherapy may be effective

Nursing Care of Clients with Paraphilias

A. DATA COLLECTION
  1. History of sexual behavior
  2. Presence of other psychosocial difficulties
  3. Level of anxiety regarding sexual behavior
  4. Pending criminal charges
  5. Why client is seeking treatment at this time
  6. Potential for violence toward others or self
B. ANALYSIS AND INTERPRETATION
  Refer to General Nursing Diagnoses for Clients with Sexual and Gender Identity Disorders: for the following diagnoses: A 1, A 2, B 1, B 2, C 1, C 2, C 3, D 1, D 2, E 1, E 2, G 2, G 3, G 4, H 1, and H 2
C. PLANNING/IMPLEMENTATION
  See Fundamental Principles When Caring for Clients with Sexual and Gender Identity Disorders
D. EVALUATION/OUTCOMES
  1. Ceases socially unacceptable behavior
  2. Seeks and continues long-term therapy
  3. Limits paraphiliac behavior to consenting adults
  4. Utilizes safer sex techniques

▼ SEXUAL DYSFUNCTION

Data Base

A. Psychopathology
  1. Inhibition or interference with the appetitive,

excitement, orgasm, or resolution phases of the sexual response cycle
   2. Dysfunction is psychogenic but it may begin with a physiologic basis
   3. Dysfunction can be lifelong or acquired
   4. Dysfunction can be generalized or situational
B. Types and behavioral/clinical findings
   1. Sexual desire disorders: deficient, absent, or extreme aversion to and avoidance of sexual activity
   2. Sexual arousal disorders: partial or complete failure to achieve a physiologic or psychologic (subjective) response to sexual activity
   3. Orgasm disorders: delay in or absence of orgasm or premature ejaculation
   4. Sexual pain disorders: recurrent or persistent genital pain before, during, or after sexual activity
C. Therapeutic interventions
   1. Treatment of underlying physiologic cause if present
   2. Sexual counseling

Nursing Care of Clients with a Sexual Dysfunction

A. DATA COLLECTION
   1. Feelings about inability to function sexually
   2. Expectations regarding sexual ability
   3. Effect of sexual dysfunction on relationship with significant other

B. ANALYSIS AND INTERPRETATION
   Refer to General Nursing Diagnoses for Clients with Sexual and Gender Identity Disorders for the following diagnoses: A 1, B 1, B 2, C 1, C 2, C 3, F 1, F 2, F 3, F 4, G 1, G 2, and G 3

C. PLANNING/IMPLEMENTATION
   1. See Fundamental Principles When Caring for Clients with Sexual and Gender Identity Disorders with the exception of D
   2. Recognize that problem is real to the client regardless of age
   3. Recognize that the desire to function sexually does not diminish with age

D. EVALUATION/OUTCOMES
   1. Reports an increased satisfaction in sexual functioning
   2. Sexual ability approaches sexual expectations

▼ GENDER IDENTITY DISORDERS

Data Base
A. Psychopathology
   1. Persistent discomfort with one's assigned gender and a feeling that it is inappropriate or inaccurate

   2. Persistent repudiation of current gender anatomy
   3. Preoccupation with activities and clothing of opposite gender
B. Behavioral/clinical findings
   1. Prepubescent gender identity disorders
      a. Has intense discomfort with own gender and desires to be the opposite sex or believes that he or she is the opposite sex
      b. Rejects anatomic structures associated with own gender
      c. Cross-dresses and participates in activities associated with opposite sex
      d. Has not reached puberty
      e. Prefers playmates of opposite sex
   2. Adolescent/adult gender identity disorders
      a. Strong desire to be the other sex
      b. Frequently cross-dresses
      c. Desires to live or be treated as the other sex
      d. Belief that one has the typical feelings and reactions of the other sex
      e. Persistent discomfort with gender
      f. Preoccupation with getting rid of primary and secondary sex characteristics
      g. Disturbance causes impairment in social and occupational relationships
   3. Transsexualism
      a. Has intense desire to exchange own sexual characteristics for those of the opposite sex
      b. Complains of discomfort wearing clothing of assigned sexual role
      c. Has anxiety and depression related to conformity with assigned sexual role
      d. Has reached puberty
      e. Can be asexual, homosexual, or heterosexual
   4. Nontranssexual type
      a. Has no intense desire to acquire sexual characteristics of opposite sex, yet a persistent feeling of discomfort with one's assigned gender
      b. Cross-dressing is practiced but without the purpose of sexual excitement
      c. Anxiety and depression are usually decreased when the person is cross-dressing
      d. Has reached puberty
      e. Can be asexual, homosexual, or heterosexual
C. Therapeutic interventions
   1. Individual or group psychotherapy
   2. Antianxiety medication if necessary

Nursing Care of Clients with Gender Identity Disorders

A. DATA COLLECTION
   1. Distress about assigned sex role
   2. Behavior, social habits, and cross-dressing inappropriate for sexual gender

3. Preoccupation with becoming, being, or behaving as the opposite sex
4. History of sexual orientation (asexual, homosexual, heterosexual)

B. ANALYSIS AND INTERPRETATION

Refer to General Nursing Diagnoses for Clients with Sexual and Gender Identity Disorders for the following diagnoses: A 1, A 2, B 1, C 1, C 2, C 3, E 1, and G 3

C. PLANNING/IMPLEMENTATION

1. See Fundamental Principles When Caring for Clients with Sexual and Gender Identity Disorders
2. Accept and understand client's discomfort with gender
3. Accept own feelings about client's cross-dressing
4. Encourage client to become involved with support groups
5. Be aware that if discomfort or depression is severe, self-mutilation and suicide are possibilities

D. EVALUATION/OUTCOMES

1. Verbalizes increased comfort with self
2. Ultimately accepts gender
3. Participates in support groups

EATING DISORDERS

Eating behavior is severely disturbed in this disorder

GENERAL NURSING DIAGNOSES FOR CLIENTS WITH EATING DISORDERS

A. Anxiety related to:
1. Low self-concept
2. Feelings of inferiority
3. Unmet dependency needs

B. Body image disturbance related to:
1. Unrealistic appraisal of body size
2. Underestimating food requirements
3. Desire for slimness

C. Ineffective family coping: compromised, related to:
1. Overprotection and unwillingness to allow client to separate (meet developmental tasks)
2. Unrealistic expectations
3. Inability to cope with client's eating disorder

D. Risk for fluid volume deficit related to inadequate intake and purging

E. Ineffective individual coping related to:
1. Deficits in self-care activities
2. Altered role performance
3. Quest for thinness
4. Delay in mastery of developmental tasks
5. Shame and guilt over secret binges

F. Alterations in health maintenance related to:

1. Inadequate health practices
2. Health beliefs
3. Alterations in self-image
4. Preoccupation with food, recipes, and preparing food for others
5. Denial of one's own hunger

G. Altered nutrition: less than body requirements related to:
1. Disturbed body image
2. Dysfunctional emotional conditioning in relationship to food
3. Self-induced vomiting and purging

H. Altered nutrition: more than body requirements related to:
1. Abnormality in amount of food consumed
2. Dysfunctional emotional conditioning in relationship to food

I. Self-esteem disturbance related to:
1. Low self-confidence
2. Feelings of inferiority
3. Unrealistic expectations of self and others

FUNDAMENTAL PRINCIPLES WHEN CARING FOR CLIENTS WITH EATING DISORDERS

A. Recognize that adolescent or adult requires:
1. Basic physiologic and safety needs be met
2. Acceptance
3. Meaningful relationships
4. Limit setting on manipulative behavior
5. Monitoring during and after meal time

B. Direct care toward helping the individual to mature by:
1. Establishing a constructive relationship
2. Promoting self-worth
3. Setting limits that are realistic
4. Being consistent in approach and in rules and regulations
5. Supporting and encouraging independence
6. Learning more effective ways of coping

▼ ANOREXIA NERVOSA

Data Base

A. Psychopathology
1. Most common in adolescent through 30-year-old population
2. More common in females
3. Avoidance of food may result from excessive concern with obesity
4. Apparent failure to separate from mother and become autonomous; unconscious fear of growing up
5. Usually triggered by an adolescent crisis

B. Behavioral/clinical findings
1. Weigh less than 85% of expected weight
2. Distorted self-image; appear fat to themselves even when emaciated
3. Intense fear of becoming fat, even though underweight
4. May have history of compulsive traits
5. Usually very manipulative
6. Usually high achievers academically
7. Frequent discord in family relationships, especially with mother
8. Often interested in food and cooking in general
9. Cessation of menses in females
10. Inability to sustain self-starvation may result in bulimic episodes (binging of food followed by self-induced vomiting)
11. Fatigue or hyperactivity
12. Feeling of fullness after small intake
13. Nausea
14. Constipation
15. Emaciation
16. Hypotension
17. Low blood glucose
18. Anemia
19. Low BMR
20. Subtypes:
    a. Restricting type: weight loss is accomplished through dieting, fasting, or excessive exercise
    b. Binge eating/purging type: weight loss is accomplished through binge eating or purging (or both); use of self-induced vomiting and misuse of laxatives, diuretics, or enemas on weekly basis
C. Therapeutic interventions
1. Unified team approach
2. Behavior modification techniques that focus on client's responsibility for weight gain
3. Time limit on meals
4. Use of nasogastric tube if weight loss is so great or fluid and electrolyte imbalance is so severe that it causes a threat to life
5. Psychotherapy focusing on self-image
6. Group therapy
7. Family therapy with all members of family involved
8. Gradual increase in calories and protein

Nursing Care of Clients with Anorexia Nervosa
A. DATA COLLECTION
1. Nutritional status, noting emaciated appearance and condition of hair
2. Weight and height
3. Signs of fluid and electrolyte imbalance
4. History of amenorrhea
5. Indulgence in excessive exercise
6. Behavior reflecting obsessiveness with food

7. History of stringent control of intake of food
8. Depressive mood
B. ANALYSIS AND INTERPRETATION
Refer to General Nursing Diagnoses for Clients with Eating Disorders for all of the diagnoses except E 5, I 1, I 2, and I 3
C. PLANNING/IMPLEMENTATION
1. Refer to Fundamental Principles When Caring for Clients with Eating Disorders
2. Develop a therapeutic environment
3. Establish a behavior modification program
4. Help client identify feelings
5. Briefly discuss dietary modification with the client in a nonthreatening manner
6. Encourage diet high in nutrient-dense foods
7. Do not focus on eating or weight loss
D. EVALUATION/OUTCOMES
1. Maintains dietary intake adequate to meet daily caloric requirements
2. Reaches and maintains appropriate body weight
3. Develops realistic body image
4. Identifies and verbalizes feelings
5. Accepts role of young adult

▼ BULIMIA NERVOSA

Data Base
A. Psychopathology
1. Most common in adolescent through 30-year-old population
2. More common in females
3. Obesity is frequently found in parents or siblings
4. Predisposition to depression
5. Discord in family relationships
6. Obsession with food results from a morbid fear of obesity and the pathologic need to binge
B. Behavioral/clinical findings
1. Compulsive eating binges characterized by rapid consumption of excessive amounts of high-caloric foods in brief periods followed by induced purging (vomiting, enemas, laxatives, or diuretics)
2. Periods of severe dieting or fasting between binges
3. Sporadic vigorous exercising between binges
4. Weight may be within normal range with frequent fluctuations above or below normal range because of alternating binges and fasts
5. Lack of control over eating during episode
6. Depression and self-deprecating thoughts follow binges
7. Impulsive
8. Extroverted
9. Possible intermittent substance abuse

10. Very concerned with body image and appearance
11. Repeated attempts to control or lose weight
12. Subtypes
    a. Purging type: engages in purging behaviors
    b. Nonpurging type: uses fasting or excessive exercise, not purging

C. Therapeutic interventions
   See Therapeutic Interventions under Anorexia Nervosa, except for 4 and 8

Nursing Care of Clients with Bulimia Nervosa

A. DATA COLLECTION

1. Behavior indicative of purging such as self-induced vomiting and use of enemas, laxatives, and diuretics
2. Obsession with excessive exercise
3. Pattern of binging
4. Overconcern with body weight and shape
5. Physiologic changes such as dental caries, dry brittle hair, and hemorrhoids as a result of binging and purging behaviors
6. Signs of fluid and electrolyte imbalances
7. Weight and height
8. History of consuming tremendous amounts of calories in a short period of time

B. ANALYSIS AND INTERPRETATION
Refer to General Nursing Diagnoses for Clients with Eating Disorders for the following diagnoses: A 1, A 2, B 1, B 3, C 2, C 3, D, E 1, E 2, E 3, E 5, F 1, F 3, H 1, H 2, H 3, I 1, I 2, and I 3

C. PLANNING/IMPLEMENTATION

1. See Fundamental Principles When Caring for Clients with Eating Disorders
2. Provide a nonjudgmental, accepting environment
3. Keep client under close observation to prevent purging
4. Encourage verbalization of feelings
5. Help client to identify feelings associated with binging and purging episodes
6. Shift focus from food, eating, and exercise to emotional issues

D. EVALUATION/OUTCOMES

1. Limits dietary intake to caloric requirements
2. Reduces episodes of binging
3. Reduces episodes of purging
4. Identifies feelings
5. Verbalizes emotions and needs

ADJUSTMENT DISORDERS

These disorders are characterized by the development of clinically significant emotional or behavioral symptoms in response to psychosocial stress

Data Base

A. Psychopathology
   1. Reaction to overwhelming environmental stress
   2. No apparent underlying mental disorder in these individuals, although present behavior may be extremely disturbed
   3. The individual seems to have the capacity to adapt to the overwhelming stress when given the time to do so
   4. Problems with distortions or interruptions in thinking processes and decision making tend to resolve themselves

B. Behavioral/clinical findings
   1. Infancy: extremely upset; demonstrating grief when separated from the mother
   2. Childhood: regression to an earlier level of development when a new sibling arrives; intense anxiety on entering school
   3. Adolescence: struggle for independence; leads to hypersensitivity and frequent episodes of heightened anxiety
   4. Adult life: heightened anxiety in response to the stresses associated with marriage, pregnancy, divorce, change of employment, purchase of a house, etc.
   5. Later life: menopause and climacteric, plan for retirement, "loss" of children to marriage, and death of a mate all serve to produce extreme stress situations
   6. Onset begins within 3 months of stressors

C. Therapeutic interventions
   Determine the underlying cause of the conflict and work toward resolution

Nursing Care of Clients with Adjustment Disorders

A. DATA COLLECTION

1. Individual's perception of problem
2. Factors impinging upon current situation
3. Individual's personal strengths and support system
4. Level of anxiety

B. ANALYSIS AND INTERPRETATION

1. Anxiety related to:
   a. Inability to handle overwhelming stress effectively
   b. Threat to self-concept
   c. Threat to security
2. Ineffective individual coping related to:
   a. Overwhelming environmental stress, which is usually resolved over time
   b. Failure of support system
   c. Developmental level
3. Chronic low self-esteem related to:
   a. Overwhelming stress
   b. Inability to cope

4. Altered role performance related to:
   a. Overwhelming stress
   b. Inability to cope
   c. Social withdrawal

C. PLANNING/IMPLEMENTATION
1. Help the client and/or parents recognize and accept that a problem exists
2. Support and avoid humiliation of the individual
3. Provide empathetic understanding
4. Encourage the identification and use of support systems
5. Attempt to minimize environmental pressures
6. Allow the client time to recover personal resources

D. EVALUATION/OUTCOMES
1. Reorganizes defenses
2. Utilizes support system
3. Verbalizes a decrease in anxiety

PERSONALITY DISORDERS

These disorders are extreme exaggerations of personality traits or styles that often define the uniqueness of the individual; under stress they manifest patterns of inflexibility, maladaptive emotional responses, and functioning impairments

Data Base
A. Psychopathology
1. Research suspects neurobiologic factors
2. Borderline states are characterized by defects in the development of the personality or by pathologic trends in its structure
3. Habitual attitudes and reaction patterns in human relationships develop early in life and form the character structure of the individual
4. In most instances these behaviors create little discomfort or stress
5. Personality disturbances are, in reality, the selection and utilization of specific defense mechanisms that are used so often that they form a life-long pattern of action that, although not normal, is neither neurotic nor psychotic
6. Premorbid personality of individuals demonstrating any of the 11 classified personality disturbances* resembles the compensatory mechanisms associated with the pathologic counterpart

B. Types and behavioral/clinical findings
1. Paranoid personality disorder
   a. Frequent use of projective mechanisms

---

*Adapted from *Diagnostic and Statistical Manual of Mental Disorders*, ed 4, revised, Washington, DC, 1994, American Psychiatric Association.

   b. Suspiciousness, fear, irritability, and stubbornness
   c. Reality testing not greatly impaired
2. Schizoid personality disorder
   a. Avoidance of meaningful interpersonal relationships
   b. Use of autistic thinking, emotional detachment, and daydreaming
   c. Introverted since childhood but maintaining fair contact with reality
3. Schizotypal personality disorder
   a. Unattached, withdrawn
   b. Affectively and intellectually diminished
   c. Frequently part of the vagabond or transient groups of society
4. Antisocial personality disorder
   a. Chronic life-long disturbances that conflict with society's laws and customs
   b. Unable to postpone gratification
   c. Randomly act out their aggressive egocentric impulses on society
   d. Do not profit from past experience or punishment; live only for the moment
   e. Have the ability to ingratiate themselves but "do not wear well"
   f. Are in contact with reality but do not seem to care about it
5. Borderline personality disorder
   a. Unstable and intense interpersonal relationships
   b. Impulsive, unpredictable behavior that is potentially self-destructive
   c. Marked mood shifts
   d. Identity disturbance
   e. Chronic feeling of emptiness
6. Histrionic personality disorder
   a. Emotional instability and hyperexcitability
   b. Extroverted and directed toward gaining attention
   c. Vain and deliberately manipulative
7. Narcissistic personality disorder
   a. Overblown sense of importance
   b. Strong need for attention and admiration
   c. Relationships marked by ambivalence
   d. Preoccupation with appearance
8. Avoidant personality disorder
   a. Social discomfort and timidity
   b. Loner; unwilling to get involved with other people
   c. Fear of negative evaluation from others
9. Dependent personality disorder
   a. Unable to make decisions
   b. Lack of self-confidence
   c. Dependent and submissive
   d. Induces others to assume responsibility
10. Obsessive-compulsive personality disorder

a. Rigidity, overconscientiousness, inordinate capacity for work

b. Driven by obsessive concerns

c. Behavior contains many rituals

11. Passive-aggressive personality disorder

a. Rather helpless and indecisive, demonstrating passive obstructionism while clinging and pouting

b. Frequent outbursts and temper tantrums when frustrated

c. Often create problems for others

d. Deleted from DSM-IV classification for further study

e. Included here as reminder of negativistic traits

C. Therapeutic interventions

1. Individual, group, and family psychotherapy

2. Crisis intervention when necessary

3. Vocational and occupational therapy

Nursing Care of Clients with Personality Disorders

A. DATA COLLECTION

1. Level of functioning with family and friends

2. Individual's perception of problem

3. Why client is seeking treatment at this time

4. Level of anxiety

5. Pending criminal charges

B. ANALYSIS AND INTERPRETATION

1. Anxiety related to:
   a. Threat to security
   b. Threat to self-concept
   c. Inability to meet role expectations
   d. Difficulty in interpersonal relationships

2. Ineffective family coping: compromised, related to:
   a. Abusive or destructive behavior
   b. Ambivalent family relationships
   c. Denial that problem exists

3. Ineffective individual coping related to:
   a. Inability to learn from experience
   b. Poorly developed or inappropriate use of defense mechanisms
   c. Inability to tolerate frustrations
   d. Inability to form meaningful relationships

4. Impaired social interactions related to:
   a. Sociocultural dissonance
   b. Altered thought processes
   c. Communication barriers
   d. Knowledge deficit of interpersonal skills

5. Social isolation related to the absence of meaningful relationships

6. Risk for violence: directed toward others, related to poor impulse control

C. PLANNING/IMPLEMENTATION

1. Maintain consistency and concern

2. Accept the individual as is; do not retaliate if provoked

3. Protect the individual from others while protecting others from the individual

4. Place realistic limits on behavior; make known what those limits are

5. Strive for consistency among health care team members

D. EVALUATION/OUTCOMES

1. Demonstrates decreased episodes of acting out

2. Verbalizes decrease in anxiety

3. Accepts and continues long-term therapy

4. Recognizes and functions within limits of personality

COMMUNITY AND HOSPITAL MENTAL HEALTH SERVICES

CONCEPTS

A. Purposes

1. To provide health promotion, prevention, assessment, treatment, and rehabilitation services for individuals and groups with emotional problems; also support for families

2. To maintain these individuals and families in the community

3. To provide hospital care within the community in those instances when the individual cannot be maintained on an outpatient basis

B. Types of settings in which services are provided

1. Outpatient services
   a. Storefront clinics
   b. Walk-in clinics in hospitals
   c. Emergency rooms
   d. Crisis intervention community mental health centers, including hot-line phone services
   e. Day-care centers/day hospitals
   f. Private offices
   g. Chemical dependency treatment centers

2. Inpatient services
   a. Specialized psychiatric hospitals
   b. General hospital psychiatric units

3. Aftercare services
   a. Foster/special care homes
   b. Halfway houses
   c. Sheltered workshops
   d. Day-care centers

C. Types of services

1. Observation and early diagnosis/identification

2. Assessment of the client's functional status

3. Crisis intervention/stabilization

4. Provide direct care services to clients, including:
   a. Individual, family, and group therapy
   b. Medications

    c. Electroconvulsive therapy
    d. Occupational therapy
    e. Recreational therapy
5. Provide a therapeutic milieu that:
    a. Supports the individual during the period of crisis
    b. Helps the individual learn new ways of coping with problems
6. Referral to proper community agencies for necessary services
7. Vocational counseling
8. Health screening
9. Provide an educational setting for various professional groups in mental health concepts and also for lay helpers and natural support networks

NURSE'S ROLE

A. Case finding and outreach to high-risk groups
B. Assessment of client's needs and the provision of support and assistance where needed
C. Formulation of nursing diagnoses and evaluation of client's progress through the administering and monitoring of therapeutic interventions and the effective management of rapidly changing situations
D. Supervising and ensuring the quality of health care practices in consultation with other professionals (e.g., physicians, psychologists, social workers, school teachers, clergy, and lay networks)
E. Active participation with the health care team, including the individual and family
F. Involvement in individual, family, and group therapy
G. Coordination of health care services for the individual and family
H. Teaching and coaching of groups within the community

PSYCHIATRIC/MENTAL HEALTH NURSING
REVIEW QUESTIONS

Personality Development

1. Which of the following is a generally accepted concept of personality development?
   1. By 2 years of age the basic personality is rather firmly set
   2. The personality is capable of change and modification throughout life
   3. The capacity for personality change decreases rapidly after adolescence
   4. By the end of the first 6 years, the personality has reached its adult parameters

2. The primary emergence of the personality is demonstrated around the age of:
   1. 6 months
   2. 9 months
   3. 24 months
   4. 48 months

3. Personality is unique for every individual because it is the result of the person's:
   1. Intellectual capacity, race, and socioeconomic status
   2. Genetic background, placement in family, and autoimmunity
   3. Biologic constitution, psychologic development, and cultural setting
   4. Childhood experiences, intellectual capacity, and socioeconomic status

4. Which relationship is of extreme importance in the formation of the personality?
   1. Peer
   2. Sibling
   3. Parent-child
   4. Heterosexual

5. For an emotional balance the individual always needs:
   1. Family, work, and play
   2. Security and social recognition
   3. Biologic satisfaction and social acceptance
   4. Individual recognition and group acceptance

6. Communication ties people to their:
   1. Social surroundings
   2. Physical surroundings
   3. Materialistic surroundings
   4. Environmental surroundings

7. The family is most important in the emotional development of the individual because it:
   1. Provides support for the young
   2. Gives rewards and punishment
   3. Helps one to learn identity and roles
   4. Reflects the mores of a larger society

8. Groups are important in the emotional development of the individual because groups:
   1. Always protect their members
   2. Are easily identified by their members
   3. Go through the same developmental phases
   4. Identify acceptable behavior for their members

9. Problems with dependence versus independence develop during the stage of growth and development known as:
   1. Infancy
   2. Toddler
   3. Preschool
   4. School age

Client Case Scenario 1: Mr. Alfred Jones, age 78, has been admitted to hospital with a diagnosis of early Alzheimer's disease. **Items 10 to 12 refer to this client case scenario.**

10. Mr. Jones tells the nurse, "I am useless to everyone, even myself." The nurse recognizes that Mr. Jones may be attempting to deal with which of Erikson's developmental tasks?
    1. Ego integrity versus despair
    2. Identity versus role diffusion
    3. Generativity versus stagnation
    4. Automony versus shame and doubt

11. It is important for the health care team to adopt a common approach to care for Mr. Jones, because he has which of the following needs?
    1. To relate to staff in a consistent manner
    2. To learn that staff cannot be manipulated
    3. To be able to accept fairly applied external controls
    4. To have sameness and consistency in his environment

12. When planning care for Mr. Jones the nurse should implement which of the following interventions?
    1. Teach him new social skills
    2. Encourage him to talk of past experiences
    3. Discuss current events with him
    4. Maintain a familiar daily routine

---

13. The basic emotional task for the toddler is:
    1. Trust
    2. Industry
    3. Identification
    4. Independence

14. During the oedipal stage of growth and development, the child:
    1. Loves and hates (ambivalence) both parents
    2. Loves the parent of the same sex and the parent of the opposite sex
    3. Loves the parent of the opposite sex and hates the parent of the same sex
    4. Loves the parent of the same sex and hates the parent of the opposite sex

15. The stage of growth and development basically concerned with role identification is the:
    1. Oral stage
    2. Genital stage
    3. Oedipal stage
    4. Latency stage

16. Play for the preschool-age child is necessary for the emotional development of:
    1. Projection
    2. Introjection
    3. Competition
    4. Independence

17. Resolution of the oedipal complex takes place when the child overcomes the castration complex and:
    1. Rejects the parent of the same sex
    2. Introjects behaviors of both parents
    3. Identifies with the parent of the same sex
    4. Identifies with the parent of the opposite sex

18. Any surgery should be delayed, if possible, because of the effects on personality development during the:
    1. Oral stage
    2. Anal stage
    3. Oedipal stage
    4. Latency stage

Client Care Scenario 2: Mrs. Annie Smith, age 89, is an elderly confused client who demonstrates aggressive episodes at times. **Items 19 to 21 refer to this client case scenario.**

19. Which of the following environments would be most appropriate for Mrs. Smith?
    1. A group orientated one
    2. One that is easily manipulated
    3. A controlled one that sets limits
    4. One that allows freedom of expression

20. The nurse recognizes that it would be most unusual for Mrs. Smith to exhibit which of the following behaviors?
    1. Resistance to change
    2. Preoccupation with personal appearance
    3. A tendency to dwell on the past and ignore the present
    4. The inability to concentrate on new activities or interests

21. Which of the following approaches would be most helpful in meeting Mrs. Smith's needs?
    1. Providing a nutritious diet high in carbohydrates and proteins
    2. Simplifying the environment as much as possible while eliminating need for choices
    3. Providing an opportunity for many alternative choices in the daily schedule to stimulate interest
    4. Developing a consistent nursing plan with fixed time schedules to provide for physical and emotional needs

---

22. Evidence of the existence of the unconscious is best demonstrated by:
    1. The ease of recall
    2. Slips of the tongue
    3. Déjà vu experiences
    4. Free-floating anxiety

23. The level of anxiety that best enhances an individual's power of perception is:
    1. Mild
    2. Panic
    3. Severe
    4. Moderate

24. A person seeing a design on the wallpaper perceives it as an animal. This is an example of:
    1. An illusion
    2. A delusion
    3. A hallucination
    4. An idea of reference

25. Sublimation is a defense mechanism that helps the individual:
    1. Act out in reverse something already done or thought
    2. Return to an earlier, less mature stage of development
    3. Exclude from the conscious things that are psychologically disturbing
    4. Channel unacceptable sexual desires into socially approved behavior

26. An example of displacement is:
    1. Imaginative activity to escape reality
    2. Ignoring unpleasant aspects of reality
    3. Resisting any demands made by others
    4. Pent-up emotions directed to other than the primary source

27. In the process of development the individual strives to maintain, protect, and enhance the integrity of the self. This is normally accomplished through the use of:
    1. Affective reactions
    2. Ritualistic behaviors
    3. Withdrawal patterns
    4. Defense mechanisms

28. A male college student who is smaller than average and unable to participate in sports becomes the life of the party and a stylish dresser. This is an example of the mechanism of:
    1. Introjection
    2. Sublimation
    3. Compensation
    4. Reaction formation

29. Mental experiences operate on different levels of awareness. The level that best portrays one's attitudes, feelings, and desires is the:
    1. Conscious
    2. Unconscious
    3. Preconscious
    4. Foreconscious

30. The ability to tolerate frustration is an example of one of the functions of the:
    1. Id
    2. Ego
    3. Superego
    4. Unconscious

31. The superego is that part of the psyche which:
    1. Contains the instinctual drives
    2. Is the source of creative energy
    3. Operates on the pleasure principle and demands immediate gratification
    4. Develops from internalizing the concepts of parents and significant others

32. Another term for the superego is:
    1. Self
    2. Ideal self
    3. Narcissism
    4. Conscience

33. The superego is that part of the self which says:
    1. I like what I want
    2. I want what I want
    3. I should not want that
    4. I can wait for what I want

Client Case Scenario 3: Mr. Laslo Czapinski, age 83, is an elderly confused client who has difficulty with English. He becomes agitated at times and strikes out at the nurses. **Items 34 to 36 refer to this client case scenario.**

34. The nurse should include which of the following goals for a therapeutic environment for Mr. Czapinski?
    1. Help the staff to help the client
    2. Assist the client to relate to others
    3. Make the hospital atmosphere more home-like
    4. Help the client become popular in a controlled setting

35. Which of the following interventions should be included in a nursing care plan for Mr. Czapinski?
    1. An extensive reeducation program
    2. Details for protective and supportive care
    3. The introduction of new leisure-time activities
    4. Plans to involve the client in group therapy sessions

36. Mr. Czapinski becomes upset in the day room. He raises his hand and threatens to strike the nurse. Which of the following interventions should the nurse first make?
    1. Tell him to stop the behavior
    2. Reach up and take hold of his arm
    3. Remove self to a safe distance from him
    4. Lead him from the room by taking him by his arm

37. A person has a mature personality if the:
    1. Ego responds to the demands of the superego
    2. Society sets demands to which the ego responds
    3. Superego has replaced and increased all the controls of the parents
    4. Ego acts as a balance between the pressures of the id and the superego

Disorders First Evident Before Adulthood

38. School phobia is usually treated by:
    1. Returning the child to school immediately
    2. Calmly explaining why attendance at school is necessary
    3. Allowing the parent to accompany the child to the classroom
    4. Allowing the child to enter the classroom before other children

39. The childhood problem that has legal as well as emotional aspects and cannot be ignored is:
    1. School phobias
    2. Fear of animals
    3. Fear of monsters
    4. Sleep disturbances

40. While talking with the nurse about the problem of not being able to make friends, a teenager begins to cry. At this time it would be most therapeutic for the nurse to:
    1. Sit quietly with the client
    2. Point out how the client can change this
    3. Tell the client that crying isn't helping
    4. Suggest that they play a game of Scrabble

41. Shortly after admission, an adolescent male client falls to the floor and has tonic and clonic movements. He does not respond verbally, but the nurse notes that he is still chewing gum. The nurse should:
    1. Remove the chewing gum
    2. Send another client for help
    3. Report and record all observation
    4. Insert a tongue blade between the teeth

42. The problem of separation anxiety initially occurs during the:
    1. Oral stage
    2. Anal stage
    3. Phallic stage
    4. Latency stage

43. A 5-year-old boy is frequently found slapping his little sister. This behavior is probably caused by:
    1. Sibling rivalry
    2. Negativistic id impulses
    3. Unresolved oedipal conflicts
    4. Overcompensation efforts of superego

44. The most common characteristic of emotionally disturbed children is that they:
    1. Respond to any stimulus
    2. Respond to little external stimulus
    3. Seem unresponsive to the environment
    4. Are totally involved with the environment

45. Autism can usually be diagnosed when the child is about:
    1. 2 years of age
    2. 6 years of age
    3. 6 months of age
    4. 1 to 3 months of age

46. The nurse should observe the autistic child for signs of:
    1. Not wanting to eat
    2. Crying for attention
    3. Catatonic-like rigidity
    4. Enjoying being with people

47. When planning activities for a child with autism, the nurse must remember that autistic children respond best to:
    1. Large group activity
    2. Loud, cheerful music
    3. Individuals in small groups
    4. Their own self-stimulating acts

48. Attention-deficit hyperactivity disorder in children is usually treated with:
    1. Haloperidol (Haldol)
    2. Methocarbamol (Robaxin)
    3. Methylphenidate hydrochloride (Ritalin)
    4. Chlorpromazine hydrochloride (Thorazine)

Delirium, Dementia, and Other Cognitive Disorders

49. The current trend in the treatment of the elderly with delirium, dementia, or other cognitive disorders is to:
    1. Provide occupational therapy
    2. Medicate during stressful periods
    3. Maintain them in the community
    4. Encourage the assumption of responsibility

50. An elderly male client on the psychiatric unit becomes upset in the day room. When attempting to deal with the situation, the nurse should:
    1. Instruct the client to be quiet
    2. Allow the client to act out until he tires
    3. Give directions in a firm, low-pitched voice
    4. Lead the client from the room by taking him by his arm

51. The nurse recognizes that dementia of the Alzheimer's type is characterized by:
    1. Aggressive acting out behavior
    2. Periodic remissions and exacerbations
    3. Hypoxia of selected areas of brain tissue
    4. Areas of brain destruction called senile plaques

52. When attempting to understand the behavior of an elderly client diagnosed with vascular dementia, the nurse recognizes that the client is probably:
    1. Not capable of using any defense mechanisms
    2. Using one method of defense for every situation
    3. Making exaggerated use of old, familiar mechanisms
    4. Attempting to develop new defense mechanisms to meet the current situation

Substance-Abuse Disorders

53. Drug abuse is best defined as:
    1. A physiologic need for a drug
    2. A psychologic dependence on a drug
    3. A compulsion to take a drug on either a continuous or periodic basis
    4. An excessive drug use inconsistent with acceptable medical practice

54. The nurse would expect an addicted client's basic personality to be marked by insecurity and:
    1. Weak id drives
    2. The need to delay gratification
    3. Infantile passion for self-gratification
    4. The use of somatoform mechanisms

Client Case Scenario 4: Jane Small, age 34, is hospitalized because of alcoholism. **Items 55 to 57 refer to this client case scenario.**

55. Jane denies that she has a problem with alcohol. The nurse understands that Jane uses denial for which of the following reasons?
    1. To reduce her feelings of guilt
    2. To live up to others' expectations
    3. To make her seem more independent
    4. To make her look better in the eyes of others

56. Jane appears suspicious of others and blames them for her personal problems. The nurse understands that the client is using this behavior because of which of the following difficulties?
    1. In telling the truth
    2. Meeting an ego ideal
    3. With dependence and independence
    4. In identifying who is creating problems

57. Jane asks if attendence at Alcoholics Anonymous is required. Which of the following would reflect the nurse's best reply?
    1. "You'll find you'll need their support."
    2. "Do you have feelings about going to these meetings?"
    3. "No, it is best to wait until you feel you really need them."
    4. "Yes, because you will learn how to cope with your problem."

58. When thinking about alcohol and drug abuse, the nurse should be aware that:
    1. Most polydrug abusers also abuse alcohol
    2. Most alcoholics become polydrug abusers
    3. Addictive individuals tend to use hostile, abusive behavior
    4. An unhappy childhood is a causative factor in many addictions

59. For clients with alcoholism, the primary rehabilitator is the:
    1. Client
    2. Nurse
    3. Physician
    4. Entire health team

60. The most important factor in rehabilitation of a client addicted to alcohol is:
    1. The availability of community resources
    2. The accepting attitude of the client's family
    3. The client's emotional or motivational readiness
    4. The qualitative level of the client's physical state

61. The most effective treatment of alcoholism is accomplished by:
    1. Individual or group psychotherapy
    2. Admission to an alcoholic unit in a hospital
    3. Active membership in Alcoholics Anonymous
    4. The daily administration of disulfiram (Antabuse)

Client Case Scenario 5: Sam Brown, age 48, is admitted to hospital. He is an alcoholic who has been drinking before admission. **Items 62 to 64 refer to this client case scenario.**

62. Sam is irritable with the nurse and seems only to wait for a friend who visits daily. One day after a visit, Sam, obviously intoxicated, tells the nurse that the friend has brought gin regularly. Sam's wife is upset and threatens to sue. Which fact would be taken into consideration in a suit?
    1. Sam needs close supervision
    2. The nurse is responsible for observing Sam's behavior
    3. Sam may have gifts brought to them without prior inspection
    4. Sam's response to his friend's visit was a clue that the nurse missed

63. Forty-eight hours after not receiving alcohol Sam asks the nurse if she sees bugs crawling on the wall. Which of the following would be the nurse's best response?

1. "No, I don't see any bugs."
2. "I will get rid of them for you."
3. "I will stay here until you are calmer."
4. "Those bugs are a part of your sickness."

64. Sam makes up stories to fill in the blank spaces in his memory. Which term most likely describes what Sam is doing?
    1. Lying
    2. Denying
    3. Rationalizing
    4. Confabulating

65. Clients with a history of alcoholism with Wernicke's encephalopathy associated with Korsakoff's syndrome are treated initially by:
    1. Providing a high-protein diet
    2. Judicious use of tranquilizers
    3. Oral administration of thorazine
    4. Intramuscular injections of thiamine

Client Case Scenario 6: Mary Coffey, age 23, is a narcotics addict who is receiving methadone hydrochloride. She is admitted to hospital for an emergency appendectomy. **Items 66 to 70 refer to this client case scenario.**

66. Mary is receiving methadone hydrochloride because it:
    1. Allows symptom-free termination of narcotic addiction
    2. Converts narcotic use from an illicit to a legally controlled drug
    3. Provides postoperative pain control without causing narcotic dependence
    4. Counteracts the depressive effects of long-term opiate usage on cardiac and thoracic muscles

67. Mary should be observed closely for which of the following signs of narcotic withdrawal?
    1. Piloerection, lack of interest in surroundings
    2. Agitation, attempts to escape from the hospital
    3. Skin dryness, scratching under incisional dressing
    4. Lethargy, refusal to participate in therapeutic exercise

68. Which of the following goals of nursing care, for Mary, would be appropriate at this time?
    1. To assess her level of drug dependency
    2. To contact and notify her family about the surgery
    3. To do preoperative teaching related to movement, deep breathing, and coughing
    4. To ensure that Mary understands the reason for and possible complications of her surgery

69. Mary may take hard drugs for which of the following reasons?
    1. To ease pain
    2. To blur reality
    3. To clear sensorium
    4. To decrease motor activity

70. Following the last dose of methadone hydrochloride, withdrawal symptoms are expected to reach a peak in:
    1. 8 to 24 hours
    2. 24 to 48 hours
    3. 48 to 72 hours
    4. 72 to 96 hours

71. The family of a client in an alcohol treatment program should be included in the treatment procedure because:
    1. Alcoholism involves the entire family
    2. Alcoholics try to hide their drinking from their families
    3. Family members will better understand the dynamics behind the drinking
    4. Family members have been most successful in providing the necessary support

Schizophrenia and Other Psychotic Disorders

72. Mental illness is evidenced when an individual:
    1. Has difficulty relating to others
    2. Has difficulty completing activities
    3. Experiences frequent periods of high anxiety
    4. Expresses little desire for work or social activities

73. Functional mental illnesses are mainly the result of:
    1. Social environment
    2. Genetic endowment
    3. Infection and inflammation
    4. Deterioration of brain tissue

74. Projection, rationalization, denial, and distortion by hallucinations and delusions are examples of a disturbance in:
    1. Logic
    2. Association
    3. Reality testing
    4. The thought process

75. A client expresses the belief that the FBI is out to kill him. This is an example of:
    1. An hallucination
    2. An error in judgment
    3. A delusion of persecution
    4. A self-accusatory delusion

Client Case Scenario 7: Mark Mattick, age 31, is suffering from schizophrenia. Currently he is experiencing a psychotic episode. **Items 76 to 78 refer to this client case scenario.**

76. Mark expresses the belief that the RCMP is out to kill him. Which of the following terms best illustrate what Mark is experiencing?
   1. An illusion
   2. A delusion
   3. Autistic thinking
   4. An hallucination

77. Mark refuses to eat because he believes that the food is being poisoned. Which of the following is the most appropriate initial nursing intervention?
   1. Taste the food in Mark's presence
   2. Suggest that food be brought in from home
   3. Convince Mark that the food is not poisoned
   4. Tell Mark that tube feedings will be started if he does not begin to eat

78. Which statement should the nurse make in order to pursue the matter of Mark's belief about poisoned food?
   1. "Why do you think the food is poisoned?"
   2. "You feel someone wants to poison you?"
   3. "Your feeling is a symptom of your illness."
   4. "You'll be safe with me. I won't let anyone poison you."

79. A disturbed client starts to repeat phrases that others have just said. This type of speech is known as:
   1. Autism
   2. Echolalia
   3. Neologism
   4. Echopraxia

80. A male client who has delusions of persecution and auditory hallucinations is admitted for psychiatric evaluation after stabbing a friend. Later, the nurse on the unit greets the client by saying, "Good evening. How are you?" The client, who has been referring to himself as "man," answers, "The man is bad." This is an example of:
   1. Dissociation
   2. Transference
   3. Displacement
   4. Reaction formation

81. The major reason for treating severe emotional disorders with tranquilizers is to:
   1. Reduce the neurotic symptoms
   2. Prevent secondary complications

3. Prevent destructiveness by the client
4. Make the client more amenable to psychotherapy

Client Case Scenario 8: Sarah McFee, age 45, has paranoid schizophrenia. **Items 82 to 85 refer to this client case scenario.**

82. Sarah has refused to eat for 36 hours. She believes that the voice of her dead father has commanded her to atone for her sins by fasting for 40 days. Which nursing intervention might interrupt Sarah's delusional system?
   1. Tell her that she has nothing to atone for
   2. Ask her to repeat exactly what the voice said
   3. Ask the physician to write an order for tube feedings
   4. Suggest other means of atonement that may be less damaging

83. Sarah has been awake for several nights. She did not have an interrupted sleep pattern prior to a transfer from a private to a four-bed room three days ago. Sarah's sleeplessness might be related to which of the following stimuli?
   1. Fear of the other clients
   2. Worry about family at home
   3. Watching for an opportunity to escape
   4. Trying to work out emotional problems

84. While the nurse is talking with another client, Sarah comes up and yells, "I hate you. You're talking about me again," and throws a glass of juice at the nurse. Which is the best nursing approach?
   1. Understand Sarah's behavior and say, "You hate me? Tell me about that."
   2. Ignore both the behavior and Sarah, clean up the juice, and talk to her when she is better
   3. Remove Sarah to an isolation room because she needs to have limits placed on her behavior
   4. Verbalize feelings of annoyance as an example to Sarah that it is more acceptable to verbalize feelings than to act out

85. Sarah approaches the nurse and states, "I am hearing voices that are saying bad things about me." Which of the following interventions should the nurse make?
   1. Simply state, "I do not hear the voices."
   2. Suggest that she join other clients playing cards
   3. Encourage Sarah not to listen to what the voices are saying
   4. State, "The staff understands that you are frightened and will stay with you while the voices are speaking."

86. Schizophrenia is considered a functional illness. This means that the:
    1. Genes of the child may carry the schizophrenic factor
    2. Brain itself undergoes actual physical change that produces the symptoms of schizophrenia
    3. Individual is predisposed to schizophrenia because of poor housing and living conditions during childhood
    4. Brain itself undergoes no physical change, but the operation of the organ is disturbed, producing the symptoms of schizophrenia

87. The affect most commonly found in the client with schizophrenia is one of:
    1. Anger and hostility
    2. Apathy and flatness
    3. Happiness and elation
    4. Sadness and depression

88. The premorbid personality of a young librarian who has now been diagnosed with a schizoid personality disorder might be described as:
    1. Rigid and controlling
    2. Schizoid and introverted
    3. Dependent and immature
    4. Suspicious and socially inadequate

89. Nursing interventions for a client diagnosed with a schizoid personality disorder should be appropriately directed toward:
    1. Convincing the client that the hospital staff is trying to help
    2. Helping the client enter into group recreational activities
    3. Helping the client learn to trust the staff through selected experiences
    4. Arranging the hospital environment so that the client's contact with other clients is limited

90. One of the primary goals in providing a therapeutic day-care environment for a client who is somewhat autistic, withdrawn, and seclusive is to:
    1. Foster a trusting relationship
    2. Administer medications on time
    3. Involve the client in a group with peers
    4. Remove the client from the family home

91. A client has delusions that the food is poisoned and therefore will not eat. The nurse tells the client that it is foolish to believe that, since the food in question comes from the same kitchen as the food for all the other clients. The nurse states, "Unless you eat, you will have to be fed by other means." This response indicates that the nurse is aware that the client has:
    1. To be reminded about needing to eat
    2. Misinterpretations that have to be corrected
    3. Created a situation the nurse cannot handle
    4. Nourishment needs and therefore has to eat

92. While watching TV in the day room, a female client who has demonstrated withdrawn, regressed behavior suddenly screams, bursts into tears, and runs out of the room to the far end of the hallway. The most therapeutic action for the nurse to take would be to:
    1. Walk to the end of the hallway where the client is standing
    2. Write up the incident in the client's chart while memory is fresh
    3. Accept the action as just being the impulsive behavior of a sick person
    4. Ask another client who was in the day room what made the client act as she did

Client Case Scenario 9: Harold Aster, age 23, is a regressed, emotionally disturbed client. **Items 93 to 95 refer to this client case scenario.**

93. Harold is seen openly masturbating. Which nursing action would be most appropriate?
    1. Restrain his hands
    2. Put Harold in seclusion
    3. Not react to the behavior
    4. State that such behavior is unacceptable

94. Harold uses his hand to eat soft foods. Which intervention should the nurse make?
    1. Place a spoon in his hand and suggest it be used
    2. Say in a joking way, "Well, I guess fingers were made before forks."
    3. Ignore the behavior and observe several additional meals before intervening
    4. Remove the food and say, "You can't have any more until you use your spoon."

95. Harold voids on the floor. The nurse should make which of the following actions?
    1. Make Harold mop the floor
    2. Restrict his fluids throughout the day
    3. Frequently toilet Harold with supervision
    4. Withhold privileges each time Harold voids on the floor

96. Observation is an important aspect of nursing care. It is especially important in the care of the withdrawn client because it:
    1. Is useful in making a diagnosis
    2. Tells the staff how ill the client is
    3. Helps in understanding the client's feelings
    4. Indicates the degree of psychic depression

Client Case Scenario 10: Karen Kim, age 16, is withdrawn and noncommunicative. She spends most of her time lying on her bed. **Items 97 to 100 refer to this client case scenario.**

97. Which nursing intervention would be the most appropriate way to help Karen accept the realities of daily living?
    1. Assist her to care for personal hygiene needs
    2. Encourage her to keep up with school studies
    3. Encourage her to join the other clients in group singing
    4. Leave her alone when there appears to be a disinterest in the activities at hand

98. Which is the best plan of nursing intervention to encourage Karen to talk?
    1. Try to get her to discuss feelings
    2. Focus on nonthreatening subjects
    3. Ask simple questions that require answers
    4. Sit and look through magazines with her

99. Which of the following is an important aspect of nursing intervention when caring for Karen?
    1. Help keep her oriented to reality
    2. Involve her in activities throughout the day
    3. Encourage her to discuss why mixing with other people is avoided
    4. Help her understand that it is harmful to withdraw from situations

100. One day Karen suddenly walks up to the nurse and shouts, "You think you're so damned perfect and good. I think you stink!" Which response should the nurse make?
    1. "You seem angry with me."
    2. "Stink? I don't understand."
    3. "Boy, you're in a bad mood."
    4. "I can't be all that bad, can I?"

101. A female client has been on the psychiatric unit for several days. She arouses anxiety and frustration in the staff and manipulates so well that she intimidates any nurse who comes near her. One morning, the client yells out at the nurse, "You've worked it so that I can't go out with the group today to bowl. You're as cunning as a fox—I hate you! Get out or I'll hit you." The best response by the nurse would be:
    1. "Tell me what I did to hurt you."
    2. "Go ahead and hit me if you have a need to."
    3. "I don't really like to hear your threats and insults. Can you tell me why you feel this way?"
    4. "You are being rude and I don't like it. Your behavior is stopping me from wanting to stay with you."

102. When there is nothing organically wrong with the organs of communication and yet the individual is unable to communicate, the condition is referred to as:
    1. A mental deficiency
    2. Dementia or delirium
    3. Chronic brain pathology
    4. A functional mental disorder

103. On being discharged, a client with psychiatric problems should be encouraged to:
    1. Go back to regular activities
    2. Call the unit whenever upset
    3. Continue in an aftercare situation
    4. Find a group that has similar problems

Disorders of Mood

104. Feelings of self-effacement are best demonstrated by a client's:
    1. Lack of initiative
    2. Quiet and monotonous voice
    3. "No one listens to me" attitude
    4. Inappropriate gestures and affect

105. The nurse is assigned to care for a 39-year-old, hyperactive, elated client who exhibits flight of ideas. The client is not eating. The nurse recognizes this may be because the client:
    1. Feels undeserving of the food
    2. Is too busy to take the time to eat
    3. Wishes to avoid the clients in the dining room
    4. Believes that at this time there is no need for food

106. A physician has been a client of the psychiatric service for the past 3 days. The client has questioned the authority of the treatment team, has advised other clients that their treatment plans are wrong, and generally has been disruptive in group therapy. The nurse's most appropriate response would be to:
    1. Ignore the client and hope the disruptive behavior will stop
    2. Tell the other clients that they should not pay attention to what the client says

3. Restrict the client's contact with other clients until the disruptive behavior ceases
4. Understand that the client is unable to control this behavior and that limits must be set

107. During periods of extreme elation and hyperactivity, the nursing staff should consider a client's nutritional needs by:
    1. Accepting the fact that the client will eat if hungry
    2. Following the client around the dining room with a tray
    3. Allowing the client to prepare own meals and eat when desired
    4. Providing the client with frequent, high-calorie feedings that can be handheld

108. When approaching a client during a period of great overactivity, it is essential to:
    1. Use a firm, warm, consistent approach
    2. Anticipate and physically control the client's hyperactivity
    3. Allow the client to choose the activities in which to participate
    4. Let the client know the staff will not tolerate destructive behavior

109. The nursing care plan for a hyperactive client should appropriately include plans to:
    1. Arouse and focus the client's interest in reality
    2. Encourage the client to talk as much as needed
    3. Persuade the client to complete any task that has been started
    4. Provide constructive channels for redirecting the client's excess energy

110. When helping the female client with personal hygiene during the manic phase of a bipolar disorder, the nurse should:
    1. Encourage her to dress attractively and in her own clothing
    2. Allow her to apply makeup in whatever manner she chooses
    3. Keep makeup away from her because she will apply it too freely
    4. Suggest that she wear hospital clothing to avoid confrontations

111. To best help meet the nutritional needs of an extremely hyperactive client during the manic phase of a bipolar disorder, the nurse should:
    1. Provide a tray in the client's room
    2. Assure the client that the food is deserved
    3. Point out that the energy the client is burning up must be replaced
    4. Order foods that the client can hold in the hand to eat while moving around

Client Case Scenario 11: Jack Johnson, age 48, is a meticulous person who has no outside interests besides his job as a machinist. He has a major depressive disorder. **Items 112 to 115 refer to this client case scenario.**

112. Which of the following would probably best describe Jack's premorbid personality?
    1. Suspicious, sensitive, aloof
    2. Dependent, immature, insecure
    3. Rigid, narrow, overly conscientious
    4. Withdrawn and seclusive, with an active fantasy life

113. Which activity would be least therapeutic for Jack?
    1. Allowing him to plan his own activities
    2. Specific, simple instructions to be followed
    3. Simple, easily completed, short-term projects
    4. Monotonous, repetitive projects and activities

114. Which nursing action would be most therapeutic when developing a nursing care plan with Jack?
    1. Allow time for his slowness when planning activities
    2. Help him focus on family strengths and support systems
    3. Encourage him to perform menial tasks to meet the need for punishment
    4. Repeat again and again that the staff views him as worthwhile and important

115. The nurse is about to discharge Jack, after 28 days of hospitalization. Which statement would demonstrate the most understanding by the nurse?
    1. "Call the unit night or day if you have problems."
    2. "I am going to miss you; we have become good friends."
    3. "I know you are really going to be all right when you go home."
    4. "This is my phone number; call me and let me know how you are doing."

116. A 23-year-old has been admitted to a psychiatric hospital after a month of unusual behavior that included eating and sleeping very little, talking and singing constantly, and frequent shopping sprees. In the hospital, the client is demanding, bossy, and sarcastic. The symptoms the client is exhibiting are usually found in clients with the diagnosis of:
    1. Mood disorder
    2. Major depression
    3. Personality disorder
    4. Schizophrenic disorder

117. The most accurate definition of "depression," as used in psychiatry, is a:
    1. Difficulty in decision making and functioning
    2. Total loss of control over emotional impulses
    3. Disturbance in mood as a reaction to the loss of a love object
    4. Disturbance in mood as a result of frustrated instinctual strivings

118. The statement that would be most appropriate for the nurse to use in interviewing a newly admitted, 35-year-old, depressed client whose thoughts focus on feelings of unworthiness and failure would be:
    1. "Tell me how you feel about yourself."
    2. "Tell me what has been bothering you."
    3. "Why do you feel so bad about yourself?"
    4. "What can we do to help you during your stay with us?"

119. An activity that would be most appropriate for a depressed client during the early part of hospitalization would be a:
    1. Game of Trivial Pursuit
    2. Project involving drawing
    3. Small dance-therapy group
    4. Card game with three other clients

120. An elderly, depressed client frequently paces the halls, becoming physically tired from the activity. To help the client reduce this activity, the nurse should:
    1. Supply the client with simple, monotonous tasks
    2. Request a sedative order from the client's physician
    3. Restrain the client in a chair reducing the opportunity to pace
    4. Place the client in a single room, thus limiting pacing to a smaller area

121. A long-term therapy goal for a female client hospitalized for a major depressive episode should be that the client will be:
    1. Able to talk about her depressed feelings
    2. Able to develop new defense mechanisms
    3. More realistic in accepting herself and others
    4. Aware of the unconscious source of her anger

Client Case Scenario 12: Judy Stanfield, age 19, has just been admitted to hospital. She has a bipolar disorder and is in the manic phase of her illness. **Items 122 to 124 refer to this client case scenario.**

122. Three new staff are being orientated to the unit. Judy comes up to them and says, "Welcome to the funny farm. I'm Jo-Jo the head Yo-Yo." Which of the following describes what is happening to Judy?
    1. She is trying to fill the "life of the party" role
    2. She is looking for attention from the new staff
    3. She is unable to distinguish fantasy from reality
    4. She is anxious over the arrival of the new staff members

123. Judy becomes vulgar and profane. What should the nurse do?
    1. State: "We do not like that kind of talk around here."
    2. Ignore it, since the client is using it only to get attention
    3. Recognize the language as part of the illness, but set limits on it
    4. State: "When you can talk in an acceptable way, we will talk to you."

124. Judy is hyperactive and elated. What could the nurse do to redirect her?
    1. Ask her to guide other clients as they clean their rooms
    2. Encourage her to tear pictures out of magazines for a scrap book
    3. Suggest that she initiate social activities on the unit for the client group
    4. Provide her with a pencil and paper and encourage her to write a short story

125. The action by the nurse that would be most therapeutic when a depressed client states, "I am no good. I'm better off dead," would be:
    1. Stating, "I think you're good; you should think of living."
    2. Stating, "I will stay with you until you are less depressed."
    3. Alerting the staff to provide 24-hour observation of the client
    4. Unobtrusively removing those articles that could be used in a suicide attempt

126. A positive nursing action when caring for a middle-aged, depressed client is to:
    1. Play a game of chess with the client
    2. Allow the client to make personal decisions
    3. Sit down next to the client as often as possible
    4. Provide the client with frequent periods of thinking time

127. The nurse is assigned to care for a middle-aged, depressed female client on a day when the client seems more withdrawn and depressed than usual. It would be most appropriate for the nurse to:

1. Remain visible to the client
2. Get the client involved in group activities
3. Ask the client, "May I sit down next to you for a while?"
4. Tell the client, "I would like to spend some time with you."

128. The nurse understands that one of the most difficult tasks for the depressed client is the expression of:
    1. Remorse and guilt
    2. Need for comforting
    3. Anger toward others
    4. Feelings of low self-esteem

129. Depressed clients seem to do best in settings where they have:
    1. Many varied activities
    2. A great deal of stimuli
    3. A simple daily schedule
    4. To make only simple decisions

130. A female client is hospitalized because of a severe depression. While at home she refused to eat, stayed in bed most of the time, and did not talk with family members. Finally, unable to cope with the problem, her husband took her to the hospital. Here the symptoms persist and she will not leave her room. The nurse caring for her attempts to talk to her, asking questions but receiving no answers. Finally, in exasperation, the nurse tells the client that if she does not respond she will be left alone. The nurse:
    1. Recognizes that the client has the right to make the decision
    2. Attempts to use reward and punishment to motivate the client
    3. Is really assaulting the client and should have refrained from this
    4. Should get her involved in group therapy rather than attempting one-to-one therapy

131. When caring for a middle-aged, female client with a major depression, who feels all her family members have been killed because she has been sinful and needs to be punished, the prime responsibility of the nurse would be to:
    1. Protect the client against any suicidal impulses
    2. Keep up the client's interest in the outside world
    3. Help the client handle her concern for family members
    4. Reassure the client that past behaviors are not being punished

132. A client admitted for suicidal ideation progresses satisfactorily and is to be discharged from the unit within a day or two. The client denies suicidal tendencies and the staff is pleased with the client's progress. One day the door to the unit is accidently left unlocked. Fifteen minutes later the client is gone and is found hanging in the bathroom. In this situation:
    1. The client's actions should have been anticipated by the nurse
    2. Suicidal clients should be observed until all symptoms of depression disappear
    3. Determined clients almost always succeed at suicide, even with constant supervision
    4. The lifting of the depression demonstrated the client's recovery, so supervision was unnecessary

133. The university health service has referred a college sophomore for admission because of an increasingly unkempt appearance and withdrawn, isolated, and depressed behavior. The referring psychiatrist notes strong suicidal tendencies. Contributing factors appear to be an abrupt ending of a romantic relationship and declining grades. The prognosis for a reasonably rapid recovery for this client is:
    1. Poor, since the client has suicidal tendencies
    2. Bad, since the client is failing in all sectors of life
    3. Fair, since the client seems intelligent enough to pull things together
    4. Good, since the onset is fairly sudden and no previous emotional problems existed

Client Care Scenario 13: Arnold Lubenkoff, age 67, has had successfully treated depressive disease for more than 10 years. Lately he has been preoccupied by suicidal thoughts and has been developing a plan of action. Arnold is admitted to hospital for reassessment. **Items 134 to 140 refer to this client case scenario.**

134. Which assessment would best aid the nurse in evaluating Arnold's potential for suicide?
    1. Ask him about plans for the future
    2. Ask other clients about suicide while in a group
    3. Ask the family if he has ever attempted suicide
    4. Ask him if suicide was ever or is now being considered

135. Which factor is most important in evaluating Arnold's risk of suicide?
    1. Presence of multiple personal problems
    2. Length of time the depression has existed
    3. Impending anniversary of the loss of a loved one
    4. Development of plans for discharge from hospital or program

136. Arnold confides to the nurse that he has been thinking of suicide. Which of the following motivations should the nurse recognize in Arnold?
    1. Wishes to frighten the nurse
    2. Wants attention from the staff
    3. Feels safe and can share his feelings with the nurse
    4. Is fearful of his own impulses and is seeking protection from them

137. Arnold is placed on suicide precautions. Which would be the most therapeutic way to provide these safety measures?
    1. Not allow him to leave his room
    2. Remove all sharp or cutting objects
    3. Give him the opportunity to ventilate feelings
    4. Assign a staff member to be with him at all times

138. The psychiatrist prescribes electroconvulsive therapy for Arnold. The nurse, when discussing electroconvulsive therapy (ECT) with Arnold, should tell him which of the following information?
    1. Sleep will be induced and treatment will not cause pain
    2. There will be a memory loss as a result of the treatment
    3. It is better not to talk about it, but he can ask any question
    4. With new methods of administration, treatment is totally safe

139. Which item should the nurse emphasize to Arnold about ECT?
    1. The treatments will make him feel better
    2. He will not be alone during the treatment
    3. A period of amnesia will follow the treatment
    4. There is no need to be afraid; the treatment does not cause pain

140. Which nursing intervention would be most appropriate after Arnold has awakened from his first ECT treatment?
    1. Bring him a lunch tray
    2. Orient him to time and place and tell him that he has just had a treatment
    3. Get him up and out of bed as soon as possible and back into the unit's routine
    4. Take his blood pressure and pulse rate every 5 minutes until he is fully awake

141. On the second day after admission, a suicidal client asks the nurse, "Why am I being observed around the clock and why is my freedom to move around the unit restricted?" The nurse's most appropriate reply would be:

1. "Why do you think we are observing you?"
2. "What makes you think that we are observing you?"
3. "We are concerned that you might try to harm yourself."
4. "Your doctor has ordered it and is the one you should ask about it."

142. One day, while shaving, a male client with the diagnosis of bipolar disorder states to the nurse, "I have hidden a razor blade and tonight I am going to kill myself." The nurse's best reply would be:
    1. "You're going to kill yourself?"
    2. "Things can't really be that bad."
    3. "I'm sure you don't really mean that."
    4. "You'd better finish shaving; it's time for lunch."

143. After 4 days on the inpatient psychiatric unit, a client on suicidal precautions tells the nurse, "Hey, look! I was feeling pretty depressed for a while, but I'm certainly not going to kill myself." The nurse's best response to this statement would be:
    1. "Kill yourself? I don't understand."
    2. "You do seem to be feeling better."
    3. "Suppose we talk some more about this."
    4. "We have to observe you until your psychiatrist tells us to stop."

144. The treatment plan for a client admitted with a severe, persistent, intractable depression and suicidal ideation would probably include:
    1. Electroconvulsive therapy
    2. Short-term psychoanalysis
    3. Nondirective psychotherapy
    4. High doses of anxiolytic-type drugs

Anxiety, Somatoform, and Dissociative Disorders

145. The defense mechanism in which emotional conflicts are expressed through motor, sensory, or somatic disability is identified as:
    1. Conversion
    2. Dissociation
    3. Compensation
    4. Psychosomatic

Client Case Scenario 14: Mary Gonzales, age 32, has a severe anxiety disorder. **Items 146 to 149 refer to this client case scenario.**

146. Mary is wringing her hands and pacing. Which intervention should the nurse make first?
    1. Get her involved
    2. Tell her to sit down
    3. Stay physically close to Mary
    4. Gently ask her what is bothering her

147. Which intervention can the nurse do to minimize Mary's psychologic stress?
    1. Learn what is of particular importance to her
    2. Explain in fine detail the procedures and therapies being used
    3. Avoid the discussion of any areas that may be emotionally charged
    4. Confidently advise her that the nurse is in charge of the situation

148. Mary is about to be discharged. A family conference is held. Which concept about anxiety should the nurse teach Mary's family?
    1. It is a totally unique experience and feeling
    2. Mary has consciously motivated thoughts and wishes
    3. Her fears are those that are related to the total environment
    4. She has a behavior pattern observed in ourselves and others

149. The nurse explains to the family that it would be unusual for Mary to handle her anxiety in the following manner:
    1. To act it out with antisocial behavior
    2. To convert it into a physical symptom
    3. To regress to earlier levels of adjustment
    4. To displace it onto less threatening objects

150. Physiologically, the nurse would expect a client's anxiety to be manifested by:
    1. Dilated pupils, dilated bronchioles, increased pulse rate, hyperglycemia, and peripheral vasoconstriction
    2. Constricted pupils, dilated bronchioles, increased pulse rate, hypoglycemia, and peripheral vasolidation
    3. Constricted pupils, constricted bronchioles, increased pulse rate, hypoglycemia, and peripheral vasodilation
    4. Dilated pupils, constricted bronchioles, decreased pulse rate, hypoglycemia, and peripheral vasoconstriction

151. Unsatisfied needs create anxiety that motivates an individual to action. This action is brought about mainly to:
    1. Reduce tension
    2. Deny the situation
    3. Remove the problem
    4. Relieve physical discomfort

152. The most appropriate way to decrease a client's anxiety is by:
    1. Avoiding unpleasant objects and events
    2. Prolonged exposure to fearful situations

    3. Acquiring skills with which to face stressful events
    4. Introducing an element of pleasure into fearful situations

Client Case Scenario 15: Sam DiPietro, age 63, has an obsessive compulsive behavior disorder. He believes that the door knobs are contaminated and refuses to touch them except with a tissue. **Items 153 to 156 refer to the client case scenario.**

153. Which intervention should the nurse make when dealing with Sam's fear of door knobs?
    1. Supply him with paper tissues to help him function until his anxiety is reduced
    2. Explain to him that his idea about doorknobs is part of his illness and is not necessary
    3. Encourage him to scrub the doorknobs with a strong antiseptic so he does not need to use tissues
    4. Encourage him to touch doorknobs by removing all available paper tissue until he learns to deal with the situation

154. Which stimulus is possibly motivating Sam to use paper towels to open doors?
    1. He is using this method to punish himself
    2. He is listening to voices telling him that the doorknobs are unclean
    3. He wants to unconsciously control unacceptable impulses or feelings
    4. He has a need to punish others by carrying out an annoying procedure

155. Which action by the nurse would most likely increase Sam's anxiety?
    1. Explore with him the nature of his anxiety
    2. Stimulate him to express his ritualistic actions regularly
    3. Encourage him to participate in his therapeutic plan of care
    4. Provide him with an environment that is both supportive and nonopinionated

156. Which intervention should be included in Sam's initial treatment plan?
    1. Deny him time for the ritualistic behavior
    2. Give him a schedule for the ritualistic behavior
    3. Determine the purpose of the ritualistic behavior
    4. Suggest a symptom substitution technique to refocus the behavior

157. The nurse could most appropriately begin to help an extremely anxious client with a sleep problem, who has been assigned to a four-bed room since admission, by saying:
    1. "You seem unable to sleep at night."
    2. "I'm going to move you to a private room."
    3. "Don't worry, you'll sleep when you're tired."
    4. "I'll get you the sedative your doctor ordered."

158. A phobic reaction will rarely occur unless the person:
    1. Thinks about the feared object
    2. Absolves the guilt of the feared object
    3. Introjects the feared object into the body
    4. Comes into contact with the feared object

159. When developing a care plan for a client with an obsessive-compulsive behavior disorder, the action that would most likely increase the client's anxiety would be:
    1. Permitting the client's ritualistic acts three times a day
    2. Having the client understand the nature of the anxiety
    3. Involving the client in establishing the therapeutic plan
    4. Providing the client with a nonjudgmental, accepting environment

Client Case Scenario 16: Sean MacFarlane, age 26, who is caught in a raging conflict between his mother and his wife, complains of pain in his right leg that has progressed to the point of paralysis. After orthopedic consultation has shown no pathology, he is referred for a psychiatric consultation and is found to have a conversion disorder. **Items 160 to 165 refer to this client case scenario.**

160. The nurse understands which of the following concepts about Sean's conversion disorder?
    1. It is an unconscious method for getting attention
    2. It is usually necessary for him to cope with the present situation
    3. It is reversible and will subside if he is helped to focus on other things
    4. It will probably be solved when he learns to deal with ongoing family conflicts

161. Sean's conflict may be caused by which of the following stimuli?
    1. Hostile feelings toward his home
    2. Ambivalent feelings toward his wife
    3. Needs to be a dependent child and an independent adult
    4. Inadequate feelings in regard to assuming the role of husband

162. Which behavior is Sean most likely to manifest?
    1. Demonstrate a spread of paralysis to other body parts
    2. Require continuous psychiatric treatment to maintain individual functioning
    3. Recover the use of the affected leg but, under stress, again develop similar symptoms
    4. Follow a rather unpredictable emotional course in the future, depending on exposure to stress

163. How would the nurse expect Sean to behave?
    1. Appear greatly depressed
    2. Exhibit free-floating anxiety
    3. Appear calm and composed
    4. Demonstrate anxiety when discussing symptoms

164. Which intervention would be most therapeutic for the nurse to make?
    1. Encourage him to try to walk
    2. Tell him there is nothing wrong
    3. Avoid focusing on his physical symptoms
    4. Help him follow through with the physical therapy plan

165. Which description best describes Sean's anxiety?
    1. Diffuse and free floating
    2. Consciously felt by him
    3. Projected onto the environment
    4. Localized and relieved by the symptom

166. The hospital or day-treatment center is often indicated for the treatment of the client with an obsessive-compulsive disorder because:
    1. It prevents the client from carrying out symptomatic rituals
    2. It allows the staff to exert control over the client's activities
    3. It resolves the client's anxiety because decision making is minimal
    4. It provides the neutral environment the client needs to work through conflicts

167. When planning care for a client with a diagnosis of conversion disorder with the chief complaint of blindness, the nurse recognizes that:
    1. It is best to ignore the client's complaints
    2. The client's behavior indicates a lack of willpower
    3. The client's symptoms are evidence of a disturbed personality
    4. If additional stress is added, the client will become permanently blind

Eating Disorders

168. The major difference between anorexia nervosa and bulimia nervosa is that the individual with bulimia nervosa:
1. Is obese and is attempting to lose weight
2. Has a distorted body image and sees the body as fat
3. Recognizes that there is a problem but is helpless to correct it
4. Is struggling with a conflict of dependence versus independence

169. A therapeutic environment for clients with bulimia nervosa would be one that is:
1. Controlling
2. Empathetic
3. Focused on food
4. Based on realistic limits

Client Case Scenario 17: Sally Berkfield, age 16, is admitted with the diagnosis of anorexia nervosa. She has lost 10 kg in 6 weeks. She is very thin but excessively concerned about being overweight. Her daily intake is 10 cups of coffee. **Items 170 to 172 refer to this client case scenario.**

170. Which nursing intervention should the nurse initially perform for Sally?
1. Explain the value of good nutrition
2. Compliment her on her lovely figure
3. Try to establish a relationship of trust
4. Explore the reasons why she does not eat

171. Which stimulus is the most likely cause of Sally's disorder?
1. A low self-esteem
2. Feelings of unworthiness
3. Anger directed at the parents
4. An unconscious fear of growing up

172. A behavior modification plan is established with Sally. Which would be an appropriate goal?
1. Eat every meal for a week
2. Gain a pound of weight a week
3. Talk about food for 1 hour a day
4. Attend a group therapy every day

Disorders of Personality

173. A person who deliberately pretends an illness is usually thought to be:
1. Neurotic
2. Malingering
3. Out of contact with reality
4. Using conversion defenses

174. The basic difference between psychophysiologic disorders and somatoform disorders is that in psychophysiologic disorders there is:
1. A feeling of illness
2. An emotional cause
3. A restriction of activities
4. An actual tissue change

Client Case Scenario 18: Donald Yarfield, age 38, has been charged with assaulting his neighbor. He has had numerous arrests in the past. He is diagnosed as having an antisocial personality disorder. **Items 175 to 177 refer to this client case scenario.**

175. Which concept about antisocial personality disorders should the nurse consider when planning care for Donald?
1. He may suffer from a great deal of anxiety
2. He probably cannot postpone gratification
3. He will rapidly learn by experience and punishment
4. He will have a great sense of responsibility toward others

176. Donald has difficulty relating to others because he may never have learned which of the following behaviors?
1. Counting on others
2. Empathizing with others
3. Being dependent on others
4. Communicating with others

177. Donald asks the nurse for her phone number so he can call her for a date. How should the nurse respond?
1. "We are not permitted to date clients."
2. "No, you are a client and I am a nurse."
3. "I like you, but our relationship is professional."
4. "It is against my professional ethics to date clients."

178. A person who habitually expresses anxiety through physical symptoms is using:
1. Projection
2. Regression
3. Conversion
4. Hypochondriasis

179. Many people control anxiety by ritualistic behavior. When taking care of these individuals it is important for the nurse to:
1. Avoid mentioning the ritual
2. Explain the meaning of the ritual
3. Allow them time to carry out the ritual
4. Prevent them from carrying out the ritual

180. The main personality problem for clients who need props to blur reality is usually:
    1. Mistrust
    2. Ego ideal
    3. Dependency
    4. Role blurring

181. A frequent finding in clients with paraphiliac sexual disorders is that they usually have:
    1. Other covert or overt emotional problems
    2. A deficiency of gonadal and pituitary hormones
    3. An inadequate physical development of the sexual organs
    4. A poor adjustment due to association with society's fringe groups

182. A nurse is orienting a new client to the unit when another client rushes down the hallway and asks the nurse to sit down to talk. The client requesting the nurse's attention is extremely manipulative and uses socially acting out behaviors when demands are unmet. The nurse should:
    1. Suggest that the client requesting attention speak with another staff member
    2. Leave the new client and talk with the other client to avoid precipitating acting out behavior
    3. Tell the interrupting client to sit down and be patient, stating, "I'll be back as soon as possible."
    4. Introduce the two clients and suggest that the client join the new client and the nurse on the tour

Client Case Scenario 19: Margaret Mumford, age 56, has an obsessive-compulsive personality disorder. She ritualistically cleans her whole house each day. **Items 183 to 185 refer to this client case scenario.**

183. Therapeutic treatment for Margaret should be directed toward helping her to do which of the following?
    1. Redirect her energy into activities to help others
    2. Learn that her behavior is not serving a realistic purpose
    3. Forget her fears by administering antianxiety medications
    4. Understand her behavior is caused by unconscious impulses that she fears

184. Which treatment would be best for Margaret?
    1. Restricting her movements
    2. Keeping her busy to distract her
    3. Calling attention to her behavior
    4. Supporting but limiting her behavior

185. In order to effectively intervene with Margaret, the nurse should understand that ritualistic behavior probably serves which purpose for her?

    1. She performs it willingly
    2. It is purposeful but useless
    3. She performs it after long urging
    4. It seems absurd but it is necessary to her

186. A client with a diagnosis of passive-aggressive personality disorder has been given a day pass from the psychiatric hospital. The client is due to return at 6 PM. At 5 PM the client telephones the nurse in charge of the unit and says, "Six o'clock is too early. I feel like coming back at 7:30." The nurse would be most therapeutic by telling the client to:
    1. Return immediately, to demonstrate control
    2. Return on time or restrictions will be imposed
    3. Come back by 6:45, as a compromise to set limits
    4. Come back as soon as possible or the police will be sent

187. Two 20-year-old female clients have become very much attached to one another and were recently found in bed together. They became angry and sarcastic when the nurse asked one of them to return to her own bed. The nurse can best handle this situation by:
    1. Asking the physician to transfer one of the clients to another unit
    2. Adopting a matter-of-fact, noncondemning attitude while setting limits on the behavior
    3. Restricting both their privileges for several days because their behavior is undesirable and immature
    4. Supervising them carefully and separating them when possible throughout the day and especially at night

188. Following an automobile accident involving a fatality and a subsequent arrest for speeding, a client has amnesia for the events surrounding the accident. This is an example of the defense mechanism known as:
    1. Projection
    2. Repression
    3. Dissociation
    4. Suppression

Crisis Situations

189. The part of the nervous system that is primarily affected during a "fight or flight" reaction is the:
    1. Central nervous system
    2. Peripheral nervous system
    3. Sympathetic nervous system
    4. Parasympathetic nervous system

190. When applying mental health principles to the care of any person with children, the nurse should be aware that:
    1. It is easier to adjust to the first child than to later ones
    2. It is pathologic to feel anger and resentment toward a child
    3. Every parent has inborn feelings of love and acceptance for children
    4. Many parents experience feelings of resentment toward their children

191. An emotional experience in childhood becomes traumatic when:
    1. The parents are harsh and restrictive
    2. The superego has not been internalized
    3. The child is unable to verbalize own feelings
    4. The ego is overwhelmed by anxiety it cannot handle

192. Strict toilet training before a child is ready will cause problems in personality development because at this age a child is learning to:
    1. Satisfy own needs
    2. Identify own needs
    3. Satisfy parents' needs
    4. Live up to society's expectations

193. When helping to resolve a crisis situation it is most important for the nurse to:
    1. Support ego strengths
    2. Encourage socialization
    3. Meet all dependency needs
    4. Involve the person in a therapy group

194. A 43-year-old, well-dressed man has been admitted to the psychiatric unit for psychiatric evaluation. He is charged with molesting a 7-year-old child. When the nurse asks him to come to dinner, he refuses. He covers his face with his hands and states, "I don't want anyone to see me. Leave me alone." The nurse's best response would be:
    1. "Certainly, I respect your wishes."
    2. "It will be easier to face other people right away."
    3. "Only the staff members know why you are here."
    4. "I hope you realize that you are the hardest judge you must face."

Client Case Scenario 20: Dominique Sarto, age 78, has been newly admitted. He is tearful and depressed. **Items 195 to 197 refer to this client case scenario.**

195. The nurse offers to walk Dominique to the evening meal. He looks at the nurse and says nothing. Which is the nurse's best response?
    1. "I'll be at the desk if you need me."
    2. "Tell me what you are feeling now."
    3. "Pull yourself together; I'll walk you to dinner."
    4. "It must be difficult to be on a psychiatric unit."

196. Dominique is visibly angry and states to the nurse, "My daughter-in-law says they can't take me home until the doctor lets me go. She doesn't understand; she is not from our culture." Which intervention should the nurse make?
    1. Ignore the statement for the present
    2. State, "You feel she doesn't want you at home."
    3. State, "The physician makes decisions about discharge."
    4. Reflect on the client's feelings about the cultural differences

197. Dominique is normally "well-adjusted" in ordinary daily living. He has become more dependent since hospitalization. This is an example of which defense mechanism?
    1. Denial
    2. Regression
    3. Compensation
    4. Reaction formation

198. A baby born with a severe bilateral cleft lip and palate is shown to the father before the mother is aware of the deformity. The father says to the nursery nurse, "Oh, what am I going to do? How could this happen to us? What is my wife going to do? It would have been better if she had never become pregnant." The most appropriate response for the nurse to make would be:
    1. "This must be very hard on you. Would it help if I went with you when the doctor talks to your wife?"
    2. "How can you say that? You have a lovely, healthy baby; the cleft lip can be fixed and then the baby will be fine."
    3. "I know that this is very difficult for you. But you can't think of yourself now. Your wife needs you. You must be strong."
    4. "I know how hard this must be for you. But believe me, you will love the baby so much, you won't even notice that there is a problem."

199. When bed rest is ordered for a multiparous client experiencing premature labor, she begins to cry and states, "I have two small children at home." The nurse should reply:
    1. "You will need someone to care for the children."
    2. "You are worried about how you will be able to manage?"
    3. "You'll be able to fix meals, and the children can go to nursery school."
    4. "Perhaps a neighbor can help out, and your husband can do the housework in the evening."

200. A young, single woman delivers a child with a severe cleft palate. The nurse recognizes the fairly typical response to a baby with a visible birth defect when the woman states:
    1. "I'm unhappy and I guess I'm being punished."
    2. "No, you must have brought me the wrong baby."
    3. "What will my parents say? What could have happened?"
    4. "I shouldn't have had this baby. Now my boyfriend will never marry me."

201. When making rounds during the night, the nurse enters the room of a client who delivered a stillborn baby during the evening and finds her crying. It would be most appropriate for the nurse to:
    1. Pull the curtain to provide privacy for the client
    2. Sit down and stay with the client, allowing her to cry
    3. Explain to the client that her feelings are normal and will pass with time
    4. Document on the chart that the client is having difficulty accepting the loss of her baby

202. A client is admitted to the psychiatric hospital under a voluntary admission status. Under this type of admission, the client:
    1. Loses civil rights for the entire hospital stay
    2. Can expect that few restrictive alternatives will apply
    3. Cannot refuse to take psychotropic drugs as prescribed by the psychiatrist
    4. Can be discharged when the maximum insurance benefits available have been used

203. A client, recently admitted for chronic abuse of drugs and alcohol, appears to have extreme difficulty participating in an art-therapy group project. The priority assessment the nurse needs to make after the group therapy is to determine if the client is experiencing a period of:
    1. Crisis
    2. Disorientation
    3. Confabulation
    4. Hallucinations

Emotional Problems Related to Physical Health and Childbearing

204. The night before surgery a client is unable to sleep despite adequate sedation. The client asks the nurse to sit for a while. Based on an understanding of the client's behavior, the nurse's response should be to:
    1. Send in a nurse's aide to provide company
    2. Stay a minute and return later in the morning
    3. Explain that nurses cannot socialize in clients' rooms
    4. Indicate that the client's inability to sleep has been noticed

Client Case Scenario 21: Milly Schwarz, age 36, is a new mother of a child with a genetic disorder that will probably significantly shorten the child's life span. **Items 205 to 208 refer to this client case scenario.**

205. When Milly first sees the baby she becomes very disturbed, pushes him away and states, "Oh take him away: I never want to see him again." In planning care, the nurse should understand which of the following about this reaction.
    1. The mother is rejecting the baby.
    2. This is a normal response to a crisis situation
    3. The mother is unable to cope with the situation
    4. She is emotionally disturbed and in need of psychiatric help.

206. Which factor about Milly's family would be most significant to the nurse in planning care?
    1. Ability to give physical care to their infant
    2. Response to family's and friends' reactions to their infant
    3. Understanding of the factors causing the genetic disorder
    4. Ability to talk about problems their infant may have in the future

207. When the nurse arrives at the client's home, Milly appears tired and is crying. Which question should the nurse ask?
    1. "Is everything all right? You look tired."
    2. "Tell me a little about your daily routine."
    3. "When did the baby have the last bottle?"
    4. "Oh, it looks like you two are having a bad day."

208. Milly cries, "What did we do to deserve this?" What would be the nurse's most therapeutic response?
    1. "Let's sit down and have a cup of coffee."
    2. "Why do you feel you are being punished?"
    3. "I know you must be upset, but it's too early to tell."
    4. "You didn't do anything; let me tell you about this disorder."

209. The parents of a child who had open-heart surgery are informed that their child is in the recovery room and is stable. The mother is crying and extremely worried. The nurse can best help allay the mother's anxiety by:
    1. Reassuring her that their child is doing well
    2. Allowing her to continue to express her feelings
    3. Bringing her and her husband to the recovery room for several minutes
    4. Encouraging them both to go have a cup of coffee and return in 2 hours

210. A female client who has had multiple hospital admissions for recurring congestive heart failure is returned to the hospital by her daughter. The client is admitted to the coronary care unit for observation. She states, "I know I'm sick, but I could really take care of myself at home." The nurse recognizes that the client is attempting to:
    1. Deny her illness
    2. Suppress her fears
    3. Reassure her daughter
    4. Maintain her independence

211. During her twelfth week of pregnancy, a client with a history of frequent spontaneous abortions says to the nurse, "Every day I wonder if I'll ever have this baby." The nurse's best response would be:
    1. "I can understand why you're worried. You will have other chances in the future."
    2. "You have the best doctors. What was the problem with your previous pregnancy?"
    3. "It's understandable for you to feel concerned that you may not carry this pregnancy to term."
    4. "Just do exactly what the doctors tell you to do. I can understand why you're worried, though."

212. A client with a chronic illness, who had been incontinent of urine at home, has not been incontinent since being hospitalized. When discussing past and present elimination patterns, the client also tells the nurse about being angry at being bedridden and unable to go anywhere or see anyone. The nurse deduces that the client's incontinence at home may have been related to:
    1. A way of maintaining control
    2. An unconscious expression of hostility
    3. A method to determine the family's love
    4. A physiologic response expected with the elderly

Drug-Related Responses

213. The aspect of electroconvulsive therapy that can result in the most serious complication is the use of:
    1. Positive pressure to inflate the alveoli
    2. Electric voltage to induce the seizures
    3. Succinylcholine chloride (Anectine) to relax muscles
    4. Methohexital sodium (Brevital sodium) to induce sleep

214. The physician has ordered imipramine (Tofranil), 75 mg tid, for a client. An appropriate nursing action in giving this drug is to:
    1. Avoid administration of barbiturates or steroids with this drug
    2. Warn the client not to eat cheese, fermenting products, and chicken liver
    3. Observe the client for increased tolerance so that the therapeutic dosage is maintained
    4. Have the client checked for intraocular pressure and provide instructions to watch for symptoms of glaucoma

215. An agitated, acting-out, delusional client is receiving large doses of haloperidol (Haldol) and the nurse is concerned, because this drug can produce untoward side effects. The nurse should be aware that the drug will be immediately stopped if the client exhibits:
    1. Jaundice
    2. Dizziness
    3. Sleepiness
    4. Extrapyramidal symptoms

216. Lithium carbonate is the drug of choice for:
    1. Acute agitation of schizophrenia
    2. Agitated phase of paranoid states
    3. Control of manic episodes of bipolar disorders
    4. Modification of the depressive phase of major depressions

217. A client is receiving lithium carbonate. While this medication is being administered, it is important that the nurse:
    1. Test the client's urine weekly
    2. Restrict the client's sodium intake
    3. Monitor the client's blood level regularly
    4. Withhold the client's other medications for 1 week

Client Case Scenario 22: Farrel Seaburg, a 52-year-old schizophrenic, is about to be discharged to a half-way house. After discharge he forgets to take his medication, and must be hospitalized again. **Items 218 to 221 refer to this client case scenario.**

218. Which medication could be given IM to Farrel every two weeks, on an outpatient basis?
    1. Trifluoperazine (Stelazine)
    2. Chlorpromazine (Largactil)
    3. Lithium carbonate (Lithazine)
    4. Prolixin deconate (Modecate)

219. Neuroleptics are the drugs of choice for Farrel because they relieve which of the following symptoms?
    1. Psychosis
    2. Depression
    3. Hyperkinesis
    4. Narcotic withdrawal

220. Which irreversible side effect of neuroleptic drugs should the nurse observe Farrel for?
    1. Torticollis
    2. Oculogyric crisis
    3. Tardive dyskinesia
    4. Pseudoparkinsonism

221. The nurse notes that Farrel sits rigidly in a chair. What other adverse effects of neuroleptics should the nurse observe him closely for?
    1. Inability to concentrate, excess salivation
    2. Uncoordinated movement of extremities, tremors
    3. Reluctance to converse, nonverbal clues indicating fear
    4. Minimal use of nonverbal expression, rambling speech

222. A common manageable side effect of neuroleptics is:
    1. Ptosis
    2. Jaundice
    3. Melanocytosis
    4. Unintentional tremors

223. A drug such as trihexyphenidyl (Artane), biperiden (Akineton), or benztropine (Cogentin) is often prescribed in conjunction with:
    1. Barbiturates
    2. Antidepressants
    3. Antipsychotic agents/neuroleptics
    4. Antianxiety agents/anxiolytics

224. Many psychiatric clients are given the drugs Cogentin or Artane in conjunction with the phenothiazine derivatives to:
    1. Reduce postural hypotension
    2. Potentiate the effect of the drug
    3. Combat extrapyramidal side effects
    4. Modify depression that often accompanies schizophrenia

Client Case Scenario 23: Theresa Donovan, age 29, has been receiving tranclypromine sulfate (Parnate) 10 mg PO bid, for the past five days, for treatment of a major depressive episode. **Items 225 to 227 refer to this client case scenario.**

225. Theresa states, "It doesn't help so what's the use of taking it." Which response by the nurse would best demonstrate an understanding of the action of this medication?
    1. Sometimes it takes 2 to 3 weeks to see an improvement."
    2. "It takes 6 to 8 weeks for this medication to have an effect."
    3. "You should have felt a response by now. I'll notify your physician."
    4. "I'll talk to the physician about increasing the dosage, and that will help."

226. Which aspect, about monamine oxidase inhibitors, should be included in teaching Theresa about the effects of this medication?
    1. Drowsiness is an expected side effect of this medication
    2. It is necessary for these clients to wear a hat outdoors and avoid the sun
    3. Clients taking this type of medication have special dietary restrictions
    4. The therapeutic level and the toxic level of these drugs are very close

227. If Theresa does not abide by her diet restrictions while taking tranclypromine sulfate, which condition will she likely develop?
    1. Generalized urticaria
    2. An occipital headache
    3. Severe muscle spasms
    4. Sudden, severe hypotension

228. When pouring liquid chlorpromazine hydrochloride (Thorazine), the nurse should:
    1. Avoid contact with skin
    2. Mix it with fruit juice immediately
    3. Administer immediately after pouring
    4. Keep it away from the face to prevent inhalation

229. Photosensitization is a side effect associated with the use of:
    1. Lithium carbonate (Lithane)
    2. Thioridazine hydrochloride (Mellaril)
    3. Methylphenidate hydrochloride (Ritalin)
    4. Chlorpromazine hydrochloride (Thorazine)

230. After 2 weeks of drug therapy, the nurse notices that the client has become jaundiced. The nurse continues to give the neuroleptic until the psychiatrist can be consulted. In situations such as this:
    1. Jaundice is a benign side effect and has little significance
    2. Jaundice is sufficient reason to discontinue the neuroleptics
    3. The blood level of neuroleptics must be maintained once established
    4. The psychiatrist's order for neuroleptics should be reduced by the nurse

231. A client receiving high-dosage chlorpromazine hydrochloride (Thorazine) has developed tremors of the hands. The nurse should:
    1. Withhold the medication
    2. Tell the client it is transitory
    3. Report the symptoms to the physician
    4. Give the client finger exercises to perform

232. When assessing a female client for adverse effects of chlorpromazine hydrochloride (Thorazine), the nurse would also:
    1. Assess her appetite and weigh her weekly
    2. Take her blood pressure and ask if she has frequent headaches
    3. Examine her sclera and question her about the color of her stools
    4. Examine her skin and ask if she has numbness or coldness of her feet

233. When monoamine oxidase inhibitors (MAOIs) are prescribed, the client should be cautioned against:
    1. Prolonged exposure to the sun
    2. Ingesting wines and aged cheeses
    3. Engaging in active physical exercise
    4. The use of medications with an elixir base

234. A standard regimen for withdrawal from secobarbital sodium (Seconal sodium) would be the administration of gradually decreasing amounts of:
    1. Lithium carbonate
    2. Phenobarbital sodium
    3. Methadone hydrochloride
    4. Chlorpromazine hydrochloride

235. Abrupt withdrawal from barbiturate use could cause a person to experience:
    1. Ataxia
    2. Urticaria
    3. Diarrhea
    4. Seizures

236. The medication used to combat an overdose of narcotics is:
    1. Dextroamphetamine (Dexedrine)
    2. Naloxone hydrochloride (Narcan)
    3. Amphetamine sulfate (Benzedrine)
    4. Caffeine sodium benzoate (Caffedrine)

237. When administered for a heroin overdose, the planned effect of naloxone hydrochloride (Narcan) is to:
    1. Compete with narcotics for receptors controlling respiration
    2. Decrease analgesia and the comatose state induced by heroin
    3. Accelerate metabolism of heroin and stimulate respiratory centers
    4. Stimulate cortical sites controlling consciousness and cardiovascular function

238. Within an hour of receiving naloxone hydrochloride (Narcan) to combat an overdose of heroin, a client is responding. Close observation of the client's status is still indicated because:
    1. The drug may cause neuropathy and seizures
    2. The combined action of the drug and heroin causes cardiac depression
    3. The narcotic effect may cause return of symptoms after the drug is metabolized
    4. Hyperexcitability and amnesia may cause the client to thrash about and become abusive

Therapeutic Relationships

239. The statement that would best describe the practice of psychiatric nursing would be:
    1. Helping people with present or potential mental health problems
    2. Assuring clients' legal and ethical rights by acting as a client advocate
    3. Focusing interpersonal skills on people with physical or emotional problems
    4. Acting in a therapeutic way with people diagnosed as having a mental disorder

240. Mentally healthy individuals can be defined as those who:
    1. Have insight into their own problems
    2. Are able to meet their own basic needs
    3. Are not exhibiting pathological symptoms
    4. Are free from both physical and emotional problems

241. Since people need some gratifying communication to learn, to grow, and to function in a group, all events that significantly curtail communication will eventually produce:
    1. Withdrawal
    2. Severe disturbances
    3. Some degree of mental deficiency
    4. Further attempts to increase communication

242. Group therapy can best help those who:
    1. Are emotionally ill
    2. Are dependent on others
    3. Feel they have a problem
    4. Have no one to listen to them

Client Case Scenario 24: Alice Hollins, age 49, is admitted for surgery. Although not physically distressed she appears apprehensive and alienated. **Items 243 to 246 refer to this client case scenario.**

243. In working with Alice, which action is the most difficult part of the nurse-client relationship?
    1. Remaining therapeutic and professional at all times
    2. Being able to understand and accept the client's behavior
    3. Developing an awareness of self and the professional role in the relationship
    4. Accepting responsibility in identifying and evaluating the real needs of the client

244. To foster sound interpersonal relationships with Alice during an initial meeting, which role should the nurse assume?
    1. Teacher
    2. Stranger
    3. Surrogate
    4. Counselor

245. Which nursing action may help Alice feel more at ease?
    1. Telling her everything is all right
    2. Giving her a copy of hospital regulations
    3. Orienting her to the environment and unit personnel
    4. Reassuring her that staff will be available if she becomes upset

246. During a one-to-one interaction with the nurse Alice states "I'm worried about going home." The nurse responds, "Tell me more about this." Which communication technique is this an example of?
    1. Focusing
    2. Clarifying
    3. Reflecting
    4. Refocusing

247. The group setting is especially conducive to therapy, since it:
    1. Fosters one-to-one relationships
    2. Creates a new learning environment
    3. Decreases the focus on the individual
    4. Confronts individual members with their shortcomings

248. When providing group therapy, the nurse must focus on:
    1. Jointly experienced stress
    2. Behavior of individual members
    3. Confrontation between members
    4. Personal feelings affecting behavior

249. Self-help groups such as AA or NA assist their members to:
    1. Set long-term goals
    2. Identify with their peers
    3. Identify the underlying cause of their behavior
    4. Deal with present behavior and changes in behavior

250. Self-help groups such as Alcoholics Anonymous are successful because they meet the client's need to:
    1. Grow
    2. Belong
    3. Be trusted
    4. Be independent

251. Self-help groups such as Alcoholics Anonymous help members to learn that:
    1. They do not need a crutch
    2. Their problems are not unique
    3. They can stand stronger together
    4. Their problems are caused by alcohol

252. The nurse sits with an elderly, depressed client twice a day, although there is little verbal communication. One afternoon, the client asks, "Do you think they'll ever let me out of here?" The nurse's best reply would be:
    1 "Why don't you ask your doctor?"
    2 "Everyone says you're doing just fine."

3. "Why, do you think you are ready to leave?"
4. "You have the feeling that you might not leave?"

Client Case Scenario 25: Jason Mulkiewich, age 48, a depressed client who is improving, is asked to join a small discussion group that meets every evening on the unit. **Items 253 to 255 refer to this client case scenario.**

253. Jason is reluctant to join. He says, "I have nothing to talk about." Which would be the nurse's best response?
    1. "Maybe tomorrow you will feel more like talking."
    2. "Could you start off by talking about your family?"
    3. "A person like you has a great deal to offer the group."
    4. "You feel you will not be accepted by the group unless you have something to say?"

254. Jason tells the group about his fear of his impending discharge from the hospital. Which would be the leader's most appropriate response?
    1. "You ought to be happy that you're leaving."
    2. "Maybe you're not ready to be discharged yet."
    3. "Maybe others in the group have similar feelings that they would share."
    4. "How many in the group feel that this member is ready to be discharged?"

255. Jason asks the nurse what "mental health" is. Which of the following is the nurse's most appropriate response?
    1 What do you think mental health is?
    2 What does the group think mental health is?
    3. Are you concerned about your own mental health?
    4. Could someone please tell Jason what mental health is?

256. The referral of discharged psychiatric clients to a psychiatric day-care facility in their own community is done primarily to assist them to:
    1. Increase social skills and awareness
    2. Get out of the house for a few hours daily
    3. Maintain goals attained during hospitalization
    4. Avoid direct confrontation with the community

257. A nurse is assigned to introduce a client who has a PhD in psychology to the other clients on the unit. The client tells the nurse, "I wish to be called Doctor." The nurse could best respond:

1. "Why do you insist on being called Doctor?"
2. "That's fine; that is how I will introduce you then."
3. "All the clients here call one another by their first names."
4. "I can't do that. It's better if the other clients do not know you are a doctor."

258. A nurse is assigned to care for a regressed 19-year-old college student newly admitted to the psychiatric unit with a 1-month history of talking to unseen people and refusing to get out of bed, go to class, or get involved in daily grooming activities. The nurse's initial efforts should be directed toward helping the client by:
    1. Providing frequent rest periods to avoid exhaustion
    2. Facilitating the client's social relationships with a peer group
    3. Reducing environmental stimuli and maintaining dietary intake
    4. Attempting to establish a meaningful relationship with the client

259. A client with a diagnosis of major depression refuses to participate in unit activities because of being "just too tired." The nursing approach that best expresses an understanding of this client's needs would be:
    1. Planning a rest period for the client during activity time
    2. Explaining why the staff believes the activities are therapeutic
    3. Helping the client express feelings of hostility toward the activities
    4. Accepting the client's behavior calmly and, without excessive comment, setting firm limits

Client Case Scenario 26: During a group session it is learned that a female member masked her depression and suicidal urges and committed suicide several days ago. **Items 260 to 262 refer to this client case scenario.**

260. What should the leaders be prepared to primarily deal with?
    1. The guilt that the group feels because they could not prevent another's suicide
    2. The lack of concern over the member's suicide expressed by some of the group
    3. The guilt, fear, and anger of the co-leaders that they failed to anticipate and prevent the suicide
    4. The fear and anxiety that some members of the group may have that their own suicidal urges may go unnoticed and unprotected

261. One client says, "I'm next. Oh, my God I'm next. They couldn't prevent hers and they can't protect me." What would be the nurse's most therapeutic response?
    1. "You are afraid you will hurt yourself?"
    2. "The other client was a lot sicker than you are."
    3. "It's different. The other client was home; you are here."
    4. "There is no need to worry. All passes will be canceled for a while."

262. One group member stands up and shouts, "Oh I know what you are thinking; you think that I should have known that she was going to kill herself. You think that I helped her plan this." Which would be the leader's best response?
    1. "It will help if you tell us the truth."
    2. "Oh, no. We all know you liked her."
    3. "You feel we're blaming you for her death?"
    4. "Helping another person to plan a suicide would not be healthy."

263. A female client on the psychiatric unit remains aloof from all other clients. The nurse with whom she has developed a friendly relationship may help her participate in some ward activity by:
    1. Finding solitary pursuits that the client can enjoy
    2. Speaking to the client about the importance of entering into activities
    3. Asking the physician to speak to the client about participating in activities
    4. Inviting another client to take part in a joint activity with the nurse and the client

264. The nurse can best reassure an elderly, depressed client who is concerned about many fears that are upsetting and frightening and expresses a feeling of having committed the "unpardonable sin" by stating:
    1. "Your family loves you very much."
    2. "You know that you are not a bad person."
    3. "You know, those ideas of yours are in your imagination."
    4. "Your ideas are part of your illness and they will change as you improve."

265. A 45-year-old physician is admitted to the psychiatric unit of a community hospital. The client is restless, loud, aggressive, and resistive during the admission procedure and states, "I will take my own blood pressure." The most therapeutic response by the nurse would be:
    1. "Right now, doctor, you are just another client."
    2. "I am sorry but I can not allow that. I must take it."
    3. "If you would rather, doctor. I'm sure you will do it OK."
    4 "If you do not cooperate, I will get the attendants to hold you down."

266. A client attending a mental health day-care unit is scheduled for several diagnostic studies. The client behavior that would be the best indicator that the client had received adequate preparation for these studies would be that the client:
    1. Requests that the tests be reexplained
    2. Repeatedly checks the appointment card
    3. Paces the hallway the morning before the tests
    4. Arrives early and waits quietly to be called for the tests

267. The most advantageous therapy for a preschool-age child with a history of physical and sexual abuse would be:
    1. Play therapy
    2. Psychodrama
    3. Group therapy
    4. Family therapy

PSYCHIATRIC / MENTAL HEALTH NURSING
ANSWERS AND RATIONALES

Personality Development

1. **2 Any behavioral therapy or learning of new methods of dealing with situations requires modifications of approach and attitudes; hence personality is always capable of change. (AN; ED; PD)**
   1 Certain personality traits are established by age 2, but not the total personality.
   3 The capacity for change exists throughout the life cycle.
   4 Accepting this theory would close the door on all future growth and development.

2. **3 Before this age the infant has not developed enough ego strength to have an identity or personality. (AN; ED; PD)**
   1 This is too early; the child has not developed enough ego strength to have a personality.
   2 Self-concept is nonexistent.
   4 The primary emergence of the personality has already occurred.

3. **3 The parameters set by birth, psychologic experiences, and the environment make each individual unique. Although other factors may impinge to a slight degree, these factors form the personality. (AN; PS; PD)**
   1 These are not inclusive; they are limited to only some aspects of personality development; race plays no part.
   2 Autoimmunity plays no part in personality development.
   4 These are not inclusive; they are limited to only some aspects of personality development.

4. **3 Children view their own worth by the response received from their parents. This sense of worth sets the basic ego strengths and is vital to the formation of the personality. (AN; ED; PD)**
   1 Peer groups come later in a child's development, but the parent-child relationship is still the most important.
   2 Although important, it is not as important as the parent-child relationship.
   4 This comes later in life, after the basic personality has been formed.

5. **4 A sense of one's self and a feeling of belonging form the basis for mental health, because they provide comfort with self and group. (AN; PS; PD)**
   1 A person could have emotional balance without all three.
   2 A person needs security but can do without social recognition.
   3 A person needs to have biologic needs met; one does not need social acceptance; the group providing acceptance may not be acceptable to society or to the individual.

6. **1 Socialization occurs through communication with others. Without some form of communication there can be no socialization. (AN; PS; PD)**
   2 People interact with other social beings, not with inanimate objects.
   3 Same as answer 2.
   4 Same as answer 2.

7. **3 Socialization, values, and role definition are learned within the family and help develop a sense of self. Once established in the family, the child can more easily move into society. (AN; ED; PD)**
   1 This is true, but not as important as identity and roles in relation to emotional development.
   2 This is only a very small aspect of the family's influence.
   4 Same as answer 2.

8. **4 Learning from others occurs in a group setting and is reinforced by group acceptance of the norms. Group pressure is peer pressure, which is more easily accepted if the individual wants to stay in the group. (AN; ED; PD)**
   1 One member of a group can be the target of hostility.
   2 This is not necessarily so; the group may not be easily identified by its members.
   3 Groups do not go through the same developmental phases as individuals.

9. **2 The toddler learns to say "no" and to express independence, yet because of human nature the child is both physically and emotionally dependent on the parents. (AN; ED; PD)**

1 The major task during infancy is development of trust.

3 This stage deals with developing a sense of initiative.

4 This stage deals with the task of industry and developing skills for working in and relating to the world.

10. **1 The sense of ego integrity comes from satisfaction with life and acceptance of what has been and what is. Despair is due to guilt or remorse over what might have been. (DC; PS; PD)**

2 During puberty adolescents attempt to find themselves and integrate values with those of society; an inability to solve conflict results in confusion and hinders mastery of future roles.

3 During early and middle adulthood the individual is concerned with the ability to produce and to care for that which is produced or created; failure during this stage leads to self-absorption or stagnation.

4 Autonomy is developed during the toddler period and corresponds to the child's ability to control the body and environment; doubt can result when made to feel ashamed or embarrassed.

11. **4 A consistent approach and consistent communication from all members of the health team help the client who has dementia remain a bit more reality oriented. (PL; PS; DD)**

1 It is the staff members who need to be consistent.

2 Clients who have this disorder do not attempt to manipulate the staff.

3 This is not needed in working with clients who have this disorder; consistency is most important.

12. **4 The client who has delirium, dementia, or another cognitive disorder will be most comfortable with the familiar and repetitive daily routine because it creates less anxiety. (PL; TC; DD)**

1 It would be beyond the client's capabilities to develop new social skills.

2 The memory impairment might make this impossible.

3 Cognitive changes would make this unrealistic.

13. **4 Testing the self both physically and psychologically occurs during the toddler stage after trust has been achieved. (AN; ED; PD)**

1 Trust is the task of infancy.

2 This task is accomplished between the ages of 6 and 12.

3 Between the ages of 3 and 6, a child starts to identify with the parent of the same sex.

14. **3 Freud's theory is that a child develops a sexualized love for the parent of the opposite sex and becomes jealous of the parent of the same sex. These thoughts result in feelings of guilt, anxiety, fear, and hate toward the parent of the same sex, which are repressed. (AN; ED; PD)**

1 Ambivalence does not occur in the oedipal stage of development.

2 The child loves the parent of the opposite sex and hates the parent of the same sex.

4 Same as answer 2.

15. **3 The child resolves oedipal conflicts by learning to identify with the parent of the same sex and accomplishes this by mimicking the role of this parent. (AN; ED; PD)**

1 This is the earliest stage of development and operates solely on the pleasure principle, largely id oriented; this stage is concerned with development of trust.

2 There is an interest shift from the anal region to the genital region, and questions about sexuality arise.

4 There is increasing sex-role development; this stage is concerned with peer-group identification.

16. **2 Values and beliefs from parents and society are expressed through the child's play world. These values become part of the child's system through the process of internalization (introjection). (AN; ED; PD)**

1 If this happened, children would learn to blame others for their own faults.

3 This would occur at a later age.

4 The environment and others in it, rather than play, influence independence.

17. **3 The child realizes that the parent of the same sex cannot be bested in a struggle for the affection of the parent of the opposite sex. The role and behavior of the same-sex parent are therefore assumed**

by the child to attract the parent of the opposite sex. (AN; ED; PD)

1 This would be a conflict, not a resolution.

2 Doing this would give rise to greater conflict and leave a fragmented self.

4 This would be in conflict with heterosexual drives.

18. **3 During the oedipal stage (between 2½ and 6 years of age) children have many fears about their bodies. Any invasive techniques done at this time can create severe emotional problems. (AN; PS; PD)**

1 If a sense of trust has been established and a caring person is allowed to spend time with the child, no damage should occur.

2 There will probably be some regression in motor skills, but the outcome is favorable upon return home.

4 The child is older and better able to deal with the surgery.

19. **3 Having poor superego control, these individuals cannot set limits for themselves and require an environment in which appropriate limits for behavior are set for them. (PL; TC; DD)**

1 This would be too stimulating for a person with socially aggressive behavior.

2 An environment that can be manipulated teaches the client nothing; it encourages a continuation of maladjustive behavior.

4 This person has too much freedom of expression and is unable to control impulses.

20. **2 The client with a delirium, dementia, or other cognitive disorder rarely expresses any concern about personal appearance. The staff must meet most of the client's needs in this area. (DC; PS; DD)**

1 Resistance to change is a symptom of this disorder.

3 The past is where these clients feel more comfortable rather than the threatening present.

4 A short attention span and little or no interest in new activities is typical of dementia.

21. **2 Clients with this disorder need a simple environment. Because of brain-cell destruction, they are unable to make choices. (PL; TC; DD)**

1 A well-balanced diet is important throughout life, not just during senescence; a diet high in carbohydrates and protein may be lacking other nutrients such as fats.

3 The client is incapable of making choices; providing many alternative choices will only increase anxiety.

4 Physical and emotional needs must be met on a continuous basis, not just at a fixed time.

22. **2 Slips of the tongue, also called "Freudian slips," are material from the unconscious that slips out in unguarded moments. (AN; ED; PD)**

1 Material in the unconscious cannot deliberately be brought back to awareness.

3 There is no evidence linking these experiences to the unconscious.

4 Free-floating anxiety is linked to the unconscious, but the best evidence of the unconscious is slips of the tongue.

23. **1 Mild anxiety motivates one to action, such as learning or emotional changes. Higher levels of anxiety tend to blur the individual's perceptions and interfere with functioning. (AN; PS; PD)**

2 Attention is severely reduced by panic.

3 The perceptual field is greatly reduced with severe anxiety.

4 The perceptual field is narrowed with moderate anxiety.

24. **1 An illusion is a misperception or misinterpretation of actual external stimuli. (DC; PS; PD)**

2 This is a false belief that cannot be changed even by evidence; it is a fixed false belief.

3 This would deal with imaginary, not real, stimuli.

4 A belief that others are talking about the person is not a visual distortion, but rather an idea of reference.

25. **4 The individual using sublimation attempts to fulfill desires by selecting a socially acceptable activity rather than one which is socially unacceptable (e.g., pursuing a career in nursing as a means of giving and receiving love). (AN; PS; PD)**

1 This would be an example of reaction formation.

2 This would be regression, not sublimation.

3 This would be an example of repression.

26. **4 When acting out against the primary source of anxiety creates even further anxiety or danger, the individual may use displacement to express feelings on a safer person or object. (AN; PS; PD)**
   1 This would be fantasy.
   2 This is an example of denial.
   3 This shows an inability to mature and accept responsibility.

27. **4 When the individual experiences a threat to self-esteem, anxiety increases and the normal defense mechanisms are used to protect the self. (AN; ED; PD)**
   1 Affective reactions are mood disorders.
   2 Ritualistic behaviors are not a normal aspect of the developmental process.
   3 Withdrawal patterns are an abnormal way of coping with stress; if carried to an extreme, behavior can become pathologic.

28. **3 By developing skills in one area the individual compensates or makes up for a real or imagined deficiency, thereby maintaining a positive self-image. (AN; PS; PD)**
   1 If the student incorporated the qualities of the college athlete, that would be introjection.
   2 This would deal more with unacceptable impulses that would pose a threat.
   4 This person is not trying to make amends for unacceptable feelings (reaction formation) but rather for a felt deficiency and a poor self-image.

29. **2 The unconscious stores past experiences and the emotional feelings associated with them. These emotional feelings influence one's perceptions, attitudes, and behavior. (AN; PS; PD)**
   1 Material in the conscious is in a state of immediate awareness.
   3 Material in the preconscious, which includes ideas and feelings, when attended to, can be made conscious.
   4 There is no such thing as the foreconscious level.

30. **2 Mediating frustration within the real world is an ego function and requires ego strengths. (AN; ED; PD)**
   1 The id is unable to tolerate frustration because it is totally involved with gratification.
   3 The superego is involved with putting pressure on the ego because the id does not tolerate frustration.

4 The unconscious does not deal with frustration.

31. **4 The superego incorporates all experiences and learning from external environments (society, family, etc.) into the internal environment. (AN; ED; PD)**
   1 This is the function of the id.
   2 The id with its drives is a source of creative energy.
   3 Same as answer 1.

32. **4 Incorporation of parental and societal values into the superego leads to the development of a sense of right and wrong. Guilt and shame are experienced when these values are broken. Thus the superego is the conscience. (AN; PS; PD)**
   1 The self is the total of the id, ego, and superego.
   2 The ideal self is how a person perceives the self to be or strives to be.
   3 Narcissism involves an excessive love of self with strong dependency needs that are impossible for others to meet.

33. **3 Conscience and a sense of right and wrong are expressed in the superego, which acts to counterbalance the id's desire for immediate gratification. (AN; ED; PD)**
   1 This does not reflect any part of the self.
   2 This is the id seeking satisfaction.
   4 A healthy ego can delay gratification and is in balance with reality.

34. **2 The therapeutic milieu is directed toward helping the client develop effective ways of dealing with interpersonal situations. (AN; TC; DD)**
   1 This would be a means of achieving the goal.
   3 The hospital atmosphere should be more structured and accepting than the client's home.
   4 This would accomplish nothing in regard to a long-term goal of functioning in society.

35. **2 Damaged brain cells do not regenerate. Care is therefore directed toward preventing further damage and providing protective and supportive care. (PL; TC; DD)**
   1 The deterioration of the brain cells makes an extensive reeducation program unrealistic.
   3 A client with this disorder may not be able to grasp, understand, or enjoy new leisure activities.

4 It is beyond the scope of the client's ability to function in a group therapy session.

36. **3 The nurse should first protect herself. The client might strike her in this instance. (IM; TC; DD)**
   1 This will sound judgmental and may upset him more.
   2 Touching him will increase his agitation and aggression.
   4 Same as answer 2.

37. **4 The mature personality does not respond to the immediate gratification demands of the id or the oppressive control of the superego because the ego is strong enough to maintain a balance between them. (AN; ED; PD)**
   1 There would be no healthy resolution of conflicts if the superego were always in control.
   2 With society in control there would be chaos, rather than maturity.
   3 This would create a rigid personality that makes impossible demands on the self.

Disorders First Evident Before Adulthood

38. **1 The longer these children stay out, the more difficult it is to get them to return to school, because more fantasies and fears develop. (AN; TC; BA)**
   2 The use of this approach rarely accomplishes anything.
   3 This will feed into the fear that the phobia is realistic.
   4 This would increase, not decrease, the fear.

39. **1 School phobia is a symptom that cannot legally be ignored for long because children must attend school. It requires intervention to alleviate the separation anxiety and/or to promote the child's increasing independence. (IM; PS; BA)**
   2 This symptom requires the parents to comfort, to reorient to reality, and to help the child regain self-control. Legally there are no requirements mandating treatment for this common childhood problem.
   3 Same as answer 2.
   4 Same as answer 2.

40. **1 Sitting quietly with the client gives the message that the nurse cares and accepts the client's feelings. (IM; PS; BA)**

2 Helping the client explore reasons is more therapeutic than giving advice.
3 This is negating feelings and the client's right to cry when upset.
4 This in effect closes the door on any further communication of feelings.

41. **3 If seizures were physiologically based, the client would not be able to continue to chew gum. This "attack" should be reported as a behavioral response, with the precipitating factors noted. (IM; TC; BA)**
   1 The chewing gum is not a danger when the client is not having a true seizure.
   2 This would probably not be necessary now.
   4 This is unsafe; it is not even used in a true seizure.

42. **1 The infant and toddler are dependent on significant others and react strongly to separation and loss, which they view as rejection and abandonment. These needs are strongest during the "taking in" or oral phase of development. (AN; PS; BA)**
   2 The child begins to exert control over the environment rather than be concerned with separation.
   3 Sexual drives for the opposite sex are dealt with and repressed; the child has already developed a sense of autonomy and is no longer as concerned with separation.
   4 The child between the ages of 6 and 12 learns a sense of self-worth through dealings with others in the environment; this age is concerned with tasks of industry such as developing skills and relating to the world; separation is not the major concern.

43. **1 Rivalry between siblings is normal and arises because one child resents the care and attention given another child. One child unconsciously wishes the other would disappear and frequently acts out negatively against the sibling. (AN; ED; BA)**
   2 This would deal more with thoughts and desires.
   3 These conflicts are directed not toward siblings but toward parents.
   4 The superego would be involved more with making amends.

44. **3 Poor interpersonal relationships, inappropriate behavior, and learning disabilities prevent these children from emotionally adapting or responding to the environment despite a possible high level of intelligence. (DC; PS; BA)**
   1 It is the lack of response to stimuli that is the clue to a child's being emotionally disturbed.
   2 This is true but not most characteristic.
   4 The exact opposite is true.

45. **1 By 2 years of age the child should demonstrate an interest in others, communicate verbally, and possess the ability to learn from the environment. Before these skills develop, autism is difficult to diagnose. (DC; KN; MH; PS; BA)**
   2 Autism can be diagnosed long before this age.
   3 Infantile autism can occur at this age but is difficult to diagnose.
   4 Same as answer 3.

46. **1 From infancy the child is nonresponsive. Not wanting to eat demonstrates a further withdrawal. (DC; TC; BA)**
   2 This is not indicative of an autistic child.
   3 This would not be characteristic of autism.
   4 Children would not be diagnosed as autistic if they enjoyed being with people.

47. **4 Autistic behavior turns inward. These children do not respond to the environment but attempt to maintain emotional equilibrium by rubbing and manipulating themselves and displaying a compulsive need for behavioral repetition. (PL; PS; BA)**
   1 Large group (or small group) activity would have little effect on the autistic child's response.
   2 These children do seem to respond to music, but not necessarily loud, cheerful music.
   3 Part of the autistic pattern is the inability to interact with others in the environment.

48. **3 This is the drug of choice in this diagnosis. It appears to act by stimulating release of norepinephrine from nerve endings in the brainstem. (AN; TC; BA)**
   1 Haldol is an antipsychotic medication.
   2 This is a muscle relaxant.
   4 Thorazine is a neuroleptic medication.

Delirium, Dementia, and Other Cognitive Disorders

49. **3 The current trend in psychiatry is to treat the clients while maintaining them in the community. This trend includes the family and community in the plan and has reduced the number of clients in institutions. (AN; PS; DD)**
   1 This might be part of the overall treatment plan but not the only aspect.
   2 This possibly would have the effect of masking the symptoms and should be used only in conjunction with psychotherapy.
   4 This would be unrealistic for most of these clients.

50. **3 Clients who are out of control are seeking control and frequently respond to simple directions stated in a firm voice. (IM; TC; DD)**
   1 "Be quiet" is an order that is nontherapeutic and is, furthermore, demeaning behavior on the part of the nurse.
   2 This would not be helping the client gain control of actions and might be frightening to other clients in the day room.
   4 This would be done only after an attempt at calming the client down had failed.

51. **4 When an elderly person's brain atrophies, some unusual deposits of iron are scattered on nerve cells. Throughout the brain, areas of deeply staining amyloid, called senile plaques, can be found; these plaques are end stages in the destruction of brain tissue. (AN; PS; DD)**
   1 This may or may not be part of the disorder.
   2 It is a chronic deterioration, not one with remissions and exacerbations.
   3 This is typical of vascular dementia, not dementia of the Alzheimer's type.

52. **3 These clients attempt to utilize defense mechanisms that have worked in the past but use them in an exaggerated manner. Because of brain-cell destruction such clients are unable to focus on one defense mechanism or develop new ones. (EV; PS; DD)**
   1 Clients with dementia will depend on old, familiar defense mechanisms.
   2 The client is not capable of focusing on one defense mechanism.
   4 The client is incapable of developing new defense mechanisms at this time.

Substance-Abuse Disorders

53. **4 The drug is not taken for medical reasons but for the favorable, pleasant, unusual, or desired effects it produces. It is often taken in doses that would be fatal if the individual had not established a tolerance to it. (AN; PS; SA)**
    1 This is true but also with psychologic dependence on the drug.
    2 This is true but also with physiologic need for the drug.
    3 It is a physiologic and psychologic need to take the drug rather than a compulsion.

54. **3 The addictive personality is marked by low self-esteem, fear of stress, and dependence with poor self-boundaries and the need for immediate gratification. (DC; PS; SA)**
    1 The client would have a strong id drive; usually the ego is weak.
    2 The client would be operating on the pleasure principle and would be unable to delay gratification.
    4 No evidence to support this.

55. **1 The client is using denial as a defense against feelings of guilt, which will reduce anxiety and protect the self. (AN; PS; SA)**
    2 Denial would deal more with the client's own expectations.
    3 Denial would help make the client seem more stable to others, not independent.
    4 This may be part of the reason, but the bigger motivating factor is to decrease guilt feelings.

56. **2 Alcoholic clients have a low self-image and overwhelming guilt feelings. They drink to relieve these feelings, but the drinking only adds to them. (AN; PS; SA)**
    1 There is no evidence of this.
    3 The problem is with low self-esteem, not dependence/independence.
    4 It is not with whom but with what that these clients have the difficulty.

57. **2 This focuses on the client's feelings rather than the organization itself. The organization is effective only when the client is able to discuss feelings openly. (IM; PS; SA)**
    1 This may or may not be true.
    3 It may be too late by that time.
    4 This is false reassurance; AA may help clients develop insight but may not be able to help them cope with their problems.

58. **1 Polydrug users abuse a variety of drugs in their search for the ultimate "high." They usually will include alcohol in their search and frequently combine their abuses. (AN; PS; SA)**
    2 This is not necessarily true.
    3 This is not necessarily so; some become very happy and outgoing.
    4 This has been mentioned as a possible causative factor but with no evidence to support it.

59. **1 According to the philosophy of Alcoholics Anonymous, clients who have problems with alcohol must identify their own need to seek help and thus become the primary rehabilitators. (AN; PS; SA)**
    2 The nurse can give support but is not the primary rehabilitator.
    3 The physician can give direction but is not the primary rehabilitator.
    4 The entire health team works for the client, but in dealing with alcoholism the client is the primary rehabilitator.

60. **3 Intrinsic motivation, stimulated from within the learner, is essential if rehabilitation is to be successful. Often clients are most emotionally ready for help when they have "hit bottom." Only then are clients motivationally ready to face reality and put forth the necessary energy and effort to change behavior. (AN; PS; SA)**
    1 This is an important factor but not the most important one.
    2 This is an important factor and a helpful one but not the most important one.
    4 Same as answer 1.

61. **3 Members find sympathy, patience, and understanding in the group. They are able to have their dependence needs met while helping others who are even more dependent than they. (AN; PS; SA)**
    1 This is helpful, but it does not have the success rate of AA.
    2 This is important for the detoxification stage, not for overall therapy.
    4 This is not getting at what is causing the alcohol problem.

62. **2 The nurse's failure to observe what was brought in for the client constituted negligence. The nurse's knowledge of the alcoholic individual would warrant checking to see what the client was consuming. (EV; TC; SA)**
   1 This is also true, but the client has no manifestations of a severe mental illness.
   3 This is not true on a substance-abuse unit.
   4 This is true, except the nurse might have believed that the friend herself had a good effect on the client.

63. **3 This addresses the emotional impact of this hallucination. The nurse's presence can reduce anxiety and provide comfort. (IM; TC; SA)**
   1 This is presenting reality but not offering the comfort of the nurse's presence.
   2 This would be entering into the hallucination.
   4 Same as answer 1.

64. **4 The individual is unaware of gaps in memory, so the use of stories is an unconscious attempt to deny or cover up the gaps. (AN; PS; SA)**
   1 Lying is a deliberate attempt to deceive rather than a face-saving device for loss of memory.
   2 Denying is blocking out of conscious awareness rather than a coverup for loss of memory.
   3 Rationalizing would be used to explain and justify the behavior rather than to cover up the loss of memory.

65. **4 Thiamine is a coenzyme in producing energy from glucose. If thiamine is not present in adequate amounts, nerve activity is diminished and damage or degeneration of myelin sheaths occurs. (AN; PA; SA)**
   1 A low-protein, not a high-protein, diet would be desirable.
   2 Use of these has a higher risk of toxic side effects in older or debilitated persons.
   3 Thorazine is a neuroleptic, which would not be used because it is severely toxic to the liver.

66. **2 Methadone can be legally dispensed; the strength of this drug is controlled and remains constant from dose to dose, which is uncertain in illicit drugs. (AN; TC; SA)**
   1 Methadone is used in the medically supervised withdrawal period to treat physical dependence on opiates; it substitutes a legal for an illegal drug.

3 Methadone is a synthetic narcotic and can cause dependence; it is only used in the treatment of heroin addiction.
   4 Methadone is not known to have this action.

67. **2 When methadone is reduced, a craving for narcotics may occur. Without narcotics, anxiety will increase, agitation will occur, and the client may try to leave the hospital to secure drugs. (EV; TC; SA)**
   1 This is not related to methadone hydrochloride reduction.
   3 This is not related to reduced methadone hydrochloride dosage.
   4 This may occur with methadone hydrochloride overdose.

68. **3 Preoperative teaching related to the surgery is a priority at this time. (PL; ED; SA)**
   1 Her drug dependence is an ongoing issue but not the most important preoperatively.
   2 The nurse can not contact Mary's family without her permission.
   4 It is the responsibility of the surgeon to ensure that she understands the reason for and possible complications of the surgery.

69. **2 The addict tries to avoid stress and reality. The drug produces a blurring of these feelings to the point that the addict becomes dependent on it. (AN; PS; SA)**
   1 Later on the psychologic effect is usually more important than the ability to ease pain.
   3 Large doses of narcotics can cause a dreamlike state.
   4 Hard drugs such as cocaine can increase motor activity.

70. **3 The symptoms of withdrawal reach a peak on the third day. (EV; PA; SA)**
   1 Symptoms begin within 8 hours and reach their peak on the third day.
   2 Symptoms become more severe on the third day.
   4 Symptoms begin to subside after the third day.

71. **1 Research indicates that alcoholism is a family disease with its roots in the family of origin. (AN; PS; SA)**
   2 Although true, this would not be a reason for including the family in the treatment program.
   3 Alcoholism is a family disease and family members do need counseling and assistance.
   4 Same as answer 3.

Schizophrenia and Other Psychotic Disorders

72. **1 Mental illness is characterized by the use of abnormal defense mechanisms or the abnormal use of normal defense mechanisms. These defenses build a wall and interrupt interpersonal relationships. (AN; PS; SD)**
    2 This is possible, but not a common factor.
    3 It is the ability or inability to handle periods of high anxiety that gives evidence of mental illness.
    4 This is possible, but may be just one factor.

73. **1 The social environment characterized by family interaction patterns and role identification and definition lays the foundation for the child's future emotional response. (AN; PE; SD)**
    2 This, as yet, has not been proved. Studies of genetic and biochemical factors continue.
    3 These would result in tissue changes and would not merely be an alteration in functioning.
    4 This is a factor in delirium, dementia, and other cognitive disorders.

74. **3 When individuals use these defense mechanisms to blur the pains of reality, they are unable to test out their feelings or differentiate the real world from their personal intrapsychic perceptions. (AN; PS; SD)**
    1 Logic is only one part of reality testing.
    2 Association is only one part of reality testing.
    4 The thought process is only one aspect of reality testing.

75. **3 A delusion of persecution is a fixed and firm belief or feeling of being harassed, in danger, or at the mercy of others. (DC; TC; SD)**
    1 Hallucinations are perceived experiences that occur in the absence of actual sensory stimulation.
    2 An error in judgment can be corrected by pointing out reality, but a delusion cannot.
    4 In this instance the person accepts blame for an act that was never committed.

76. **2 A delusion is a fixed, false personal belief that is not founded in reality. (AN; PS; SD)**
    1 An illusion would be a misinterpretation of a sensory stimulus.
    3 Autistic thinking is a distortion in the thought process associated with schizophrenic disorders.

4 An hallucination is a perceived experience that occurs in the absence of an actual sensory stimulus.

77. **3 Clients cannot be argued out of delusions, so the best approach is a simple statement of reality. (IM; TC; SD)**
    1 This would be a form of entering into the client's delusions; the client would only feel that a particular part was free of poison.
    2 This may reinforce the delusion that the hospital food is poisoned.
    4 Threats are always poor nursing intervention no matter how exasperated the nurse feels.

78. **2 It is important to help the client focus on feelings, and this is the only response that does this. (IM; PS; SD)**
    1 "Why" calls for a conclusion rather than exploring the issue; the client may not have the answer.
    3 Although this is true, it is not something the client is ready to understand; it is a closed statement.
    4 This is false reassurance and not realistic; the client is still concerned as to what will happen when the nurse is not there.

79. **2 Echolalia is repetition of another person's remarks, words, or statements. It occurs when individuals are fearful of saying their own words and therefore just echo the words of others. (DC; PS; SD)**
    1 This is a thought process connected with associative looseness.
    3 This is when new words are coined or old words take on private symbolic meanings.
    4 Echopraxia is the reflecting of observed movements rather than of speech.

80. **1 Talking in the third person reflects poor ego boundaries and a dissociation from the real self. (AN; PS; SD)**
    2 Transference is the movement of emotional energy and feelings from one person to another.
    3 Displacement is the attempt to reduce anxiety by transferring the emotions associated with one object or person to another.
    4 Reaction formation is the expression of an emotion opposite the one really felt.

81. **4 Tranquilizers reduce anxiety levels and make clients more amenable to looking at new approaches to handling stress. (AN; PS; SD)**
    1 They are used to treat severe emotional illness, not neurotic symptoms.
    2 They cannot prevent any secondary complications.
    3 The major tranquilizers are used to treat psychotic symptoms, which may include destructive behavior; however, this is not the major reason for their administration.

82. **4 If clients feel a need to be punished, it is best to permit them to engage in controlled activities that expiate guilt feelings. (IM; PS; SD)**
    1 The client cannot be talked out of her delusion; she must believe within herself that she has nothing to atone for.
    2 This would do nothing to interrupt the delusional system; it would support the hallucination.
    3 A procedure such as this would reinforce her belief of the need to be punished.

83. **1 Since the client has paranoid feelings that other people are out to do harm, assignment to a four-bed room would be very threatening. (EV; TC; SD)**
    2 This seems unlikely since it appears to have started with the transfer to a four-bed room.
    3 This is possible but unlikely; planning an escape is not usually part of the schizophrenic pattern of behavior.
    4 This is possible but not likely; clients with schizophrenia have difficulty working out problems.

84. **4 The nurse's response provides an example to the client that feelings can be expressed by words rather than by action. This response also demonstrates that the nurse cares enough to set limits on behavior. (IM; TC; SD)**
    1 The nurse would be accepting physical abuse, which is never done.
    2 The behavior and the client should never be ignored; the client needs limits set on behavior now.
    3 The nurse is punishing the client rather than trying to focus on what is happening at this time to cause the behavior.

85. **4 When the client's perceptions are especially frightening, the nurse must let the client know that the fears are recognized as real and frightening even if the nurse does not share these perceptions. Staying with the client will convey concern as well as reduce the fears. (IM; PS; SD)**
    1 This is nontherapeutic; the voices are real to the client.
    2 The client will be unable to play cards because of a reduced ability to concentrate when the voices are speaking.
    3 This is nontherapeutic; the client is unable to separate the voices from reality.

86. **4 Although there are many theories, none have been consistently documented. No organic pathology has yet been identified in schizophrenia. Behavioral responses learned in childhood cause the individual to distort events and relationships and lose the ability to relate to the world. (AN; PS; SD)**
    1 This would be an organic rather than a functional illness.
    2 This would be an organic rather than a functional illness, and there is no evidence that the brain undergoes any change in schizophrenia.
    3 This might be a factor, but there is no proof that it is true because we do not know what causes schizophrenia.

87. **2 Disinterest in or fear of personal involvement creates distancing behavior and lack of response to the environment. (DC; PS; SD)**
    1 These may or may not be present.
    3 These would be more commonly found in the manic phase of a bipolar disorder.
    4 Same as answer 1.

88. **4 These clients usually display social inadequacy and suspiciousness of others. (DC; PS; SD)**
    1 Reserve and reclusive behaviors would be manifested; therefore, this option is incorrect.
    2 These qualities are descriptive of the disorder, not the premorbid personality.
    3 The client held a responsible job before becoming sick.

89. **3 Demonstrating that the staff can be trusted is a vital initial step in the therapy program. (IM; TC; SD)**

1 Even proof would not convince the client with a schizoid personality that the feelings of distrust are false.

2 The client is not ready to enter group activities yet and will not be until trust is established.

4 This would not be realistic even if it were possible; limiting contact does not develop trust.

90. 1 **An interpersonal relationship based on trust must be established before clients can be helped back to reality. (PL; PS; SD)**

2 This is an important part of the treatment and care, but of lesser importance than a trusting relationship.

3 Socialization would come at a later time in therapy.

4 There is nothing to indicate an urgency to remove the client from the home.

91. 3 **You cannot argue a client out of a delusion. Statements made by the nurse show a lack of knowledge and constitute a threat, which is a form of assault. (EV; PS; SD)**

1 There is no indication that the client needed a reminder to eat.

2 A person cannot be argued out of a delusion.

4 Everyone needs nourishment, but threats accomplish little.

92. 1 **This lets the client know the nurse is available if needed. It also demonstrates an acceptance of the client. (IM; TC; SD)**

2 Although it is important to note the incident on the chart, it does not take precedence over letting the client know the nurse is there if needed.

3 This is an avoidance technique; it shows a lack of acceptance of the client as a person.

4 Another client's perception of the incident may or may not be valid.

93. 4 **The nurse sets limits on behavior; accepts the client but rejects the behavior. (IM; TC; SD)**

1 It would be unrealistic as well as cruel to do this.

2 This is a punishment rather than a setting of limits.

3 The nurse has a responsibility to the other clients to limit the behavior.

94. 1 **The client needs limits set. This response by the nurse sets limits and rejects the behavior but accepts the client. (IM; PS; SD)**

2 This does not help raise the client to a functioning level.

3 This serves no useful purpose; inappropriate behavior should be dealt with when first noted.

4 This is a punishing action; it shows no support or acceptance of the client.

95. 3 **The client is voiding on the floor not to express hostility but because of confusion. Taking the client to the toilet frequently limits voiding in inappropriate places. (PL; TC; SD)**

1 This is a form of punishment for something the client cannot control.

2 This is not realistic; it will have no effect on the problem.

4 If the client were doing this to express hostility, such action would be useful; but not when the client is unable to control the behavior.

96. 3 **By observing behavior, the nurse is able to understand the client's feelings better. Behavior usually serves a purpose and is directed toward satisfaction of needs. (DC; TC; SD)**

1 It is only one of the many aspects that are part of making a diagnosis; this is true in the care of all clients, not just the withdrawn individual.

2 Observation alone is insufficient to make this judgment; however, it would allow the staff to individualize the nursing care plan to suit the client's needs.

4 It is more important to have insight into what the person may be feeling rather than the degree of depression.

97. 1 **Assisting clients with grooming keeps them in contact with reality and allows them to see that staff members care enough to help. It also places value on appearance. (IM; PS; SD)**

2 This would be a long-term goal.

3 A one-to-one relationship would be best initially.

4 The client may withdraw even more.

98. 2 **Nursing care involves a steady attempt to draw the client into some response. This can best be accomplished by focusing on nonthreatening subjects that do not demand a specific response. (IM; TC; SD)**

1 The client is not ready yet to discuss feelings, so the first step is to focus on nonthreatening subjects.

3 Questions like these do not allow a person to explore feelings.

4 By doing this, the nurse is showing acceptance of the client but is doing nothing to encourage communication.

99. **1 Keeping the withdrawn client oriented to reality prevents the client from withdrawing even further into a private world. (PL; TC; SD)**
2 A gradual involvement in selected activities would be best.
3 The client would be unable to tell anyone why this is so.
4 This would be futile at this time.

100. **1 This response reflects on the client's feelings rather than focusing on the verbalization. (EV; TC; SD)**
2 This response focuses on the statement rather than on the feeling behind the statement.
3 This response dismisses the client's feelings.
4 This response puts the client on the defensive and asks for verification that the nurse is indeed a good person; it fails to focus on the feeling behind the statement.

101. **3 This shows acceptance for the client yet sets firm limits on the behavior. (IM; TC; SD)**
1 This puts the focus on the nurse rather than on what is behind the outburst.
2 The nurse accepts the client but should not accept physical abuse from the client.
4 This statement not only rejects the behavior but also attacks the client.

102. **4 Inner psychic stress and environmental difficulties can interfere with the function of organically sound organs, resulting in a loss of ability to communicate. (AN; PS; SD)**
1 Mental deficiency results when there are changes in brain tissue.
2 These problems are usually associated with changes in brain tissue.
3 This problem is associated with changes in brain tissue.

103. **3 Close follow-up and continued monitoring of medication, behavior, and emotional state are necessary to enable the client to maintain a positive behavioral change. (PL; TC; SD)**
1 This would depend on what the client's regular activities were.
2 This would encourage dependence.
4 A self-help group might or might not be effective.

Disorders of Mood

104. **3 This attitude conveys to others that the client feels too insignificant for anyone to listen. (DC; PS; MO)**
1 Initiative and self-effacement are two different factors.
2 This is indicative of feelings of sadness, not self-effacement.
4 The affect associated with self-effacement is not inappropriate because it matches the inner feelings of depression.

105. **4 Hyperactive clients frequently will not take the time to eat because they are overinvolved in everything that is going on. (AN; TC; MO)**
1 This is indicative of a depressive episode.
3 The client is unable to sit long enough with the other clients to eat a meal; this is not conscious avoidance.
4 The client probably gives no thought to food because of overinvolvement with the activities in the environment.

106. **4 Clients out of control need controls set for them. The staff must understand that the client is not deliberately trying to disrupt the unit. (PL; TC; MO)**
1 Ignoring the client will not stop the disruptive behavior; the nurse has a responsibility to the other clients.
2 This is demeaning the client in the eyes of the other clients, and does not deal with the problem directly.
3 This may be a last resort taken to solve the problem but should not be used until other alternatives are explored.

107. **4 Hyperactive clients burn up large quantities of calories, which must be replenished. Since these clients will not take the time to sit down to eat, providing them with food they can carry with them sometimes helps. (PL; PA; MO)**
1 The client will probably not be aware of any hunger and could go without food for a dangerously long time.
2 This is an exercise in futility for the nurse.
3 The client is not presently capable of preparing food.

108. **1 This will help reduce the client's anxiety, thereby reducing hyperactivity. (PL; TC; MO)**

2 It is not possible physically to control hyperactivity.

3 The client is not capable of choosing activities at this time.

4 The client is not capable of controlling overactive behavior; setting verbal limits will not be effective.

109. 4 **The hyperactive client is usually rather easily distracted, so the excess energy can be redirected into constructive channels. (PL, TC; MO)**

1 There is nothing to indicate at this time that the client is not in touch with reality.

2 The client will talk a great deal with no encouragement.

3 The client will not be able to stay long enough with one thing to finish it.

110. 1 **Having these clients wear personal clothing helps keep them more in touch with reality. (IM; PS; MO)**

2 This may set the client up as a target of ridicule by the other clients.

3 The client will need help with makeup, since these clients usually go to extremes with it.

4 This is not helping the client learn new and better ways to deal with situations.

111. 4 **The hyperactive client will frequently eat hand foods that do not require sitting down to eat. (IM; TC; MO)**

1 The client will most likely ignore the tray.

2 Unworthy feelings are part of a depressive episode.

3 It is unlikely that the client would understand or care about this piece of information.

112. 3 **From the history the nurse can determine that the client's contacts were limited, schedule fixed, and demands on self quite rigid. (AS; PS; MO)**

1 The symptoms described are not characteristically noted in this disorder.

2 Same as answer 1.

4 Same as answer 1.

113. 1 **Severely depressed clients are not motivated to take action or to plan ahead. They are unable to direct their energy on the environment. (PL; PS; MO)**

2 This would be helpful to a severely depressed client, whose attention span is limited.

3 This would be helpful to a severely depressed client because it requires little thought and provides gratification and satisfaction.

4 This would be helpful for a person with depression as well as for the mentally retarded.

114. 1 **Routines should be kept simple and no demands should be made that the client cannot meet. The client is depressed, and all reactions will be slow. Putting pressure on the client will only increase anxiety and feelings of worthlessness. (PL; TC; MO)**

2 The client will have to focus on personal strengths, not on family strengths.

3 This would feed into the client's feelings of unworthiness and frustration.

4 Feelings of worth must come from within the individual; the nurse must reassure the client through actions, not words.

115. 1 **This response demonstrates an understanding that the newly discharged client needs to have the support of the therapeutic unit when discharged. The client needs to feel that in a crisis the staff will be there for support. (IM; TC; MO)**

2 The role of the nurse was not to become a good friend but to aid the client in becoming a functioning being again.

3 This response provides false reassurance; the nurse could not know this.

4 This is unprofessional and blurs the roles of nurse and client.

116. 1 **Hyperactive behavior in individuals such as this is typical of the manic flight of ideas associated with mood disorders. (DC; PS; MO)**

2 Depression, loss of interest in usual activities, and poor appetite are more indicative of a major depression.

3 The symptoms are more indicative of a mood than a personality disorder.

4 A flat affect and apathy are more indicative of a schizophrenic disorder.

117. 3 **Depression is a disturbance in the mood or affect (classified as a mood disorder) that usually develops when the person suffers a real or imagined loss. (AN; TC; MO)**

1 The degree of depression will determine the extent to which a person can function.

2 There is not a total loss of control, and the loss of control may be only part of the clinical picture.

4 This may also be true, but it is not the most accurate description.

118. 1 **The nurse must base nursing intervention on a client's problems. Since major depression is due to the client's feelings of self-rejection, it is important for the nurse to have the client identify these feelings before a plan of action can be taken. (DC; PS; MO)**

2 This is asking the client to draw a conclusion; the client may be unable to do so at this time.

3 Asking why does not let a client explore feelings; it usually elicits an "I don't know" response.

4 This is beyond the scope of the client's abilities at this time; clients would rather have the nurse tell them how staff can help them than help themselves.

119. 2 **An art-type project that could be worked on successfully at one's own pace would be important. (IM; PS; MO)**

1 This would require too much concentration and increase the client's feelings of despair.

3 This is used mostly for severely regressed clients, and at this point it may not be appropriate for this client.

4 Same as answer 1.

120. 1 **These clients can usually be fairly easily distracted by planned involvement in repetitious, simple tasks. (IM; TC; MO)**

2 This should be employed only if the client's restlessness cannot be controlled with other measures and physical exhaustion creates a danger for the client.

3 This would be abusive treatment for a client with a need to pace and would reinforce the client's belief that punishment was required for redemption.

4 The client may perceive this isolation as a punishment, and it would not allow for observation by the staff.

121. 3 **A major part of depression involves an inability to accept the self as it is, which leads to making demands on others to meet unrealistic needs. (PL; TC; MO)**

1 A short-term goal would be to talk about the client's depressed feelings; a long-term goal would be to look at what is causing those feelings.

2 Developing new defense mechanisms is not the priority because they tend to help the client avoid reality.

4 This is not important or crucial to the client's recovery.

122. 4 **The client's behavior demonstrates increased anxiety. Since it was directed toward the new staff, it was probably precipitated by their arrival. (AN; PS; MO)**

1 The client is not filling the "life-of-the-party" role; the client is resorting to previous coping behavior in the face of extreme stress.

2 This is possible, but the remark is more indicative of increased anxiety.

3 The client is aware of what is going on and who everyone is at this time.

123. 3 **Recognizing the language as part of the illness makes it easier to tolerate, but limits must be set for the benefit of the staff and other clients. Setting limits also shows the client that the nurse cares enough to stop the behavior. (IM; TC; MO)**

1 This statement shows little understanding or tolerance of the illness.

2 Ignoring the behavior is a form of rejection; the client is not using the behavior for attention.

4 This statement demonstrates a rejection of the client and little understanding of the illness.

124. 2 **Physical activity will help utilize some of the excess energy without requiring the client to make decisions or forcing other clients to deal with the behavior. (IM; TC; MO)**

1 The client needs guidance and would not be able to guide others.

3 The client would greatly disrupt the unit because of the excess activity and bossiness associated with this disorder.

4. The client's extreme activity would limit concentration or task completion.

125. 3 **This is the most therapeutic approach. The staff member also provides special attention to help the client meet dependency needs and reduce a self-defeating attitude. (PL; TC; MO)**

1 This response negates the client's feelings and cuts off further communication.

2 This is unrealistic because the nurse cannot be with the client constantly until the depression lifts.

4 The priority is 24-hour observation of the client; removing articles that could provide a means for suicide would also be done.

126. 3 **This gives the client the nonverbal message that someone cares and views the client as being worthy of attention and concern. (IM; PS; MO)**

1 The concentration required for chess is too much for the client at this time.

2 The client is incapable of making decisions at this time.

4 Depressed clients often have too much thinking time.

127. **4 Telling the client the nurse wants to spend time communicates that the client is worthy of the nurse's time and that the nurse cares. (IM; PS; MO)**

1 This does not show the acceptance and care that sitting with the client would.

2 The client may be unable, at this point, to expend energy on anything outside the self.

3 It is unlikely that the client would respond to the nurse because of feeling unworthy and depressed.

128. **3 The client is very dependent, and such individuals can never get enough attention to meet their dependent needs. This unfulfilled need causes anger, which the client has problems expressing for fear of losing the people on whom the client is dependent. (AN; PS; MO)**

1 The client is well able to express remorse and guilt.

2 The client is expressing the need for comfort.

4 The client is well able to express feelings of low self-esteem.

129. **3 Depression is usually both emotional and physical, so a simple daily routine is the least stressful and least anxiety producing. (PL; TC; MO)**

1 A depressed client has limited interest in any activities; too many activities may increase the anxiety.

2 Too many stimuli increase the anxiety in a depressed client.

4 Such a client may be incapable of making even simple decisions.

130. **3 The nurse's response really was a threat by attempting to put pressure on the client to speak or be left alone. (IM; TC; MO)**

1 The statement reflects an insensitivity to, rather than a recognition of, the client's rights.

2 This is not reward and punishment, which is used in behavior modification therapy.

4 The client is not ready at this stage for group involvement; the nurse must start with a one-to-one relationship.

131. **1 Suicidal impulses take priority, and the client must be stopped from acting on them while treatment is in progress. (AN; TC; MO)**

2 This has a very low order of priority.

3 Safety is the primary responsibility.

4 Reassurance will not necessarily decrease the client's feeling; safety is the priority.

132. **1 The nurse failed to use knowledge regarding suicidal clients and did not protect the client from this ever present danger. This failure could be legally defined as negligence. (EV; TC; MO)**

2 Clients need observation even after the depression has lifted, especially when plans for discharge are pending.

3 Constant supervision would help prevent suicide; the unit was left unlocked and the client was not under constant supervision.

4 Clients are in greater danger of suicide when they are coming out of depression.

133. **4 Past level of success demonstrates ego strengths that can be built on. (AN; PS; MO)**

1 This constitutes only a crisis situation, not necessarily a poor prognosis.

2 The client's premorbid personality must be fairly sound because the client is in the second year of college and thus has achieved some success.

3 Intelligence has little to do with recovery, but the client's ego strengths play a big part.

134. **4 Directness is the best approach at the first interview, because this sets the focus and concern and lets the nurse know what the client is feeling now. (EV; TC; MO)**

1 At this point the client is most likely unable to think past the present, much less deal with future plans; too general a question.

2 This may be helpful during the course of treatment, but initially the direct approach with the client is best.

3 This would be one resource for input; but regarding suicide, it is best to approach the client directly.

135. 3 **The anniversary frequently reemphasizes the feeling of loss and abandonment and serves to heighten the current feelings of depression and hopelessness.** (EV; TC; MO)

1 This would be an important consideration, but the anniversary of the loss of a loved one would take precedence.

2 Length of time has less influence than the anniversary of a loss.

4 Suicide risk may still be a factor at this time but less than at the anniversary of a loss.

136. 4 **Clients frequently report suicidal feelings so the staff will have the chance to stop them. They are really asking, "Do you care enough to stop me?"** (DC; TC; MO)

1 This could be true but is an unlikely motivation for the behavior.

2 Same as answer 1.

3 This may be true; but, more important, the client is seeking help and protection.

137. 4 **Emotional support and close surveillance can demonstrate the staff's caring and their attempt to prevent acting out of suicidal ideation.** (IM; TC; MO)

1 This would be punishment for a client who still may find a way to carry out a suicide attempt in the room.

2 This would be routinely done; by itself it is not necessarily therapeutic.

3 This is not a suicide precaution.

138. 1 **Clients fear this therapy because of the expected pain. If they are reassured that they will be asleep and have no pain, there will be less anxiety and more cooperation.** (IM; PS; MO)

2 Permanent loss does not occur.

3 Clients may not be able to realize their own fears and thus do not ask questions; this statement cuts off future communication.

4 No treatment requiring anesthesia is totally safe.

139. 2 **The staff's presence provides continued emotional support and helps relieve anxiety.** (IM; PS; MO)

1 They may not make the client better; this would be false reassurance.

3 Not all clients experience amnesia, and the amnesia passes; placing emphasis on amnesia will increase fear.

4 This will be part of explaining the treatments; the focus should not be on fear but on having someone present.

140. 2 **Clients are confused when they awaken after electroconvulsive therapy. They have a loss of recent memory, so it is important to orient them to time, place, and situation.** (IM; TC; MO)

1 This would be a later action, if the client asked for food.

3 This would not be appropriate for a client who has just awakened after a treatment.

4 This is not necessary. Routine postoperative vital signs are adequate.

141. 3 **This statement helps the client realize that staff members care and feel that the client is worthy of care.** (IM; PS; MO)

1 This is a response that places the client on the defensive.

2 This is an inappropriate response to a rather obvious situation.

4 This is an evasive tactic by the nurse.

142. 1 **The client is asking for help to prevent suicide. This response focuses on feelings and does not challenge or deny them.** (IM; PS; MO)

2 This response negates the client's feelings and interprets the situation for the client.

3 This response denies the client's feelings and does not follow through on what the client is saying.

4 This response ignores the client's cry for help and does not follow through on what the client is expressing.

143. 3 **This encourages the client to talk about feelings without really setting the focus for the discussion.** (EV; TC; MO)

1 This would make the client wonder where the nurse had been for 4 days.

2 This cuts off any further communication of feelings; it ignores what the client has expressed to the nurse.

4 This shifts the responsibility of care to the psychiatrist rather than dealing with it directly.

144. 1 **Electroconvulsive therapy, which interrupts established patterns of behavior, helps relieve symptoms and limits possible suicide attempts in clients with severe, intractable depressions that do not respond to antidepressant medication.** (AN; PS; MO)

2 The client's depressed mood would greatly limit participation in psychotherapy; feelings precipitated by therapy may lead to suicidal acting out.

3 Psychotherapy is directed toward helping the person learn new coping mechanisms and better ways of dealing with problems; the depressed client needs direction to accomplish this.

4 These are antianxiety medications that would not ordinarily be used for clients with depression.

Anxiety, Somatoform, and Dissociative Disorders

145. 1 **The defense mechanism is called conversion because the individual actually reduces emotional anxiety by converting it to a physical disability. (AN; PS; AX)**

2 In dissociation there is separation of certain mental processes from the consciousness as though they belonged to another; a dissociative-type reaction is expressed as amnesia, fugue, multiple personality, aimless running, depersonalization, sleepwalking, etc.

3 This is a mechanism used to make up for a lack in one area by emphasizing capabilities in another.

4 This just identifies the term used to describe mind and body; it is not a defense mechanism.

146. 3 **By staying physically close, the nurse conveys to the client the message that someone cares enough to be there and that the client is a person worth caring for. (IM; PS; AX)**

1 This would not be an initial nursing intervention.

2 Sitting still will increase the tension the client is experiencing.

4 The client is incapable of telling anyone what the problem is.

147. 1 **Providing support, understanding, and acceptance of feelings that the client is experiencing is essential for reducing stress. (IM; PS; AX)**

2 This would most likely have the effect of increasing anxiety.

3 The hospital provides the client with a safe, accepting environment in which to face problems and discuss emotionally charged areas.

4 This is unrealistic; the nurse cannot be present at all times. Concerns about the nurse's absence would increase anxiety.

148. 4 **Anxiety is a normal human response, causing both physical and emotional changes that everyone experiences when faced with stressful situations. (IM; PS; AX)**

1 Anxiety is experienced to a greater or lesser degree by every person.

2 Anxiety does not operate from the conscious level.

3 The fear may be related to a specific aspect of, rather than the total environment.

149. 1 **Acting out anxiety with antisocial behavior is most commonly found in individuals with personality rather than anxiety disorders. (DC; TC; AX)**

2 This is an example of a conversion disorder.

3 Regression is an attempt during periods of stress to return to behavior that has been satisfying and is appropriate at an earlier stage of development.

4 This is an example of a phobic disorder.

150. 1 **The "fight or flight" responses of the autonomic nervous system would be stimulated and result in these findings. (EV; PA; AX)**

2 The pupils would dilate, not constrict, and the blood glucose would increase, not decrease

3 The "fight or flight" response is not characterized by constricted pupils, constricted bronchioles, and hypoglycemia.

4 The pulse rate would be increased, and the blood glucose would increase, not decrease.

151. 1 **When tension is reduced, anxiety diminishes and the person feels more comfortable, safe, and secure. (AN; PA; AX)**

2 There would be less anxiety if the person were able to deny the situation.

3 This is what the person hopes will happen but it does not.

4 This action would have an effect on psychologic rather than physical discomfort.

152. 3 **Learning a variety of coping mechanisms helps reduce anxiety in stressful situations. (PL; PS; AX)**

1 A person must learn to cope with unpleasant objects and events.

2 Prolonged exposure would increase anxiety to possibly uncontrollable levels.

4 Fearful situations can never be viewed as pleasurable.

153. **1 The client is using this compulsive behavior to control anxiety and needs to continue with it until the anxiety is reduced and more acceptable methods are developed to handle it. (IM; TC; AX)**
2 This would not reduce the client's anxiety since he is aware that doorknobs are not contaminated but cannot stop the compulsive act.
3 Same as answer 2.
4 This would greatly increase anxiety; compulsive behavior is a defense that cannot be interrupted until new defenses are learned.

154. **3 By carrying out the compulsive ritual, the client unconsciously tries to control the situation so that unacceptable impulses and feelings will not be acted on. (AN; PS; AX)**
1 This mechanism does not operate on a conscious level.
2 Hallucinations are not part of a phobic disorder.
4 They feel no need to punish others.

155. **2 This sets an unrealistic limit that would increase anxiety by removing a defense the client needs. (AN; PS; AX)**
1 This is done in therapy as the client's condition improves. Insight is slowly developed to minimize anxiety.
3 This would increase self-esteem and self-control, not increase anxiety.
4 This would reduce, not increase, anxiety, because the client would feel free to express feelings.

156. **2 This action limits the ritualistic behavior but does not attempt to extinguish it entirely. (PL; PS; AX)**
1 Taking away all of the client's ritualistic behaviors would be ineffective and serve to increase anxiety.
3 This is one of the goals to be accomplished during the client's hospitalization, not in the initial phase.
4 This action is an appropriate intervention during the working phase of the nurse-client intervention, not the initial phase.

157. **2 The client is too anxious to sleep in a four-bed room and should simply be moved to a private room. (IM; PS; AX)**
1 Just talking about the problem will not improve it; quietly moving the client to a private room would be better intervention at this time.

3 This is false reassurance.
4 This probably would not help since it would not relieve the client's anxiety.

158. **4 In phobias the individual transfers anxiety to a rather safe inanimate object. Therefore the anxiety and resulting feelings will only be precipitated when in direct contact with the object. (AN; PS; AX)**
1 It is not thinking about the feared object that causes anxiety; it is the possibility of having to come into contact with it.
2 It is the guilt or fear within the person, not the object, that must be dealt with.
3 It is not possible to introject the feared object within the body.

159. **1 This sets an unrealistic limit that would increase anxiety by removing a defense the client needs. (AN; PS; AX)**
2 This is done in therapy as the client's condition improves. Insight is slowly developed to minimize anxiety.
3 This would increase self-esteem and self-control, not increase anxiety.
4 This would reduce, not increase, anxiety, because the client would feel free to express feelings.

160. **2 The client is caught between two equally compelling needs, and movement or sight is impossible. Paralysis or blindness justifies to the client the inability to move in any direction. (DC; PS; AX)**
1 It is an unconscious method of solving a conflict.
3 It is necessary for the client to focus on the problem causing the disorder, not on other things.
4 It is more important that the client learn how to deal with personal feelings before dealing with family conflicts.

161. **3 Needing to be dependent while wanting to be independent creates a struggle that makes all movement psychologically difficult. Symptoms develop and remove psychologic choice, making movement physically impossible. (DC; PS; AX)**
1 It is unlikely the feelings would involve the home; rather the people in the home.
2 This is a part of the picture but not the total picture.
4 Same as answer 2.

162. **3 The conversion type of defense tends to be a learned behavioral response that the individual will use when put under stress.** (AN; PS; AX)
1 This is not a likely occurrence if the client learns to deal with problems.
2 Psychiatric treatment may be needed at different times throughout life but usually not on a continuous basis.
4 Based on studies of this disorder, it usually returns when the client is under severe stress.

163. **3 The client with a conversion disorder literally converts the anxiety to the symptom. Once the symptom develops, it acts as a defense against the anxiety and the client is diagnostically almost anxiety free.** (DC; PS; AX)
1 In a conversion disorder the reactions the nurse would expect to encounter are not in proportion to the disability; therefore the client would not be greatly depressed.
2 The conflict is resolved by the paralysis of the legs; therefore the anxiety is under control.
4 Just the opposite is true.

164. **3 The physical symptoms are not the client's major problem and therefore should not be the focus for care. This is a psychologic problem, and the focus should be on this level.** (PL; PS; AX)
1 This would be focusing on the physical symptoms of the conflict; the client is not ready to give the symptom up.
2 The disorder operates on an unconscious level but is very real to the client; this response denies feelings.
4 Psychotherapy would have to come before physical therapy.

165. **4 The client's anxiety results from being unable to choose psychologically between two conflicting actions. The conversion to a physical disability removes the choice and therefore reduces the anxiety.** (AN; PS; AX)
1 The anxiety is put under control by the conversion to a physical disability.
2 The anxiety is decreased, and the conversion disorder operates on an unconscious level.
3 The anxiety is internalized into a physical symptom.

166. **4 These clients can better work through their underlying conflicts when demands are reduced and the routine is simple.** (AN; PS; AX)

1 Preventing these clients from carrying out rituals can precipitate panic reactions.
2 The intent of therapy should be to help the client gain control, not to enable others to do the controlling.
3 Since anxiety stems from unconscious conflicts, a controlled environment alone is not enough to effect resolution.

167. **3 The symptoms are problematic to the client and thus have caused emotional pain that is beyond conscious control.** (PL; PS; AX)
1 Ignoring the client's complaints will increase anxiety.
2 Willpower does not enter into it; a conversion disorder operates on an unconscious level.
4 There is no evidence that this will occur.

Eating Disorders

168. **3 These clients hide food, eat excessively in private, and purge in secret; attempts to hide their behavior indicate that they are aware of and are ashamed of their behavior.** (AN; PS; EA)
1 Clients with bulimia nervosa are frequently not obese.
2 This is associated with clients with anorexia nervosa.
4 Same as answer 2.

169. **4 Realistic guidelines reduce anxiety, increase feelings of security, and increase compliance with the therapeutic regimen.** (PL; TC; EA)
1 A controlling environment would set up a power struggle between these clients and the nurse.
2 These clients need realistic rules and regulations that they recognize as helpful, not empathy.
3 This would not be therapeutic; focusing on food generally results in a power struggle between these clients and the nurse.

170. **3 The problem is psychologic. Therefore the initial approach by the nurse should be directed toward establishing trust.** (IM; TC; EA)
1 The client is not ready for this information.
2 The client is convinced of being overweight; complimenting the client's lovely figure would not change the client's self-perception.
4 This would be an initial nursing intervention after trust had been established.

171. 4 Clients with anorexia nervosa are struggling between the dependency of childhood and the demands of adulthood. (AN; PS; EA)

1 A distortion of body image rather than a low self-esteem is the problem.
2 These clients feel fat, not unworthy.
3 These clients are not angry at anyone.

172. 2 A goal focuses on where the client should be after certain actions are taken; these clients need to gain weight. (AN; TC; EA)

1 This could set up a struggle between the client and the nurse; the focus of care should not be on the actual intake of food
3 These clients talk freely about food; this would not be therapeutic.
4 Behavior modification techniques work much better than group therapy; these clients lack insight and would focus on food, not eating.

Disorders of Personality

173. 2 When the individual consciously pretends an illness with no physical basis, it is called malingering. (DC; PS; PR)

1 People using neurotic defenses really believe they are sick.
3 A person out of contact with reality is unable to pretend an illness.
4 The use of conversion defenses is not a conscious act.

174. 3 The psychophysiologic response (hyperfunction or hypofunction) creates actual tissue change. Somatoform disorders are unrelated to organic changes. (AN; PS; PR)

1 There is a feeling of illness in both instances.
2 There is an emotional component in both instances.
4 There may be a restriction of activities in both instances.

175. 2 Individuals with this personality disorder tend to be self-centered and impulsive. They lack judgment and self control and do not profit from their mistakes. (AN; PS; PR)

1 Generally, just the opposite is true.
3 These people never learn from their mistakes, experiences, and punishment.
4 These people are too self-centered to have a sense of responsibility to anyone.

176. 2 The lack of superego control allows the ego and the id to control the behavior.

Self-motivation and self-satisfaction are of paramount concern. (AN; PS; PR)

1 They count on others to extricate them from the problems they find themselves faced with.
3 These people are extremely dependent on others.
4 These people are usually charming on the surface and can easily "con" people into doing what they want.

177. 3 Accepts the client as a person of worth rather than being cold or implying rejection. However, the nurse maintains a professional rather than a social role. (IM; TC; PR)

1 This is shifting responsibility from the issue at hand to the institution.
2 This does not respond to the statement; the client is aware of their roles.
4 This avoids the real issue and elevates the nurse to a higher social order.

178. 3 The development of physical symptoms without a physical cause is an anxiety-reducing mechanism known as conversion. (AN; PS; PR)

1 Blaming others in the environment for failure and mistakes is not converting anxiety into physical symptoms.
2 Going back to an earlier state when one felt safer and more secure is not converting anxiety into physical symptoms.
4 This is a continued concern about health characterized by anxiety and an unrealistic interpretation of real or imaginary symptoms as indication of serious illness.

179. 3 Clients prevented from using ritualistic behavior to control anxiety will be deprived of their defense and have no way of relieving tension. (PL; TC; PR)

1 The client's behavior should never be ignored; it is important to accept and support these clients during this time.
2 This would not decrease the ritualistic behavior.
4 Preventing ritualistic behavior will only increase anxiety.

180. 3 When props are needed to blur reality, the individual is not able to rely on the self to test out situations, and therefore dependence on others or props increases. (AN; PS; PR)

1 The person who mistrusts has not learned to trust the environment; however, the person does not necessarily need props.

2 The person with an ego ideal would not need props to blur reality.

4 Role blurring is not a problem requiring a prop.

181. **1 Clients with these sexual disorders usually have many other emotional problems that may be overt or covert in nature. (DC; PS; PR)**

2 There is no proof of a deficiency of these hormones.

3 There is normal development of sexual organs in individuals with paraphiliac sexual disorders.

4 This has no basis in fact.

182. **3 This sets realistic limits on behavior without rejecting the client. (IM; PS; PR)**

1 This would constitute a rejection of the person rather than the behavior.

2 This would encourage further manipulation of the staff by the client.

4 The other client is entitled to a special time with the nurse; this is inconsistent limit setting on the part of the nurse.

183. **4 Helping clients understand that a behavior is being used to control impulses usually makes them more amenable to psychotherapy. (IM; TC; PR)**

1 Part of treatment may include activities to help the client, not others.

2 The client usually understands this already.

3 This would only mask symptoms and would not get at the root of what is bothering the client.

184. **4 Accepting these clients and their symptomatic behavior sets the foundation for the nurse-client relationship. Setting limits provides external controls and helps lower anxiety. (PL; TC; PR)**

1 Restricting movements would have no effect other than to increase anxiety.

2 This will only increase their anxiety and increase their use of the behavior.

3 This is unrealistic.

185. **4 The client's exact compliance in carrying out the compulsive ritual relieves anxiety, at least temporarily. Furthermore, it meets a need and is necessary to the client. (AN; PS; PR)**

1 The person cannot stop the activity; it is not under voluntary control.

2 The compulsive act is purposeless repetition and useful only in that it decreases anxiety for the client.

3 Urging has no effect on trying to have the client start or stop the ritualistic behavior.

186. **2 This sets limits, points out reality, and places responsibility for behavior on the client. (IM; PS; PR)**

1 This is a punishing response and endangers the trust relationship.

3 Clients such as this need limits set; changing the time shows inconsistency.

4 The nurse using this response is showing inconsistency, endangering the trust relationship, and using a threat to gain control.

187. **2 Everyone has the right to personal sexual preference, but limits must be set on acting-out behavior within the hospital. (IM; TC; PR)**

1 This would be a punishing attitude, especially for the client who would be transferred.

3 Limits would need to be set; punishment is inappropriate.

4 This is not a realistic approach to the situation.

188. **3 Dissociation is defined as handling emotional conflicts, or internal or external stressors, by a temporary alteration of consciousness or identity. (AN; PS; PD)**

1 Projection is attributing one's own unacceptable feelings and thoughts to others.

2 Repression is unconsciously keeping unacceptable feelings out of awareness.

4 Suppression is consciously keeping unacceptable feelings and thoughts out of awareness.

Crisis Situations

189. **3 The sympathetic nervous system reacts to stress by releasing epinephrine, which prepares the body to fight or flee by increasing the heart rate, constricting peripheral vessels, and increasing oxygen supply to the muscles. (AN; PA; CS)**

1 Although the brain responds to stress, it is the sympathetic nervous system that is primarily affected.

2 The sympathetic and parasympathetic nervous systems are both part of the peripheral nervous system; the sympathetic nervous system is primarily affected; the parasympathetic nervous system does not play a role in the fight or flight reaction.

4 This has an effect opposite to that of the sympathetic nervous system.

190. **4** **Feelings of resentment toward children by parents is a normal response. To relieve feelings of guilt and shame, it is vital to help parents realize this. (IM; PS; CS)**
    1 The first child causes the greatest amount of adjustment in one's life.
    2 These are normal feelings.
    3 This is an untrue generalization.

191. **4** **The ego develops during childhood as a result of positive experiences. When the situation in childhood is such that severe anxiety is unresolved, the ego seems to be permanently traumatized and is unable to recover totally. (AN; PS; CS)**
    1 This in itself would not necessarily be traumatic unless abuse was also present.
    2 This would have no effect.
    3 This is a normal occurrence; children are often unable to verbalize their feelings and play therapy is utilized for that reason.

192. **2** **Toddlers struggle to identify their own needs. Too early and too strict toilet training results in ambivalence because toddler's needs and physical abilities are in conflict with parental demands. Toddlers are faced with giving up these needs or risking parental disapproval. (AN; PS; CS)**
    1 Children are involved from birth in satisfying their own needs.
    3 Children are involved from birth in satisfying their parents' needs, but toilet training is really the first time a conflict develops.
    4 A child has no interest in society's expectations.

193. **1** **A person able to cope with life situations usually has developed fairly strong ego defenses. In a crisis situation the individual frequently just needs support to regroup strengths and reestablish the ability to cope. (IM; PS; CS)**
    2 Socialization would be part of recovery, not the crisis stage.
    3 This is not possible or realistic.
    4 This might have the effect of increasing anxiety, thereby making the crisis situation worse.

194. **4** **The client is in the hospital for treatment and evaluation, not judgment of behavior. Because the client feels people are judging, it is important to point out that at this time the only one filling this role is the client. (IM; TC; CS)**
    1 This statement ignores feelings and does not help the client deal with the situation.

    2 This may or may not be true and could be false reassurance.
    3 The nurse does not know this to be a fact.

195. **4** **This statement lets the client know the nurse realizes the client is having difficulty without asking direct questions or focusing on specific behavior. (IM; TC; CS)**
    1 This is an avoidance technique.
    2 This response is stated more like an order than an offering of an opportunity to express feelings.
    3 This would be negating the client's feelings.

196. **2** **Identifying and accepting feelings help to open lines of communication. (IM; PS; CS)**
    1 This does not allow the client to explore feelings with an accepting person.
    3 This is avoiding the real issue.
    4 This focuses on only one aspect of the statement; it does not allow exploration of feelings.

197. **2** **During a crisis one may regress to a stage provoking less anxiety in an attempt to cope with an unacceptable situation. (AN; PS; CS)**
    1 Clients may use denial during an illness, but this would not make them dependent and demanding.
    3 This is a normal defense mechanism; it is not used specifically during times of illness.
    4 This compensatory mechanism would cause a person to try to make amends, not become more dependent and demanding.

198. **1** **Identifying feelings and providing support during stressful times are both ways of demonstrating concern during a crisis. (IM; PS; CS)**
    2 This is not a supportive or insightful reply.
    3 This is an inappropriate reply that may instill guilt feelings; the father as well as the mother need support through this crisis.
    4 Same as answer 2.

199. **1** **The therapeutic regimen includes bed rest; peace of mind can best be achieved if the children are adequately cared for. (IM; PS; CS)**
    2 This explores feelings without including the therapeutic regimen.
    3 Complete bed rest has been prescribed.
    4 This is giving solutions rather than exploring the situation with the client.

200. **2** **Denial or disbelief and shock are considered initial responses of grieving. There is**

a feeling of guilt and inadequacy when a child is born with a defect or abnormality. (DC; PS; CS)

1 It would be unusual for a client initially to verbalize feelings of punishment or guilt so directly.

3 A sense of shame and guilt is voiced later; after denial, disbelief, and shock.

4 It would be unusual for a client to use rationalization and voice it so obviously.

201. **2 This action demonstrates recognition of the client's behavior as a normal response to the situation.** (IM; PS; CS)

1 This may make the client feel that the behavior is wrong or is annoying others.

3 This closes off communication and does not allow the client to talk about feelings.

4 This may be done later; the need to respond to the client's feelings is the priority at this time.

202. **4 This is a true statement since the client was admitted under a voluntary status and is responsible for the cost of hospitalization.** (AN; TC; CS)

1 This would not be true if the client was admitted voluntarily.

2 Same as answer 1.

3 Same as answer 1.

203. **1 The client's behavior indicates that a problem is occurring in response to the therapy group. The nurse should assess whether participating in the group is creating a crisis for the client.** (DC; TC; CS)

2 There are no data to suggest the client is disoriented.

3 There are no data to suggest the client is using confabulation.

4 There are no data to suggest the client is hallucinating.

Emotional Problems Related to Physical Health and Childbearing

204. **4 Insomnia is often caused by anxiety. By stating an observation about the client's activity, the nurse communicates both concern and a recognition that there may be more covert problems that the client wishes to verbalize.** (IM; PS; EP)

1 This denies the client's request and serves to cut off communication.

2 Same as answer 1.

3 Same as answer 1.

205. **2 The usual initial response to a crisis situation such as this is denial that it could occur and that she and her husband could produce a less than normal child. The mother's response is her way of dealing with the reality of the situation.** (EV; PS; CS)

1 Although the mother initially rejected her baby, time and coping may help her accept the anomaly.

3 First reactions to a child with a congenital anomaly cannot be judged as final.

4 The mother's reaction is a normal part of the grief response.

206. **4 When the parents can verbalize a recognition that their infant may have present or future problems, it usually signifies that they are beginning to face reality.** (EV; PS; CS)

1 This is not a problem specifically related to an infant with a genetic disorder. It is therefore not the most significant factor for the nurse working with this particular family.

2 Although this may have an effect on the parents' reaction to their infant, it is probably not critically significant to the nurse at this time.

3 This would be after the fact for this infant; it is not the most significant factor to be considered by the nurse at this time.

207. **2 This provides for collection of more data.** (DC; PS; CS)

1 This implies that things are not well, and the mother may be to blame.

3 This could make the mother feel guilty about not meeting her baby's needs.

4 This is a negative comment that closes communication.

208. **1 Sitting down shows the client that the nurse cares enough to spend time. It also opens up channels of communication.** (IM; PS; CS)

2 The nurse sets dimensions on the mother's feelings; this does not promote free expression of feelings.

3 This statement provides false hope; the possibility of the diagnosis has been introduced.

4 This statement ignores the mother's need to express feelings; it takes a cognitive approach to the problem.

209. **3 This action provides the best reassurance as long as the parents know what to expect in the recovery room.** (IM; PS; EP)

1 If a recovery room visit were not possible, this would be the next best action.

2 This action might increase the mother's anxiety; seeing her child would be more therapeutic.

4 There is an immediate need to reduce the parents' anxiety; having coffee will not meet this need.

210. **4 The client's statement is really saying, "I can manage this myself. I am capable."** (DC; PS; EP)

1 Nothing in the statement can be interpreted as denial; the client has stated, "I know I'm sick."

2 None of the information given would lead to this conclusion.

3 The statement would not be reassuring to the family member who brought the client to the hospital and who probably is more reassured having the client hospitalized.

211. **3 This response recognizes fearful feelings. It also permits further communication.** (IM; PS; EP)

1 This response does not recognize feelings; instills fear by implying that this pregnancy may not go to term, for which there is no evidence.

2 This response does not recognize feelings of fear and changes the focus of the conversation.

4 This response closes off communication and may increase anxiety and guilt.

212. **2 Incontinence without a physiologic basis is an act of hostility that the individual uses to deal with anxiety-producing situations.** (AN; PS; EP)

1 Incontinence is often seen as a symbol of regression and loss of control.

3 Incontinence is rarely the result of conscious effort.

4 Incontinence is not a necessary complication of age and inactivity; it can be prevented by a bladder-training program.

Drug-related Responses

213. **3 Succinylcholine chloride temporarily paralyzes the muscles, including those of respiration. Therefore some artificial means of respiration is necessary until the drug is metabolized and excreted.** (AN; PA; DR)

1 This prevents the complication of respiratory acidosis.

2 The most significant therapeutic factor in ECT is the seizure itself.

4 Brevital sodium decreases the occurrence of fractures; the drug is rapidly excreted with few side effects.

214. **4 The development of glaucoma is one of the side effects of imipramine (Tofranil), and the client should be alerted to the symptoms.** (IM; TC; DR)

1 This is true of monamine oxidase inhibitors (MAOIs).

2 Tofranil is not an MAOI.

3 This would be essential for a person being treated with lithium.

215. **1 Jaundice signifies liver function interference and requires stopping the medication.** (EV; TC; DR)

2 This symptom usually subsides after several weeks of treatment.

3 Same as answer 2.

4 These symptoms usually require that the dose be reduced; if symptoms do not subside, the drug is stopped.

216. **3 Lithium carbonate does not impair intellectual activity, consciousness, or range or quality of emotional life. However, it can control the manic phase of a bipolar disorder.** (AN; PA; DR)

1 Lithium is not used for schizophrenia.

2 Lithium is not used for agitated paranoid states.

4 Lithium is not used for major depressions except with a history of at least one manic episode or a family history of manic disorders.

217. **3 Lithium carbonate alters sodium transport in nerve and muscle cells and causes a shift toward intraneuronal metabolism of catecholamines. Since the range between therapeutic and toxic levels is very small, the client's serum lithium level should be monitored closely.** (EV; PA; DR)

1 This is not necessary or useful.

2 Sodium restriction may cause electrolyte imbalance and lithium toxicity.

4 This is not necessary; it would depend on what the client was receiving.

218. **4 This medication can be given IM every 2 weeks for clients who cannot be relied**

upon to take oral medications; it allows them to live in the community while keeping the symptoms under control. (PL; TC; DR)

1 This medication must be taken on a daily basis.
2 Same as answer 1.
3 This medication is not used for the treatment of schizophrenia.

219. 1 **The neuroleptics modify the behavior of psychotic clients so they can more effectively cope with the environment and benefit from therapy. (AN; TC; DR)**
2 Antidepressants are used for depression.
3 Ritalin is used to treat children with attention deficit hyperactivity disorders; neuroleptics decrease the severity of psychotic symptoms.
4 Neuroleptics are contraindicated during narcotic withdrawal.

220. 3 **This occurs as a late and persistent extrapyramidal complication of long-term chlorpromazine therapy. It can take many forms (e.g., torsion spasm, opisthotonos, oculogyric crisis, drooping of the head, protrusion of the tongue). (EV; TC; DR)**
1 This is reversible with administration of Cogentin and Benadryl.
2 Same as answer 1.
4 Same as answer 1.

221. 2 **Acute dystonic reactions, parkinsonian syndrome, dyskinesia, and akathisia are observable side effects of chlorpromazine hydrochloride therapy. (EV; TC; DR)**
1 After the first few days of treatment, Thorazine has no effect on concentration or other mental abilities; there would be a decrease, not an increase, in salivation.
3 These are not side effects of neuroleptics.
4 Same as answer 3.

222. 4 **Unintentional tremors are one of the extrapyramidal side effects of the neuroleptics and are considered common and manageable. (EV; PA; DR)**
1 This is not a common side effect.
2 This is a severe but not a common occurrence; periodic liver function tests should be done.
3 This is not applicable; an excessive number of melanocytes is not a side effect.

223. 3 **These drugs are used to control the extrapyramidal (parkinsonism-like) symptoms that often develop as a side effect of neuroleptic therapy. (AN; TC; DR)**

1 Barbiturates do not have extrapyramidal side effects, which would respond to these drugs.
2 Antiparkinsonian drugs such as Cogentin are not usually prescribed in conjunction with antidepressants; gastrointestinal tract depression can result in paralytic ileus.
4 There is no documented use of these drugs with antianxiety agents because they do not have extrapyramidal side effects.

224. 3 **These drugs control the extrapyramidal (parkinsonism-like) symptoms associated with the neuroleptics and are classified as antiparkinsonian drugs. (EV; TC; DR)**
1 These have no effect on postural hypotension.
2 These drugs do not potentiate phenothiazine derivatives.
4 These drugs have no effect on depression.

225. 1 **Improvement is usually seen within 48 hours to 3 weeks with this monamine oxidase inhibitor (MAOI). (IM; TC; DR)**
2 This is not true; this medication works within 48 hours to 3 weeks.
3 The client may need a longer time to see an effect from this medication.
4 Same as answer 2.

226. 3 **Wine, aged cheese, and other foods with a high tyramine level must be avoided. (PL; TC; DR)**
1 This is not an expected side effect but can occur as an adverse reaction.
2 No photosensitivity has been reported in clients on this medication.
4 This is not true for this medication.

227. 2 **An occipital headache is the beginning of a hypertensive crisis that results from excessive tyramine. (EV; TC; DR)**
1 This is unrelated to the ingestion of tyramine.
3 These are unrelated to the ingestion of tyramine.
4 Excessive tyramine would cause a rise in blood pressure, not a drop.

228. 1 **The liquid concentrate is a highly irritating substance on contact with skin and eyes and can cause uncomfortable dermatologic conditions. (IM; TC; DR)**
2 This is not necessary; leaving it unmixed provides greater assurance that the client will ingest the full dose of Thorazine.
3 This is not necessary for drug stability.
4 There is no indication for this precaution.

229. 4 Clients taking chlorpromazine should be told to stay out of the sun. Photosensitivity makes the skin more susceptible to burning. (IM; TC; DR)
1 Photosensitivity is not a side effect of lithium.
2 Photosensitivity is reported as being extremely rare with this drug.
3 Photosensitivity is not reported with the use of Ritalin.

230. 2 Liver damage is a well-documented toxic side effect of the neuroleptics. By continuing to administer the drug, the nurse failed to use professional knowledge in the performance of responsibilities as outlined in the Nurse Practice Act. (EV; PA; DR)
1 This is false; liver damage, indicated by jaundice, is a well-documented side effect.
3 This is false; blood levels must be reduced when signs of liver damage are present.
4 The neuroleptics should be stopped, not reduced; liver damage is a well-documented toxic side effect.

231. 3 The physician is responsible for medication orders but depends on the nurse's observations before making decisions. (EV; TC; DR)
1 This is not a severe enough symptom to warrant withholding the drug.
2 It is a reaction to the Thorazine and must be treated.
4 This would have no effect on the tremors.

232. 3 This checks functioning of the liver; liver damage may occur from use of the drug. Cholestatic hepatitis with obstructive jaundice is the most frequent form of liver disturbance and can be identified by yellow sclerae and clay-colored stools. (EV; TC; DR)
1 Anorexia is not a side effect of Thorazine; clients frequently gain weight.
2 Hypertension and headaches do not occur.
4 Numbness and coldness of the feet do not occur.

233. 2 The monoamine oxidase inhibitors can cause a hypertensive crisis if food or beverages that are high in tyramine are ingested. (IM; TC; DR)
1 This would be important for clients taking one of the phenothiazines.
3 This is not contraindicated.

4 An elixir base only makes the medications more palatable; alcohol, not wine, is used in elixirs.

234. 2 The withdrawal regimen is usually gradually decreasing doses of a barbiturate to prevent the severe symptoms associated with barbiturate withdrawal. (PL; TC; DR)
1 This drug is used in the treatment of mood disorders.
3 This drug is used for narcotic addiction withdrawal.
4 This drug is contraindicated in the presence of central nervous system depressants.

235. 4 This is a serious side effect that may happen with abrupt withdrawal from barbiturates. (EV; TC; DR)
1 This is not associated with barbiturate withdrawal.
2 Same as answer 1.
3 Same as answer 1.

236. 2 Naloxone hydrochloride (Narcan) is a narcotic antagonist that counteracts and reverses the respiratory depressive action of narcotics without causing sedation or analgesia; nalorphine (Nalline) could also be used but can precipitate a severe withdrawal reaction. (AN; TC; DR)
1 This is a CNS stimulant with no therapeutic use for a narcotic overdose.
3 Same as answer 1.
4 Same as answer 1.

237. 1 Narcan is used when narcotic-induced apnea occurs. It competes for CNS receptor sites, thus acting as a narcotic antagonist. (EV; PA; DR)
2 This is not the specific action of this drug; it prevents respiratory arrest.
3 Narcan does not accelerate the metabolism of heroin; it competes for CNS receptor sites.
4 An adverse reaction is cardiovascular irritability.

238. 3 When Narcan is metabolized and its effects are diminished, the respiratory distress caused by the original drug overdose returns. (EV; TC; DR)
1 There is no known report of this.
2 Narcan counteracts the respiratory depression from heroin overdose.
4 This is not a known effect after use of Narcan.

Therapeutic Relationships

239. **1 An important aspect of the role of the psychiatric nurse is primary, secondary, and tertiary intervention to prevent emotional disequilibrium. (AN; PS; TR)**
  2 This is only a small part of the role of the psychiatric nurse, a role usually shared with others on the health team.
  3 Same as answer 2.
  4 This is only a part of the role of the psychiatric nurse, since psychiatry is concerned with people with varying degrees of mental and emotional disorders.

240. **2 It is the inability to meet these needs that will cause a person to become mentally ill. (DC; PS; TR)**
  1 This is not necessary to be mentally healthy.
  3 To be considered mentally healthy a person must be more than just free from illness.
  4 This would rule out most of the population.

241. **2 The individual who cannot communicate cannot test reality. Without this connection to others or reality, severe emotional problems will develop. (AN; PS; TR)**
  1 Lack of communication can lead to isolation and withdrawal, but this response is too narrow because a variety of problems usually develop.
  3 Without the stimulation of communication, mental dullness or slowness will occur, not mental deficiency.
  4 There is a frustration and inability to foster communication.

242. **3 Sharing problems with others who have similar problems, thoughts, and feelings helps the individual learn new ways of coping. (AN; PS; TR)**
  1 Emotional illness is not enough; the person must recognize that a problem exists and help is necessary.
  2 All people are dependent on others to some degree; this would not be a criterion for group therapy.
  4 This might be partly true, but the person should still feel the need for help in coping with a problem.

243. **3 The nurse's major tool in psychiatric nursing is the therapeutic use of self. Psychiatric nurses must learn to be aware of their own feelings and how they affect the situation. (EV; TC; TR)**
  1 This may be true, but an awareness of self still seems the most difficult.
  2 This may be true but is not part of the nurse-client relationship.
  4 This implies that the nurse is working alone in planning care for the client.

244. **2 The role of stranger is the initial role in any relationship. (PL; PS; TR)**
  1 If the nurse moves in too quickly, future relationships may be severely hampered.
  3 Same as answer 1.
  4 Same as answer 1.

245. **3 Orienting the client to the hospital provides knowledge that may reduce the strangeness of the environment, and introducing staff members lets the client know who will be providing care. (IM; PS; TR)**
  1 This may be false reassurance, because no one can guarantee that everything will be all right.
  2 This would be part of orienting the client to the unit.
  4 This implies that staff members are available only if the client becomes upset.

246. **1 This response invited the client to explore the issue in more depth by focusing on it. (IM; PS; TR)**
  2 Clarifying is a technique used to ask the client to give an example to better understand the nature of the client's statement.
  3 Reflecting is a technique used to either reiterate the content or the feeling message; in content reflection, the nurse repeats basically the same statement; in feeling reflection, the nurse verbalizes what seems to be implied about feelings in the comment.
  4 This is incorrect; refocusing is to bring the subject back to a previous point; there is no information that this was discussed previously.

247. **2 The group setting provides the individual with the opportunity to learn that others share the same problems and needs. The group also provides an arena where new, healthier methods of relating to others can be tried. (PL; PS; TR)**
  1 Groups promote interaction among many people, rather than one-to-one relationships.
  3 The focus is still on the individual, but more on the individual's learning how to relate to others.
  4 This may happen from time to time with support given to the individual by the group, but it is not a main function of the group.

248. **4 Group therapy should focus on the present and how current problems and feelings are affecting current behavior. In the group setting the individual members have the opportunity to receive feedback on their behavior. (PL; PS; TR)**
1 The nurse focuses not on the stress itself, but on how to deal with the stress.
2 The focus is the feelings behind the behavior with which others can identify.
3 The nurse must protect individual group members from confrontation until certain that they are strong enough to deal with it.

249. **4 Self-help groups deal with behavior and changes in behavior rather than the underlying causes of behavior. Small steps are encouraged and when attained are reinforced by the group. (AN; TC; TR)**
1 On the contrary, they deal with 1 day at a time.
2 Help to identify with the people in the group is not necessary because they all share the same problem and identify readily.
3 This is not the purpose of this group.

250. **2 Self-help groups are successful because they support a basic human need for acceptance. A feeling of comfort and safety and a sense of belonging may be achieved in a nonjudgmental, supportive, sharing experience with others. (AN; TC; TR)**
1 If the client had a need to grow, AA would probably not be able to meet this need.
3 AA would not meet the client's need to be trusted.
4 On the contrary, AA meets dependency needs rather than focusing on independence.

251. **2 Sharing problems with others who are also open and concerned because of similar problems can reduce guilt and shame and begin to increase ego strengths. (EV; TC; TR)**
1 AA is viewed by some as a crutch in itself.
3 Although AA is a support group, it is a self-help support group.
4 Their problem drinking is usually caused by how they feel about themselves.

252. **4 The nurse's response urges the client to reflect on feelings and encourages the communication of feeling tones. (IM; PS; TR)**
1 This is shifting responsibility from the nurse to the doctor; it is an evasion technique.

2 This is not what the client is asking the nurse; it closes the door to further communication.
3 "Why" asks the client to draw a conclusion, which this client may not be able to do.

253. **4 This is a reflection of feelings that allows the client to either validate or correct the nurse. (IM; PS; TR)**
1 This delays confronting the problem and avoids exploring feelings.
2 This is a response that gives advice and does not allow the client to explore feelings.
3 This is an uncalled-for statement that does not allow the client to explore feelings.

254. **3 This permits the client to see that personal feelings are not unique but are shared by others. (IM; TC; TR)**
1 This statement makes the client worry about not feeling happy.
2 This is a nonsupportive remark to a realistic fear of leaving the safe hospital and going back to where problems must be dealt with.
4 How the others feel about whether the client is ready to be discharged is totally irrelevant.

255. **1 This response allows the group as a whole to explore the common issue of concern. (IM; PS; TR)**
2 This response would be appropriate in one to one therapy.
3 This is a closed question to Jason that doesn't include the group.
4 This response would encourage a dialogue between two group members but would exclude the rest of the group.

256. **3 The day-care center provides the client with a therapeutic setting for a few hours daily during the transitional stage between hospital and total discharge. (AN; PS; TR)**
1 This would have little or no effect on social skills.
2 Day-care treatment would meet this goal, but that is not its primary purpose.
4 This does help during the transition stage, but it is not the primary goal of day care.

257. **2 The client has the right to make this decision and the staff should accept the client's wishes. (IM; PS; TR)**
1 The client is a doctor, and the nurse's statement attacks the client's self-concept.
3 It helps support clients' dignity by addressing them as they wish.
4 For whom is it better—the staff, the other clients, or the client?

258. **4 The first step in a nursing care plan should be the establishment of a meaningful relationship because it is through this relationship that the client can be helped. (AN; PS; TR)**
1 Encouraging this behavior would not be therapeutic.
2 This would be a long-term goal.
3 Reduction of stimuli may limit the hallucinations, but there is no evidence the client is not eating meals.

259. **4 The client is expressing hostility symbolically by not being cooperative. The client has a right to feel this way. If members of the staff criticize, it will only increase the client's feeling of guilt. (IM; PS; TR)**
1 This would allow the client to manipulate the environment.
2 This will not change the client's mind about the activities. This response does not show an understanding of the client's needs.
3 This will only serve to increase feelings of guilt because the client is unaware of the hostility.

260. **4 Ambivalence about life and death plus the introspection commonly found in clients with emotional problems would lead to increased anxiety and fear in the group members. (PL; TC; TR)**
1 This will probably be a secondary goal of the group leader.
2 It is not a primary goal; but this lack of concern should also be explored later on to see what is behind such apparent indifference, which may be a mask to cover feelings.
3 These feelings must be handled within the support and supervisory systems for the staff; the other group members are the primary concern.

261. **1 This statement recognizes the importance of feelings and provides an opening so the client may talk about them. (EV; TC; TR)**
2 The client is not going to believe this, and it is not helping the client express feelings.
3 The nursing goal is to help people function outside the hospital environment, not be afraid to leave it.
4 A statement like this avoids the real issue and solves nothing.

262. **3 This puts the focus on feelings, not on a statement of what did or did not happen. (IM; TC; TR)**
1 This statement implies that the client may have had some part in causing another person's death.
2 This statement does not give the client an opportunity to explore feelings.
4 This statement closes the door to any further communication of feelings or fears.

263. **4 Bringing another client into a set situation would be the most therapeutic, least threatening approach. (IM; TC; TR)**
1 At this point in time, it would not be therapeutic to allow the client to remain with solitary pursuits.
2 Explanations will not necessarily change behavior.
3 This transfers nursing responsibility to the physician.

264. **4 This statement points out reality while accepting the fact that the client believes the feelings and thoughts are real. (IM; PS; TR)**
1 This is false reassurance that the nurse does not know as fact.
2 The client does not know this and believes the opposite to be true.
3 This is reality but it is not a supportive response.

265. **2 This simply states facts without getting involved in role conflict. (IM; PS; TR)**
1 Being a doctor is a big part of this client's self-esteem, and by this remark the nurse is threatening that self-esteem.
3 Firm, consistent limits need to be set and the nurse-client role established.
4 Threats will only make the situation worse and set the tone for future nurse-client interactions.

266. **4 The client's early arrival indicates an expected degree of anxiety; the quiet waiting indicates that the client has been told what to expect. (EV; ED; TR)**
1 This would indicate an inadequate explanation or the inability of the client to remember the explanation that had been given.
2 This indicates a high degree of anxiety that may denote a fear of the tests because they were not adequately explained.
3 Same as answer 2.

267. 1 It is the most effective method for the child to play out feelings; when feelings are allowed to surface, the child can then learn to face them by controlling, accepting, or abandoning them; through this process, the child can experience growth. (AN; PS; TR)

2 This is not child specific and generally is more suited for adolescents, young adults, and adults.

3 Same as answer 2.

4 Same as answer 2.

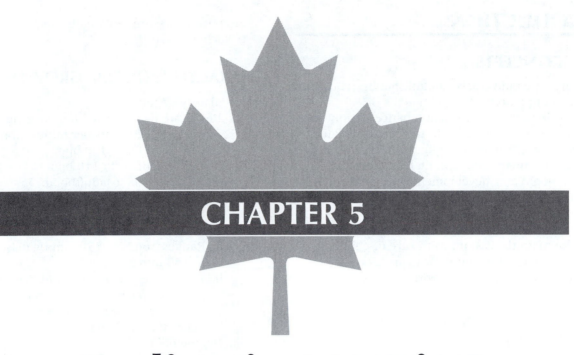

CHAPTER 5

Pediatric Nursing

Pediatric nursing encompasses the care of well children and those who are acutely and chronically ill, stressing both preventive and restorative interventions. This section is divided into the descriptive age groups of childhood; that is, infancy, toddlerhood, preschool years, school-age years, and adolescence. Principles of growth and development, age-specific achievements, health maintenance objectives, and disease-related states are discussed for each age category. Such an organization attempts to present the nursing of children as one that incorporates their physical and psychologic needs toward optimum promotion of health.

INTRODUCTION

BASIC CONCEPTS

A. Children are individuals, not little adults, who must be seen as part of a family
B. To provide total health maintenance, family-centered care is the objective in the care of children
C. Children are influenced by genetic factors, home and environment, and parental attitudes
D. Chronologic and developmental ages of children are the most important contributing factors influencing their care
E. Prevention of illness and maintenance of health are the main thrusts in health care of children
F. Play is a natural medium for expression, communication, and growth in children

HUMAN GROWTH AND DEVELOPMENT

PRINCIPLES OF GROWTH

A. Traditional definition of growth is limited to physical maturation
B. Integrated definition includes functional maturation
C. Growth is complex with all aspects closely related
D. Growth is measured both quantitatively and qualitatively over a period of time
E. Although the rate is not even, growth is a continuous and orderly process
   1. Infancy: most rapid period of growth
   2. Preschool to puberty: slow and uniform rate of growth
   3. Puberty: (growth spurt) second most rapid growth period
   4. After puberty: decline in growth rate till death
F. There are regular patterns in the direction of growth and development, such as the cephalocaudal law (from head to toe) and the proximodistal law (from center of body to periphery)
G. Different parts of the body grow at different rates
   1. Prenatally: head grows the fastest
   2. During the first year: elongation of trunk dominates
H. Both rate and pattern of growth can be modified, most obviously by nutrition
I. There are critical or sensitive periods in growth and development, such as brain growth during uterine life and infancy
J. Although there are specified sequences for achieving growth and development, each individual proceeds at own rate
K. Development is closely related to the maturation of the nervous system; as some primitive reflexes disappear, they are replaced by a voluntary activity such as grasp

CHARACTERISTICS OF GROWTH

A. Circulatory system
   1. Heart rate decreases with increasing age
      a. Infancy: 120 beats per minute (bpm)
      b. One year: 80 to 120 bpm
      c. Childhood: 70 to 110 bpm
      d. Adolescence to adulthood: 55 to 90 bpm (after maturity, women have slightly higher pulse rate than men)
   2. Blood pressure increases with age
      a. Ranges from 40 to 70 mm Hg diastolic to 65 to 140 mm Hg systolic
      b. These levels increase about 2 to 3 mm Hg per year starting at age 7 years
      c. Systolic pressure in adolescence: higher in males than in females
   3. Hemoglobin
      a. Highest at birth, 170 g/L; then decreases to 100 to 150 g/L by 1 year
      b. Fetal hemoglobin (60% to 90% of total hemoglobin) gradually decreases during the first year to less than 5%
      c. Gradual increase in hemoglobin level to 145 g/L between 1 and 12 years of age
      d. Level higher in males than in females
B. Respiratory system
   1. Rate decreases with increase in age
      a. Infancy: 30 to 40 per minute
      b. Childhood: 20 to 24 per minute
      c. Adolescence and adulthood: 16 to 18 per minute
   2. Vital capacity
      a. Gradual increase throughout childhood and adolescence, with a decrease in later life
      b. Capacity in males exceeds that in females
   3. Basal metabolism
      a. Highest rate is found in the newborn
      b. Rate declines with increase in age; higher in males than in females
C. Urinary system
   1. Premature and full-term newborns have some inability to concentrate urine
      a. Specific gravity (newborn): 1.001 to 1.02
      b. Specific gravity (others): 1.001 to 1.03
   2. Glomerular filtration rate greatly increased by 6 months of age
   3. Glomerular filtration rate reaches adult values between 1 and 2 years of age
   4. Glomerular filtration rate gradually decreases after 20 years of age
D. Digestive system
   1. Stomach size is small at birth; rapidly increases during infancy and childhood

2. Peristaltic activity decreases with advancing age
3. Blood glucose levels gradually rise from 4.2 to 4.5 mmol/L of blood in infancy to 5.3 to 5.6 mmol/L during adolescence
4. Premature infants have lower blood glucose levels than do full-term infants
5. Enzymes are present at birth to digest proteins and a moderate amount of fat, but only simple sugars (amylase is produced as starch is introduced)
6. Secretion of hydrochloric acid and salivary enzymes increases with age until adolescence; then decreases with advancing age
E. Nervous system
   1. Brain reaches 90% of total size by 2 years of age
   2. All brain cells are present by end of the first year, although their size and complexity will increase
   3. Maturation of the brainstem and spinal cord follows cephalocaudal and proximodistal laws
F. Impact on medications
   1. Pediatric dosages differ from adult medication dosages as a result of differences in physiology
      a. Immature liver function
      b. Immature kidney function
      c. Decreased gastric function
      d. Decreased plasma protein concentration
      e. Altered body composition
         (1) Decreased fat
         (2) Increased water
   2. Calculate dosage based on body surface area (m^2) or weight (mg/kg) to ensure that the child receives the correct drug dosage within a safe therapeutic range
   3. Dosage can also be calculated based on body weight, although it is not as accurate as surface area
      a. For most drugs the difference in calculated dosage is not significant
      b. Children at either higher or lower growth chart percentiles will have the greatest difference
   4. Child must be closely monitored for signs and symptoms of toxicity. Long-term dosages change as the result of growth

PLAY

Functions of Play

A. Educational
B. Recreational
C. Physical development
D. Social and emotional adjustment
   1. Learn moral values
   2. Develop the idea of sharing
E. Therapeutic

Types of Play

A. Active, physical
   1. Push-and-pull toys
   2. Riding toys
   3. Sports and gym equipment
B. Manipulative, constructive, creative, or scientific
   1. Blocks
   2. Construction toys such as erector sets
   3. Drawing sets
   4. Microscope and chemistry sets
   5. Books
   6. Computer programs
C. Imitative, imaginative, and dramatic
   1. Dolls
   2. Dress-up costumes
   3. Puppets
   4. Music
D. Competitive and social
   1. Games
   2. Role playing
   3. Digital games

Criteria for Judging the Suitability of Toys

A. Safety
B. Compatibility
   1. Child's age
   2. Level of development
   3. Experience
C. Usefulness
   1. Challenge to development of the child
   2. Enhancing social and personality development
   3. Increasing motor and sensory skills
   4. Developing creativity
   5. Expressing emotions
   6. Achieving mastery/knowledge
   7. Implementing therapeutic procedures

Criteria for Judging the Nonsuitability of Toys

A. Unsafe
B. Beyond the child's level of growth and development
C. Overstimulating; frustrating
D. Limited uses and transient value (see play for each age group)
E. Foster isolation from peer group
F. Violence

THE FAMILY

STRUCTURE OF THE FAMILY

A. The basic unit of a society
B. Composition varies, although one member is usually recognized as head
C. Usually share common goals and beliefs
D. Roles change within the group and reflect both the individual's and the group's needs

E. Status of members determined by position in family in conjunction with views of society

FUNCTIONS OF THE FAMILY

A. Reproduction: group developed to reproduce and rear members of a society
B. Maintenance to provide
   1. Basic needs, clothing, housing, food, and medical care
   2. Social, psychologic, and emotional support for family members
   3. Protection, because immaturity of young children necessitates that care be given by adults
   4. Status: child is a member of a family that is also a part of the larger community
   5. Buffer to the world
C. Socialization
   1. Child is "acculturated" by introduction to social situations and instruction in appropriate social behaviors
   2. Self-identity develops through relationships with other family members
   3. Child learns appropriate sex roles and responsibilities
D. Growth of individual members toward maturity and independence

THE FAMILY OF AN INFANT OR CHILD WITH SPECIAL NEEDS

MEETING THE NEEDS OF THE FAMILY OF AN INFANT OR CHILD WITH SPECIAL NEEDS

A. Recognize that members of the family will exhibit a variety of responses, such as grief and mourning, chronic grief, and excessive use of defense mechanisms
B. Understand the stages of chronic grief
   1. Shock and disbelief: parents tend to:
      a. Learn about the deformity but deny the facts
      b. Feel inadequate and guilty
      c. Feel insecure in their ability to care for the child
      d. "Doctor shop" in hope of finding solutions
   2. Awareness of the special needs: parents tend to:
      a. Feel guilty, angry, and depressed
      b. Envy well children: closely related to bitterness and anger
      c. Search for clues or reasons why this happened to them
      d. Reject and feel ambivalent toward the child
   3. Restitution or recovery phase: parents tend to:
      a. See the child's special needs in proper perspective

b. Function more effectively and realistically
c. Socially and emotionally accept the child
d. Reintegrate family life without centering it around the child

C. Help parents and siblings gain awareness of the child's special needs
   1. Learning cannot take place until awareness of the problem exists
   2. Help the parents develop an awareness through their own realization of the problem rather than identifying problem for them
   3. Help the parents see the problem by drawing attention to certain manifestations such as failure to walk or talk
   4. Allow family to acknowledge difficulty at own pace, if reasonable
D. Help the family understand the child's potential ability and assist them in setting realistic goals
   1. Help family feel a sense of adequacy in parenting by emphasizing good care, identifying small steps in learning process of child, and acquainting them with parents of children with similar problems
   2. Teach family how to work with their child in simple childhood tasks of sitting, walking, talking, toileting, feeding, and dressing
   3. Teach family how to stimulate the child's learning of new skills
E. Encourage the parents to treat the child as normally as possible
   1. Encourage them to avoid overprotection and to use consistent, simple discipline
   2. Help them become aware of the effects of this child on siblings, who may resent the excessive attention given to this child
F. Provide the family with an outlet for own emotional tensions and needs
   1. Acquaint them with organizations, especially groups of parents who have children with similar problems
   2. Be a listener, not a preacher
   3. Assist siblings who may fear the possibility of giving birth to children with similar problems or fear catching the illness
G. Teach parents the importance of follow-up and long-term medical supervision
H. Evaluate clients' response and revise plan as necessary

GENERAL NURSING DIAGNOSES FOR THE FAMILY OF A CHILD WITH SPECIAL NEEDS

A. Risk for altered parent infant/child attachment related to:
   1. Loss of image of ideal child

2. Child's physical condition that limits handling or fondling
3. Inability of parents to meet child's special needs
B. Risk for caregiver role strain
C. Family coping: potential for growth, related to child's ability and care
D. Decisional conflict related to:
   1. Need for medical therapies
   2. Proposed care for child
E. Risk for disorganized infant behavior related to:
   1. Pain
   2. Oral/motor problems
   3. Invasive procedures
F. Diversional activity deficit related to inadequate support systems to provide respite
G. Fatigue related to care requirements of child with special needs
H. Anticipatory grieving related to:
   1. Loss of image of ideal child
   2. Projected death of child
   3. Loss of future roles (e.g., parent, grandparent)
I. Altered parenting related to:
   1. Unrealistic expectations of child
   2. Knowledge deficit
J. Situational low self-esteem related to loss of image of ideal child
K. Spiritual distress related to decisions regarding conflicts over the cessation or continuation of treatment

THE INFANT

GROWTH AND DEVELOPMENT

A. 1 month
   1. Physical
      a. Weight: gains about 150 to 210 g weekly during the first 6 months of life
      b. Height: grows about 2.5 cm a month for the first 6 months of life
      c. Head circumference: grows about 1.5 cm a month for the first 6 months of life
   2. Motor
      a. Assumes flexed position with pelvis high, but knees not under abdomen, when prone
      b. Holds the head parallel with the body when suspended in prone position
      c. Can turn the head from side to side when prone; lifts head momentarily from bed
      d. Asymmetric posture dominates, such as tonic neck reflex
      e. Primitive reflexes still present
   3. Sensory
      a. Follows a light to midline
      b. Eye movements coordinated most of the time
      c. Visual acuity 20/100 to 20/50

4. Socialization and vocalization
   a. Watches face intently while being spoken to
   b. Utters small, throaty sounds
B. 2 to 3 months
   1. Physical: posterior fontanel closed
   2. Motor
      a. Holds the head erect for a short time and can raise chest supported on the forearms
      b. Bears some weight on legs when held in standing position
      c. Actively holds rattle but will not reach for it
      d. Grasp, tonic neck, and Moro reflexes are fading
      e. Step or dance reflex disappears
      f. Plays with fingers and hands
   3. Sensory
      a. Follows a light to the periphery
      b. Has binocular coordination (vertical and horizontal vision)
      c. Listens to sounds
   4. Socialization and vocalization
      a. Smiles in response to a person or object
      b. Laughs aloud and shows pleasure in making sounds
      c. Cries less
C. 4 to 5 months
   1. Physical
      a. Birth-weight doubles
      b. Drools because salivary glands are functioning but child does not have sufficient coordination to swallow saliva
   2. Motor
      a. Balances the head well in a sitting position
      b. Can sit when the back is supported; knees will be flexed and back rounded
      c. Symmetric body position predominates
      d. Can sustain a portion of own weight when held in a standing position
      e. Reaches for and grasps an object with the whole hand
      f. Can carry hand or an object to the mouth at will
      g. Reaches for attractive objects but misjudges distances
      h. Can roll over from abdomen to back
      i. Lifts head and shoulders at a 90° angle when prone
      j. Primitive reflexes (e.g., grasp, tonic neck, and Moro) have disappeared
      k. Neurologic reflexes
         (1) Landau (from 6 to 8 months to 12 to 24 months): when infant is suspended in a horizontal prone position, the head is raised, legs and spine are extended
         (2) Parachute (7 to 9 months, persists indefinitely): when the infant is suspended in a horizontal prone position

and suddenly thrust forward, hands and fingers extend forward as if to protect from falling

3. Sensory
   a. Recognizes familiar objects and people
   b. Has coupled eye movements; accommodation is developing
4. Socialization and vocalization
   a. Coos and gurgles when talked to
   b. Definitely enjoys social interaction with people
   c. Vocalizes displeasure when an object is taken away

D. 6 to 7 months
1. Physical
   a. Weight: gains about 90 to 150 g weekly during second 6 months of life
   b. Height: grows about 1.25 cm a month
   c. Head circumference: grows about 0.5 cm a month
   d. Teething may begin with eruption of two lower central incisors, followed by upper incisors
2. Motor
   a. Can turn over equally well from stomach or back
   b. Sits fairly well unsupported, especially if placed in a forward-leaning position
   c. Lifts head off table when supine
   d. Can transfer a toy from one hand to the other
   e. Can approach a toy and grasp it with one hand
   f. Plays with feet and puts them in mouth
   g. When lying down, lifts head as if trying to sit up
   h. Transfers everything from hand to mouth
3. Sensory
   a. Has taste preferences
   b. Will spit out disliked food
4. Socialization and vocalization
   a. Begins to differentiate between strange and familiar faces and shows "stranger anxiety"
   b. Makes polysyllabic vowel sounds
   c. Vocalizes "m-m-m-m" when crying
   d. Cries easily on slightest provocation but laughs just as quickly

E. 8 to 9 months
1. Motor
   a. Sits steadily alone
   b. Has good hand-to-mouth coordination
   c. Developing pincer grasp, with preference for use of one hand over the other
   d. Crawls, may go backward at first
   e. Pulls self to standing position and stands holding onto furniture
2. Sensory
   a. Depth perception is increasing
   b. Displays interest in small objects
3. Socialization and vocalization
   a. Shows anxiety with strangers by turning or pushing away and crying
   b. Definite social attachment is evident: stretches out arms to loved ones
   c. Is voluntarily separating self from mother by desire to act on own
   d. Reacts to adult anger: cries when scolded
   e. Has imitative and repetitive speech, using vowels and consonants such as "Dada"
   f. No true words as yet, but comprehends words such as "bye-bye"
   g. Responds to own name

F. 10 to 12 months
1. Physical
   a. Weight: birth-weight triples
   b. Height: birth-length increases by 50%
   c. Head and chest circumference are equal
   d. Upper and lower lateral incisors usually have erupted, for total of six to eight teeth
2. Motor
   a. Stands alone for short times
   b. Creeps (creeping is more advanced because the abdomen is supported off the floor)
   c. Walks with help: moves around by holding onto furniture
   d. Can sit down from a standing position without help
   e. Can eat from a spoon and a cup but needs help; prefers using fingers
   f. Can play pat-a-cake and peek-a-boo
   g. Can hold a crayon to make a mark on paper
   h. Helps in dressing, such as putting arm through sleeve
3. Sensory
   a. Visual acuity 20/50+
   b. Amblyopia may develop with lack of binocularity
   c. Discriminates simple geometric forms
4. Socialization and vocalization
   a. Shows emotions such as jealousy, affection, anger
   b. Enjoys familiar surroundings and will explore away from mother
   c. Fearful in strange situation or with strangers; clings to mother
   d. May develop habit of "security" blanket
   e. Can say two words besides Dada or Mama with meaning
   f. Understands simple verbal requests, such as, "Give it to me."

PLAY DURING INFANCY (SOLITARY PLAY)

A. Safety is chief determinant in choosing toys (aspirating small objects is one cause of accidental death)
B. Mostly used for physical development
C. Toys need to be simple because of short attention span
D. Visual and auditory stimulation is important
E. Suggested toys
   1. Rattles
   2. Soft, stuffed toys
   3. Mobiles
   4. Push-pull toys
   5. Simple musical toys
   6. Strings of big beads and large snap toys
   7. Unbreakable mirrors
   8. Weighted or suction toys
   9. Squeeze toys
   10. Teething toys
   11. Cloth or thick-paged books with textures
   12. Activity boxes
   13. Simple take-apart toys
   14. Nested boxes and fitting forms

HEALTH PROMOTION DURING INFANCY

Feeding Milestones

A. At birth the full-term infant has sucking, rooting, and swallowing reflexes
B. Newborn feels hunger and indicates desire for food by crying; expresses satiety by contentedly falling asleep
C. At 1 month the infant has strong extrusion reflex
D. At about 6 months the infant is able to pick up finger foods and begin to use a cup
E. By 6 to 7 months the infant is developmentally ready to chew
F. By 8 to 9 months the infant can hold a spoon and play with it during feeding
G. By 9 months the infant can hold own bottle
H. By 12 months the child usually can drink from a cup, though a bottle may be preferred to satisfy the urge to suck

Infant Nutrition

A. Nutrition as it affects growth
   1. Birth weight usually doubled by 5 months of age and tripled by 1 year (small babies may gain more weight in a shorter period)
   2. Growth during the first year should be charted to observe for comparable gain in length, weight, and head circumference
   3. Generally, growth charts demonstrate the percentile of the child's growth rate (below the fifth and above the ninety-fifth percentile are considered abnormal)
   4. Percentiles of growth curves must be seen in relation to:
      a. Deviation from a steady rate of growth
      b. Hereditary factors of parents (size and body shape)
      c. Comparison of height and weight
   5. Satisfactory rate of growth judged by:
      a. Weight and length (overweight and underweight constitute malnutrition)
      b. Muscular development
      c. Tissue tone and turgor
      d. General appearance and activity level
      e. Amount of crying and needed sleep
      f. Presence or absence of illness
      g. Mental status and behavior in relation to norms for the age
B. Proper feeding essential to growth and development
   1. General good nutrition that promotes growth but prevents overweight
   2. Prevention of nutritional deficiencies
   3. Prevention of gastrointestinal disturbances, such as vomiting or constipation
   4. Establishment of good eating habits later in life
   5. Consistency of foods should progress from liquid to semisoft to soft to solids as the dentition and jaw develop

Guidelines for infant feedings

A. Breast milk is the most desirable complete diet for the first 6 months but may require supplements of fluoride, iron, and vitamin D
B. Iron-fortified commercial formula is an acceptable alternative to breastfeeding
C. Breast milk or commercial formula is recommended for the first year, but after this age the infant can be given homogenized vitamin D-fortified whole milk; the use of milk with reduced fat content (skimmed or low fat) is not recommended because increased quantities of solids would be required to supply the caloric needs, leading to overfeeding, and the high solute load would place excessive demands on the immature kidneys; in addition, essential fatty acids are missing
D. Solids can be introduced at 4-6 months; the first food is often commercially prepared iron-fortified infant cereals; rice is usually introduced first because of its low allergenic potential; infant cereals should be continued until 18 months of age
E. With the exception of infant cereals, the order of introducing other foods is variable; recommended sequence is weekly introduction of other foods such as fruits and vegetables, and then meats
F. First solid foods are strained, puréed, or finely mashed
G. Finger foods such as toast, teething crackers, noncitrus soft fruits, and cooked vegetables can be introduced at 6-7 months; parents should be strongly cautioned to watch for choking

H. Chopped table food or commercially prepared junior foods can be started by 9 to 12 months
I. Diluted apple juice should be offered from a cup to reduce development of nursing bottle caries; the use of a cup is suggested at 6 months
J. Method
    1. Introduce one food at a time, usually at intervals of 4 to 7 days, to allow for identification of food allergies
    2. Feed when the baby is hungry, after a few sucks of breast milk or formula, early in the day
    3. Begin spoonfeeding by placing food on back of the tongue, because of the infant's natural tendency to thrust tongue forward
    4. Use a small spoon with straight handle; begin with 5-10 ml of food; gradually increase to 60 ml per feeding
    5. As the amount of solid food increases, the quantity of milk needs to be decreased to approximately 900 ml daily to prevent overfeeding
    6. Never introduce foods by mixing them with the formula in the bottle
K. Weaning
    1. Giving up the bottle or breast for a cup is psychologically significant, because it requires the relinquishing of a major source of pleasure
    2. Usually, readiness develops during second half of the first year because of:
       a. Pleasure from receiving food by a spoon
       b. Increasing desire for more freedom
       c. Acquiring more control over body and the environment
    3. Weaning should be gradual, replacing only one bottle at a time with a cup and finally ending with the nighttime bottle
    4. If breastfeeding must be terminated before 5 or 6 months of age, a bottle should be used to allow for the infant's continued sucking needs; after about 6 months wean directly to a cup
L. Diseases or conditions during infancy requiring possible dietary modifications
    1. Diarrhea: decreased fat and carbohydrate
    2. Constipation: increased fluids, add prune juice or strained fruit, change in type of carbohydrate
    3. Celiac disease (malabsorption syndrome): results from gluten sensitivity; diet should be low in gluten, which is found in wheat, rye, barley, and oat grains, so these grains are eliminated and rice and corn are substituted
    4. Allergy: individual diet modification according to specific food sensitivity; e.g., if milk allergy exists, substitute forms of soybean or meat formula preparations are used
    5. Lactose intolerance: lactose-free diet used with Nutramigen as a milk substitute

    6. Refer to Inborn Errors of Metabolism for other disorders
    7. SIDS: position on side, not stomach, after meals

Immunizations

A. Schedule of recommended routine immunizations
    1. Diphtheria, pertussis, and tetanus, polio with hemophilus DPTP-HIB (penta) combined in one injection
       a. DPTP-HIB given at 2, 4, 6, 18 months
       b. DPTP (Quad) without the HIB given as a booster once between the fourth birthday and before entry to grade one
       c. Diphtheria, pertussis and tetanus vaccinations given early as no passive immunity from mother exists
       d. Pertussis vaccine not given after preschool dose as the risk of the illness is less than the side-effects of the vaccine
       e. Tetanus induces immunity for about 10 years
       f. Polio given as injectable, inactivated polio virus IPV (Salk), rather than oral Sabin
       g. Immunizations against hemophilus have significantly decreased the incidence of meningitis in children
    2. Measles, mumps, and rubella vaccine (MMR)
       a. Given once at about 12 months
       b. Natural immunity from mother exists until approximately 12 to 15 months
       c. The only live vaccine administered
       d. Rubella given to prevent the illness in women during the first trimester of pregnancy
       e. Later immunizations of rubella are not given if pregnancy is suspected, and pregnancy should be prevented for three months following the immunization
    3. Hepatitis B vaccine
       a. Given in grade 5, at about 10 or 11 years of age
       b. Can be acquired individually for usually exempt children
    4. Tetanus, diphtheria TD
       a. Combined and given in grade 9, at about 14 or 15 years of age
       b. Following this booster, may be given at 5-year intervals in the event of a contaminated wound
B. Factors influencing the administration of immunizations
    1. Immunizations are not mandatory in Canada, but are highly recommended and are monitored by the regional community health nurse or by the physician
    2. Admistration of immunizations is governed provincially, and variations exist
    3. Administration of immunizations to immuno-suppressed children are assessed on an individual basis

4. The benefit from being protected by the immunization is believed to greatly outweigh the risk from the disease
5. Presence of maternal antibodies
6. Administration of blood transfusion or immune serum globulin within 3 months
7. High fever, serious illness (common cold is not a contraindication)
8. Diseases in which immunity is impaired
9. Immunosuppressive therapy in child or family member
10. Generalized malignancy such as leukemia
11. Anaphylactic reaction to egg protein, bovine, porcine, equine, or other products
12. Neurologic problems such as convulsions during administration of pertussis vaccine
13. Allergic reaction to a previously administered vaccine or a substance in the vaccine such as preservatives or neomycin
14. Live virus vaccines are usually not given to any child with an altered immune system

Injury Prevention

A. Accidents are one of the leading causes of death during infancy
   1. Mechanical suffocation causes most accidental deaths in children under 1 year of age
   2. Aspiration of small objects and ingestion of poisonous substances occur most often during second half of the first year and into early childhood
   3. Trauma from rolling off a bed or falling down stairs can occur at any time
B. Teaching is an essential aspect of prevention
   1. Birth to 4 months
      a. Aspiration
         (1) Not as great a danger to this age group but should begin practicing safeguards early (refer to 4 to 7 months)
         (2) Inform parents about the irritation of the respiratory tract caused by baby powder; encourage its proper use and storage if they insist on use
      b. Suffocation
         (1) Keep all plastic bags stored away from infant's reach; discard large plastic garment bags after tying in a knot
         (2) Do not cover mattress or pillows with plastic
         (3) Use a firm mattress, no pillows, and loose blankets
         (4) Make sure crib design follows regulations and mattress fits snugly
         (5) Position crib away from other furniture
         (6) Do not tie pacifier on string around infant's neck
         (7) Remove bibs at bedtime

         (8) Keep crib away from other furniture and cords from window blinds
         (9) Drowning: never leave infant alone in bath
      c. Falls
         (1) Always raise crib rails; tie rails to crib if malfunctioning
         (2) Never leave infant on a raised, unguarded surface
         (3) When in doubt about where to place child, use the floor
         (4) Restrain child in the infant seat and never leave unattended while the seat is resting on a raised surface
         (5) Avoid using a high chair until child is old enough to sit well and restrain in chair
      d. Poisoning
         Not as great a danger to this age group but should begin practicing safeguards early (refer to 4 to 7 months)
      e. Burns
         (1) Pretest bath water and warmed formula and food
         (2) Do not pour hot liquids when infant is close by, such as sitting on lap
         (3) Beware of cigarette ashes that may fall on infant
         (4) Do not leave infant in the sun for more than a few minutes, use hats and sunscreens
         (5) Wash flame-retardant clothes according to label directions
         (6) Use cool mist vaporizers
         (7) Do not keep child alone in parked car
         (8) Check surface heat of car restraint
      f. Motor vehicles
         (1) Transport infant (even newborn) in a specially constructed rear-facing car seat with appropriate restraints
         (2) Do not place infant on the seat or in the lap
         (3) Do not place a carriage or stroller behind a parked car
      g. Bodily damage
         (1) Avoid sharp, jagged-edged objects
         (2) Keep diaper pins closed and away from infant
   2. 4 to 7 months
      a. Aspiration
         (1) Keep buttons, beads, and other small objects out of infant's reach
         (2) Use pacifier with one-piece construction and loop handle
         (3) Keep floor free of any small objects
         (4) Do not feed infant hard candy, nuts, food with pits or seeds, or whole hot dogs
         (5) Inspect toys for removable parts
         (6) Avoid balloons as playthings

b. Suffocation
May begin to teach swimming as part of water safety

c. Falls
(1) Restrain in high chair
(2) Keep crib rails raised to full height

d. Poisoning
(1) Make sure that paint for furniture or toys does not contain lead
(2) Place toxic substances on a high shelf and/or locked cabinet
(3) Hang plants or place on a high surface rather than on floor
(4) Avoid storing large quantities of cleaning fluids, paints, pesticides, and other toxic substances
(5) Discard used containers of poisonous substances
(6) Do not store toxic substances in food containers
(7) Know telephone number of local poison control center

e. Burns
(1) Always check bath water and adjust household hot-water temperature to 49° C or lower
(2) Place hot objects (cigarettes, candles, incense) on high surfaces

f. Motor vehicles
(Refer to birth to 4 months)

g. Bodily damage
(1) Give toys that are smooth and rounded, made of wood or plastic
(2) Avoid long, pointed objects as toys

3. 8 to 12 months
a. Aspiration
(refer to 4 to 7 months)

b. Suffocation
(1) Keep doors of ovens, dishwashers, refrigerators, and front-loading clothes washers and dryers closed at all times
(2) If storing an unused appliance, such as a refrigerator, remove the door
(3) Fence swimming pools; always supervise when near any source of water, such as cleaning buckets
(4) Keep bathroom doors closed

c. Falls
Fence stairways at top and bottom if child has access to either end

d. Poisoning
(1) Administer medications as a drug, not as a candy
(2) Do not administer adult medications unless prescribed by a physician
(3) Replace medications and poisons

immediately after use; replace caps properly if a child protector cap is used
(4) Advise parents regarding proper use of syrup of ipecac if ordered

e. Burns
(1) Place guards in front of any heating appliance, fireplace, or furnace
(2) Keep electrical wires hidden or out of reach
(3) Place plastic guards over electrical outlets; place furniture in front of outlets
(4) Keep hanging tablecloths out of reach
(5) Do not allow infant to play with electrical appliances

f. Motor vehicles
(1) Do not use adult seat or shoulder belt without infant car seat
(2) Do not allow infant to crawl behind a parked car
(3) If infant plays in a yard, have the yard fenced or use a playpen

g. Bodily damage
(1) Do not allow infant to use a fork for self-feeding
(2) Use plastic cups or dishes
(3) Check safety of toys and toybox
(4) Protect from animals
(5) Use caution with automatic door closures
(6) Install safety devices for toy boxes

PARENTAL GUIDANCE

A. First 6 months
1. Understand each parent's adjustment to newborn, especially mother's postpartal emotional needs
2. Teach infant care, assist parents to understand infant's individual needs and temperament, that infant expresses wants through crying, and that trust is established by meeting the infant's needs
3. Encourage parents to establish a schedule that meets the family's needs
4. Help parents understand infant's need for stimulation in environment
5. Support parent's pleasure in seeing child's growing friendliness and social response, especially smiling
6. Plan anticipatory guidance for safety
7. Stress need for immunization against disease
8. Prepare for introduction of solid foods

B. Second 6 months
1. Prepare parents for child's "stranger anxiety"
2. Encourage parents to allow child to cling to mother or father and avoid long separation from either

3. Guide parents concerning discipline because of infant's increasing mobility
4. Teach accident prevention because of child's advancing motor skills and curiosity
5. Encourage parents to leave child with suitable parental substitute to allow some free time
6. Discuss readiness for weaning

HEALTH PROBLEMS FIRST NOTED DURING INFANCY

(Problems may continue past 12 months of age and through childhood)

Hospitalization

A. Reactions to parental separation (begins later in infancy: refer to the Toddler)
B. General problems in care of the infant
   1. Small size
      a. Body warmth and temperature control
      b. Maintenance of fluids: prone to edema, dehydration, and electrolyte imbalance
         (1) Infants have a higher percentage of extracellular fluid than do adults, which can be quickly excreted
         (2) Infants' kidneys are unable to concentrate urine
   2. Immature organ systems
      a. Primary defense mechanisms just developing: loss of antibodies from fetal life increases the infant's susceptibility to infection
         (1) Antibody levels lowest at 6 weeks to 2 months of age; then infants begin to develop their own system
         (2) Problem subsides as infants grow older
      b. Blood vessels still developing; increased fragility causes hemorrhage
      c. Some essential enzymes (e.g., glucuronyl transferase, which is necessary for conjugation of bilirubin) still developing: more chance for jaundice and brain damage

GENERAL NURSING DIAGNOSES FOR INFANTS WITH HEALTH PROBLEMS

A. Ineffective airway clearance related to:
   1. Accumulation of secretions
   2. Immobility
   3. Fatigue
B. Risk for altered parent infant/child attachment related to:
   1. Possible loss of child
   2. Child's physical condition that limits handling or fondling
   3. Inability of parents to meet child's health needs

C. Anxiety related to:
   1. Strange environment
   2. Perception of impending event
   3. Separation
   4. Anticipated discomfort
   5. Knowledge deficit
   6. Discomfort
   7. Difficulty breathing
   8. Feelings of powerlessness
D. Risk for aspiration related to:
   1. Disease process
   2. Impaired swallowing
   3. Immature cough reflex
   4. Availability of foreign objects
E. Risk for disorganized infant behavior related to:
   1. Pain
   2. Intrusive procedures
   3. Separation from support systems
F. Interrupted breastfeeding related to:
   1. Mother-infant separation
   2. Inability of infant to suck
G. Risk for caregiver role strain related to:
   1. Inadequate support systems
   2. Family member illness
   3. Unfamiliarity with resources
H. Ineffective family coping: compromised, related to:
   1. Situational crisis
   2. Temporary family disorganization
I. Diversional activity deficit related to lack of sensory stimulation and altered mobility
J. Altered family processes related to:
   1. Situational crisis
   2. Knowledge deficit
   3. Temporary family disorganization
   4. Inadequate support systems
K. Fear related to:
   1. Separation from support systems
   2. Uncertain prognosis (parental)
   3. Perceived inability to control events (parental)
L. Risk for fluid volume deficit related to:
   1. Inability to concentrate urine
   2. Higher percentage of extracellular to intracellular water
M. Anticipatory grieving (parental) related to:
   1. Expected loss
   2. Gravity of infant's physical status
N. Risk for infection related to:
   1. Immature immune system
   2. Impaired skin integrity
   3. Presence of infective organisms
O. Risk for injury related to:
   1. Use of specific therapies and appliances
   2. Incapacity for self-protection
   3. Immobility
P Knowledge deficit related to anxiety

Q. Pain related to:
   1. Disease process
   2. Interventions
R. Altered parenting related to:
   1. Separation
   2. Skill deficit
   3. Family stress
   4. Knowledge deficit
   5. Interrupted parent-infant bonding
S. Powerlessness related to health care environment
T. Sensory perceptual alteration: tactile related to protective environment
U. Risk for impaired skin integrity related to:
   1. Immature structure and function
   2. Immobility
V. Sleep-pattern disturbance related to:
   1. Excessive crying
   2. Frequent assessment
   3. Therapies
   4. Interventions
   5. Fear of child's prognosis
W. Spiritual distress (parental) related to:
   1. Inadequate support systems
   2. Challenged belief and value system because of moral/ethical implications of therapy

CHROMOSOMAL ABERRATIONS

GENERAL NURSING CARE OF INFANTS AND CHILDREN WITH CHROMOSOMAL ABERRATIONS

A. DATA COLLECTION
   1. Identify chromosomal abnormality
   2. Determine functional limitations
   3. Parental perceptions of child
   4. Child's health status

B. ANALYSIS AND INTERPRETATION
   1. Ineffective airway clearance related to:
      a. Nasal obstruction
      b. Excessive thick secretions
      c. Impaired musculature
   2. Risk for aspiration related to:
      a. Impaired swallowing
      b. Nasogastric tube feedings
      c. Impaired gag reflex
   3. Body image disturbance related to:
      a. Unrealistic self-expectations
      b. Sterility (Turner's and Klinefelter's syndromes)
      c. Lack of pubertal changes (Turner's and Klinefelter's syndromes)
   4. Impaired verbal communication related to cognitive impairment
   5. Fear related to hospitalization
   6. Knowledge deficit related to cognitive or sensory impairment

   7. Altered nutrition: potential for more than body requirements related to immobility
   8. Chronic low self-esteem related to:
      a. Unrealistic self-expectations
      b. Sterility (Turner's and Klinefelter's syndromes)
      c. Lack of pubertal changes (Turner's and Klinefelter's syndromes)
   9. Risk for impaired skin integrity related to:
      a. Immobility
      b. Dermatologic changes (Down syndrome)
   10. Refer to General Nursing Diagnoses for the Family of a Child with Special Needs and General Nursing Diagnoses for Infants with Health Problems

C. PLANNING/IMPLEMENTATION
   1. Provide emotional support to parents
   2. Encourage genetic counseling appropriate for type of problem
   3. Assist parents in setting realistic expectations and goals for the child
   4. Refer for careful testing of intellectual functioning for guidance to parents
   5. Refer to Nursing Care of Children Who Are Developmentally Disabled
   6. Refer to Meeting the Needs of the Family of an Infant or Child with Special Needs

D. EVALUATION/OUTCOMES
   1. Child is able to breathe without obstruction
   2. Child does not aspirate
   3. Child is able to communicate with caregivers
   4. Child expresses feelings and concerns
   5. Child demonstrates understanding of procedures
   6. Child consumes adequate calories for growth and development
   7. Child exhibits behavior indicative of positive self-image
   8. Child does not exhibit signs of skin breakdown

▼ TRISOMY 21 (DOWN SYNDROME)

Data Base
A. Types
   1. Trisomy 21: frequently associated with advanced parental age (40 to 44 years of age—1%; over 45 years of age—2%); can occur in all age groups
   2. Translocation 15/21: translocated chromosome transmitted most often by the mother who is a carrier; age not a factor
   3. Mosaicism: mixture of normal cells and cells that are trisomic for 21 (usually leads to a less severe phenotype)
B. Clinical findings
   1. Small, rounded skull with a flat occiput

2. Inner epicanthic folds and oblique palpebral fissures
3. Speckling of the iris (Brushfield's spots)
4. Small nose with a depressed bridge (saddle nose)
5. Protruding, sometimes fissured, tongue
6. Small, sometimes low-set, ears
7. Short, thick neck
8. Hypotonic musculature (protruding abdomen, umbilical hernia)
9. Hyperflexible and lax joints
10. Simian line (transverse crease on the palmar side of the hand)
11. Broad, short, and stubby hands and feet
12. Delayed or incomplete sexual development (men with Down syndrome usually are infertile)
13. Cardiac deficits, especially atrial in origin

Nursing Care of Infants and Children with Trisomy 21

A. Prevent infection, especially respiratory
B. Provide activity consistent with abilities and limits
C. Provide physical supervision and habilitation
D. Refer to General Nursing Care of Infants and Children with Chromosomal Aberrations

▼ TRISOMY 18

Data Base

A. Types
  1. Trisomy
  2. Translocation
  3. Mosaicism
B. Clinical findings
  1. Several physical anomalies of the head, ears, mandible, hands, feet, heart, and kidneys
  2. Failure to thrive and short survival; if survive, severe developmental disability

Nursing Care of Infants and Children with Trisomy 18

A. Because of short survival, prepare the parents for loss of their child
B. Refer to General Nursing Care of Infants and Children with Chromosomal Aberrations

▼ TURNER SYNDROME (GONADAL DYSGENESIS)

Data Base

A. Chromosome monosomy (XO karyotype) in females
B. Clinical findings
  1. Congenital malformations such as short stature, webbed neck, infantile genitalia, and developmental failure of secondary sex characteristics at puberty
  2. Usually normal intelligence; problems in directional sense and space-form recognition

Nursing Care of Infants and Children with Turner Syndrome

A. Prepare child for lack of pubertal changes and need for hormonal replacement
B. Counsel with emphasis on adoption rather than on the person's inability to conceive
C. Refer to General Nursing Care of Infants and Children with Chromosomal Aberrations

▼ KLINEFELTER SYNDROME

Data Base

A. Sex-chromosomal abnormality of XXY in males
B. Clinical findings
  1. Physical characteristics: tall; skinny; long legs and arms; small, firm testes; gynecomastia; and poorly developed secondary sex characteristics at puberty
  2. Behavioral disorders and developmental disability often present

Nursing Care of Infants and Children with Klinefelter Syndrome

A. Counsel with emphasis on positive aspects such as adoption or donor insemination
B. Recognize that emotional problems may require lifelong counseling
C. Refer to General Nursing Care of Infants and Children with Chromosomal Aberrations

GASTROINTESTINAL MALFORMATIONS

▼ CLEFT LIP

Data Base

A. Failure of union of embryonic structure of face
  1. Fusion of maxillary and premaxillary processes
  2. Occurs between 5 and 8 weeks of fetal life
B. Cause unknown; evidence of hereditary influence and relationship to maternal smoking
  1. Incidence in general population is 1 in 700 births
  2. If one infant is born with a cleft lip or palate but no history of the anomaly in family, the chance of occurrence in the next infant is about 4%
  3. If a history of either anomaly exists in one parent, there is about a 4% chance that the first infant will have the defect

C. More common in males
D. Classification
  1. Bilateral or unilateral; if unilateral, more common on the left side
  2. Can be of several degrees; complete cleft usually continuous with cleft palate
E. Clinical findings
  1. Difficulty feeding because the infant cannot form a vacuum with the mouth to suck, but may be able to breastfeed (sometimes the breast fills the cleft, making sucking easier)
  2. Mouth breathing results in:
    a. Increased swallowed air, causing a distended abdomen, pressure against the diaphragm
    b. Mucous membranes of the oropharynx become dried and cracked with increased risk of infection
F. Therapeutic interventions—surgical repair
  1. Performed soon after birth—further modification may be necessary
  2. Aids infant's ability to suck
  3. Helps parents with the visible aspects of the defect
  4. Multidisciplinary team

Nursing Care of Infants with a Cleft Lip

A. DATA COLLECTION
  1. Feeding behaviors; does infant consume adequate calories for growth without excessive energy expenditure
  2. Check mucous membranes for dryness, signs of infection
  3. Observe parent/infant interaction and the effect of facial defect on bonding

B. ANALYSIS AND INTERPRETATION
  1. Refer to General Nursing Diagnoses for the Family of a Child with Special Needs and General Nursing Diagnoses for Infants with Health Problems
  2. Risk for disorganized infant behavior related to pain and discomfort and need to restrict sucking
  3. Risk for injury related to surgical incision and developmental age
  4. Altered nutrition: less than body requirements related to feeding difficulties
  5. Risk for altered parenting related to visible physical defect
  6. Altered family processes related to having an infant with a physical defect
  7. Sensory-perceptual alteration related to inability to suck

C. PLANNING/IMPLEMENTATION
  1. Preoperative nursing care
    a. Feed in an upright position
    b. Feed with a soft large-holed nipple or rubber-tipped syringe or cleft lip or palate nurser

c. Burp frequently because of swallowed air
    d. Teach parents to give water after each feeding to cleanse the infant's mouth
    e. Prevent infection from irritation of the lip
      (1) Restrain infant's arms, if needed
      (2) Provide a pacifier to increase sucking pleasure
  2. Postoperative nursing care
    a. Maintain a patent airway
      (1) Problem because of edema of the nose, tongue, and lips combined with the infant's habit of breathing through the mouth
      (2) Proper equipment such as laryngoscope, endotracheal tube, and suction at or near the bedside
    b. Cleanse the suture line to prevent crust formation and eventual scarring
    c. Prevent crying, because of pressure on suture line (encourage the parent to stay with the infant); restrict the use of a soother
    d. Place the infant in supine position with arm or elbow restraints
      (1) Change position to the side or sitting up to prevent hypostatic pneumonia
      (2) Remove restraints only when supervised
    e. Feed (same as before surgery)
    f. Support the parents by accepting and treating the infant as normal
  3. Refer to Meeting the Needs of the Family of an Infant or Child with Special Needs

D. EVALUATION/OUTCOMES
  1. Infant consumes adequate calories for growth and development
  2. Family accepts infant despite visible handicap
  3. Surgical site heals without trauma
  4. Infant is comforted by other means because unable to suck until suture line is healed
  5. Family is able to meet needs of infant

▼ CLEFT PALATE

Data Base

A. Failure of union of embryonic structure of face; fusion of palatal structures between 9 and 12 weeks; may involve the soft or hard palate and may extend into the nose, forming an oronasal passageway
B. Cause unknown; evidence of hereditary influence (refer to Data Base B1, B2, and B3 under Cleft Lip)
C. More common in females
D. Clinical findings
  1. Infection, especially aspiration pneumonia
  2. Speech
    a. Palate is needed to trap air in the mouth

b. Tonsils usually not removed because they provide an additional mechanism to trap air

c. The child will need a speech appliance to help prevent guttural sounds if repair is delayed beyond speech development

3. Dental development
   a. Excessive dental caries
   b. Malocclusion from displacement of the maxillary arch

4. Hearing problems caused by recurrent otitis media (eustachian tube connects the nasopharynx and middle ear and easily transports foreign material to ear)

E. Therapeutic interventions—surgical repair
   1. Age for repair is usually after the child has grown but before speech is well developed; between 6 months and 3 years
   2. Multidisciplinary-team approach, including speech therapist

Nursing Care of Infants and Children with a Cleft Palate

A. DATA COLLECTION

1. Feeding behaviors; child must consume adequate calories for growth and development
2. Respiratory status; child at increased risk for aspiration pneumonia
3. Parent/child interaction
4. Oral hygiene
5. Possible hearing impairment; child has frequent otitis media

B. ANALYSIS AND INTERPRETATION

1. Risk for disorganized infant behavior related to pain and discomfort and need to restrict sucking
2. Altered family processes related to having a child with a physical defect
3. Risk for infection related to aspiration potential and otitis media
4. Risk for injury related to surgical incision and developmental age
5. Altered nutrition: risk for less than body requirements related to feeding difficulties
6. Refer to General Nursing Diagnoses for the Family of a Child with Special Needs and General Nursing Diagnoses for Infants with Health Problems

C. PLANNING/IMPLEMENTATION

1. Preoperative nursing care: same as for infants with cleft lip except:
   a. Feed upright to prevent aspiration
   b. Feed by gavage if necessary
   c. Encourage early use of spoon and cup
   d. Teach parents the need for proper dental hygiene and the importance of regular dental supervision

2. Postoperative nursing care: same as for infants with cleft lip except:
   a. When maintaining a patent airway, try to avoid use of suction that traumatizes the operative site
   b. Place the child in a prone Trendelenburg position to prevent aspiration and promote postural drainage
   c. Avoid trauma to suture line by telling child not to rub tongue on roof of mouth
   d. Provide liquid diet; no milk, because of curd formation on suture line
   e. Avoid the use of straw or spoon
   f. Recognize the need for emotional support of the parents is greater, since recovery is longer and the prognosis uncertain
3. See Meeting the Needs of the Family of an Infant or Child with Special Needs

D. EVALUATION/OUTCOMES

1. Child consumes adequate calories for growth and development
2. Child has decreased number of infections (pneumonia, otitis media)
3. Surgical site heals without trauma
4. Family is able to meet the needs of child

▼ TRACHEOESOPHAGEAL ANOMALIES

Data Base

A. Occurrence is 1 in 800 to 5000 births
B. Usually low birth weight
C. May be associated with other anomalies
D. Most commonly, the proximal esophagus ends in a blind pouch and the distal esophagus is connected to the trachea or primary bronchus
E. Classification
   1. Absence of the esophagus
   2. Atresia of the esophagus without a tracheal fistula
   3. Tracheoesophageal fistula
   4. The most common type of anomaly is proximal esophageal atresia combined with distal tracheoesophageal fistula
F. Clinical findings
   1. Excessive drooling
   2. Excessive mucus in nasopharynx causing cyanosis, which is easily reversed by suctioning
   3. Choking, sneezing, and coughing during feeding, with regurgitation of formula through the mouth and nose
   4. Inability to pass a catheter into the stomach
G. Therapeutic intervention—surgical repair
   Can be done in one procedure or several, depending on infant's condition and severity of defect

Nursing Care of Infants with Tracheoesophageal Anomalies

A. DATA COLLECTION

1. Three C's of tracheoesophageal fistula
   a. Coughing
   b. Choking
   c. Cyanosis
2. Monitor for signs of respiratory distress
3. Observe parent/infant interaction

B. ANALYSIS AND INTERPRETATION

1. Ineffective airway clearance related to physical defect
2. Anxiety related to inability to swallow, surgical pain
3. Risk for disorganized infant behavior related to pain and discomfort and need to restrict oral intake
4. Risk for injury related to surgical procedure
5. Altered family processes related to having an infant with a disability
6. Impaired swallowing related to physical defect
7. Impaired skin integrity if esophagostomy is performed
8. Refer to General Nursing Diagnoses for the Family of a Child with Special Needs and General Nursing Diagnoses for Infants with Health Problems

C. PLANNING/IMPLEMENTATION

1. Preoperative nursing care
   a. Keep NPO
   b. Maintain in upright position
   c. Suction oropharynx to remove accumulated secretions
   d. Observe for signs of respiratory distress
   e. Change position to prevent pneumonia
   f. Monitor intake and output
2. Postoperative nursing care
   a. Frequently suction mouth and pharynx
   b. Provide high humidity to liquefy thick secretions
   c. Change position to prevent pneumonia; position upright to prevent aspiration
   d. Perform proper care of chest tubes if used
   e. Maintain nutrition by oral, parenteral, or gastrostomy method
   f. Provide a pacifier if oral feedings are contraindicated
   g. Provide comfort and physical contact, because hospital stay is usually long
3. See Meeting the Needs of the Family of an Infant or Child with Special Needs

D. EVALUATION/OUTCOMES

1. Airway is maintained and infant does not aspirate secretions
2. Infant receives adequate calories for growth and development

3. The surgical site is not injured
4. Infant rests calmly
5. Family demonstrates ability to care for infant
6. Infant alert when awake
7. Family able to list potential complications

▼ INTESTINAL OBSTRUCTION

Data Base

A. Congenital life-threatening obstruction of the intestines
B. Classification
   1. Mechanical: constricted or occluded lumen
   2. Muscular: interference with normal muscular contraction
C. Clinical findings
   1. Abdominal distention
   2. Absence of stools, especially meconium in the newborn (meconium ileus)
   3. Vomiting of bile-stained material; may be projectile
   4. Cyanosis and weak grunting respirations from abdominal distention, causing the diaphragm to compress the lungs
   5. Paroxysmal pain
   6. Weak, thready pulse
D. Therapeutic interventions—surgical repair
   1. Either by single-staged or multistaged procedures if defect is severe
   2. Prevention of pneumonia
   3. Supportive nutritional therapy; gastrostomy tube

Nursing Care of Infants with an Intestinal Obstruction

A. DATA COLLECTION

1. Protruding abdomen indicative of distention
2. Visible peristaltic waves often indicate pathologic state
3. Absence of bowel movements

B. ANALYSIS AND INTERPRETATION

1. Risk for disorganized infant behavior related to pain and discomfort and need to restrict oral intake
2. Altered family processes related to having an infant with a defect
3. Risk for injury related to inability to evacuate rectum
4. Altered nutrition: less than body requirements related to inability to feed
5. Refer to General Nursing Diagnoses for Infants with Health Problems

C. PLANNING/IMPLEMENTATION

1. Preoperative nursing care
   a. Keep NPO

b. Monitor intake and output

c. Observe for signs of dehydration

d. Maintain nasogastric suction

2. Postoperative nursing care: dependent on type of surgery performed

   a. Keep operative sites clean and dry, especially after passage of stool

   b. Position infant on side rather than abdomen to prevent pulling legs up under the chest

   c. Care of colostomy: prevent excoriation of skin by frequent cleansing, the use of a barrier cream on the skin surrounding the colostomy, or the use of an ostomy appliance

   d. Instruct the parents about colostomy care (include avoidance of tight diapers and clothes around the abdomen)

   e. See Meeting the Needs of the Family of an Infant or Child with Special Needs

D. EVALUATION/OUTCOMES

1. Infant achieves normal bowel function

2. Infant consumes sufficient calories for growth and development

3. Family demonstrates ability to care for infant

▼ ANORECTAL ANOMALIES (IMPERFORATE ANUS)

Data Base

A. Most common intestinal anomaly

B. Failure of the membrane separating the rectum from the anus to absorb during eighth week of fetal life

C. Fistulas within the vagina, urinary tract, or scrotum are common

D. Classification

   1. Low anomalies
Puborectalis muscle, internal and external sphincter present and well developed with normal function

   2. Intermediate anomalies

     a. Rectum at or below puborectalis muscle

     b. Rectal opening anterior in perineum

     c. May be persistent opening to genitourinary tract

   3. High anomalies

     a. Rectum ends above puborectalis muscle

     b. Absence of internal and external sphincters

E. Clinical findings

   1. Failure to pass meconium stool

   2. Inability to insert a thermometer, catheter, or small finger into the rectum

   3. Abdominal distention

F. Therapeutic interventions

   1. Immediate surgical correction unless fistula is present

2. Possible colostomy with multistaged surgical repair

Nursing Care of Infants and Children with Anorectal Anomalies

A. DATA COLLECTION

1. Digital examination of rectum for patency

2. Passage of meconium

3. Absent or hyperactive bowel sounds

B. ANALYSIS AND INTERPRETATION

1. Risk for disorganized infant behavior related to pain and discomfort and need to restrict oral intake

2. Altered family processes related to having a child with a defect

3. Risk for injury related to inability to evacuate rectum

4. Altered nutrition: less than body requirements related to inability to feed

5. Refer to General Nursing Diagnoses for the Family of a Child with Special Needs and General Nursing Diagnoses for Infants with Health Problems

C. PLANNING/IMPLEMENTATION

See Planning/Implementation under Intestinal Obstruction

D. EVALUATION/OUTCOMES

1. Child achieves bowel function

2. Child consumes sufficient calories for growth and development

3. Family demonstrates ability to care for child

▼ PYLORIC STENOSIS

Data Base

A. Congenital hypertrophy of muscular tissue of the pyloric sphincter, usually asymptomatic until 2 to 4 weeks after birth

B. Five times more common in males than females

C. Classification

   1. Grossly enlarged circular muscle of pylorus

   2. Narrowed opening between stomach and duodenum

   3. Inflammation and edema can result in total obstruction

D. Clinical findings

   1. Vomiting, progressively projectile

   2. Non–bile-stained vomitus

   3. Constipation

   4. Dehydration and weight loss

   5. Distention of the epigastrium, visible peristalsis, and palpable olive-shaped mass in the right upper quadrant

E. Therapeutic intervention—surgical repair
The Fredet-Ramstedt (pylorotomy) procedure: longitudinal splitting of the hypertrophied muscle

Nursing Care of Infants with Pyloric Stenosis
A. DATA COLLECTION
1. Feeding history-vomiting, yet eager to feed
2. Failure to gain weight
3. Presence of projectile vomiting
4. No evidence of pain or discomfort
5. Upper abdominal distention
6. Palpable olive-shaped mass in epigastrium just to the right of umbilicus
7. Visible peristaltic waves in RUQ

B. ANALYSIS AND INTERPRETATION
1. Risk for disorganized infant behavior related to pain and discomfort and need to restrict oral intake
2. Altered family processes related to having a child with a life-threatening illness
3. Altered nutrition: less than body requirements related to vomiting
4. Fluid volume deficit and electrolyte alterations related to vomiting
5. Refer to General Nursing Diagnoses for Infants with Health Problems

C. PLANNING/IMPLEMENTATION
1. Preoperative nursing care
   a. Keep NPO
   b. Monitor intake and output
   c. Monitor for signs of dehydration
2. Postoperative nursing care
   a. Same as for any abdominal surgery
   b. Teach parents the specific feeding method
      (1) Give small, frequent feedings and feed slowly
      (2) Hold the infant in a high Fowler's position during feeding and place on the right side after feeding with head of bed slightly elevated
      (3) Bubble frequently during feeding and avoid handling afterward
3. See Meeting the Needs of the Family of an Infant or Child with Special Needs

D. EVALUATION/OUTCOMES
1. Infant maintains hydration
2. Infant consumes adequate calories for growth and development
3. Family demonstrates ability to care for infant

▼ MEGACOLON (HIRSCHSPRUNG'S DISEASE)

Data Base
A. Absence of parasympathetic ganglion cells in a portion of the bowel, which causes enlargement of the bowel proximal to the defect

B. Four times more common in males than females
C. Classification
1. Length of involved bowel varies from only internal sphincter to entire colon
2. Rectosigmoid colon the most commonly affected site
D. Clinical findings
1. Symptoms may occur gradually
2. Constipation or passage of ribbonlike or pellet-like stool
3. Intestinal obstruction
E. Therapeutic intervention—surgical
1. Removal of aganglionic portion of the bowel
2. Colostomy if necessary

Nursing Care of Infants and Children with Megacolon
A. DATA COLLECTION
1. Thorough elimination history
   a. Onset of constipation
   b. Character of stools—ribbonlike, foul smelling
   c. Nutritional/hydration status
2. Poor feeding habits; fussiness; irritability
3. Abdominal distention
4. Current nutrition/hydration status

B. ANALYSIS AND INTERPRETATION
1. Risk for disorganized infant behavior related to pain and discomfort associated with condition and treatment
2. Constipation related to defective bowel motility
3. Altered family processes related to situational crisis (hospitalized child)
4. Refer to General Nursing Diagnoses for the Family of a Child with Special Needs and General Nursing Diagnoses for Infants with Health Problems

C. PLANNING/IMPLEMENTATION
1. Teach parents the correct procedure for enemas if indicated (point out danger of water intoxication)
2. Use only isotonic solutions
3. Prepare isotonic saline by using 5 ml table salt to 500 ml of tap water
4. Use the following suggested amounts of fluid for enemas:

Age	Amount (ml)
Infant	120 to 240
2 to 4 years	240 to 360
4 to 10 years	360 to 480
11 years	480 to 720

5. Postoperative nursing care: dependent on type of surgery performed
6. See Meeting the Needs of the Family of an Infant or Child with Special Needs

D. EVALUATION/OUTCOMES
1. Child is able to have regular, painless, soft bowel movements
2. Child and family can demonstrate colostomy care

DIAPHRAGMATIC MALFORMATIONS

▼ DIAPHRAGMATIC HERNIA

Data Base
A. Failure of the pleuroperitoneal cavity to close completely during embryonic life
B. High mortality; a surgical emergency in immediate newborn period
C. Classification
1. Most of abdominal organs may be found in the thorax
2. Respirations compromised by increased contents in the chest—interferes with newborn's normal diaphragmatic breathing
D. Clinical findings
1. Severe respiratory difficulty with cyanosis
2. Relatively large chest, especially on the affected side
3. Failure of affected side of the chest to expand during respiration, absence of breath sounds
4. Relatively small abdomen
E. Therapeutic interventions
1. Respiratory support
   a. Position head and thorax higher than abdomen and feet
   b. Nasogastric suction for stomach decompression
2. Surgical repair

Nursing Care of Infants with Diaphragmatic Hernia
A. DATA COLLECTION
1. Monitor respiratory status
2. Observe for irritability/pain on increased distress
B. ANALYSIS AND INTERPRETATION
1. Activity intolerance related to:
   a. Generalized weakness
   b. Hypoxia
2. Risk for aspiration related to depressed cough and gag reflexes
3. Risk for disorganized infant behavior related to pain and discomfort and need to restrict oral intake
4. Ineffective breathing pattern related to interference with diaphragmatic breathing
5. Altered family processes related to situational crisis (critically ill infant)
6. Risk for infection related to incision and increased secretions
7. Altered nutrition: less than body requirements related to lack of energy to suck and chew
8. Pain related to difficulty in breathing
9. Refer to General Nursing Diagnoses for the Family of a Child with Special Needs and General Nursing Diagnoses for Infants with Health Problems
C. PLANNING/IMPLEMENTATION
1. Support parents because of critical nature of the condition
2. Gastric suction to remove secretions and swallowed air from the stomach and intestine before and after surgery
3. Preoperatively position the infant on affected side with the head elevated to allow full expansion of the unaffected side
4. Postoperatively feed the infant
5. Care of chest tubes
6. Administer analgesics as required
D. EVALUATION/OUTCOMES
1. Infant is able to maintain oxygenation
2. Infant will not show evidence of pain/irritability
3. Parents will be able to verbalize feelings about serious nature of infant's condition

CARDIAC MALFORMATIONS

▼ CARDIAC DEFECTS

Data Base
A. Normal circulatory changes that occur at or shortly after birth
1. Pulmonary circulation rapidly increases
2. Decreased oxygen concentration results in closure of the foramen ovale, ductus arteriosus, and ductus venosus
B. Classification of cardiac defects
1. Acyanotic: shunt from left to right side of heart
   a. No abnormal communication between pulmonary and systemic circulation
   b. If a connection within the heart chambers exists, pressure forces blood from the arterial (left) to the venous (right) side of the heart, where it is reoxygenated
2. Cyanotic: shunt from the right to left side of the heart
   a. Abnormal connection between the pulmonary and systemic circulations
   b. Venous or unoxygenated blood enters the systemic circulation
   c. Polycythemia (increase in the number of red blood cells) occurs as the body tries to compensate for inadequate supply of oxygen

d. Squatting or knee-chest position is preferred because it decreases venous return by constricting the femoral veins, which have a very low oxygen content; consequently a smaller volume of this blood enters the right ventricle so that the blood shunted into the aorta has a higher oxygen content; it also increases systemic vascular resistance, which diverts right ventricular blood from the aorta into the pulmonary artery, increasing pulmonary blood flow; this increases the amount of oxygenated blood in the left side of the heart and eventually into systemic circulation

e. Compensation and the nature of the defect cause clubbing of fingers and toes, retarded growth, and increased viscosity of blood; can lead to congestive heart failure

C. General clinical findings
1. Dypsnea, especially on exertion
2. Feeding difficulty and failure to thrive, often first signs discovered by the parent
3. Stridor or choking spells
4. Heart rate over 200, respiratory rate about 60 in the infant
5. Recurrent respiratory tract infections
6. In the older child, poor physical development, delayed milestones, and decreased exercise tolerance
7. Cyanosis, squatting, and clubbing of fingers and toes
8. Heart murmurs
9. Excessive perspiration

D. General therapeutic interventions
1. Surgical intervention
2. Pharmacologic approach: cardiac glycosides to increase the efficiency of heart action
   a. Positive inotropic effect is achieved by increasing the permeability of muscle membranes to the calcium and sodium ions required for contraction of muscle fibrils
      (1) Forceful contraction during systole improves peripheral tissue perfusion
      (2) Chamber emptying allows additional venous blood to enter the cardiac chambers during diastole
   b. Negative chronotropic effect is achieved through an action mediated by the vagus nerve that slows firing of the sinoatrial (SA) node and impulse transmission through the atrioventricular (AV) node (negative dromotropic action)
   c. Drug preparations have the same qualitative effect on heart action but differ in potency, rate of absorption, amount absorbed, onset of action, and speed of elimination

      (1) Digitalis: longer onset, peak action, and half-life
      (2) Digoxin (Lanoxin): rapid onset and peak action and short half-life; drug of choice in children, especially because the risk of toxicity is lessened by the shorter half-life
   d. Digitalization
      (1) Provides an initial loading dose for acute effect on the enlarged heart
      (2) After desired effect is achieved, the dosage is lowered to maintenance level, replacing the drug metabolized and excreted each day
   e. Adverse effects
      (1) Most frequent: nausea, vomiting, headache, drowsiness, insomnia, vertigo, confusion; all attributable to drug action at central nervous system (CNS) sites; oral forms also cause nausea and vomiting by irritation of the gastric mucosa
      (2) Bradycardia attributable to drug-induced slowing of SA node firing
      (3) Dysrhythmias are first evidence of toxicity in one third of clients; premature nodal or ventricular impulses; varying degrees of heart block caused by drug action that slows transmission of impulses through the AV node
      (4) Xanthopsia (yellow vision) caused by drug effect on the visual cones
      (5) Gynecomastia (mammary enlargement) in males resulting from the estrogen-like steroid portion of digitalis glycosides
   f. Considerations during therapy
      (1) Premature contractions elevate the audible apical rate and mask the pacemaker conduction rate; apical pulse is taken before administration and drug is withheld when pulse rate drops to 110 to 90 in infants and below 70 in older children
      (2) Immaturity of hepatic and renal systems in premature and newborn infants or depressed hepatic or renal function in children may result in accumulation
      (3) Because potassium ions are required for interaction of digitalis glycosides with sodium-potassium–dependent membranes, the lowering of serum potassium ions may foster digitalis toxicity
      (4) Because calcium ions act synergistically with digitalis on myocardial membranes, an elevation of serum calcium ion levels may increase sensitivity of cardiac muscle to digitalis action

g. Drug interactions
   (1) Phenobarbital, phenytoin, and phenyl-butazone, by induction of hepatic microsomal enzymes, accelerate metabolism of digitalis glycosides; serum levels are lower when drugs are used concomitantly
   (2) Diuretics that cause hypokalemia may contribute to the incidence of serious dysrhythmias when administered concurrently with digitalis glycosides; supplemental potassium may be used for replacement of losses, or potassium-sparing diuretics may be prescribed to prevent potassium ion losses

▼ ACYANOTIC DEFECTS

Ventricular Septal Defect (VSD)

A. Abnormal opening between the two ventricles
B. Severity of the defect depends on size of the opening
C. High pressure in the right ventricle causes hypertrophy, with development of pulmonary hypertension
D. Low, harsh murmur heard throughout systole
E. Specific therapeutic intervention—closure of the opening at the septum
F. Prognosis—a single membranous defect has less than a 5% mortality rate; multiple muscular defects can have a mortality risk of 20%

Atrial Septal Defect (ASD)

A. Types
   1. The hole is in the center of the septum
   2. There is inadequate development of the endocardial cushions
   3. The superior portion of the atrial septum fails to form near the junction of the atrial wall with the superior vena cava
B. Murmur heard high on the chest, with fixed splitting of the second heart sound
C. Specific therapeutic intervention—closure of the opening at the septum
D. Prognosis—this defect has less than a 1% operative mortality

Patent Ductus Arteriosus (PDA)

A. Failure of the fetal connection between the aorta and pulmonary artery to close
B. Blood shunted from the aorta back to the pulmonary artery; may progress to pulmonary hypertension and cardiomegaly
C. Machinery-type murmur heard throughout the heartbeat in the left second or third interspace
D. Specific therapeutic intervention—closure of the opening between the aorta and the pulmonary artery; in critically ill newborns, pharmacologic closure may be attempted with a prostaglandin inhibitor (e.g., indomethacin, Indocid)
E. Prognosis—this defect has less than a 1% mortality

Coarctation of the Aorta

A. In utero, failure of aorta to develop completely; stricture usually occurs below level of the aortic arch
B. Increased systemic circulation above the stricture: bounding radial and carotid pulses, headache, dizziness, epistaxis
C. Decreased systemic circulation below the stricture: absent femoral pulses, cool lower extremities
D. Increased pressure in aorta above the defect causes left ventricular hypertrophy
E. Murmur may or may not be heard
F. Specific therapeutic intervention—resection of the defect and anastomosis of ends of the aorta
G. Prognosis—this defect has less than a 5% mortality in children with isolated coarctation

Aortic Stenosis

A. Narrowing of the aortic valve
B. Causes increased workload on the left ventricle, and the lowered pressure in the aorta reduces coronary artery flow
C. Specific therapeutic intervention—division of the stenotic valves of the aorta
D. Prognosis—this defect has a significant (greater than 20%) mortality in critically ill newborns; older children have a lower mortality risk

Pulmonary Stenosis

A. Narrowing of the pulmonary valve
B. Causes decreased blood flow to the lungs and increased pressure to the right ventricle
C. Specific therapeutic intervention—valvotomy or balloon angioplasty
D. Prognosis—this defect has less than a 2% mortality

▼ CYANOTIC DEFECTS

Tetralogy of Fallot

A. Four associated defects
   1. Pulmonary valve stenosis
   2. Ventricular septal defect (VSD), usually high on the septum
   3. Overriding aorta, receiving blood from both ventricles, or an aorta arising from the right ventricle
   4. Right ventricular hypertrophy
B. Specific therapeutic interventions
   1. Palliative treatment procedures performed to increase pulmonary blood flow

Repair procedure: subclavian artery to pulmonary artery anastomosis

2. Complete repair: closure of the ventricular septal defect and resection of the infundibular stenosis, possibly with a pericardial patch to enlarge the right ventricular outflow tract

C. Prognosis—this defect has a 5% to 10% surgical repair mortality

Transposition of the Great Vessels

A. Aorta arises from the right ventricle, and pulmonary artery arises from the left ventricle

B. Incompatible with life unless there is a communication between the two sides of the heart, such as an atrial septal defect, ventricular septal defect, or patent ductus arteriosus

C. Specific therapeutic interventions
1. Palliative treatment procedures performed to prevent pulmonary vascular resistance and congestive heart failure until the child is able to tolerate complete repair
   a. Repair procedure: enlargement of an existing atrial septal defect by pulling a balloon through the defect (balloon septostomy) during a cardiac catheterization
   b. Pulmonary artery banding if a ventricular septal defect is present to decrease blood flow to the lungs and increase shunting of oxygenated blood intraventricularly to the aorta
   c. Pharmacologic dilation of a patent ductus arteriosus with use of prostaglandins (e.g., Prostin VR)
   d. Surgical creation of an atrial septal defect
2. Complete repair
   a. Closure of ventricular septal defect (VSD) (directing left ventricular blood through VSD into aorta, pulmonic valve closed and conduit made from right ventricle to pulmonary artery) results in physiologic normal circulation but requires revision as child grows; procedure of choice for infants with transposition of the great vessels, VSD, and severe pulmonic stenosis
   b. Removing the entire atrial septum and creating a new atrial septum from existing pericardium or a prosthesis that tunnels or baffles blood for more effective oxygenation, with creation of two new functionally correct atrial chambers
   c. Transposing the great vessels to their correct anatomic placement with reimplantation of the coronary arteries

D. Prognosis—this defect has a 5% to 10% surgical mortality

Tricuspid Atresia

A. Absence of the tricuspid valve

B. Incompatible with life unless there is a communication between the right and left sides of the heart, such as atrial septal defect, ventricular septal defect, or patent ductus arteriosus

C. Specific therapeutic interventions
1. Palliative treatment procedures: same as for tetralogy of Fallot
2. Complete repair: conversion of the right atrium into an outlet for the pulmonary artery, which involves placing a tubular conduit with a valve between the two and closing the atrial septal defect; physiologically corrects tricuspid atresia by preventing any mixing of systemic blood in the left atrium and shunting the entire venous blood to the lungs for oxygenation

D. Prognosis—this defect has a surgical mortality greater than 10%

Truncus Arteriosus

A. Single great vessel arising from the base of the heart, serving as a pulmonary artery and aorta

B. Systolic murmur is heard, and a single semilunar valve produces a loud second heart sound that is not split

C. Specific therapeutic interventions
1. Palliative treatment: banding the pulmonary arteries as they arise from the truncus to decrease blood flow to lungs
2. Complete repair: Rastelli's operation: excising pulmonary arteries from aorta and attaching them to the right ventricle by means of a prosthetic valve conduit; septal defects also repaired

D. Prognosis—this defect requires complex repair and has a mortality of 10%

General Nursing Care of Infants and Children with Cardiac Malformations

A. **DATA COLLECTION**
1. Cyanosis, pallor, diaphoresis
2. Apical pulse, peripheral pulses, presence of murmurs
3. Respirations, dyspnea, frequency of colds
4. Blood pressure, cardiac rhythm
5. Chest abnormalities

B. **ANALYSIS AND INTERPRETATION**
1. Potential/actual oxygen deprivation
2. Risk for disorganized infant behavior related to pain and discomfort
3. Body-image disturbance related to having a physical defect
4. Risk for caregiver role strain related to caring for ill child
5. Decreased cardiac output related to structural defect

6. Altered family processes related to having a child with a heart condition
7. Altered growth and development related to inadequate oxygen and nutrients to tissues and limited socialization with peers
8. Risk for infection related to debilitated physical status
9. Risk for injury (complications) related to cardiac condition and therapies
10. Social isolation related to inability to participate in active play
11. Refer to General Nursing Diagnoses for the Family of a Child with Special Needs and General Nursing Diagnoses for Infants with Health Problems

C. PLANNING/IMPLEMENTATION

1. Check safe dosage range of digoxin; usually prescribed in micrograms (1000 µg = 1 mg)
2. Take the apical pulse prior to administering the drug
3. Observe for signs of digitalis toxicity
4. Teach the parents home administration of digoxin
   a. Give digoxin at regular intervals, usually every 12 hours, such as 8 AM and 8 PM
   b. Plan the times so that the drug is given 1 hour before or 2 hours after feedings
   c. Use a calendar to mark off each dose that is given or post a reminder, such as a sign on the refrigerator
   d. Have the prescription refilled before the medication is completely used
   e. Administer the drug carefully by slowly squirting it in the side and back of the mouth
   f. Do not mix it with other foods or fluids because refusal to consume these results in inaccurate intake of the drug
   g. If the child has teeth, give water after administering the drug; whenever possible, brush the teeth to prevent tooth decay from the sweetened liquid
   h. If a dose is missed and more than 6 hours have elapsed, withhold the dose and give the next dose at the regular time; if less than 6 hours have elapsed, give the missed dose
   i. If the child vomits within 15 minutes of receiving the digoxin, repeat the dose once; if more than 15 minutes have elapsed, do not give a second dose
   j. If more than two consecutive doses have been missed, notify the physician
   k. Do not increase or double the dose for missed doses
   l. If the child becomes ill, notify the physician immediately
   m. Keep digoxin in a safe place, preferably a locked cabinet, at room temperature
   n. In case of accidental overdose of digoxin, call the nearest poison control center immediately
5. Help the parents cope with symptoms of the disease
   a. During dyspneic/cyanotic spell, place the child in a side-lying knee-chest position, with the head and chest elevated
   b. Keep the child warm; encourage rest and sleep
   c. Decrease the child's anxiety by remaining calm
   d. Feed the child slowly; allow frequent burping
   e. Administer small, frequent meals
   f. Introduce solids and spoonfeeding early
   g. Encourage the anorexic child to eat
   h. Encourage parents to include others in child's care to prevent exhaustion
   i. Provide teaching for parents of infant with cardiac catheterization
6. Foster growth-promoting family relationships
   a. Encourage family members to discuss their feelings about each other and the child's defect
   b. Maintain expectations from all siblings as equally as possible
   c. Provide consistent discipline to prevent behavioral problems
   d. Encourage acceptable pursuits for the child
   e. Discuss school entry with the teacher and school nurse
   f. Guide parents to the eventual hazards of fostering overdependency
   g. Help the parents feel adequate in their maternal-paternal roles by emphasizing growth and developmental progress of the child
   h. Help the parents foster the child's development by stimulating the child to age-appropriate goals consistent with the child's activity tolerance
   i. Provide social experiences for the child
7. Preoperative assessment areas necessary for planning postoperative care
   a. Keep a sleep record so care can be organized around the child's usual rest pattern
   b. Avoid constipation and straining after surgery
      (1) Assess the child's elimination pattern
      (2) Know words the child uses
      (3) Have the child practice using a bedpan
   c. Record the level of activity and list favorite toys or games that require gradually increased exertion
   d. Determine the child's fluid preferences for postoperative maintenance; maintain adequate fluid intake

e. When recording vital signs, always indicate the child's activity at the time of measurement

f. Observe the child's verbal and nonverbal responses to pain

8. Prepare the child physically and emotionally for surgery

   a. Main assessment factor in preparation of the child is the developmental and chronologic age

      (1) Explanation of the heart differs according to age of the child

      (2) Children 4 to 6 years of age know that the heart is in the chest, describe it as valentine shaped, and characterize its function by the sound of "tick tock"

      (3) Children 7 to 10 years of age do not see the heart as valentine shaped, know it has veins, have an idea of its function (e.g., "It makes you live"), but do not understand the concept of pumping

      (4) Children over 10 years of age have a concept of veins, valves, circulation, and why death occurs when the heart stops

   b. Preparation is based on the principle that fear of the unknown increases anxiety

   c. The same nurse should participate in preoperative and postoperative preparation as a source of support for the child and parents

   d. Nurse must know what equipment is usual after open or closed heart surgery

   e. Let the child play with equipment such as stethoscope, blood pressure machine, SaO_2 monitor, oxygen mask, suction, and syringes

   f. For the young child, especially the preschooler, use dolls and puppets to describe procedures

   g. Preparation for cardiac catheterization prior to surgery is essential as well

   h. For the young child, talk about the size of the bandage; for the older child, discuss the actual incision

   i. Familiarize the child with the postoperative environment, such as the post-anesthesia unit and intensive care unit, stressing the strange noises

   j. Have the child practice coughing, using blow bottles, and breathing with an incentive spirometer

   k. Explain to the child why coughing and moving are necessary even though they may be uncomfortable

   l. Explain to the child what tubes may be used and what they will look like

9. Specifics of postoperative care are similar to those for any major surgery

10. Help the child and family adjust to correction of the cardiac defect

    a. Improved physical status is often difficult for the child who has become accustomed to the sick role and its secondary gains

    b. Improved physical status of the child is also difficult for the parents, since it reduces child's dependency

    c. The child may have difficulty learning to relate to peers and siblings on a competitive basis

    d. The child can no longer use the disability as a crutch for educational and social shortcomings

    e. Parental expectations must be adjusted to accommodate the child's new physical vigor and search for independence

11. See Meeting the Needs of the Family of an Infant or Child with Special Needs

D. EVALUATION/OUTCOMES

1. Child chooses and participates in appropriate activities for energy and developmental levels

2. Child experiences less dyspnea

3. Child participates in age-appropriate activities

4. Child consumes sufficient nutrients for growth and development

5. Child remains free of infection

6. Family discusses fears

7. Family demonstrates home care for child

8. Child discusses disorder and feelings about limitations

9. Child learns positive adaptation strategies

NEUROLOGIC MALFORMATIONS

▼ SPINA BIFIDA

Data Base

A. Malformation of the spine in which the posterior portion of the laminae of the vertebrae fails to close; most common site is the lumbosacral area

B. Associated defects include weakness or paralysis below the defect, bowel and bladder dysfunction, clubfeet, dislocated hip, and hydrocephalus

C. Arnold-Chiari syndrome: defect of the occipitocervical region with swelling and displacement of the medulla into the spinal cord

D. Classifications

1. Spina bifida occulta: defect only of the vertebrae; spinal cord and meninges are intact

2. Meningocele: meninges protrude through the vertebral defect

3. Meningomyelocele: meninges and spinal cord protrude through the defect; most serious type

E. Clinical findings
  1. Degree of neurologic dysfunction directly related to level of defect, extent of defect
  2. Defective nerve supply to bladder affects sphincter and muscle tone
  3. Frequently poor anal sphincter control
F. Therapeutic management
  1. Multidisciplinary approach promoting rehabilitation
  2. Surgical repair of the sac to maintain existing neurologic function and prevent infection

Nursing Care of Infants and Children with Spina Bifida

A. DATA COLLECTION
  1. Condition of the myelomeningocele sac, presence of CSF leakage
  2. Level of neurologic involvement
  3. Elimination
     a. Urine: dribble or stream, quantity of output
     b. Altered anal reflexes
  4. Monitor head circumference and fontanels at least daily

B. ANALYSIS AND INTERPRETATION
  1. Altered family processes related to the birth of a child with a physical defect
  2. Risk for infection related to exposed myelomeningocele sac, immobility
  3. Risk for impaired skin integrity related to paralysis, incontinence
  4. Risk for trauma related to spinal cord lesion
  5. Refer to General Nursing Diagnoses for the Family of a Child with Special Needs and to General Nursing Diagnoses for Infants with Health Problems

C. PLANNING/IMPLEMENTATION
  1. Protect against infection because breakdown of the sac leaves the spinal cord open to the environment
     a. Area must be kept clean, especially from urine and feces
     b. Sterile gauze soaked in sterile normal saline is maintained over the sac
     c. Avoid pressure on sac
  2. Maintain function through proper position: place in prone position, hips slightly flexed and abducted, feet hanging free of mattress
  3. Because of restriction in position, feed child in prone position; establish eye contact and encourage parents to visit and feed the child
  4. Foster elimination in the infant with a neurogenic bladder:
     a. Use the Credé method or slight pressure against the abdomen for complete emptying of the bladder
     b. While the infant is prone, apply pressure to the abdomen above the symphysis pubis

with the sides of the fingers and counterpressure with the thumbs against the buttocks
  5. Postoperative nursing care
     a. Measure head circumference to determine whether hydrocephalus is occurring
     b. Monitor for signs of increased intracranial pressure
  6. See Meeting the Needs of the Family of an Infant or Child with Special Needs
     a. Family planning with multidisciplinary team for immediate and long-term care

D. EVALUATION/OUTCOMES
  1. Remains free of infection
  2. Meningeal sac remains intact
  3. No signs of skin breakdown
  4. Family demonstrates home care for child
  5. Maintain existing neurologic function

▼ HYDROCEPHALUS

Data Base
A. Abnormal accumulation of cerebrospinal fluid within the ventricular system
B. Classifications
  1. Noncommunicating: obstruction within the ventricles such as congenital malformation, neoplasm, or hematoma
  2. Communicating: inadequate absorption of cerebrospinal fluid (CSF) resulting from infection, trauma, or obstruction by thick arachnoid membrane or meninges
C. Clinical findings
  1. Increasing head size in the infant because of open sutures and bulging fontanels
  2. Prominent scalp veins and taut, shiny skin
  3. "Sunset" eyes (sclera visible above iris), bulging eyes, and papilledema of retina
  4. Head lag, especially important after 4 to 6 months
  5. Increased intracranial pressure: projectile vomiting not associated with feeding, irritability, anorexia, high shrill cry, seizures
  6. Damage to the brain because increased pressure decreases blood flow to the cells, causing necrosis
D. Therapeutic interventions
  1. Relief of hydrocephalus
     a. Removal of the obstruction if that is the cause
     b. Mechanical shunting of CSF to another area of the body—ventricular peritoneal shunt: catheter passed subcutaneously to the peritoneal cavity
  2. Treatment of complications
  3. Management of problems related to effect on psychomotor problems

Nursing Care of Infants and Children with Hydrocephalus

A. DATA COLLECTION

1. Head circumference/fontanels
2. Signs of increased intracranial pressure

B. ANALYSIS AND INTERPRETATION

1. Altered family process related to having a seriously ill child
2. Risk for infection related to shunt
3. Risk for injury related to increased intracranial pressure
4. Risk for skin breakdown related to immobility
5. Refer to General Nursing Diagnoses for the Family of a Child with Special Needs and General Nursing Diagnoses for Infants with Health Problems

C. PLANNING/IMPLEMENTATION

1. Prevent breakdown of scalp, infection, and damage to spinal cord
   a. Place the infant in a Fowler's position to facilitate draining of fluid; infant should be positioned supine to 20-degree elevation and neutral midline
   b. When holding the infant, support the neck and head
   c. Observe shunt site (abdominal site in peritoneal procedure) for infection
2. Monitor for increasing intracranial pressure
   a. Carefully observe neurologic signs
   b. Measure head circumference, palpate anterior fontanel
   c. Use minimal sedatives or analgesics, which can mask symptoms
   d. Check the valve frequently for patency
3. Promote adequate nutrition
   a. Monitor for vomiting, irritability, lethargy, and anorexia, because these will decrease the intake of nutrients
   b. Perform all care before feeding to prevent vomiting; hold infant if possible
   c. Observe for signs of dehydration
4. Keep eyes moist and free of irritation if eyelids incompletely cover corneas; use Isopto-tears or NaCl drops
5. Postoperative nursing care: similar to that for cardiac surgery with the addition of:
   a. Place the infant or child on bed rest after surgery, with minimal handling to prevent damage to shunt
   b. Support parents
      (1) Continued shunt revisions are usually necessary as growth occurs
      (2) Usually very concerned about developmental delay
   c. Observe for brain damage by assessing and recording milestones during infancy

   d. Teach parents
      (1) Pumping of the shunt, if indicated by physician
      (2) Signs of increasing intracranial pressure
      (3) Evidence of dehydration, measure urine output
6. See Meeting the Needs of the Family of an Infant or Child with Special Needs

D. EVALUATION/OUTCOMES

1. Child does not exhibit signs of hydrocephalus
2. Child does not become infected
3. There are no signs of skin breakdown
4. Family can demonstrate home care for child

GENITOURINARY MALFORMATIONS

▼ EXSTROPHY OF THE BLADDER

Data Base

A. Absence of portion of abdominal wall and bladder wall, causing the bladder to appear to be turned inside out and outside the abdominal cavity

B. May be accompanied by defects such as inguinal hernia, epispadias, undescended testes, or short penis in boys and a cleft clitoris or absent vagina in girls

C. Occurs three times more frequently in males than females

D. Clinical findings
   1. Lower urinary tract is exposed
   2. Constant seepage of urine leading to skin breakdown and infection
   3. Progressive renal failure may result from infection and obstruction

E. Therapeutic interventions
   1. Plastic surgery
   2. Closure of the bladder within 48 hours if possible; final repair attempted before school age
   3. Ileal conduit (also called ureteroileal cutaneous ureterostomy): a small section of the ileum or colon is resected, and the remaining bowel is reanastomosed; one end of the resected bowel is sutured closed and the other end is attached to a small opening in the lower abdomen, forming a stoma; the distal ends of the ureters are severed from the bladder and attached to the ileum, which acts like a bladder, although there is no voluntary control in the regulation of voiding; the child wears an ileostomy appliance over the stoma, which collects the continuously flowing urine
   4. Cutaneous ureterostomy: the ureters are attached directly to the abdominal wall, usually

at a site proximal to the level of the kidneys; two collecting appliances are worn over the bilateral openings

Nursing Care of Infants and Children with Exstrophy of Bladder

A. DATA COLLECTION
1. Condition of skin
2. Renal function; urine output
3. Parental interaction with child

B. ANALYSIS AND INTERPRETATION
1. Altered family processes related to loss of image of ideal child
2. Risk for infection related to structural alterations
3. Risk for impaired skin integrity related to incontinence
4. Refer to General Nursing Diagnoses for the Family of a Child with Special Needs and General Nursing Diagnoses for Infants with Health Problems

C. PLANNING/IMPLEMENTATION
1. Help the parents to accept the disorder and the long-term sequelae
2. Scrupulously clean the area around the bladder and apply sterile petrolatum gauze
3. Use loose clothing to avoid pressure over the area
4. Change clothing frequently because of odor
5. Care for the urine-collecting appliance; change frequently
6. See Meeting the Needs of the Family of an Infant or Child with Special Needs

D. EVALUATION/OUTCOMES
1. No signs of skin breakdown
2. No evidence of infection
3. Renal function remains within normal limits
4. Family can verbalize care of child

▼ DISPLACED URETHRAL OPENING

Data Base

A. Urethral opening is abnormally located
B. In males severity varies, depending on distance from the tip of the penis and involvement of additional penile deformities
C. Classification
1. Hypospadias
a. In males the urethra opens on the lower surface of the penis from just behind the glans to the perineum (placement varies)
b. In females the urethra opens into the vagina
2. Epispadias
a. Occurs only in males
b. Urethra opens on dorsal surface of the penis; often associated with exstrophy of the bladder

3. Defect can be a sign of ambiguous genitalia
D. Clinical findings
1. Procreation may be interfered with in severe cases
2. Increased risk of urinary tract infection
E. Therapeutic interventions—surgery
1. Repair of the defect
2. Repair may be performed in several stages

Nursing Care of Infants and Children with a Displaced Urethral Opening

A. DATA COLLECTION
1. Parental knowledge of defect
2. Origin of urinary stream

B. ANALYSIS AND INTERPRETATION
1. Risk for disorganized infant behavior related to pain and discomfort
2. Body image disturbance related to perception of physical defect
3. Pain related to:
a. Response to deformity
b. Postoperative response
4. Social isolation related to:
a. Frequent hospitalization
b. Body-image disturbance
5. Refer to General Nursing Diagnoses for the Family of a Child with Special Needs and General Nursing Diagnoses for Infants with Health Problems

C. PLANNING/IMPLEMENTATION
1. Provide the parents with an explicit explanation of child's future functioning
2. Prepare child for surgery; the boy needs help in coping with anatomic difference from peers and the adjustments to voiding in the sitting position
3. See Meeting the Needs of the Family of an Infant or Child with Special Needs

D. EVALUATION/OUTCOMES
1. Child will not exhibit physiologic signs of pain
2. Child/parents will verbalize effects of the defect and correction
3. Child/parents will maintain peer interactions

SKELETAL MALFORMATIONS

▼ CLUBFOOT

Data Base

A. Foot has been twisted out of normal shape or position
B. Most common type: talipes equinovarus: foot is fixed in plantar flexion (downward) and deviated medially (inward)

C. Clinical findings
1. Deformity is readily apparent at birth
2. Deformity may be rigid or flexible
D. Therapeutic interventions
1. Treatment is most successful when started early in infancy because delay causes muscles and bones of legs to develop abnormally, with shortening of tendons
2. Nonsurgical treatment: gentle, repeated manipulation of the foot with casting; done every few days for 1 to 2 weeks then at 1- to 2-week intervals
3. Surgical treatment: done if nonsurgical treatment not effective
   a. Tight ligaments released
   b. Tendons lengthened or transplanted
4. Follow-up care of the client
   a. Extended medical supervision is required because there is a tendency for this deformity to recur (considered cured when the child is able to wear normal shoes and walk properly)
   b. Care emphasizes muscle reeducation (by manipulation) and proper walking
   c. Heels and soles of braces or shoes prescribed following correction must be kept in repair
   d. Corrective shoes may have sole and heel lifts on lateral border to maintain proper position

Nursing Care of Infants and Children with Clubfoot
A. DATA COLLECTION
1. Parental understanding and compliance with treatment regimen
2. Skin and circulation of affected limb
B. ANALYSIS AND INTERPRETATION
1. Risk for injury related to knowledge deficit and use of corrective devices
2. Risk for impaired skin integrity related to use of corrective devices
3. Refer to General Nursing Diagnoses for the Family of a Child with Special Needs and General Nursing Diagnoses for Infants with Health Problems
C. PLANNING/IMPLEMENTATION
1. Observe toes for signs of circulatory impairment; make sure toes are visible at the end of the cast
2. Watch for signs of weakness and wear of the cast, especially if the child is allowed to walk on it
3. Teach parents all the necessary care and emphasize the need for follow-up, which may be prolonged

4. Need to replace cast frequently to accommodate growth
5. For other areas of cast care, see Congenital Hip Dysplasia
6. See Meeting the Needs of the Family of an Infant or Child with Special Needs
D. EVALUATION/OUTCOMES
1. Parents can demonstrate home care
2. Skin remains intact

▼ CONGENITAL HIP DYSPLASIA

Data Base
A. Imperfect development of hip—can affect femoral head, acetabulum, or both
B. Head of the femur does not lie deep enough within the acetabulum and slips out on movement
C. Occurs in females seven times more often than in males
D. Classification
1. Acetabular dysplasia
   a. Mildest form
   b. Femoral head remains in acetabulum
2. Subluxation
   a. Most common form
   b. Femoral head partially displaced
3. Dislocation
   a. Femoral head not in contact with acetabulum
   b. Displaced posteriorly and superiorly
E. Clinical findings
1. Limitation in abduction of leg on the affected side
2. Asymmetry of gluteal, popliteal, and thigh folds
3. Audible click when abducting and externally rotating the hip on the affected side: Ortolani's sign
4. Apparent shortening of the femur: Galeazzi's sign
5. Waddling gait and lordosis when the child begins to walk
F. Therapeutic interventions
1. Directed toward enlarging and deepening the acetabulum by placing the head of the femur within the acetabulum and applying constant pressure
2. Proper positioning: legs slightly flexed and abducted
   a. Pavlik harness
   b. Frejka pillow: a pillow splint that maintains abduction of the legs
   c. Bryant's (Gallow's) traction
   d. Spica cast: from the waist to below the knees
   e. Brace
3. Surgical intervention such as open reduction with casting

Nursing Care of Infants and Children with Congenital Hip Dysplasia

A. DATA COLLECTION

1. Limb shorter on affected side
2. Positive Ortolani's test (hip click)
3. Restricted abduction of hip on affected side

B. ANALYSIS AND INTERPRETATION

1. Altered family processes related to having a child with a physical defect
2. Altered growth and development related to immobilization
3. Impaired physical mobility related to immobilizing device
4. Risk for injury related to:
   a. Corrective device
   b. Immobility
5. Refer to General Nursing Diagnoses for the Family of a Child with Special Needs and General Nursing Diagnoses for Infants with Health Problems

C. PLANNING/IMPLEMENTATION

1. Respiratory problems: hypostatic pneumonia
   a. Change position frequently from back to stomach
   b. Teach parents postural drainage and exercises for child, such as blowing bubbles to increase lung expansion
   c. Encourage parents to seek immediate medical care if the child develops congestion or cough
2. Infection and excoriation of skin
   a. Observe for circulation to toes, pedal pulses, and blanching
   b. Do not let the child put small toys or food inside cast
   c. Use gauze strips inside cast as a scratcher
   d. Alert parents to signs of infection, such as odor
   e. Protect cast edges with adhesive tape or waterproof material, especially around perineum
   f. Use diapers and plastic lining to minimize soiling of cast by feces and urine
3. Constipation from immobility
   a. Teach parents to observe for straining on defecation and constipation
   b. Increase fluids and fiber to prevent constipation
4. Nutrition
   a. Provide small, frequent meals because of inflexibility of cast around waist (a window may be made over the abdominal area to allow for expansion with meals)
   b. Adjust calorie intake, because less energy expenditure can lead to obesity
5. Transportation and positioning
   a. Use wagon or stroller with back flat or mechanic's creeper
   b. Use back seat of car with lap belt around waist
   c. Protect child from falling when positioned
   d. Never pick up child by the bar between the legs of the cast (use two people to provide adequate body support if necessary)
6. Meet emotional needs
   a. Use touch as much as possible; small children can be picked up and cuddled
   b. Stimulate and provide for play activities appropriate to age
7. Provide parents with help and support
   a. Give written instructions
   b. Schedule routine home visits with telephone counseling available
   c. Stress need for follow-up care because treatment may be prolonged
   d. Prepare parents for the possible use of an abduction brace after the cast is removed
8. When a spica cast is applied see Fractures in Medical-Surgical Nursing (Chapter 6) for care of the client with a cast
9. See Meeting the Needs of the Family of an Infant or Child with Special Needs

D. EVALUATION/OUTCOMES

1. Child can move about and control environment
2. Child remains free of injury
3. Parents can discuss special needs and demonstrate home care
4. Child is able to regain prior movement (crawling/walking) when device is removed

INBORN ERRORS OF METABOLISM

Inherited disorders caused by absence of a substance essential to cellular metabolism

Characterized by abnormal fat, protein, or carbohydrate metabolism

Usually inherited as autosomal recessive trait

▼ PHENYLKETONURIA (PKU)

Data Base

A. Lack of the enzyme phenylalanine hydroxylase, which changes phenylalanine (essential amino acid) into tyrosine
B. Clinical findings
   1. Developmental disability from damage to the nervous system by buildup of phenylalanine, often noticed by 4 months of age

2. Strong musty odor in urine from phenylacetic acid
3. Absence of tyrosine reduces the production of melanin and results in blond hair and blue eyes
4. Fair skin is susceptible to eczema

C. Therapeutic interventions
1. Guthrie blood test: testing should be done after protein ingestion; if testing is done during initial 24 hours, it should be repeated by the third week of life
2. Early detection is essential
3. Dietary: low-phenylalanine: for infants use a milk substitute and restrict foods to those low in this amino acid
   a. Use of phenylalanine-free formulas for children over 3 years of age
   b. Dietary restrictions of phenylalanine through adolescence
   c. Individuals with phenylketonuria who become pregnant must consume a low-phenylalanine diet
4. Treat eczema; see Atopic Dermatitis (Eczema)

▼ GALACTOSEMIA

Data Base

A. Missing enzyme that converts galactose to glucose
B. Clinical findings
1. Jaundice develops
2. Weight loss/vomiting
3. Hepatosplenomegaly
4. Cataracts
C. Therapeutic interventions
1. Early detection: test for galactosemia at birth; Beutler test (method similar to Guthrie test for PKU)
2. Dietary reduction of lactose: use a soy-based formula as a milk substitute and restrict foods to those low in lactose (usually continued until the child is 7 to 8 years of age), followed by a dietary modification throughout life

▼ CONGENITAL HYPOTHYROIDISM

Data Base

A. Failure of embryonic development of the thyroid gland or inborn enzyme defect in the formation of thyroxine
B. Clinical findings
1. Prolonged physiologic jaundice, feeding difficulties, inactivity (excessive sleeping, little crying), anemia, problems resulting from hypotonic abdominal muscles (constipation, protruding abdomen, and umbilical hernia)
2. Appears at 3 to 6 months of age in formula-fed babies; may be delayed in breastfed babies
3. Impaired development of nervous system leads to developmental disability; level depends on degree of hypothyroidism and interval before therapy is begun
4. Decreased growth and decreased metabolic rate resulting in increased weight
5. Characteristic infant facies: short forehead; wide, puffy eyes; wrinkled eyelids; broad, short, upturned nose; large, protruding tongue; hair is dry, brittle, and lusterless with low hairline
6. Skin is mottled because of decreased heart rate and circulation
7. Skin is yellowish from carotenemia resulting from decreased conversion of carotene to vitamin A
C. Therapeutic interventions
1. Detection: neonatal screening for thyroxine (T_4) and thyroid-stimulating hormone (TSH)
   a. Test is done when indicated
   b. Performed by heel-stick blood test
2. Treatment: replacement therapy with thyroid hormone; if therapy begun before 3 months of age, chances for normal growth and development are increased

General Nursing Care of Infants and Children with Inborn Errors of Metabolism

A. DATA COLLECTION
1. Verification of test results
2. Parents' understanding of disorder
3. Growth and development

B. ANALYSIS AND INTERPRETATION
1. Body image disturbance related to dietary restrictions
2. Altered family processes related to:
   a. Situational crisis
   b. Genetic illness
3. Anticipatory grieving related to loss of perfect child
4. Altered growth and development related to changes in metabolism
5. Knowledge deficit related to special dietary needs
6. Altered nutrition: less than body requirements related to restrictive diet
7. Refer to General Nursing Diagnoses for the Family of a Child with Special Needs and General Nursing Diagnoses for Infants with Health Problems

C. PLANNING/IMPLEMENTATION
1. Help parents to understand the disease and the role of diet and medications

2. Refer parents for genetic counseling
3. Specific nursing care for children with hypothyroidism
   a. Instruct parents regarding administration of thyroid replacement and signs of overdose (rapid pulse, dyspnea, insomnia, irritability, sweating, fever, and weight loss)
   b. Teach parents to take pulse
4. See Meeting the Needs of the Family of an Infant or Child with Special Needs

D. EVALUATION/OUTCOMES
1. Child achieves satisfactory growth and development
2. Child consumes adequate nutrients for growth
3. Child/family verbalizes necessity of diet and acceptable modifications
4. Child/family verbalizes and demonstrates prescribed diet/medications

HEALTH PROBLEMS THAT DEVELOP DURING INFANCY

(Problems may continue past 12 months of age and through childhood)

▼ INTUSSUSCEPTION

Data Base
A. Telescoping of one portion of the intestine into another; occurs most frequently at the ileocecal valve
B. Males affected two times more frequently than females
C. Usually occurs between 3 to 12 months of age
D. Classification
   1. Ileocecal: invagination at the ileocecal valve; most common type
   2. Ileoileal: one part of ileum invaginates on another section of the ileum
   3. Colocolic: one part of the colon invaginates on another section of the colon
E. Clinical findings
   1. Healthy, well-nourished infant or child who wakes up with severe paroxysmal abdominal pain, evidenced by kicking and drawing legs up to the abdomen
   2. One or two normal stools, then bloody mucus stool ("currant jelly-like" stool)
   3. Palpation of sausage-shaped mass
   4. Other signs of intestinal obstruction usually present
F. Therapeutic interventions
   1. Medical reduction by hydrostatic pressure (barium enema)
   2. Surgical reduction; sometimes with intestinal resection

Nursing Care of Infants and Children with Intussusception

A. DATA COLLECTION
1. Sudden, acute, intermittent abdominal pain
2. Vomiting
3. Red "currant jelly-like" stools
4. Tender, distended abdomen

B. ANALYSIS AND INTERPRETATION
1. Pain related to invaginating bowel
2. Altered family processes related to having a child with life-threatening illness
3. Altered nutrition: less than body requirements related to:
   a. Decreased intake
   b. Increased peristalsis
4. Risk for fluid volume deficit related to:
   a. Vomiting
   b. Diarrhea
5. Refer to General Nursing Diagnoses for the Family of a Child with Special Needs and General Nursing Diagnoses for Infants with Health Problems

C. PLANNING/IMPLEMENTATION
1. Same as for any abdominal surgery
2. Make provisions for frequent parental visits because the problem usually occurs when the child is 6 to 8 months of age and separation anxiety is acute
3. See Meeting the Needs of the Family of an Infant or Child with Special Needs

D. EVALUATION/OUTCOMES
1. Child does not show physiologic manifestation of pain
2. Family can verbalize feelings about the illness
3. Child consumes sufficient nutrients for growth
4. Child does not exhibit signs of dehydration

▼ FAILURE TO THRIVE (FTT)

Data Base
A. The term used to describe infants and children whose weight and sometimes height fall below the fifth percentile for their age
B. Persistent deviation from established growth curve
C. Classification
   1. Organic (OFTT): result of a physical cause, such as congenital heart defects, neurologic lesions, microcephaly, chronic urinary tract infection, malabsorption syndrome, gastroesophageal reflux, renal insufficiency, endocrine dysfunction, or cystic fibrosis
   2. Nonorganic (NFTT): caused by psychosocial factors, problem being between the child and the primary caregiver; in this situation the lack of physical growth is secondary to the lack of emotional and sensory stimulation (other

terms include maternal deprivation, environmental deprivation, and deprivation dwarfism)

3. Idiopathic (IFTT): unexplained by the usual organic or environmental etiologies but usually classified as NFTT

4. Nonorganic and idiopathic failure to thrive account for the majority of FTT

D. Clinical findings

1. Organic: identifiable physical cause of the growth failure

2. Nonorganic

a. Characteristics of nonorganic FTT in children

(1) Growth failure: below the fifth percentile in height and weight

(2) Developmental disability: social, motor, adaptive, language

(3) Apathy

(4) Poor hygiene

(5) Withdrawn behavior

(6) Feeding or eating disorders, such as vomiting, anorexia, pica, rumination

(7) No fear of strangers (at the age when stranger anxiety is normal)

(8) Avoidance of eye-to-eye contact

(9) Wide-eyed gaze and continual scan of the environment ("radar gaze")

(10) Stiff and unyielding or flaccid and unresponsive

(11) Minimal smiling

b. Characteristics of the parent providing care

(1) Difficulty perceiving and assessing the infant's needs

(2) Frustrated and angered at the infant's dissatisfied response

(3) Frequently under stress and in crisis, with emotional, social, and financial problems

(4) Often with marital disturbances (e.g., absent spouse or one who gives little emotional support)

(5) Tend to lead lonely, solitary lives with few outside interests or friends

(6) Experienced poor parenting as a child

E. Therapeutic interventions

1. Provide sufficient nutrients to achieve a rate of growth greater than expected

2. Treat underlying cause

a. Coexisting medical problems

b. Parent-child relationship

Nursing Care of Infants and Children with Failure to Thrive

A. DATA COLLECTION

1. Accurate height and weight and daily weight

2. Feeding behavior

3. Parent-child behavior/interactions

4. Developmental level

B. ANALYSIS AND INTERPRETATION

1. Altered growth and development related to:

a. Physiologic factors

b. Physical neglect

c. Social neglect

2. Altered nutrition: less than body requirements related to feeding, eating disorders, malabsorption of nutrients

3. Altered parenting related to:

a. Knowledge deficit

b. Poverty

c. Infant's failure to develop

4. Refer to General Nursing Diagnoses for the Family of a Child with Special Needs and General Nursing Diagnoses for Infants with Health Problems

C. PLANNING/IMPLEMENTATION

1. Provide a consistent caregiver who can begin to satisfy routine needs

2. Provide optimum nutrients

a. Make feeding a priority goal

b. Keep an accurate record of intake to determine daily calories

c. Weigh daily and record to ascertain weight gain

3. Introduce a positive feeding environment

a. Assign one nurse for feeding

b. Maintain a calm, even temperament; be persistent

c. Provide a quiet, unstimulating environment

d. Hold the young child for feeding

e. Maintain eye-to-eye contact with the child

f. Talk to the child by giving appropriate directions and praise for eating

g. Follow the child's rhythm of feeding

h. Establish a structured routine and follow it consistently

4. Increase stimulation appropriate to the child's present developmental level

5. Provide the parent an opportunity to talk

6. When necessary, relieve the parent of child-rearing responsibilities until able and ready emotionally to support the child

7. Demonstrate proper infant care by example, not lecturing (allow the parent to proceed at own pace)

8. Supply the parent with emotional support without fostering dependency

9. Promote the parent's self-respect and confidence by praising achievements with child

D. EVALUATION/OUTCOMES

1. Child demonstrates a positive response to interventions

2. Child steadily gains weight
3. Parents demonstrate the ability to care for the child

▼ SUDDEN INFANT DEATH SYNDROME (SIDS; INFANT CRIB DEATH)

Data Base

A. A definite syndrome with unknown cause
B. The number one cause of death in infants between 1 week and 1 year of age; incidence of 1.4 in every 1000 live births
C. Peak age of occurrence: healthy infants 2 to 4 months of age—90% occur by 6 months
D. Higher incidence in:
    1. Males
    2. Premature infants
    3. Multiple births
    4. Newborns with low Apgar scores
    5. Infants with CNS disturbances
    6. Infants with respiratory disorders such as bronchopulmonary dysplasia
    7. Infants sleeping on abdomen
    8. Infants using soft, moldable pillows and/or mattresses
E. Feeding habits not significant; breastfeeding does not prevent SIDS
F. May be a greater incidence in siblings of children with SIDS
G. Pulmonary edema and intrathoracic hemorrhages found on autopsy
H. Clinical findings
    1. Sudden, unexplained death of an infant under 1 year of age
    2. Frothy, blood-tinged fluid fills mouth and nose
I. Therapeutic interventions
    1. Avoid implying wrongdoing, abuse, or neglect
    2. Support parents
    3. Be nonjudgmental about parents' attempts at resuscitation

Nursing Care of Families of Infants with Sudden Infant Death Syndrome

A. DATA COLLECTION
    1. Parental knowledge of SIDS
    2. Parental support system
B. ANALYSIS AND INTERPRETATION
    1. Family coping: potential for growth related to successfully coping with loss
    2. Ineffective family coping: disabling related to situational crisis
    3. Altered family processes related to disruption of life-style
    4. Dysfunctional grieving related to loss of child
    5. Risk for altered parenting of other children related to grief
C. PLANNING/IMPLEMENTATION
    1. Know signs of SIDS to distinguish it from child neglect or abuse; do or say nothing that instills guilt in the parents
    2. Reassure the parents that they could not have prevented the death or predicted its occurrence
    3. Reinforce that an autopsy should be done on every child to confirm diagnosis
    4. Visit the parents at home to discuss the cause of death and help them with their guilt and grief
    5. Refer the parents to a national SIDS parent group
    6. Teach parents suggested positioning
D. EVALUATION/OUTCOMES
    1. Family exhibits positive coping behavior
    2. Family members avail themselves of support services
    3. Family exhibits positive bereavement behavior
    4. Parents maintain supportive relationship with other children

▼ APNEA OF INFANCY (AOI)

Data Base

A. Apnea of 15 seconds or less is normal at any age
B. Pathologic apnea lasts at least 20 seconds
C. May be symptomatic of sepsis, seizures, upper airway abnormalities, gastroesophageal reflux, hypoglycemia, or impaired regulation of sleep or feeding
D. No cause identified in 50% of cases
E. Less than 7% of SIDS cases
F. Clinical findings
    1. Usually presents as an apparent life-threatening event
    2. Is associated with cyanosis, marked pallor, hypotonia, or bradycardia
G. Therapeutic interventions
    1. Continuous home monitoring of cardiorespiratory rhythm
    2. Use of respiratory stimulant medication such as theophylline
    3. Treatment discontinued when child has gone 2 to 3 months without a significant number of alarms or with apneic episodes that did not require intervention

Nursing Care of Infants with Apnea
A. DATA COLLECTION
    1. Parental fears and concerns
    2. Knowledge about cardiopulmonary resuscitation (CPR) and home monitoring

3. Description of apparent life-threatening event

B. ANALYSIS AND INTERPRETATION
1. Ineffective breathing pattern related to periods of apnea
2. Caregiver role strain related to constant monitoring
3. Ineffective family coping: compromised; related to prolonged need for monitoring that exhausts supportive capacity of parents
4. Altered family processes related to constant monitoring
5. Fear related to possible loss of child
6. Anticipatory grieving related to loss of perfect child
7. Knowledge deficit related to home monitoring, CPR
8. Refer to General Nursing Diagnoses for the Family of a Child with Special Needs and General Nursing Diagnoses for Infants with Health Problems

C. PLANNING/IMPLEMENTATION
1. Monitor type and quality of apneic episodes
2. Teach parents about home monitoring
3. Teach parents how to stimulate/resuscitate infant
4. Assist parents to identify support system

D. EVALUATION/OUTCOMES
1. Parents can demonstrate proper use of equipment for home monitoring
2. Parents demonstrate CPR
3. Parents verbalize fears
4. Family identifies support system

▼ DIARRHEA

Data Base
A. Frequent, watery stools caused by increased peristalsis resulting from a variety of causes, local or systemic
B. Classification
1. Acute: sudden change in frequency and consistency of stools
2. Chronic: persists longer than 2 weeks
C. Clinical findings
1. Frequent, watery stools
2. Loss of fluids and electrolytes
3. If fluid loss is severe
   a. Weight loss greater than 10% (severe dehydration)
   b. Poor skin turgor and dry mucous membranes
   c. Depressed fontanels and sunken eyeballs
   d. Decreased urine output, increased specific gravity, and increased hematocrit
   e. Irritability, stupor, seizures from loss of intracellular water and decreased plasma volume

f. Metabolic acidosis, which decreases available bicarbonate

D. Therapeutic interventions
1. In severe diarrhea correct fluid and electrolyte imbalance
2. Identify the causative agent and institute proper therapy (antibiotics are used if a bacterial agent is present)

Nursing Care of Infants and Children with Diarrhea
A. DATA COLLECTION
1. Assess diarrhea: number, volume, characteristics
2. State of hydration
3. Possible source of infection

B. ANALYSIS AND INTERPRETATION
1. Altered family processes related to having a child with a defect
2. Risk for infection related to presence of infectious organisms
3. Altered nutrition: less than body requirements related to increased losses
4. Risk for impaired skin integrity related to frequent loose stools
5. Fluid volume deficit related to losses in stools
6. See General Nursing Diagnoses for Infants with Health Problems

C. PLANNING/IMPLEMENTATION
1. Isolate the infant until stool culture results are reported as negative
2. Explain to the parents why antibiotics and an increase in food are ineffective in treating viral diarrhea
3. Teach parents progressive increase in diet: alterations in diet may control mild diarrhea
   a. Clear fluids to decrease inflammation of the intestinal mucosa
   b. If tolerated, use half-strength formula
   c. Regular diet of bland foods
   d. Daily weights

D. EVALUATION/OUTCOMES
1. Child consumes sufficient calories and fluids
2. No evidence of skin breakdown
3. Child and family do not spread infection
4. Family can discuss illness and home care of child

▼ VOMITING

Data Base
A. Common symptom in childhood, usually minor and of short duration
B. Associated hazard: aspiration with risk of asphyxiation, atelectasis, or pneumonia
C. Forcible ejection of stomach contents: usually associated with nausea

D. Causes
   1. Most commonly caused by infection
   2. Response to allergen, drug ingestion
   3. Recurrent or prolonged vomiting may be caused by increased intracranial pressure
E. Clinical findings
   1. One or more episodes of regurgitation or emesis
   2. If vomiting is severe
      a. Dehydration
      b. Tetany and convulsions in severe alkalosis resulting from hypokalemia and hypocalcemia
      c. Metabolic alkalosis from loss of hydrogen ions
F. Therapeutic intervention—correction of underlying disorder

Nursing Care of Infants and Children with Vomiting

A. DATA COLLECTION
   1. Amount and character of vomiting
   2. Circumstances preceding vomiting
   3. Child's behavior
B. ANALYSIS AND INTERPRETATION
   1. Altered nutrition: less than body requirements related to vomiting
   2. Fluid volume deficit related to losses with vomiting
   3. See General Nursing Diagnoses for Infants with Health Problems
C. PLANNING/IMPLEMENTATION
   1. Maintain in side-lying or prone position with body inclined at 30 degrees at all times
   2. Do not disturb infant after feeding
   3. If associated with gastroesophageal reflux or cardiac sphincter problems:
      a. Thicken the consistency of foods given
      b. Provide small volume feedings every 2 to 3 hours
D. EVALUATION/OUTCOMES
   1. Child does not show evidence of dehydration
   2. Child consumes adequate nutrients for growth and development
   3. Parents verbalize feelings about illness

▼ COLIC

Data Base

A. Paroxsymal abdominal pain or cramping
B. More common in infants of less than 3 months
C. May be caused by cow's milk sensitivity, but often no cause is found
D. May be associated with excessive swallowing of air, size of nipple opening or shape of nipple, too rapid feeding or overfeeding, tenseness or anxiety in the primary caregiver, maternal diet
E. Clinical findings
   1. Pulling up of arms and legs
   2. Red-faced crying over long periods of time
   3. Presence of excessive gas
F. Therapeutic intervention—correction of the underlying cause when identified

Nursing Care of Infants with Colic

A. DATA COLLECTION
   1. Characteristics of the cry (duration and intensity)
   2. Diet of breastfeeding mother or type of formula/food intake
   3. When the attacks occur in relationship to feeding
   4. Activity of caregiver around time of attack
   5. Measures to relieve crying and their effectiveness
   6. Posture of children when cuddled
   7. Acceptance of cuddling by primary caregiver
   8. Activities of success/frustration
B. ANALYSIS AND INTERPRETATION
   1. Ineffective family coping: compromised, related to alterations in family life-style and relationships related to infant's discomfort
   2. Knowledge deficit related to infant feeding practices
   3. Pain related to abdominal cramping
   4. Altered sleep patterns related to:
      a. Pain
      b. Interrupted sleep from infant crying
   5. Refer to General Nursing Diagnoses for the Family of a Child with Special Needs and General Nursing Diagnoses for Infants with Health Problems
   6. See Nursing Diagnoses for Infants with Diarrhea
C. PLANNING/IMPLEMENTATION
   1. Watch the parent feed the infant before attempting to counsel
   2. Provide smaller, frequent feedings
   3. Teach the parent to bubble the infant frequently and to position on the side or abdomen after feeding
   4. Encourage the mother to take time away from the infant
   5. Reassure mother that the condition is not life-threatening, the infant will gain weight, the condition will eventually subside, she is not a bad parent
   6. Alternative therapeutics (e.g., massage therapy, vibrating sounds/motions)
   7. Review stress management techniques and resources
D. EVALUATION/OUTCOMES
   1. Child has decreased pain episodes

2. Parents and child are rested and ready for day's activities
3. Parents demonstrate proper feeding practices
4. Family can discuss the impact of the infant's colic
5. Pattern episodes with dietary changes

▼ CONSTIPATION

Data Base

A. Hard, dry stools that are difficult to pass or are infrequent
B. Usually a result of diet, although may have a psychologic component
C. May be indicative of Hirschsprung's disease
D. Classification
   1. Obstipation: long periods between defecation
   2. Encopresis: constipation with fecal soiling
E. Clinical findings
   1. "Stool withholding" behavior
   2. Pain on defecation
F. Therapeutic interventions
   1. Dietary: increased fiber and fluid
   2. If mineral oil is used, it should not be given with foods, because it decreases the absorption of nutrients
   3. Enemas should be avoided; bowel retraining should be instituted

Nursing Care of Infants and Children with Constipation

A. DATA COLLECTION
   1. History of bowel habits, diet
   2. Stool characteristics, frequency
   3. Parent/child knowledge of elimination
   4. Cultural patterns or environment

B. ANALYSIS AND INTERPRETATION
   1. Constipation related to inadequate fluid and fiber intake
   2. Altered nutrition: less than body requirements related to inadequate intake of fiber
   3. Pain related to:
      a. Bowel distention
      b. Alteration in bowel motility
   4. See General Nursing Diagnoses for Infants with Health Problems

C. PLANNING/IMPLEMENTATION
   1. Teach parents to provide foods with fiber and avoid those that bind
   2. Teach parents to increase amount of fluid given to infant/child
   3. Place infant in knee-chest position if abdominal distention or cramping is present
   4. Cuddle infant to provide comfort as necessary
   5. Teach child stool elimination patterns (e.g., take time to sit)

D. EVALUATION/OUTCOMES
   1. Child consumes appropriate amount of fiber
   2. Child drinks increased fluid
   3. Child does not experience pain with defecation
   4. Child defecates in response to physiologic messages and more frequently

▼ RESPIRATORY TRACT INFECTIONS

Data Base

A. Frequent cause of morbidity
B. Young children have four to five infections per year
C. Children between 6 months and 3 years react more severely
D. Classification
   1. Acute infection may be bacterial or viral
   2. Acute nasopharyngitis (common cold)
   3. Pneumonia
   4. Bronchitis
   5. Tonsillitis
   6. Epiglottitis
   7. Acute laryngotracheobronchitis (croup)
E. Clinical findings
   1. Infection
      a. Elevated temperature
      b. Purulent discharge from nose, ears, lungs
      c. Enlarged cervical lymph nodes
   2. Cough
   3. Wheeze
   4. Cyanosis
F. Therapeutic interventions
   1. Supportive therapy
   2. Treat underlying cause if infectious

Nursing Care of Infants and Children with Respiratory Tract Infections

A. DATA COLLECTION
   1. Respirations: rate, depth, ease, and rhythm
   2. Color: cyanosis
   3. Lungs: adventitious sounds
   4. Nasal discharge
   5. Presence of sputum
   6. Posture
   7. Pyrexia
   8. Cough
   9. Characteristics of cry

B. ANALYSIS AND INTERPRETATION
   1. Ineffective airway clearance related to:
      a. Mechanical obstruction
      b. Inflammation
      c. Increased secretions
      d. Pain
   2. Ineffective breathing pattern related to:
      a. Inflammatory process
      b. Pain

3. Risk for injury related to presence of infective organisms
4. Pain related to:
   a. Inflammatory process
   b. Excessive coughing
5. See General Nursing Diagnoses for Infants with Health Problems

C. **PLANNING/IMPLEMENTATION**
1. Increase fluid intake
   a. Prevents dehydration from fever and perspiration
   b. Loosens thickened secretions
2. Increase humidity and coolness
   a. Liquifies secretions
   b. Decreases the febrile state and inflammation of the mucous membrane
   c. Causes vasoconstriction and bronchiolar dilation
3. Promote nasal and pulmonary drainage
   a. Clean the nares with a bulb syringe
   b. Suction the oronasal pharynx
   c. Perform postural drainage, clapping, and vibrating
4. Provide rest by decreasing stimulation
5. Increase oxygen
6. Never use tongue blade to visualize posterior pharynx in children with epiglottitis or croup. Laryngospasm is likely in this circumstance with croup as well as epiglottitis
7. If a tracheotomy is necessary see Medical-Surgical Nursing (Chapter 6) for Nursing Care of Clients with a Tracheotomy
8. Prepare for X-ray

D. **EVALUATION/OUTCOMES**
1. Child rests and sleeps with unlabored respirations
2. Airway remains clear
3. Child shows decreasing severity of symptoms
4. Child does not exhibit physiologic signs of pain

▼ OTITIS MEDIA

Data Base
A. Acute infection of the middle ear; causative organism usually *Streptococcus pneumoniae*, *Haemophilus influenzae*, or *Staphylococcus aureus*
B. One of most common diseases of early childhood
C. Highest incidence between ages 6 months to 2 years
D. Classification
   1. Otitis media: inflammation of middle ear without reference to cause or pathogenesis
   2. Acute otitis media: rapid, short onset of signs and symptoms lasting about 3 weeks
   3. Otitis media with effusion: middle ear inflammation with fluid present

4. Subacute otitis media: lasts more than 3 weeks
5. Chronic otitis media with effusion: lasts more than 3 months
E. Clinical findings
   1. Acute otitis media
      a. Pain: infant frets and rubs ear or rolls head from side to side
      b. Drum bulging, red, may rupture; no light reflex
   2. Otitis media with effusion
      a. No pain or fever, but "fullness" in the ear
      b. Drum appears gray, bulging
      c. Possible loss of hearing from scarring of the drum
F. Therapeutic interventions
   1. Antibiotic therapy
   2. Surgery including myringotomy or insertion of tympanotomy tubes

Nursing Care of Infants and Children with Otitis Media
A. **DATA COLLECTION**
1. Pain
2. Signs and symptoms of infection
3. Allergies

B. **ANALYSIS AND INTERPRETATION**
1. Altered family processes related to having child with an infection
2. Risk for infection related to:
   a. Inadequate treatment
   b. Infectious organism
3. Risk for injury related to:
   a. Inadequate treatment
   b. Infectious organism
4. Pain related to pressure caused by inflammatory process
5. See General Nursing Diagnoses for Infants with Health Problems

C. **PLANNING/IMPLEMENTATION**
1. Teach parents proper administration of antibiotics; stress importance of full course of therapy
2. Teach parent proper instillation of ear drops
   a. If the child is under 3 years of age, pull the auricle down and back
   b. For an older child, pull the auricle up and back
3. Minimize recurrence
   a. Eliminate environmental allergens
   b. Feed in upright position
4. Encourage medical follow-up to check for complications such as chronic hearing loss, mastoiditis, or possible meningitis

D. **EVALUATION/OUTCOMES**
1. Child sleeps and rests without signs of discomfort
2. Child remains free from infection
3. Family verbalizes importance of antibiotic therapy

▼ MENINGITIS

Data Base

A. Most common CNS infection of infants and children
B. Inflammation of the meninges
C. Classification
   1. Bacterial: caused by pus-forming bacteria, especially meningococcus, pneumococcus, and influenza bacillus
   2. Tuberculous: caused by tubercle bacillus
   3. Viral or aseptic: caused by a wide variety of viral agents
D. Clinical findings
   1. Opisthotonos: rigidity and hyperextension of the neck
   2. Headache
   3. Irritability and high-pitched cry
   4. Signs of increased intracranial pressure
   5. Fever, nausea, and vomiting
E. Therapeutic intervention—massive doses of intravenous antibiotics

Nursing Care of Infants and Children with Meningitis

A. DATA COLLECTION

   1. Fever
   2. Headache, irritability
   3. Vomiting
   4. Seizures
   5. Nuchal rigidity

B. ANALYSIS AND INTERPRETATION

   1. Altered family processes related to having a child with a serious illness
   2. Risk for infection related to presence of infective organisms
   3. Risk for injury related to presence of infection
   4. Refer to General Nursing Diagnoses for Infants with Health Problems

C. PLANNING/IMPLEMENTATION

   1. Provide for rest
   2. Decrease stimuli from the environment (control light and noise)
   3. Position on the side with head gently supported in extension
   4. Institute respiratory isolation/universal precautions
   5. Maintain fluid balance because of meningeal edema
      a. Record intake and output carefully
      b. Correct any deficits
      c. Monitor IV fluid
      d. Daily weights
   6. Provide emotional support for parents, since child usually becomes ill suddenly
   7. Administer antibiotic therapy as prescribed

D. EVALUATION/OUTCOMES

   1. Child shows decreasing severity of illness
   2. Family verbalizes fears regarding child's prognosis
   3. Prevention of sequelae

▼ FEBRILE SEIZURES

Data Base

A. Caused by elevation of temperature
B. Usually occur in children between 6 months and 3 years of age
C. Affects 3% to 5% of children in this age group
D. Classification
   1. Simple seizure
      a. Brief
      b. Generalized
   2. Complex seizure
      a. Prolonged
      b. May have focal features
E. Clinical findings
   1. Associated with disease outside the CNS
   2. Fever usually exceeds 38.8° C; seizures occur on rise
   3. 25% of children have a recurrence
F. Therapeutic interventions
   1. Control seizure with medication
   2. Reduce temperature
   3. Treat underlying cause
G. Some evidence of familial tendency

Nursing Care of Infants and Children with Febrile Seizures

A. DATA COLLECTION

   1. Description of seizure
   2. History of present illness
   3. Cultural practices
   4. Parental interventions

B. ANALYSIS AND INTERPRETATION

   1. Ineffective airway clearance related to decreased level of consciousness
   2. Risk for aspiration related to seizures
   3. Risk for injury related to environmental hazards and lack of knowledge
   4. See General Nursing Diagnoses for Infants with Health Problems

C. PLANNING/IMPLEMENTATION

   1. Reduce fever with antipyretic drugs
   2. General seizure precautions
      a. Protect the child from injury; do not restrain; pad crib rails; do not use tongue blade
      b. Place in side-lying position to prevent aspiration

c. Record the time of seizure, duration, and body parts involved

d. Suction the nasopharynx and administer oxygen after the seizure as required

e. Observe the degree of consciousness and behavior after the seizure

f. Provide rest after the seizure

3. Teach parents to give antipyretics at first sign of increased temperature

4. For further discussion of seizure disorders, see Medical-Surgical Nursing (Chapter 6)

5. Teach fever management techniques (e.g., fans, fluids, bathing)

D. EVALUATION/OUTCOMES

1. Airway remains clear
2. Child does not aspirate
3. Child does not injure self during seizure

▼ ATOPIC DERMATITIS (ECZEMA)

Data Base

A. Atopic manifestation of a specific allergen that may have an emotional component

B. Most common during first 2 years of life

C. Majority of children with infantile form have a family history of allergies

D. Classification

1. Infantile: begins between 2 and 6 months of age; spontaneous remission by 3 years

2. Childhood: occurs at 2 to 3 years of age; 90% manifest the disease by 5 years

3. Preadolescent and adolescent: begins at about 12 years and continues into adulthood

E. Clinical findings

1. Erythema and edema from dilation of capillaries
2. Papules, vesicles, and crusts
3. Itching that may precipitate infection from scratching
4. Periods of remission and exacerbation
5. Seen mostly on cheeks, scalp, neck, and flexor surfaces of arms and legs

F. Therapeutic interventions

1. Relieve pruritis
2. Hydrate skin
3. Reduce inflammation
4. Prevent or control secondary infection

Nursing Care of Infants and Children with Atopic Dermatitis

A. DATA COLLECTION

1. Family history for allergies
2. Environmental or dietary factors associated with previous exacerbations
3. Skin lesions: distribution, type, presence of secondary infection
4. Parent/child attitude toward lesions

B. ANALYSIS AND INTERPRETATION

1. Altered family processes related to:
   a. Child's discomfort/appearance
   b. Lengthy therapy
2. Risk for infection related to skin impairment
3. Impaired skin integrity related to eczematous lesions
4. Sleep pattern disturbance related to:
   a. Physical discomfort
   b. Schedule of therapies
5. See General Nursing Diagnoses for Infants with Health Problems

C. PLANNING/IMPLEMENTATION

1. Support the parents—this long-term problem is often discouraging, since the infant is difficult to comfort

2. Place mittens on hands or restrain if necessary to keep the infant from scratching when unsupervised, but provide supervised, unrestrained play periods

3. Pick up frequently since the infant is irritable, fretful, and anorectic

4. Avoid using wool clothing or blankets or any furry toys

5. Provide the parent with a list of foods permitted and omitted on an elimination or restricted diet

6. Instruct the parent how to apply topical ointments/antihistamines prescribed

D. EVALUATION/OUTCOMES

1. Child does not scratch
2. Affected areas remain free from infection
3. Child rests/sleeps adequate amount for age
4. Family demonstrates correct performance of procedures

▼ HUMAN IMMUNODEFICIENCY VIRUS (HIV) AND ACQUIRED IMMUNODEFICIENCY SYNDROME (AIDS)

Data Base

A. Infection with human immunodeficiency virus (HIV)

B. Viral infection occurs either:

1. Vertically from an HIV-infected mother to child (breastfeeding has been identified as a source of the virus)

2. Horizontally by sexual contact or parenteral exposure to blood

C. Immunosuppression results from decreased number of CD4 T cells as well as functional defects in B cells

D. Three populations of pediatric clients

1. Children exposed in the perinatal period

2. Children who have received blood products prior to 1987
3. Adolescents who are infected after engaging in high-risk behavior

E. Clinical findings
1. Failure to thrive
2. Lymphocytic interstitial pneumonitis (LIP)
3. Hepatosplenomegaly
4. Diffuse lymphadenopathy
5. Chronic diarrhea
6. Pulmonary lymphoid hyperplasia
7. Eczema
8. *Pneumocystis carinii* pneumonia
9. Developmental failure
10. Neurologic involvement

F. Therapeutic interventions
1. Use of medication to control disease progression; (AZT, Retrovir, didanosine, Videx, zovirax)
2. Routine injections of gamma globulin
3. Immunizations for immunocompromised children are administered following individual assessments
4. Prevention and management of secondary infections
5. Treatment of pain
6. Nutritional support

Nursing Care of Infants and Children with AIDS

A. DATA COLLECTION
1. Family support; who is able to care for child
2. History to determine source of infection
3. Health status

B. ANALYSIS AND INTERPRETATION
1. Body image disturbance related to having a serious illness
2. Altered family processes related to having a child with a life-threatening disease
3. Anticipatory grieving related to having a child with a potentially fatal illness
4. Risk for infection related to impaired immune response
5. Refer to General Nursing Diagnoses for the Family of a Child with Special Needs and General Nursing Diagnoses for Infants with Health Problems

C. PLANNING/IMPLEMENTATION
1. Prevent transmission of virus
   a. Blood and body secretion precautions
   b. Education of child and parent about modes of transmission/universal precautions
2. Support child and family
3. Monitor child for signs and symptoms of sepsis and other complications
4. See Meeting the Needs of the Family of an Infant or Child with Special Needs

D. EVALUATION/OUTCOMES
1. Child does not transmit the HIV infection
2. Child remains free of opportunistic infection
3. Child has positive interpersonal relationships
4. Family can demonstrate appropriate care for child
5. Family demonstrates positive bereavement behavior

▼ EMOTIONAL DISORDERS

For common emotional disorders of infancy see Disorders Usually First Evident in Infancy, Childhood, or Adolescence in Mental Health/Psychiatric Nursing (Chapter 4)

THE TODDLER

GROWTH AND DEVELOPMENT

Developmental Timetable

A. 15 months
1. Motor
   a. Walks well alone by 14 months, with a wide-based gait
   b. Creeps upstairs
   c. Builds tower of two blocks
   d. Drinks from a cup and can use a spoon
   e. Enjoys throwing objects and picking them up
2. Vocalization and socialization
   a. Can use four to six words including name
   b. Has learned "no," which may be said while doing a requested demand

B. 18 months
1. Physical
   a. Growth has decreased and appetite lessened—"physiologic anorexia"
   b. Anterior fontanel is usually closed
   c. Abdomen protrudes, larger than chest circumference
2. Motor
   a. Runs clumsily
   b. Climbs stairs or up on furniture
   c. Imitates strokes in drawing
   d. Drinks well from a cup, manages a spoon well
   e. Builds tower of three to four cubes
3. Vocalization and socialization
   a. Says 10 or more words
   b. Has new awareness of strangers
   c. Begins to have temper tantrums
   d. Very ritualistic, has favorite toy or blanket, thumb-sucking may be at peak

C. 2 years
1. Physical
   a. Weight—about 11 to 12 kg

b. Height—about 80 to 82 cm

c. Teeth—16 temporary

2. Motor

   a. Gross motor skills quite refined

   b. Can walk up and down stairs, both feet on one step at a time, holding onto rail

   c. Builds tower of six to seven cubes or will make cubes into a train

3. Sensory

   a. Accommodation well developed

   b. Visual acuity 20/40

4. Vocalization and socialization

   a. Vocabulary of about 300 words

   b. Uses short, two- to three-word phrases, also pronouns

   c. Obeys simple commands

   d. Still very ritualistic, especially at bedtime

   e. Can help undress self and pull on simple clothes

   f. Shows signs of increasing autonomy and individuality

   g. Does not share possessions, everything "mine"

D. 30 months

1. Physical

   a. Full set of 20 temporary teeth

   b. Decreased need for naps

2. Motor

   a. Walks on tiptoe

   b. Stands on one foot momentarily

   c. Builds tower of eight blocks

   d. Copies horizontal or vertical line

   e. May attend to own toilet needs

3. Vocalization and socialization

   a. Beginning to see self as a separate individual from reflected appraisal of significant others

   b. Still sees other children as "objects"

   c. Increasingly independent, ritualistic, and negativistic

Major Learning Events

A. Toilet training: most important task of the toddler

1. Physical maturation must be reached before training is possible

   a. Sphincter control adequate when the child can walk

   b. Able to retain urine for at least 2 hours

   c. Usual age for bowel training: 24 to 30 months

   d. Daytime bowel and bladder control: during second year

   e. Night control: by 3 to 4 years of age

2. Psychologic readiness

   a. Aware of the act of elimination

   b. Able to inform the parent of the need to urinate or defecate

   c. Desire to please the parent

3. Process of training

   a. Usually begin with bowel, then bladder

   b. Accidents and regressions frequently occur

4. Parental response

   a. Choose a specific word for the act

   b. Have a specific time and place

   c. Do not punish for accidents

B. Need for independence without overprotection; the parents should:

1. Be consistent: set realistic limits

2. Reinforce desired behavior

3. Be constructive, geared to teach self-control

4. Punish immediately after a wrongdoing

5. Punish appropriately

Play During Toddlerhood (parallel play)

A. The child plays alongside other children but not with them

B. Mostly free and spontaneous, no rules or regulations

C. Attention span is still very short, and change of toys occurs at frequent intervals

D. Safety is important; there is danger of:

1. Breaking a toy through exploration and ingesting small pieces

2. Ingesting lead from lead-based paint on toys

3. Being burned by potentially flammable toys

E. Imitation and make-believe play begins by end of the second year

F. Suggested toys

1. Play furniture, dishes, cooking utensils

2. Play telephone

3. Puzzles with a few large pieces

4. Pedal-propelled toys, such as tricycle

5. Straddle toys and rocking horse

6. Clay, sandbox toys, crayons, finger paints

7. Pounding toys, blocks

8. Push-pull toys

HEALTH PROMOTION FOR TODDLERS AND PRESCHOOLERS

Childhood Nutrition

A. Nutritional objectives

1. Provide adequate nutrient intake to meet continuing growth and development needs

2. Provide a basis for support of psychosocial development in relation to food patterns, eating behavior, and attitudes

3. Provide sufficient calories for increasing physical activities and energy needs

B. Diet: calorie and nutrient requirements increase with age

1. Increased variety in types and textures of foods

2. Increased involvement in the feeding process, stimulation of curiosity about food environment, language learning

3. Consideration for the child's appetite, choices, motor skills
C. Possible nutritional problem areas
   1. Anemia: increase foods containing iron (e.g., enriched cereals, meat, egg, green vegetables)
   2. Obesity or underweight: increase or decrease calories; maintain core foods
   3. Low intake of calcium, iron, vitamins A and C; usually caused by dietary fads
   4. Often omitting breakfast
   5. Influence of commercialism on selection of foods and emphasis on fast foods, "empty-calorie" snacks, and high-carbohydrate convenience foods

Injury Prevention

A. Leading cause of death in children over 1 year of age
B. Children under 5 years of age account for over half of all accidental deaths during childhood
C. More than half of accidental child deaths are related to automobiles and fire
D. Accidents can be viewed in terms of the child's growth and development, especially curiosity about the environment
   1. Motor vehicle
     a. Walking or running, especially chasing after objects thrown into the street
     b. Poor perception of speed, lack of experience to foresee danger
     c. Child often unseen because of small size; can be run over by a car backing out of the driveway, or when playing in leaves or snow
     d. Failure to restrain in a car (sitting in a person's lap, improper use of seat belts rather than appropriate car restraint)
   2. Burns
     a. Investigating: pulls a pot off the stove, plays with matches, inserts an object into wall socket
     b. Climbing: reaches the stove, oven, ironing board and iron, cigarettes on the table
   3. Poisons
     a. Learning new tastes and textures, puts everything into mouth
     b. Developing fine motor skills: able to open bottles, cabinets, jars
     c. Climbing to previously unreachable shelves and cabinets
   4. Drowning
     a. Child and parents do not recognize the danger of water
     b. Child is unaware of inability to breathe under water
   5. Aspirating small objects and putting foreign bodies in ear or nose
     a. Puts everything in mouth
     b. Very interested in body and newly found openings
   6. Fractures
     a. Climbing, running, and jumping
     b. Still developing sense of balance
E. Prevention, through parent education and child protection, is the goal

HEALTH PROBLEMS MOST COMMON IN TODDLERS

Hospitalization

A. Toddler experiences basic fear of loss of love, fear of unknown, fear of punishment
B. Immobilization and isolation represent additional crises to the toddler
C. Stages of separation anxiety: the specific response of toddler
   1. Protest
     a. Prolonged loud crying, consoled by no one but the parent or usual caregiver
     b. Continually asks to go home
     c. Rejection of the nurse or any other stranger
   2. Despair
     a. Alteration in sleep pattern
     b. Decreased appetite and weight loss
     c. Diminished interest in environment and play
     d. Relative immobility and listlessness
     e. No facial expression or smile
     f. Unresponsive to stimuli
   3. Detachment or denial
     a. Cheerful, undiscriminating friendliness
     b. Lack of preference for parents

GENERAL NURSING DIAGNOSES FOR TODDLERS WITH HEALTH PROBLEMS

A. Anxiety related to:
   1. Strange environment
   2. Perception of impending event (specify)
   3. Separation
   4. Anticipated discomfort
   5. Knowledge deficit
   6. Discomfort
   7. Difficulty breathing
   8. Feelings of powerlessness
B. Family coping: potential for growth related to successful parenting
C. Ineffective family coping: compromised, related to situational crisis
D. Ineffective individual coping: compromised, related to situational crisis

E. Diversional activity deficit related to:
1. Lack of sensory stimulation
2. Frequent or prolonged hospitalization
F. Altered family processes related to:
1. Situational crisis
2. Knowledge deficit
3. Temporary family disorganization
4. Inadequate support systems
G. Fear related to:
1. Separation from support systems
2. Uncertain prognosis
H. Anticipatory grieving (parental) related to:
1. Expected loss (specify)
2. Gravity of child's physical status
I. Impaired home-maintenance management related to:
1. Knowledge deficit
2. Inadequate support system
J. Risk for injury related to:
1. Use of specific therapies and appliances
2. Incapacity for self-protection
3. Immobility
K. Pain related to:
1. Disease process
2. Interventions
L. Parental role conflict related to:
1. Illness of child
2. Inability to care for child
M. Risk for altered parenting related to:
1. Separation
2. Skill deficit
3. Family stress
4. Cultural variations
N. Risk for altered parent/infant/child attachment related to:
1. Inability of parents to meet child's needs
2. Separation
3. Illness of child
O. Feeding, bathing/hygiene, dressing/grooming, toileting self-care deficit related to developmental level or altered cultural practices
P. Sensory-perceptual alteration (tactile) related to protected environment
Q. Risk for impaired skin integrity related to:
1. Immature structure and function
2. Immobility
R. Sleep-pattern disturbance related to:
1. Excessive crying
2. Frequent assessment
3. Therapies
S. Spiritual distress (parental) related to:
1. Inadequate support systems
2. Decisions regarding "right to life" conflicts
T. See General Nursing Diagnoses for the Family of a Child with Special Needs

GENERAL NURSING CARE OF TODDLERS WITH HEALTH PROBLEMS

A. Prevents separation anxiety
1. Encourage the parents to stay with the child in hospital or to visit frequently
2. Provide a consistent caregiver
3. Provide individual attention, physical touch, sensory stimulation, and affection
4. Prepare the parents for the child's reaction to separation
5. Involve the parents in the child's care as much as possible
6. If a parent is unable to visit, establish phone contact
7. Establish routine similar to the child's home routine
8. Provide the child with favorite items from home; e.g., a blanket, a toy, a bottle, or a pacifier
9. Maintain the child's familiarity with home by talking about the parents, having the child listen to a tape recording of family members' voices, and showing photographs of family members
10. When family members leave, stay with child for comfort and to reassure parents
11. Associate the parents' visits with familiar events, such as "Mommy is coming after lunch"
12. Encourage the parents to visit at frequent intervals for shorter times, rather than one long visit
B. Prepare parents and the child for hospitalization
1. Give primary consideration to maintaining the parent-child relationship by limiting separation
2. Based on assessment, establish routines and rituals that the child is accustomed to in the areas of:
   a. Toilet training
   b. Feeding
   c. Bathing
   d. Sleep patterns
   e. Recreational activities
3. Prepare the parent for regression of the child to previous modes of behavior and loss of newly learned skills
4. Avoid teaching the child new skills during hospitalization
5. Allow the child's release of tension, especially aggression, through play (banging a drum, knocking blocks over, scribbling on paper)
6. Recognize that only minimal advance preparation of the child for hospitalization is possible, since cognitive ability to grasp verbal explanation is limited

▼ BURNS

(See Medical-Surgical Nursing [Chapter 6] for additional information)

Data Base
A. Second and third most common cause of death by trauma in individuals less than 15 years of age for boys and girls, respectively
B. Causative agents
  1. Thermal: flame; hot water
  2. Chemical
  3. Electrical
  4. Radiation
C. Classification
  1. Superficial (first degree)
    a. Tissue damage minimal
    b. Pain predominant symptom
  2. Partial thickness (second degree)
    a. Involves epithelium and part of corium
    b. Severity and rate of healing depend on the amount of damaged corium
    c. Very painful
  3. Full thickness (third degree)
    a. All layers of skin destroyed
    b. Systemic effects can be life-threatening
    c. Requires skin grafting
D. Clinical findings
  1. Local response
    a. Edema formation
    b. Fluid loss from nonprotected skin
    c. Circulatory stasis occurs; usually restored within 24 to 48 hours in partial-thickness burns
  2. Systemic response
    a. "Burn shock" causes a precipitous drop in cardiac output; returns to normal in 24 to 36 hours
    b. Metabolic rate greatly increased
E. Therapeutic interventions
  1. Stop the burning process
    a. Remove from source of danger
    b. Remove smoldering clothes
    c. For superficial burns, immerse the affected area in cool water
  2. Administer prompt first aid
    a. Maintain a patent airway
    b. For first-degree burns, cleanse the area, apply sterile dressing soaked in sterile saline if possible
    c. Do not apply creams, butter, or any household remedies
    d. Do not give oral fluids for severe burns (more than 10% of body)
  3. Transport the client to a proper health care facility

    a. Children are hospitalized with burns of 5% to 12% of body surface or more
    b. Child's large body surface in proportion to weight results in greater potential for fluid loss
    c. Shock: primary cause of death in first 24 to 48 hours
    d. Infection: primary cause of death after initial period
  4. Treat fluid and electrolyte loss
    a. Greatest in first 24 to 48 hours because of tissue damage
    b. Immediate replacement of both fluids and electrolytes is essential
    c. Determination of hematocrit, hemoglobin, and chemistries should be done daily to provide a guide for replacement

Nursing Care of Children with Burns
A. DATA COLLECTION
  1. Wound assessment/classification
  2. Vital signs
  3. Fluid balance
  4. Nutritional needs
  5. Respiratory status
  6. Pain
B. ANALYSIS AND INTERPRETATION
  1. Body image disturbance related to:
    a. Perception of appearance
    b. Mobility
  2. Altered family processes related to situational crisis (seriously injured child)
  3. Risk for infection related to:
    a. Injured skin
    b. Pathogenic organisms
  4. Altered nutrition: less than body requirements related to increased metabolic need
  5. Pain related to:
    a. Skin trauma
    b. Therapies
  6. Impaired physical mobility related to:
    a. Pain
    b. Impaired joint movement
  7. Impaired skin integrity related to thermal injury
  8. Anxiety related to therapeutic interventions
  9. See General Nursing Diagnoses for Toddlers with Health Problems
  10. See Meeting the Needs of the Family of an Infant or Child with Special Needs
C. PLANNING/IMPLEMENTATION
  1. Monitor fluids and electrolytes
    a. Administer prescribed fluids accurately, both time and volume
    b. Accurate measurement of intake and output is critical (daily weights, diaper count, and weight)

2. Maintain isolation
   a. The child has feelings of guilt and punishment
   b. Children under 5 years of age rarely understand the reason for isolation
   c. Furthers separation between parents and the child
   d. Encourage the child to express feelings
3. Compensate for touch deprivation
   a. Touch, a child's main means of comfort and security, is now painful
   b. Pleasurable touch must be reestablished (apply lotion to unaffected areas)
   c. Maximize the use of other senses to promote security and comfort
4. Provide for adequate nutrition
   a. High in protein, vitamins, and calories
   b. The child is frequently anorectic because of discomfort, isolation, emotional depression
   c. Provide the child's food preferences when feasible; do not force eating or use it as a weapon; encourage parent participation
   d. Alter the diet as needs change, especially when high-calorie foods are no longer needed and can cause obesity
5. Prevent contractures
   a. Make moving a game; use play that uses the affected part, such as throwing a ball for arm movement
   b. Provide for functional body alignment; place the child so attention is focused on an object that will keep the body in specific position
   c. Do passive exercises during bath or whirlpool
   d. Give analgesics before exercise
6. Meet child's emotional needs
   a. Allow the child to play with gown, mask, gloves, and bandages so that they are less strange
   b. Prepare the child for baths and whirlpool treatments, which can be frightening and painful
   c. Allow child to reenact treatments and care on a doll to work through feelings
   d. Help child deal with changes in body
      (1) For the younger child, more of a concern to parents (whose reactions are communicated to the child)
      (2) For the older child, especially the adolescent, body appearance is of great concern
      (3) Emphasize what can be done to improve looks (plastic surgery, wigs, appropriate clothing, makeup)
7. Help limit pain
   a. Assess extent of pain by observing behavior of the young child, as well as verbal complaints
   b. Distinguish pain from fear of dark, being left alone, or being in strange surroundings
   c. Administer analgesics before procedures; often narcotics may be required
8. See Meeting the Needs of the Family of an Infant or Child with Special Needs
9. See General Nursing Care of Toddlers with Health Problems
10. Teach prevention of burn injuries
    a. Educate children regarding fire safety
       (1) Tell the child to leave the house as soon as smoke is smelled or flames are seen, without stopping to retrieve a pet or toy
       (2) Involve all members of the family in fire drills
       (3) Demonstrate "stop, drop, and roll," rather than running, if clothes are on fire
    b. Educate parents especially in regard to the child's growth and development and specific dangers at each age level
    c. Help parents prevent fires in the home
       (1) Teach cautious use of heaters, barbecue, and fireplace; place shield in front of heating unit; use childproof lighters
       (2) Supervise children at all times
       (3) Maintain integrity of the electrical system
       (4) Regulate water heater to safe level
       (5) Use and maintain smoke detectors
       (6) Maintain escape route

D. EVALUATION/OUTCOMES
1. Wound heals without infection
2. Child exhibits only minimal evidence of pain
3. Child consumes an adequate amount of fluids and nutrients
4. Burn heals with minimal scarring
5. Joints remain flexible and functional
6. Child verbalizes feelings and concerns about appearance
7. Family members set realistic goals for selves, child, and others

▼ POISONING

A. Ingestion of a toxic substance or an excessive amount of a substance
B. More than 90% of poisonings occur in the home
C. Highest incidence occurs in children under 4
D. Improper storage is the major contributing factor to poisonings

General Nursing Care of Children with Poisoning
A. DATA COLLECTION
1. Vital signs
2. Need for respiratory or cardiac support
3. Treat other symptoms such as seizures
4. See Clinical Findings under type of poisoning

B. ANALYSIS AND INTERPRETATION
1. Altered family processes related to sudden hospitalization and emergency aspects of illness
2. Fear related to sudden hospitalization and treatment (multiple injections for lead poisoning)
3. Risk for injury related to sources of toxic substances in the environment
4. Risk for injury related to presence of toxic substance in the body
5. Risk for poisoning related to immature judgment of child
6. See General Nursing Diagnoses for Toddlers with Health Problems

C. PLANNING/IMPLEMENTATION
1. Terminate the exposure
   a. Empty the mouth of pills, plant parts, or other material
   b. Thoroughly flush eyes with tap water if they were involved
   c. Flush skin and wash with soap and soft cloth
   d. Remove clothing, especially if pesticide, acid, alkali, or hydrocarbon involved
   e. Bring the victim into fresh air if an inhalation poisoning
   f. Give water to dilute ingested poison, if not contraindicated
2. Identify that a poisoning has occurred
   a. Call the local poison control center, emergency facility, or physician for immediate advice regarding treatment
   b. Save all evidence of poison (container, vomitus, urine, plant, etc.)
   c. Be alert to signs and symptoms of potential poisoning in absence of other evidence
3. Do not induce vomiting
   a. If the person is comatose, in severe shock, or convulsing or has lost the gag reflex; these conditions can increase the risk of aspiration
   b. If the poison is a low-viscosity hydrocarbon; once aspirated, it can cause a severe chemical pneumonitis
   c. If the poison is a strong corrosive (acid or alkali), emesis of the corrosive redamages the mucosa of the esophagus and pharynx
4. Remove the poison
   a. Dilute with water
   b. Induce vomiting except as contraindicated by administering ipecac syrup (for 6- to 12-month-olds give 10 ml of ipecac syrup with 250-350 ml of water, for 1- to 2-year-olds give 15 ml of ipecac syrup with 250-500 ml of water; over 12 years of age give 30 ml of ipecac syrup with 500 ml of water); if vomiting does not occur repeat once in 20 minutes for those over 12 months of age; for those under 12 months of age ipecac is not repeated
   c. Administer activated charcoal 1 g per kg 30 to 60 minutes after inducing vomiting
   d. Prepare appropriate equipment for potential medical use, such as gastric lavage
5. Whether vomiting is spontaneous or induced, prevent aspiration
   a. Keep the child's head lower than the chest
   b. When alert, place the head between the legs
   c. When unconscious, position on the side
6. Observe for latent symptoms and complications of poisoning
   a. Monitor vital signs
   b. Treat as appropriate (e.g., institute seizure precautions, keep warm and position correctly in case of shock, reduce temperature if hyperpyretic)
7. Support the child and parent
   a. Keep calm and quiet
   b. Do not admonish or accuse the child or parent of wrongdoing
8. See Specific Nursing Care under Type of Poisoning
9. See General Nursing Care of Toddlers with Health Problems
10. Teach prevention of poisoning
   a. Assess possible contributing factors in the occurrence of an accident, such as discipline, parent-child relationship, developmental ability, environmental factors, and behavior problems
   b. Institute anticipatory guidance for possible future accidents based on the child's age and maturational level
   c. Refer to a visiting nurse agency for evaluation of the home environment and the need for safety measures
   d. Provide assistance with environmental manipulation when necessary
   e. Educate the parents regarding safe storage of all substances
   f. Teach children the hazards of ingesting non-food items without supervision
   g. Caution against keeping large amounts of drugs on hand, especially children's varieties
   h. Discourage transferring drugs to containers without safety caps
   i. Discuss problems of discipline and children's noncompliance

D. EVALUATION/OUTCOMES
1. Child recognizes and does not ingest harmful substances
2. Child is treated without complications
3. Child receives medication with minimal distress
4. Toxin is eliminated from body
5. Child expresses feelings and concerns

6. Parents express confidence in care
7. Parents and child have knowledge concerning prevention of future poisoning

▼ ACETAMINOPHEN POISONING

Data Base

A. One of the most common drugs taken by children
   1. Toxic dose 150 mg/kg body weight
   2. Therapeutic use of 150 mg/kg/day for several days has resulted in toxicity
B. Clinical findings—symptoms of overdose
   1. Profuse diaphoresis
   2. Nausea and vomiting
   3. Pallor
   4. Weakness
   5. Pain in right upper quadrant
   6. Slow, weak pulse
   7. Confusion
   8. Decreased urine output
   9. Jaundice
   10. Coagulation abnormality
   11. Coma
   12. Liver failure
C. Therapeutic interventions
   1. Induce vomiting with ipecac syrup, lavage
   2. Administer IV fluid
   3. Administer an antidote (acetylcysteine, Mucomyst)

Specific Nursing Care of Children with Acetaminophen Poisoning

A. Identify ingested substance and amount
B. Monitor the electrocardiograph
C. Measure intake and output
D. Measure and record the vital signs frequently
E. Obtain blood for hepatic and renal function tests
F. Support the child and family
G. See General Nursing Care of Children with Poisoning

▼ SALICYLATE TOXICITY AND POISONING

Data Base

A. Toxic dose: 300 to 500 mg per kilogram of body weight or 7 adult aspirins (28 baby aspirin) for a 9-kg child
B. Clinical findings
   1. Mild salicylate toxicity (items i to k are of little value in small children)
      a. Diaphoresis
      b. Nausea
      c. Vomiting
      d. Dehydration
      e. Delirium
      f. Oliguria
      g. Hyperpnea
      h. Hyperpyrexia
      i. Ringing in the ears
      j. Dizziness
      k. Disturbances of hearing and vision
   2. Salicylate poisoning
      a. Hyperventilation: confusion, coma
      b. Metabolic acidosis: anorexia, sweating, increased temperature
      c. Bleeding, especially if chronic ingestion
C. Therapeutic interventions
   1. Induce vomiting, gastric lavage, activated charcoal, saline cathartics
   2. IV fluids
   3. Vitamin K if bleeding
   4. Peritoneal dialysis in severe cases

SPECIFIC NURSING CARE OF CHILDREN WITH SALICYLATE POISONING

A. Identify the salicylate overdose
B. Assess blood gases and serum electrolyte concentration frequently
C. Administer sodium bicarbonate, electrolytes, and vitamin K as indicated
D. Place on a cooling blanket
E. See General Nursing Care of Children with Poisoning

▼ PETROLEUM DISTILLATE POISONING

Data Base

A. Distillates include kerosene, turpentine, gasoline, lighter fluid, furniture polish, metal polish, benzene, naphthalene, some insecticides, and cleaning fluid
B. Clinical findings
   1. Gagging, choking, and coughing
   2. Nausea
   3. Vomiting
   4. Alterations in sensorium, such as lethargy
   5. Weakness
   6. Respiratory symptoms of pulmonary involvement
      a. Tachypnea
      b. Cyanosis
      c. Substernal retractions
      d. Grunting
C. Therapeutic interventions
   Vomiting *should not* be induced: aspiration is a particular danger because of the risk of a chemical pneumonia
D. Gastric lavage

Specific Nursing Care of Children with Petroleum Distillate Poisoning

A. Identify ingestion of distillates

B. Prevent further irritation
  1. Avoid causing emesis
  2. Implement gastric lavage only as ordered
C. See General Nursing Care of Children with Poisoning

▼ CORROSIVE CHEMICAL POISONING

Data Base

A. Corrosive chemicals include oven and drain cleaners, electric dishwasher granules, and strong detergents
B. Clinical findings
  1. Severe burning pain in the mouth, throat, and stomach
  2. White, swollen mucous membranes; edema of the lips, tongue, and pharynx (respiratory obstruction)
  3. Violent vomiting; hemoptysis; hematemesis
  4. Signs of shock
  5. Anxiety and agitation
C. Therapeutic intervention—*never* induce vomiting because regurgitation of the substance will cause further damage to the mucous membranes

Specific Nursing Care of Children with Corrosive Chemical Poisoning

A. Identify ingestion
B. Maintain a patent airway
  1. Examine the pharynx for burns
  2. Observe for respiratory difficulty
  3. Provide an airway if necessary; have emergency equipment available
  4. Administer steroids if prescribed
C. Prevent further irritation
  1. Avoid causing emesis
  2. Dilute with water if advised
  3. Give nothing by mouth except as ordered and tolerated
D. Provide comfort and support to the child and family
  1. Administer analgesics as needed
  2. Remain with the child
  3. Keep parents informed of the child's progress
E. See General Nursing Care of Children with Poisoning

▼ LEAD POISONING (PLUMBISM)

Data Base

A. A prevalent, significant, preventable health problem that causes neurologic and intellectual damage from even low levels of lead
B. Blood lead concentration should be less than 2 μmol/L
C. Associated with increased levels of lead in the environment

  1. Most common source is lead-based paint
  2. Soil, dust, or drinking water with lead
  3. Parental occupations, hobbies
D. Clinical findings (chronic ingestion)
  1. Loss of weight, anorexia
  2. Abdominal pain, vomiting
  3. Constipation
  4. Anemia, pallor, listlessness, fatigue
  5. Lead line on teeth and long bones
  6. Behavioral changes (impulsiveness, irritability, hyperactivity, or lethargy)
  7. Headache, insomnia, joint pains
  8. Brain damage, convulsions, death
E. Therapeutic interventions
  1. Objective: reduce concentration of lead in the blood and soft tissue by promoting its excretion and deposition in bones
    a. Calcium disodium edetate (Calcium Disodium Versenate)
      (1) Urine lead content monitored; peak excretion in 24 to 48 hours
      (2) Adverse effects: acute tubular necrosis, malaise, fatigue, numbness of extremities, GI disturbances, fever, pain in muscles and joints
    b. Dimercaprol (BAL)
      (1) Generally used in conjunction with calcium disodium edetate
      (2) Adverse effects: local pain at the site of injection; may cause persistent fever in children receiving therapy; rise in blood pressure accompanied by tachycardia after injection
    c. D-penicillamine (Cuprimine)
      (1) Oral chelating agent
      (2) Increases urinary excretion
      (3) Adverse effects: transient decrease in white blood cells and platelets; rash; enuresis; abdominal pain
  2. Prevention of further ingestion

Specific Nursing Care of Children with Lead Poisoning

A. Determine environmental exposure
B. Screen children at risk by recognizing clinical findings, especially behavior changes
C. Plan preparation of the child and rotation of injection sites if therapeutic intervention includes IM chelating agents
D. Observe child carefully and closely
E. Plan discharge and follow-up care of the child
F. Prevent future lead poisoning by parental and child education, appropriate environment, and supervision of child and siblings
G. See General Nursing Care of Children with Poisoning

▼ FRACTURES

(See Medical-Surgical Nursing [Chapter 6] for additional information)

Data Base

A. An interruption in the integrity of a bone
B. In children, bones are more easily injured; fractures can result without major injury to surrounding tissue
C. Healing occurs rapidly in children; rapidity of healing is inversely related to the age of the child
D. Classification
   1. Bend: bone is bent, not broken
   2. Buckle or torus fracture: bone is compressed; appears as a bulge
   3. Greenstick fractures: incomplete break and bending of a long bone, occurs in young children because the bones are soft and not fully mineralized
   4. Complete fractures: bone fragments are divided; may be connected by a periosteal hinge
      a. Transverse
      b. Oblique
      c. Spiral
E. Clinical findings
   1. Generalized swelling
   2. Pain or tenderness
   3. Diminished function or use of part
F. Therapeutic interventions
   1. Splints
   2. Bryant's traction for fractured femur
      a. Legs are suspended vertically via skin traction with buttocks slightly off bed and upper body maintaining countertraction
      b. Generally used for children under 2 years of age or 13.5 kg
   3. Skeletal/traction for older children
   4. Casts

Nursing Care of Children with Fractures

A. DATA COLLECTION
   1. Assess for the five Ps associated with fractures
      a. Pain and point of tenderness
      b. Pulse distal to fracture site
      c. Pallor
      d. Paresthesia; sensation distal to fracture site
      e. Paralysis; movement distal to fracture site
   2. Mechanism of injury

B. ANALYSIS AND INTERPRETATION
   1. Fear related to:
      a. Discomfort
      b. Unfamiliar apparatus
      c. Strange environment
   2. Risk for injury related to:
      a. Immobility
      b. Traction apparatus or cast
   3. Pain related to physical injury
   4. Impaired physical mobility (specify) related to musculoskeletal impairment
   5. Risk for impaired skin integrity related to unrelieved pressure
   6. See General Nursing Diagnoses for Toddlers with Health Problems

C. PLANNING/IMPLEMENTATION
   1. Relieve pain by administering medication as ordered
   2. Monitor neurovascular status of distal extremity
   3. Provide activity to keep child occupied and entertained
   4. Maintain traction
      a. Keep child positioned flat on back
      b. Maintain line of pull and freehanging weights
   5. See General Nursing Care of Toddlers with Health Problems

D. EVALUATION/OUTCOMES
   1. Neurovascular status in affected extremity remains intact
   2. Child experiences minimal discomfort
   3. Skin remains intact
   4. Joints remain flexible and muscles retain tone
   5. Child plays and readily interacts with others

▼ ASPIRATION OF FOREIGN OBJECTS

Data Base

A. Obstruction of the airway by a foreign object
B. Most common in children 1 to 3 years of age
C. Leading cause of fatal injury in children less than 1 year of age
D. Foods that cause asphyxiation include hot dogs, round candy, peanuts, grapes, and popcorn
E. Foreign body can lodge anywhere from larynx to bronchi
F. Classification
   1. Partial obstruction has time interval (hours to days) without symptoms
   2. Complete obstruction is an emergency
G. Clinical findings
   1. Complete obstruction
      a. Substernal retractions
      b. Inability to cough or speak
      c. Increased pulse and respiratory rate
      d. Cyanosis
   2. Partial obstruction
      a. Wheeze
      b. Stridor
      c. Persistent respiratory infection
H. Therapeutic interventions
   1. If incomplete obstruction, do not intervene;

allow child to continue coughing until object is dislodged

2. Immediate first aid if object is completely obstructing the trachea
   a. Try to pull the object out if possible without forcing it further down
   b. Turn the small child upside down (head lower than chest) and deliver four quick, sharp back blows with the heel of the hand; turn the child over and deliver four quick chest thrusts using the technique for CPR
   c. Abdominal thrust for children aged 1 year and older (Heimlich maneuver): grasp the victim from behind around the upper abdomen and squeeze, forcing the diaphragm up
3. Medical removal by bronchoscopy
4. Surgical relief by a tracheotomy below level of the object

Nursing Care of Children Who Aspirate Foreign Objects

A. DATA COLLECTION
1. Color
2. Breathing pattern
3. Absence of speech

B. ANALYSIS AND INTERPRETATION
1. Ineffective airway clearance related to obstruction
2. Anxiety related to:
   a. Parents' perceived threat to life of child
   b. Child's inability to breathe
3. Risk for suffocation related to knowledge deficit of risk factors
4. See General Nursing Diagnoses for Toddlers with Health Problems

C. PLANNING/IMPLEMENTATION
1. Keep small objects such as balloons, hard candies, buttons, and batteries out of the child's reach
2. Inspect larger toys for removable objects
3. Teach the child not to run or laugh with food or fluid in the mouth
4. Avoid giving young children foods easily aspirated, such as nuts or hot dogs
5. Teach the child to chew food well before swallowing
6. See General Nursing Care of Toddlers with Health Problems

D. EVALUATION/OUTCOMES
1. Parents and child verbalize feelings about the child's condition
2. Parents verbalize knowledge of the danger of small objects/food
3. Child's airway remains clear

▼ CHILD ABUSE

Data Base
A. One of the most significant social problems affecting children
B. Majority of abused children are under 4 years of age
C. About 70% to 80% of abuse is by parents or other relatives
D. Intentional physical abuse or neglect, emotional abuse or neglect, and sexual abuse of children
E. Parental characteristics
   1. Their own childhood included abuse
   2. Difficulty controlling aggressive impulses
   3. Low self-esteem and lack of identity
   4. Tend to be young, immature, and dependent
   5. Frequently expect the child to provide them with nurturing and love
   6. Tend to be socially isolated, depressed, lonely people, yearning for love and understanding
   7. Have no outside resources for emotional support or relief from responsibility, especially in time of crisis, thus they take out their frustration on the child
F. Child characteristics
   1. Temperament
   2. Physically demanding
   3. Emotionally dependent
   4. Premature development
   5. Special needs
G. Environmental characteristics
   1. Atmosphere of chronic stress
   2. Presence of alcohol or substance abuse
H. Classification
   1. Neglect—most common form of maltreatment
      a. Emotional neglect
      b. Physical neglect
      c. Emotional abuse
   2. Physical abuse—minor physical abuse responsible for more reported cases than major physical abuse (which results in increased mortality)
   3. Sexual abuse
      a. Incest
      b. Molestation
      c. Exhibitionism
      d. Child pornography/prostitution
      e. Pedophilia
I. Clinical findings
   1. Physical evidence of abuse/previous injuries
   2. Conflicting stories about injury
   3. Inappropriate parental response
   4. Inappropriate response of child
J. Therapeutic interventions
   1. Treat injury
   2. Identify and protect child from further abuse

Nursing Care of Children Who Are Abused

A. DATA COLLECTION

1. History of injury
2. Physical examination
3. Evidence of past injuries
4. Parent-child interaction
5. Developmental level of child
6. Drawing/playing discussion and observation

B. ANALYSIS AND INTERPRETATION

1. Fear related to:
   a. Negative interpersonal interaction
   b. Repeated maltreatment
   c. Powerlessness
2. Altered parenting related to:
   a. Abusive or neglectful caregivers
   b. Situational characteristics
3. Risk for trauma related to characteristics of:
   a. Child
   b. Caregiver(s)
4. See General Nursing Diagnoses for Toddlers with Health Problems

C. PLANNING/IMPLEMENTATION

1. Be alert for clues that indicate child abuse or neglect
   a. The child has many unexplained injuries, scars, bruises
   b. Parents offer inconsistent stories explaining child's injuries when questioned
   c. Emotional response of parents is inconsistent with the degree of the child's injury
   d. Parents may resist or fail to be present for questioning
   e. The child exhibits physical signs of neglect: malnourished, dehydrated, unkempt
   f. The child cringes when physically approached and appears unduly afraid
   g. The child responds in a manner that indicates avoiding punishment rather than gaining reward
   h. The child has excessive interest in sexual matters
   i. The child has a sexually transmitted disease
2. Be aware of child abuse laws; most states mandate reporting
3. Recognize that the main objective is to protect the child from further abuse
4. Focus on helping parents with their own dependency needs
   a. Group therapy
   b. Home visiting
   c. Foster grandparents
5. Help parents learn to control frustration through other outlets
6. Educate parents about the child's normal needs and development, new modes of discipline, and realistic expectations

7. Provide emotional support and therapy for the child since abused children frequently grow up to be abusing parents

D. EVALUATION/OUTCOMES

1. Child is free of injury or neglect
2. Child engages in positive relationships with caregivers
3. Parents demonstrate appropriate parenting activities

▼ DEVELOPMENTAL DISABILITY

Data Base

A. Causes
   1. Infection and intoxication—congenital rubella, syphilis, maternal alcohol or drug consumption, chronic lead ingestion, and kernicterus (high bilirubin level)
   2. Injury to the brain suffered during the prenatal, perinatal, or postnatal periods; intracranial hemorrhage, anoxia, physical injury
   3. Inadequate nutrition and metabolic or endocrine disorders such as PKU or hypothyroidism
   4. Unknown prenatal influences, including cerebral and cranial malformations such as microcephalus and hydrocephalus
   5. Low birth weight or prematurity
   6. Chromosomal abnormalities such as Down syndrome and Fragile X syndrome
B. Conditions that may lead to a false diagnosis of developmental disability
   1. Emotional disturbance, such as autism or maternal deprivation
   2. Sensory problems, such as deafness or blindness
   3. Cerebral dysfunctions, such as cerebral palsy, learning disorders, hyperkinesia, seizure disorders
C. Definition: a fundamental difficulty in learning and performing daily life skills including conceptual, practical, and social intelligence that manifests before the age of 18 years
D. Clinical findings
   1. Delayed milestones
      a. Infant fails to suck
      b. Head lag after 4 to 6 months of age
      c. Slow in learning self-help; slow to respond to new stimuli
      d. Slow or absent speech development
   2. Mental abilities are concrete: abstract ability is limited
   3. Lack power of self-appraisal
   4. Does not learn from errors
   5. Cannot carry out complex instructions
   6. Does not relate with peers: more secure with adults

7. Comforted by physical touch
8. Learns rote responses and socially acceptable behavior
9. May repeat words (echolalia)
10. Short attention span, but usually attracted to music

E. Therapeutic interventions
1. Prevent causes that damage brain cells such as hypoxia, untreated PKU
2. Identify condition early
3. Minimize long-term consequences
   a. Treatment of associated problems
   b. Infant stimulation
   c. Parent education

Nursing Care of Children Who Are Developmentally Disabled

A. DATA COLLECTION
1. Developmental screening
2. Associated illnesses/risk factors

B. ANALYSIS AND INTERPRETATION
1. Altered family processes related to having a child with developmental disability
2. Altered growth and development related to impaired cognitive function
3. See General Nursing Diagnoses for the Family of a Child with Special Needs

C. PLANNING/IMPLEMENTATION
1. Always consider the child's developmental, not chronologic, age
   a. Educate the parent regarding developmental age
   b. Near adolescence, sexual feelings accompany maturation and need to be explained according to the child's cognitive ability
2. Set realistic goals; teach by simple steps for habit formation rather than for understanding or transference of learning
   a. Break down the process of skills learning into simple steps that can be easily achieved
   b. Ensure each step is learned completely before teaching the child the next step
   c. Recognize that behavior modification is a very effective method of teaching these children
   d. Praise accomplishments to develop the child's self-esteem
   e. Keep discipline simple, geared toward learning acceptable behavior rather than developing judgment
   f. Recognize that routines are the foundation of the child's life-style; hospital routines should be based on the child's normal schedule
   g. See Meeting the Needs of the Family of an Infant or Child with Special Needs

D. EVALUATION/OUTCOMES
1. Child performs activities of daily living at optimum level
2. Family members make realistic decisions based on their needs and capabilities

▼ CEREBRAL PALSY

Data Base

A. Nonspecific term for a neuromuscular disability or difficulty in controlling voluntary muscles (caused by damage to some portion of the brain, with associated sensory, intellectual, emotional, or seizure disorders)
B. Characteristics of cerebral palsy
   1. Affects young children, usually becoming evident before 3 years of age
   2. Nonprogressive, but persists throughout life
   3. Some motor dysfunction always present
   4. Mental deficiency may be present
   5. Language deficit may be present
   6. Strabismus
C. Major causes
   1. Anoxia of the brain caused by a variety of insults at or near the time of birth
   2. Congenital or neonatal infection of the central nervous system
   3. Trauma
   4. Prematurity
   5. Cerebral vascular accident
D. Classification (based on predominant clinical manifestations)
   1. Spastic type: hypertonicity with poor control of posture, balance, and coordinated movements; impairment of gross and fine motor skills
   2. Dyskinetic type: abnormal involuntary movement
      a. Athetosis; characterized by slow, wormlike, writhing movements
      b. Involvement of mouth and throat results in drooling
   3. Ataxic type: wide-based gait, rapid repetitive movements performed poorly
   4. Mixed type: combination of spasticity and athetosis
   5. Rigid tremor and atonic types: uncommon with deformities and lack of active movement, have poor prognosis
E. Clinical findings
   1. Delayed gross motor development
   2. Difficulty in feeding, especially sucking and swallowing
   3. Abnormal motor performance
   4. Asymmetry in motion or contour of body
   5. Delayed motor development and speech

6. Reflex abnormalities—hyperreflexia
7. Any of the muscular abnormalities listed under classification

F. Therapeutic interventions
1. Multidisciplinary approach
2. Mobility devices
3. Surgery to correct spastic muscle imbalance
4. Medications, such as skeletal muscle relaxants and anticonvulsants
5. Physiotherapy and occupational and speech therapy

Nursing Care of Children with Cerebral Palsy

A. DATA COLLECTION
1. Presence of prenatal/perinatal risk factors
2. Poor feeding
3. Muscle rigidity
4. Tenseness or hypotonia
5. Delayed developmental milestones

B. ANALYSIS AND INTERPRETATION
1. Body image disturbance related to:
   a. Physical disability
   b. Appearance
2. Altered family processes related to the birth of a child with special needs
3. Fatigue related to increased energy expenditure
4. Risk for injury related to neuromuscular and cognitive-perceptual impairments
5. Impaired physical mobility related to neuromuscular impairment
6. Feeding, bathing/hygiene, dressing/grooming, toileting self-care deficit related to impaired neuromuscular development
7. Impaired verbal communication related to neuromuscular impairment
8. See General Nursing Diagnoses for Toddlers with Health Problems
9. See General Nursing Diagnoses for the Family of a Child with Special Needs

C. PLANNING/IMPLEMENTATION
1. Feeding
   a. Recognize drooling results from difficulty in swallowing
   b. Use a spoon and blunt fork, with plate attached to the table, for easier self-feeding
   c. Provide child with increased calories because of excessive energy expenditure, increased protein for muscle activity, and increased vitamins (especially B_6) for amino acid metabolism
2. Relaxation
   a. Provide rest periods in an area with few stimuli
   b. Set limits and control activity level
3. Safety
   a. Protect from accidents resulting from poor balance and lack of muscle control

b. Provide helmet for protection against head injuries
c. Restrain the child when up, and restrain in bed if indicated
4. Play
   a. Keep safety as main objective
   b. Do not overstimulate; should have educational value, appropriate to child's developmental level and ability
5. Elimination
   a. Recognize difficulty in toilet training is because of poor muscle control
   b. Provide special bowel and bladder training
6. Speech
   a. Recognize poor coordination of lips, tongue, cheeks, larynx, and poor control of diaphragm make formation of words difficult
   b. Refer for speech therapy
7. Breathing
   a. Recognize poor control of the intercostal muscles and diaphragm causes the child to be prone to respiratory tract infection
   b. Protect the child from exposure to infection as much as possible; be alert for symptoms of aspiration pneumonia
8. Dental problems
   a. Recognize problems in muscular control affect development and alignment of teeth
   b. Explain that frequent dental caries occur and that there is a great need for dental supervision and care
   c. Teach the parent to brush the child's teeth if muscular dysfunction present
9. Vision
   a. Recognize that common ocular problems such as strabismus and refractive errors may be related to poor muscular control
   b. Look for such disorders to prevent further problems such as amblyopia
10. Hearing
    a. Recognize hearing problems may be present, depending on the basic cause of the brain damage
    b. Encourage parents to have child's hearing checked periodically
11. See General Nursing Care of Toddlers with Health Problems
12. See Meeting the Needs of the Family of an Infant or Child with Special Needs

D. EVALUATION/OUTCOMES
1. Family provides a safe environment for the child
2. Child consumes adequate nutrients for growth
3. Child is able to communicate needs to caregiver
4. Family verbalizes effect of child's disability on family
5. Child is able to move around environment

6. Child performs self-care activities within capabilities
7. Child exhibits behavior indicative of positive self-image

▼ HEARING DISORDERS

Data Base

A. Causes
   1. Maternal factors: rubella, syphilis
   2. Perinatal: anoxia, kernicterus, prematurity, excessive noise
   3. Postnatal: mumps, otitis media, head trauma, drugs such as gentamycin
B. Classification
   1. Conductive: loss from damage to middle ear
      a. Accounts for about 80% of reduced hearing
      b. Conductive loss of 30 dB or more may require a hearing aid
   2. Sensorineural: damage to inner ear structures of the auditory nerve
      a. Distortion in clarity of words
      b. Problem in discrimination of sounds
   3. Mixed conductive-sensorineural
   4. Central auditory imperception
      a. Not explained by other three causes
      b. The child hears but does not understand
C. Clinical findings
   1. Lack of the Moro reflex in response to a sharp clap
   2. Failure to respond to loud noise
   3. Failure to locate a source of sound at 60-100 cm after 6 months of age
   4. Absence of babble by 7 months of age
   5. Inability to understand words or phrases by 12 months of age
   6. Use of gestures rather than verbalization to establish wants
   7. History of frequent respiratory tract infections and otitis media
D. Therapeutic interventions
   1. Conductive loss
      a. Antibiotics for acute otitis media
      b. Tympanostomy tubes for chronic otitis media
      c. Hearing aids to amplify sounds
   2. Sensorineural
      a. Cochlear implants
      b. Hearing aids of less value
   3. Central auditory imperception—may not respond to any therapy

Nursing Care of Children with Impaired Hearing

A. DATA COLLECTION

   1. Identify children whose history places them at risk

   2. Response to auditory stimuli
   3. Failure to develop intelligible speech by 24 months

B. ANALYSIS AND INTERPRETATION

   1. Altered family processes related to:
      a. Situational crisis
      b. Difficulty in communication
   2. Altered growth and development related to defective communication
   3. Risk for injury related to cognitive-perceptual impairment
   4. Sensory-perceptual alteration (auditory) related to hearing impairment
   5. Impaired verbal communication related to loss of hearing before speech is established
   6. See General Nursing Diagnoses for Toddlers with Health Problems
   7. See General Nursing Diagnoses for the Family of a Child with Special Needs

C. PLANNING/IMPLEMENTATION

   1. Observe for manifestations beginning at birth
   2. Face the child to facilitate lip reading
   3. Do not walk back and forth while talking
   4. Have a good light on speaker's face
   5. Be level with the child's face and speak toward the unaffected ear
   6. Always enunciate and articulate carefully
   7. Do not talk too loudly, especially if the loss is sensorineural
   8. Use facial expressions, since verbal intonations are not communicated
   9. Encourage active play to build self-confidence
   10. Teach sign language
   11. Early intervention to promote speech retention/development
   12. See General Nursing Care of Toddlers with Health Problems
   13. See Meeting the Needs of the Family of an Infant or Child with Special Needs

D. EVALUATION/OUTCOMES

   1. Child obtains and uses hearing aid
   2. Child/family use effective communication techniques
   3. Parents and child demonstrate a positive relationship
   4. Child engages in activities appropriate to developmental level
   5. Child has a safe environment

▼ VISUAL DISORDERS

Data Base

A. Functional definition of blindness: visual loss of acuity to read print; must use braille, may have light perception

B. Strabismus: imbalance of the extraocular muscles causing a physiologic incoordination of the eye
   1. A cause of blindness: amblyopia develops in the weak eye from disuse
   2. Must be corrected before 4 years of age to prevent blindness
   3. Treatment
      a. To force the weak eye to fixate: patch the unaffected and exercise the weak eye
      b. Surgery to lengthen or shorten the extraocular muscles
C. Causes other than strabismus
   1. Maternal: albinism, congenital cataracts, rubella, galactosemia, gonorrhea
   2. Perinatal: retrolental fibroplasia
   3. Postnatal: trauma, diabetes, syphilis, tumor
D. Clinical findings
   1. Delayed motor development
   2. Rocking for sensory stimulation
   3. Squinting, rubbing eyes
   4. Sitting close to television, holding book close to face
   5. Clumsiness, bumping into objects
E. Therapeutic interventions
   1. Surgical intervention
      a. Strabismus
      b. Cataracts
      c. Detached retina repair
      d. Enucleation
   2. Corrective lenses

Nursing Care of Children with Impaired Vision
A. DATA COLLECTION
   1. Identify those children at risk
   2. Observe for behavior indicative of vision loss
   3. Screen children for visual acuity and signs of ocular disorders
B. ANALYSIS AND INTERPRETATION
   1. Altered family processes related to situational crisis
   2. Altered growth and development related to sensory/perceptual alterations (visual)
   3. Risk for injury related to cognitive-perceptual impairment
   4. See General Nursing Diagnoses for Toddlers with Health Problems
   5. See General Nursing Diagnoses for the Family of a Child with Special Needs
C. PLANNING/IMPLEMENTATION
   1. Be aware of early signs of visual problems
   2. Explain and encourage parents to follow treatments for strabismus and other conditions
   3. Always talk so the child can hear clearly
   4. Use noise so the child can locate your position
   5. Help the child learn through other senses, especially touch, with play activities

   6. Facilitate eating
      a. Arrange food on the plate and teach the child its location
      b. Provide finger foods when possible
      c. Provide a light spoon and deep bowl so the child can feel weight of food on spoon
   7. See Meeting the Needs of the Family of an Infant or Child with Special Needs
   8. See General Nursing Care of Toddlers with Health Problems
D. EVALUATION/OUTCOMES
   1. Child engages in appropriate activities for level of development
   2. Parents and child demonstrate a positive relationship
   3. Child remains free from injury

▼ LYME DISEASE

(See Medical-Surgical Nursing [Chapter 6] for additional information)

Data Base
A. Caused by spirochete transmitted by ticks
B. Three stages of infection
   1. Tick bite at time of inoculation
   2. Development of erythematous papule that enlarges radially, resulting in a large, circumferential ring with a raised, edematous, doughnut-like border
   3. Systemic involvement of neurologic, cardiac, and musculoskeletal systems, which appears several weeks after the cutaneous phase is completed
C. Clinical findings
   Symptoms depend on which organ system is involved after the initial cutaneous phase
D. Therapeutic interventions
   1. Antibiotics used for treatment in the second phase will prevent most disease progression
   2. Neurologic symptoms are treated with oral prednisone or antibiotics when present less than 24 hours
   3. Cardiac symptoms are treated with daily prednisone and aspirin
   4. Musculoskeletal pain treated with aspirin, prednisone, and/or nonsteroidal antiinflammatory drugs

Nursing Care of Children with Lyme Disease
A. DATA COLLECTION
   1. Observe for tick bite
   2. Observe for signs and symptoms associated with erythematous papule and system involvement

B. ANALYSIS AND INTERPRETATION
1. Fear related to uncertain prognosis
2. Pain related to disease process
3. See General Nursing Diagnoses for Toddlers with Health Problems

C. PLANNING/IMPLEMENTATION
1. Teach caregivers to dress child appropriately for the woods and to examine children for ticks
2. Support child and family
3. See General Nursing Care of Toddlers with Health Problems

D. EVALUATION/OUTCOMES
1. Child will report pain at an acceptable level
2. Child will verbalize feelings about disease process

▼ CELIAC DISEASE

Data Base

A. Known as gluten-induced enteropathy and celiac sprue
B. Chronic intestinal malabsorption and inability to digest gluten, a protein found mostly in wheat, rye, oats, and barley
C. Usually begins in infancy or toddler stage, but later in breastfed infants
D. Progression of illness
1. Fat absorption affected in early stage of disease
2. Protein, carbohydrate, mineral, and electrolyte absorption then affected
3. Growth failure, muscle wasting finally occur
E. Clinical findings
1. Progressive malnutrition
   a. Muscle wasting
   b. Anorexia
   c. Distended abdomen
2. Secondary deficiencies: anemia and rickets
3. Steatorrhea: fatty, foul, frothy, bulky stools
4. Celiac crisis: severe episode of dehydration and acidosis from diarrhea
F. Therapeutic intervention—dietary
1. Low in glutens; no wheat, rye, oats, or barley
2. High in calories and protein
3. Low fat
4. Small, frequent feedings; adequate fluids
5. Vitamin supplements, all in water-miscible form
6. Supplemental iron

Nursing Care of Children with Celiac Disease
A. DATA COLLECTION
1. Nutritional assessment
2. Parent/child for knowledge of diet regimen

B. ANALYSIS AND INTERPRETATION
1. Risk for injury related to knowledge deficit (diet and food composition)

2. Alteration in nutrition: less than body requirements related to impaired intestinal absorption
3. See General Nursing Diagnoses for Toddlers with Health Problems
4. See Nursing Diagnoses for the Family of a Child with Special Needs

C. PLANNING/IMPLEMENTATION
1. Protect the child from infection
2. Teach parents dietary restrictions
3. Explain need for frequent follow-up supervision, home visits
4. See General Nursing Care of Toddlers with Health Problems
5. See Meeting the Needs of the Family of an Infant or Child with Special Needs

D. EVALUATION/OUTCOMES
1. Parent/child verbalizes correct dietary information
2. Child consumes adequate calories for growth and development

▼ CYSTIC FIBROSIS

Data Base

A. Autosomal recessive disorder affecting the exocrine glands
B. Most common serious pulmonary and genetic disease of children
C. Increased viscosity of mucous gland secretions is responsible for most clinical findings
1. Elevation in sweat electrolytes
2. Pancreas: becomes fibrotic, with a decreased production of pancreatic enzymes (late complication—diabetes) resulting in deficiencies of:
   a. Lipase: causes steatorrhea (fatty, foul, bulky stools)
   b. Trypsin: causes increased nitrogen in stool
   c. Amylase: inability to break down polysaccharides
3. Rectal prolapse
4. Sweat glands: high electrolyte content of sodium and chloride (three to five times higher than normal); chloride levels above 60 mEq/L are diagnostic
5. Respiratory system: increased viscous mucus in the trachea, bronchi, and bronchioles resulting in:
   a. Obstruction, interfering with expiration (emphysema)
   b. Infection
6. Liver: possible cirrhosis from biliary obstruction, malnutrition, or infection; portal hypertension leads to esophageal varices
7. Sexual organs: infertility possible

D. Clinical findings
1. Based on pathophysiology listed in C above
2. Similar to celiac disease
3. Some early manifestations during infancy
   a. Meconium ileus at birth (about 15%)
   b. Failure to regain normal 10% weight loss at birth
   c. Presence of cough or wheezing during first 6 months of age
4. Because of respiratory involvement, there may be clubbing of fingers, barrel-shaped chest, cyanosis, distended neck veins
5. Cardiac enlargement, particularly right ventricular hypertrophy (cor pulmonale)

E. Therapeutic interventions
1. Pulmonary problems
   a. Chest physiotherapy
   b. Bronchodilators
   c. Antibiotic therapy as indicated
2. Gastrointestinal problems
   a. Pancreatic enzyme supplements
   b. Balanced nutritional intake

Nursing Care of Children with Cystic Fibrosis

A. DATA COLLECTION
1. Pulmonary assessment
2. GI observation
3. Failure to thrive

B. ANALYSIS AND INTERPRETATION
1. Activity intolerance related to:
   a. Imbalance between oxygen supply and demand
   b. Ineffective airway clearance
2. Ineffective airway clearance related to secretion of thick, tenacious mucus
3. Ineffective breathing pattern related to mechanical tracheobronchial obstruction
4. Altered family processes related to situational crisis (child with a chronic illness)
5. Altered nutrition: less than body requirements related to inability to digest nutrients
6. See General Nursing Diagnoses for Toddlers with Health Problems
7. See General Nursing Diagnoses for the Family of a Child with Special Needs

C. PLANNING/IMPLEMENTATION
1. Prevent respiratory tract infections
   a. Postural drainage, percussion, vibrating
   b. Aerosol therapy
   c. Use of expectorants and antibiotics
   d. Avoid antitussives and antihistamines
2. Promote optimal nutrition
   a. Replacement of pancreatic enzymes, given with cold food in middle of meal
   b. Replacement of fat-soluble vitamins in water-miscible form
   c. High-protein diet of easily digested food, normal fat, high calories
3. Promote mobility and activity
   a. Encourage activity and regular exercise
   b. Help the child regulate activity to own tolerance
4. Promote a positive body image
   a. Help child deal with barrel-shaped chest, poor weight gain, thin extremities, bluish coloring, smell of stools, poor posture
   b. Encourage good hygiene and select clothes that compensate for protuberant abdomen and emaciated extremities
5. Provide for emotional support and counseling for child and family
   a. Long-term problem causing emotional stresses
   b. Illness can become a major controlling factor in the family
      (1) The child begins to recognize that wheezing brings attention and uses this knowledge
      (2) Parents can deal with such behavior by recognizing false attacks and using consistent discipline
   c. Encourage the family to join the Cystic Fibrosis Foundation
   d. Refer family for genetic counseling
6. See General Nursing Care of Toddlers with Health Problems
7. See Meeting the Needs of the Family of an Infant or Child with Special Needs

D. EVALUATION/OUTCOMES
1. Child rests quietly and engages in activity suitable to developmental level
2. Child is able to clear airway of mucus
3. Child breathes easily
4. Family demonstrates ability to care for child
5. Child consumes adequate calories for growth and development

▼ IRON DEFICIENCY ANEMIA

Data Base
A. A prevalent nutritional disorder among children; caused by lack of adequate sources of dietary iron
1. Infant usually has iron reserve for 6 months
2. Premature infant lacks reserve
3. Children receiving only milk have no source of iron
B. Insidious onset: usually diagnosed because of an infection or chronic GI problems
C. Causes
1. Decreased intake of iron (deficiencies of vitamin B_{12}, folic acid, proteins, or vitamin C may also cause anemia)

2. Increased destruction
3. Increased loss
D. Clinical findings
   1. Pallor, weakness
   2. Slow motor development
   3. Poor muscle tone
   4. Hemoglobin level below normal for age
E. Therapeutic interventions
   1. Food sources rich in iron
   2. Iron replacement
      a. Oral iron sources
         (1) Drug: ferrous sulfate (Fer-in-Sol) most absorbable form of iron
         (2) Adverse effects: nausea, vomiting; fatalities in children who ingest enteric-coated tablets, thinking they are candy
         (3) Drug interactions: ferrous sulfate binds tetracycline and decreases absorption; magnesium trisilicate decreases absorption of iron
      b. Parenteral iron sources
         (1) Jectofer for IM use and Infed for IV use
         (2) Adverse effects: tissue staining (use Z tract for intramuscular injection), fever, lymphadenopathy, nausea, vomiting, arthralgia, urticaria, severe peripheral vascular failure, anaphylaxis, secondary hematochromatosis

Nursing Care of Children with Iron Deficiency Anemia

A. DATA COLLECTION
   1. Nutritional history
   2. History of chronic infection
   3. Eating habits
      a. Pica
      b. Ingestion of lead
   4. Bowel habits/blood in stools
   5. Family history of hematologic disorder

B. ANALYSIS AND INTERPRETATION
   1. Activity intolerance related to generalized weakness
   2. Altered nutrition: less than body requirements related to knowledge deficit of appropriate foods
   3. See General Nursing Care of Toddlers with Health Problems

C. PLANNING/IMPLEMENTATION
   1. Prevent development of anemia
      a. Teach pregnant women the importance of their iron intake
      b. Encourage feeding of iron-fortified infant formula or breastfeeding
      c. Encourage feeding iron-fortified infant cereal
      d. Introduce foods high in iron

2. Provide for good nutrition and proper administration of supplemental iron
   a. Vitamin C aids absorption
   b. Hydrochloric acid aids absorption
   c. Oxalates, phosphate, and caffeine decrease absorption
   d. Use a straw because some liquid preparations stain teeth
   e. Discolors stools; may cause gastric irritation or constipation

D. EVALUATION/OUTCOMES
   1. Child engages in appropriate activities
   2. Child consumes adequate nutrients for correction of anemia
   3. Parents can verbalize nutritional requirements of child

▼ SICKLE CELL ANEMIA

Data Base

A. Autosomal disorder affecting hemoglobin
B. Defective hemoglobin causes red blood cells to become sickle shaped and clump together under reduced oxygen tension
C. Classification
   1. Sickle cell anemia: homozygous for sickle cell gene
   2. Sickle cell trait: heterozygous for sickle cell gene
D. Clinical findings
   1. Vasoocclusive crisis (pain episode): most common and non–life-threatening
      a. Results from sickled cells obstructing blood vessels, causing occlusion, ischemia, and potential necrosis
      b. Symptoms include fever, acute abdominal pain (visceral hypoxia), hand-foot syndrome, priapism, and arthralgia without an exacerbation of anemia
   2. Splenic sequestration crisis
      a. Results from the spleen pooling large quantities of blood, which causes a precipitous drop in blood pressure and ultimately shock
      b. Acute episode occurs most commonly in children between 8 months and 5 years of age; can result in death from anemia and cardiovascular collapse
      c. Chronic manifestation is termed functional asplenia
   3. Aplastic crisis: diminished red blood cell production
      a. May be triggered by a viral or other infection
      b. Profound anemia results due to rapid destruction of red blood cells combined with a decreased production

4. Hyperhemolytic crisis: increased rate of red blood cell destruction
   a. Characterized by anemia, jaundice, and reticulocytosis
   b. Rare complication that frequently suggests a coexisting abnormality such as glucose-6-phosphate dehydrogenase deficiency
5. Stroke: sudden and severe complication with no related illnesses
   a. Sickled cells block the major blood vessels in the brain
   b. Repeat strokes in 60% of children who have experienced previous one
6. Chest syndrome: clinically similiar to pneumonia
7. Overwhelming infection
   a. Streptococcus pneumonia
   b. *Haemophilus influenzae* type B

E. Therapeutic interventions
   1. Prevention of sickling phenomenon
      a. Adequate oxygenation
      b. Adequate hydration
      c. Administration of hydroxyurea to limit sickling
   2. Treatment of crisis
      a. Rest
      b. Hydration/electrolyte replacement
      c. Pain management
      d. Antibiotic therapy
      e. Blood products
      f. Oxygen

Nursing Care of Children with Sickle Cell Anemia

A. DATA COLLECTION
1. Vital signs
2. Neurologic signs
3. Vision/hearing
4. Location and intensity of pain

B. ANALYSIS AND INTERPRETATION
1. Body image disturbance related to:
   a. Retarded growth and maturation
   b. Limited activity tolerance
   c. Chronic illness
2. Fear related to:
   a. Unfamiliar environment
   b. Separation from support system
3. Pain related to tissue ischemia
4. Altered tissue perfusion (cardiovascular) related to decreased oxygen tension
5. See General Nursing Diagnoses for Toddlers with Health Problems
6. See General Nursing Diagnoses for the Family of a Child with Special Needs

C. PLANNING/IMPLEMENTATION
1. Prevent crisis
   a. Avoid infection, dehydration, and other conditions causing strain on body, which precipitates a crisis; prophylactic use of pneumococcal, meningococcal, and *Haemophilus* flu vaccines
   b. Avoid hypoxia: treat respiratory tract infections immediately
   c. Avoid dehydration
      (1) May cause a rapid thrombus formation
      (2) Daily fluid intake should be calculated according to body weight (130 to 200 ml per kilogram)
      (3) During crisis, fluid needs to be increased, especially if the child is febrile
2. During crisis provide for:
   a. Adequate hydration (may need IV therapy)
   b. Proper positioning, careful handling
   c. Exercise as tolerated (immobility promotes thrombus formation and respiratory problems)
   d. Adequate ventilation
   e. Control of pain; use narcotics; schedule to prevent pain
   f. Blood transfusions for severe anemia
3. Provide for genetic counseling
   a. Disorder associated with black or Mediterranean heritage
   b. Parents need to know the risk of having other children with trait or disease
   c. If both parents are carriers, each pregnancy has 25% chance of producing a child with the disease
   d. Screen young children for the disorder, since clinical manifestations usually do not appear before 6 months of age
4. See General Nursing Care of Toddlers with Health Problems
5. See Meeting the Needs of the Family of an Infant or Child with Special Needs

D. EVALUATION/OUTCOMES
1. Child reports minimal pain
2. Child verbalizes feelings about disease process
3. Child demonstrates positive body image
4. Child does not exhibit signs of sickling

▼ ß-THALASSEMIA (COOLEY ANEMIA)

Data Base
A. Autosomal disorder with varied expressivity
B. Basic defect seems to be a deficiency in the synthesis of ß-chain polypeptides, which results in a decreased rate of production of the globin molecule
C. Classification
   1. Thalassemia trait: heterozygous, mild anemia

2. Thalassemia intermedia: splenomegaly, severe anemia
3. Thalassemia major: severe anemia; incompatible with life without transfusion support

D. Clinical findings
1. Severe anemia
2. Unexplained fever
3. Poor feeding
4. Markedly enlarged spleen
5. Enlarged abdomen, reflecting significant hepatomegaly
6. Impaired physical growth
7. Exercise intolerance
8. Headache
9. Listlessness
10. Anorexia

E. Therapeutic interventions
1. Use of blood transfusions to maintain adequate hemoglobin levels
2. Transfusions greatly increase the risk of hemosiderosis (excessive iron storage in various tissues of the body, especially the spleen, liver, lymph glands, heart, and pancreas) and hemochromatosis (excessive iron storage with resultant cellular damage)
3. Iron-chelating agents such as deferoxamine (Desferal) are given to reduce iron storage
4. Bone marrow transplantation

Nursing Care of Children with ß-Thalassemia (Cooley Anemia)

A. DATA COLLECTION
1. Family history
2. Significant anemia

B. ANALYSIS AND INTERPRETATION
1. Activity intolerance related to generalized weakness
2. Body image disturbance related to:
   a. Retarded growth and maturation
   b. Limited activity tolerance
   c. Chronic illness
3. Altered family processes related to situational crisis (child with a disability/serious illness)
4. Fear related to:
   a. Unfamiliar environment
   b. Separation from support system
5. Anticipatory grieving related to perceived potential loss of child
6. See General Nursing Diagnoses for Toddlers with Health Problems
7. See General Nursing Diagnoses for the Family of a Child with Special Needs

C. PLANNING/IMPLEMENTATION
1. Be alert for signs and symptoms in older infants or young children of Mediterranean descent
2. Prevent infection
   a. Avoid contact with persons who have infections
   b. Administer prophylactic antibiotics
3. Prevent complications
   a. Carry out careful observation during transfusion
   b. Administer folic acid
   c. Avoid activities that increase risk of fractures
   d. Observe for signs of cholecystitis in the adolescent
4. Assist the child in coping with the disorder and its effects
   a. Explore the child's feelings about being different from other children
   b. Emphasize the child's abilities and focus on realistic endeavors
   c. Encourage quiet activities, creative efforts, and "thinking" games
   d. Emphasize good hygiene and grooming
   e. Encourage interaction with peers
   f. Help plan therapies and medical care so they do not interfere with the child's regular activities and social interaction
   g. Assist the child with vocational planning
   h. Introduce the child to other children who have adjusted well to this or a similar disorder
5. Support the parents
   a. Explore feelings of guilt regarding the hereditary nature of the disease
   b. Emphasize the need for the child to lead as normal a life as possible
   c. Help the family deal with the potentially fatal nature of the disease
6. Prevent the occurrence of ß-thalassemia
   a. Refer for genetic counseling
   b. Reinforce and clarify counseling information
7. See General Nursing Care of Toddlers with Health Problems
8. See Meeting the Needs of the Family of an Infant or Child with Special Needs

D. EVALUATION/OUTCOMES
1. Child participates in appropriate activities for energy level
2. Parents demonstrate ability to care for child
3. Child verbalizes feelings about disease/hospitalization
4. Parents verbalize seriousness of illness
5. Child demonstrates positive body image

▼ PINWORMS

Data Base
A. A common intestinal parasite in children
B. Children reinfest themselves by fingers-to-anus-to-mouth route

C. Crowded conditions such as classrooms and day-care centers increase risk of transmission
D. Can also be infested by breathing airborne ova
E. Clinical findings
1. Severe pruritus of the anal area
2. Vaginitis
3. Irritability and insomnia
4. Poor appetite and weight loss
5. Eosinophilia
6. Pinworm eggs isolated from the perianal area; cellophane-tape test done first thing in the morning before the first bowel movement
F. Therapeutic interventions
1. Mebendazole (Vermox)
a. Selectively and irreversibly inhibits uptake of glucose and other nutrients of pinworms
b. Adverse effects: occasional, transient abdominal pain and diarrhea
c. Should be given to all family members
2. Piperazine adipate (Entacyl)
a. Paralyzes musculature of pinworms and roundworms by curarelike action
b. Within 3 days pinworms are passed active and alive; roundworms paralyzed and alive
3. Pyrantel pamoate (Combatrin)
a. Blocks neuromuscular transmission in roundworms, hookworms, pinworms
b. Adverse effects: anorexia, nausea, vomiting, diarrhea, abdominal cramps, headache, dizziness, drowsiness, rash
4. Pyrvinium pamoate (Vanquin)
a. Inhibits respiratory enzymes and anaerobic metabolism to inactivate pinworms, threadworms
b. Adverse effects: nausea, vomiting, abdominal cramps; cyanine-dye origin of the drug colors stool, emesis, and most materials bright red or orange

Nursing Care of Children with Pinworms
A. DATA COLLECTION
1. Assess the perineal area for signs of inflammation
2. Perform the cellophane-tape test
B. ANALYSIS AND INTERPRETATION
1. Pain related to severe itching in the rectal area
2. Risk for impaired skin integrity related to irritation of the perianal area
3. See General Nursing Diagnoses for Toddlers with Health Problems
C. PLANNING/IMPLEMENTATION
1. Prevent reinfestation
a. Do not allow the child to scratch the anus; child may need to wear mittens
b. Keep fingernails short
c. Place a tight diaper or underpants on child

d. Wash anal area thoroughly at least once a day
e. Change child's clothes daily; wash in hot water
f. Air out bedroom, dust and vacuum house thoroughly
2. Teach parents about administration of medication
a. Overdose will not produce a quicker recovery
b. Stools may turn bright red from medication
c. Additional series of medication may be used depending on medication; frequently 2 weeks after initial dose
D. EVALUATION/OUTCOMES
1. Perianal skin intact
2. Stool specimen is free of pinworm infestation

▼ EMOTIONAL DISORDERS

For common emotional disorders of the toddler see Disorders Usually First Evident in Infancy, Childhood, or Adolescence in Mental Health/Psychiatric Nursing (Chapter 4)

THE PRESCHOOLER

GROWTH AND DEVELOPMENT
Developmental Timetable
A. 3 years
1. Physical
a. Usual weight gain 1.8 to 2.7 kg
b. Usual height gain 7.5 cm
2. Motor
a. Jumps off bottom step
b. Rides a tricycle using pedals
c. Walks upstairs alternating feet
d. Builds tower of 9 or 10 cubes
e. Constructs three-block bridge
f. Can unbutton front or side button
g. Usually toilet trained at night
3. Sensory: visual acuity 20/30
4. Vocalization and socialization
a. Vocabulary of about 900 words; uses three- to four-word sentences
b. May have normal hesitation in speech pattern
c. Uses plurals
d. Begins to understand ideas of sharing and taking turns
5. Mental abilities
a. Beginning understanding of the past, present, future, or any aspect of time
b. Stage of magical thinking

B. 4 years
1. Physical
   a. Height and weight increases are similar to previous year
   b. Length at birth is doubled
2. Motor
   a. Skips and hops on one foot
   b. Walks up and down stairs like an adult
   c. Can button buttons and lace shoes
   d. Throws ball overhand
   e. Uses scissors to cut outline
3. Vocalization and socialization
   a. Vocabulary of 1500 words or more
   b. May have an imaginary companion
   c. Tends to be selfish and impatient, but takes pride in accomplishments
   d. Exaggerates, boasts, and tattles on others
4. Mental abilities
   a. Unable to conserve matter
   b. Can repeat four numbers and is learning number concept
   c. Knows which is the longer of two lines
   d. Has poor space perception
C. 5 years
1. Physical: height and weight increases are similar to previous year
2. Motor
   a. Gross motor abilities well developed
   b. Can balance on one foot for about 10 seconds
   c. Can jump rope, skip, and roller skate
   d. Can draw a picture of a person
   e. Prints first name and other words as learned
   f. Dresses and washes self
   g. May be able to tie shoelaces
3. Sensory
   a. Minimal potential for amblyopia to develop
   b. Color recognition is well established
4. Vocalization and socialization
   a. Vocabulary of about 2100 words
   b. Talks constantly
   c. Asks meaning of new words
   d. Generally cooperative and sympathetic toward others
   e. Basic personality structure is well established
5. Mental abilities (*Piaget's phase* of intuitive thought)
   a. Beginning understanding of time in terms of days as part of a week
   b. Beginning understanding of conversation of numbers
   c. Has not mastered the concept that parts equal a whole regardless of their appearance

Play During Preschool Years (cooperative play)

A. Loosely organized group play where membership changes readily, as do rules
B. Through play, the child deals with reality, learns control of feelings, and expresses emotions more through words than through actions
C. Play is still physically oriented but is also imitative and imaginary
D. Increasing sharing and cooperation among preschool children, especially 5-year-old children
E. Suggested toys (same principles as discussed before)
1. Puppets
2. Additional dress-up clothes, dolls, house, furniture, small trucks, animals, etc.
3. Painting sets, coloring books, paste, and cut-out sets
4. Illustrated books
5. Puzzles with large pieces and more shapes
6. Tricycle, swing, slide, and other playground equipment

HEALTH PROMOTION FOR PRESCHOOLERS

See Health Promotion for Toddlers and Preschoolers in the Toddler Section

HEALTH PROBLEMS MOST COMMON IN PRESCHOOLERS

Hospitalization

A. Reaction of the child
1. Fears about body image are now greater than fear of separation
2. The fears include:
   a. Intrusive experiences: needles, thermometer, otoscope
   b. Punishment and rejection
   c. Pain
   d. Castration and mutilation
B. If possible, parents can be helped to prepare the child beforehand, since increased cognitive and verbal ability makes explanations possible

GENERAL NURSING DIAGNOSES FOR PRESCHOOLERS WITH HEALTH PROBLEMS

A. Anxiety related to:
1. Strange environment
2. Perception of impending event
3. Anticipated discomfort
4. Knowledge deficit
5. Discomfort
6. Difficulty breathing
7. Feelings of powerlessness
B. Family coping: potential for growth related to successful parenting

C. Ineffective family coping: compromised, related to situational crises
D. Ineffective individual coping related to situational crises
E. Diversional activity deficit related to:
   1. Lack of sensory stimulation
   2. Frequent or prolonged hospitalization
F. Altered family processes related to:
   1. Situational crisis
   2. Knowledge deficit
   3. Temporary family disorganization
   4. Inadequate support system
G. Fear related to:
   1. Separation from support systems
   2. Uncertain prognosis
   3. Potential change in body
H. Anticipatory grieving (parental) related to:
   1. Expected loss
   2. Gravity of child's physical status
I. Impaired home maintenance management related to:
   1. Knowledge deficit
   2. Inadequate support systems
J. Risk for injury related to:
   1. Use of specific therapies and appliances
   2. Incapacity for self-protection
   3. Immobility
K. Pain related to:
   1. Disease process
   2. Interventions
L. Parental role conflict related to:
   1. Sick child
   2. Inability to care for child
M. Risk for altered parenting related to:
   1. Separation
   2. Skill deficit
   3. Family stress
N. Feeding, bathing/hygiene, dressing/grooming, toileting self-care deficit related to:
   1. Fatigue
   2. Pain
   3. Developmental level
   4. Limitations of treatment modalities
O. Sensory-perceptual alterations (tactile) related to protected environment
P. Risk for impaired skin integrity related to immobility
Q. Sleep pattern disturbance related to:
   1. Excessive crying
   2. Frequent assessment
   3. Therapies
R. Spiritual distress (parental) related to:
   1. Inadequate support systems
   2. Decisions regarding life or death conflicts
S. See General Nursing Diagnoses for the Family of a Child with Special Needs

GENERAL NURSING CARE OF PRESCHOOLERS WITH HEALTH PROBLEMS

A. Begin preparing for hospitalization a few days before but not too early because of the child's poor concept of time
B. Clarify cause and effect because of the child's phenomenalistic thinking (in the child's mind, proximity of two events relates them to each other)
C. Explain routines of hospital admission but not all procedures at one time, because this would be overwhelming
D. Recognize play is an excellent medium for preparation (use dolls, puppets, make-believe equipment, dress-up doctor and nurse clothes)
E. Provide time for play as an outlet for fear, anger, and hostility, as well as a temporary escape from reality
F. Keep verbal explanation as simple as possible and always honest
G. Add details about procedures, drugs, surgery, and the like as the child's cognitive level and personal experiences increase
H. Link to supports and resources
I. See Nursing Care under each disorder

▼ LEUKEMIA

Data Base
A. The most common type of childhood cancer; prognosis is improving; familial history
B. Peak incidence: 2 to 6 years of age
C. Malignant neoplasm of blood-forming organs
D. In children, overproduction of immature leukocytes: blast-cell or stem-cell leukemia
E. Classification
   1. Acute lymphocytic: about 85% of incidence; better prognosis than for myelogenous
   2. Acute myelogenous or acute nonlymphoid: about 10% incidence; poorer prognosis
   3. Others: 5% incidence
F. Clinical findings
   1. Caused by overproduction of immature nonfunctional cells
   2. Anemia: pallor, weakness, irritability
   3. Infection: fever
   4. Tendency toward bleeding: petechiae and bleeding into joints
   5. Pain in joints caused by seepage of serous fluid
   6. Tendency toward easy fracture of bones
   7. Enlargement of spleen, liver, lymph glands
   8. Abdominal pain and anorexia resulting in weight loss
   9. Necrosis and bleeding of gums and other mucous membranes

10. Later symptoms: CNS involvement and frank hemorrhage
G. Therapeutic interventions
   1. Induce remission by chemotherapy (see Pharmacology related to neoplastic disorders)
      a. Prednisone (Deltasone): steroid
      b. Vincristine (Oncovin): plant alkaloid
      c. Methotrexate (Methotrexate): folic acid antagonist
      d. L-asparaginase (Asparaginase): enzyme
      e. 6-mercaptopurine (Purinethol): purine antagonist
      f. Cyclophosphamide (Cytoxan): alkylating agent
      g. Doxorubicin hydrochloride (Adriamycin): cytotoxic antibiotic
   2. Prevent CNS involvement by use of irradiation and intrathecal methotrexate, because leukemic cells invade the brain, but most antileukemic drugs do not pass the blood-brain barrier
   3. Transfusions to replace and provide needed blood factors such as red blood cells, platelets, and white blood cells
   4. Bone marrow transplantation

Nursing Care of Children with Leukemia

A. DATA COLLECTION
   1. Hematologic status
      a. Anemia
      b. Thrombocytopenia
      c. Neutropenia
   2. Activity level
   3. Exposure to infectious diseases
   4. Complications of therapy/disease process

B. ANALYSIS AND INTERPRETATION
   1. Activity intolerance related to:
      a. Anemia
      b. Reduced energy and fatigue
   2. Body image disturbance related to:
      a. Loss of hair
      b. Moon face
      c. Debilitation
   3. Altered family processes related to situational crisis (child with life-threatening disease)
   4. Fear related to:
      a. Diagnostic tests
      b. Procedures
   5. Anticipatory grieving related to perceived potential loss of child
   6. Risk for infection related to:
      a. Decreased immune response
      b. Use of chemotherapy
   7. Risk for injury (including hemorrhage) related to:
      a. Decreased strength and endurance

   b. Pain and discomfort
   c. Decreased platelets
   8. Altered nutrition: less than body requirements related to loss of appetite
   9. Pain related to physiologic effect of neoplasia and treatment
   10. Impaired physical mobility related to:
      a. Decreased strength and endurance
      b. Pain and discomfort
      c. Neuromuscular impairment
   11. Risk for impaired skin integrity related to:
      a. Immobility
      b. Administration of antimetabolites
      c. Disease process
   12. Refer to General Nursing Diagnoses for the Family of a Child with Special Needs and General Nursing Diagnoses for Preschoolers with Health Problems

C. PLANNING/IMPLEMENTATION
   1. Encourage adjustment to chronic illness; stress need for normal life-style
   2. Deal with the child's idea of death: discussion should be appropriate to level of understanding
      a. Preschooler: concept that death is reversible; greatest fear is separation
      b. Child 6 to 9 years of age: concept that death is personified; a person actually comes and removes the child
      c. Child over 9 years of age: adult concept of death as irreversible and inevitable
   3. Be alert for and attempt to support the child experiencing side effects of drugs
      a. Cytoxan: severe nausea, vomiting, cystitis, and alopecia
      b. Vincristine: constipation, alopecia, neurotoxicity
      c. Methotrexate: oral and rectal ulcers
   4. Prevent infection by hand washing; avoid contact with people who have active infections and avoid crowded places
   5. Handle the child carefully because of pain and hemorrhage; administer analgesics for pain
   6. Provide gentle oral hygiene; soft, bland foods; increased liquids
   7. Provide for frequent rest periods, quiet play
   8. See General Nursing Care of Preschoolers with Health Problems
   9. See Meeting the Needs of the Family of an Infant or Child with Special Needs

D. EVALUATION/OUTCOMES
   1. Child participates in developmental, age-appropriate activities
   2. Child repeats information accurately
   3. Child exhibits no physiologic signs of pain
   4. Child and family demonstrate understanding of procedures

5. Family and child discuss fears, concerns, and needs
6. Child is not exposed to infectious diseases
7. Child does not exhibit signs of bleeding/injury
8. Child ambulates without difficulty
9. Child consumes adequate calories for growth
10. Child expresses feelings about altered body image
11. Child does not exhibit signs of skin impairment

▼ WILMS TUMOR (NEPHROBLASTOMA)

Data Base
A. Most common malignant neoplasm of the kidney in children
B. Estimated occurrence 1 in 10,000 live births
C. May be associated with congenital anomalies
   1. Aniridia (congenital absence of iris)
   2. Hemihypertrophy
   3. Genitourinary: hypospadias, cryptorchidism
D. Clinical findings
   1. Swelling or nontender mass in abdomen; confined to one side of midline
   2. Weight loss
   3. Fever
   4. Hematuria occurs in less than 25%
   5. Fatigue and malaise
   6. Hypertension occasionally occurs
   7. Other symptoms associated with compression of neighboring organs or metastasis (lungs: cough, dyspnea, shortness of breath, waistline increases)
E. Therapeutic interventions
   1. Surgery: should be scheduled soon after confirmation of renal mass
      a. Tumor, kidney, and associated adrenal gland removed; precautions taken not to rupture the capsule of the tumor
      b. Contralateral kidney inspected
      c. Regional lymph nodes and organs inspected and biopsied; when indicated, they are removed
      d. When bilateral kidney involvement, partial nephrectomy is done on the less affected side
   2. Radiation therapy: indicated for all children except those in stage I with favorable histology
   3. Chemotherapy
      a. Indicated for all stages
      b. Drugs used include actinomycin D (Cosmegan), vincristine (Oncovin), and doxorubicin hydrochloride (Adriamycin)
      c. Treatment continued for 6 to 15 months

4. Prognosis
   a. Stages I and II with localized tumor: 90% cure with multimodal therapy
   b. When metastasis present: 50% survival

Nursing Care of Children with Wilms Tumor
A. DATA COLLECTION
1. Manifestations of Wilms tumor
   a. Abdominal mass or swelling; firm, nontender; does not cross midline
   b. Anemia
   c. Weight loss
2. Symptoms of compression
3. Signs of metastasis
   a. Dyspnea
   b. Cough
   c. Shortness of breath

B. ANALYSIS AND INTERPRETATION
1. Anxiety related to:
   a. Fear of the unknown
   b. Strange environment
2. Altered family processes related to situational crisis (child with a serious illness)
3. Risk for infection related to:
   a. Lowered body defenses
   b. Abdominal surgery
4. Risk for injury related to presence of encapsulated tumor
5. Altered nutrition: less than body requirements related to loss of appetite
6. See Nursing Care of Children with Leukemia
7. See General Nursing Diagnoses for Preschoolers with Health Problems

C. PLANNING/IMPLEMENTATION
1. Preoperative
   a. Handle and bathe carefully to prevent trauma to the abdomen, which may result in rupture of the tumor capsule
   b. Place sign over bed: "Do not palpate abdomen"
   c. Prepare parents and child for large size of incision and drainage
   d. Monitor blood pressure
   e. Begin teaching family about chemotherapy and radiation therapy
2. Postoperative
   a. Monitor blood pressure carefully
   b. Monitor intake and output to assess function of remaining kidney
   c. Encourage child to turn, cough, and deep breathe to prevent pulmonary complications
   d. Teach parents to identify untoward reactions from chemotherapy and radiation therapy
3. See Nursing Care of Children with Leukemia

4. See General Nursing Care of Preschoolers with Health Problems
5. See Meeting the Needs of the Family of an Infant or Child with Special Needs

D. EVALUATION/OUTCOMES
1. Child and family discuss disease process and therapy
2. Family demonstrates understanding of the disorder, therapies, and expected outcomes
3. Child does not exhibit signs of infection
4. Tumor capsule does not rupture
5. Child consumes adequate calories for growth

▼ NEPHROTIC SYNDROME (MINIMAL CHANGE NEPHROTIC SYNDROME)

Data Base
A. Pathology: abnormal, increased permeability of the glomerular basement membrane to plasma albumin
B. Cause unknown
C. Peak incidence: 2 to 7 years of age
D. Classification
  1. Minimal change nephrotic syndrome (80% incidence)
  2. Secondary nephrotic syndrome
  3. Congenital nephrotic syndrome (usually die by second year of life)
E. Clinical findings
  1. Proteinuria
  2. Hypoalbuminemia: poor general health, loss of appetite
  3. Hyperlipemia
  4. Generalized dependent edema, especially genital, periorbital, and abdominal (ascites)
  5. May also see symptoms usually associated with nephritis
    a. Hematuria
    b. Hypertension
F. Therapeutic interventions
  1. Supportive therapy
  2. Diet: salt restrictions
  3. Corticosteroid therapy
    a. Response to therapy usually within 7 to 21 days
    b. Lower dose or gradually discontinue when satisfactory response noted
  4. Immunosuppressant therapy for children who do not respond to steroids or those who have frequent relapses (e.g., Cyclosporine [Sandimmune])

Nursing Care of Children with Nephrotic Syndrome
A. DATA COLLECTION
1. Vital signs/blood pressure
2. Fluid balance; fluid restrictions
3. Urine studies
  a. Specific gravity
  b. Albumin
4. Daily weight/abdominal girth
5. Edema

B. ANALYSIS AND INTERPRETATION
1. Activity intolerance related to fatigue
2. Body image disturbance related to change in appearance
3. Altered family processes related to situational crisis (child with a serious illness)
4. Risk for fluid volume deficit related to protein and fluid loss
5. Risk for infection related to:
  a. Presence of infective organisms
  b. Lowered body defenses
6. Altered nutrition: less than body requirements related to loss of appetite
7. Risk for impaired skin integrity related to:
  a. Edema
  b. Lowered body defenses
8. See General Nursing Diagnoses for Preschoolers with Health Problems
9. See General Nursing Diagnoses for the Family of a Child with Special Needs

C. PLANNING/IMPLEMENTATION
1. Infection: both disease state and drug therapy increase susceptibility
  a. Protect the child from others who are ill
  b. Teach parents the signs of impending infection and encourage them to seek medical care
2. Malnutrition caused by loss of protein and poor appetite
  a. Provide regular diet; discourage the use of salt and salty foods
  b. Encourage the child to select foods from high-protein choices
  c. Restrict fluids if ordered
3. Respiratory difficulty caused by ascites
  a. Place in a Fowler's position to decrease pressure against the diaphragm
  b. Monitor vital signs
4. Discomfort caused by edema, pressure areas
  a. Provide some relief by positioning and giving skin care
  b. Support the genitalia if edematous
5. Change in body image caused by edema and steroids
  a. Recognize that this becomes a greater problem as the child gets older
  b. Emphasize clothes, hairdo, etc., that make the child attractive
  c. Stress that "diets" will not help weight loss

6. Behavioral changes such as irritability and depression
   a. Help parents understand that mood swings are influenced by physical condition
   b. Encourage the child to participate in own care
   c. Encourage diversionary activities that provide satisfaction
7. See General Nursing Care of Preschoolers with Health Problems
8. See Meeting the Needs of the Family of an Infant or Child with Special Needs

D. EVALUATION/OUTCOMES
1. Child engages in activities appropriate to capabilities
2. Family can demonstrate care of child
3. Child does not exhibit signs of hypovolemia
4. Child exhibits no signs of infection
5. Child consumes adequate calories for growth and development
6. Child discusses feelings and concerns
7. Child exhibits no sign of skin redness or breakdown

▼ URINARY TRACT INFECTION (UTI)

Data Base

A. Very common in females because of anatomy of the lower urinary tract: urethra is short and meatus is close to the anus
B. Peak incidence occurs at 2 to 6 years of age
C. Classification
   1. Bacteriuria
      a. Asymptomatic
      b. Symptomatic
   2. Recurrent UTI
   3. Relapse UTI
   4. Urethritis
   5. Cystitis
   6. Ureteritis
   7. Pyelonephritis
   8. Ureteral reflux
D. Clinical findings
   1. Children under 2 years of age; symptoms mimic gastrointestinal disorders
   2. Enuresis or daytime incontinence
   3. Dysuria/urgency
   4. Increased frequency of urination
E. Therapeutic interventions
   1. Eliminate infection
   2. Identify and correct structural anomalies if present
   3. Prevent recurrence
   4. Preserve renal function

Nursing Care of Children with Urinary Tract Infections

A. DATA COLLECTION
1. Discomfort on urination
2. Urinary frequency
3. Urine sample

B. ANALYSIS AND INTERPRETATION
1. Altered family processes related to a child with a mild disease with potential for renal damage
2. Risk for injury related to:
   a. Kidney damage from chronic infection
   b. Knowledge deficit of medication administration
3. See General Nursing Diagnoses for Preschoolers with Health Problems

C. PLANNING/IMPLEMENTATION
1. Teach prevention
   a. Cleanse genitalia (front to back)
   b. Void when necessary as opposed to holding urine in bladder
   c. Increase fluids, particularly those that acidify urine
   d. Identify asymptomatic infections
2. See General Nursing Care of Preschoolers with Health Problems

D. EVALUATION/OUTCOMES
1. Child exhibits no sign of infection
2. Family administers medication correctly
3. Family understands condition
4. Child receives follow-up care

▼ ASTHMA

Data Base

A. Reversible obstructive process characterized by increased responsiveness and inflammation of the airway as a result of exposure to a substance that has been inhaled or ingested or that has contacted the skin
B. Spasms of bronchi and bronchioles
C. Edema of mucous membranes
D. Increased secretions
E. Respiratory acidosis from buildup of carbon dioxide
F. Classification
   1. Intermittent: child symptom free for extended periods of time
   2. Chronic: child requires frequent or continuous medical therapy
G. Clinical findings
   1. Wheezing, especially on expiration
   2. Labored breathing, cough, increased secretions
   3. Flaring nares, distended neck veins
H. Therapeutic interventions
   1. Bronchodilators
      a. Theophylline derivatives

(1) Drugs
  (a) Aminophylline
  (b) Theophylline
(2) Actions
  (a) Act directly on the bronchial smooth muscle to decrease spasm, relax smooth muscle of the vasculature
  (b) Direct stimulatory effect on the myocardium increases cardiac output, which improves blood flow to kidneys
  (c) Direct action on the renal tubules provides diuretic effect by increasing excretion of sodium and chloride ions
(3) Adverse effects: oral forms cause gastric irritation
b. ß-adrenergic agonists
(1) Epinephrine hydrochloride: drug of choice in respiratory emergency, such as status asthmaticus
(2) Salbutamol (Ventolin), fenoterol hydrobromide (Berotec), metaproterenol (Alupent), terbutaline (Brethine)
(3) Actions
  (a) Effect is on the beta-adrenergic receptors in the bronchi; relaxes smooth muscle and increases respiratory volume
  (b) Inhalants cause vasoconstriction, which reduces congestion or edema
(4) Adverse effects: cardiac palpitation; overuse of inhalants may cause "congestive rebound"
c. Cromolyn sodium (Intal): acts primarily by preventing release of mediators of type I allergic reactions (histamine, slow-reacting substance of anaphylaxis) from sensitized mast cells; prophylactic use by inhaling capsule contents lessens bronchoconstriction
d. Adverse effects common to bronchodilator group: anxiety, nervousness, tremors, nausea, vomiting, headache, dizziness
2. Corticosteroids
a. Antiinflammatory effect diminishes the inflammatory component of asthma and reduces airway obstruction
b. Used in status asthmaticus; however, less often for long-term control because of side effects

Nursing Care of Children with Asthma
A. DATA COLLECTION
1. Chest shape
2. Type of breathing
3. History of current and previous attacks

4. Precipitating events/environmental factors
5. Knowledge of and compliance with drug therapy
B. ANALYSIS AND INTERPRETATION
1. Activity intolerance related to imbalance between oxygen supply and demand
2. Body image disturbance related to perception of physiologic changes
3. Ineffective breathing pattern related to:
   a. Bronchiolar edema
   b. Increased mucus secretions
   c. Bronchiolar constriction
4. Altered family processes related to situational crisis (illness of child)
5. Sleep pattern disturbance related to:
   a. Illness
   b. Separation
6. Social isolation related to:
   a. Hospitalization
   b. Confinement to home
7. Risk for suffocation related to interaction between individual and environmental allergen
8. See General Nursing Diagnoses for Preschoolers with Health Problems
9. See General Nursing Diagnoses for the Family of a Child with Special Needs
C. PLANNING/IMPLEMENTATION
1. Recognize that cumulation of drug can occur unless dosage is regulated
2. Administer parenteral drugs slowly over a 4- to 5-minute period to avoid peripheral vasodilation (hypotension, facial flushing), cerebral vascular constriction (headache, dizziness), cardiac palpitation, and precordial pain
3. Teach parents how to give antispasmodic drugs and bronchodilators and why they must be given even if child does not have an attack
4. Teach parents postural drainage, need for increased fluids, and the use of a cool mist humidifier to provide high humidity in home to promote good respiratory hygiene
5. Improve ventilating capacity
   a. Position in a high-Fowler's, leaning slightly forward (orthopneic position)
   b. Teach breathing exercises, controlled breathing, relaxation exercises
6. Teach parents that a controlled environment can limit attacks
   a. Keep environment as allergen free as possible
   b. Avoid exertion, exposure to cold air, and people with infections
   c. Avoid emotional factors that precipitate attacks as much as possible
7. See General Nursing Care of Preschoolers with Health Problems

8. See Meeting the Needs of the Family of an Infant or Child with Special Needs

D. EVALUATION/OUTCOMES
1. Child engages in appropriate activities
2. Child breathes without dyspnea
3. Child is able to manage secretions
4. Family copes with symptoms and effects of disease
5. Child verbalizes feelings about physiologic effects and disease
6. Child obtains sufficient sleep to feel rested
7. Child maintains family and peer-group relationships
8. Child participates in therapeutics as prescribed

▼ MUCOCUTANEOUS LYMPH NODE SYNDROME (KAWASAKI DISEASE)

Data Base

A. Acute febrile illness of unknown cause; principally involving the cardiovascular system, with extensive perivasculitis of arterioles, venules, capillaries, including the coronary arteries; panvasculitis and perivasculitis of the main coronary arteries may cause stenosis or obstruction with aneurysm formation, pericarditis, interstitial myocarditis and endocarditis, and phlebitis of the larger veins
B. Geographic and seasonal outbreaks
C. Clinical findings
   1. Fever for 5 or more days
   2. Bilateral congestion of the ocular conjunctiva without exudation
   3. Changes of the mucous membranes of the oral cavity, such as erythema, dryness, and fissuring of lips, oropharyngeal reddening, or "strawberry tongue"
   4. Changes in the extremities, such as peripheral edema, peripheral erythema and desquamation of the palms and soles, particularly periungual peeling
   5. Polymorphous rash, primarily of the trunk
   6. Cervical lymphadenopathy
D. Therapeutic interventions
   1. Primarily supportive and directed toward controlling fever, preventing dehydration, and minimizing possible cardiac complications
   2. Intravenous gamma globulin
   3. Large doses of aspirin
   4. Monitoring the cardiac status

Nursing Care of Children with Kawasaki Disease

A. DATA COLLECTION
1. Cardiac status; signs of congestive heart failure

2. Daily weight; intake and output
3. Symptom identification

B. ANALYSIS AND INTERPRETATION
1. Anxiety related to concern for child's prognosis
2. Pain related to disease process
3. Risk for impaired skin integrity related to:
   a. Edema
   b. Desquamation
4. See General Nursing Diagnoses for Preschoolers with Health Problems
5. See General Nursing Diagnoses for the Family of a Child with Special Needs

C. PLANNING/IMPLEMENTATION
1. Administer aspirin to control fever; assess for early signs of toxicity
2. Provide optimal nutrition
3. Administer analgesics for joint pain if needed in addition to aspirin
4. Observe for allergic reaction to and side effects of IV gamma globulin
5. Monitor for any signs of heart disease, especially dysrhythmias
6. See General Nursing Care of Preschoolers with Health Problems
7. See Meeting the Needs of the Family of an Infant or Child with Special Needs

D. EVALUATION/OUTCOMES
1. Parents and child can discuss concerns about the illness
2. Child exhibits no sign of impaired skin integrity
3. Child does not report the presence of pain

▼ TONSILLECTOMY AND ADENOIDECTOMY

Data Base

A. Not done routinely, since lymphoid tissue helps prevent invasion of organisms
B. Indications for surgical removal
   1. Recurrent tonsillitis or otitis media
   2. Enlargement that interferes with breathing or swallowing
C. Contraindications for removal
   1. Occasional infections that clear up rapidly
   2. Cleft palate, hemophilia, or debilitating disease such as leukemia
D. Clinical findings—complications after surgery
   1. Hemorrhage: first 24 hours
      a. Frequent swallowing, bright-red blood in the vomitus
      b. Restlessness
      c. Increased pulse rate, pallor
   2. Hemorrhage from sloughing of tissue: 5 to 10 days after surgery

Nursing Care of Children Following a Tonsillectomy and/or Adenoidectomy

A. DATA COLLECTION
1. Swallowing ability
2. Pain
3. Bleeding

B. ANALYSIS AND INTERPRETATION
1. Ineffective airway clearance related to discomfort when swallowing and coughing
2. Altered family processes related to situational crisis
3. Fear related to:
   a. Discomfort
   b. Unfamiliar surroundings
   c. Separation from support people
4. Risk for fluid volume deficit related to vomiting
5. Knowledge deficit related to unfamiliar routine and environment
6. Risk for altered nutrition: less than body requirements related to:
   a. Difficulty swallowing
   b. Nausea and vomiting
7. Pain related to surgical incision
8. See General Nursing Diagnoses for Preschoolers with Health Problems

C. PLANNING/IMPLEMENTATION
1. Keep the child positioned on the abdomen or side with head turned to the side
2. After surgery give child cool liquids, not red in color and not thick or mucus producing
3. Ask the child to talk; provide assurance that it is possible
4. Apply ice collar to decrease edema
5. Administer analgesics as necessary for comfort
6. See General Nursing Care of Preschoolers with Health Problems

D. EVALUATION/OUTCOMES
1. Child is able to manage secretions
2. Child reports minimal pain
3. Family can demonstrate care of child
4. Child/family can discuss surgery/healing process
5. Child does not exhibit signs of dehydration
6. Family verbalizes postoperative/discharge instructions
7. Child consumes adequate calories for growth and healing

▼ EMOTIONAL DISORDERS

For common emotional disorders of the preschooler see Disorders Usually First Evident in Infancy, Childhood, or Adolescence in Mental Health/Psychiatric Nursing (Chapter 4)

SCHOOL-AGED CHILDREN

GROWTH AND DEVELOPMENT

Developmental Timetable

A. Physical growth
   1. Permanent dentition, beginning with 6-year molars and central incisors at 7 or 8 years of age
   2. Tends to look lanky because bone development precedes muscular development
      a. 6 years: height and weight gain slower, 5 cm and 2 to 3 kg
      b. 7 years: continues to grow, 5 cm and 2.5 kg a year
      c. 8 to 9 years: continues to grow, 5 cm and 3 kg a year
      d. 10 to 12 years: slow growth in height compared to rapid weight gain, 6.25 cm and 4.5 kg a year; pubescent changes may begin to appear, especially in females
B. Motor
   1. Refinement of coordination, balance, and control occurs
   2. Motor development necessary for competitive activity becomes important
C. Sensory: visual acuity of 20/20
D. Mental abilities
   1. Readiness for learning, especially in perceptual organization: names months of year, knows right from left, can tell time, can follow several directions at once
   2. Acquires use of reason and understanding of rules
   3. Trial-and-error problem solving becomes more conceptual rather than action oriented
   4. Reasoning ability allows greater understanding and use of language
   5. Concrete operations (Piaget): knows that quantity remains the same even though appearance differs

Play During School-aged Years

A. Play activities vary with age
B. Number of play activities decreases while the amount of time spent in one particular activity increases
C. Likes games with rules because of increased mental abilities
D. Likes games of athletic competition because of increased motor ability
E. Should learn how to work as well as play, with a beginning appreciation for economics and finances
F. In beginning of school years, boys and girls play together but gradually separate into gender-oriented type of activities

G. Suggested play for 6- to 9-year olds
1. More housekeeping toys that work, doll accessories, paper-doll sets, simple sewing machine, and needlework
2. Simple work and number games (i.e., calling for increased skills)
3. Physically active games such as hopscotch, jump rope, climbing trees
4. Collections and hobbies such as stamp collecting and building simple models
5. Bicycle riding
H. Suggested play for 9- to 12-year olds
1. Handicrafts of all kinds
2. Model kits, collections, hobbies
3. Archery, dart games, chess, jigsaw puzzles
4. Sculpturing materials such as pottery clay
5. Science toys, magic sets

HEALTH PROBLEMS MOST COMMON IN SCHOOL-AGED CHILDREN

Hospitalization

A. Reactions of the school-aged child
1. Usually handles separation well but prefers parents to be near
2. Fears the unknown, especially when dependency or loss of control is expected; fears bodily harm, especially disfigurement
3. Possesses realistic concept of death by 9 to 10 years of age
4. Self-image about reaction to pain is important; may use avoidance to deal with physical discomfort
5. Wants to know scientific rationale for treatments and procedures
B. If possible parents can be helped to prepare the child beforehand, since increased cognitive and verbal ability makes explanations possible

GENERAL NURSING DIAGNOSES FOR SCHOOL-AGED CHILDREN WITH HEALTH PROBLEMS

A. Anxiety related to:
1. Strange environment
2. Perception of impending event
3. Anticipated discomfort
4. Knowledge deficit
5. Discomfort
6. Difficulty breathing
7. Feelings of powerlessness
B. Family coping: potential for growth related to successful parenting
C. Ineffective family coping: compromised, related to situational crises
D. Ineffective family coping related to situational crises

E. Diversional activity deficit related to:
1. Lack of sensory stimulation
2. Frequent or prolonged hospitalization
F. Altered family processes related to:
1. Situational crisis
2. Knowledge deficit
3. Temporary family disorganization
4. Inadequate support system
G. Fear related to:
1. Separation from support systems
2. Uncertain prognosis
3. Potential change in body
H. Anticipatory grieving (parental) related to:
1. Expected loss
2. Gravity of child's physical status
I. Impaired home maintenance management related to:
1. Knowledge deficit
2. Inadequate support systems
J. Risk for injury related to:
1. Use of specific therapies and appliances
2. Incapacity for self-protection
3. Immobility
K. Pain related to:
1. Disease process
2. Interventions
L. Parental role conflict related to:
1. Sick child
2. Inability to care for child
M. Risk for altered parenting related to:
1. Separation
2. Skill deficit
3. Family stress
N. Feeding, bathing/hygiene, dressing/grooming, toileting self-care deficit related to:
1. Fatigue
2. Pain
3. Developmental level
4. Limitations of treatment modalities
O. Sensory-perceptual alterations (tactile) related to protected environment
P. Risk for impaired skin integrity related to immobility
Q. Sleep pattern disturbance related to:
1. Excessive crying
2. Frequent assessment
3. Therapies
R. Spiritual distress (parental) related to:
1. Inadequate support systems
2. Decisions regarding life or death conflicts
S. See General Nursing Diagnoses for the Family of a Child with Special Needs

GENERAL NURSING CARE OF SCHOOL-AGED CHILDREN WITH HEALTH PROBLEMS

A. Begin preparing child for hospitalization before admission if possible

B. Explain diagnostic modalities and treatments at level of child's understanding
C. Involve child and parents in planning care
D. Provide time for play as an outlet for fear, anger, and hostility, as well as a temporary escape from reality
E. Keep verbal explanation as simple as possible and always honest
F. Add details about procedures, drugs, surgery, and the like as the child's cognitive level and personal experiences increase
G. Encourage and allow child to express feelings, emotions, and fears
H. Provide for tutoring if absence from school is prolonged
I. Encourage visits from siblings and peers and the formation of new peer relationships
J. Recognize that although play is diversional, this age group enjoys games with challenge and skill
K. Allow dependency but foster independence as much as possible
L. See Nursing Care under each disorder

▼ DIABETES MELLITUS

Data Base

A. Peak incidence of Early Onset Insulin Dependent Diabetes Mellitus Type I in the school-aged group
B. Differences in diabetes in children and adults
   1. Onset
      a. Rapid in children
      b. Insidious in adults
   2. Obesity
      a. Not a factor in children
      b. Predisposing factor in adults
   3. Dietary treatment
      a. Rarely adequate for children
      b. May be beneficial for some adults
   4. Oral hypoglycemics
      a. Contraindicated for children
      b. May be beneficial for some adults
   5. Insulin
      a. Almost universally necessary in children
      b. May be beneficial for some adults
   6. Hypoglycemia and ketoacidosis
      a. Quite frequent in children
      b. More uncommon in adults
   7. Degenerative vascular changes
      a. Develop after adolescence in children
      b. May be present at the time of diagnosis in adults
C. Classification
   1. Idiopathic
      a. Insulin dependent (IDDM): onset usually in childhood but can be anytime

   b. Non-insulin dependent (NIDDM): appears to involve resistance to insulin action and defective glucose-mediated insulin secretion
   c. Maturity-onset diabetes of youth (MODY): autosomal dominant disorder; structurally abnormal insulin with decreased activity
   2. Secondary: caused by exogenous factors; usually reversible if primary disorder corrected
D. Clinical findings
   1. Juvenile onset diabetes is always type I insulin-dependent diabetes mellitus (IDDM); not the same disease process as type II non–insulin-dependent diabetes mellitus (NIDDM)
   2. Onset: rapid, obvious
   3. Child usually thin, underweight
   4. Increased thirst, fluid intake, appetite, and urinary output (polydipsia, polyphagia, polyuria)
   5. Hyperglycemia: ketoacidosis or diabetic coma
      a. Causes
         (1) Decreased insulin
         (2) Emotional stress
         (3) Fever
         (4) Infection
         (5) Increased food intake
      b. Symptoms
         (1) Weakness, drowsiness
         (2) Lack of appetite, thirst
         (3) Abdominal and/or generalized pain
         (4) Acetone breath, flushing
         (5) Late signs: Kussmaul breathing (deep, rapid respirations), cherry-red lips, loss of consciousness, death
   6. Hypoglycemia: insulin-therapy related
      a. Causes
         (1) Overdose of insulin
         (2) Decreased food intake
         (3) Excessive physical exercise: increases muscle activity and movement of glucose into muscle cells
      b. Symptoms
         (1) Sweating, pallor
         (2) Numbness, trembling, chilliness
         (3) Unsteadiness, nervousness, irritability
         (4) Hunger
         (5) Hallucinations
         (6) Late signs: convulsions, coma, death
E. Therapeutic interventions
   1. Control calorie, carbohydrate, fat, and protein intake
   2. Insulin (see Pharmacology Related to the Endocrine System)
   3. Exercise
   4. Hyperglycemia: hospitalization with administration of fluids and insulin
   5. Hypoglycemia: immediate supply of readily available glucose followed by a complex carbohydrate or protein

Nursing Care of Children with Diabetes Mellitus

A. DATA COLLECTION

1. Knowledge of disease management
2. Blood glucose monitoring
3. Signs of hypoglycemia/hyperglycemia
4. Superimposed illnesses; GI, respiratory
5. Early signs of complications

B. ANALYSIS AND INTERPRETATION

1. Body image disturbance related to perceived body changes (insulin dependence)
2. Risk for injury related to:
   a. Hypoglycemia
   b. Insulin deficiency
3. Knowledge deficit (diabetic management) related to newly diagnosed diabetes
4. Altered nutrition: less than body requirements related to altered ability/inability to use nutrients
5. Powerlessness related to diagnosis of chronic illness
6. Self-esteem disturbance related to:
   a. Need to restrict diet
   b. Need for insulin injections
   c. Feeling of being different from peers
7. See General Nursing Diagnoses for School-aged Children with Health Problems
8. See General Nursing Diagnoses for the Family of a Child with Special Needs

C. PLANNING/IMPLEMENTATION

1. Explain to the parents and the child the differences between Type I and Type II diabetes mellitus. They may have previous experience with Type II diabetes on which to base the comparison
2. Teach factors that affect insulin requirements and signs of hyperglycemia (diabetic coma) and hypoglycemia (insulin reaction)
   a. Give family a written list explaining symptoms
   b. Emphasize that a simple or complex carbohydrate (candy containing sugar or milk) can be given if insulin reaction is suspected
   c. Emphasize the need for close medical supervision
3. Teach need for prevention of infection
   a. Good skin care, frequent baths
   b. Properly fitting shoes
   c. Prompt treatment of any small cut
   d. Protection from undue exposure to illness
4. Encourage a well-balanced diet based on the guidelines promoted by the Canadian Diabetic Association (CDA)
5. Help plan exercise, medication, and diet according to child's requirements and preferences

6. Teach parents and child how to do blood glucose and urine testing to increase independence
7. Teach parents and child how to administer insulin (by injection or pump)
   a. The child should be taught as early as motor and mental abilities allow, usually by 7 to 9 years of age
   b. Explanations should be simple; diagrams for rotating sites should be used
   c. Periodic observation by an adult should be routine to discover faulty or careless technique
8. Allow child to make choices when possible for sense of control
9. Teach parents and child the importance of preventing the use of tobacco products
10. See General Nursing Care of School-aged Children with Health Problems
11. See Meeting the Needs of the Family of an Infant or Child with Special Needs

D. EVALUATION/OUTCOMES

1. Child exhibits no signs of hypoglycemia
2. Child maintains blood glucose levels within acceptable range
3. Child demonstrates a positive self-image
4. Child consumes adequate calories for growth and development
5. Parents and child demonstrate ability to care for needs associated with diabetes
6. Child verbalizes being in control of therapeutic regimen

▼ HEMOPHILIA

Data Base

A. Defect in clotting mechanism of blood
B. Genetic disorder; X-linked recessive transmission
C. Usually occurs in males
D. Classification
   1. Factor VIII deficiency (classic hemophilia): hemophilia A
   2. Factor IX deficiency (Christmas disease): hemophilia B
E. Clinical findings
   1. Prolonged bleeding from any wound
   2. Bleeding into the joints (hemarthrosis), resulting in pain, deformity, and retarded growth
   3. Intracranial hemorrhage
   4. Severity of bleeding
      a. Mild
         (1) Factor VIII activity of 5% to 50%
         (2) Bleeding with severe trauma or surgery
      b. Moderate
         (1) Factor VIII activity of 1% to 5%
         (2) Bleeding with trauma

c. Severe
(1) Factor VIII activity of 1%
(2) Spontaneous bleeding without trauma
5. Anemia
F. Therapeutic interventions
1. Control of bleeding
2. Prevention of bleeding with use of factor replacement
a. Drugs that replace deficient coagulation factors
(1) Factor VIII concentrate from recombinant DNA (cryoprecipitate)
(2) Factor IX complex contains factors II, VII, IX, X (concentrated)
b. Adjunctive measures
(1) Aminocaproic acid (Amicar): inhibits the enzyme that destroys formed fibrin and increases fibrinogen activity in clot formation
(2) Fibrinogen: maintains plasma fibrinogen levels required for clotting materials
(3) Thrombin: supplies physiologic levels of natural material at superficial bleeding sites to control bleeding

Nursing Care of Children with Hemophilia

A. DATA COLLECTION

1. Parent/child knowledge of disease process and injury prevention
2. Joint bleeding
3. Mobility of joints

B. ANALYSIS AND INTERPRETATION

1. Body image disturbance related to:
   a. Perception of self as different
   b. Inability to participate in selected activities
2. Altered family processes related to situational crisis (child with a chronic illness, fear of HIV)
3. Risk for infection related to frequent transfusions
4. Risk for injury (hemorrhage) related to deficient blood clotting
5. Knowledge deficit related to:
   a. Disease process
   b. Home management
   c. Activity limitations
6. Impaired mobility related to effects of hemorrhages into joints and other tissues
7. Pain related to bleeding into joints/tissues
8. See General Nursing Diagnoses for School-aged Children with Health Problems
9. See General Nursing Diagnoses for the Family of a Child with Special Needs

C. PLANNING/IMPLEMENTATION

1. Instruct the child and parents in the treatment of bleeding, especially of joints

a. Immobilization of the area
b. Compression of the area
c. Elevation of the body part
d. Application of cool compresses
2. Provide for appropriate activity that lessens the chance of trauma, which is often difficult because boys are so physically active
3. Select safe toys and inform parents to safe-proof house to minimize injuries; secure throw rugs
4. Avoid use of aspirin or ibuprofen
5. Control joint pain so the child uses extremities to prevent muscle atrophy
6. Provide counseling, because disease is genetic and parents need assistance
7. Encourage parents to treat the child as normally as possible, avoiding overprotection or overpermissiveness
8. See General Nursing Care of School-aged Children with Health Problems
9. See Meeting the Needs of the Family of an Infant or Child with Special Needs

D. EVALUATION/OUTCOMES

1. Child exhibits no sign of injury
2. Child reports minimal pain
3. Child maintains full range of motion of joints
4. Child/family demonstrates knowledge of disease process, home management, and activity limitations
5. Child participates in desired activities
6. Family and child have positive interactions

▼ RHEUMATIC FEVER

Data Base

A. Collagen disease: characterized by damage to connective tissue and usually blood vessels
B. Classification
1. Autoimmune reaction to group A, ß-hemolytic streptococcal pharyngitis
2. Self-limited; involves joints, skin, brain, and heart
C. Clinical findings
1. Heart: mitral and aortic stenosis may occur
2. Joints: edema, inflammations, and effusion, especially in knees, elbows, hips, shoulders, and wrists
3. Skin: erythematous macule with a clear center and wavy demarcated border usually on trunk and proximal extremities
4. Neurologic: chorea
5. Low-grade fever, epistaxis, abdominal pain, arthralgia, weakness, fatigue, pallor, anorexia, and weight loss
D. Therapeutic interventions
1. Antibiotic therapy to eradicate organism and prevent recurrence

2. Prevention of permanent cardiac damage
3. Palliation of other symptoms

Nursing Care of Children with Rheumatic Fever

A. DATA COLLECTION

1. Child/parent compliance with drug regimen
2. Symptom development
3. Nutritional intake
4. Activity level

B. ANALYSIS AND INTERPRETATION

1. Activity intolerance related to decreased cardiac output
2. Decreased cardiac output related to disease process
3. Fatigue related to decreased cardiac output
4. Risk for injury related to autoimmune response
5. Altered nutrition: less than body requirements related to:
   a. Anorexia
   b. Fatigue
6. Pain related to inflammation of joints
7. Risk for impaired skin integrity related to disease process
8. Impaired physical mobility related to joint pain
9. See General Nursing Diagnoses for School-aged Children with Health Problems
10. See General Nursing Diagnoses for the Family of a Child with Special Needs

C. PLANNING/IMPLEMENTATION

1. Encourage bed rest to reduce workload of the heart
2. Encourage child to do schoolwork and keep up with class
3. Stimulate the development of quiet hobbies and collections
4. Gradually increase activities over a period of weeks to months
5. Handle painful joints carefully
6. Maintain proper body alignment to prevent deformities
7. Monitor need for pain medication and administer when necessary
8. Encourage an increased intake of nutritious fluids
9. Provide small, frequent, nutritious meals
10. Emphasize abilities rather than limitations
11. Maintain child's status in home and school by keeping channels of communication open during illness
12. Help parents with home problems that may have served as predisposing factors
13. See General Nursing Care of School-aged Children with Health Problems
14. See Meeting the Needs of the Family of an Infant or Child with Special Needs

D. EVALUATION/OUTCOMES

1. Child does not exhibit cardiac damage
2. Cardiac output remains within normal limits
3. Child consumes adequate calories for growth
4. Child's skin remains intact
5. Child does not exhibit decreased mobility
6. Child reports minimal pain
7. Child has sufficient energy for desired activities
8. Child participates in desired activities

▼ JUVENILE RHEUMATOID ARTHRITIS

Data Base

A. Inflammatory disease of unknown cause
B. Slight tendency to run in families
C. Two peak ages of onset: 2 to 5 and 9 to 11 years of age
D. Females affected somewhat more frequently than males
E. Classification
   1. Systemic onset
   2. Monoarticular or pauciarticular: involves a few joints; usually less than five
   3. Polyarticular: simultaneous involvement of four or more joints
F. Clinical findings
   1. Joint enlargement
      a. Stiffness, pain, and limited motion, especially in morning on awakening
      b. Spindle-fingers: thick proximal joint with slender tip
   2. Low-grade fever
   3. Erythematous rash on the trunk and extremities
   4. Weight loss, fatigue, weakness
   5. Tachycardia
   6. Enlargement of the spleen, liver, and lymph nodes
G. Therapeutic interventions
   1. Medications
      a. Nonsteroidal antiinflammatory drugs (NSAIDs)
         (1) Fever reduction in hours
         (2) Pain reduction in days, weeks
         (3) Antiinflammatory effects in 30 to 37 days
      b. Corticosteroids and aspirin
      c. Cytotoxic drugs: reserved for clients with severe debilitating disease unresponsive to NSAIDs and corticosteroids
         (1) Cyclophosphamide (Cytoxan)
         (2) Azathioprine (Imuran)
         (3) Chlorambucil (Leukeran)
         (4) Methotrexate
   2. Physical therapy

Nursing Care of Children with Juvenile Rheumatoid Arthritis

A. DATA COLLECTION

1. Physical health
2. Status of involved joints
3. Physical restrictions
4. Pain
5. Child's response to disease process

B. ANALYSIS AND INTERPRETATION

1. Body image disturbance related to:
   a. Perception of self as different
   b. Inability to participate in selected activities
2. Altered family processes related to having a child with a chronic illness
3. Pain related to joint inflammation
4. Impaired physical mobility related to discomfort
5. Feeding, bathing/hygiene, dressing/grooming, toileting self-care deficit related to:
   a. Pain
   b. Musculoskeletal impairment
6. See General Nursing Diagnoses for School-aged Children with Health Problems
7. See General Nursing Diagnoses for the Family of a Child with Special Needs

C. PLANNING/IMPLEMENTATION

1. Emphasize that medication must be taken regularly, even in periods of remission, to decrease inflammation and pain
2. Promote proper body alignment and provide passive range of motion
3. Encourage a warm bath in the morning to decrease stiffness and increase mobility
4. Encourage exercises such as swimming
5. Encourage parents to accept the child's illness but to limit the use of the disease to foster dependency or control relationships
6. Teach the family why aspirin is given in large dosages
7. Encourage use of enteric-coated aspirin if there is GI irritability
8. Observe for signs of aspirin toxicity as demonstrated by tinnitus, vertigo, nausea, vomiting, sweating, and other signs of salicylate poisoning
9. See General Nursing Care of School-aged Children with Health Problems
10. See Meeting the Needs of the Family of an Infant or Child with Special Needs

D. EVALUATION/OUTCOMES

1. Child is able to move with minimum discomfort
2. Child engages in activities suitable to interests, capabilities, and development
3. Family demonstrates appropriate care for child
4. Child is involved in self-care to maximum capabilities
5. Child verbalizes positive body image

SKIN INFECTIONS

▼ PEDICULOSIS (LICE)

Data Base

A. Highly infectious infestation of head, body, or pubic hair
B. Nits (grayish-white, oval eggs) attach to hair
C. Severe itching may lead to secondary infection
D. Treatment: special shampoo, use of a fine-toothed comb to remove nits, teach child/parents not to share head gear or brushes/combs
E. Watch for allergies to treatments or toxicity

▼ SCABIES

Data Base

A. Produced by itch mite
B. Female burrows under the skin to lay eggs (usually in folds of skin)
C. Intensely pruritic: scratching can lead to secondary infection with the development of papules and vesicles
D. Treatment: all members of the family must be treated, since it is highly contagious
   1. Must wear clean clothes
   2. Must wash with sulfur or other special soap

▼ RINGWORM (FUNGAL DISEASE)

Data Base

A. Scalp (tinea capitis)
   1. Reddened, oval or round areas of alopecia
   2. Treated topically or orally with an antifungal drug
   3. Head should be covered to prevent spread of infection
B. Feet (athlete's foot, tinea pedis)
   1. Scaly fissures between toes, vesicles on sides of feet, pruritus
   2. Particularly common in summer; contracted in swimming areas and gymnasium locker rooms
   3 Treated by application of topical antifungal agents, encouraging the use of cotton socks or bare feet

▼ INTERTRIGO

Data Base

A. Excoriation of any adjacent body surfaces
B. Caused by moisture and chafing that can complicate to involve a fungal infection
C. Teach parents the specifics of treatment
   1. Area to be kept clean and dry

2. Avoid the use of rubber or plastic pants
3. Change disposable or cloth diapers as soon as they are wet
4. Avoid the use of cornstarch as it provides a medium for microorganisms
5. Attempt to expose the diaper area to air as often as possible
6. Use topical antifungal medications as prescribed, often alternating with low-potency topical steroids to treat inflammation

---

▼ IMPETIGO

Data Base

A. Bacterial infection of skin by streptococci or staphylococci
B. Highly contagious; other areas of body frequently become infected
C. Treatment: antibiotics systemically and locally; isolate child; keep from scratching other areas of the body

Nursing Care of Children with Skin Infections

A. DATA COLLECTION

1. Type of skin lesion
2. Pain
3. Parental knowledge of cause/treatment

B. ANALYSIS AND INTERPRETATION

1. Body image disturbance related to perceived appearance
2. Altered family processes related to situational crisis (child with a skin disorder)
3. Infection related to impairment of skin integrity
4. Pain related to skin lesions
5. Impaired skin integrity related to:
   a. Somatic factors
   b. Environmental agents
6. Risk for impaired skin integrity related to:
   a. Mechanical trauma
   b. Depressed defense mechanisms
7. Sleep pattern disturbance related to discomfort from skin lesions
8. Social isolation related to self-concept disturbance
9. See General Nursing Diagnoses for School-aged Children with Health Problems

C. PLANNING/IMPLEMENTATION

1. Keep nails short to prevent injury from scratching
2. Administer medications to limit pruritus
3. Encourage daily bathing with tepid water; dry thoroughly
4. Prevent spread of infection to other members of the family
   a. Prevent direct contact between children

b. Keep oozing lesions covered
c. Prevent athlete's foot; do not walk barefooted; dry feet carefully; wear lightweight shoes to decrease heat; disinfect shoes and socks
5. Teach proper hair care
6. Encourage frequent bathing and change of clothes
7. Encourage completion of the full regimen of antimicrobial medication
8. Avoid use of strong alkalis such as bleach in clothes washing, double-rinse diapers
9. Keep area clean and dry, rinse wastes from skin
10. Expose area to light and air
11. Apply bland ointment at night
12. Encourage screening in schools to identify the source of infection
13. See General Nursing Care of School-aged Children with Health Problems

D. EVALUATION/OUTCOMES

1. Child does not exhibit signs of discomfort
2. Family demonstrates appropriate skills to care for child
3. Infection is confined to primary site
4. Child verbalizes feelings and concerns
5. Skin lesions are confined to primary sites
6. Child avoids causative agents
7. Child is sufficiently rested for daily activities
8. Child maintains customary activities and relationships

▼ REYE SYNDROME

Data Base

A. Acute toxic encephalopathy associated with characteristic organ involvement
B. Fever, profoundly impaired consciousness, disordered hepatic function
C. Usually follows viral illness, influenza, or varicella
D. Associated with aspirin administration
E. A 91% decline in occurrence in children less than 5 years of age because of reduced use of aspirin
F. A 75% decline in occurrence in children over 5 years of age
G. Classification
   1. Stage I: Vomiting, lethargy, drowsiness
   2. Stage II: Disorientation, delirium, aggressiveness and combativeness, central neurologic hyperventilation (or sometimes shallow breathing), hyperactive reflexes, and stupor
   3. Stage III: Obtundity, coma, hyperventilation, cerebral decortication
   4. Stage IV: Deepening coma; decerebrate rigidity; loss of ocular reflexes; large, fixed pupils; divergent eye movements

5. Stage V: Seizures, loss of deep tendon reflexes, flaccidity, respiratory arrest

H. Clinical findings
  1. Prodromal symptoms
    a. Malaise
    b. Cough
    c. Rhinorrhea
    d. Sore throat
  2. Worsening cerebral signs as seen in the clinical stages

I. Therapeutic interventions
  1. Early diagnosis with aggressive therapy
  2. Treatment: determined by the clinical stage of the disease
    a. Stage I treatment is primarily supportive and directed toward restoring blood sugar levels, controlling cerebral edema, correcting acid-base imbalances, and eliminating factors known to increase intracranial pressure
    b. Stages II through V require invasive support, intracranial pressure monitoring, and tracheal intubation with controlled ventilation; a radical approach is curarization and sedation

Nursing Care of Children with Reye Syndrome

A. DATA COLLECTION
  1. Monitoring of vital signs; neurologic status
  2. Fluid volume
  3. Level of consciousness
  4. Signs of impaired coagulation (related to hepatic dysfunction)

B. ANALYSIS AND INTERPRETATION
  1. Risk for aspiration related to:
    a. Vomiting
    b. Decreased level of consciousness
  2. Altered breathing pattern related to increased intracranial pressure
  3. Altered family processes related to situational crisis (acute illness of child)
  4. Fear (parental) related to sudden critical nature of illness
  5. Risk for fluid volume deficit related to intractable vomiting
  6. Risk for injury related to:
    a. Disorientation
    b. Delirium
    c. Impaired coagulation
  7. Parental role conflict related to sudden illness of child
  8. See General Nursing Diagnoses for School-aged Children with Health Problems

C. PLANNING/IMPLEMENTATION
  1. Assess vital signs and neurologic status continuously
  2. Assist with numerous invasive procedures

  3. Explain all therapies to the child (if alert) and parents
  4. Monitor intake and output and invasive equipment (intracranial line, hemodynamic monitoring)
  5. Keep parents informed of child's progress
  6. Include parents in child's care whenever possible
  7. Support the family, who will be frightened by the sudden and critical nature of the illness
  8. Foster dissemination of information concerning the role of aspirin in relation to viral disease and the development of Reye syndrome
  9. See General Nursing Care of School-aged Children with Health Problems

D. EVALUATION/OUTCOMES
  1. Parents can verbalize questions and concerns about child's status
  2. Child does not aspirate
  3. Child exhibits no sign of physical injury
  4. Child maintains fluid balance
  5. Child's breathing pattern returns to baseline
  6. Parents interact appropriately with child
  7. Parents participate in care of child

▼ LEGG-CALVÉ-PERTHES DISEASE (COXA PLANA)

Data Base

A. A disturbance of circulation to the femoral capital epiphysis producing an ischemic aseptic necrosis of the femoral head, epiphysis, and acetabulum

B. Cause unknown

C. Classification
  1. Age range: 3 to 12 years of age
    a. Most common in males 4 to 8 years of age
    b. More common in Caucasians
  2. In 10% to 15% of incidences, both hips are involved
  3. Most children have skeletal ages below chronologic age

D. Clinical findings
  1. Insidious onset
  2. Persistent pain in the affected hip(s)
  3. Limitation of movement in the affected hip(s)
  4. Limp

E. Therapeutic interventions
  1. Aim is to keep the head of the femur in the acetabulum and maintain a full range of motion
  2. Conservative therapy must be continued for 2 to 4 years, whereas surgical correction returns the child to normal activities in 3 to 4 months
  3. Use of non–weight-bearing devices such as an abduction brace, leg casts, or a leather harness sling that prevents weight bearing on the affected limb

4. Use of abduction-ambulation braces or casts after a period of bed rest and traction
5. Surgical reconstructive and containment procedures

Nursing Care of Children with Legg-Calvé-Perthes Disease

A. DATA COLLECTION
1. Pain
2. Level of joint dysfunction
3. Parent/child knowledge of disease process/therapy

B. ANALYSIS AND INTERPRETATION
1. Body image disturbance related to:
   a. Perception of self as different
   b. Inability to participate in selected activities
2. Altered family processes related to situational crisis (child with a temporary but extensive disability)
3. Risk for injury related to:
   a. Musculoskeletal impairment
   b. Unaccustomed use of appliance
4. Impaired physical mobility related to:
   a. Pain
   b. Use of non–weight-bearing devices
5. See General Nursing Diagnoses for School-aged Children with Health Problems
6. See General Nursing Diagnoses for the Family of a Child with Special Needs

C. PLANNING/IMPLEMENTATION
1. Instruct the child and parents regarding what constitutes non–weight-bearing (e.g., no standing or kneeling on the affected leg)
2. Educate the child and parents regarding correct use of appliances
3. Assist the child and family in selecting activities according to the child's age, interests, and physical limitations
   a. Quiet games
   b. Hobbies such as collections, model building, crafts, indoor gardening
4. Encourage peer interaction
5. Involve the child in planning activities and therapy
6. Help the child determine alternatives to weight-bearing activity (e.g., scorekeeping, sideline "coach")
7. Help the child devise explanations for appliances and the inability to participate actively with peers
8. See General Nursing Care of School-aged Children with Health Problems
9. See Meeting the Needs of the Family of an Infant or Child with Special Needs

D. EVALUATION/OUTCOMES
1. Child does not exhibit signs of physical injury
2. Child reports minimal pain
3. Child is able to participate in activities with immobilizing device
4. Family demonstrates ability to care for child

▼ EMOTIONAL DISORDERS

For common emotional disorders of the school-aged child see Disorders Usually First Evident in Infancy, Childhood, or Adolescence in Mental Health/Psychiatric Nursing (Chapter 4)

THE ADOLESCENT

GROWTH AND DEVELOPMENT
Developmental Timetable
A. Physical growth: includes the physical changes associated with puberty such as secondary sexual characteristics
B. Pubertal growth spurt
   1. Females between 10 and 14
      a. Weight gain 7 to 25 kg, mean 17.5 kg
      b. Approximately 95% of mature height achieved by the onset of menarche or skeletal age of 13 years; height gain 5 to 25 cm, mean 20.5 cm
   2. Males between 12 and 16 years
      a. Weight gain 7 to 30 kg, mean 23.7 kg
      b. Approximately 95% of mature height achieved by skeletal age of 15 years; height gain 10 to 30 cm, mean 27.5 cm
C. Mental abilities
   1. Abstract thinking
      a. New level of social communication and understanding
         (1) Can comprehend satire and double meanings
         (2) Can say one thing and mean another
      b. Can conceptualize thought; more interested in exploring ideas than facts
      c. Can appreciate scientific thinking, problem solve, and theoretically explore alternatives
   2. Perception
      a. Can appreciate nonrepresentational art
      b. Can understand that the whole is more than the sum of its parts
   3. Learning
      a. Much longer span of attention
      b. Learns through inference, intuition, and surmise, rather than repetition and imitation
      c. Enjoys regressing in terms of language development by using jargon to suit changing moods

D. Social patterns
1. Peer-group identity
   a. One of the strongest motivating forces of behavior
   b. Extremely important to be part of the group and like everyone else in every way
   c. Clique formation; usually based on common denominators such as social class, ethnic group, or special interests
2. Personal development
   a. Major goal is development of a self-identity
   b. Adolescents may develop crushes and worship many idols
   c. Time of sexual exploration and questioning of one's sexual role
3. Independence
   a. By 15 or 16 years of age, adolescents feel they should be treated as adults
   b. Ambivalence: adolescent wants freedom but is not happy about corresponding responsibilities and frequently yearns for more carefree days of childhood
   c. Parental ambivalence and discipline problems are common as parents try to allow for increasing independence but continue to offer constructive guidance and enforce discipline

HEALTH PROMOTION DURING ADOLESCENCE

Adolescent Nutrition

A. Nutritional objectives
1. Provide optimum nutritional support for demands of rapid growth and high energy expenditure
2. Support development of good eating habits through variety of foods, regular pattern, good quality snacks (high in protein; low in refined carbohydrate, primarily sugar)
B. Nutrient needs increased in all respects, so adequate intake of all nutrients should form basis of diet
C. Possible nutritional problems
1. Low intakes of calcium, vitamin A and C, iron in girls
2. Anemia: increase foods containing iron
3. Obesity or underweight: decrease or increase calories as needed
4. Nutritional deficiencies related to:
   a. Psychologic factors: food aversions, emotional problems
   b. Fear of overweight: crash diets, mainly in girls; cultural pressure
   c. Fad diets: caused by misinformation; need for sound counseling
   d. Poor choice of snack foods: usually high in sugar; use more fruit and protein forms

   e. Irregular eating pattern
5. Additional stress of pregnancy: need high protein and calorie intake
D. Nutrition education may be made through association with teenagers' concerns about physical appearance, figure control, complexion, physical fitness, athletic ability

Injury Prevention

A. Appropriate education regarding sexual maturity, reproduction, and sexual behavior
B. Driver education
C. Education regarding use and abuse of drugs, especially alcohol
D. Education on health hazards associated with smoking

Areas Needing Health Guidance During Adolescence

A. Accidents: leading cause of death, with motor vehicle accidents causing the most fatalities
B. Homicide and suicide: next two causes of death among this age group
C. Drug abuse
D. Delinquency
E. Alcoholism
F. Pregnancy
G. Obesity
H. Acne
I. Anorexia nervosa and bulimia nervosa
J. Orthopedic problems
K. Cancer

HEALTH PROBLEMS MOST COMMON IN ADOLESCENTS

Hospitalization

A. Reaction of the adolescent
1. Increased need for privacy, sense of control, and independence
2. Increased concern for mutilation, disfigurement, and loss of function; needs to be like peers; body image important
3. Concerned about separation from peers and possible loss of status in group
B. Parents and medical/nursing team can help prepare the adolescent for hospitalization by providing full explanations and answering questions completely and honestly

GENERAL NURSING DIAGNOSES FOR ADOLESCENTS WITH HEALTH PROBLEMS

A. Anxiety related to:
1. Strange environment
2. Perception of impending event (specify)

3. Separation from family/peer group
4. Anticipated discomfort
5. Knowledge deficit
6. Feelings of powerlessness

B. Risk for aspiration related to:
   1. Disease process
   2. Impaired swallowing

C. Body image disturbance related to:
   1. Change in body characteristics
   2. Perceived developmental imperfections

D. Family coping: potential for growth related to:
   1. Successful parenting
   2. Resolution of situational crisis

E. Ineffective family coping: compromised, related to situational crisis

F. Ineffective individual coping related to situational crisis

G. Diversional activity deficit related to:
   1. Frequent or prolonged hospitalization
   2. Separation from peer group

H. Altered family processes related to:
   1. Situational crisis
   2. Knowledge deficit
   3. Temporary family disorganization
   4. Inadequate support system

I. Fear related to:
   1. Separation from support system
   2. Uncertain prognosis
   3. Body-image disturbance

J. Anticipatory grieving related to expected loss of life or limb or severity of illness

K. Impaired home maintenance management related to:
   1. Knowledge deficit
   2. Inadequate support system

L. Risk for injury related to:
   1. Use of specific therapies and appliances
   2. Incapacity for self-protection
   3. Immobility

M. Knowledge deficit related to new medical regimen

N. Risk for noncompliance with therapy and health teaching related to:
   1. Perceived invulnerability
   2. Denial of illness
   3. Desire not to be different from peers

O. Pain related to:
   1. Disease process
   2. Interventions

P. Parental role conflict related to:
   1. Ill child
   2. Inability to care for child

Q. Altered parenting related to:
   1. Separation
   2. Skill deficit
   3. Family stress

R. Risk for impaired skin integrity related to radiotherapy

S. Sleep pattern disturbance related to:
   1. Frequent assessment
   2. Therapies

T. Spiritual distress related to:
   1. Inadequate support system
   2. Decisions regarding life or death conflicts

U. See General Nursing Diagnoses for Adolescents with Health Problems

V. See General Nursing Diagnoses for the Family of a Child with Special Needs

GENERAL NURSING CARE OF ADOLESCENTS WITH HEALTH PROBLEMS

A. Involve the adolescent in planning care
B. Answer questions honestly and directly
C. Be as open as possible concerning feelings, care, and prognosis
D. Foster independence as much as possible
E. Provide for contact with peers
F. Encourage compliance with health program
G. Arrange for continuity in schoolwork
H. Recognize that problems of adolescence are magnified by an illness during this period of development
I. Encourage involvement of positive support systems
J. Accept the adolescent's self-appraisal but point out reality
K. Encourage use of clothing or makeup to minimize perceived shortcomings
L. See Meeting the Needs of the Family of an Infant or Child with Special Needs
M. See Nursing Care under specific diseases in this chapter, Childbearing and Woman's Health Nursing (Chapter 3), Mental Health/Psychiatric Nursing (Chapter 4), and Medical-Surgical Nursing (Chapter 6)

▼ SCOLIOSIS

Data Base

A. Lateral curvature of the spine usually associated with a rotary deformity that eventually causes cosmetic and physiologic alterations in the spine, chest, and pelvis

B. Cause in 70% of cases is "idiopathic"; probably transmitted as an autosomal dominant trait with incomplete penetrance

C. Most common spinal deformity

D. More frequent in adolescent girls during growth spurt

E. Classification
   1. Nonstructural scoliosis: curve is flexible and corrects by bending

2. Structural scoliosis: curve fails to straighten on side-bending: characterized by changes in the spine and its supporting structures

F. Clinical findings

1. Prominence of one hip
2. Deformity of the rib cage
3. Prominence of one scapula
4. Difference in shoulder or scapular height
5. Curve in the vertebral spinous process alignment
6. Breasts appear unequal in size
7. Other clues
   a. Clothes do not fit right
   b. Skirt hems are uneven

G. Therapeutic interventions

1. Screening for scoliosis
2. Diagnosis: confirmed by x-ray examination
3. Interventions depend on severity of the curvature
   a. Exercise can be used in nonstructural scoliosis
   b. Mild to moderate curvature
      (1) Braces
         (a) Milwaukee brace, an individually adapted steel and leather brace that extends from a chin cup and neck pads to the pelvis, where lumbar pads rest on the hips
         (b) Low profile or underarm brace
      (2) Treatment
         (a) Worn 23 hours a day
         (b) The child is gradually weaned from the brace over a 1- to 2-year period
         (c) Brace then worn only at night until the spine is mature
         (d) Electrical stimulation to the convex side of the curvature may prevent progression of the scoliosis
   c. More severe curves usually require surgery: techniques consist of spinal realignment and straightening by way of external or internal fixation and instrumentation combined with bony fusion (arthrodesis) of the realigned spine
      (1) Harrington rods
      (2) Luque segmental instrumentation
      (3) Dwyer instrumentation
   d. Most severe scoliotic curvatures require traction devices and exercises for a time before spinal fusion to provide partial correction and more flexibility

Nursing Care of Adolescents with Scoliosis

A. DATA COLLECTION

1. Have the child stand erect, clothed only in underpants (and bra if older girl) and observe from behind; note asymmetry of the shoulders and hips
2. Have the child bend forward so the back is parallel with the floor; observe from the side, noting asymmetry or prominence of the rib

B. ANALYSIS AND INTERPRETATION

1. Body image disturbance related to:
   a. Perceived alteration in body structure
   b. Altered appearance when using supportive devices
2. Altered family processes related to situational crisis (child with a structural defect)
3. Altered growth and development related to disease process
4. Risk for injury related to use of supportive devices
5. Knowledge deficit related to disorder
6. Impaired physical mobility related to use of supportive devices
7. Risk for impaired skin integrity related to:
   a. Presence of brace
   b. Use of electrical stimulation
8. Pain related to medical/surgical therapies
9. See General Nursing Diagnoses for Adolescents with Health Problems
10. See General Nursing Diagnoses for the Family of a Child with Special Needs

C. PLANNING/IMPLEMENTATION

1. Check spinal alignment
2. Reinforce and clarify explanations provided by the orthopedist in regard to:
   a. Appliance
   b. Plan of care
   c. Activities allowed or restricted
   d. Child's and parents' responsibilities in therapy
3. Examine skin surfaces in contact with the brace or electrical stimulator for signs of irritation; implement corrective action to treat or prevent skin breakdown
4. Help in selection of the appropriate wearing apparel to wear over the brace to minimize altered appearance and footwear to maintain proper balance
5. Prepare for surgery if required
6. See General Nursing Care for Adolescents with Health Problems

D. EVALUATION/OUTCOMES

1. Family members demonstrate appropriate care and support of child
2. Child demonstrates proper use of brace
3. Parent/child verbalize understanding of disorder and treatment plan
4. Child verbalizes feelings and concerns
5. Skin does not break down
6. Child engages in activities appropriate to limitations and developmental level
7. Child reports minimal pain

▼ BONE TUMORS

Data Base

A. Less than 1% of all malignant neoplasms
B. More common in children than adults; peak ages 15 to 19 years
C. Classification
  1. Osteogenic sarcoma
    a. Most frequent bone tumor in children
    b. Primary tumor site: diaphysis (shaft) of a long bone, especially the femur
    c. Arises from osteoid tissue
  2. Ewing sarcoma
    a. Most frequent sites: shaft of the long and trunk bones, especially the femur, tibia, fibula, humerus, ulna, vertebra, scapula, ribs, pelvic bones, and skull
    b. Arises from medullary tissue (marrow)
D. Clinical findings
  1. Symptoms
    a. Localized pain in the affected site
    b. Limp
    c. Voluntary curtailment of activity
    d. Inability to hold heavy objects
    e. Weight loss
    f. Frequent infections
  2. Diagnosis
    a. X-ray examination
    b. Computerized tomography (bone)
    c. Bone scan
    d. Bone marrow aspiration
    e. Surgical biopsy (Ewing sarcoma)
E. Therapeutic interventions
  1. Osteogenic sarcoma: amputation of the affected bone followed by high-dose methotrexate or preoperative and postoperative use of chemotherapy with en bloc resection of the primary tumor followed by a prosthetic replacement
  2. Ewing sarcoma: intensive irradiation of the involved bone and chemotherapy

Nursing Care of Adolescents with Bone Tumors

A. DATA COLLECTION

1. Parent/child knowledge about disease process/therapy
2. Pain at affected site
3. Functional status of involved area
4. Inflammation, lymph nodes
5. Systemic involvement

B. ANALYSIS AND INTERPRETATION

1. Anxiety related to diagnosis and treatment
2. Body image disturbance related to altered physical appearance following amputation and other therapies
3. Ineffective individual coping related to medical/surgical interventions
4. Decisional conflict related to variety of treatment modalities
5. Altered family processes related to:
  a. Hospitalization
  b. Child with a life-threatening disease
6. Fear related to knowledge deficit (surgical/medical care)
7. Anticipatory grieving (adolescent) related to possible loss of limb
8. Anticipatory grieving (parental) related to perceived loss of child
9. Pain related to:
  a. Disease process
  b. Medical therapies
10. Impaired physical mobility related to amputated extremity
11. Social isolation related to:
  a. Disease process
  b. Body image
12. See General Nursing Diagnoses for Adolescents with Health Problems
13. See General Nursing Diagnoses for the Family of a Child with Special Needs

C. PLANNING/IMPLEMENTATION

1. Prepare the child and family for surgery
  a. Employ straightforward honesty
  b. Avoid disguising the diagnosis with terms such as "infection"
  c. Emphasize lack of alternatives if amputation is planned
  d. Answer questions regarding information presented by the surgeon and clarify any misconceptions
  e. Avoid overwhelming the child or parents with too much information
2. Prepare the child and family for radiotherapy (Ewing sarcoma)
  a. Explain the procedure
  b. Remain with the child during the procedure
  c. Explain the undesirable side effects of radiotherapy
  d. Suggest and/or implement measures to reduce the physical effects of radiotherapy, such as selecting loose-fitting clothing over the irradiated areas to decrease additional irritation, protection of the area from sunlight and sudden changes in temperature (avoid ice packs, heating pads)
3. Prepare the child and family for chemotherapy
  a. Impress on the child the importance of therapy
  b. Explain the probable side effects of antimetabolites (e.g., nausea, hair loss)
4. Assist the child in adjusting to his or her disability; focus on abilities
  a. Assist the child in becoming adept at using the appliances

b. Help the child select clothing to camouflage the prosthesis

c. Encourage good hygiene, grooming, and sex-appropriate items to enhance appearance, such as a wig (for hair loss from antimetabolites), makeup, attractive (sex-appropriate) clothing

d. Allow the child time and opportunity to go through the grief process

e. Allow for expression of feelings regarding the loss and the undesirable effects of chemotherapy

f. Help the child cope with the side effects of chemotherapy and irradiation

g. Allow dependence but encourage independence

5. Support the child and family

a. Allow for expression of feelings

b. Clarify misconceptions and provide technical information as needed

c. Impress upon both child and family the need for continuing normal activities, interactions, and behaviors

6. See General Nursing Care of Adolescents with Health Problems

7. See Meeting the Needs of the Family of an Infant or Child with Special Needs

D. EVALUATION/OUTCOMES

1. Parents and child demonstrate understanding of disease process

2. Parents and child demonstrate understanding of therapies and side effects

3. Family expresses feelings about the potential loss of child

4. Child readily discusses concerns and asks appropriate questions

5. Child and family adjust to loss of limb

6. Child resumes former contacts and activities commensurate with limitations

7. Child reports minimal pain

8. Child/family make appropriate decisions regarding care

9. Child/family demonstrate positive coping skills

▼ EMOTIONAL DISORDERS

For common emotional disorders of the adolescent see Disorders First Evident in Infancy, Childhood, or Adolescence in Mental Health/Psychiatric Nursing (Chapter 4)

▼ OTHER HEALTH PROBLEMS

Many problems of adolescence are similar to those of adults; see specific areas in Childbearing and Women's Health Nursing (Chapter 3) and Medical-Surgical Nursing (Chapter 6) for further discussion

PEDIATRIC NURSING
REVIEW QUESTIONS

Growth and Development

1. When teaching a mother how to prevent accidents while caring for her 6-month-old, the nurse should emphasize that at this age children can usually:
   1. Sit up
   2. Roll over
   3. Crawl lengthy distances
   4. Stand while holding onto furniture

2. In terms of preventive teaching for the parents of a 1-year-old, the nurse would speak to them about:
   1. Accidents
   2. Toilet training
   3. Adequate nutrition
   4. Sexual development

Client Case Scenario 1: Trevor is a 15-month-old who has a chronic renal disorder that has resulted in numerous prolonged hospitalizations. He has been diagnosed with maternal deprivation. **Items 3 to 6 refer to this client case scenario.**

3. Which of the following is a characteristic of maternal deprivation that Trevor most likely manifested?
   1. Extreme activity
   2. Susceptibility to illness
   3. Responsiveness to stimuli
   4. Tendency toward overeating

4. Which of the following is the major depriving factor in long-term hospitalization that Trevor has most likely experienced?
   1. Lack of play objects
   2. Lack of multisensory stimulation
   3. Care provided by a consistent caregiver
   4. Absence of interaction with the primary caregiver

5. In reference to maternal deprivation, which of the following responses should the nurse consider unusual in Trevor?
   1. Lack or slowness of weight gain
   2. Limited emotional response to stimuli
   3. Excessive crying and clinging when approached
   4. Looking at ceiling lights rather than at persons caring for him

6. Trevor's nurse should be aware that studies of children who have suffered prolonged maternal deprivation early in life demonstrate that these children have which of the following difficulties?
   1. Have difficulty trusting
   2. Recall past experiences vividly
   3. Are particularly conscious of time
   4. Establish warm relationships with a mother substitute

7. The primary task to be accomplished between 12 and 15 months of age is to learn to:
   1. Walk erect
   2. Use a cup
   3. Climb stairs
   4. Say simple words

8. A 15-month-old infant is playing in the playpen. The nurse observing the infant's activities evaluates the infant's ability with physical tasks to be at the age-related norm when the infant:
   1. Builds a tower of six blocks
   2. Walks across the playpen with ease
   3. Throws all the toys out of the playpen
   4. Stands in the playpen holding onto the sides

9. A father brings his 18-month-old son to the clinic. He asks the nurse why his son is so difficult to please, has temper tantrums, and annoys him by throwing food from the table. The nurse should explain that:
   1. Toddlers need to be disciplined at this stage to prevent the development of antisocial behaviors
   2. The child is learning to assert independence, and his behavior is considered normal for his age
   3. This is the usual way that a toddler expresses his needs during the initiative stage of development
   4. It is best to leave the child alone in his crib after calmly telling him why his behavior is unacceptable

Client Case Scenario 2: Rebecca, a 2-year-old, and her mother are consulting the community health nurse. **Items 10 to 13 refer to this client case scenario.**

10. The nurse observes Rebecca at play in the clinic. She realizes that at this age, Rebecca could be expected to exhibit which of the following?
    1. Builds houses with blocks
    2. Is extremely possessive of toys
    3. Attempts to stay within the lines when coloring
    4. Amuses herself with a picture book for 15 minutes

11. When observing Rebecca, the nurse would expect her to engage in which type of play?
    1. Parallel play
    2. Solitary play
    3. Competitive play
    4. Tumbling-type play

12. Rebecca's mother asks the nurse when it would be appropriate to take her to the dentist for dental prophylaxis. What is the nurse's most appropriate response?
    1. Before starting school
    2. Between 2 and 3 years of age
    3. When Rebecca begins to lose deciduous teeth
    4. The next time another family member goes to the dentist

13. Rebecca's mother says that Rebecca consistently says "no" every time she is offered fluids. Considering Rebecca's development, how could the nurse assist the mother to increase Rebecca's fluid intake?
    1. Distract her with some food
    2. Be firm and hand her the glass
    3. Offer her a choice of two things to drink
    4. Let Rebecca see that she is making her mother angry

---

14. A 2-year-old boy, admitted to the hospital for further surgical repair of a clubfoot, is standing in his crib crying. The child refuses to be comforted and calls for his mother. As the nurse approaches the crib the child screams louder. The nurse, recognizing that this behavior is typical of the stage of protest, decides to:
    1. Pick him up and carry him around the room
    2. Fill the basin with water and proceed to bathe him
    3. Sit by his crib and bathe him later when his anxiety decreases
    4. Skip the bath since a child this upset does not really need a bath

15. When evaluating a 3-year-old's developmental progress, the nurse should recognize that development is delayed when the child is unable to:
    1. Copy a square
    2. Hop on one foot
    3. Catch a ball reliably
    4. Use a spoon effectively

16. The nurse should attempt to involve a preschool-age child in therapeutic play to give the child the opportunity to:
    1. Meet other children on the unit
    2. Work out ways of coping with fears
    3. Learn to accept the hospital situation
    4. Forget the reality of the situation for a while

17. The nurse plans to talk to a mother about toilet training a toddler, knowing that the most important factor in the process of toilet training is the:
    1. Child's desire to be dry
    2. Ability of the child to sit still
    3. Parent's willingness to work at it
    4. Approach and attitude of the parent

18. A mother asks the nurse what to do when her toddler has temper tantrums. The nurse suggests that the mother allow the child another way of expressing anger such as by the use of a:
    1. Ball and bat
    2. Punching bag
    3. Pounding board
    4. Wad of clay or Play-Doh

19. A mother tells the nurse that the pediatrician has expressed concern that her 4-year-old child exhibits developmental delays. The mother expresses readiness to place her child in a preschool program for children with developmental disabilities. The nurse should:
    1. Praise the mother for her acceptance and encourage her plan
    2. Advise the mother to have the pediatrician help choose an appropriate program
    3. Ask the mother for more specific information related to the developmental delays
    4. Tell the mother that this is probably a premature action since developmental delays often disappear

20. The nurse should encourage two 6-year-old boys in the playroom to play with:
    1. Clay
    2. Checkers
    3. A board game
    4. An erector set

Client Case Scenario 3: Bradley is a preschool child who has been brought to the community health clinic for assessment. **Items 21 to 24 refer this client case scenario.**

21. Bradley is a preschool age child. The nurse tells Bradley's mother that he will likely role play as a part of socialization. Which rationale explains why?
   1. Role playing teaches children about stereotypes.
   2. Role playing encourages Bradley to express himself.
   3. This behavior helps Bradley to think about possible careers.
   4. This behavior provides Bradley with guidelines for adult behaviors.

22. Bradley is having difficulty relating with the other children in the play area. It is important for the nurse to realize which behavior is expected of this age group?
   1. Engaging in parallel or solitary play
   2. Being almost totally dependent on parents
   3. Exaggerating and boasting to impress others
   4. Having fierce temper tantrums and negativism

23. The nurse explains to Bradley's mother that at this age, children have a fear of which of the following?
   1. Pain
   2. Death
   3. Isolation
   4. Intrusive procedures

24. The nurse explains to Bradley's mother that as he is a preschool aged child, he is not yet capable of accomplishing which of the following?
   1. Tying shoelaces
   2. Abstract thought
   3. Making decisions
   4. Hand-eye coordination

25. A 9-year-old who is in bed convalescing becomes very bored and irritable. The nurse plans activities that a school-age child would like and suggests the child:
   1. Play chess
   2. Start a collection
   3. Do arithmetic puzzles
   4. Watch game shows on TV

26. Postoperatively, to help relieve the anxiety of a young school-age child, the nurse should:
   1. Allow the child time to talk about feelings
   2. Tell a story about a child with similar surgery
   3. Ask the mother to room with the child for a few days
   4. Provide the child with bandages, tape, and a doll

27. An 11-year-old young male has gained weight. His mother is concerned that her son, who loves sports, may become obese. The nurse:
   1. Advises an increase in activity
   2. Urges a decreased caloric intake
   3. Explains this is normal for a preadolescent
   4. Discusses the relationship of genetics and weight gain

Emotional Needs Related to Health Problems

28. To help parents cope with the behavior of young school-aged children, the nurse suggests that it could help if they would:
   1. Avoid asking specific questions
   2. Write a list of expectations to avoid confusion
   3. Be consistent and firm about established rules
   4. Allow the child to set up his or her own routines

29. Prior to administering a well-tolerated gastrostomy tube feeding to an infant, which of the following nursing actions would be most appropriate when considering the infant's needs?
   1. Irrigate the tube
   2. Slowly instill 5 ml of water
   3. Provide the baby with a pacifier
   4. Place the infant in a low Fowler's position

30. Which of the following nursing actions would be most appropriate in considering the needs of a 13 year old who has been diagnosed with insulin dependent diabetes mellitus?
   1. Reinforce the need to act responsibly
   2. Discourage independent decision-making
   3. Assure the child his activities need not change
   4. Encourage parental involvement in management of care

31. Prior to surgery to relieve an intestinal obstruction, a 3-month-old is kept NPO and has a nasogastric tube in place. To calm, as well as meet the infant's developmental needs best, the nurse should:
   1. Allow the infant to suck on a pacifier
   2. Allow the infant to hold onto a favorite toy
   3. Hang a brightly colored mobile in the infant's crib
   4. Place the infant on the abdomen and permit crawling

Client Case Scenario 4: Casey is a 6-year-old who has been admitted with suspected child abuse. **Items 32 to 34 refer to this client case scenario.**

32. Casey begins to suck his thumb on admission. His social worker says this is unusual behavior for him. Which should the nurse do about this behavior?
    1. Accept the thumb-sucking
    2. Distract him by playing checkers
    3. Report this behavior to the physician
    4. Tell him thumb-sucking causes buckteeth

33. Casey's nurse is aware that the best legal definition of assault is which of the following?
    1. Threats to do bodily harm to the person of another person
    2. The application of physical force to another person without lawful justification
    3. A legal wrong committed by one person against the property of another person
    4. A legal wrong committed against the public and punishable by law through the courts

34. It is also important for Casey's nurse to understand the legal definition of battery. Which statement defines battery?
    1. A legal wrong committed by one person against the property of another
    2. Maligning the character of an individual while threatening to do bodily harm
    3. The application of force to the person of another person without lawful justification
    4. Doing something that a reasonable person with the same education or preparation would not do

35. During the second week of hospitalization, a 2-year-old girl does not express interest in her mother when she visits, but readily goes to all of the nurses. Which statement best explains this situation? The child:
    1. Has established a routine and feels safe
    2. Is repressing her feelings for her mother
    3. Has given up fighting and accepts the separation
    4. Feels better physically so her behavior has improved

Client Case Scenario 5: Richard is a toddler who has been admitted to hospital for a series of investigations. He has extensive eczema of his face and arms. **Items 36 to 38 refer to this client case scenario.**

36. Richard has scratched his eczema, despite the nurse's requests to stop scratching, to the point

where he is bleeding. The nurse restrains his arms to the sides of the crib, saying "Now you're tied so you won't be able to scratch anymore." Which explanation best describes this nurse's action?
    1. The nurse has merely done the job with considerable accountability.
    2. The nurse has used actions that can be interpreted as assault and battery.
    3. Richard's skin had to be protected, and the nurse acted in a prudent manner.
    4. Richard was told not to scratch and the nurse had rightly expected him to understand and cooperate.

37. Richard is to have a painful procedure performed. Richard's parents ask if they can stay with him for the procedure. The nurse should assess their attendance based on which of the following?
    1. The type of procedure to be performed
    2. An individual assessment of the parents
    3. Attendance should be permitted if the child desires their presence
    4. An understanding that attendance is of no benefit to the child or parents

38. When Richard's parents go home for the night, he screams loudly and is inconsolable. The nurse puts his crib in a storeroom and closes the door until he stops crying 30 to 45 minutes later. Which statement best describes this situation?
    1. Richard needed to have limits set to control the crying
    2. Richard had a right to remain in the room with the other children
    3. Keeping Richard segregated alone for more than 30 minutes was too long
    4. The other children had to be considered, so Richard needed to be removed

39. Which of the following fears are typical of a 5-year-old child?
    1. Fear of separation
    2. Fear of bodily harm
    3. Belief in death's finality
    4. Belief in the supernatural

40. When the nurse brings a dinner tray to a 4-year-old girl with pneumonia, the child says, "I'm too sick to feed myself." The nurse should respond:
    1. "Let it go until you feel better."
    2. "Try to eat as much as you can."
    3. "Wait 5 minutes and I will help you."
    4. "Be a big girl and don't act like a baby."

41. A hospitalized 5-year-old is apathetic about eating. Which of the following nursing actions would most likely increase the child's interest in eating?
    1. Asking the parents to visit at mealtime
    2. Giving only the foods the child likes best
    3. Providing diversional activity at mealtime
    4. Eliminating all between-meal nourishment

42. A 14-year-old is severely hurt while on a skateboard and develops muscle contractures in all the limbs. The adolescent refuses to move, so the nurse should encourage movement by:
    1. Allowing friends to visit every day
    2. Explaining that some pain is inevitable
    3. Setting strict limits to increase the adolescent's security
    4. Permitting the adolescent to make decisions regarding care

Respiratory

Client Case Scenario 6: Sally is a 2-year-old who has a barky cough, and has been diagnosed with laryngotrachealbronchitis (croup). **Items 43 to 46 refer to this client case scenario.**

43. Which nursing action would be most important when preparing for Sally's admission?
    1. Arrange for a quiet room
    2. Pad the side rails of her croup tent
    3. Set up a cot so that a parent can stay
    4. Obtain a tracheostomy set for the bedside

44. Which would be the highest priority nursing action when caring for Sally?
    1. Initiate measures to reduce fever
    2. Constantly assess respiratory status
    3. Provide support to reduce apprehension
    4. Ensure delivery of 40% humidified oxygen

45. Today is Sally's third day of hospitalization. She had been inconsolably crying and screaming, but now she is lying quietly in her croup tent. Which of the following stages of separation is Sally most likely exhibiting?
    1. Denial
    2. Despair
    3. Mistrust
    4. Rejection

46. Sally is well and is to be discharged. Her mother asks the nurse why Sally persists in saying "no" to everything. The nurse explains to Sally's mother that this negativism is helping Sally to meet a two-year-old's need for which of the following?
    1. Trust
    2. Attention
    3. Discipline
    4. Independence

Client Case Scenario 7: Jason is a 6-year-old boy who has been admitted with pneumonia. **Items 47 to 50 refer to this client case scenario.**

47. Which criterion is the physician most likely to use to select the drugs to be used for Jason's pneumonia?
    1. Jason's toleration of the drug
    2. Selectivity of the causative organism
    3. Sensitivity of the causative organism
    4. Jason's physician's preference for the drug

48. Which of the following would be of immediate priority in Jason's nursing care?
    1. Rest
    2. Exercise
    3. Nutrition
    4. Elimination

49. Jason is anxious about his hospitalization. Which of the following nursing actions would be most likely to assist Jason?
    1. Read Jason a story
    2. Give Jason a jigsaw puzzle
    3. Put Jason in a room by himself
    4. Give Jason a toy car to play with

50. When Jason's dinner tray arrives, he tells the nurse "I want you to feed me." Which of the following should the nurse recognize this statement to reflect?
    1. Anorexia
    2. Regression
    3. Immaturity
    4. Temper tantrum

51. A mother talks to the nurse about her sick infant, and she is disturbed because she did not realize the baby was ill. A major indication of illness in an infant is:
    1. Profuse perspiration
    2. Longer periods of sleep
    3. Grunting and rapid respirations
    4. Desire for increased fluids during the feedings

52. The nurse teaching a mothers' class tells them that the best way to position their infants during the first couple of weeks of life is to lay them on their:
    1. Backs with their heads flat
    2. Right or left sides with their heads flat
    3. Backs with their heads slightly elevated
    4. Stomachs with their heads slightly elevated

53. A 7-year-old is admitted for surgery. Preoperatively it is essential that the nurse:
    1. Observe the child's ASO titer
    2. Provide the child with a favorite toy
    3. Check for loose teeth and report the findings to the physician
    4. Encourage a parent to stay until the child goes to the operating room

54. A distressed toddler is admitted to the hospital because of sudden hoarseness and continuous, somewhat unintelligible speech. In talking with the mother, the nurse will be particularly concerned about:
    1. Retropharyngeal abscess
    2. Acute respiratory tract infection
    3. Undetected laryngeal abnormality
    4. Respiratory tract obstruction due to a foreign body

55. A newborn is admitted to the intensive care nursery with the diagnosis of choanal atresia. The nurse is aware that choanal atresia is an anomaly located in the:
    1. Anal area
    2. Nasopharynx
    3. Intestinal tract
    4. Pharynx and larynx

56. An infant is in the pediatric recovery room after open heart surgery for the repair of a ventricular septal defect. A nursing priority should be to:
    1. Monitor the infant's urinary output
    2. Assess the infant's pulmonary status
    3. Determine the status of the operative site
    4. Check the patency of the intravenous catheter

Client Case Scenario 8: Amanda is a 6-month-old infant who has cystic fibrosis. **Items 57 to 60 refer to this client case scenario.**

57. Which of the following initial presentations were likely noticed by Amanda's nurse in the newborn nursery?
    1. Excessive crying
    2. Sternal retractions
    3. Increased heart rate
    4. Abdominal distention

58. Amanda has a predisposition to bronchitis. Which statement best explains this predisposition?
    1. Neuromuscular irritability that causes spasm and constriction of the bronchi
    2. Increased salt content in saliva that can irritate and necrose mucous membranes in nasopharynx

3. The associated heart defects of cystic fibrosis that cause congestive heart failure and respiratory depression
    4. Tenacious secretions that obstruct the bronchioles and respiratory tract and provide a favorable medium for growth of bacteria.

59. Amanda is to have chest physiotherapy done every 4 hours. When is the best time to schedule her treatments?
    1. After every feeding
    2. Before every feeding
    3. During every feeding
    4. Midway between every feeding

60. Which of the following combinations of medications are essential to Amanda's treatment?
    1. A steroid and an antimetabolite
    2. Pancreatic enzymes and antibiotics
    3. Aerosol mists, decongestants, and fat-soluble vitamins
    4. Antibiotics, a multivitamin preparation, and cough drops

---

Client Case Scenario 9: James Linetz, the father of three young children, is diagnosed as having tuberculosis, but is asymptomatic. **Items 61 to 63 refer to this client case scenario.**

61. Which of the following will be used to treat members of James's family who react positively to the tuberculin test?
    1. BCG vaccine
    2. INH and PAS
    3. Old tuberculin
    4. Purified protein derivative of tuberculin

62. James is to have prophylactic drug therapy. For how long is he likely to be treated after his last exposure?
    1. 1 year
    2. 5 years
    3. 3 weeks
    4. 6 months

63. James's children have been exposed to tuberculosis, but do not show any evidence of the illness. What is the most likely situation for them?
    1. They will be considered immune.
    2. They should be treated with INH and PAS.
    3. They are usually given massive doses of penicillin.
    4. They will be examined by X-ray every 6 months.

---

64. The earliest clinical sign of idiopathic respiratory distress syndrome in a young infant is usually:
    1. Flaccidity
    2. Bradypnea
    3. Hypoxemia
    4. Sternal retractions

65. The most critical factor in the immediate care of an infant after repair of a cleft lip would be the:
    1. Prevention of vomiting
    2. Maintenance of a patent airway
    3. Administration of parenteral fluids
    4. Administration of drugs to reduce oral secretions

66. It is expected that, after a thoracotomy, lung expansion will recur within:
    1. 1 hour
    2. 4 hours
    3. 12 to 48 hours
    4. 48 to 72 hours

67. Following a tonsillectomy, the nurse initially suspects postoperative bleeding when the child:
    1. Snores noisily
    2. Becomes pale
    3. Complains of thirst
    4. Swallows frequently

68. When caring for the child with cystic fibrosis the nurse should:
    1. Prevent coughing
    2. Perform postural drainage
    3. Encourage active exercise
    4. Provide small, frequent feedings

Client Case Scenario 10: Shauna is a 3-year-old who has asthma. **Items 69 to 72 refer to this client case scenario.**

69. Shauna's initial treatment is to be aminophylline IV, for 20 minutes every 8 hours. Which of the following actions should the nurse implement with administration of the drug?
    1. Assess Shauna's vital signs
    2. Place Shauna in a croup tent
    3. Check Shauna's temperature
    4. Administer oxygen to Shauna

70. Shauna is placed on oxygen therapy and is given prednisone, 15 mg PO bid. Which of the following objectives are important for this child?
    1. Prevent exposing Shauna to infection
    2. Have Shauna rest as much as possible
    3. Check Shauna's eosinophil count daily
    4. Keep Shauna NPO except for her medications

71. During her nap, Shauna wets the bed. Which would likely be the best approach by the nurse?
    1. Tell her to help with remaking the bed
    2. Change her clothes and make no issue of it
    3. Change her bed, and put a rubber sheet on it
    4. Explain that big girls should be able to call the nurse

72. Which statement should be included when the nurse is planning discharge teaching for Shauna?
    1. Avoid foods high in fat
    2. Increase the usual calorie intake
    3. Avoid exertion and exposure to cold
    4. Stay in the house for at least 2 weeks

Reproductive and Genitourinary

73. The nurse explains to the parent group that the most important complication of mumps in post-pubertal males is:
    1. Sterility
    2. Hypopituitarism
    3. Decrease in libido
    4. A decrease in androgens

74. One of the earliest signs of sexual maturity in young girls that occurs about the age of 12 years is:
    1. Attention to grooming
    2. Interest in the opposite sex
    3. An increase in the size of the breasts
    4. The appearance of axillary and pubic hair

75. A physician orders the following for a young child with the diagnosis of Wilms' tumor. The nurse should question the physician regarding orders related to preparation for:
    1. An IVP
    2. A renal biopsy
    3. A nephrectomy
    4. An abdominal CT scan

76. The best choice for a between-meal nourishment for a preschool-age child hospitalized with a urinary infection would be:
    1. Skim milk
    2. Fresh fruit
    3. Hard candy
    4. Creamed soup

77. The most important nursing intervention for a 3-year-old child with a diagnosis of nephrosis is:
    1. Encouraging fluids
    2. Regulating the diet
    3. Preventing infection
    4. Maintaining bed rest

78. After a circumcision on a 6-month-old infant, the most essential nursing action during the initial postoperative period is to assess the infant for:
    1. Infection
    2. Hemorrhage
    3. Shrill, piercing cry
    4. Decreased urinary output

Client Case Scenario 11: Lindsay is a 5-year-old child with glomerulonephritis. **Items 79 to 82 refer to this client case scenario.**

79. Which of the following manifestations of glomerulonephritis were most likely included in Lindsay's presentation with this illness?
    1. Polyuria, high fever
    2. Oliguria, hypotension
    3. Dehydration, hematuria
    4. Hypertension, circumocular edema

80. The nurse needs to recognize when planning nursing care that Lindsay will need help in recognizing necessary restrictions. Which of the following is one of these restrictions?
    1. Daily doses of IM penicillin
    2. A bland diet high in protein
    3. Bed rest for at least 4 weeks
    4. Isolation from children with infections

81. Lindsay's mother asks the nurse why Lindsay is being weighed every morning. Which would be the best reply?
    1. "It is the best way to measure Lindsay's fluid balance."
    2. "When weight gain ceases it indicates the disease process is over."
    3. "It gives the doctors a good idea of how much protein is being lost."
    4. "The dietitian plans the daily caloric intake according to the daily weight change."

82. Lindsay's parents are very concerned about activity restrictions after discharge. The nurse should indicate that after the urinary findings return to normal, restrictions will likely include which of the following?
    1. Lindsay must not play active games
    2. Activity must be limited for 1 month
    3. Lindsay must remain in bed for 2 weeks
    4. Lindsay may return to pre-illness activities

Neuromuscular

83. A viral disease caused by one of the smallest human viruses that infect the motor cells of the anterior horn of the spinal cord is:
    1. Rubella
    2. Rubeola

    3. Chickenpox
    4. Poliomyelitis

84. When picked up by the mother or the nurse, an 8-month-old infant screams and seems to be in pain. The nurse notes the behavior and talks to the mother about:
    1. Accidents and injuries and the importance of their prevention
    2. Any other behavior of the infant that may have been noticed by the mother
    3. The food and specific vitamins that should be given to infants, including vitamins C and D
    4. Limiting the play time and activities that this infant has with other children in the family

85. A mother expresses concerns that her 9-month-old infant no longer has the same strong grasp that was present shortly after birth. The nurse should discuss with the mother that:
    1. It would be advisable to have a neurologic examination
    2. Failure of this response may be related to developmental disability
    3. This response is usually replaced by voluntary activity at 5 to 6 months of age
    4. The infant needs additional sensory stimulation to aid in the return of this response

86. Which of the following findings would the nurse find most unusual in a full-term infant?
    1. A small amount of lanugo over the back
    2. Both testes descended well into scrotum
    3. Ears containing cartilage with a firm pinna
    4. Square window sign (wrist forms a 90° angle)

Client Case Scenario 12: Curtis is a 3-year-old who has had a fever for several days, has held his neck rigid, and has been vomiting. **Items 87 to 89 refer to this client case scenario.**

87. The mother informs the nurse that Curtis has had a febrile convulsion. The nurse informs the physician, who is unconcerned. The nurse takes no further action. Curtis later has a convulsion that results in neurologic impairment. Which statement best describes the legal status of the nurse?
    1. The physician's decision takes precedence over the nurse's concern
    2. The nurse's action was inadequate in ensuring the safety of the child
    3. The physician is totally responsible for the client's health history and treatment regimen
    4. High temperatures are common in children, and this situation presented little cause for undue concern

88. Curtis's mother asks the nurse for information about febrile convulsions. Which information should guide the nurse's reply?
    1. These may occur in minor illnesses
    2. The cause is usually readily identified
    3. Usually occur after 3 years of life
    4. Occur more frequently in females than males

89. Which of the following would be the priority nursing action when Curtis is having a grand mal seizure?
    1. Start oxygen at 10 L by mask
    2. Insert a padded tongue blade
    3. Restrain Curtis to prevent injury to soft tissue
    4. Protect Curtis from harm from the environment

Client Case Scenario 13: Matthew, a newborn, is diagnosed with communicating hydrocephalus. **Items 90 to 93 refer to this client case scenario.**

90. Which of the following statements is correct when explaining the disorder of communicating hydrocephalus to Matthew's parents?
    1. "Too much cerebrospinal fluid is produced within the ventricles of the brain."
    2. "The cerebrospinal fluid is prevented from proper absorption by a blockage in the ventricles of the brain."
    3. "The part of the brain surface that normally absorbs cerebrospinal fluid after its production is not functioning adequately."
    4. There is a flow of cerebrospinal fluid between the brain cells and the ventricles, which do not empty properly into the spinal cord."

91. Which of the following might be an outcome if Matthew's hydrocephalus is untreated?
    1. CSF dilutes blood supply, causing cells to atrophy
    2. Increasing head size necessitates more oxygen and nutrients than normal blood flow can supply
    3. Hypertonic CSF disturbs normal plasma concentration, depriving nerve cells of vital nutrients
    4. Gradually increasing size of the ventricles compresses the brain against the bony cranium; anoxia and decreased blood supply result

92. Matthew has had a ventriculoperitoneal shunt inserted. What should the nurse include when explaining his prognosis to his parents?
    1. The prognosis is excellent and the shunt is permanent

2. The shunt may need to be revised as the child grows older
3. If any brain damage has occurred, it is reversible during the first year of life
4. Hydrocephalus usually is self-limiting by 2 years of age and then the shunt is removed

93. During Matthew's postoperative period, which nursing action would best meet his major developmental need?
    1. Give Matthew a pacifier
    2. Put a mobile over Matthew's crib
    3. Provide Matthew with a soft, cuddly toy
    4. Warm Matthew's formula before feeding

---

94. Studies of young children institutionalized for some time indicate that they show signs of developmental delay. Which of the following abilities is least likely affected by this delay?
    1. Sense of hearing
    2. Ability to understand
    3. Ability for self-expression
    4. Neuromuscular development

95. A 10-month-old is brought to the emergency room for a head injury after falling down the stairs. An immediate CT scan is ordered. In preparing a 10-month-old for a CT scan the nurse should:
    1. Shave the infant's head
    2. Administer prescribed sedative
    3. Start the prescribed intravenous infusion
    4. Give the infant an explanation of the procedure

96. Which of the following actions would be the most appropriate when a child develops cyanosis early during a tonic-clonic seizure?
    1. Insert an oral airway
    2. Use a padded tongue blade
    3. Administer oxygen by mask
    4. Observe without intervening

97. When performing a physical assessment of a newborn with Down syndrome, the nurse should carefully evaluate the infant's:
    1. Heart sounds
    2. Anterior fontanel
    3. Pupillary reaction
    4. Lower extremities

Client Case Scenario 14: Amy is an infant who has been born with a meningomyelocele. **Items 98 to 101 refer to this client case scenario.**

98. Which of the following nursing actions would provide the best support for Amy's parents?
    1. Discourage them from talking about Amy
    2. Encourage them to express their worries and fears
    3. Tell them not be worry because the defect can be repaired
    4. Show them postoperative photographs of babies who had similar defects

99. Which should be the primary nursing goal before Amy's defect is surgically corrected?
    1. Prevent infection
    2. Prevent damage to the sac
    3. Observe for increasing paralysis
    4. Observe for bowel and bladder dysfunction

100. What postoperative nursing care should be included after closure of Amy's meningomyelocele?
    1. Strict limitation of leg movement
    2. Decrease of environmental stimuli
    3. Measurement of head circumference daily
    4. Observation of serous drainage from the nares

101. Amy is to be catheterized for a sterile urine specimen. Her mother expresses fear that this procedure may traumatize Amy psychologically. Which statement would reassure Amy's mother?
    1. Her fear is justified and the nurse will obtain a "clean catch" specimen
    2. She has every right to refuse the catheterization since her concerns are realistic
    3. Her concern is appropriate but the need for a sterile specimen is a higher priority
    4. The procedure, though slightly uncomfortable, should not have any damaging effect

102. A 7-year-old child with cerebral palsy is required to wear braces and shoes in bed for at least 8 hours a day, following a tendon-lengthening procedure. This is to:
    1. Encourage ambulation as soon as possible
    2. Continue the child's acceptance of physical restraints
    3. Stretch the child's ligaments and strengthen muscle tone
    4. Maintain hip and knee alignment and prevent footdrop

103. A school-age child with cerebral palsy and diminished sensation in the legs should be taught special safety precautions, including to:

1. Test the temperature of water in any water-related activity
2. Tighten straps and buckles more than usual on braces when ambulating
3. Set the clock two times during the night to awaken and change position
4. Look down at the lower extremities when crutch walking to determine proper positioning of the legs

104. When planning long-term care for a child with cerebral palsy, it is important for the nurse to recognize that the:
    1. Illness is not progressively degenerative
    2. Child probably has some degree of intellectual impairment
    3. Effects of cerebral palsy are unstable and unpredictable
    4. Child should have genetic counseling before planning a family

105. One of the major behavioral characteristics of children with attention-deficit disorders is their:
    1. Overreaction to stimuli
    2. Continued use of rituals
    3. Delayed speech development
    4. Inability to use abstract thought

Client Case Scenario 15: Darryl is an 8-year-old who is febrile and has been diagnosed with meningococcal meningitis. **Items 106 to 108 refer to this client case scenario.**

106. Which of the following nursing actions should the nurse employ to reduce Darryl's fever?
    1. Discourage oral liquids
    2. Measure output every hour
    3. Limit exposure to prevent shivering
    4. Monitor vital signs every 10 minutes

107. Which of the following manifestations should the nurse observe for in Darryl?
    1. Palatal paralysis and glossitis
    2. Identifying purpuric skin rash
    3. Low-grade nature of the fever
    4. Continual tremors of the extremities

108. Which of the following is the most serious complication that could result from Darryl's meningitis?
    1. Epilepsy
    2. Blindness
    3. Peripheral circulatory collapse
    4. Communicating hydrocephalus

109. A 13-year-old, who has stepped on a nail is seen by the nurse in the emergency room. When the

nurse asks the adolescent if he has been immunized against tetanus, the reply is affirmative. The adolescent is readmitted with a diagnosis of tetanus a few days later. Legally:
1. Hospital protocol should govern treatment in emergency room care
2. The nurse's judgement was adequate in view of the client's symptoms
3. Assessment by the nurse was incomplete and the treatment was inadequate
4. The possibility of tetanus could not have been foreseen, since the adolescent had been immunized

110. Nursing care for an adolescent admitted with tetanus following a puncture wound should be primarily directed toward:
1. Decreasing external stimuli
2. Maintaining body alignment
3. Encouraging high intake of fluid
4. Carefully monitoring urinary output

111. Which of the following may occur with late correction of monocular strabismus?
1. Dyslexia
2. Loss of peripheral vision
3. Amblyopia in the weak eye
4. Diminished vision in both eyes

Client Case Scenario 16: Ryan is a 4-year-old who has been diagnosed with lead poisoning. **Items 112 to 115 refer to this client case scenario.**

112. Which of the following statements suggest the most likely etiology of lead poisoning in children?
1. Passive caregivers who fail to supervise children
2. The availability of sources of environmental lead
3. Clearly understood to be caused by the child's ingestion of nonfood substances
4. Unknown, but groups at high risk include children with pica and those exposed to environmental hazards

113. Although lead poisoning affects various organ systems, which of Ryan's systems will suffer irreversible side effects?
1. Urinary system
2. Skeletal system
3. Hematologic system
4. Central nervous system

114. Ryan is to receive painful injections. Which nursing action might best relieve the discomfort of the injections?

1. Applying warm soaks to the affected area
2. Giving Ryan a cool tub bath following each injection
3. Massaging the affected area vigorously after each injection
4. Having Ryan ambulate with assistance immediately following each injection

115. In Ryan's case, which would likely be the nursing diagnosis of highest priority?
1. Constipation related to the ingestion of lead
2. Risk for injury related to the ingestion of lead
3. Altered growth and development related to inadequate parenting
4. Altered nutrition, less than body requirements, related to decreased iron intake

Skeletal

Client Case Scenario 17: Paul is a 3-month-old infant who has a congenital hip dislocation. **Items 116 to 118 refer to this client case scenario.**

116. Paul was initially diagnosed in the newborn nursery. Which presentation was most likely?
1. Depressed dance reflex
2. Asymmetry of the gluteal folds
3. Limitation in adduction of the leg
4. Shortening of the leg on the unaffected side

117. Paul has had a spica cast applied from below his axilla to below his knee. In order to prevent a serious complication, which of the following actions should be taught to Paul's parents?
1. Feed Paul a low-calorie diet
2. Change Paul's diapers frequently
3. Limit Paul's movement to prevent cast damage
4. Seek immediate medical care if Paul develops a cough

118. Which of the following nursing actions should accompany elevation of Paul's head while he is in the spica cast?
1. Place folded diapers at the edge of the cast
2. Limit his position to 1 hour at a maximum
3. Use at least two pillows under Paul's shoulders
4. Raise the entire mattress and spring at the head of the bed

119. A week-old infant is postoperative after a club-foot casting. The nurse notes that the infant's respiratory rate is less than 30 breaths per minute, is unconcerned, and takes no action. Subsequently, the infant requires emergency care for respiratory distress. Legally:
    1. Respirations in young infants are often irregular and a drop is rarely important
    2. Most infants experience slow respirations with skeletal deformities or discomfort
    3. A reading outside normal parameters is significant and should have been reported
    4. The respiratory tract is underdeveloped in young infants and the respiratory rate is not significant

120. While caring for a young child in Bryant's traction, the nurse should be aware that this traction:
    1. Is skin traction to the affected leg
    2. Is used to allow the child to turn from side to side
    3. Is attached to a pin placed in the affected femur
    4. Is skin traction and elevates the hips slightly from the bed

121. A 9-year-old has a fractured femur and a full leg cast has been applied. The nurse should immediately notify the physician if assessment demonstrates:
    1. A pedal pulse of 90
    2. An increased urinary output
    3. An inability to move the toes
    4. A cast that is still damp and warm after 4 hours

122. Following orthopedic surgery, a 15-year-old complains of pain and is given 15 mg of codeine sulfate as ordered q 3 to 4 hours prn. Two hours after being given this medication the adolescent complains of severe pain. The nurse should:
    1. Report that the adolescent has an apparent idiosyncrasy to codeine
    2. Tell the adolescent that additional medication cannot be given for 1 more hour
    3. Request that the physician evaluate the adolescent's need for additional medication
    4. Administer another dose of codeine within 30 minutes, since it is a relatively safe drug

Client Case Scenario 18: Andrea is a 12-year-old with scoliosis. Items 123 to 126 refer to this client case scenario.

123. Andrea's parents did not accompany her during her admission. Andrea offered to sign the permission for treatment. An adolescent:
    1. Does not have the legal capacity to give consent

    2. Is not able to make an acceptable or intelligent choice
    3. Is able to give voluntary consent when parents are not available
    4. Will most likely be unable to choose between alternatives when asked to consent

124. The nurse explains to Andrea that proper exercise and avoidance of fatigue are essential components of care. Which sport would best meet Andrea's needs?
    1. Golf
    2. Bowling
    3. Swimming
    4. Badminton

125. To assist with curvature correction, Andrea is fitted with a brace. The nurse should explain to Andrea and her parents that the length of time the brace must be worn varies, but is usually worn until which situation occurs?
    1. The iliac crests are at equal levels
    2. Pain on prolonged standing diminishes
    3. Several months after the cessation of bone growth
    4. The curvature of the spine is completely straightened

126. Andrea's developmental task, according to Erikson, is to acquire an identity. Which of the following is a characteristic of a developmental task?
    1. Tasks occur with precise rhythm
    2. There is no uniform time for learning a task
    3. Tasks are learned at the same age in children
    4. Most developmental tasks are learned by school age

Endocrine

Client Case Scenario 19: Nigel is an 11-year-old child who has just been diagnosed with insulin dependent diabetes mellitus. Items 127 to 130 refer to this client case scenario.

127. Nigel is to receive a combination of isophane suspension (NPH) and regular insulin at 0700h. Which of these will be responsible for Nigel's response prior to lunch at noon?
    1. The regular insulin rather than the isophane suspension (NPH)
    2. Decreasing effects of the regular and the isophane suspension (NPH) insulin
    3. Increasing effects of the regular and the isophane suspension (NPH) insulin
    4. Decreasing effects of the regular and increasing effects of the isophane suspension (NPH) insulin

128. Which of the following statements should be included when teaching Nigel about the dietary portion of the management of diabetes mellitus?
    1. Eat all meals at home
    2. Weigh all food on a gram scale
    3. Always carry a concentrated form of glucose
    4. Have the parent prepare food separately from the rest of the family

129. Which of the following statements by Nigel would indicate to the nurse that he has a need for cognitive learning?
    1. "What is diabetes?"
    2. "Can I still play hockey?"
    3. "How do I give myself an injection?"
    4. "When do I test my blood for glucose?"

130. Which of the following objectives would be most important when the nurse is planning a teaching program for Nigel and his parents?
    1. The child is taught to give injections before being discharged
    2. The parents receive instruction about blood glucose monitoring
    3. The child's activity be limited and the parents understand the need for this
    4. The parents and child be helped to understand their feelings about diabetes

131. A 10-year-old is diagnosed with lymphocytic (Hashimoto's) thyroiditis. The nurse should explain to the parents and child that this condition is:
    1. Chronic
    2. Inherited
    3. Often fatal
    4. Probably temporary

132. An evening snack of crackers and cheese is planned for a child receiving NPH (Humulin N) insulin. The nurse understands that this will provide:
    1. Added calories to help the child gain weight
    2. Encouragement for the child to stay on a diet
    3. High-carbohydrate nourishment for immediate utilization
    4. Nourishment with a latent effect to counteract late insulin activity

133. In reviewing the pathophysiology of diabetes mellitus with an 8-year-old, newly diagnosed child, the nurse's plan should take into consideration that:
    1. The child is in the abstract level of cognition
    2. Peer influence will decrease in importance to the child

3. The child will respond favorably to opportunities to participate in self care
    4. The child's current developmental task involves achieving a sense of identity

134. A 14-year-old who has been on prolonged steroid therapy develops a cushingoid appearance. A nursing assessment of this child would probably reveal:
    1. Increased linear growth
    2. Loss of hair, including body hair
    3. Hypotension and hyponatremia
    4. Thin extremities with truncal obesity

Client Case Scenario 20: Malika is a 3-month-old infant with congenital hypothyroidism. **Items 135 to 137 refer to this client case scenario.**

135. Which would likely be the outcome if Malika has not yet received medical care for this disorder?
    1. Myxedema
    2. Thyrotoxicosis
    3. Some developmental disability
    4. Hyperreactive deep tendon reflexes

136. Malika is to receive thyroxine sodium 0.35 mg qd PO. The medication is available in elixir form, 0.25 mg/ml. Which quantity of medication should the nurse administer?
    1. 0.6 ml
    2. 0.8 ml
    3. 1.0 ml
    4. 1.4 ml

137. On discharge, Malika's mother asks the nurse what she should do to prevent accidents with Malika. What should the nurse include in the teaching plan?
    1. Remove all tiny objects from the floor
    2. Cover electric outlets with safety plugs
    3. Keep crib rails up to the highest position
    4. Remove poisonous substances from low areas

Integumentary

138. A viral infection characterized by a red, blotchy rash and Koplik's spots in the mouth is:
    1. Mumps
    2. Rubella
    3. Rubeola
    4. Chickenpox

139. A viral disease that begins with respiratory inflammation and skin rash and may result in grave complications is:
    1. Rubella
    2. Rubeola
    3. Yellow fever
    4. Chickenpox

140. Under certain circumstances the virus that causes chickenpox can also cause:
    1. Athlete's foot
    2. Herpes zoster
    3. German measles
    4. Infectious hepatitis

141. When teaching parents at the school about communicable diseases, the nurse reminds them that these diseases are serious, and that encephalitis can be a complication of:
    1. Pertussis
    2. Chickenpox
    3. Poliomyelitis
    4. Scarlet fever

142. Chickenpox can sometimes be fatal to children who are receiving:
    1. Insulin
    2. Steroids
    3. Antibiotics
    4. Anticonvulsants

143. Which of the following skin infections is most likely to lead to glomerulonephritis?
    1. Scabies
    2. Impetigo
    3. Intertrigo
    4. Herpes simplex

144. An infection caused by the yeast *Candida albicans,* often occurring in infants and debilitated individuals, is:
    1. Thrush
    2. Dysentery
    3. Malta fever
    4. Typhoid fever

Client Case Scenario 21: Jared is a 15-year-old teenager who has received partial thickness burns of the face and chest in a house fire. **Items 145 to 147 refer to this client case scenario.**

145. For which of the following should the nurse observe primarily in Jared for the first 24 hours?
    1. Wound sepsis
    2. Pulmonary distress
    3. Effects of immobility
    4. Fluid and electrolyte imbalance

146. Which of the following rationales would guide the nurse in deciding to administer Jared's analgesics intravenously instead of intramuscularly?
    1. Intramuscular injections increase the risk of tissue irritation
    2. Intravenous injections reduce severe pain more effectively
    3. Intravenous injections bypass impaired peripheral circulation
    4. Intramuscular injections provide for more prolonged relief of pain

147. Jared develops a minor infection and is prescribed tetracycline (Achromycin). He is anorexic, lethargic, and irritable. Which of the following rationales might indicate why the nurse should discuss this with the physician?
    1. Jared needs a higher food intake to fight the infection
    2. Anemia is a frequent occurrence after infection and treatment with antibiotics
    3. Concurrent bladder infection may be present as an extension of his gram-negative infection
    4. Generalized physical symptoms and behavior problems may indicate drug-induced liver damage

148. A mother asks the nurse how to tell the difference between measles (rubeola) and German measles (rubella). The nurse tells the mother that with rubeola the child has:
    1. A high fever and Koplik's spots
    2. A rash on the trunk with pruritus
    3. Nausea, vomiting, and abdominal cramps
    4. Symptoms similar to a cold, followed by a rash

Gastrointestinal

Client Case Scenario 22: Kathleen is a 6-year-old girl who reports anal itching and is suspected to have pinworms. **Items 149 to 152 refer to this client case scenario.**

149. For which complication of pinworm infestation should the nurse observe?
    1. Hepatitis
    2. Stomatitis
    3. Appendicitis
    4. Encephalitis

150. The nurse is asked to teach Kathleen's mother to perform a cellophane tape test. Which would be the most effective time to perform this test?
    1. Just following a BM
    2. Immediately after meals

3. At bedtime before bathing
4. Early morning before arising

151. The nurse is to administer mebendazole (Vermox) to Kathleen for 3 consecutive days. To which family members should this drug also be administered?
    1. Kathleen's younger brother who is 1-year-old
    2. All members of Kathleen's family who test positive
    3. All people using the same toilet facilities as Kathleen
    4. Kathleen's mother, father, and siblings even though they are symptom free

152. After administration of the drug, what should the nurse teach Kathleen's mother to observe?
    1. Convulsions
    2. Hypertension
    3. Intestinal bleeding
    4. Worms in the stool

Client Case Scenario 23: Josh is a 2-year-old child who was born with a unilateral cleft lip and palate. He is being readmitted for a palate repair. **Items 153 to 156 refer to this client case scenario.**

153. Which of the following would be the most important factor in preparing Josh for his hospitalization?
    1. Gratification of Josh's wishes
    2. Josh's previous hospitalization
    3. Never leaving Josh with strangers
    4. Assurance of affection and security

154. Prior to the repair of a unilateral cleft lip and palate, feeding will probably be:
    1. Limited to IV fluids
    2. With a soft, large altered nipple
    3. Accomplished per gastrostomy tube
    4. Facilitated by the use of a spoon or medicine dropper

155. Which of the following nursing actions would have been included for Josh following his cleft lip repair?
    1. Using a spoon to administer oral feedings
    2. Cleansing the suture line to prevent infection
    3. Allowing Josh to suck on a pacifier to prevent crying
    4. Positioning Josh on the abdomen to avoid aspiration

156. Why will Josh be unable to use a toothbrush postoperatively?
    1. The suture line might be injured

2. Josh would probably have no teeth
3. The toothbrush might be frightening to Josh
4. Josh would not be accustomed to a brush at home

157. Parents can predispose their children to problems with nutrition by using food in early childhood as a means of:
    1. Socializing
    2. Acculturation
    3. Teaching discipline
    4. Reward and punishment

158. The major influence on eating habits of the early school-aged child is the:
    1. Availability of food selections
    2. Smell and appearance of food
    3. Example of parents at mealtime
    4. Food preferences of the peer group

159. The nurse recognizes that a newborn infant, a client following a cholecystectomy, and a client on anticoagulant therapy following a myocardial infarction have a common nutrient-related problem associated with the:
    1. Neuromuscular function of thiamin
    2. Blood-clotting function of vitamin K
    3. Calcium-absorbing function of vitamin D
    4. Hemoglobin-forming function of iron and vitamin B_{12}

160. An 8-month-old infant has a gastrostomy tube and is given 240 ml of tube feeding q4h. One of the primary nursing responsibilities is to:
    1. Open the tube 1 hour before feeding
    2. Position on the right side after feeding
    3. Give 10 ml of normal saline before and after feeding
    4. Elevate the tube 30 cm above the level of the mattress

161. Which of the following suggestions would assist in confirming a suspected diagnosis of pinworms?
    1. Ask the parent to collect stools for 3 consecutive days for culture
    2. Instruct the parent to do an anal cellophane tape test early in the morning
    3. Have the parent bring in the child's stools for visual examination for 3 days
    4. Assist the parent to schedule a hypersensitivity test of the child's blood serum

Client Case Scenario 24: Celia is an 8-year-old with cystic fibrosis. **Items 162 to 165 refer to this client case scenario.**

162. Celia is very small for her age. Which manifestation of cystic fibrosis explains why?
    1. She has an extremely poor appetite
    2. She has developed muscular and bony atrophy from lack of activity
    3. She secretes less than normal amounts of pituitary growth hormone
    4. She is unable to absorb nutrients because of lack of pancreatic enzymes

163. Celia's stools are foul-smelling and frothy, characteristic of cystic fibrosis. Which component of the stool results in this characteristic?
    1. Undigested fat
    2. Sodium and chloride
    3. Semidigested carbohydrates
    4. Lipase, trypsin, and amylase

164. Celia's nurse needs to be aware that with cystic fibrosis, muscle wasting, and malnutrition often result in which of the following complications?
    1. Anal fissures
    2. Rectal prolapse
    3. Intussusception
    4. Meconium ileus

165. As Celia gets older, which of the following objectives will be most important for her nurses to help her develop?
    1. A positive body image
    2. Fine muscle coordination
    3. The ability to manage her diet
    4. Acceptance of possible sterility

Client Case Scenario 25: Samantha is a 2-week-old infant who has been admitted to hospital for the repair of a pyloric stenosis. **Items 166 to 168 refer to this client case scenario.**

166. Which of the following should be assessment priorities for the nurse collecting data about Samantha?
    1. Quality of cry
    2. Quality of stool
    3. Signs of dehydration
    4. Coughing and gagging after feeding

167. Which of the following explains why Samantha's emesis is not bile-stained?
    1. The bile duct is also obstructed
    2. The obstruction is above the opening of the common bile duct
    3. The sphincter of the bile duct is connected to the hypertrophied pyloric muscle
    4. The obstruction of the cardiac sphincter prevents bile from entering the esophagus

168. Which of the following postoperative orders might be expected after Samantha has a surgical repair of her pyloric stenosis?
    1. Thickened formula 24 hours after surgery
    2. Withholding all feedings for the first 24 hours
    3. Additional glucose feedings after the first 24 hours
    4. Diluted formula feeding 24 hours after surgery

169. Which of the following instructions should the nurse give regarding bottle feeding to the parent of a healthy infant?
    1. "Burp the baby five to six times during each feeding for the first month."
    2. "You should burp your baby at the end of the feeding only. Babies can become confused at having their feeding stopped."
    3. "Burp your baby periodically during the feeding. If the baby has been crying, you can burp before starting."
    4. "With new infants we recommend burping every 5 to 10 minutes. That gets your baby used to a routine and lets you see how much formula is being taken."

170. A parent brings a week-old infant into the clinic because the infant regurgitates with each feed. The nurse instructs the parent to:
    1. Keep the infant prone following feedings
    2. Prevent the infant from crying for prolonged periods
    3. Administer a minimum of 240 ml of formula at each feeding
    4. Keep the infant in a semisitting position, particularly after feedings

171. Nursing care for an infant after the surgical repair of a cleft lip should include:
    1. Keeping the baby NPO
    2. Keeping the infant from crying
    3. Placing the infant in a semisitting position
    4. Spoonfeeding for the first 2 days after surgery

172. Exposure to hepatitis B may occur in hospitals because of:
    1. Careless handling of feces by staff
    2. Increasing use of ventilating systems
    3. Needle sticks and mucous membrane exposure
    4. Early diagnosis and improved treatment of hepatitis A

173. One symptom common in children with celiac disease is stools that are:
    1. Small, pale, mucoid
    2. Large, frothy, dark green

3. Large, pale, foul smelling
4. Moderate, green, foul smelling

Client Case Scenario 26: Bryan is an infant who has been diagnosed with phenylketonuria, PKU. **Items 174 to 177 refer to this client case scenario.**

174. Which statements should the nurse include when teaching Bryan's parents about this disorder?
    1. A low-phenylalanine diet is required
    2. Phenylalanine is not necessary for growth
    3. Phenylalanine can be administered to correct the deficiency
    4. Other amino acids can be increased to substitute for phenylalanine

175. Which of the following is true regarding Bryan's screening for PKU?
    1. Bryan's blood is tested for high levels of phenylalanine
    2. A urine test is done after 6 weeks on infant formula
    3. Bryan's blood is tested to detect phenylalanine deficiency
    4. A 24-urine collection is tested for the presence of phenylalanine

176. Which statement should the nurse be aware of when assisting Bryan's parents to understand this disorder?
    1. Treatment for PKU includes life-long medications
    2. Developmental disability occurs if PKU is not treated
    3. PKU is transmitted by an autosomal dominant gene
    4. Bryan will be unusually susceptible to infections if not treated.

177. Bryan's mother asks the nurse, "How long will Bryan have to be on this special diet?" Which response by the nurse would be most appropriate?
    1 "No one knows, but why don't you discuss it with your doctor?"
    2. "Usually, if the child does well for 1 year, regular foods can gradually be introduced."
    3. "Unfortunately, this is a life-long problem and dietary management must always be maintained."
    4. "As of now, research shows that a child needs to be on this diet at least until adolescence and possibly longer."

178. Dietary treatment of children with PKU includes a:
    1. Protein-free diet
    2. Phenylalanine-free diet

3. Low-phenylalanine diet
4. Dietary supplement for phenylalanine

179. The nurse plans to discuss childhood nutrition with parents of children with Down syndrome in an attempt to minimize a common nutritional problem encountered in children with Down syndrome, namely:
    1. Rickets
    2. Obesity
    3. Anemia
    4. Rumination

180. In a 3-month-old infant with bile-stained vomitus and abdominal distention, the nurse should observe for:
    1. Bounding pulse and hypotonicity
    2. High-pitched cry and weak thready pulse
    3. Paroxysmal pain and grunting respirations
    4. Constant severe pain and absence of stools

181. The behavior of an infant with colic is usually suggestive of:
    1. An allergic response to certain proteins in milk
    2. Inadequate peristalsis resulting in constipation
    3. Paroxysmal abdominal pain due to excessive gas
    4. A protective mechanism designed to rid the GI tract of foreign proteins

Client Case Scenario 27: Marcie Collins has brought her 6-month-old infant, Chelsea, to the well-baby clinic. **Items 182 to 185 refer to this client case scenario.**

182. Marcie asks the nurse how she should introduce pureed food to Chelsea. Which reply would be the most appropriate?
    1. "Mix the pureed food in with the formula twice a day."
    2. "Introduce one food at a time, usually at intervals of 4 to 7 days."
    3. "Give the pureed foods by spoon after the infant has had formula."
    4. "Keep the formula intake fairly constant regardless of the solid food intake."

183. What solid foods should the nurse suggest Marcie introduce to Chelsea?
    1. Rice infant cereal and fruit
    2. Sweets, such as fruits and puddings
    3. Meat first, then add fruit and vegetables
    4. Cereal and a soft-boiled egg for breakfast

184. As part of the newborn assessment, the nurse reviews Chelsea's birth records. Which of the following data might indicate Chelsea may require special attention?
    1. Birth weight of 3500 g
    2. The Apgar score at birth was 3
    3. The infant has a positive Babinski reflex
    4. Cloudy fluid was suctioned from her stomach at birth

185. Which of the following statements should the nurse include when teaching Marcie about the importance of play during infancy? Play is:
    1. Initiated by the child
    2. A way of teaching how to share
    3. More important than in later years
    4. Mostly used for physical development

Fluid and Electrolytes

Client Case Scenario 28: Erin is a 5-month-old infant who has severe diarrhea, and is admitted with a fluid and electrolyte imbalance. **Items 186 to 189 refer to this client case scenario.**

186. Which of the following represents an essential nursing action in the care of Erin?
    1. Force fluids orally
    2. Take daily weights
    3. Replace lost calories
    4. Keep body temperature below 37.8° C

187. Which of the following statements best explains why the maintenance of fluid and electrolyte balance is more critical in Erin than in an adult?
    1. Cellular metabolism is less stable than in adults
    2. The proportion of water in the body is less than in adults
    3. Renal function is immature in children below 4 years of age
    4. The daily fluid requirement per unit of body weight is greater than in adults

188. Erin has an intravenous initiated. Which of the following is a priorty reason for close observation of the rate of flow?
    1. Avoid IV infiltration
    2. Replace all fluids lost
    3. Prevent increased output
    4. Prevent cardiac overload

189. Erin is to receive 500 ml of IV fluid per 24 hours. Using a minidrip IV set, with a drop rate of 60 drops per ml, at what rate should the IV infuse?
    1. 8 drops per minute
    2. 13 drops per minute
    3. 21 drops per minute
    4. 24 drops per minute

190. The physician orders a tap-water enema for a 6-month-old child. The nurse considers that a tap-water enema could:
    1. Result in loss of necessary nutrients
    2. Cause a fluid and electrolyte imbalance
    3. Increase the child's fear of intrusive procedures
    4. Result in shock from a sudden drop in temperature

191. The physician orders an isotonic enema for a 2-year-old with constipation. The nurse is aware that the maximum amount of fluid to be given a small child without a physician's specific order is:
    1. 100 to 150 ml
    2. 155 to 250 ml
    3. 255 to 350 ml
    4. 355 to 500 ml

192. An 18-month-old is to receive 1000 ml 5% dextrose and normal saline, IV, in 24 hours. The drop factor of the minidropper is 60 gtt/ml. The nurse should regulate the IV to run at:
    1. 21 drops per minute
    2. 34 drops per minute
    3. 38 drops per minute
    4. 42 drops per minute

193. Of primary importance when the nurse plans for the discharge of a child following a sickle cell crisis (pain episode) is the child's need for:
    1. A high caloric diet
    2. Rigorous exercise and play
    3. At least 14 hours' sleep per day
    4. Ingestion of large quantities of liquids

194. Which of the following statements best explains the acid-base imbalance that occurs in a child experiencing a severe asthma attack?
    1. Metabolic alkalosis caused by excessive production of acid metabolites
    2. Respiratory alkalosis caused by the accelerated respirations and loss of carbon dioxide
    3. Respiratory acidosis caused by the impaired respirations and increased formation of carbonic acid
    4. Metabolic acidosis caused by the kidneys' inability to help compensate for the increased carbonic acid formed

Client Case Scenario 29: Robby is a dehydrated infant who has been vomiting for the last 3 hours. **Items 195 to 197 refer to this client case scenario.**

195. Which of the following might be a complication of Robby's vomiting?
    1. Tetany
    2. Acidosis
    3. Alkalosis
    4. Hyperactivity

196. Robby has an intravenous initiated. Which is the most critical factor for the nurse to consider in the administration of IV fluids to an infant?
    1. Assurance of sterility
    2. Calculation of the total necessary intake
    3. Maintenance of the prescribed rate of flow
    4. Maintenance of the fluid at body temperature

197. On admission, Robby's mother indicates that he has colic. Which of the following suggestions by the nurse might assist Robby's mother with coping during his episodes of colic?
    1. Give her son a warm bath to calm him down
    2. Arrange for some time away from her son each day to rest
    3. Provide her son with warm sweetened tea when he begins to cry
    4. Sit comfortably in a quiet, darkened room to hold her son when he cries

198. A child has been admitted for surgery to correct a congenital megacolon. Enemas are ordered preoperatively to cleanse the bowel. The nurse should use:
    1. Tap water
    2. Soap suds
    3. Isotonic saline
    4. Hypertonic phosphate

Cardiovascular

199. The nurse doing a newborn assessment counts the infant's cord vessels. In a normal infant there are:
    1. Two vessels: one vein and one artery
    2. Three vessels: two veins and one artery
    3. Three vessels: one vein and two arteries
    4. Four vessels: two veins and two arteries

200. A disorder, following a *Streptococcus* infection, characterized by swollen joints, fever, and the possibility of endocarditis and death is:
    1. Tetanus
    2. Measles
    3. Rheumatic fever
    4. Whooping cough

201. Among the last signs of heart failure in the infant and child is:
    1. Orthopnea
    2. Tachypnea
    3. Tachycardia
    4. Peripheral edema

202. A young child has coarctation of the aorta. When taking the child's vital signs, the nurse can expect to observe:
    1. Notching of the clavicle
    2. Bounding femoral pulses
    3. Weak, thready radial pulses
    4. Higher BP in upper extremities

203. When observing a newborn with Down syndrome, the nurse should be aware that a common defect associated with this condition is:
    1. Deafness
    2. Hydrocephaly
    3. Muscular hypertonicity
    4. Congenital heart defect

Client Case Scenario 30: Jamie is an infant diagnosed with a patent ductus arteriosus (PDA), an acyanotic congenital heart defect. **Items 204 to 207 refer to this client case scenario.**

204. Which of the following symptoms of acyanotic heart defects should the nurse observe for in Jamie?
    1. Polycythemia
    2. Severe retarded growth
    3. Clubbing of fingers and toes
    4. The presence of an audible heart murmur

205. Which of the following descriptions by the nurse would best assist Jamie's parents to understand the pediatric cardiologist's explanation of patent ductus arteriosus?
    1. A narrowing of the pulmonary artery
    2. An enlarged aorta and pulmonary artery
    3. A connection between the pulmonary artery and the aorta
    4. An abnormal opening between the right and left ventricles

206. Jamie has his PDA ligated surgically. Which of the following best indicates why gavage feeding is indicated for weak infants following repair of a congenital heart defect?
    1. Vomiting is prevented
    2. The feeding can be given quickly, so handling is minimized
    3. The amount of food given can be more accurately regulated
    4. It conserves the infant's strength and does not depend on the swallowing reflex

207. Without appropriate treatment for his congenital cardiac anomaly, which would Jamie most likely have developed?
1. Developmental disability
2. Delayed physical growth
3. Cyanosis without physical exertion
4. Significant essential hypertension

Client Case Scenario 31: Sarah is a 5-year-old who has been admitted for surgical repair of tetralogy of Fallot, a cyanotic heart defect. **Items 208 to 211 refer to this client case scenario.**

208. Which of the following groups of defects make up the disorder tetrology of Fallot?
1. Right ventricular hypertrophy, atrial and ventricular defects, and mitral valve stenosis
2. Origin of the aorta from the right ventricle and of the pulmonary artery from the left ventricle
3. Right ventricular hypertrophy, ventricular septal defect, stenosis of pulmonary artery, and overriding aorta
4. Abnormal connection between the pulmonary artery and the aorta, right ventricular hypertrophy, and atrial septal defects

209. Which of the following presentations should the nurse expect to find in Sarah?
1. Anemia
2. An elevated hematocrit
3. Absence of pedal pulses
4. Edema in the extremities

210. Sarah has polycythemia. For which characteristic of her heart anomaly is this compensating?
1. Low BP
2. Cardiomegaly
3. Low iron level
4. Tissue hypoxia

211. Sarah undergoes surgery to repair her cardiac defects. Which of the following is it essential that the nurse prevent postoperatively?
1. Crying
2. Coughing
3. Constipation
4. Unnecessary movement

Blood and Immunity

212. Which of the following terms describes bacterial cells that have been modified?
1. A toxin
2. A toxoid
3. A vaccine
4. An antitoxin

213. A child comes to the hospital after exposure to diphtheria and is given antitoxin. This type of immunity is known as:
1. Active natural immunity
2. Active artificial immunity
3. Passive natural immunity
4. Passive artificial immunity

214. Which of the following types of immunity describes immunity by antibody formation during the course of an illness
1. Active natural immunity
2. Active artificial immunity
3. Passive natural immunity
4. Passive artificial immunity

215. Occasionally infants are born without an immune system. They can live normally with no apparent problems during their first months after birth because:
1. Exposure to pathogens during this time can be limited
2. Limited antibodies are produced by the infant's colonic bacteria
3. Antibodies are passively received from the mother through the placenta and breast milk
4. Limited antibodies are produced by the fetal thymus during the eighth and ninth months of gestation

Client Case Scenario 32: David is a pale, lethargic 1-year-old who has been admitted with a hemogloblin level of 50 g/L. **Items 216 to 219 refer to this client case scenario.**

216. Which of the following values represents an expected hemoglobin for David?
1. 90-100 g/L
2. 100-159 g/L
3. 150-170 g/L
4. 170-200 g/L

217. David is diagnosed with iron deficiency anemia. Which of the following contributes most to iron deficiency anemia in young children?
1. Blood disorders
2. Overfeeding of milk
3. Lack of adequate iron reserves from the mother
4. Introduction of solid foods too early for proper absorption

218. Which of the following nutrients, combined with iron, are required to produce red blood cells?
1. Calcium and vitamins
2. Vitamin D and riboflavin

3. Proteins and ascorbic acid
4. Carbohydrates and thiamine

219. Which of the following actions by David's mother should the nurse encourage?
    1. Immediately begin the weaning process
    2. Take the infant to the metabolic clinic for a checkup
    3. Give the infant finger foods such as raisins and chopped meat
    4. Put a large hole in the nipple and put baby food in with the milk

220. Using live virus vaccines against measles is contraindicated in children receiving corticosteroid, antineoplastic, or irradiation therapy because these children may:
    1. Have had the disease or have been immunized previously
    2. Be unlikely to need this protection during their shortened life span
    3. Be susceptible to infection because of their depressed immune response
    4. Have an allergy to rabbit serum, which is used as a basis for these vaccines

221. Which of the following boosters are generally received by a preschool child if they have received all of the primary immunizations?
    1. Diphtheria, polio, tetanus, pertussis
    2. Pertussis, hemophilus, polio, tetanus
    3. Measles, mumps, rubella, hemophilus
    4. Tetanus, polio, hemophilus, diphtheria

222. When reviewing the immunization schedule for a 12-month-old, the nurse would expect that the infant had been previously immunized against:
    1. Pertussis, tetanus, polio, and measles
    2. Polio, pertussis, tetanus, and diphtheria
    3. Measles, mumps, rubella, and tuberculosis
    4. Measles, rubella, polio, tuberculosis, and pertussis

223. Which of the following statements best explains the body's response to immunization?
    1. Lipid agents are formed by the body against antigens
    2. Protein antigens are formed in the blood to fight invading antibodies
    3. Protein substances are formed by the body to destroy or neutralize antigens
    4. Blood antigens are aided by phagocytes in defending the body against pathogens

224. The measles immunization is usually routinely given at 12 months of age because of the:

1. Increased hazard of side effects in infants
2. Presence of maternal antibodies during the first year
3. Rare incidence of measles infection prior to 12 months of age
4. Interference it causes with effectiveness of pertussis, diphtheria, and tetanus immunizations

Client Case Scenario 33: Tyson is a 6-year-old who has sickle cell anemia. He has been admitted with a vasoocclusive crisis. **Items 225 to 228 refer to this client case scenario.**

225. Which of the following problems can result in sickling of the red blood cells in a child with sickle cell anemia?
    1. Hypoxia
    2. Hypocalcemia
    3. Hemodilution
    4. Thrombocytopenia

226. Which of the following nursing actions could prevent thrombus formation in Tyson's capillaries?
    1. Administer oxygen
    2. Ensure Tyson maintains bed rest
    3. Increase fluids by mouth and use a humidifier
    4. Administer ordered heparin or other anticoagulants

227. Which of the following objectives will prevent crisis in both sickle cell anemia and celiac disease?
    1. Limitation of activity
    2. Protection from infection
    3. Careful observation of all vital signs
    4. High-iron, low-fat, high-protein diet

228. Which of the following should be priority nursing concerns in the care of Tyson?
    1. Nutrition and hydration
    2. Nutrition and antibiotics
    3. Hydration and pain management
    4. Pain management and antibiotics

Client Case Scenario 34: Terry is a toddler who has classical hemophilia. **Items 229 to 232 refer to this client case scenario.**

229. Which of the following statements is true regarding Terry's disorder?
    1. Hemophilia is an autosomal dominant disorder in which the woman carries the trait
    2. Hemophilia follows regular laws of Mendelian inherited disorders such as sickle cell anemia
    3. This disorder can be carried by either male or female but occurs in the sex opposite that of the carrier
    4. Hemophilia is an X-linked disorder in which the mother is usually the carrier of the illness but is not affected by it

230. Terry has some internal bleeding. At which of the following sites is it most common for a child with hemophilia to bleed?
    1. Joints
    2. Intestines
    3. Cerebrum
    4. Ends of the long bones

231. Which of the following blood products is most likely to be given to Terry?
    1. Albumin
    2. Fresh frozen plasma
    3. Factor VIII concentrate
    4. Factor II, VII, IX, X complex

232. Terry's parents ask if their other children will be affected by the disorder. Which of the following statements should guide the nurse in her response?
    1. All the girls will be normal and the other son a carrier
    2. All the girls will be carriers and one half the boys will be affected
    3. Each son has a 50% chance of being affected and each daughter a 50% chance of being a carrier
    4. Each son has a 50% chance of being either affected or a carrier, and the girls will all be carriers

233. Infants receive immunizations made up of attenuated viruses. This means that these immunizations:
    1. Contain active antibodies
    2. Contain passive antibodies
    3. Cause the development of active antibodies
    4. Cause the development of passive antibodies

234. A child is to receive a blood transfusion. If an allergic reaction to the blood occurs, the nurse's first intervention should be to:
    1. Call the physician
    2. Slow the flow rate
    3. Stop the blood immediately
    4. Relieve the symptoms with an ordered antihistamine

235. Anemia, a nutritional problem encountered in children and adults, involves several different nutrients. The nutrients include proteins, iron, vitamin B_{12}, and:
    1. Calcium
    2. Thiamine
    3. Folic acid
    4. Carbohydrates

236. The food that the nurse would emphasize to the mother of a 2-year-old as the best source of iron to be included in the diet daily is:
    1. Milk
    2. Lamb
    3. Orange juice
    4. Mineral-fortified cereal

237. During a period of heavy play activity, a first grader with a known history of anemia complains of feeling woozy. The school nurse's best initial response would be to:
    1. Check the child's pulse and blood pressure
    2. Have the child sit until the dizziness subsides
    3. Use spirits of ammonia to prevent the child from fainting
    4. Assist the child to the nurse's room and place the child in a supine position

238. Infants with sickle cell anemia may not be diagnosed as having this disorder because of:
    1. The absence of any respiratory disorders
    2. General good health and an excellent growth curve
    3. The presence of fetal hemoglobin during the first year of life
    4. Compensation of increased hematocrit and hemoglobin if well fed

239. A child receiving chemotherapy for the treatment of cancer of the bone is at risk for mouth lesions from the chemotherapy. The nurse teaching the child and the mother should stress the importance of:
    1. Frequent rinsing with undiluted mouthwash
    2. Use of foam-tipped applicators for mouthcare
    3. Brushing three times a day with a toothbrush
    4. Frequent mouth rinsing with hydrogen peroxide

Client Case Scenario 35: Scott is a 4-year-old, newly diagnosed with acute lymphocytic leukemia. **Items 240 to 243 refer to this client case scenario.**

240. Scott's laboratory results indicate that he is neutropenic. Which of the following has resulted in neutropenia?
    1. Overwhelming infection
    2. Increased internal bleeding
    3. Increased immature cell growth
    4. Decreased intake of iron-rich nutrients

241. In considering the usual presentation of leukemia, which of the following manifestations might cause the most concern about Scott?
    1. Marked fatigue, pallor
    2. Multiple bruises, petechiae
    3. Enlarged lymph nodes, spleen, and liver
    4. Marked jaundice and generalized edema

242. When Scott brushes his teeth, he has some bloody expectorant. Which of the following nursing actions would be the most appropriate?
    1. Secure a smaller toothbrush for Scott's use
    2. Tell Scott to be more careful when brushing his teeth
    3. Record and report the incident without alarming Scott
    4. Rinse Scott's mouth with half-strength hydrogen peroxide

243. Scott is scheduled to receive cranial radiation. The nurse should explain to Scott's parents that this is being done for which of the following reasons?
    1. Improve the quality of life
    2. Reduce the risk of systemic infection
    3. Avoid metastasis to the lymphatic system
    4. Prevent central nervous system involvement

Drug-Related Responses

Client Case Scenario 36: Linda is a 9-year-old who is scheduled for orthopedic surgery tomorrow morning. **Items 244 to 246 refer to this client case scenario.**

244. On admission, Linda's mother hands the nurse a bottle of capsules and says, "These are for Linda's allergies. Would you make sure she takes one at nine o'clock?" What would be the nurse's best response?
    1. "One capsule at 9 PM? Of course, I will give it to her."
    2. "Did you ask the doctor if she should have this tonight?"
    3. "I am certain the doctor knows about your daughter's allergy."

    4. "I will ask your daughter's doctor to write an order so I can give this medication to her."

245. Linda's physician has ordered atropine, gr 1/300 IM preoperatively. The vial reads "atropine 0.4 mg/ml." Which would be the correct quantity to administer to Linda?
    1. 0.5 ml
    2. 1.0 ml
    3. 0.25 ml
    4. 0.75 ml

246. Following surgery, Linda receives codeine sulphate for an analgesic. About 8 hours later, she reports itching. Which drug might relieve this discomfort?
    1. Wydase, hyaluronidase
    2. Macrobid, nitrofurantoin
    3. Entrophen, acetylsalicylic acid
    4. Chlor-Tripolon, chlorpheneramine

247. When administering a parenteral iron preparation to a child, the nurse should:
    1. Apply ice packs to the site after the injection
    2. Rotate injections among the four extremities
    3. Firmly massage the site after withdrawal of the needle
    4. Change needles after drawing the drug into the syringe

248. A client who is 18 weeks pregnant and her 6-year-old child are prescribed tetracycline (Achromycin). Which of the following drug effects might cause the nurse to question the order?
    1. Changes in the bone structure of young children and pregnant women
    2. Persistent vomiting when given to small children and pregnant women
    3. Tooth enamel defects in children under 8 years of age and in the maturing fetus
    4. Lower red blood cell production at times in their development when anemia is a common problem

249. A 4-year-old has a seizure disorder and has been taking phenytoin (Dilantin) for 3 years. An important nursing measure for the child would be to:
    1. Offer the urinal frequently
    2. Check for pupillary reaction
    3. Observe for flushing of the face
    4. Administer scrupulous oral hygiene

250. A toddler is found playing with an open bottle of medication, and the mother is directed by the nurse to administer syrup of ipecac. Which of the following actions suggested by the nurse will enhance the effect of syrup of ipecac?
    1. Stimulating the gag reflex
    2. Resting until vomiting occurs
    3. Drinking 2 to 3 glasses of water
    4. Actively playing until vomiting occurs

251. A 9-year-old is about to have surgery. The physician orders meperidine (Demerol), 20 mg, IM preoperatively. The container reads "50 mg/ml." The nurse should administer:
    1. 0.4.ml
    2. 0.6 ml
    3. 0.8 ml
    4. 1.0 ml

Client Case Scenario 37: Charlie is a 7-year-old with acute leukemia. He is prescribed a chemotherapy regime that includes prednisone and methotrexate. **Items 252 to 254 refer to this client case scenario.**

252. Which of the following is the primary reason for using prednisone in the treatment of Charlie's acute leukemia?
    1. Decrease inflammation
    2. Enhance the drug effect
    3. Suppress mitosis in lymphocytes
    4. Increase appetite and sense of well-being

253. For which of the following side effects of prednisone should Charlie's nurse observe?
    1. Alopecia
    2. Anorexia
    3. Weight loss
    4. Mood changes

254. By prescribing methotrexate, Charlie's physician hopes to achieve which method of action?
    1. Acting as an antibiotic to control the spread of infected white blood cells
    2. Intervening in mitosis, thus inhibiting the growth of the malignant cells
    3. Depressing bone marrow function, thus decreasing white blood cell production
    4. Competing for essential structural components, thus inhibiting white blood cell production

255. Following a tonsillectomy, an 8-year-old is complaining of pain in the throat. The pain medication that would be best for the child at this time would be:
    1. Aspirin, 300 mg
    2. Tylenol, 300 mg
    3. Demerol, 50 mg
    4. Phenobarbital, 15 mg

256. Which of the following statements best explains the overall objective of drug therapy with lead poisoning?
    1. Reduce the concentration of lead in the blood and tissues
    2. Reverse the central nervous system effects of the uptake
    3. Enhance excretion of the lead from the osseous tissue
    4. Promote the transfer of the lead from the bones to the blood

257. Based on developmental norms for a 5-year-old, the nurse should withhold a scheduled dose of digoxin (Lanoxin) elixir and notify the physician if the child's apical pulse rate is below:
    1. 80 beats per minute
    2. 90 beats per minute
    3. 100 beats per minute
    4. 110 beats per minute

258. An 8-year-old with juvenile rheumatoid arthritis is receiving salicylate therapy. During the salicylate therapy the nurse should observe the child for:
    1. Nausea, dizziness, edema, headache
    2. Constipation, deafness, nausea, headache
    3. Gastric distress, nausea, vomiting, tinnitus
    4. Diarrhea, gastric distress, edema of the face

259. Which of the following drug classifications includes salicylates?
    1. Analgesic and sedative
    2. Antipyretic and hypnotic
    3. Antibiotic and antipyretic
    4. Analgesic and antipyretic

260. A 7-year-old female develops a urinary tract infection. The physician orders a sulfonamide preparation. A major nursing responsibility when administering this drug is to:
    1. Weigh the child daily
    2. Give milk with the medication
    3. Monitor the temperature frequently
    4. Administer the drug at the prescribed times

261. An adolescent is started on a chemotherapeutic drug regime that includes prednisone, vincristine, and L-asparaginase. Which of the following side effects of these drugs would likely cause this client the most immediate concern?
1. Anemia
2. Alopecia
3. Constipation
4. Growth retardation

262. A combination of drugs, which includes vincristine (Oncovin) and prednisone, is prescribed for a child with leukemia. Because of their toxicity the nurse should expect:
1. Anemia and fever
2. Irreversible alopecia
3. Neurologic symptoms
4. Intergumentary symptoms

PEDIATRIC NURSING
ANSWERS AND RATIONALES

Growth and Development

1. 2 **Muscular coordination and perception are developed enough at 6 months so the infant can roll over. If unaware of this ability of the infant, the mother could leave the child unattended for a moment to reach for something and the child could roll off the crib. (IM; ED; GD)**
  1 Sitting up unsupported is accomplished by most children at 7 to 8 months.
  3 Crawling takes place at about 9 months of age.
  4 Standing by holding on to furniture is accomplished by most children between 8 and 10 months.

2. 1 **Because of the infant's increasing mobility, high level of oral activity, and relative lack of fear or appreciation for danger, accidents are the primary cause of death in children above 1 year of age. (IM; ED; GD)**
  2 This is too early for discussions about toilet training.
  3 This is best discussed with the mother prenatally or soon after delivery.
  4 This is too early for discussions of psychosexual development.

3. 2 **Infants who have experienced maternal deprivation usually exhibit failure to thrive (i.e., weight below third percentile, developmental delay, clinical signs of deprivation, and malnutrition). These physical and emotional factors predispose the infant to a variety of illnesses. (DC; PS; ED)**
  1 Infants who have experienced maternal deprivation are usually quiet and nonresponsive.
  3 Responsiveness to stimuli is limited or nonexistent.
  4 Weight below the third percentile is characteristic.

4. 4 **The child experiencing long-term hospitalization is forced to relate to a variety of significant adults instead of to a single figure providing mothering. The lack of continuity creates anxiety. (AN; PS; GD)**
  1 Even with sufficient play objects, the child will still suffer from the lack of a mother figure.
  2 Even with sufficient sensory stimulation, the young child will still suffer from the lack of a mother figure.
  3 Consistent caregivers do not deprive hospitalized children.

5. 3 **Excessive crying and clinging are the usual responses of an infant who expects to be comforted, not one who has experienced prolonged separation from a parent because of illness. (DC; PS; EH)**
  1 Prolonged hospitalization and separation from parenting can cause delayed growth or even death in infants.
  2 Withdrawing active attention is the infant's way to "turn off" and may be learned from multiple failures in interactions with stimuli.
  4 Inattentiveness to focus may be learned from failure to gain response from humans in previous experiences.

6. 1 **A child learns to trust others by having his needs met in infancy. A child who has been maternally deprived is unlikely to have developed trust. (AN; PS; GD)**
  2 Studies do not address this issue.
  3 Same as answer 2.
  4 These children have difficulties forming attachments to people.

7. 1 **Walking is the primary developmental task of this age group. The other choices are not applicable to this age group. (AN; ED; GD)**
  2 The ability to drink from a cup is achieved between 6 and 12 months of age.
  3 A child learns to climb stairs at around 18 months of age.
  4 Learning to walk takes precedence over learning to talk; speaking is not a primary task at this age.

8. **2 At 15 months, strength and balance have improved, and an infant can stand and walk alone. (EV; ED; GD)**
   1 This is not usually true until the child is 2 years old.
   3 Infants are very capable of throwing toys.
   4 Children 9 to 12 months of age can stand with support.

9. **2 The psychosocial need during the early toddler age is the development of autonomy. The toddler objects strongly to discipline. (AN; ED; GD)**
   1 This is untrue; excessive discipline leads to feelings of shame and self-doubt, the major crisis at this stage of development.
   3 The sense of initiative is attained during the preschool age, not during the toddler age.
   4 It is frightening for a child to be left alone; it leaves the child with feelings of rejection, isolation, and insecurity.

10. **2 Common developmental norms of the toddler, who is struggling for independence, are inability to share easily, egotism, egocentrism, and possessiveness. (DC; PS; GD)**
    1 This task is too advanced for toddlers and more accurate for preschoolers.
    3 This is true of 4-year-olds.
    4 One characteristic of toddlers is their short attention span; 15 minutes is too much to expect.

11. **1 Rebecca is still dependent on the mother, is narcissistic, and still plays alone, but is aware of others playing nearby. (DC; ED; GD)**
    2 Solitary play or onlookers' play is characteristic of the 1- to 2-year-old.
    3 Competitive play would be seen in school-age children.
    4 Tumbling-type play is not a commonly accepted term used to refer to how play incorporates other children.

12. **2 Rebecca should be taken to the dentist between 2 and 3 years of age, when most of the 20 deciduous teeth have erupted. (IM; ED; GD)**
    1 This is too late.
    3 Same as answer 2.
    4 This is too indefinite.

13. **3 Children who are expressing negativism need to have a feeling of control. One way of achieving this within reasonable limits is for the parent or caregiver to provide a choice of two items, rather than force one on the child. (IM; ED; GD)**
    1 This will not achieve the goal of giving fluids.
    2 This will probably not be successful with a toddler; it will probably end in disaster.
    4 This will complicate the situation and further inhibit the child's willingness to take fluids.

14. **3 The nurse recognizes the child's protest over the mother's absence and tries to comfort by staying near until the child feels more relaxed. The bathing can be postponed until the child has had time to test out the environment and is less anxious. (IM; ED; GD)**
    1 This may frighten the child more.
    2 This action does not attempt to relieve the child's anxiety and will probably cause it to increase.
    4 This is probably true, although the nurse has not attempted to reduce anxiety.

15. **4 This is a task expected of the 3-year-old. (DC; ED; GD)**
    1 This is a task expected of the 4- or 5-year-old.
    2 This is a task expected of the 4-year-old.
    3 Same as answer 2.

16. **2 Because their verbal ability is limited, children act out their feelings via play. (IM; PS; GD)**
    1 Therapeutic play does not necessarily involve other children.
    3 Acceptance of the hospital situation is not as important as dealing with feelings.
    4 The child needs to cope with feelings rather than forget them.

17. **4 The parents' attitude, approach, and understanding of the child's physical and psychologic readiness are essential to letting the child proceed at his or her own pace with appropriate interventions by the parent. (PL; ED; GD)**
    1 This will not be the major motivation for toilet training.
    2 Although this will definitely be a factor, it is not a major one.
    3 This, of course, is a factor; but the major factor is the child, who is strongly influenced by the parents' attitudes and approach.

18. **3 A pounding board is a safe toy for toddlers, since it is fairly large, easy to manipulate, and sturdy. A pounding board provides a way for anger to be sublimated. (IM; PS; GD)**
   1 The child's motor and hand-eye coordination is too immature for using this.
   2 This would be appropriate for an older child with more mature motor coordination to compensate for a moving object.
   4 This is not as safe since toddlers may eat clay or Play-Doh.

19. **3 More information is needed; developmental delay suggests some milestone for age is not being met at the average time; it is not synonymous with developmental disability. (DC; ED; GD)**
   1 This would be inappropriate as more information must be obtained.
   2 Although the physician may help, it is not yet known if such a program is needed.
   4 The nurse does not know this without more information.

20. **4 Six-year-olds are aware of their hands as tools and enjoy building simple structures. (IM; ED; GD)**
   1 This is more appropriate for preschoolers.
   2 This is more useful for an older, school-age child, with a longer attention span and a better ability to follow instructions.
   3 Same as answer 2.

21. **2 Role playing encourages expression of feelings through behavior, since children's ability to verbalize feelings is limited. (AN; PS; GD)**
   1 This may occur, but it is not a purpose of role playing.
   3 The preschooler is too young to think about careers.
   4 Although preschoolers may try to imitate adults, providing guidelines for adult behavior is premature.

22. **3 Four-year-olds boast, exaggerate, and are impatient, noisy, and selfish. (EV; PS; GD)**
   1 Four-year-olds engage in more advanced cooperative play.
   2 This is highly unusual for 4-year-olds as they are striving toward more initiative and less dependence.
   4 The tendency toward tantrums and negativism should have waned by 4 years of age.

23. **4 Fear of mutilation and intrusive procedures is most common at this age because of fantasies and active imagination. These children also connect illness with being bad and view intrusion as punishment. (IM; PS; GD)**
   1 A child this age usually has little previous contact with pain and therefore little experience upon which to base fear.
   2 Death is seen as reversible and not final.
   3 Fear of isolation from peers is a problem for school-age children and adolescents.

24. **2 Piaget stresses that age 7 is the turning point in mental development. New forms of organization appear at this age that mark the beginning of logic, symbolism, and abstract thought. (AN; ED; GD)**
   1 A 5-year-old is capable of tying laces.
   3 A toddler is capable of making simple decisions.
   4 An infant is capable of hand-eye coordination.

25. **2 School-age children have an interest in hobbies or collections of various kinds as a means of gathering information and knowledge about the world in which they live. (PL; ED; GD)**
   1 This is too advanced for a normal 9-year-old.
   3 This would not interest a 9-year-old.
   4 These would probably not interest a 9-year-old.

26. **4 Since young children have difficulty verbalizing their fears or anxiety, play is a therapeutic way for these feelings to be expressed. The school-age child also likes to role play. (IM; PS; GD)**
   1 A child this age is unable to express feelings entirely through words.
   2 Young school-age children are still somewhat egocentric and therefore interested in their own experiences and sensations.
   3 This may be helpful for a toddler or preschooler.

PEDIATRIC ANSWERS

27. **3 Normally there may be a weight gain caused by the influence of hormones prior to the growth spurt. Also, 10- to 12-year-olds eat an adult-size meal without the increased metabolic needs of adolescence. (IM; ED; GD)**

1 Before advising increased activity, the nurse would need to assess the client's present activity level.

2 This weight gain is normal and adequate calorie intake is needed for the growth spurt occurring in adolescence.

4 Family eating patterns appear to have more effect on weight than do genetics.

Emotional Needs Related to Health Problems

28. **3 Because of a short attention span and distractibility, the specific limit setting consistently employed is crucial toward providing an environment that promotes concentration, prevents confusion, and minimizes conflicts for the child. (IM; PS; EH)**

1 Questions are appropriate as long as judgments are not made about the answers.

2 Some children have difficulty reading.

4 Parents need to manipulate the child's environment so it is simplified, controlled, and predictable.

29. **3 A pacifier should be given during the feeding to help the infant associate sucking with feeding and the sense of fullness. (IM; PS; EH)**

1 Irrigation may be used to reestablish patency of a blocked tube.

2 Instilling water after the feeding clears the tube.

4 Upright rather than semi-Fowler's position is essential to prevent regurgitation or reflux and subsequent aspiration.

30. **3 It is most important for an adolescent to be an active part of the peer group. Assure adolescent that activities do not need to change; allow continued peer membership. (IM; PS; EH)**

1 This will not meet a 13 year old's emotional needs.

2 A 13 year old will not need to make decisions.

4 Although this may be needed, it is unlikely to provide for the 13 year old's needs.

31. **1 Sucking is a primary need of infancy. It decreases anxiety and does not interfere with gastric decompression. (IM; PS; EH)**

2 This would be more helpful if the client were a toddler.

3 This will probably not help to calm the infant.

4 This will probably increase the pain from abdominal distention.

32. **1 Regression is normal in times of stress. It is a transient need that should be accepted, since it helps reduce anxiety. (IM; PS; EH)**

2 Distraction works only as long as it is employed.

3 This behavior is unrelated to medical progress.

4 Cause (thumb sucking) and future effect (buckteeth) will not be meaningful to a 6-year-old child.

33. **1 Assault is a threat or an attempt to do violence to another. (IM; ED; EH)**

2 This is not the appropriate legal definition of assault.

3 Assault implies harm to persons rather than property.

4 This definition is too broad to describe assault.

34. **3 Battery means touching in an offensive manner or the actual injuring of another person. (IM; ED; EH)**

1 Battery refers to harm against persons instead of property.

2 Battery refers to actual bodily harm rather than threats of physical or psychologic harm.

4 This definition is too broad to describe battery.

35. **2 Detachment is the result of trying to escape the emotional pain of desiring the mother by repressing feelings for her. (EV; PS; EH)**

1 This interpretation is not appropriate to the situation cited.

3 This conclusion cannot be drawn from the situation cited.

4 This response lacks insight.

36. **2 Assault is a threat or an attempt to do violence to another, and battery means touching an individual in an offensive manner or the actual injuring of another person. (EV; PS; EH)**

1 The nurse's behavior demonstrates anger and has not taken into account the growth and developmental needs of this age.

3 Although the behavior (scratching) needs to be decreased, this can be done through mittens so as not to immobilize a child of this age.

4 A 3-year-old does not have the capacity to understand cause (scratching) and effect (bleeding).

37. **2 If able to handle personal anxiety and give comfort to the child, parents can be a real help to the staff as well as the child. If the parents are extremely anxious, their anxiety can be transmitted, making the child even more anxious. (DC; PS; EH)**
   1 It is how the parents cope with the situation, rather than the situation itself, that helps determine how helpful their presence may be.
   3 Toddlers have limited experience with pain and will not likely be aware of a need for the parents prior to the procedure.
   4 Parents can be helpful to the child and the staff; they often want to participate in the child's care.

38. **2 A client cannot legally be isolated unless there is a threat of danger involved either to the client or to other clients. (EV; ED; EH)**
   1 This is a reaction to separation from the mother, which is common at this age. Limits are inappropriate.
   3 The action is illegal; not permitted for any length of time.
   4 Crying, although irritating, will not harm the other children.

39. **2 Fear of mutilation is typical of the older preschooler. (AN; PS; EH)**
   1 Toddlers and preschool children under 5 years of age fear separation from their parents.
   3 Preschoolers do not view death as final.
   4 Preschoolers have fantasies about supernatural beings. These fantasies may include bodily harm.

40. **3 A few minutes will be enough time for the child to begin self-feeding. The nurse should provide both physical and emotional support, since the child's request for help indicates the need for dependence during a period of stress. (IM; PS; EH)**
   1 It may be a while until the child feels better; in the meantime, adequate nourishment to provide for healing is needed.
   2 This does not provide the child the help that may be needed.
   4 A nurse should never make a statement like this; it can cause stress, feelings of guilt, and embarrassment to a sick child.

41. **1 Dinner is frequently a family activity. Having the parents visit during meals may provide the child with additional emotional, social, and physical support, resulting in an improved nutritional intake. (PL; TC; EH)**
   2 If given full rein, a young child will not select the most nutritional foods.
   3 This will further inhibit the child's nutritional intake.
   4 This may not influence the child's overall intake.

42. **4 Decision making fosters and supports independence, a developmental need of the adolescent. It also increases a sense of self-worth and control. (IM; PS; EH)**
   1 This does not ensure movement but social interaction.
   2 Although this may be true, it is not motivating.
   3 Limit setting meets the security needs of young children.

Respiratory

43. **4 A patent airway is the first priority, and necessary equipment must be immediately available. (PL; PA; RE)**
   1 Although this would be helpful, it is not the priority.
   2 Convulsions are not necessarily associated with croup; respiratory promotion is the priority.
   3 Although appropriate, this is not the priority.

44. **2 Laryngeal spasms can occur abruptly; patency of airway is determined by constant assessment for symptoms of respiratory distress. (DC; PA; RE)**
   1 This is important, but maintenance of respiration has priority.
   3 Same as answer 1.
   4 Same as answer 1.

45. **2 The second stage of separation anxiety is despair, in which the child is depressed, lonely, and disinterested in the surroundings. (EV; PS; EH)**
   1 The third stage of separation, denial or detachment, is a more advanced stage than that demonstrated in the situation.
   3 Separation anxiety does not include a stage of mistrust.
   4 Separation anxiety does not include a stage of rejection.

PEDIATRIC ANSWERS

46. **4 Sally is in Erikson's stage of acquiring a sense of autonomy. The negativism is the result of the child's need to express her will and test out her environment. (IM; ED; GD)**

1 This is the developmental task achieved in infancy.

2 Although this is a factor, toddlers assert themselves in an attempt to attain more autonomy.

3 Children do not assert themselves to obtain discipline.

47. **3 When the causative organism is isolated, it is tested for antimicrobial susceptibility (sensitivity) to various antimicrobial agents. When an organism is sensitive to a medication, the medication is capable of destroying the organism. (DC; TC; RE)**

1 Although this is considered, the selection of drugs is based primarily on the ability of the drug to destroy the specific organism.

2 This is an inappropriate answer.

4 Although the physician's preference is considered, the selection of drugs is based primarily on the ability of the drug to destroy the specific organism.

48. **1 Rest reduces the need for oxygen and minimizes metabolic needs during the acute, febrile stage of the disease. (AN; TC; RE)**

2 The child with pneumonia is usually confined to bed and needs to reduce activity to conserve oxygen.

3 This is not a priority, and Jason will be anorectic during the febrile phase.

4 Elimination is not usually a problem except as a result of immobility.

49. **1 Nonstrenuous, diversional activities involving interpersonal relationships with another person provide better support and resting conditions than does more active play. (PL; PA; RE)**

2 A jigsaw puzzle is too complicated for a 6-year-old and does not provide the human contact needed.

3 This will probably increase Jason's anxiety and does not provide the human contact needed.

4 Although a toy car may be appropriate for a 6-year-old, it does not provide the human contact needed.

50. **2 Regression is the retreat to a past level of behavior as a way of minimizing stress or controlling anxiety. Increased dependence, such as being fed by another person, is a form of regression. (AN; PS; EH)**

1 Although Jason may be anorexic, this statement more likely reflects a psychological need.

3 Jason's statement does not reflect immaturity.

4 Jason's statement can hardly be construed as a temper tantrum.

51. **3 Grunting and rapid respirations are abnormal behaviors in an infant. Grunting is a compensatory mechanism whereby an infant attempts to keep air in the alveoli to increase arterial oxygenation; increased respirations increase oxygen and carbon dioxide exchange. (DC; TC; RE)**

1 Sweating in infants is usually scanty because of immature functioning of the exocrine glands; profuse sweating is rarely seen in the sick infant.

2 This is not necessarily a sign of illness.

4 This is not necessarily indicative of illness.

52. **2 This allows air to circulate around the drying cord and permits the drainage of secretions if the infant regurgitates. (IM; ED; RE)**

1 This could result in aspiration if regurgitation occurs.

3 Same as answer 1.

4 This position has been associated with the incidence of SIDS and should be avoided.

53. **3 School-age children lose their primary teeth, which could be aspirated during surgery. The anesthesiologist must take special precautions to maintain client safety. (IM; TC; RE)**

1 There is no reason to obtain an ASO titer on the client.

2 This is a comforting gesture but is not essential.

4 This is important but not essential and not always possible.

54. **4 Respiratory tract obstructions usually occur in the larynx, trachea, or major bronchi (usually right). Hoarseness may indicate vocal cord injury. Unintelligible speech may indicate an interference in the flow of air out of the respiratory tract and/or obstruction or injury to the larynx. (DC; TC; RE)**
    1 A retropharyngeal abscess would not produce the clinical signs listed.
    2 Acute respiratory infection usually has a gradual onset.
    3 In view of the sudden onset of clinical signs and the age of the child, this is unlikely.

55. **2 Choanal atresia is a lack of an opening between one or both of the nasal passages and the nasopharynx. (AN; PA; RE)**
    1 Rectal atresia involves the rectum's ending in a pouch and the normal anal canal's opening into the other (nonconnected) end of the rectum.
    3 Atresias associated with the GI tract include esophageal and intestinal atresia involving the ileum, jejunum, or colon.
    4 An atresia involving the pharynx and larynx is not commonly seen, and is not choanal atresia.

56. **2 A patent airway and adequate pulmonary ventilation are always priorities after surgery. (DC; PA; RE)**
    1 It is too soon for output to be a priority; however, it certainly must be assessed later.
    3 This is important, but adequate ventilation is the priority.
    4 The IV lines would be checked once the airway, breathing, and circulation are determined to be functioning well.

57. **4 The first usual indication of cystic fibrosis is meconium ileus. The small intestine is blocked with a thick, tenacious, mucilaginous meconium, usually near the ileocecal valve. This causes intestinal obstruction with abdominal distention, vomiting, and fluid and electrolyte imbalance. (DC; PA; RE)**
    1 This does not have special significance in cystic fibrosis.
    2 This is not an early sign of cystic fibrosis.
    3 Same as answer 1.

58. **4 Cystic fibrosis is characterized by an overproduction of viscid mucus by exocrine glands in the lungs. The mucus traps bacteria and foreign debris that adheres to the lining and cannot be expelled by the**
cilia, thus obstructing the airway and favoring growth of organisms and infection. **(AN; PA; RE)**
    1 Neuromuscular irritability of the bronchi does not occur in cystic fibrosis.
    2 Although there is increased sodium and chloride in the saliva, it does not irritate or necrose mucous membranes.
    3 Cardiac defects are not associated with cystic fibrosis.

59. **4 Pulmonary hygiene is done midway between feedings to lessen vomiting and increase drainage for suctioning. (IM; TC; RE)**
    1 Doing pulmonary hygiene at this time may cause the infant to vomit the feeding.
    2 Doing pulmonary hygiene at this time will tire the infant and possibly lead to an impaired nutritional intake.
    3 This is inadvisable; the infant may vomit and nutritional intake will be impaired.

60. **2 Pancreatic enzymes are given as replacement because of the lack of their production by the pancreas. Antibiotics are prescribed to prevent and control respiratory tract infection. (PL; TC; GI)**
    1 These are not indicated in the treatment of cystic fibrosis.
    3 Mists may be used but are not as vital as pancreatic enzymes and antibiotics; fat-soluble vitamins must be given in water-miscible preparations; decongestants provide little relief.
    4 These may be used but are not specific for cystic fibrosis.

61. **2 Isoniazid (INH) is the most potent tuberculostatic drug available at this time. It is given in conjunction with rifampin or with paraaminosalicylic acid (PAS), since a regimen involving two or more drugs is found to be more effective. (PL; TC; RE)**
    1 Bacille Calmette-Guérin (BCG) vaccine is the only successful vaccine for tuberculosis to date, but greater protection is afforded by daily prophylactic administration of INH.
    3 Old tuberculin is one type of skin test used to detect tuberculosis.
    4 Purified protein derivative (PPD) is a widely used skin test for detecting tuberculosis.

62. **1 Tubercle bacilli multiply in caseous lesions, which have a poor vascular supply. These areas receive lower levels of the drugs, and as a result therapy must be prolonged. (PL; TC; RE)**
    2 This time period is too long.
    3 The length of therapy is insufficient to eradicate the bacilli.
    4 Because lower levels of drug reach caseous lesions, longer treatment periods are needed.

63. **2 Family members who have been exposed are at high risk and should receive prophylactic therapy with INH and PAS. (PL; TC; RE)**
    1 Symptoms generally do not contribute significantly to a diagnosis of tuberculosis.
    3 Tubercle bacilli are not responsive to penicillin treatment.
    4 Too frequent; in addition prophylactic therapy should be started.

64. **4 The atelectasis that occurs with RDS increases the effort of breathing for the infant. The retractions of the sternum with inspiration demonstrate the increased work of breathing as well as the immaturity of the musculature and the cartilaginous skeleton. (DC; PA; RE)**
    1 The flaccidity of the infant is a later sign.
    2 The infant would have tachypnea rather than bradypnea, in an attempt to increase oxygenation.
    3 Hypoxemia is a later sign, as the child is unable to maintain an adequate gas exchange.

65. **2 These children frequently have difficulty in handling secretions as well as breathing after surgery. Nursing measures such as using the partial side-lying position or gently aspirating secretions from the mouth or nasopharynx may be necessary to prevent aspiration and respiratory complications. (IM; TC; RE)**
    1 Although this is important, maintaining a patent airway is essential.
    3 Fluids are usually administered carefully by mouth.
    4 This is not necessary.

66. **3 Following a thoracotomy, negative intrathoracic pressure is reestablished and the alveoli reexpand within 12 to 48 hours. (EV; PA; RE)**
    1 This time is inadequate for reexpansion to occur.
    2 This time is inadequate for expecting reexpansion.
    4 In most instances, reexpansion will occur sooner than 48 hours; 72 hours is too prolonged.

67. **4 The seeping of blood from the operative site increases secretions, which the child adapts to by swallowing frequently. (EV; TC; RE)**
    1 Snoring can be expected in a child who is postoperative from a tonsillectomy.
    2 This may be a later sign of hemorrhage. Frequent swallowing would be an initial sign.
    3 The child has been NPO for an extended time and is not able to ingest fluids easily because of a sore throat; the child will probably be thirsty.

68. **2 In cystic fibrosis the mucous glands secrete thick mucoid secretions that accumulate, reducing ciliary action and mucus flow. Expectoration is greatly hindered. Postural drainage promotes the removal of mucopurulent secretions by means of gravity. (IM; PA; RE)**
    1 Coughing should be encouraged.
    3 The nurse should encourage activities appropriate for the child's physical capacity; this will include helping the child conserve energy during acute phases of illness.
    4 This is not necessary with cystic fibrosis.

69. **1 Xanthines can cause either hypotension or tachycardia. It would be essential for the nurse to monitor her cardiovascular response to the drug. This is best done by assessing her baseline vital signs prior to and with administration. (IM; PA; RE)**
    2 Moisture is often contraindicated for children with asthma.
    3 Temperature changes are not related to aminophylline administration.
    4 Oxygen therapy is not associated with drug administration.

70. **1 Prednisone causes atrophy of the thymus; decreases the number of lymphocytes, plasma cells, and eosinophils in the blood; and decreases the formation of antibodies. Therefore it reduces the individual's resistance to certain infectious processes and**

viral diseases. Also, prednisone is an anti-inflammatory drug that masks infection. (IM; TC; DR)

2 The child will limit own activity based upon the respiratory status.

3 Eosinophil counts are often consistently elevated in children with asthma.

4 The child will need adequate hydration to assist with loosening and removing mucus from the lungs.

71. **2 Bed-wetting accidents are not uncommon in this age group, especially during hospitalization when regression may occur. Therefore the best approach is to ignore the event. (IM; PS; GD)**

1 The child may interpret this as punishment. Punishment for regressive behavior is inappropriate.

3 Rubber sheets are contraindicated; they would hold moisture close to the skin.

4 This may tend to make the child feel guilty for the behavior.

72. **3 Cold can precipitate bronchospasm, and increased exercise depletes oxygen. (PL; ED; RE)**

1 Treatment of asthma does not involve a high-fat diet.

2 Although increased calories may be needed to support the child during a coexisting bacterial infection in the acute stage, by discharge a return to usual habits is indicated.

4 Asthma is a chronic condition. Return to usual activities after the acute stage is essential for normal growth and development.

Reproductive and Genitourinary

73. **1 Mumps can cause orchitis (inflammation of the testes) in males and oophoritis (inflammation of the ovaries) in females. Although rare, both can render the post-pubescent child sterile. (IM; TC; RG)**

2 This symptom is not associated with mumps.

3 Same as answer 2.

4 Same as answer 2.

74. **4 The hypothalamic-pituitary-gonadal-adrenal mechanism is responsible for the physiologic and structural changes that occur at puberty. In girls the adrenal glands secrete**

androgens that are responsible for the appearance of axillary and pubic hair, generally between 11 and 14 years of age. Menarche usually occurs 2 years after initial pubescent changes. (DC; PA; RG)

1 This is not an indicator of sexual maturity.

2 This is not an indicator of early sexual maturity in females.

3 This is not an appropriate indicator of sexual maturity in females.

75. **2 Renal biopsy is an invasive procedure. In early stages, Wilms' tumor is encapsulated. Any disruption of the tumor capsule would allow metastasis. (EV; TC; RG)**

1 IVP is helpful in making a diagnosis.

3 Surgical removal of the involved kidney is the preferred treatment, not diagnosis.

4 Abdominal CT scan is helpful in making a diagnosis.

76. **1 A bland, high-protein, high-carbohydrate snack provides adequate nutrition in the face of infection and fever. In addition, the child should have an increased fluid intake. (PL; PA; RG)**

2 This does not provide the protein needed for the healing process.

3 These are empty calories.

4 This is too heavy for a between-meal snack and contains fats, which are not helpful in the healing process.

77. **3 Infection is a constant threat because of a poor general state of nutrition, a tendency toward skin breakdown in edematous areas, corticosteroid therapy, and lowered immunoglobulin levels. (IM; TC; RG)**

1 Fluid monitoring, not encouraging, is important in determining whether restriction is indicated.

2 The nurse should encourage intake of foods with high nutritional value and restrict salt during massive edema; the priority is preventing infection.

4 Bed rest may be used for severe stages, but generally ambulation is encouraged.

78. **2 This is an extremely vascular area and the infant must be closely observed for bleeding. (IM; TC; RG)**
    1 It is too soon to observe for signs of infection.
    3 Generally the infant is not too uncomfortable after circumcision; this may, with other signs, be indicative of central nervous system difficulty.
    4 Urinary output is assessed, but is not the most essential nursing action in the initial postoperative period.

79. **4 The decreased filtration of plasma in the glomeruli results in an excess accumulation of water and sodium, producing edema that is first evident around the eyes. Hypertension is thought to be due to hypervolemia, although its exact cause is unclear. (DC; TC; RG)**
    1 Neither of these is a sign of acute glomerulonephritis.
    2 Oliguria is not found with acute glomerulonephritis. The client is usually hypertensive.
    3 Although hematuria is found, dehydration is not a sign of acute glomerulonephritis.

80. **4 During the acute stage, anorexia and the loss of protein lower the child's resistance to infection. (PL; TC; RG)**
    1 Antibiotics are not necessary for all children with acute glomerulonephritis, only those with persistent streptococcal infections.
    2 A bland diet is not necessary, and high protein should be avoided.
    3 Bed rest is necessary only during the most acute stage; 4 weeks is too long.

81. **1 Daily changes in weight are good indicators of fluid changes; loss or gain of muscle and fat do not usually cause apparent daily fluctuations in weight. (IM; ED; RG)**
    2 Disease cessation would be associated with weight loss, not gain.
    3 Protein molecules do not weigh enough to be reflected in the child's weight on a daily basis.
    4 It is not beneficial to plan the child's daily caloric intake on weight loss or gain.

82. **4 When urinary findings are normal, such as no evidence of hematuria or proteinuria, the child may resume pre-illness activities. (EV; TC; RG)**
    1 This restriction is unnecessary.
    2 Same as answer 1.
    3 Bed rest is unnecessary at this stage.

Neuromuscular

83. **4 The virus for polio damages the anterior horn cells of the spinal cord with a typical irregular and asymmetric pattern. The cervical and lumbar regions contain more anterior horn cells, and therefore the extremities are more frequently affected than the trunk. (AN; PA; NM)**
    1 The virus for rubella does not affect the motor cells of the anterior horn of the spinal cord.
    2 The virus for rubeola does not affect the motor cells of the anterior horn of the spinal cord.
    3 The virus for chickenpox does not affect the motor cells of the anterior horn of the spinal cord.

84. **2 When taking a health history, any areas of concern should be explored fully before a nursing diagnosis is made. (DC; PS; NM)**
    1 The nurse needs to gather more data to be able to determine the basis for the problem.
    3 Data are inadequate to focus immediately on nutrition.
    4 More data are needed before recommendations can be made.

85. **3 Touching the palms of the hands causes flexion of the fingers (grasp reflex); this usually lessens after 3 months of age. (IM; ED; NM)**
    1 These changes are consistent with normal growth and development. Neurological examination is not needed.
    2 The data do not support making this comment and would cause needless concern.
    4 Sensory stimulation at this age is directed toward experiences to add new motor, language, and social skills, not at primitive reflexes.

86. **4 The angle the wrist forms with the arm decreases as gestation increases; the angle is zero at term. (DC; ED; NM)**
    1 Lanugo is characteristic of premature infants. At term, infants have at least half of their back devoid of lanugo.
    2 Term infants usually have descended testes.
    3 In immature infants the ears contain little cartilage and are very springy when folded; at term the ears contain cartilage and the pinna is firm.

87. **2 Since part of a nurse's responsibility is to foresee potential harm and prevent risks, it is imperative that the nurse not only take a health history and perform a phys-**

ical assessment on each client, but act to
ensure the safety of the client. (EV; TC; NM)
1 This is not true and cannot be accepted as a
rationale for inaction.
3 The nurse and physician share interdependent
roles in the assessment and care of clients.
4 High temperatures are common in children
but are nonetheless a valid cause for concern.

88. 1 **Febrile convulsions are not necessarily
associated with major neurologic problems but often accompany fever. Such
convulsions may be partially accounted
for by the overall brain immaturity in
children. (PL; ED; NM)**
2 The cause of febrile convulsions is still uncertain.
3 Febrile convulsions are more common in the
infant and young toddler.
4 Boys are affected about twice as often as girls.

89. 4 **The nurse should remain, observe, and
protect the child from injury during the
seizure activity. (IM; TC; NM)**
1 Useless until the seizure is over; child is apneic during seizure.
2 Contraindicated; attempts at inserting a
tongue blade are futile; this could damage the
child's teeth and jaws.
3 Never restrain an individual during a seizure;
fractured bones or torn muscles and ligaments
can result.

90. 3 **This is what occurs in communicating
hydrocephalus. (IM; ED; NM)**
1 This is often caused by a choroid plexus tumor
and does not interfere with the flow of cerebrospinal fluid through the ventricles.
2 This reflects the pathophysiologic process of
noncommunicating hydrocephalus.
4 This is an inaccurate answer; brain cells and
the spinal cord are not involved.

91. 4 **Cellular destruction occurs as the brain is
compressed against the skull. This occludes
blood vessels and deprives the cells of oxygen. (AN; PA; NM)**
1 The increased CSF does not dilute the blood
supply; pressure on vessels diminishes the blood
supply, causing atrophy and death of cells.
2 Oxygen deprivation occurs when blood vessels are occluded secondary to the pressure in
the skull caused by hydrocephalus.
3 Hydrocephalus results when CSF is produced

in too great quantities or is not adequately circulated or absorbed; there is no change in the
fluid tonicity.

92. 2 **Shunts need to be revised; as the child
grows, the length of tubing needs to be
changed. The shunts are also prone to
malfunction and may need revision. (IM;
ED; NM)**
1 Although treatment of hydrocephalus by shunt
replacement is quite successful, there is danger
of malfunction and infection of the shunt.
3 Damage to brain cells is irreversible.
4 Hydrocephalus necessitates treatment for the
life of the child. It is not self-limiting.

93. 1 **Sucking meets oral needs, which are primary during infancy. (IM; PS; GD)**
2 Matthew is probably too young to focus well
on a mobile.
3 Matthew is not yet developmentally capable
of enjoying a soft, cuddly toy.
4 This is not a developmental need.

94. 1 **Hearing is a sense that is not greatly
influenced by emotional response in the
young child. (AN; PA; NM)**
2 The emotional trauma of institutionalization may influence the child's cognitive development.
3 The trauma of institutionalization may also
result in speech and other expressive delays.
4 Institutionalized children often manifest
delays in neuromuscular development.

95. 2 **A 10-month-old is unable to comply with
directions to remain still and may be
extremely frightened by the equipment
used. (IM; TC; NM)**
1 This is not necessary; head must remain still
but need not be shaved.
3 This is not necessary unless a contrast medium
is being used.
4 The child is too young to understand details.

96. 4 Cyanosis is expected because the child will not breathe until the tonic-clonic phase of the convulsion is over. Observation and prevention of injury are the priorities at this time. (IM; TC; NM)

1 Insertion of a foreign body into the mouth during the tonic-clonic phase of a convulsion may cause injury.
2 Same as answer 1.
3 This is useless until the child breathes.

97. 1 Cardiac anomalies often accompany other genetic problems such as Down syndrome; 30% to 40% of these infants have congenital heart defects. (DC; PA; NM)

2 No need for special evaluation; routine assessment would be sufficient.
3 Same as answer 2.
4 Same as answer 2.

98. 2 This helps and encourages parents to put their fears and feelings into words. Once these sentiments are expressed, they can at least be examined and dealt with. (IM; PS; EH)

1 This would not assist the parents in coping with the problem. Neither would it demonstrate the supportive and empathetic roles of the nurse.
3 This response lacks insight. Parents will worry about their infant anyway.
4 This may or may not be helpful.

99. 2 A meningomyelocele sac is thinly covered and can be partially open, allowing a portal of entry for organisms directly to the CNS. The sac should be protected. (AN; TC; NM)

1 Although this is always an important nursing measure, care of the sac is even more important.
3 Although observation of paralysis is an important nursing measure, care of the meningomyelocele sac is of primary importance.
4 A meningomyelocele will influence the client's ability to control these functions, but control is not developed until the toddler and preschool years.

100. 3 The surgical closure of the sac decreases absorptive surface and eliminates a route by which the spinal fluid drains. Skull bones are soft and will expand as fluid increases with hydrocephalus. (EV; TC; NM)

1 Most infants with meningomyelocele are partially or completely paralyzed in the lower extremities; careful range-of-motion exercises are one of the important parts of nursing care for these infants.
2 There is no reason to decrease environmental stimuli for infants with hydrocephalus unless they also have seizures.
4 This is not expected since damage to the meninges of the brain is not a factor in the surgical treatment of meningomyelocele.

101. 4 Amy is not in a developmental stage where fears related to sexuality are present. These concerns are not age appropriate. (IM; ED; GD)

1 A "clean catch" at this age is often contaminated; the physician ordered a catheterization.
2 The mother does have the right to refuse but concerns are not realistic for this age infant.
3 The mother's concern is not appropriate for the developmental age of the infant.

102. 4 Braces are used to enable the spastic child to control motions. They also prevent deformities from poor alignment. (AN; PA; NM)

1 Early ambulation is promoted by maintaining muscle strength and tone.
2 Since the child is at the age when self-reliance is important (Erikson's stage of industry versus inferiority) and is dependent on the braces for self-care, it is unlikely that they would be rejected.
3 Exercises are used to stretch ligaments and improve muscle strength and tone.

103. 1 Clients whose thermoreceptive senses are impaired are unable to detect changes or degrees of temperature. They must be taught to test the temperature in any water-related activity to prevent scalding and burning. (IM; ED; NM)

2 Overtightening straps and buckles may lead to circulatory impairment and/or skin breakdown.
3 The child with cerebral palsy normally has uncontrolled movement of voluntary muscles that makes it unnecessary to reposition on a schedule.
4 This is dangerous, as this action alters the center of gravity; with practice the child will be able to place the legs in the appropriate position for walking without looking down.

104. **1 The damage is fixed. It does not progressively increase. (AN; PA; NM)**
  2 Although intellectual impairment may be present in some children with cerebral palsy, it cannot be assumed that all children with this disorder are mentally retarded.
  3 Cerebral palsy is a nonprogressive chronic condition.
  4 The etiology of cerebral palsy is related to anoxia in the prenatal, perinatal, or postnatal periods and is not genetic.

105. **1 A practically universal characteristic of these children is distractibility. They are highly reactive to any extraneous stimuli such as noise and movement and are unable to inhibit their responses to such stimuli. (AN; PS; NM)**
  2 Repetition in language or movement may be seen; rituals are uncommon.
  3 Delayed development of language skills is seen in varying degrees and may include dyslexia (reading difficulty), dysgrammatism (speaking difficulty), dysgraphia (writing difficulty), or delayed talking.
  4 Learning disabilities associated with minimal brain dysfunction are manifested in a variety of ways; loss of abstract thought is not a universal characteristic.

106. **3 Shivering increases the metabolic rate, which intensifies the body's need for oxygen and raises the body temperature. (PL; TC; NM)**
  1 Fluids should be encouraged.
  2 Although monitoring output will provide information about the child's level of hydration, it is more important to take affirmative action toward preventing increases in fever.
  4 Monitoring vital signs is not as important as taking affirmative action to prevent increases in fever.

107. **2 Meningococcal meningitis is identified by its epidemic nature and purpuric skin rash. (DC; TC; NM)**
  1 This is not characteristic of meningococcal meningitis.
  3 The fever of meningitis is usually high.
  4 Same as answer 1.

108. **3 Peripheral circulatory collapse (Waterhouse-Friderichsen syndrome) is a serious complication of meningococcal meningitis due to bilateral adrenal hemorrhage. The resultant acute adrenocortical insufficiency causes profound shock, petechiae and ecchymotic lesions, vomiting, prostration, and hypotension. (AN; TC; NM)**
  1 Although this may occur, it is controllable and not as serious as peripheral circulatory collapse.
  2 Although this may occur, it is not as serious a complication as peripheral circulatory collapse.
  4 Although this may occur, it is rare and not as serious as peripheral circulatory collapse.

109. **3 The nurse's data collection was not adequate because no questions were asked concerning the recency of the previous tetanus inoculation. The nurse failed to support the life and well-being of a client. (EV; TC; NM)**
  1 This is usually a clinical decision.
  2 The nurse's assessment was not thorough in regard to determining the recency of immunization.
  4 It was essential to determine the recency of the immunization; for a "tetanus-prone" wound, like a puncture from a rusty nail, some form of tetanus immunization is usually given.

110. **1 The slightest stimulation sets off a wave of very severe and very painful muscle spasms involving the whole body. Nerve impulses cross the myoneural junction and stimulate muscle contraction due to the presence of exotoxins produced by *Clostridium tetani*. (PL; TC; NM)**
  2 Body alignment is not an important consideration in tetanus.
  3 Oral intake of fluids may not be possible because of excessive secretions and laryngospasm.
  4 Monitoring output is not a major nursing concern with tetanus.

111. **3 Amblyopia is reduced visual acuity that may occur when an eye weakened by strabismus is not forced to function. (AN; TC; NM)**
  1 The lack of binocularity could result in impaired depth and spatial perceptions, not dyslexia.
  2 Depth and spatial perceptions are impaired when vision in one eye is severely impaired.
  4 Only vision in the affected eye will be diminished.

112. **4 The exact reason is unknown, but three factors appear to influence it: a child prone to pica, lead in the environment, and a lack of supervision. (DC; PA; NM)**
   1 The role of the caregiver is only one of the three etiologic factors.
   2 The environment is only one of the three etiologic factors.
   3 A child prone to pica is only one of the three etiologic factors.

113. **4 Damage to the central nervous system is irreversible. (AN; PA; NM)**
   1 Damage to kidneys is reversible with treatment.
   2 Skeletal changes are not significant and are reversible as lead leaves the body.
   3 Effects of lead in bone marrow are reversible when lead is mobilized for excretion in urine or deposition in bone by chelation therapy.

114. **1 Applying moist or dry heat relieves muscle pain through vasodilation, increasing circulation to the area and facilitating drug absorption. (AN; TC; NM)**
   2 This will prolong the discomfort by slowing the rate of absorption of the drug by vasoconstriction.
   3 This will cause more discomfort when the injection site is tender.
   4 Movement will most likely be difficult and cause more discomfort.

115. **2 Irreversible neurologic and intellectual damage are the most serious consequences of lead intoxication because of cortical atrophy and lead encephalopathy; protecting the child from injury is the priority. (AN; TC; NM)**
   1 Although constipation can occur, it is not the priority.
   3 Although this could be true, there is not enough information to conclude that altered parenting is the etiology of this nursing diagnosis.
   4 Anemia occurs because lead is toxic to the biosynthesis of heme, not because of an inadequate intake of iron.

116. **2 Gluteal folds should be symmetric, as should all planes and folds of the body. An abnormality of the hips will cause asymmetry and/or a shorter leg on the affected side. (DC; PA; SK)**
   1 The dance reflex is not affected.
   3 In congenital hip dysplasia there is usually a limited abduction of the leg at the hip.
   4 The affected side is shorter.

117. **4 Hypostatic pneumonia can develop from decreased activity. Also the cast prevents full chest expansion. (IM; ED; SK)**
   1 This is not necessary or desirable.
   2 Soiling of the cast with excreta, although problematic, is not a serious complication.
   3 Cast damage, although problematic, is not a serious complication.

118. **4 Pillows under the head or shoulders of a child in a spica cast will thrust the chest forward against the cast, causing discomfort and respiratory distress. Therefore, when elevation of the head is desired, the entire mattress and spring should be raised at the head of the bed. (IM; TC; SK)**
   1 This will not help in any way.
   2 There is no reason to place a time limit on this position.
   3 This will thrust the chest forward against the cast, causing discomfort and respiratory distress.

119. **3 A respiratory rate below 30 in the young infant is not within the normal range; normal is 30 to 60 breaths per minute; a drop below 30 per minute is a significant change and should have been reported. (EV; TC; SK)**
   1 Regularity of respiration is not the concern, the drop in rate is the significant data.
   2 This is untrue; more likely respirations will accelerate when discomfort is increased.
   4 The respiratory tract is fully developed, and respiratory rate is a cardinal sign of the infant's well-being.

120. **4 The principle of Bryant's traction is bilateral 90° hip flexion. It is skin traction applied to the legs to decrease the fracture, maintain alignment, and immobilize both legs. (AN; TC; SK)**
   1 Bryant's traction is always applied bilaterally.
   2 Bryant's traction requires the supine position.
   3 Skeletal traction is applied to a pin in the affected extremity.

121. **3 A plaster cast is not flexible and can inhibit circulation. Cold toes, loss of sensation in toes, pain, and inability to move toes should be reported to the physician immediately. (EV; TC; SK)**
   1 The normal pulse for a 9-year-old ranges from 70 to 110.
   2 This may be related to increased fluid intake.
   4 It takes 24 to 48 hours for a plaster cast to dry.

122. **3 The nurse made the assessment that the medication was ineffective in relieving the child's pain for the duration ordered. This information should be communicated to the physician for evaluation. (IM; TC; SK)**

1 There are no data to support this. The amount of medication was probably inadequate for the client's pain tolerance level.

2 The nurse should not ignore the client's need for pain relief.

4 The physician's order is for administration only every 3 to 4 hours. Legally it can be given only within these guidelines.

123. **1 An individual is legally unable to sign a consent until the age of consent. The only exception is the emancipated minor, a minor who is self-sufficient or married. (AN; ED; EH)**

2 Although the adolescent is capable of intelligent choices, it is the legality, not the acceptability or intelligence of the choice, that is at issue.

3 Parents or guardians are legally responsible under all circumstances unless the adolescent is an emancipated minor.

4 Adolescents have the capacity to choose between alternatives, but not the legal right in this situation.

124. **3 The hyperextension required in swimming aids in strengthening back muscles and increases deeper respirations, both of which are necessary prior to surgery and/or wearing a brace or cast. (IM; TC; SK)**

1 This will not be especially therapeutic for a child with this condition.

2 Same as answer 1.

4 Same as answer 1.

125. **3 Continuing growth causes changes in muscle, bone structure, and position. Adolescents have a rapid growth spurt. The brace is worn for 6 months after physical maturity, which is proved by x-ray examination to show cessation of bone growth. (IM; ED; SK)**

1 This is not an appropriate criterion for removal of the brace.

2 Pain is not usually a symptom of scoliosis.

4 The brace is used to halt the progression of the curvature, not correct it.

126. **2 Although there is a time range, there is no specific time for a developmental task. (AN; ED; GD)**

1 Tasks are more often learned in spurts than in a uniform, predictable rhythm.

3 Children differ in the ages at which they learn tasks.

4 The entire life cycle requires the learning of developmental tasks.

Endocrine

127. **4 Peak action of regular insulin is 2 to 4 hours; peak action of isophane suspension (NPH) insulin is 6 to 8 hours. (AN; PA; EN)**

1 Regular insulin duration is 6 to 8 hours.

2 Regular insulin onset is 30 minutes to 1 hour; isophane suspension (NPH) insulin onset is 1 to 2 hours.

3 The regular insulin effects will be decreasing.

128. **3 An insulin-dependent diabetic client must carry a source of concentrated glucose (glucose tablets, sugar-containing candy such as Lifesavers) as a rapid source of carbohydrate in the event of signs of hypoglycemia; this should be followed by a complex carbohydrate and a protein. (IM; ED; EN)**

1 This is an unrealistic and unnatural pattern for an adolescent.

2 This is an unnecessary and a time-consuming procedure.

4 The client should be made to feel a part of the family; the diabetic diet will have foods that will be nutritious for the entire family.

129. **1 The acquiring of knowledge or understanding aids in developing concepts rather than skills or attitudes and is a basic learning task in the cognitive domain. (AN; ED; EN)**

2 The acquiring of values and self-realization are in the affective domain.

3 The acquiring of skills and tasks is psychomotor learning.

4 Same as answer 3.

130. **4** Helping families understand their feelings about diabetes is essential in assisting them to develop positive attitudes for optimal control of the disease and promotion of a normal life for the child. (PL; PS; EN)
    1 This is important; however, if feelings are not dealt with first, compliance with insulin injections is less likely.
    2 Instruction in specific psychomotor tasks should be preceded by an assessment of the family's acceptance of the diagnosis and knowledge about the disease.
    3 The client should participate in activities normal for the age group. Adequate exercise is an important part of the treatment regimen for diabetes.

131. **4** The goiter associated with this disease (Hashimoto's disease) is usually transient and regresses spontaneously in a year or two; the client is usually euthyroid but may be slightly hypo- or hyperthyroid. (IM; ED; EN)
    1 This is not a chronic disease.
    2 There seems to be a strong genetic predisposition, but no mode of inheritance has been identified.
    3 This is not a fatal disorder; it can be controlled with a medical regimen.

132. **4** A bedtime snack is needed for the evening. Humulin N insulin lasts for 24 to 28 hours. Protein/carbohydrate ingestion prior to sleep prevents hypoglycemia during the night, when the action of Humulin N insulin will still be high. (PL; PA; EN)
    1 There are no data to indicate such a need; a bedtime snack is routinely provided to help cover long-acting insulin during sleep.
    2 The snack is important for diet/insulin balance during the night, not encouragement.
    3 The snack must contain mainly protein-rich foods to help cover the long-acting insulin during sleep.

133. **3** An 8-year-old is in the stage of industry and strives to complete assigned tasks. (PL; ED; EN)
    1 This is true of an older age group (adolescent).
    2 Peer influences increase rather than decrease as a child grows.
    4 This is true in the period of adolescence.

134. **4** There are both an increased appetite with increased deposition of fat in the stomach and trunk and muscle wasting, which causes thin extremities. (DC; PA; EN)
    1 Increased excretion of calcium causes a retarded linear growth with a short stature.
    2 Because of the excess production of androgens, virilization and hirsutism occur.
    3 Increased salt and water retention cause hypernatremia and hypertension.

135. **3** Congenital hypothyroidism is the result of insufficient secretion by the thyroid gland due to an embryonic defect. The decreased thyroid hormone has been affecting the infant since before birth during cerebral development, so it is likely that some developmental disability will have occurred. Treatment prior to 3 months would have prevented damage (DC; TC; EN)
    1 Congenital hypothyroidism does not become myxedema.
    2 This is a term for hyperthyroidism.
    4 Hyperthyroidism results in hyporeactive deep tendon reflexes.

136. **4** $\dfrac{0.35 \text{ mg}}{0.25 \text{ mg}} \times \dfrac{X \text{ ml}}{1 \text{ ml}} = 1.4 \text{ ml}$

    (AN; TC; DR)
    1 This is too low.
    2 Same as answer 1.
    3 Same as answer 1.

137. **3** By 4 months of age infants are able to turn over and can easily fall from an inadequately guarded height. (IM; TC; GD)
    1 Although infants are capable of putting small things in their mouth, they are not yet able to crawl and would probably not be placed on the floor.
    2 At 4 months of age infants are not yet able to explore the environment to the point that electric outlets pose a problem.
    4 Infants are still too small and have not yet developed motor capabilities to get into containers of poison.

Integumentary

138. **3** Rubeola, or measles, is generally a viral-induced childhood disease, diagnosed on or about the second day by the presence of Koplik's spots on the oral mucosa. (DC; TC; IT)

1 Neither a rash nor Koplik's spots occurs with mumps.

2 Rubella is manifested by a rash, but not by Koplik's spots.

4 Chickenpox is manifested by a maculopapular rash; no Koplik's spots are present.

139. **2 Rubeola, or measles, produces coldlike respiratory symptoms and, after 3 or 4 days, a dark-red macular or maculopapular skin rash. Complications include convulsions in young children and secondary infection with hemolytic streptococci, pneumococci, or staphylococci. Such infection can result in otitis media and pneumonia, which are especially dangerous in children under 2 years of age. (AN; PA; IT)**

1 This is the most benign communicable disease; complications are rare.

3 Yellow fever does not have respiratory complications.

4 Chickenpox does not usually include respiratory inflammation, although pneumonia may occur as a complication.

140. **2 Invasion of the posterior (dorsal) root ganglia by the same virus that causes chickenpox can result in herpes zoster, or shingles. This may be due to reactivation of a previous chickenpox virus that has lain dormant in the body or by fresh contact with an individual who has chickenpox. (DC; PA; IT)**

1 Athlete's foot is caused by a fungus.

3 German measles is caused by a virus, but not the herpesvirus.

4 Hepatitis type A is caused by a virus, but not the herpesvirus.

141. **2 Chickenpox, mumps, and rubeola are all caused by a virus and may be followed by encephalitis. (IM; ED; IT)**

1 Pertussis is caused by a bacterium and does not result in encephalitis.

3 Although polio is caused by a virus, it does not result in encephalitis.

4 Scarlet fever is caused by a bacterium and does not result in encephalitis.

142. **2 Steroids have an antiinflammatory effect. It is believed that resistance to certain viral diseases, including chicken-**
pox, is greatly decreased when the child is taking steroids regularly. (EV; TC; IT)

1 There is no known correlation between chickenpox and insulin.

3 Since chickenpox is viral, antibiotics would have no effect.

4 There is no known correlation between chickenpox and anticonvulsants.

143. **2 Impetigo is a bacterial infection of the skin caused by streptococci or staphylococci. Group A hemolytic streptococci can cause rheumatic fever and glomerulonephritis. (AN; PA; IT)**

1 This infectious condition of the skin is a result of infestation by mites; it is not associated with rheumatic fever or glomerulonephritis.

3 Intertrigo is a superficial dermatitis in the folds of the skin; it is not associated with rheumatic fever or glomerulonephritis.

4 This is a viral condition; not associated with rheumatic fever or glomerulonephritis.

144. **1 Thrush, also called moniliasis, usually affects the mucous membranes of the oral cavity, causing painful white patches. Individuals with immunologic deficiencies, those receiving prolonged antibiotic therapy, and infants are particularly susceptible to this organism. (AN; TC; IT)**

2 This is usually caused by an amoeba or a bacterium; it is not common in infants.

3 This is not caused by yeast and is not common in *Candida* or in infants.

4 This is not caused by yeast, nor does it occur often in infants.

145. **2 Inhalation burns are usually present with facial burns, regardless of the depth; the immediate threat to life is asphyxia from irritation and edema of the respiratory passages and lungs. (DC; TC; IT)**

1 Although wound sepsis is a possible complication, it would not be evident until the third to fifth day.

3 The effects of immobility would not likely manifest in the first 24 hours. The airway is the first priority.

4 Fluid losses can be extremely high but reach their maximum about the fourth day; the initial priority is the airway.

146. 3 **Damage to tissues interferes with stability of peripheral circulation, precluding the use of intramuscular medications. (PL; TC; IT)**
    1 This is not a consideration in this situation.
    2 Mode of administration does not alter effectiveness of drug.
    4 Same as answer 2.

147. 4 **Tetracycline is potentially hepatotoxic, since it is metabolized in the liver. Signs of hepatotoxicity are lethargy, anorexia, behavioral changes, jaundice, and fatty necrosis. (EV; TC; DR)**
    1 This is a nursing role.
    2 Anemia may cause fatigue but is unassociated with withdrawal and irritability.
    3 Common symptoms of bladder infection include burning upon urination, frequency or hesitancy, abdominal pain, and low-grade fever.

148. 1 **Rubeola signs and symptoms include a high fever, photophobia, Koplik's spots (white patches on mucous membranes of the oral cavity), and a rash. Rubella usually does not cause a high fever, runs a 3 to 6-day course, and never causes Koplik's spots. (DC; ED; IT)**
    2 The rash spreads over most of the body.
    3 These symptoms are not associated with rubeola.
    4 Some symptoms may be similar to those of a severe cold, but are associated with high fever.

Gastrointestinal

149. 3 **The worm attaches itself to the bowel wall in the cecum and appendix and can damage the mucosa, causing appendicitis. (DC; TC; GI)**
    1 The pinworm does not migrate to the liver.
    2 Although pinworms (and their ova) are ingested by mouth, they do not attach there; inflammation of the mouth is not a complication of pinworm.
    4 The pinworm does not migrate to the central nervous system.

150. 4 **The adult pinworm lives in the rectum or colon and emerges onto the perirectal skin during hours of sleep, depositing her eggs during this time. (IM; TC; GI)**
    1 Pinworms attach to the bowel wall and do not emerge from the rectum at this time.
    2 Same as answer 1.
    3 Same as answer 1.

151. 4 **All household members should be treated at the same time unless they are younger than 2 years or pregnant. (PL; TC; GI)**
    1 This drug is not recommended for children under the age of 2.
    2 Positive testing is not a criterion for administration.
    3 This is not a significant criterion for administration of medication since eggs are airborne.

152. 4 **This is the expected response since medication causes death of the worm. (EV; TC; DR)**
    1 Convulsions do not occur as a result of this medication.
    2 Hypertension does not occur as a result of this medication.
    3 Neither the drug nor the worms cause intestinal bleeding.

153. 4 **The 2-year-old is still attached to and dependent on the parents. Fear of separation is a great stress. (PL; PS; EH)**
    1 This is neither possible nor desirable.
    2 He will not remember previous hospitalizations.
    3 This is not possible in a health care setting.

154. 2 **These children often have difficulty forming a vacuum. A soft nipple that has been altered to enlarge the opening will often allow enough of a vacuum to result in an adequate flow of formula. (PL; PS; EH)**
    1 Feeding can be accomplished with special equipment; IV feedings do not supply ample calories
    3 It is not necessary to feed this child with a gastrostomy tube.
    4 The use of a spoon or dropper would not provide enough formula to satisfy the infant. In addition, the child would not be able to satisfy a need to suck.

155. 2 **Meticulous care of the suture line is necessary to prevent infection and to provide the best cosmetic effect. (PL; PA; GI)**
    1 This is contraindicated because it can disrupt the suture line; the child can be fed using an asepto syringe with a rubber tip.
    3 This is contraindicated because it puts tension on the suture line and may cause disruption of the sutures.
    4 In this position the child might rub the face on the sheet and disrupt the surgical repair of the cleft lip.

156. 1 **A priority during the immediate postoperative period is protecting the operative site.** (AN; TC; GI)
2 Normal 2-year-olds have about 16 teeth; although tooth development may not be normal in these children, they usually have them.
3 A toothbrush should be a familiar sight to a 2-year-old, not a frightening one.
4 Two-year-olds can brush their teeth.

Gastrointestinal

157. 4 **If food is used early as praise or punishment, the older child or adult will undereat or overeat at times of stress to decrease anxiety.** (DC; PS; GI)
1 Eating is a social as well as a nutritional process.
2 This does not usually cause nutritional problems.
3 Unless discipline involves food, this will not create eating problems.

158. 3 **The early school-age child has become a cooperative member of the family and will mimic parents' attitudes and food habits readily.** (AN; ED; GI)
1 This does not have a major influence on later eating habits.
2 This certainly has some influence, though not major, on later eating habits.
4 The peer group does not become highly influential until later school age and during adolescence.

159. 2 **The infant lacks the ability to produce vitamin K because of a lack of bacteria in the intestine; following a cholecystectomy the client has an interference with the absorption of the fat-soluble vitamin K because of the disruption in bile flow; the client on anticoagulants experiences an inhibition of vitamin K–dependent activation of clotting factors.** (AN; PA; GI)
1 This is not a common nutritional problem with these clients.
3 Same as answer 1.
4 Same as answer 1.

160. 2 **Positioning on the right side after feeding facilitates digestion because the pyloric sphincter is on this side and gravity aids in emptying the stomach.** (IM; PA; GI)
1 Feeding may proceed immediately after opening the tube. Leaving the tube open may facilitate drainage of gastric contents.
3 It is standard procedure to flush the tube after the feeding to ensure that all the formula gets into the stomach; not necessary before feeding. Normal saline will not be used.
4 The usual height for elevation of the gastrostomy tube when feeding an infant is 6 to 8 inches.

161. 2 **Pinworms emerge nocturnally to lay eggs in the perianal area; eggs are caught on transparent tape in the morning before toileting.** (IM; TC; GI)
1 A culture will not reveal the presence of parasites.
3 Ova cannot be seen with the naked eye; the parasite is rarely observed in the stool.
4 There is no such test to diagnose pinworms.

162. 4 **Production of tenacious mucus in the pancreatic ducts prevents the flow of digestive enzymes into the intestines. Thus fats, proteins, and (to a lesser extent) carbohydrates cannot be digested and absorbed.** (EV; PA; GI)
1 Anorexia is not a usual problem found with cystic fibrosis.
2 These are not problems associated with cystic fibrosis.
3 Cystic fibrosis does not influence the secretion of growth hormone.

163. 1 **Because of a lack of the pancreatic enzyme lipase, fats remain unabsorbed and are excreted in excessive amounts in the stool.** (AN; PA; GI)
2 This does not cause the foul smell of stools.
3 Same as answer 2.
4 These are the pancreatic enzymes, whose passage into the intestine is prevented by blocked pancreatic ducts.

164. 2 **Rectal prolapse is the most common GI complication and is due to wasting of perirectal supporting tissues, secondary to malnutrition.** (AN; PA; GI)
1 Anal fissures may or may not occur with cystic fibrosis.
3 Intussusception is not associated with cystic fibrosis.
4 Meconium ileus, associated with cystic fibrosis in newborns, prevents passage of meconium.

165. **1 Children with cystic fibrosis have a characteristic underweight, frail appearance. They may become sensitive to their appearance as they grow older. (PL; PA; GI)**
    2 Engaging in usual childhood activities between attacks should promote development of fine muscle coordination.
    3 There is little dietary management in the treatment of cystic fibrosis.
    4 Sterility is not associated with cystic fibrosis.

166. **3 Hypertrophy of the pyloric sphincter, at the distal end of the stomach, causes partial and then complete obstruction. Nonprojectile vomiting progresses to projectile vomiting, which rapidly leads to dehydration. (DC; TC; GI)**
    1 The infant's cry is not affected by pyloric stenosis; there does not appear to be pain associated with this condition, except for the pain of hunger.
    2 The quality of the stool is not usually affected by pyloric stenosis.
    4 This can be expected with a tracheoesophageal fistula, but not with pyloric stenosis.

167. **2 The pyloric sphincter is located at the junction between the stomach and duodenum. The common bile duct enters the duodenum below the junction. Therefore, a hypertrophied pyloric sphincter obstructs the entry of bile into the stomach. (AN; TC; GI)**
    1 The bile duct is not obstructed in pyloric stenosis.
    3 The bile duct enters into the duodenum and is not involved with pyloric stenosis.
    4 The area obstructed in pyloric stenosis is the pyloric sphincter, between the stomach and duodenum.

168. **4 Initial feedings of glucose in water or electrolyte solutions are given 4 to 6 hours after surgery. When clear fluids are retained, usually within 24 hours, diluted formula feedings are begun. (PL; TC; GI)**
    1 The formula should be diluted 24 hours after surgery in an attempt to gradually return the infant to a full feeding schedule.
    2 This is not necessary.
    3 Same as answer 2.

169. **3 This is usually sufficient if no problems exist with sucking or palate; too frequent burping is confusing. (IM; ED; GI)**
    1 Excessive burping may confuse a new infant.
    2 Sucking too long without burping may result in regurgitation because of swallowed air.
    4 Same as answer 1.

170. **4 Reflux results from an incompetent cardiac sphincter, which allows a reflux of gastric contents into the esophagus and eventual regurgitation. Placing the infant in an upright position keeps the gastric contents in the stomach by gravity as well as limits the pressure against the cardiac sphincter. (IM; ED; GI)**
    1 This will promote regurgitation.
    2 This will probably have little effect on reflux.
    3 This will promote vomiting since it is too much formula for a week-old infant.

171. **2 Crying should be prevented, since it places tension on the suture line. Frequently an appliance called a Logan bow is taped to the cheeks to relax the operative site, which helps prevent trauma. (IM; TC; GI)**
    1 This is not necessary or desirable.
    3 The infant may also be positioned on the side and on the back with surveillance.
    4 The feeding method of choice is by a rubber-tipped syringe or dropper.

172. **3 Hepatitis B virus is in the blood during the late incubation and acute stages of the disease. It may also persist in the carrier state for years. It is transmitted when the blood of an infected individual comes in contact with the blood or mucous membranes of another individual. Posttransfusion hepatitis has been reduced now that the surface antigen of hepatitis B (HBS Ag) and the antibody to hepatitis B core antigen tests are performed on blood donors and on the blood of carriers of type B virus (PL; TC; GI)**
    1 Hepatitis A is principally transferred through oral-fecal routes.
    2 Ventilating systems do not transmit this virus.
    4 This is unrelated to hepatitis B.

173. **3 This is due to the fact that celiac clients have a gluten-induced enteropathy and are unable to absorb fats from the intestinal tract. (DC; TC; GI)**

1 Stools are large and fatty or frothy, not mucoid.
2 Although stools are large and frothy, they lack color because of incomplete absorption.
4 Stools are foul smelling, in large quantities, and without color because of incomplete absorption.

174. **1 It is hoped that reducing dietary phenylalanine will prevent brain damage. Diets are planned to attempt to maintain the serum phenylalanine level between 5 and 10 mg/100 ml. (IM; ED; GI)**
2 Phenylalanine is essential for normal growth and development of the brain.
3 Phenylalanine does not need to be supplemented.
4 There are no substitutes; phenylalanine is one of the essential amino acids.

175. **1 A blood test reliably detects abnormally high levels of phenylalanine as early as 4 days, provided that the infant has been fed formula. (DC; ED; GI)**
2 Testing after 6 weeks exposes the infant to toxic effects.
3 Phenylketonuria demonstrates an inability to metabolize phenylalanine, resulting in an excess amount, not a deficiency.
4 This test is not done.

176. **2 In PKU the absence of the hepatic enzyme phenylalanine hydroxylase prevents normal metabolism (hydroxylation to tyrosine) of the amino acid phenylalanine. The increased fluid levels of phenylalanine in the body and the alternate metabolic by-products (phenylketones) are associated with severe developmental disability (exact mechanism not known). (PL; ED; GI)**
1 Medications are not part of therapy.
3 PKU is transmitted by an autosomal recessive gene.
4 PKU is not associated with dysfunctions of the immune system.

177. **4 Maintaining low phenylalanine levels is recommended until brain growth is almost completed, usually by adolescence. (IM; ED; GI)**
1 This is untrue and is not helpful to the parents.

2 Dietary management is necessary until the child is an adolescent or older.
3 Same as answer 2.

178. **3 Because phenylalanine is an essential amino acid, it must be provided in quantities sufficient for promoting growth while maintaining safe blood levels. (PL; TC; GI)**
1 All proteins do not contain phenylalanine.
2 Phenylalanine is an essential amino acid and cannot be totally removed from the diet.
4 In PKU phenylalanine accumulates in the blood, causing irreversible CNS damage; additional phenylalanine must be avoided.

179. **2 Obesity is a very common nutritional problem in children with Down syndrome; it is thought to be related to excessive caloric intake and impaired growth. (PL; TC; GI)**
1 This is a nutritional disorder related to vitamin D deficiency; it is not especially encountered in these children.
3 This is the most common nutritional problem in children (iron deficiency); it is not especially encountered in these children.
4 This is a psychiatric eating disorder of infancy characterized by repeated regurgitation without gastrointestinal illness; it is not usually encountered in these children.

180. **3 Paroxysmal pain is related to peristaltic action. Abdominal distention pushes up the diaphragm, causing respiratory distress characterized by grunting respirations. (DC; PA; GI)**
1 These symptoms do not usually accompany intestinal obstruction.
2 These symptoms are not characteristic of intestinal obstruction.
4 The pain of intestinal obstruction is paroxysmal.

181. **3 The traditional efforts to explain and treat colic center on control of gas in the intestinal tract that is causing the paroxysmal pain. (EV; PA; GI)**
1 Allergic responses may cause flatus, but diet changes rarely prevent colic attacks.
2 Colic is thought to be caused by excessive fermentation and gas production.
4 The exact cause of colic is not known.

182. **2 The introduction of one new food at a time permits the identification of any food allergies that might be present; multiple new foods make the identification of the causative food more difficult. (IM; TC; GI)**
    1 This can create feeding problems; if the infant does not like a food taste it may be associated with the formula.
    3 Solid foods should be given when the infant is hungry to encourage intake.
    4 Formula intake should be decreased as solid food intake increases or the infant will be receiving excessive calories.

183. **1 The first solid foods added to the infant's diet should be easily digestible, such as fruits and cereals, and provide rich sources of iron, such as fortified cereals. (IM; ED; GI)**
    2 Sweets have less nutritional value and may make an infant less accepting of other foods later.
    3 Meats are more difficult to digest and so are added later.
    4 Egg white is added very late because of the allergic reactions associated with it.

184. **2 An Apgar score of 3 indicates neonatal distress and should signal the nurse that the infant requires close supervision and support. (EV; TC; GD)**
    1 Average birth weight is about 3200 g.
    3 A positive Babinski is normal through the age of 2 years.
    4 Infants often swallow in utero.

185. **4 Play during infancy (solitary) promotes physical development. For example, mobiles strengthen eye movement, large beads promote fine finger movement, and soft toys encourage tactile sense. (AN; ED; GD)**
    1 Play during infancy is usually initiated by the parent.
    2 Children do not begin to share until the pre-school years.
    3 Play is important throughout childhood.

Fluid and Electrolytes

186. **2 Weight is the best indicator of fluid loss if measured each day at the same time, on the same scale, and with the same amount of clothing. (EV; PA; FE)**

1 In cases of severe diarrhea, an IV is usually employed until the diarrhea is controlled; oral fluids are gradually added as tolerated.
3 Because of the diarrhea, food will not be properly absorbed.
4 This temperature is not unusual in infants.

187. **4 The extracellular body fluid represents 40% at birth, 25% at 2 years of age, and 20% at maturity. Another measurement is percentage of total body weight, which is 80% at birth, 63% at 3, and approximately 60% at 12 years. (AN; PA; FE)**
    1 Cellular metabolism in children is not less stable than in adults.
    2 The proportion of total body water in children (up to 2 years) is 20% greater than in adults.
    3 Renal function is immature during infancy only.

188. **4 If the circulation is overloaded with too much fluid or the rate is too rapid, the stress on the heart becomes too great and cardiac overload may occur. (PL; TC; FE)**
    1 This is important, but an infiltrated IV is not as serious a complication.
    2 Although fluid replacement is important, prevention of cardiac problems from fluid overload is critical.
    3 Increased output is not the primary consideration.

189. **3** $\dfrac{\text{Amount of fluid} \times \text{Drop rate}}{\text{Time (in minutes)}}$

    $$\frac{500 \times 60}{24 \times 60} = 21 \text{ drops}$$

    (AN; PA; FE)
    1 This would be too slow to infuse the desired amount.
    2 Same as answer 1.
    4 This would be too rapid; the fluid would run out before 24 hours had elapsed.

190. **2 Tap-water enemas are hypotonic and are contraindicated; they may cause increased absorption of fluid via the bowel and may upset the balance of fluid in the body. There also is interference with potassium ion balance; this electrolyte can be lost via the large intestine. (EV; TC; FE)**
    1 The enema would remove only waste products from the bowel.
    3 Fear of intrusive procedures is typical of preschoolers.

4 The temperature of the water should be regulated so this does not occur.

191. **3 No more than 350 ml of solution should be administered to an infant or child unless ordered, since fluid and electrolyte balance in an infant or child is easily disturbed. (PL; PA; FE)**
   1 This quantity may be ordered for a small infant.
   2 This quantity may be ordered for an older or larger infant.
   4 This quantity is too large for small children.

192. **4** $\dfrac{\text{Total milliliters to be infused} \times \text{Drop factor}}{\text{Total time to be infused in minutes}}$

   $\dfrac{1000 \times 60}{1440} = \dfrac{60{,}000}{1440} = 41.6\ \text{drops/minute}$

   (AN; TC; FE)
   1 Calculations show this is too low to deliver 1000 ml in 24 hours.
   2 Same as answer 1.
   3 Same as answer 1.

193. **4 Dehydration promotes the sickling of erythrocytes. Increased fluid intake minimizes the chance that a sickle cell pain episode will occur. (PL; ED; FE)**
   1 This is not necessary or helpful in sickle cell anemia.
   2 Rigorous exercise will cause sickling because of decreased oxygen.
   3 This is not necessary.

194. **3 The restricted ventilation accompanying an asthmatic attack limits the body's ability to blow off carbon dioxide. As carbon dioxide accumulates in the body fluids, it reacts with water to produce carbonic acid (H_2CO_3); the result is respiratory acidosis. (AN; PA; FE)**
   1 The problem basic to asthma is respiratory, not metabolic.
   2 Respiratory alkalosis is caused by exhaling large amounts of carbon dioxide; asthma causes carbon dioxide retention.
   4 Asthma is a respiratory problem, not a metabolic one; metabolic acidosis can result from a gain of nonvolatile acids or a loss of base bicarbonate.

195. **3 In excessive vomiting there is an increased loss of hydrogen ions (hydrochloric acid), which leads to a lowered serum pH (metabolic alkalosis) and an excess of base bicarbonate. (DC; TC; FE)**
   1 Although some calcium is lost through vomiting, it is highly unusual that the infant would develop tetany.
   2 This is caused by a retention of hydrogen ions and a loss of base bicarbonates. In vomiting, base bicarbonates are retained and hydrogen ions are lost.
   4 Hyperactivity is not associated with vomiting.

196. **3 An infant's intravascular compartment is fairly limited and cannot accommodate large volumes of fluid administered in a short time. Equipment such as minidroppers, volume control chambers, and infusion pumps should be used, since they help control or limit the volume of fluid to be infused. (PL; TC; FE)**
   1 This is important for everyone receiving IV fluids.
   2 This is the physician's role.
   4 IV fluids can be administered at room temperature.

197. **2 Peak crying times are early evening and night, which exhaust the mother. She needs time away from Robby to rest and should be encouraged to hire a sitter or make some arrangements for time alone. (IM; ED; EH)**
   1 This is unlikely to assist Robby's mother with coping.
   3 Providing Robby with many treatments, including this one, may not be effective; children do outgrow colic, so parents need support to help them manage until that time.
   4 Treatment is usually based on relieving abdominal cramping by stimulating peristalsis; quiet environments may help prevent, not treat, the problem.

PEDIATRIC ANSWERS

198. 3 Isotonic saline is compatible with body fluids. It is neither hypertonic nor hypotonic, so it does not cause a change in osmotic pressure and upset the balance of intracellular and extracellular fluid and electrolytes. (IM; TC; FE)

1 This hypotonic solution might cause fluid and electrolyte imbalance.

2 Soap-suds enemas are water with added soap products and are therefore usually hypotonic; this can cause fluid shifts and overloads.

4 This solution would cause excess fluid loss and therefore be dangerous.

Cardiovascular

199. 3 There are three vessels; one vein carries oxygenated blood to the fetus, and two arteries return deoxygenated blood to the placenta. (EV; PA; CV)

1 The umbilical cord has three vessels; a cord with two vessels is frequently associated with congenital abnormalities.

2 This is the right number of vessels, but there are two arteries and one vein.

4 The umbilical cord has three vessels, not four.

200. 3 Rheumatic fever is an inflammatory disease involving the joints, heart, CNS, and subcutaneous tissue. It is believed to be an autoimmune process that causes connective tissue damage. (DC; PA; CV)

1 Tetanus is not caused by a streptococcal infection and does not include the symptoms listed.

2 Measles is caused by a virus and does not include the symptoms listed.

4 Whooping cough is not caused by a streptococcal infection and does not include the symptoms listed.

201. 4 In heart failure there is a decrease in the blood flow to the kidneys, causing sodium and water reabsorption and resulting in peripheral edema. The peripheral edema indicates severe cardiac decompensation. (DC; PA; CV)

1 This may be an early attempt by the body to compensate for decreased cardiac output.

2 Same as answer 1.

3 Same as answer 1.

202. 4 Coarctation of the aorta is a narrowing, usually in the thoracic segment, causing decreased blood flow below the constriction and increased blood volume above it. (EV; PA; CV)

1 This has nothing to do with coarctation of the aorta.

2 In coarctation of the aorta, femoral pulses would be weak or absent, and blood pressure in the lower extremities would be decreased.

3 In coarctation of the aorta, radial pulses would be full and bounding.

203. 4 Babies with Down syndrome have a high incidence of congenital heart defects, especially atrial defects. (PL; PA; CV)

1 Deafness is not usually a problem in Down syndrome.

2 Infants with Down syndrome usually do not have a problem with hydrocephaly.

3 The muscles of infants with Down syndrome are usually hypotonic.

204. 4 In acyanotic heart disease there is a narrowing of the vessels and/or pinpoint holes in the septum of the heart that cause a murmuring sound as the blood is pumped through. (DC; PA; CV)

1 This is not a common clinical finding in acyanotic heart disease.

2 This is not a common finding in acyanotic heart disease; tissue perfusion is usually adequate to support growth.

3 Clubbing is a common finding in cyanotic heart disease.

205. 3 In the fetus, oxygenated blood is shunted directly into the systemic circulation via the ductus arteriosus, a connection between the pulmonary artery and the aorta. Normally after birth the increased oxygen tension causes a functional closure of the ductus arteriosus. Occasionally, particularly in premature infants, this vessel remains open and is known as patent ductus arteriosus. (IM; ED; CV)

1 This is known as pulmonic stenosis.

2 This is not the problem in patent ductus arteriosus.

4 Patent ductus arteriosus does not involve ventricular septal defects.

206. 4 Gavage feeding is preferred for weak infants, those with respiratory distress or poor sucking-swallowing coordination, and those who are easily fatigued because of physical stress such as surgery. (AN; TC; CV)

1 This is not a reason for instituting gavage; however, vomiting may be lessened with gavage feeding since the amount and rapidity of feeding can be controlled.

2 Feeding the infant quickly is not desirable; vomiting with aspiration may occur.

3 The amount can be regulated with bottle-feeding as well.

207. **2 Oxygen is necessary for growth of cells. Decreased oxygen in the developing child causes a slow growth rate. (DC; ED; CV)**

1 Developmental disabilities are not common in children with congenital heart anomalies.

3 Cyanosis is not characteristic of most children with cardiac anomalies, only of those with serious hypoxia.

4 Essential hypertension is high blood pressure without a know cause, and is not associated with cardiac anomalies.

208. **3 Tetralogy of Fallot classically consists of four defects. Three of them are anatomic: ventricular septal defect, pulmonic stenosis, and overriding aorta. The fourth defect, right ventricular hypertrophy, is secondary to increased resistance to blood flow in that ventricle. (AN; PA; CV)**

1 Right ventricular hypertrophy is correct, the other anomalies are not.

2 These are the characteristics of transposition of the great vessels.

4 Same as answer 1.

209. **2 Polycythemia, reflected in an elevated hematocrit level, is a direct attempt of the body to compensate for the decrease in oxygenation to all body cells caused by the mixture of oxygenated and unoxygenated circulating blood. (DC; PA; CV)**

1 This is not characteristic of cyanotic heart disease in children.

3 This is characteristic of coarctation of the aorta, an acyanotic heart disease.

4 Edema is not a common finding in cyanotic heart disease.

210. **4 Decreased tissue oxygenation stimulates erythropoiesis, resulting in excessive production of red blood cells. (EV; PA; CV)**

1 This would not be a direct cause of polycythemia.

2 Same as answer 1.

3 This may or may not affect the production of red blood cells.

211. **3 Forceful evacuation results in the child's taking a deep breath, holding it, and straining (Valsalva's maneuver). This increased intrathoracic pressure puts excessive strain on the heart sutures. (PL; TC; CV)**

1 Crying is not a problem after cardiac surgery; it may, in fact, help prevent respiratory complications.

2 Coughing and deep breathing are essential for the prevention of postoperative respiratory complications.

4 Activity is gradually increased postoperatively.

Blood and Immunity

212. **3 The injected microbes in the vaccine have been so modified that they do not cause active infection but still elicit an immune response. (AN; PA; BI)**

1 This is a poisonous substance released from bacterial cells.

2 This is a modified toxin, whose poisonous properties are destroyed but that is still capable of producing antibodies.

4 This is an antibody capable of neutralizing a specific toxin.

213. **4 In passive artificial immunity, an antibody made in another organism is injected into the infected or presumed infected person to provide immediate immunity to the invading organism. (IM; PA; BI)**

1 This type of immunity requires the child to acquire the illness

2 This occurs with immunization.

3 Passive natural immunity is acquired from the mother and is effective only during the first few months of the child's life.

214. **1 In active natural immunity, the infected person's immune system responds to the invading organism by producing antibodies specific for the invader. (AN; PA; BI)**

2 Active artificial immunity is acquired by the injection of antigens, after which the individual develops antibodies.

3 Passive natural immunity is acquired by the fetus from the mother.

4 Passive artificial immunity is acquired through injection of antibodies.

215. **3** **Antibodies received in utero through the placenta and in the newborn via mother's milk provide the baby with immunity against most viral, bacterial, and fungal infections during the first several weeks after birth. Then, as the titer of maternal antibodies drops and is not replaced by the child's own antibodies, prolonged and repeated infection occurs.** (EV; PA; BI)
 1 This is not enough to prevent infections in these children.
 2 Bacteria do not produce antibodies.
 4 This probably does not occur in children born without an immune system.

216. **2** **This is the normal hemoglobin range for a one-year-old child.** (AN; PA; BI)
 1 This hemoglobin is too low, and is associated with anemia.
 3 A newborn's hemoglobin is about 17 g/L, but will have fallen by one year of age.
 4 This hemoglobin is too high.

217. **2** **Milk is a very poor source of iron. If fed in large amounts to the exclusion of solid foods after 4 to 6 months of age, iron deficiency anemia results.** (AN; TC; BI)
 1 Anemia is a blood disorder.
 3 Iron stores received from the mother in the last trimester are usually adequate for the infant's first 4 to 5 months.
 4 Lack of absorption and early introduction of solid foods are not commonly the cause of anemia in infants.

218. **3** **Proteins are essential for the synthesis of the blood proteins, albumin, fibrinogen, and hemoglobin. Ascorbic acid influences the removal of iron from ferritin (making more iron available for production of heme) and influences the conversion of folic acid to folinic acid.** (PL; PA; BI)
 1 These are not involved in building red blood cells.
 2 Same as answer 1.
 4 Same as answer 1.

219. **3** **A diet of milk only is not sufficient to meet iron needs. Raisins and meat are high in iron, and finger foods are appropriate for toddlers.** (IM; ED; BI)
 1 Weaning from the bottle is not the issue; supplementary iron intake is.

 2 Although medical care and monitoring will be required, the metabolic clinic is not the appropriate referral.
 4 This is not appropriate for a 1-year-old, nor is it necessary or desirable.

220. **3** **Corticosteroids (e.g., cortisol) cause involution of lymphatic tissue and resultant depression of the immune response. Antineoplastic drugs or high-energy radiation preferentially destroys tissues with high mitotic rates, including lymphatic tissue and bone marrow, where antibody production and other immune responses take place.** (EV; TC; BI)
 1 This is an inappropriate answer; it is no more true for these children than for other children.
 2 This is not a reason to withhold immunizations.
 4 The measles vaccine does not contain rabbit serum.

221. **1** **Suggested immunizations for normal preschool children include DTPT and HiB.** (IM; PA; BI)
 2 The tuberculin test is not an immunization.
 3 Same as answer 4.
 4 Rubella vaccine is normally given between 12 and 15 months of age and is not repeated.

222. **2** **The recommended immunization schedule for infants is administration of diphtheria, pertussis, tetanus, and polio.** (EV; PA; BI)
 1 Measles vaccine is not usually administered until the child is 12 months old.
 3 Measles, mumps, and rubella vaccines are not given until 12 months; tuberculosis vaccine is not routinely administered to children.
 4 Measles and rubella vaccines are not usually given until 12 months of age; tuberculosis vaccine is not given routinely to children.

223. **3** **The body's immune system constructs proteins called antibodies that possess a specificity toward another protein called the antigen. The antibody may neutralize or damage the antigen and thus render it harmless.** (IM; ED; BI)
 1 Antibodies are protein substances.
 2 Antibodies are produced to fight antigens.
 4 Antigens are harmful to the body.

224. **2 Maternal antibodies to measles infection persist in the infant until approximately 15 months of age.** (PL; PA; BI)
    1 Side effects are no more common for infants than for toddlers.
    3 This is true, but vaccination is delayed due to the presence of maternal antibodies.
    4 This has not been found to be true.

225. **1 Under conditions of decreased oxygen the relatively insoluble hemoglobin S changes its molecular structure to form long, slender crystals and eventually the crescent, or sickled, shape.** (AN; TC; BI)
    2 This will not influence the sickling process.
    3 Hemodilution helps prevent sickling and is accomplished by encouraging fluids.
    4 The platelets are not involved in sickle cell anemia.

226. **3 Sickling is related to the concentration of hemoglobin within the cell. Since hypertonicity of the blood plasma increases the intracellular concentration of hemoglobin, dehydration promotes sickling.** (IM; TC; BI)
    1 This will not prevent thrombus formation.
    2 The condition determines the activity level; although bed rest may be necessary during a pain episode, complete bed rest is rarely necessary.
    4 Anticoagulants do not help prevent thrombus formation in sickle cell anemia.

227. **2 Both cause poor resistance to infection. With sickling it is due to low oxygen levels, and with celiac disease it is due to malnourishment and immunologic defects.** (IM; ED; BI)
    1 Activity does not need to be limited in celiac disease; strenuous activity should be limited in sickle cell anemia.
    3 Vital signs will not be abnormal except during a crisis in either condition.
    4 This specific diet is not particularly helpful for either sickle cell anemia or celiac disease.

228. **3 Hydration is necessary to promote and maintain hemodilution; pain in the area of involvement is a major problem in vasoocclusive crises and demands priority care.** (PL; TC; BI)

    1 Although hydration is a major concern, nutrition is not.
    2 Neither of these factors are priority concerns in a vasoocclusive crisis.
    4 Although antibiotics may be ordered to treat any preexisting infection that may have precipitated the crisis, it would be a medical, not a nursing, decision; pain management is a major nursing concern.

229. **4 Hemophilia is carried on the X chromosome but is recessive. Therefore the female is the carrier (an unaffected XO and an affected XH). If the male receives the affected XH (XHYO), the disease is manifest.** (IM; ED; BI)
    1 Hemophilia is a sex-linked recessive disorder.
    2 Hemophilia is carried by the female. Regular laws of Mendelian inheritance are not sex-specific.
    3 Only females carry the trait.

230. **1 Bleeding is greatly influenced by activity. Therefore weight-bearing joints, especially the knees, are the most common site of hemorrhage.** (AN; PA; BI)
    2 This area is usually protected from the trauma of direct force.
    3 This area is fairly well protected by the skull and less likely to be injured.
    4 Bleeding from bones themselves is not common without other associated trauma.

231. **3 Factor VIII is the missing plasma component necessary to control bleeding in classic hemophilia.** (AN; PA; BI)
    1 Factor VIII, the missing component, would not be provided by this blood derivative.
    2 Although fresh frozen plasma does contain factor VIII, it is an insufficient amount and a high volume is required.
    4 Same as answer 1.

232. **3 The mating of a carrier female (XOXH) and an unaffected male (XOYO) results in the following possible offspring: a carrier female (XOXH), an unaffected female (XOXO), an unaffected male (XOYO), or an affected male (XHYO).** (IM; ED; BI)
    1 For each child there is a 50% chance of being normal.
    2 For each child there is a 50% chance of being affected.
    4 Males cannot carry the trait; females have a 50% chance of being carriers.

233. **3 An attenuated virus is an inactivated antigen that causes a protective active response in the individual (the development of antibodies). (AN; PA; BI)**
  1 An immunization contains antigens, not antibodies.
  2 Same as answer 1.
  4 Passive antibodies are produced by another person; for example, maternal antibodies that cross the placenta to the fetus.

234. **3 The child is having an allergic reaction, and flow of blood should be stopped immediately to prevent serious complications. (IM; TC; BI)**
  1 Physician should be called after blood has been stopped.
  2 Slowing the rate of infusion will not halt the allergic reaction to the blood.
  4 This is dangerous as an initial action because the degree of allergic reaction cannot be determined at this time; blood must be stopped.

235. **3 Folic acid acts as a necessary coenzyme in the formation of heme, the iron-containing protein in hemoglobin. (AN; PA; BI)**
  1 Calcium is not involved in the production of red blood cells.
  2 This is a coenzyme in carbohydrate metabolism.
  4 The production of red blood cells does not involve carbohydrates.

236. **4 Fortified cereal is a rich source of iron that is easily digested by children. (IM; ED; BI)**
  1 Milk is a poor source of iron.
  2 Lamb contains iron in smaller amounts and is not as easily digestible as cereal.
  3 Orange juice does not contain iron.

237. **2 The child's immediate physical safety takes priority. The child must sit down to avoid falling. Later the child can be placed in the supine position. (IM; TC; BI)**
  1 Immediate physical safety takes priority over further assessment.
  3 The subjective symptom of dizziness alone does not warrant this; immediate physical safety takes priority.
  4 Although gravity promotes cerebral blood flow in this position, immediate physical safety takes priority; walking at this time would be unsafe.

238. **3 High levels of fetal hemoglobin prevent sickling of red blood cells. The newborn has from 44% to 89% fetal hemoglobin, but this rapidly decreases during the first year. (AN; PA; BI)**
  1 Respiratory difficulties are not associated with sickle cell anemia except as a consequence of hypoxia during a crisis.
  2 The diagnosis of sickle cell anemia is made on the basis of hematologic tests; general health and growth are not affected initially.
  4 These will not affect the diagnosis of sickle cell anemia.

239. **2 Foam is soft, so it will not damage the oral mucosa. (PL; ED; BI)**
  1 This may irritate the oral mucosa and should always be diluted.
  3 This will injure the oral mucosa.
  4 This will irritate the mucosa and has an offensive taste.

240. **3 The extensive growth of lymphoblasts suppresses the normal growth of red cells, white cells, and platelets. (DC; PA; BI)**
  1 Infection is a result of, not the cause of, leukopenia.
  2 Internal bleeding does not cause neutropenia.
  4 Iron-intake deficit will not result in neutropenia.

241. **4 Marked jaundice generally indicates liver damage or excessive hemolysis and is not a sign of leukemia unless hepatic damage from late effects of the disease or drugs has occurred. Edema is not a manifestation of the disease, because the pathophysiology does not involve transport of fluids. (DC; PA; BI)**
  1 Marked fatigue and pallor are the result of anemia associated with leukemia.
  2 Multiple bruises and petechiae are due to thrombocytopenia associated with leukemia.
  3 Enlarged lymph nodes, spleen, and liver are due to the infiltration of these organs with leukemic cells.

242. **3 Because of the increased capillary fragility and decreased platelet counts that accompany leukemia, even the slightest trauma can cause hemorrhage. Therefore the toothbrush can produce gingival hemorrhage, and the physician should be informed of this happening; this may also assist in defining the diagnosis. (IM; TC; BI)**
  1 It would be wiser to eliminate the use of a toothbrush and use a sponge-type applicator; therefore this is not necessary.

2 It cannot be assumed that a 4-year-old would follow such direction In addition, being more careful may not prevent gingival hemorrhage in a child with leukemia.

4 This is appropriate if oral mucosal bleeding continues or oral ulcers develop, not for a one-time incident.

243. **4 Radiation destroys leukemic cells in the brain because chemotherapeutic agents are poorly absorbed through the blood-brain barrier. (AN; PA; BI)**

1 This is not the primary reason for the treatment; it is a curative measure.

2 This is inaccurate; this is not the reason for cranial radiation.

3 This is inaccurate; ALL is an abnormality of the bone marrow and lymphatic system.

Drug-related Responses

244. **4 By law, a nurse cannot administer medications without a prescription from a physician. This is a dependent function of the nurse. (IM; TC; DR)**

1 The nurse cannot distribute medication without a physician's order.

2 The nurse must get a physician's order for the medication and cannot accept the parent's information alone.

3 The nurse should not assume that the physician is aware of the problem.

245. **1 Convert grains to milligrams (gr 1/300 = 0.2 mg); then use the formula:**

$$\frac{0.2 \text{ mg}}{0.4 \text{ mg}} \times \frac{X \text{ ml}}{1 \text{ ml}}$$

$$0.4 \text{ X} = 0.2$$

$$\text{X} = 0.5 \text{ ml (This will contain the desired dose of 0.2 mg atropine.)}$$

(AN; TC; DR)

2 This amount is too much according to calculations.

3 This amount is too little according to calculations.

4 Same as answer 2.

246. **4 Chlorpheniramine (Chlor-Tripolon) is an antihistamine that prevents histamine from reaching its site of action by competing for the receptors. (IM; TC; DR)**

1 Hyaluronidase is a mucolytic enzyme that promotes diffusion and absorption of injected fluids, exudates, and transudates.

2 Nitrofurantoin is an antibacterial agent used for urinary infections.

3 This is a salicylate.

247. **4 Residual medication on the needle may stain the skin during penetration. (IM; TC; DR)**

1 This action would constrict blood vessels and impair absorption.

2 Deep penetration is necessary; only the gluteal muscles should be used because of their size and the decreased visibility of staining.

3 This should be avoided. This action might cause seepage of drug through the needle track, with subsequent tissue irritation and staining.

248. **3 The tetracyclines are not recommended during periods of tooth development (children under 8 years of age or in pregnant women during the latter half of pregnancy) because they may permanently discolor teeth yellow, gray, or brown. (EV; TC; DR)**

1 Tetracycline does not interfere with bone structure of school-age children or pregnant women.

2 This is not an expected complication of tetracycline.

4 Anemia is not a common condition for 6-year-olds.

249. **4 A common side effect of long-term phenytoin (Dilantin) therapy is hyperplasia of the gingiva. (IM; TC; DR)**

1 Dilantin does not affect urinary output.

2 Dilantin does not influence pupillary response.

3 Dilantin does not cause flushing.

250. **3 Ipecac exerts its effect through direct stimulation of the vomiting control center and local irritation of the gastric mucosa; ipecac's effects are enhanced through dilution of the drug in large quantities of fluid. (IM; TC; DR)**

1 Ipecac works by stimulating the vomiting control center and local gastric irritation.

2 Resting has no effect on drug efficiency.

4 The child should be kept calm and quiet.

251. 1 $\dfrac{20 \text{ mg}}{50 \text{ mg}} \times \dfrac{X}{1 \text{ ml}}$

     $50 X = 20$

     $X = 0.4 \text{ ml}$

     (AN; TC; DR)

     2 This calculation is too high.
     3 Same as answer 2.
     4 Same as answer 2.

252. 1 **Prednisone is a synthetic glucocorticoid that has an active antiinflammatory effect by stabilizing lysosomal membranes and thus inhibiting proteolytic enzyme release.** (AN; PA; DR)

     2 Prednisone does not enhance the action of methotrexate.
     3 Prednisone does not affect mitosis, but inhibits proteolytic enzyme release.
     4 Although prednisone increases the appetite and creates a sense of well-being, these are not the reasons it is administered.

253. 4 **Euphoria and mood swings may result from steroid therapy.** (EV; TC; DR)

     1 Alopecia does not result from steroid therapy.
     2 An increased appetite, not anorexia, results from steroid therapy.
     3 Weight gain, not weight loss, results from steroid therapy.

254. 2 **Generally, antineoplastic drugs act by interfering with, or inhibiting, synthesis of DNA in malignant cells.** (AN; PA; DR)

     1 Malignant cells are not infected, in the normal sense of the term; therefore this drug does not act in this manner.
     3 Bone marrow depression is a side effect of this drug, not a desired action.
     4 This is the activity of the malignant cells themselves.

255. 2 **Acetaminophen relieves pain and does not cause bleeding tendencies, as does aspirin. The correct dose for this age is 300 mg.** (EV; TC; DR)

     1 Aspirin increases the clotting time and should be avoided.
     3 Demerol may be given, although a narcotic is not usually necessary for children after tonsillectomy; however, 50 mg would be the normal dose for an adult.
     4 Phenobarbitol will not relieve the pain; it will only sedate the client.

256. 1 **Drug therapy reduces the toxic lead from the blood and other tissues to produce a complex for renal excretion.** (AN; TC; DR)

     2 CNS effects are not reversible.
     3 Lead is excreted by the kidneys.
     4 This is one goal, but not the overall objective.

257. 1 **The purpose of digoxin (Lanoxin) is to slow and strengthen the apical rate. The normal apical rate for a child of 5 years is 90 to 110 beats per minute. If the apical rate is already slow (10 to 20 beats below normal), administration of the drug could lower the apical rate to an unsafe level.** (EV; TC; DR)

     2 This is a low normal rate.
     3 This is within the normal range of the heart rate of 5-year-olds and does not necessitate withholding Lanoxin.
     4 Same as answer 3.

258. 3 **Salicylates in large doses cause irritation of the gastric mucosa (gastric distress, nausea, vomiting) and also affect the CNS (tinnitus, dizziness, disturbance in hearing and vision).** (EV; TC; DR)

     1 Although nausea, dizziness, and severe headache may be associated with salicylate ingestion, edema is not.
     2 Constipation is not a common problem associated with salicylates.
     4 Edema is not a problem associated with salicylates.

259. 4 **Salicylates act as analgesics by reducing inflammation. Salicylates act as antipyretics by affecting the heat-regulating center in the hypothalamus and increasing the elimination of heat through peripheral blood vessel dilation and evaporation of increased perspiration.** (AN; TC; DR)

     1 Salicylates have no capacity to act as a sedative and calm individuals.
     2 Salicylates have no capacity to act as a hypnotic and induce sleep.
     3 Salicylates have no capacity to destroy or control a microorganism's effect.

260. **4 To maintain the desired blood level, the drug must be given in the exact amount at the times directed. If the blood level of the drug falls, the organisms have an opportunity to build up resistance to the drug. (PL; TC; DR)**

1 Weighing a client is important with drugs that affect fluid balance.

2 Giving medication with milk or meals is important with drugs that cause GI distress.

3 Monitoring temperature would be important with antipyretic drugs.

261. **2 A side effect of vincristine is alopecia. To adolescents, who are very concerned with identity, this represents a tremendous threat to their self-image. (PL; ED; DR)**

1 Anemia is not likely to affect self-image.

3 Constipation, although very serious, does not threaten a child's self-image.

4 This will not be immediately obvious.

262. **3 Vincristine is highly neurotoxic, causing paresthesias, muscle weakness, ptosis, diplopia, paralytic ileus, vocal cord paralysis, and loss of deep tendon reflexes. (EV; TC; DR)**

1 Anemia can occur, but neither drug should cause fever.

2 Alopecia is reversible with cessation of the drug.

4 Integumentary symptoms are not usually a problem.

PEDIATRIC ANSWERS

CHAPTER 6

Medical-Surgical Nursing

Medical-surgical nursing is concerned with those aspects of nursing care that are related to the physical and emotional needs of clients with specific types of health problems. The concepts, principles, and skills included here will assist the practitioner in all aspects of nursing care.

Medical-surgical content has been developed by using a systems approach with examples of major diseases. The areas covered include a general conceptual introduction; preoperative and postoperative care; and cardiovascular, respiratory, gastrointestinal, genitourinary, endocrine, neurologic, musculoskeletal, and integumentary systems. The format for each section follows a similar pattern, beginning with a review of anatomy and physiology, related pharmacology, and related procedures and moving into the major diseases. A data base that may include such topics as etiology and pathophysiology, clinical findings, and therapeutic interventions begins the discussion of each disease process. Nursing care is presented in the nursing process format, which includes the familiar steps of data collection, analysis and interpretation, planning/implementation, and evaluation/outcomes.

GROWTH AND DEVELOPMENT

▼ THE YOUNG ADULT (AGED 20 TO 44 YEARS)

Data Base

A. Physiologic development
 1. Physical maturation occurs
 2. Muscle strength and coordination peak
 3. Biorhythms become established
 4. Sexuality
     a. Established sex drive remains high for men
     b. Female sex drive reaches a peak during later phase of young adulthood
     c. Physiologically optimal period for childbearing
 5. Basal metabolic rate (BMR) decreases at rate of 2% to 4% per decade after 20 years of age
B. Psychosocial development
 1. Mental abilities reflect formal operations (see Growth and Development of the Adolescent in Pediatric Nursing)
 2. Resolving the developmental crisis of intimacy versus isolation
 3. Establishing new family relationships and parenting patterns
 4. Establishing the self in, and advancing in, a chosen occupation
C. Health problems
 1. Accidents and adverse effects (suicides, motor vehicles, and homicides) are the leading causes of death in Canadians in this age group
 2. Circulatory system (ischemic heart diseases, high blood pressure)
 3. Malignancies involving the reproductive organs
 4. Sexually transmitted diseases
 5. Chemical dependency and abuse
 6. Fertility regulation
 7. Periodontal disease
 8. Unbalanced diet
 9. Spousal abuse
 10. Intimacy problems

GENERAL NURSING CARE OF YOUNG ADULTS

A. DATA COLLECTION

 1. Obtain history of drug and alcohol use, sexual practices, and family relationships
 2. Determine baseline height and weight and dietary history
 3. Measure vital signs to establish baseline
 4. Question client about health practices related to cancer prevention and detection

B. ANALYSIS AND INTERPRETATION

 1. Risk for infection related to sexual activity
 2. Risk for injury related to chemical impairment
 3. Ineffective management of therapeutic regimen (individual) related to feelings of invincibility
 4. Noncompliance related to denial or to fear of diagnosis/prognosis
 5. Altered nutrition: risk for more than body requirements related to consumption of fast food and junk food
 6. Parental role conflict related to caring for elderly parents
 7. Altered sexuality patterns related to:
     a. Increased sex drives
     b. Sexual preference
     c. Establishment of a family
 8. Altered tissue perfusion related to dietary indiscretions

C. PLANNING/IMPLEMENTATION

 1. Encourage attendance at safety programs to promote accident prevention (e.g., defensive driving, self-defense)
 2. Increase public awareness of problems and availability of crisis counseling, support groups, and other community resources (e.g., hot lines, Alcoholics Anonymous, family planning clinics)
 3. Teach safer sex practices
 4. Promote awareness that optimal diet is essential to achieving and maintaining optimal health; encourage nutritional evaluation and consultation
 5. Teach the Canada's Food Guide to Healthy Eating* (Fig. 6-1)
 6. Teach dietary guidelines
     a. Eat a variety of foods from the four food groups
     b. Eat foods rich in calcium and iron (especially women and children)
     c. Eat moderate amounts of protein, balancing intake of plant and animal sources
     d. Eat more complex carbohydrates, fiber, and natural sugars
     e. Choose lower-fat foods more often since diets high in fat have been associated with heart disease and certain types of cancer
     f. Choose lower-fat dairy products, leaner meats, and foods prepared with little or no fat
     g. Eat less meat with high fat content
     h. Limit intake of salt and sodium
     i. Use alcohol and caffeine in moderation. For adults, no more than 1 alcoholic drink a day and no more than 7 drinks a week.

*Health and Welfare Canada (1992). Ottawa: Minister of Supply and Services. (Catalogue No. H39-252/1992E)

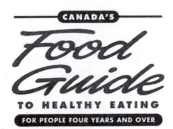

Different People Need Different Amounts of Food

The amount of food you need every day from the 4 food groups and other foods depends on your age, body size, activity level, whether you are male or female and if you are pregnant or breast-feeding. That's why the Food Guide gives a lower and higher number of servings for each food group. For example, young children can choose the lower number of servings, while male teenagers can go to the higher number. Most other people can choose servings somewhere in between.

Grain Products
5-12
SERVINGS PER DAY

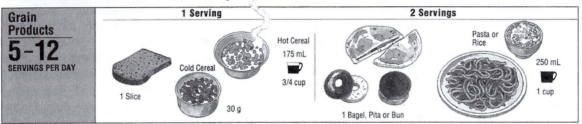

1 Serving

1 Slice
Cold Cereal
30 g
Hot Cereal
175 mL
3/4 cup

2 Servings

1 Bagel, Pita or Bun
Pasta or Rice
250 mL
1 cup

Vegetables & Fruit
5-10
SERVINGS PER DAY

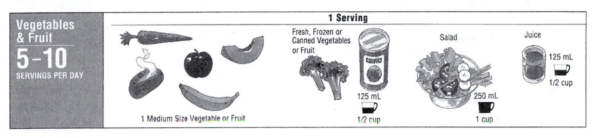

1 Serving

1 Medium Size Vegetable or Fruit
Fresh, Frozen or Canned Vegetables or Fruit
125 mL
1/2 cup
Salad
250 mL
1 cup
Juice
125 mL
1/2 cup

Milk Products
SERVINGS PER DAY
Children 4–9 years: 2–3
Youth 10–16 years: 3–4
Adults: 2–4
Pregnant & Breast-feeding Women: 3–4

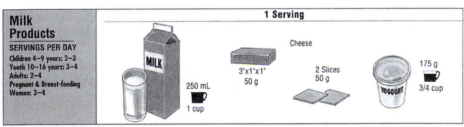

1 Serving

MILK
250 mL
1 cup
Cheese
3"x1"x1"
50 g
2 Slices
50 g
175 g
YOGOURT
3/4 cup

Other Foods

Taste and enjoyment can also come from other foods and beverages that are not part of the 4 food groups. Some of these foods are higher in fat or Calories, so use these foods in moderation.

Meat & Alternatives
2-3
SERVINGS PER DAY

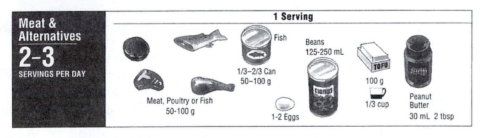

1 Serving

Meat, Poultry or Fish
50-100 g
Fish
1/3–2/3 Can
50–100 g
1-2 Eggs
Beans
125-250 mL
Tofu
100 g
1/3 cup
Peanut Butter
30 mL 2 tbsp

Enjoy eating well, being active and feeling good about yourself. That's VITALIT

FIGURE 6-1 Canada's Food Guide.© Catalogue No. H39-252/1992E. No changes permitted. Reprint permission not required. Minister of Supply and Services, Canada, 1992.

Limit caffeine intake from all sources to no more than the equivalent of 4 cups of coffee a day

   j. Describe 1-serving equivalents
     (1) Grain products—175 ml hot cereal; 30 g ready-to-eat cereal; 1 slice of bread; 125 ml cooked rice or pasta; ½ bagel or pita
     (2) Vegetables and fruits—1 medium-sized potato, carrot, tomato, apple, banana, orange, or peach; 1 small apricot or plum; 125 ml fresh, frozen, or canned vegetable or fruit; or 125 ml vegetable or fruit juice
     (3) Milk products—250 ml milk; 50 g cheese or 2 slices processed cheese; or 175 g yogurt
     (4) Meat and alternatives—50 to 100 g meat, poultry, or fish; 1 to 2 eggs; 125 ml beans; 100 g tofu; or 30 ml peanut butter

7. Maintain recommended daily caloric intake
   a. 2000 calories daily for sedentary women and some older adults
   b. 2200 calories daily for children, teenage girls, active women, and many sedentary men; pregnant or breastfeeding women require additional calories
   c. 2800 calories daily for teenage boys, many active men, and some very active women
8. Assist client to examine options for caring for elderly parents
9. Teach breast and testicular self-examination techniques and encourage regular medical checkups

D. EVALUATION/OUTCOMES
1. Establishes safe health care practices
2. Maintains ideal body weight
3. Maintains blood pressure within normal limits
4. Remains free from infection

▼ THE MIDDLE-AGED ADULT (AGED 45 TO 59 YEARS)

Data Base
A. Physiologic development
1. Greater diversity in physiologic conditioning resulting from established life-style
2. Early signs of aging (e.g., wrinkling, thinning hair, decreased muscle tone and nerve function)
3. Decreased BMR with subsequent weight gain unless caloric intake is reduced
4. Decreased production of sexual hormones
   a. Menopause (See Chapter 3, Childbearing and Women's Health Nursing)
   b. Male climacteric; may pass unnoticed, especially in those with high self-esteem;

symptoms may include diminished potency, less forceful ejaculation, thinning and greying hair, fatigue, and depression

B. Psychosocial development
1. Cognitive abilities enhanced because of motivation and past experiences
2. Resolving developmental crisis of generativity versus stagnation
3. Adjusting to changes in family caused by aging parents and growing or returning children
4. Maintaining satisfactory status of one's career
5. Accepting physical changes associated with advancing age
6. Developing social and civic activities that are personally satisfying

C. Health problems
1. Cardiovascular and circulatory system diseases (high blood pressure, myocardial infarction, angina)
2. Malignancies of respiratory and reproductive systems
3. Intestinal/rectal cancer
4. Suicide
5. Alcoholism
6. Diabetes
7. Sexual dysfunction
8. Presbyopia
9. Depression
10. Unbalanced or inadequate diet

GENERAL NURSING CARE OF MIDDLE-AGED ADULTS

A. DATA COLLECTION
1. Determine cardiovascular status
   a. Vital signs and peripheral pulses
   b. Peripheral edema and shortness of breath
   c. Chest pain
2. Measure visual acuity
3. Obtain history of alcohol use, sexual patterns, and family relationships
4. Determine baseline height and weight and dietary history
5. Question client about leisure activities and retirement plans

B. ANALYSIS AND INTERPRETATION
1. Risk for activity intolerance related to diminished physiologic conditioning
2. Risk for caregiver role strain related to aging parents
3. Ineffective individual coping related to chronic health problems
4. Anticipatory grieving related to altered family relationships and/or altered job status
5. Altered nutrition: risk for more than body requirements related to:

a. Sedentary life-style

b. Dietary indiscretions

6. Altered sexuality patterns related to decreased hormonal production

7. Altered tissue perfusion related to dietary indiscretions

C. PLANNING/IMPLEMENTATION

1. Reinforce importance of regular exercise to prevent cardiovascular and neuromusculo-skeletal disease

2. Stress dietary changes: reduction of calories, fats and protein; increased calcium and fiber

3. Encourage individuals to identify new interests, and to anticipate and plan for retirement

4. Emphasize need for regular medical evaluations as well as self-evaluations

5. Encourage attendance at self-help groups to stop substance dependency (e.g., smoking, alcohol, weight control)

6. Increase awareness of the relationship between an unbalanced diet and disease

7. Encourage individuals to follow Canada's Food Guide

8. Assist client to establish appropriate communication with sexual partner

D. EVALUATION/OUTCOMES

1. Maintains ideal body weight

2. Maintains blood pressure within normal limits

3. Establishes healthy dietary pattern

4. Participates in exercise regimen

5. Develops coping skills to manage stress

▼ THE OLDER-AGED ADULT (AGED 60 TO 74 YEARS)

Data Base

A. Physiologic development

1. Slowing of reaction time

2. Loss of sensory acuity

3. Diminished muscle tone and strength

4. Increased diversity in health status and function resulting from prior life-style and development of chronic health problems

B. Psychosocial development

1. Cognitive abilities may be affected by cardiovascular disease

2. Adjusting to retirement: some individuals experience a loss of self-esteem, whereas others enjoy the freedom to explore other interests

3. Coping with altered economic status; adjusting to fixed income

4. Resolving death of parents and possibly spouse

5. Accepting separation from their children and their families

C. Health problems

1. Ischemic heart disease

2. Malignancies of respiratory, reproductive, and intestinal systems

3. Presbyopia

4. Cerebrovascular insufficiency

5. Hearing loss

6. Respiratory disease

7. Depression

8. Diabetes

9. Osteoporosis/osteoarthritis

10. Unbalanced or inadequate diet

GENERAL NURSING CARE OF OLDER ADULTS

A. DATA COLLECTION

1. Determine cardiovascular status

a. Vital signs and peripheral pulses

b. Peripheral edema

c. Shortness of breath

d. History of chest pain

e. Changes in sensation

2. Measure visual and auditory acuities

3. Obtain history relative to warning signs of cancer

4. Identify coping skills and support systems

B. ANALYSIS AND INTERPRETATION

1. Risk for caregiver role strain related to illness of significant other

2. Ineffective individual coping related to fear of disability

3. Impaired gas exchange related to respiratory system changes

4. Risk for injury related to:

a. Sensory perceptual alterations

b. Weakness

5. Altered nutrition: risk for less than body requirements related to:

a. Physiologic anorexia

b. Lack of interest in food preparation

6. Sensory perceptual alteration (visual and auditory) related to changes in visual and/or hearing acuity

7. Social isolation related to:

a. Loss of hearing

b. Changes in peer group

c. Death of spouse or friends

8. Altered tissue perfusion related to cardiovascular changes

C. PLANNING/IMPLEMENTATION

1. Encourage individuals to maintain a schedule of regular medical, dental, and visual examinations to control or prevent health problems

2. Assess living conditions for possible hazards that could cause accidents

3. Refer widows and widowers to appropriate self-help groups as necessary
4. Encourage individuals to anticipate and plan for retirement and to develop new interests and support systems
5. Encourage nutritional assessment and consultation to prevent nutrient deficiencies and to provide for diet modifications with aging
6. Encourage individuals to follow Canada's Food Guide

D. EVALUATION/OUTCOMES
1. Participates in a supervised exercise program
2. Verbalizes fears to health care providers
3. Remains free from injury
4. Develops satisfying interpersonal relationships
5. Consumes nutritionally adequate diet

▼ THE SENIOR ADULT (AGED 75+ YEARS)

Data Base
A. Physiologic development
1. Diminished sensation and reaction time (e.g., narrowed visual field, hearing loss)
2. Increased sensitivity to cold because of decreased subcutaneous tissue, decreased thyroid functioning, and impaired circulation
3. Decreased enzyme secretion in and motility of the gastrointestinal (GI) tract
4. Decreased glomerular filtration rate
5. Decreased cardiac output
6. Arteriosclerotic changes with diminished elasticity of blood vessels
7. Decreased lung capacity
8. Demineralization and other degenerative skeletal changes, particularly in weight-bearing bones
9. Muscle atrophy
B. Psychosocial development
1. Cognitive abilities not necessarily affected by age, but may be impaired as a result of disease, leading to diminished awareness
2. Resolving the developmental crisis of ego integrity versus despair
3. Adjusting to the death of important others
4. Adapting to decreased physical capacity and changes in body image
5. Adjusting to the economic burden of a fixed income
6. Recognizing the inevitability of death
7. Reminiscing increasingly about the past
C. Health problems
1. Cardiovascular disease
2. Cardiac dysrhythmias and heart failure
3. Cerebrovascular insufficiency

4. Cancer
5. Pneumonia and influenza
6. Accidents (e.g., falls, hip fractures)
7. Resistance to changes in environment
8. Impaired nutritional intake
9. Cataracts, glaucoma, hearing loss
10. Depression

GENERAL NURSING CARE OF SENIOR ADULTS

A. DATA COLLECTION
1. Determine cardiovascular status
   a. Vital signs and peripheral pulses
   b. Peripheral edema
   c. Shortness of breath
   d. History of chest pain
   e. Changes in sensation
2. Identify neurologic deficits
   a. Level of consciousness
   b. Orientation
   c. Motor function
   d. Sensory function
3. Determine respiratory function
   a. Respiratory rate
   b. Respiratory characteristics: rhythm, depth, use of accessory muscles
   c. Breath sounds
   d. Vital capacity
   e. Arterial blood gases
4. Review nutritional status
   a. Dietary history
   b. Body weight
   c. Skin condition
   d. Serum protein and albumin levels
5. Assess the individual's ability to cope with the environment
6. Review prescription medications

B. ANALYSIS AND INTERPRETATION
1. Impaired gas exchange related to decreased vital capacity
2. Risk for injury related to neurologic deficits
3. Altered nutrition: less than body requirements related to:
   a. Decreased appetite
   b. Decreased taste
   c. Poor-fitting dentures
   d. Depression
4. Risk for peripheral neurovascular dysfunction related to age-related changes
5. Relocation stress syndrome related to inability to maintain own home
6. Self-care deficit related to altered motor/sensory function
7. Altered tissue perfusion related to cardiovascular changes

C. PLANNING/IMPLEMENTATION

1. Encourage individuals to maintain a schedule of regular medical supervision
2. Promote maximum degree of independence
3. Initiate appropriate referrals for individuals requiring assistance with activities of daily living
4. Open channels of communication for reality orientation, reminiscing, and emotional support
5. Refer to social service and other resources that can provide economic assistance when necessary
6. Ensure that prosthetic devices (e.g., dentures, corrective lenses, eye prosthetics, braces, limbs) fit comfortably and do not cause irritation; teach proper care of such devices
7. Assess for side effects of medications
8. Encourage following Canada's Food Guide

D. EVALUATION/OUTCOMES

1. Assists in self-care activities
2. Remains free from injury
3. Uses community resources to maximize independence
4. Maintains nutritionally adequate diet
5. Maintains social relationships

INFECTION

REVIEW OF PHYSIOLOGY

Resistance

A. Nonspecific resistance: that is directed against all invading microbes; varies considerably from one species to another and even among individuals of same species
   1. Body surface barriers
      a. Intact skin and mucosa
      b. Cilia and secretion of mucus
   2. Antimicrobial secretions
      a. Oil of skin: contains fatty acids effective against many bacteria and fungi
      b. Tears: contain lysozyme, a bactericidal (gram-positive) enzyme
      c. Gastric juice: contains highly bactericidal hydrochloric acid
      d. Vaginal secretions: low pH acts to inhibit microbial growth
   3. Internal antimicrobial agents
      a. Interferon: antiviral substance produced within the cells in response to a viral attack; inhibits viral growth and multiplication
      b. Properdin: protein agent in blood that destroys certain gram-negative bacteria and viruses
      c. Lysozyme: destroys mainly gram-positive bacteria
   4. Phagocytosis: part of the role of the reticuloendothelial system
      a. Phagocytes: cells in the blood that ingest and destroy microbes
         (1) Microphages: polymorphonuclear leukocytes, of which the neutrophils are the most active; in the inflammatory response they pass through the intact capillary wall (diapedesis) into the intercellular area
         (2) Macrophages
            (a) Fixed (sessile) macrophages: phagocytes lining the capillary endothelium and sinuses of the liver (Kupffer cells), spleen, bone marrow, lymph nodes, and other organs where they remove microbes from the blood
            (b) Wandering macrophages (histiocytes): blood monocytes that enter the tissues (via diapedesis) and devour intercellular debris, including debilitated microphages
B. Specific resistance: that directed against a specific pathogen (foreign protein) or its toxin
   1. Antigen: any substance, including allergens, that stimulates production of antibodies when introduced into the body; typically, antigens are foreign proteins, the most potent being microbial cells and their products
      a. B lymphocytes: derive from stem cells and differentiate into plasma cells in the presence of antigens; provide humoral immunity; a specific antigen provokes the production of a specific antibody (homologous antibody), which is considered to be ineffective against any other antigen
      b. T lymphocytes: derive from stem cells and are responsible for cellular immunity; involved in delayed hypersensitivity responses, graft rejection, and acquired immunodeficiency syndrome (AIDS)
      c. Memory cells: large population of antibodies that develop on first encounter with an antigen; they become somewhat dormant until stimulated by subsequent encounters with the antigen; this phenomenon explains the dramatic rise in antibody titer following a booster shot of a vaccine (anamnestic reaction)
   2. Antibody: immune substance produced by plasma cells; antibodies are gamma globulin molecules and are commonly referred to as immunoglobulin (Ig)
      a. Chemical structure: made up of four polypeptide chains in two pairs

b. Classification: there are five major classes of antibodies
   (1) Immunoglobulin G (IgG) antibodies: most important class, making up more than 80% of the total immunoglobulins; only immunoglobulin that passes the placental barrier, providing natural passive immunity to the newborn
   (2) Immunoglobulin A (IgA) antibodies: present in blood, mucus, and human milk secretions; play an important role against respiratory pathogens
   (3) Immunoglobulin M (IgM) antibodies: first antibodies to be detected after an injection of antigen; bactericidal for gram-negative bacteria under specific conditions
   (4) Immunoglobulin D (IgD) antibodies: present in small numbers in normal individuals; specific immunologic role presently under investigation
   (5) Immunoglobulin E (IgE) antibodies: responsible for hypersensitivity and allergies; these antibodies exist tightly bound to the surface of mast cells (large basophilic connective tissue cells)
       (a) On introduction of their homologous antigens (allergens), they cause the mast cells to release histamine and other pharmacologic agents
       (b) Release of histamine and other pharmacologic agents causes the symptoms of hypersensitivity reactions
       (c) This process explains relief of symptoms by administration of antihistamines
3. Antigen-antibody reactions
   a. Agglutination: clumping together of cells and specific antigens by homologous antibodies called agglutinins
   b. Cytolysis: disruption or dissolution of cells (lysis) by homologous antibodies called cytolysins or lysins
   c. Opsonization: rendering of bacteria and other cells susceptible to phagocytosis by homologous antibodies called opsonins
   d. Neutralization (viral): rendering of viruses noninfective by homologous antibodies called neutralizing antibodies
   e. Neutralization (toxin): chemical neutralization of a toxin by homologous antibodies called antitoxins
   f. Precipitation: formation of an insoluble complex (precipitate) in the reaction between a soluble antigen and its homologous antibodies called precipitins

4. Complement-fixation: group of blood serum proteins needed in certain antigen-antibody reactions; both the complement and the antibody must be present for a reaction to occur

Immunity

A. Species immunity: certain species are naturally immune to specific microorganisms (e.g., humans are immune to distemper, dogs are immune to measles)
B. Active immunity: antibodies formed in the body
   1. Natural active immunity: antibodies formed by the individual during the course of the disease; in some instances the antibodies provide lifelong immunity (e.g., measles, chickenpox, yellow fever, smallpox)
   2. Artificial active immunity: use of a vaccine or toxoid to stimulate formation of homologous antibodies; revaccination (booster shot) is often needed to sustain antibody titer (anamnestic effect)
      a. Killed vaccines: antigenic preparations containing microbes grown in the laboratory separated from growth medium and killed by heat or a chemical agent; usually injected subcutaneously; less often given by intramuscular or oral routes (e.g., pertussis vaccine, typhoid vaccine)
      b. Live vaccines: antigenic preparations containing microbes weakened (attenuated) by drying, continued and prolonged passage through culture media or animals (to induce mutations), or by other means; typically such vaccines are more antigenic than killed preparations; (e.g., oral [Sabin] poliomyelitis vaccine, measles vaccine)
      c. Toxoids: antigenic preparations composed of inactivated bacterial toxins (generally an exotoxin treated with formaldehyde) (e.g., tetanus toxoids, diphtheria toxoids)
C. Passive immunity: antibodies acquired from an outside source
   1. Natural passive immunity: passage of preformed antibodies from the mother through the placenta or colostrum to the baby; therefore during the first few weeks of life the newborn is immune to certain diseases to which the mother has active immunity
   2. Artificial passive immunity: injection of antisera derived from immunized animals or humans; antisera (antiserums) provide immediate and often complete protection in susceptible exposed persons and also are of value in treatment (e.g., diphtheria antitoxin, tetanus antitoxin); individuals may be hypersensitive to certain sera such as horse serum, and pretesting for hypersensitivity must be carried out before administration

REVIEW OF MICROBIOLOGY
Pathology of Infection

A. Definition: invasion of the body by pathogenic microorganisms (pathogens) and the reaction of the tissues to their presence and to the toxins generated by them

B. Types
  1. Local, focal, or systemic
     a. Local infection: one in which the etiologic agent is limited to one locality of the body, such as a boil; often a local infection may have systemic repercussions such as fever and malaise
     b. Focal infection: a local infection such as an abscess from which the organisms themselves spread to other parts of body (e.g., a tooth abscess that continues to seed organisms into the blood)
     c. Systemic infection: one in which the infectious agent is spread throughout the body (e.g., typhoid fever)
  2. Acute or chronic
     a. Acute infection: one that develops rapidly, usually resulting in a high fever and severe sickness
     b. Chronic infection: one that develops slowly, with mild but longer-lasting symptoms; sometimes an acute infection may become chronic and vice versa
  3. Primary or secondary
     a. Primary infection: initial infection, unrelated to other health problems
     b. Secondary infection: occasioned when invaders (or opportunists) take advantage of the weakened defenses resulting from the primary infection (e.g., staphylococcal pneumonia as a sequela of measles)
  4. Bacteremia: presence of nonmultiplying bacteria in the blood
  5. Septicemia: bacterial cells actively multiplying in the blood
  6. Toxemia: presence of microbial toxins in the blood
  7. Viremia: presence of viruses in the blood

C. Source and transmission of pathogens
  1. Source: ultimate source (or reservoir) of almost all pathogens is human or animal; human sources include:
     a. Persons exhibiting symptoms of disease
     b. Carriers: persons who harbor a pathogen in the absence of a discernible clinical disease
        (1) Types of carriers
           (a) Healthy carriers: those who have never had the disease in question
           (b) Incubatory carriers: those in the incubation period of a disease
           (c) Chronic carriers: those who have recovered from a disease but continue to harbor pathogens
        (2) Diseases commonly spread by carriers
           (a) Tuberculosis
           (b) Diphtheria
           (c) Meningitis
           (d) Pneumonia
           (e) Typhoid fever
  2. Transmission
     a. Direct
        (1) Body or body fluid contact
        (2) Droplets (droplet infection)
     b. Indirect
        (1) Food
        (2) Water
        (3) Air
        (4) Soil
        (5) Fomites
        (6) Vectors (e.g., insects)
           (a) Mechanical transfer: insects' feet
           (b) Biologic transfer: microbe undergoes part of its life cycle in the insect's body
  3. Portals of entry and exit
     a. Portal of entry: where microbes enter the body
        (1) Nose
        (2) Mouth
        (3) Urogenital tract
        (4) Skin: wounds, abrasions, and insect bites
     b. Portal of exit: where microbes leave the body
        (1) Nose
        (2) Mouth
        (3) Feces
        (4) Urine
        (5) Vaginal discharges
        (6) Pus and exudates
        (7) Vomitus
        (8) Blood
  4. Susceptible host
     a. Developmental level: extremes of age
     b. Inadequate nutritional status
     c. Coexisting disease
     d. Prior immunity

D. Development
  1. Definitions
     a. Pathogenicity: ability of a microbe to cause disease
     b. Virulence: degree of pathogenicity
  2. Determinants of pathogenicity
     a. Chemical products
        (1) Exotoxins: heat-labile proteins readily released from bacterial cell; most dead-

ly of all biologic poisons (e.g., botulism, tetanus, and diphtheria)

   (2) Endotoxins: heat-stable lipopolysaccharide-protein complexes released from gram-negative bacteria; less deadly than exotoxins (e.g., typhoid fever and dysentery)

   (3) Other toxic products

     (a) Hemolysins: these destroy the red blood cells (RBCs; erythrocytes)

     (b) Leukocidins: these destroy the white blood cells (WBCs; leukocytes)

     (c) Coagulase: clots blood plasma

     (d) Hyaluronidase: dissolves intercellular cement

     (e) Kinases: dissolve clots or inhibit their formation

     (f) Collagenase: disintegrates collagen

  b. Cellular destruction: some microbes damage tissues and cause disease by direct mechanical injury to the cells, particularly intracellular parasites (e.g., viruses and rickettsiae)

  c. Capsules: increase virulence apparently by making microbes possessing them less vulnerable to destruction by phagocytosis

Types of Pathogens

Bacteria

A. Definition: bacteria are unicellular microbes without chlorophyll

B. Some examples of medically important bacteria

  1. Eubacteriales ("true bacteria"): typically unicellular microbes having a rigid cell wall; the morphologic types are:

  a. Rod-shaped bacilli: variations of the rod shape may be curved or clubbed (some of the gram-positive rods form endospores)

  b. Spheric cocci

  c. Eubacteriales are divided into five families based on shape, Gram stain, and endospore formation

   (1) Gram-positive cocci include

     (a) Diplococci: occurring predominantly in pairs (e.g., *Diplococcus pneumoniae*)

     (b) Streptococci: occurring predominantly in chains (e.g., *Streptococcus pyogenes*)

     (c) Staphylococci: occurring predominantly in grapelike bunches (e.g., *Staphylococcus aureus*)

   (2) Gram-negative cocci include *Neisseria gonorrhoeae* and *Neisseria meningitidis*

   (3) Gram-negative rods include enterobacteria such as *Escherichia*, *Salmonella*, and *Shigella* species

   (4) Gram-positive rods that do not produce endospores include *Corynebacterium diphtheriae*

   (5) Gram-positive rods producing endospores include *Bacillus anthracis*, *Clostridium botulinum*, and *Clostridium tetani*

  2. Actinomycetales (actinomycetes): moldlike microbes with elongated cells, frequently filamentous (e.g., *Mycobacterium tuberculosis* and *Mycobacterium leprae*)

  3. Spirochaetales (spirochetes): flexuous, spiral organisms (e.g., *Treponema pallidum*)

  4. Mycoplasmatales (mycoplasmas): delicate, nonmotile microbes displaying a variety of sizes and shapes

  a. Commonly referred to as pleuropneumonia-like organisms (PPLO)

  b. Mycoplasmas are the smallest organisms known that are capable of growth and reproduction outside living cells

C. Bacterial cell

  1. Size: from 0.5 to 15 mm

  2. Cell wall: gram-positive species are rich in muramic acid and low in lipids; the opposite is true of the gram-negative species

  3. Capsule: a thickened protective material (generally a polysaccharide) that is secreted by the cell, thereby protecting it from being phagocytized and increasing its virulence (e.g., *Diplococcus pneumoniae*)

  4. Spores: the inactive resistant structures into which bacterial protoplasm can transform under adverse conditions (under favorable conditions a spore germinates into an active and growing vegetative cell)

  a. The endospores are resistant to heat, desiccation, and other antimicrobial agents

  b. Spore formers *Clostridium tetani* and *Clostridium botulinum* are difficult to destroy; therefore their destruction is used to set the standards of sterilization for the hospital and food industries

  5. Flagella: organelles of locomotion possessed by all motile bacteria; some species have one flagellum (monotrichous), whereas others have flagella over their entire surface (peritrichous)

  6. Reproduction: bacteria reproduce by binary fission, an asexual process dividing the cell into new daughter cells; bacteria are also able to conjugate and exchange genetic material (recombination)

D. Growth needs

  1. Nutrition

  a. Autotrophic organisms: may do well on simple diet of carbon dioxide, inorganic salts, and water

b. Heterotrophic organisms: demand organic nutrients
  (1) Saprophytes: derive nourishment from dead or decaying organic matter
  (2) Parasites: derive nourishment from living tissue; obligate parasites cannot be cultured except in living tissue

2. Culturing
  a. Culture: growth of large numbers of microbes on suitable food media
  b. Culture media: food substances in or on which cultures are grown (e.g., broth, agar, milk)
  c. Colony: cluster of millions of microbes, presumably all descendants from a single bacterium, visible to naked eye
  d. Ways in which cultures are studied
    (1) Smears made and organisms studied microscopically either with or without staining
    (2) Cultural characteristics observed
      (a) Media most favorable to growth
      (b) Appearance of colonies: color, shape, and texture, whether large or small, smooth or rough, opaque or translucent
      (c) Molecular oxygen requirement: anaerobic, aerobic, or facultative

E. Biochemical reactions
  1. Fermentation: anaerobic oxidation reactions by which some organisms use carbohydrates to generate energy-rich adenosine triphosphate (ATP) molecules; various kinds of fermentation reactions are useful for identifying different groups of microorganisms
    a. Nonfermenters
    b. Fermenters that produce only acid
    c. Fermenters that produce acid and gas (e.g., *Escherichia coli*, a normal inhabitant of the intestinal tract)
    d. Lactose fermenters (e.g., *Escherichia coli* and other nonpathogens in the intestinal tract)
    e. Nonlactose fermenters (e.g., *Shigella* and *Salmonella* pathogens in the intestinal tract)
  2. Urea-splitting reaction: identifies organisms as:
    a. Urease-positive organisms: contain enzyme urease, which catalyzes conversion of urea to ammonia (e.g., *Proteus* bacilli, which are the gram-negative, normal inhabitants of the intestinal tract)
    b. Urease-negative organisms: do not contain urease so cannot convert urea to ammonia (e.g., *Salmonella* and *Shigella*, pathogens in the intestinal tract)
F. Hydrogen ion concentration (pH): majority of bacteria grow and are cultured best at a pH of about

7.5; most fungi (molds and yeasts) are cultured best at a pH of about 5
G. Oxygen use
  1. Obligate aerobes: organisms that cannot grow without free (molecular) oxygen
  2. Obligate anaerobes: organisms that cannot grow in the presence of free (molecular) oxygen
  3. Facultative: organisms that can grow with or without free oxygen
H. Temperature
  1. Psychrophiles: organisms growing best at low temperatures of 10° to 20° C
  2. Mesophiles: organisms growing best at middle temperatures of 20° to 45° C; this range includes human pathogens that have an optimum temperature of 37° C
  3. Thermophiles: organisms growing best at high temperatures of 45° to 65° C
I. Staining: artificial coloration to facilitate visualization and identification of tissues and microorganisms
  1. Gram stain: gram-positive organisms retain the crystal violet color when treated with ethyl alcohol; gram-negative organisms are decolorized with ethyl alcohol
  2. Acid-fast stain: after being stained with carbolfuchsin, acid-fast organisms resist decolorization with dilute acid alcohol and do not take counterstain (usually methylene blue); non–acid-fast organisms decolorize and take counterstain
J. Pathogenicity: some 2000 species of bacteria, most of which are harmless; those causing disease (pathogens) are usually heterotrophic mesophiles

Viruses
A. Definition: obligate intracellular parasite of unknown relationship to other forms of life
B. Characteristics: virions (virus particles)—range in size from 1 to 350 nanometers (nm); 1 nm equals 1 billionth of a meter or 1/1000 of a millimeter; some cuboidal and others rod-shaped; unlike rickettsiae and chlamydiae, composed of either ribonucleic acid (RNA) or deoxyribonucleic acid (DNA), not both
C. Classification
  1. Animal viruses: some contain RNA and others DNA; divided into 14 categories on the basis of particle size, symmetry, and nucleic acid content
  2. Plant viruses: contain RNA
  3. Bacterial viruses: most contain DNA; those that destroy bacterial cells called bacteriophages
D. Culturing: being obligate parasites, viruses demand living tissues such as embryonated hen's eggs, tissue cultures, and animal inoculation

E. Pathogenicity: viruses cause cancer in animals and cause Burkitt's lymphoma, mumps, rubeola, rubella, smallpox, chickenpox, herpes simplex, encephalitis, yellow fever, AIDS, and many other infections in humans

Fungi

A. Definition: higher protists; include morels, truffles, cup fungi, mildews, mushrooms, puffballs, smuts, rusts, molds, and yeasts (molds and yeasts are of medical concern)

B. Molds: fuzzy growths of interlacing filaments called hyphae
   1. Hyphae: filaments of a mold; in some species hyphae are divided by partial septa and appear to be multicellular, whereas in others they are nonseptate
   2. Mycelium: tuft of interwoven hyphae
   3. Spores: means by which molds reproduce; a single spore in the proper environment gives rise to a new mycelium; spores produced sexually and asexually

C. Yeasts: organisms that usually are single-celled and usually reproduce by budding
   1. Yeast cell: round or ovoid and much larger and more complex than bacterial cell
   2. Reproduction: usually by the asexual process of budding, but many species also reproduce sexually by means of ascospores
   3. True yeasts: reproduce sexually as well as asexually (by budding); many species, such as *Saccharomyces cerevisiae* (baker's yeast), convert glucose into alcohol and carbon dioxide (alcoholic fermentation); *Candida albicans*, another type of yeast, causes "thrush" in humans (this yeast is part of the normal flora but may become an opportunistic pathogen in persons with low resistance)
   4. Pathogenicity: certain species of molds cause infection, particularly those belonging to the class Fungi Imperfecti (Deuteromycetes), which account for diseases such as athlete's foot, ringworm of the scalp and axillary regions, and systemic mycosis

PHYSICAL AND CHEMICAL CONTROL OF MICROORGANISMS

Definition of Terms

A. Disinfection: removal or destruction of pathogenic microbes

B. Sterilization: removal or destruction of all microbes

Physical Methods

A. Heat sterilization
   1. Moist heat
      a. Steam under pressure (autoclave): usually operated at 121° C; time needed for procedure depends on material(s) being sterilized
      b. Boiling water: object(s) to be sterilized immersed in water and boiled for 15 minutes; because some spores resist boiling, this procedure is not suitable for surgical instruments
   2. Dry heat (hot-air oven)
      a. Operating temperature: 154° to 170° C (usually for 2 hours)
      b. Items sterilized: petrolatum gauze dressings and other items that might be damaged by steam or water
   3. Pasteurization: disinfection of milk and other substances by moderate heat; pathogenic organisms killed and microbial development considerably delayed (thus retarding spoilage)
      a. Holding method: heating to 63° C for 30 minutes, followed by rapid cooling
      b. Flash method: heating to 71.7° C for not less than 15 seconds, followed by rapid cooling

B. Radiation: all types of radiation injurious to microbes
   1. Gamma rays: used to sterilize food and drugs
   2. Ultraviolet light: used to inhibit the microbial population of air in operating rooms, nurseries, laboratories, school rooms, and food establishments (the disadvantage of ultraviolet light is that it has little penetration power)

C. Filtration: removal of microbes from liquids by means of porous materials (diatomaceous earth, porcelain); used to sterilize drugs, culture media, and certain other heat-sensitive substances

D. Refrigeration: low temperature inhibits microbial multiplication; used for food preservation

E. Hypertonicity: by their osmotic effects, hypertonic solutions inhibit microbial multiplication (e.g., brine and syrups)

F. Desiccation (drying): removal of water; bacterial spores and certain vegetable cells are resistant to such treatment; commonly used in food preservation

Chemical Methods (for body surfaces and inanimate objects)

A. Definitions: many terms used to describe action of chemical agents on microorganisms; in actual practice such terms often have little meaning because of variables
   1. Antiseptic: inhibits microbial growth
   2. Disinfectant: destroys pathogenic microbes
   3. Germicide: destroys pathogenic microbes
   4. Bactericide: destroys bacteria
   5. Fungicide: destroys fungi
   6. Viricide: destroys viruses

B. Conditions (variables) affecting action of chemical agents

1. Type and number of microbes: microbes respond differently to different agents; spores are resistant to most agents
2. Concentration: typically the greater the concentration of chemical, the greater the effect
3. Time: a certain time needed for maximum effect
4. Temperature: a rise usually hastens action
5. Organic matter: presence inhibits action

C. Evaluation: various tests used to evaluate antiseptics and disinfectants; all have limitations
   1. Phenol coefficient: bactericidal activity of a chemical agent in relation to the bactericidal action of phenol
   2. Culture inhibition: filter paper disks impregnated or saturated with chemical agent placed on agar plates previously inoculated with test organism; clear zone observed around disk (following incubation) if agent is inhibitory to organism (this is the same procedure used in determining the sensitivity of a culture to chemotherapeutic agents)

D. Commonly used chemical agents
   1. Ethyl alcohol (70%)
   2. Isopropyl alcohol (80%)
   3. Benzalkonium chloride (Zephiran) (1:1000)
   4. Hydrogen peroxide (3%)
   5. Silver nitrate (1%)
   6. Iodine and iodine-releasing compounds
   7. Chlorine and chlorine-releasing compounds
   8. Substituted phenols
   9. Cresols
   10. Ethylene oxide

PHARMACOLOGIC CONTROL OF INFECTION

Definition of Terms

A. Bactericidal effect: capable of destroying bacteria at low concentrations (e.g., disrupt building of cell membrane or wall, allow leak of cytoplasm)
B. Bacteriostatic effect: slows reproduction of bacteria; natural physiologic mechanisms are required for phagocytic abolition of the bacteria
C. Superinfection: emergence of microorganism growth (e.g., yeast and fungi) when natural protective flora is destroyed by antiinfective drug
D. Bacterial resistance: a natural characteristic of an organism or one acquired by mutation preventing destruction by a drug to which it was previously susceptible

Antibiotics

A. Description
   1. Drugs used to destroy bacteria (bactericidal effect) or inhibit bacterial reproduction (bacte-

riostatic effect); the net result is to control infection and restore homeostasis to the human organism
   2. Available in oral, parenteral (IM, IV), and topical, including ophthalmic, preparations

B. Antibiotic sensitivity: determined by two general techniques
   1. Paper disks: multilobed disk impregnated with different antibiotics placed on surface of inoculated plate; zones of inhibition (following incubation) surround lobes containing antibiotics to which microbe is sensitive
   2. Tube dilution: antibiotic in question diluted out in growth broth and tubes then inoculated with the organisms in question; minimal inhibitory concentration (MIC) determined (following incubation) by noting minimal concentration preventing growth

C. Examples
   1. Penicillins: interfere with bacterial cell wall synthesis; broad spectrum
      a. Amoxicillin (Amoxil)
      b. Ampicillin (Ampicin)
      c. Carbenicillin indanyl sodium (Geopen oral)
      d. Methicillin sodium (Staphcillin)
      e. Nafcillin sodium (Unipen)
      f. Penicillin G sodium (Crystapen)
      g. Penicillin G procaine (Axercillin)
      h. Penicillin V potassium (Nadopen-V)
   2. Cephalosporins: interfere with bacterial cell wall synthesis; broad spectrum
      a. First-generation cephalosporins
         (1) Cefazolin sodium (Ancef, Gen-Cefazolin)
         (2) Cephalexin (Cephalex)
         (3) Cephalothin sodium (Keflin)
      b. Second-generation cephalosporins
         (1) Cefaclor (Ceclor)
         (2) Cefamandole nafate (Mandol)
      c. Third-generation cephalosporins
         (1) Cefotaxime sodium (Claforan)
         (2) Moxalactam disodium (Moxam)
   3. Erythromycins: along with similar drugs, inhibit mRNA synthesis of bacterial protein
      a. Clindamycin HCl (Dalacin C)
      b. Erythromycin (Kenral)
      c. Lincomycin HCl (Lincocin)
   4. Tetracyclines: inhibit bacterial protein synthesis by blocking tRNA attachment to ribosomes; broad spectrum
      a. Chlortetracycline HCl (Aureomycin)
      b. Demeclocycline HCl (Declomycin)
      c. Doxycycline (Doxycin)
      d. Oxytetracycline (Terramycin)
      e. Tetracycline (Achromycin, Sumycin)

5. Aminoglycosides: disrupt bacterial protein synthesis by providing a substitute for essential nucleotide required by mRNA; broad spectrum
   a. Gentamicin sulfate (Cidomycin)
   b. Kanamycin sulfate (Anamid)
   c. Neomycin sulfate (Mycifradin)
   d. Streptomycin sulfate
   e. Tobramycin sulfate (Nebcin)
6. Polymyxin group: decreases bacterial cell membrane permeability
   a. Colistimethate sodium (Coly-Mycin M)
   b. Polymyxin B sulfate (Aerosporin)
7. Chloramphenicol: inhibits bacterial protein synthesis by interfering with mRNA activity; broad spectrum
   Chloromycetin
D. Major side effects
   1. Depressed appetite (altered taste sensitivity)
   2. Nausea, vomiting (normal flora imbalance)
   3. Diarrhea (normal flora imbalance)
   4. Suppressed absorption of a variety of nutrients including fat; protein; lactose; vitamins A, D, K, and B_{12}; and the minerals calcium, iron, and potassium (normal flora imbalance)
   5. Increased excretion of water-soluble vitamins and minerals (normal flora imbalance)
   6. Superinfection (normal flora imbalance)
   7. Allergic reactions, anaphylaxis (hypersensitivity)
   8. Nephrotoxicity (direct kidney toxic effect)
   9. Tetracyclines
      a. Hepatotoxicity (direct liver toxic effect)
      b. Phototoxicity (degradation to toxic products by ultraviolet rays)
      c. Hyperuricemia (impaired kidney function)
      d. Enamel hypoplasia, dental caries, and bone defects in children under 8 years of age (drug binds to calcium in tissue)
   10. Aminoglycosides
      a. Ototoxicity (direct auditory [eighth cranial] nerve toxic effect)
      b. Leukopenia (decreased WBC synthesis)
      c. Thrombocytopenia (decreased platelet synthesis)
      d. Headache (neurotoxicity)
      e. Confusion (neurotoxicity)
      f. Peripheral neuropathy (neurotoxicity)
      g. Optic neuritis (irritation of optic [second cranial] nerve)
      h. Respiratory paralysis (neuromuscular blockade)
   11. Chloramphenicol
      a. Blood dyscrasias (bone marrow depression)
      b. Fever, rash, urticaria (hypersensitivity)
      c. Jaundice (direct liver toxic effect)
E. Nursing care
   1. Assess client for history of drug allergy

2. Instruct client regarding:
   a. How to take the drug (frequency, relation to meals)
   b. How to dispose of unused drugs
   c. Completing the prescribed course of therapy
   d. Symptoms of allergic response
   e. Side effects, including superinfection; suggest ingestion of yogurt or food supplements containing *Lactobacillus acidophilus* when dairy products cannot be tolerated; suggest nutritional consultation when drug therapy may have an impact on client's nutritional status
3. Shake liquid suspensions to mix thoroughly
4. Administer most preparations 1 hour before meals or 2 hours after meals for best absorption
5. Administer at equal intervals around the clock to maintain blood levels
6. Assess vital signs during course of therapy
7. Cephalosporins: false positive urine glucose results have occurred with Clinitest and Fehling's and Benedict's solutions
8. Tetracyclines
   a. Avoid use during last half of pregnancy or by children younger than 8 years of age
   b. Assess for potentiation of oral anticoagulant effect
   c. Teach client to avoid direct sunlight
   d. Advise client to avoid dairy products, antacids, or iron preparations, because they reduce effectiveness
9. Aminoglycosides and polymyxins: assess for potentiation of neuromuscular blocking agent, general anesthetic, or parenterally administered magnesium effects
10. Chloramphenicol
   a. Assess blood work before and during therapy
   b. Assess for potentiation of phenytoin, oral antidiabetic agent, and coumarin anticoagulant effects
11. Evaluate client's response to medication and understanding of teaching

Antifungals

A. Description
   1. Used to treat systemic and localized fungal infections
   2. Act either to destroy fungal cells (fungicidal) or to inhibit the reproduction of fungal cells (fungistatic)
   3. Available in oral, parenteral (IV), topical, vaginal, and intrathecal preparations
B. Examples
   1. Amphotericin B (Fungizone): disrupts fungal cell membrane permeability
   2. Fluconazole (Diflucan): disrupts fungal cell membrane function

3. Griseofulvin (Grisactin): disrupts fungal nucleic acid synthesis
4. Nystatin (Mycostatin, Nilstat): disrupts fungal cell membrane permeability

C. Major side effects
1. Nausea, vomiting (irritation to gastric mucosa)
2. Headache (neurotoxicity)
3. Fever, chills (blood dyscrasias)
4. Paresthesia (neurotoxicity)

D. Nursing care
1. Assess vital signs during course of therapy
2. Review proper method of application with client
3. Amphotericin B
   a. Use infusion control device for IV administration
   b. Protect solution from light during IV infusion
   c. Monitor blood work during therapy; potential hypokalemia as well as increased urinary excretion of magnesium
4. Griseofulvin
   a. Assess for antagonism if client is taking oral anticoagulants
   b. Instruct client to avoid direct exposure to sunlight
5. Topical preparations
   a. Instruct client to wash drug-stained clothing with soap and water
   b. Instruct client to report signs of local irritation
6. Evaluate client's response to medication and understanding of teaching

Antiparasitics

A. Description
1. Used to treat parasitic diseases
2. Act by interfering with parasite metabolism and reproduction; helminthic (pinworm and tapeworm) as well as protozoal (amebiasis and malaria) infestations respond well to this class of drugs
3. Available in oral, parenteral (IM, SC, IV), vaginal, and rectal preparations

B. Examples
1. Anthelmintics
   a. Mebendazole (Vermox)
   b. Piperazine
   c. Pyrivinium pamoate (Vanquin)
2. Amebicides
   a. Chloroquine HCl (Aralen)
   b. Emetine HCl
   c. Metronidazole (Flagyl)
3. Antimalarials
   a. Chloroquine HCl (Aralen)
   b. Hydroxychloroquine sulfate (Plaquenil)
   c. Primaquine phosphate
   d. Pyrimethamine (Daraprim)
   e. Quinine sulfate

C. Major side effects
1. Anthelmintics
   a. Gastrointestinal irritation (direct tissue irritation)
   b. CNS disturbances (neurotoxicity)
   c. Skin rash (hypersensitivity)
2. Amebicides
   a. Gastrointestinal irritation (direct tissue irritation)
   b. Blood dyscrasias (decreased RBCs, WBCs, platelet synthesis)
   c. Skin rash (hypersensitivity)
   d. Headache (neurotoxicity)
   e. Dizziness (CNS effect)
3. Antimalarials
   a. Nausea, vomiting (irritation to gastric mucosa)
   b. Blood dyscrasias (decreased RBCs, WBCs)
   c. Visual disturbances (impairment of accommodation; retinal and corneal changes)

D. Nursing care
1. Administer drug with meals to decrease GI irritability
2. Assess vital signs during course of therapy
3. Monitor blood work during therapy
4. Instruct client regarding proper hygiene to prevent spread of disease
5. Use safety precautions (supervise ambulation) if CNS effects are manifested
6. Antimalarials: encourage frequent visual examinations
7. Evaluate client's response to medication and understanding of teaching

Antituberculars

A. Description
1. Single drug therapy is usually limited to use of isoniazid for prevention of tuberculosis
2. Administered in combination (first-line and second-line drugs) over a prolonged time period to reduce the possibility of mycobacterial drug resistance
3. Available in oral and parenteral (IM) preparations

B. Examples
1. First-line drugs
   a. Ethambutol (Myambutol)
   b. Isoniazid (INH, Nydrazid)
   c. Rifampin (Rifadin, Rimactane)
2. Second-line drugs: inhibit mycobacterial cell metabolism
   a. Pyrazinamide (PMS-Pyrazinamide, Tebrazid)
3. Third-line drugs
   a. Capreomycin sulfate (Capastat)
   b. Cycloserine (Seromycin)
   c. Ethionamide (Trecator S.C.)

4. Alternatives: increase activities of ethambutol and isoniazid; most effective in first weeks of treatment
   a. Aminosalicylic acid (PAS [parasal sodium], Teebacin Acid)
   b. Capreomycin (Capastat)
   c. Cycloserine (Seromycin)
   d. Pyrazinamide (Tebrazid)
   e. Streptomycin
C. Major side effects
   1. GI irritation (direct tissue irritation)
   2. Suppressed absorption of fat and B complex vitamins, especially folacin and B_{12}; depletion of vitamin B_6 by isoniazid

TABLE 6-1 Precautions to prevent the spread of microorganisms

Category	Indications	Conditions	Room	Gown
UNIVERSAL/ STANDARD PRECAUTIONS	Used for all clients regardless of diagnosis when there is contact with: 1. Blood 2. Body fluid 3. Secretions 4. Excretions 5. Non-intact skin 6. Mucous membranes	Used for all clients, particularly those with acquired immunodeficiency syndrome (AIDS) and hepatitis type B	Private room indicated if personal hygiene is inadequate	Indicated if soiling with blood, body fluid, secretions, or excretions is likely (e.g., during client care activities that are associated with splashes of blood)
TRANSMISSION-BASED PRECAUTIONS*				
AIRBORNE PRECAUTIONS	Prevents transmission of droplet nuclei less than or equal to 5 microns or dust particles that contain the pathogen. These nuclei and particles remain suspended in the air for an extended period	Tuberculosis, varicella, rubeola	Negative-pressure isolation room with at least six air exchanges per hour. Door must be kept closed	See Universal/Standard Precautions
DROPLET PRECAUTIONS	Prevents transmission of particle droplets greater than 5 microns that are dispersed by coughing, sneezing, talking, or suctioning. These droplets travel up to 1 meter before settling to the floor or other surfaces	*Haemophilus influenzae* type B, meningitis, *Streptococcus pneumoniae* pneumonia, mycoplasmal pneumonia, streptococcal pharyngitis, scarlet fever, pertussis, rubella, mumps	Private room; clients infected with the same organism may share a room	See Universal/Standard Precautions
CONTACT PRECAUTIONS a. Direct b. Indirect	Prevents transmission of epidemiologically important microorganisms by direct contact with client's skin or indirect contact with contaminated items or surfaces	*Clostridium difficile* enteric infection, enterohemorrhagic *Escherichia coli*, shigella, hepatitis type A, herpes simplex virus, cellulitis, scabies	Private room; clients infected with the same organism may share a room	See Universal/Standard Precautions. Don gown when first entering room if contact with client or items in room is likely

*Used in addition to standard precautions for clients with documented or suspected infection with highly transmittable or epidemiologically important pathogens.

3. Dizziness (CNS effect)
4. CNS disturbances (direct CNS toxic effect)
5. Liver disturbances (direct liver toxic effect)
6. Blood dyscrasias (decreased RBCs, WBCs, platelet synthesis)
7. Streptomycin: ototoxicity (direct auditory [eighth cranial] nerve toxic effect)

8. Ethambutol: visual disturbances (direct optic [second cranial] nerve toxic effect)

D. Nursing care
1. Support natural defense mechanisms of client; encourage intake of foods rich in the immune-stimulating nutrients such as vitamins A, C, and E, and the minerals selenium and zinc

Gloves	Mask and Eye	Handwashing	Precautions
Required for touching blood, body fluids, secretions, excretions, contaminated items or surfaces, mucous membranes, and non-intact skin	Required if splashes of blood, body fluids, secretions, or excretions are likely	Required after touching blood, body fluids, secretions, excretions, or contaminated articles whether gloves were worn or not. Hands must be washed when gloves are removed, before contact with another client and before touching a noncontaminated item or surface	Discard items contaminated with blood, body fluids, secretions, or excretions in a biohazard receptacle or handle equipment in a manner that will prevent transfer of microorganisms. Disinfect and sterilize reusable items. Dispose of used needles and other sharp devices in properly labeled, puncture-resistant container. Never recap used needles. Use ventilation devices instead of mouth-to-mouth resuscitation.
See Universal/Standard Precautions	See Universal/Standard Precautions. Use particulate respirators such as HEPAmask (high efficiency particulate air filter respirator) when client has a known or suspected diagnosis of tuberculosis. People susceptible to varicella or rubeola should not enter the room	See Universal/Standard Precautions	See Universal/Standard Precautions. Confine client to room; transport only if absolutely essential; during transport have client wear a surgical mask to minimize droplet nuclei dispersal
See Universal/Standard Precautions	See Universal/Standard Precautions	See Universal/Standard Precautions	See Universal/Standard Precautions. See Airborne Precautions
See Universal/Standard Precautions. Apply gloves when entering room; change gloves after contact with substances such as feces or wound drainage that have high concentrations of microorganisms	See Universal/Standard Precautions	See Universal/Standard Precautions	See Universal/Standard Precautions. Confine client to room. Transport only if absolutely essential; during transport maintain precautions to limit transmission of microorganisms. If possible, equipment such as a stethoscope or sphygmomanometer should be used only for the infected client

2. Obtain sputum specimens for acid-fast bacillus
3. Monitor blood work during therapy
4. Instruct the client to take the drugs regularly as prescribed; reinforce need for medical supervision
5. Offer client emotional support during therapy
6. Use safety precautions (supervise ambulation) if CNS effects are manifested
7. Instruct client regarding nutritional side effects and encourage foods rich in B complex vitamins
8. Encourage client to avoid use of alcohol during therapy
9. Ethambutol: encourage frequent visual examinations
10. Rifampin: instruct client that body fluids may appear orange-red
11. Streptomycin: encourage frequent auditory examinations
12. Evaluate client's response to medication and understanding of teaching

Antivirals

A. Description
  1. Used to provide prophylaxis when exposure to viral infection has occurred
  2. Prevent entrance of the virus into host cells
  3. Available in oral, parenteral (IV), and topical, including ophthalmic, preparations
B. Examples
  1. Acyclovir sodium (Zovirax)
  2. Amantadine HCl (Symmetrel)
  3. Idoxuridine (Herplex)
  4. Interferon (Roferon-A, Intron-A)
  5. Vidarabine (Vira-A)
C. Major side effects
  1. Central nervous system (CNS) stimulation (direct CNS effect)
  2. Orthostatic hypotension (depressed cardiovascular system)
  3. Dizziness (hypotension)
  4. Constipation (decreased peristalsis)
  5. Nephrotoxicity (direct kidney toxic effect)
  6. Local irritation (direct local tissue effect)
D. Nursing care
  1. Assess vital signs during course of therapy
  2. Support natural defense mechanisms of client; encourage intake of foods rich in the immune-stimulating nutrients, such as vitamins A, C, and E, and the minerals selenium and zinc
  3. Encourage intake of high-fiber foods to reduce potential of constipation
  4. Monitor disease symptoms and laboratory data
  5. Evaluate client's response to medication and understanding of teaching

Sulfonamides

A. Description
  1. Antiinfective drugs used primarily to treat urinary tract infections
  2. Act by substituting a false metabolite for paraaminobenzoic acid (PABA) required in the bacterial synthesis of folic acid
  3. Available in oral, parenteral (IM, SC, IV), and topical, including ophthalmic, preparations
B. Examples
  1. Sulfamethizole
  2. Sulfamethoxazole (Gantanol)
  3. Sulfasalazine (Kennal)
  4. Sulfisoxazole (Novosoxazole)
  5. Combination product: trimethoprim and sulfamethoxazole (Bactrim, Septra)
C. Major side effects
  1. Nausea, vomiting; decreased absorption of folacin (irritation of gastric mucosa)
  2. Skin rash (hypersensitivity)
  3. Malaise (decreased RBCs)
  4. Blood dyscrasias (decreased RBCs, WBCs, platelet synthesis)
  5. Crystalluria (drug precipitation in acidic urine)
  6. Stomatitis (GI irritation)
  7. Headache (CNS effect)
  8. Photosensitivity (hypersensitivity)
  9. Allergic response, anaphylaxis (hypersensitivity)
D. Nursing care
  1. Assess client for history of drug allergy
  2. Promote increased fluid intake
  3. Caution client to avoid direct exposure to sunlight
  4. Assess vital signs during course of therapy
  5. Maintain alkaline urine
  6. Monitor blood work during therapy; potential for megaloblastic anemia caused by folacin deficiency
  7. Assess for potentiation of oral anticoagulant and oral hypoglycemic effects
  8. Evaluate client's response to medication and understanding of teaching

GENERAL NURSING CARE OF CLIENTS AT RISK FOR INFECTION

A. DATA COLLECTION

  1. Obtain history to identify factors affecting chain of infection (see Source and Transmission of Pathogens under Pathology of Infection)
     a. Microorganism or etiologic agent
     b. Source or reservoir
     c. Portal of exit from host
     d. Mode of transmission
     e. Portal of entry to body
     f. Susceptible host

2. Obtain baseline vital signs
3. Monitor baseline WBC
4. Review results of culture and sensitivity tests

B. ANALYSIS AND INTERPRETATION

1. Risk for fluid volume deficit related to increased fluid loss associated with fever
2. Hyperthermia related to infectious process
3. Risk for infection related to impaired immune response

C. PLANNING/IMPLEMENTATION

1. Decrease host susceptibility
   a. Use hygienic practices to maintain skin and mucous membranes as first line of defense
   b. Reinforce or maintain natural protective mechanisms such as coughing, pH of secretions, resident flora
   c. Maintain nutrition and encourage rest and sleep to promote tissue repair and production of lymphocytes and antibodies
   d. Educate client about immunizations
2. Use principles of asepsis
   a. Medical asepsis
      (1) Denotes absence of infectious organisms (pathogens)
      (2) Limits the growth and spread of microorganisms by confining them to a specific area
      (3) Contamination occurs if pathogens are transferred to a previously clean site or article
   b. Surgical asepsis
      (1) Denotes absence of all microorganisms and spores
      (2) Prevents microorganisms from entering a specific area
      (3) Contamination occurs if a sterile article:
         (a) Touches an unsterile article
         (b) Is placed outside a 2.5 cm inside border of a sterile field
         (c) Is below waist level or above shoulder level
         (d) Is beyond the field of vision
         (e) Rests on a wet, permeable surface, which enables contamination by capillary action
         (f) Is exposed to airborne microorganisms
3. Limit or eliminate the microbiologic agent
   a. Disinfection and sterilization (see Physical and Chemical Control of Microorganisms)
   b. Administration of antimicrobial agents (see Pharmacologic Control of Infection)
4. Prevent transmission
   a. Employ hand-washing techniques
      (1) Before client contact; after client contact
      (2) Use friction, soap, and warm water to loosen and remove microorganisms

b. Use standard precautions (Table 6-1)
   (1) Standard precautions are used for all clients regardless of their diagnosis or presumed infection status
   (2) Standard precautions apply to blood, all body fluids, secretions, and excretions regardless of whether or not they contain visible blood; they also apply to non-intact skin and mucous membranes
   (3) The basic tenets of infection control are preserved in standard precautions, including hand washing and use of gloves, masks, eye protection, and gowns as appropriate for client contacts where splashing or soiling is likely to occur
c. Use transmission-based precautions (Table 6-1): employed in addition to standard precautions; designed for clients documented or suspected to be infected with highly transmissible or epidemiologically important pathogens; precautions may be combined for diseases that have multiple routes of transmission
   (1) Airborne precautions: designed to reduce the risk of transmission of airborne droplet nuclei (5 microns or smaller) or dust particles containing infectious agents; microorganisms can remain suspended in the air and are dispersed by air currents; transmission occurs when these droplets are inhaled by a susceptible host
   (2) Droplet precautions: designed to reduce the transmission of large particle droplets (greater than 5 microns); droplets are dispersed by coughing, sneezing, or talking, and during procedures such as suctioning; these droplets do not remain suspended in the air and generally travel 1 meter or less; transmission occurs when these droplets are deposited on a host's conjunctiva, nasal mucosa, or mouth
   (3) Contact precautions
      (a) Direct contact precautions: designed to reduce the transmission of microorganisms by skin-to-skin contact and physical transfer of microorganisms; transmission occurs when there is physical contact between a susceptible host and an infected or colonized person
      (b) Indirect contact precautions: designed to reduce the transmission of microorganisms by contaminated inanimate objects; transmission

occurs when a susceptible host contacts a contaminated intermediate object in the client's environment
   d. Correctly dispose of contaminated material
     (1) Use impervious bags or double-bagging technique to dispose of contaminated material
     (2) Do not recap or break needles after administering injections; use rigid container for disposal
  5. Monitor vital signs
  6. Employ measures to decrease body temperature as prescribed
   a. Tepid bath
   b. Antipyretics
   c. Hypothermia blanket
  7. Ensure adequate fluid intake

D. EVALUATION/OUTCOMES
1. Complies with medical regimen
2. Establishes health practices that enhance immunity
3. Maintains body temperature within normal range
4. Maintains fluid balance
5. Becomes infection free
6. Remains free from infection

FLUID, ELECTROLYTE, AND ACID-BASE BALANCE

FLUID AND ELECTROLYTE BALANCE
Basic Concepts

A. Total volume of fluid and total amount of electrolytes in body normally remain relatively constant
B. Volume of blood plasma, interstitial fluid, and intracellular fluid, and the concentration of electrolytes in each, remain relatively constant
C. Fluid balance and electrolyte balance are interdependent
D. Intake must equal output
E. Fluid and electrolyte balance maintained primarily by mechanisms that adjust output to intake; secondarily by mechanisms that adjust intake to output
F. Fluid balance is also maintained by a physical mechanism that controls movement of water between fluid compartments (osmosis)
G. The average adult contains about 40 L of water, comprising 60% of body weight; 25 L intracellular, 15 to 17 L extracellular
H. Extracellular fluid divided among:
  1. Interstitial fluid: 10 to 12 L
  2. Plasma: 3 L
  3. Small fluid compartments: 1 L (e.g., fluid,

aqueous humor, serous and synovial fluid, lymphatic channels)
  4. Gastrointestinal tract: 1 L at any given time for all gastrointestinal organs
I. All body fluids are related and mix well with each other: plasma becomes interstitial fluid as it filters across the capillary wall; interstitial fluid can return to the capillary by osmosis or enter lymphatic channels, becoming lymph; interstitial fluid and intracellular fluid are in osmotic equilibrium across the cell membranes, regulated by the sodium ion (Na^+) concentration of interstitial fluid and the potassium ion (K^+) concentration of intracellular fluid
  1. Mechanism of fluid flow between plasma and interstitial fluid involves several forces
   a. Blood hydrostatic pressure
   b. Blood osmotic pressure
   c. Interstitial fluid hydrostatic pressure
   d. Interstitial fluid osmotic pressure
  2. Blood hydrostatic pressure, interstitial fluid osmotic pressure, and interstitial fluid hydrostatic pressure (normally a negative value) tend to move fluid out of the blood in the capillaries and into the interstitial fluid
  3. Blood osmotic pressure moves fluid back into the capillary blood from the interstitial fluid
  4. Starling's law of the capillaries states that equal amounts of water move back and forth between blood and interstitial fluid only when the blood hydrostatic pressure plus the interstitial fluid osmotic pressure equals the blood osmotic pressure; under these conditions fluid balance exists between the blood and interstitial fluid
   a. Blood gains liquid from interstitial fluid whenever the blood hydrostatic pressure plus the interstitial fluid hydrostatic pressure plus the interstitial fluid osmotic pressure is less than the blood osmotic pressure
   b. Blood loses liquid to interstitial fluid whenever blood osmotic pressure is less than blood hydrostatic pressure plus interstitial fluid hydrostatic pressure plus interstitial fluid osmotic pressure
J. Chemically, extracellular fluid and intracellular fluid are strikingly different: sodium is the main cation of extracellular fluid; potassium is the main cation of intracellular fluid; chloride is the main anion of extracellular fluid; phosphate is the main anion of intracellular fluid; protein concentration is much higher in intracellular fluid than in interstitial fluid (Table 6-2)
K. Chemically, plasma and interstitial fluid are almost identical except that plasma contains slightly more electrolytes, considerably more proteins, somewhat more sodium, and fewer chloride ions than interstitial fluid (Table 6-2)

TABLE 6-2 Average concentrations of major ions in extracellular and intracellular fluids (usually expressed in milliosmols per liter [mOsm/L] of H_2O)

Ion	Intracellular fluid	Extracellular fluid	
		Plasma	Interstitial
Na^+	10	144.0	137.0
K^+	141	5.0	4.7
Cl^-	4	107.0	112.7
HCO_3^-	10	27.0	28.3
Ca^{++}	0	2.5	2.4
Mg^{++}	31	1.5	1.4
$SO_4^=$	1	0.5	0.5
Phosphates ($H_2PO_4^-$, $HPO_4^=$)	11	2.0	2.0
Proteins	4	1.2	0.2

Major Ions (Electrolytes)

A. Cations ($^+$)
  1. Sodium (Na^+)
     a. Most abundant cation in extracellular fluid
     b. Sodium pump in most body cells pumps sodium out of intracellular fluid
     c. Regulates cell size by osmotically drawing water from the cells to balance flow of water into the cells as a result of osmotically active intracellular proteins
     d. Action potential of nervous and muscle fibers requires sodium; sodium is basic to the communication between nerves and muscles
     e. Helps to regulate acid-base balance by exchanging hydrogen ions for sodium ions in the kidney tubules; excess hydrogen ions (acid) are excreted
  2. Potassium (K^+)
     a. Most abundant cation of intracellular fluid
     b. Potassium pump brings potassium into cells of the body
     c. Resting polarization and repolarization of nerve and muscle fibers depend on potassium
        (1) If potassium concentration of extracellular fluid rises above normal (hyperkalemia), the force of the contracting heart weakens; with extremely high concentrations the heart will not contract
        (2) If potassium concentration of extracellular fluid drops below normal (hypokalemia), the resting polarization in nerve and muscle fibers increases, resulting in weakness and eventual paralysis
  3. Calcium (Ca^{++})
     a. Forms salts with phosphates, carbonate,

and fluoride in bones and teeth to make them hard
     b. Required for correct functioning of nerves and muscles
        (1) If calcium concentration rises above normal levels (hypercalcemia), nervous system becomes depressed and sluggish
        (2) If calcium concentration falls below normal levels (hypocalcemia), nervous system becomes extremely excitable, resulting in cramps and tetany
     c. Calcium is required for blood clotting, acting as a cofactor in the formation of prothrombin activator and thrombin
  4. Magnesium (Mg^{++})
     a. Cofactor for many enzymes involved in energy metabolism
     b. Normal constituent of bone
B. Anions ($^-$)
  1. Chloride (Cl^-)
     a. Most abundant anion in extracellular fluid
     b. Helps balance sodium
     c. Major component of gastric secretions
  2. Bicarbonate (HCO_3^-)
     a. Part of bicarbonate buffer system
     b. Reacts with a strong acid to form carbonic acid and a basic salt, thus limiting the drop in pH
  3. Phosphate ($H_2PO_4^-$ and $HPO_4^=$)
     a. Part of phosphate buffer system
     b. Functions in cellular energy metabolism: phosphate + ADP —>ATP (the energy currency of the cell)
     c. Combines with calcium ions in bone, providing hardness
     d. Involved in structure of genetic material, DNA and RNA

Major Avenues by Which Water Enters and Leaves the Body

A. Water enters the body through digestive tract both in liquids (drinking) and in foods (preformed water)
B. Water is formed in the body by metabolism of foods (oxidative water)
C. Water leaves the body via kidneys (as urine), intestines (with feces), and lungs and skin (insensible water losses)

Mechanisms that Maintain Total Fluid Volume

A. Osmoreceptor system
  1. Regulates water output volume to balance fluid intake volume
  2. Most important mechanism for regulation of water output because other fluid losses through the skin, lungs, and gastrointestinal

system have no feedback mechanism relative to water loss

3. Cells in the hypothalamus synthesize antidiuretic hormone (ADH), which is then stored in the posterior pituitary before release into the circulation

4. Osmoreceptors respond to dehydration by increasing the frequency of nerve impulses to the posterior pituitary, resulting in an increase in the amounts of ADH released; this increases water reabsorption in the kidney tubules and decreases urinary output

5. Osmoreceptors respond to overhydration by decreasing nerve impulses to the posterior pituitary, which decreases the release of ADH, resulting in an increase in urinary output

B. Interaction of the circulatory system
   1. Regulation of blood volume (extracellular fluid volume)
   2. Increased fluid intake increases the blood volume
   3. Increased blood volume results in an increase in cardiac output, blood pressure, and therefore glomerular filtration
   4. Increased glomerular filtration results in an increase in urinary output and a decrease in blood volume

C. Regulation of fluid intake: thirst mechanism
   1. Dehydration of cells in the thirst center of the hypothalamus gives rise to thirst sensation
   2. Thirst sensations are also induced by dryness of the oral mucosa
   3. Fluid intake stretches the stomach and moistens the mouth and throat; these sensations cancel thirst sensation before the actual hydration of body fluids

D. Various factors such as hyperventilation, hypoventilation, vomiting, diarrhea, and circulatory failure may alter the volume of fluid lost

Mechanisms that Maintain Electrolyte Concentrations

A. Aldosterone feedback mechanism
   1. Adrenal cortex secretes the steroid hormone aldosterone when extracellular fluid sodium concentrations decrease or potassium concentrations increase
   2. Aldosterone stimulates kidney tubules to reabsorb sodium; potassium reabsorption decreases as sodium reabsorption increases; sodium is salvaged while potassium is excreted
   3. This mechanism helps preserve normal sodium and potassium concentrations in extracellular fluid
   4. Secondary effects of aldosterone
      a. Chloride conserved with sodium
      b. Water conserved because it is reabsorbed by osmosis as tubules reabsorb salt

B. Parathyroid regulation of calcium
   1. Parathyroid glands secrete parathormone when extracellular fluid calcium concentrations decrease
   2. Parathormone stimulates the release of calcium from bone, calcium reabsorption in the small intestine (vitamin D required), and calcium reabsorption in kidney tubules
   3. Increased extracellular fluid calcium concentrations result in decreased secretion of parathormone and gradual loss of excess calcium

ACID-BASE BALANCE

Basic Concepts

A. Healthy survival depends on the body's maintaining a state of acid-base balance; more specifically, healthy survival depends on the maintenance of a relatively constant, slightly alkaline pH of blood and other fluids

B. When the body is in a state of acid-base balance, it maintains a stable hydrogen ion concentration in body fluids; specifically, blood pH remains relatively constant between 7.35 and 7.45

C. The body has three devices or mechanisms for maintaining acid-base balance; named in order of the speed with which they act, they are the buffer mechanism, the respiratory mechanism, and the renal or urinary mechanism

D. A state of uncompensated acidosis exists if blood pH decreases below 7.35

E. A state of uncompensated alkalosis exists if blood pH increases above 7.45

F. The pH of body fluids shifts below the ideal of 7.35 to 7.45 for several reasons
   1. Glucose, used by almost all body cells, is oxidized; as a result, energy, water, and carbon dioxide are produced; the CO_2 combines with the water to produce carbonic acid (H_2CO_3)
   2. Metabolism of sulfur amino acids results in formation of sulfuric acid
   3. Metabolism of phospholipids and phosphoproteins results in formation of phosphoric acid
   4. Muscle metabolism under anaerobic conditions produces lactic acid
   5. Rapid weight loss results in extra fat metabolism, producing ketone bodies that include alpha keto acids
   6. The acid produced by the normal mechanisms just mentioned requires neutralization to avoid acidosis, coma, and death

Buffer Mechanisms for Maintaining Acid-Base Balance

A. The buffer mechanism consists of chemicals called buffers, which are present in the blood and other body fluids and which combine with relatively strong acids or bases to convert them to weaker acids or bases; hence, buffers function to prevent marked changes in blood pH levels when either acids or bases enter the blood

B. A buffer is often referred to as a buffer pair because it consists of not one but two substances; the chief buffer pair in the blood consists of the weak acid, carbonic acid (H_2CO_3), and its basic salts, collectively called base bicarbonate ($B \bullet HCO_3$); sodium bicarbonate ($NaHCO_3$), is by far the most abundant base bicarbonate present in blood plasma

C. When the body is in a state of acid-base balance, blood contains 27 mEq base bicarbonate per liter and 1.35 mEq carbonic acid per liter; usually this is written as a ratio, referred to as the base bicarbonate/carbonic acid ratio:

$$\frac{27 \text{ mEq B}\bullet\text{HCO}_3}{1.35 \text{ mEq H}_2\text{CO}_3} = \frac{20}{1}$$

D. Whenever the base bicarbonate/carbonic acid ratio of blood equals 20/L, blood pH equals 7.4

E. Base bicarbonate buffers nonvolatile acids that are stronger than carbonic acid; it reacts with them to convert them to carbonic acid and a basic salt
   1. Buffering does not prevent blood pH from decreasing, but it does prevent it from decreasing as markedly as it would without buffering
   2. Buffering removes some sodium bicarbonate from blood and adds some carbonic acid to it; this necessarily decreases the base bicarbonate/carbonic acid ratio, which in turn necessarily decreases the pH of blood as it flows through capillaries (from its arterial level of about 7.4 to its venous level of about 7.38)
   3. Anything that decreases the blood's base bicarbonate/carbonic acid ratio necessarily decreases blood pH and thus tends to produce acidosis; the corollary is also true; anything that increases the base bicarbonate/carbonic acid ratio necessarily increases blood pH and thus tends to produce alkalosis

F. Other buffer systems in body fluids
   1. Protein buffer
      a. Most plentiful; three fourths of all chemical buffering power lies in proteins of the body fluids
      b. Provides support to other buffering systems such as bicarbonate buffer and phosphate buffer
   2. Phosphate buffer system
      a. One sixth the neutralizing ability of bicarbonate buffer in extracellular fluid
      b. More important in intracellular fluids, where its concentration is considerably higher
      c. Helps to buffer pH of urine in kidney tubules

   3. Hemoglobin buffer system: buffers intracellular fluid of the erythrocyte

G. Bicarbonate buffer is the most important buffer in human body fluids because its components, base bicarbonate and carbonic acid, are actively and constantly regulated by the action of the respiratory and urinary systems

Respiratory Mechanism for Maintaining Acid-Base Balance

A. Respiratory system controls acid-base balance by controlling rate of carbon dioxide (CO_2) exhalation from lungs; during normal body metabolism CO_2 is produced, which reacts with water to form carbonic acid, resulting in a decrease in pH (as acidity increases, pH decreases); when the respiratory system blows CO_2 out of the body, carbonic acid breaks down into CO_2 and water, resulting in an increase in pH (as acidity decreases, pH increases)
   1. Conditions impairing the ability of the respiratory system to blow off CO_2 will result in a buildup of CO_2 in the body; excess CO_2 combines with water to form carbonic acid and hydrogen ions, resulting in a decrease in pH
   2. Signs of respiratory acidosis include dyspnea, irritability, tachycardia, and cyanosis
   3. Common causes include emphysema, pneumonia, asthmatic attack, atelectasis, pneumothorax, respiratory depression from drug overdose

B. Respiratory alkalosis as a result of failure of mechanism
   1. Hyperventilation blows off too much CO_2 from the body, causing an excessive breakdown of carbonic acid, resulting in an increase of pH
   2. Signs of respiratory alkalosis include deep or deep and rapid breathing, lightheadedness, tetany, convulsions, and unconsciousness
   3. Common causes include hysteria, prolonged crying, and mechanical ventilation

C. Respiratory compensation for metabolic imbalance
   1. In metabolic acidosis the respiratory system compensates by hyperventilation in an attempt to blow off CO_2 and raise the pH
   2. In metabolic alkalosis the respiratory system compensates by decreasing the rate and depth of breathing in an attempt to retain CO_2 and decrease the pH

Renal Mechanism for Maintaining Acid-Base Balance

A. The renal mechanism is the most effective device the body has for maintaining acid-base balance; unless it operates adequately, acid-base balance cannot be maintained

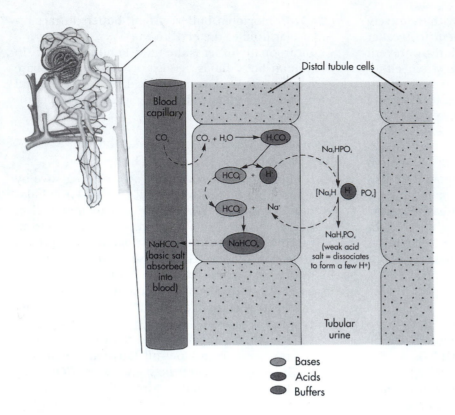

FIGURE 6-2 Acidification of urine and conservation of base by the distal renal tubular excretion of hydrogen ions (H^+) from the urine and the reabsorption of sodium ions (Na^+) into the blood in exchange for the H^+ excreted into it. (From Thibodeau GA and Patton KT: *Anatomy and physiology,* ed 2, St. Louis, 1993, Mosby.)

FIGURE 6-3 Acidification of urine by the tubular excretion of ammonia (NH_3). An acid (glutamine) leaves the blood, enters a tubule cell, and is deaminized to form ammonia. The ammonia is excreted into the urine, where it combines with hydrogen to form the ammonium ion (NH_4^+). In exchange for NH_4^+ the tubule cell reabsorbs Na^+. (From Thibodeau GA and Patton KT: *Anatomy and physiology,* ed 2, St. Louis, 1993, Mosby.)

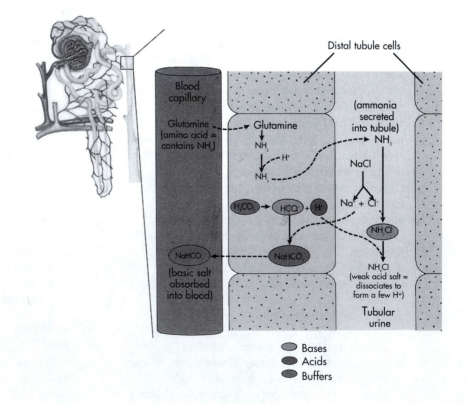

B. The renal mechanism for maintaining acid-base balance makes the urine more acidic and the blood more alkaline; this neutralizes the constant production of acid products from cells; the mechanism consists of two functions performed by the distal renal tubule cells, both of which remove hydrogen ions from blood to urine and in exchange reabsorb sodium ions from tubular urine to blood
   1. Distal tubule cells secrete hydrogen ions and reabsorb sodium ions (Fig. 6-2)
   2. Distal tubule cells form ammonia, which combines with hydrogen ions they have secreted to form ammonium ions (NH_4^+) which are excreted in the urine in exchange for sodium ions, which are reabsorbed into the blood (Fig. 6-3)
C. The distal tubule functions produce the following results:
   1. They increase blood's sodium bicarbonate content and decrease its carbonic acid content, thereby increasing the base bicarbonate/carbonic acid ratio and blood pH
   2. They acidify urine (decrease urine pH)
D. Metabolic acidosis as a result of failure of mechanism
   1. Excess acid, other than carbonic acid, which is a respiratory acid, accumulates in the body beyond the body's ability to neutralize it
   2. Signs of metabolic acidosis include weakness, malaise, headache, disorientation, deep rapid breathing, fruity odor to breath, coma
   3. Common causes include diabetes mellitus, salicylate poisoning, severe diarrhea, vomiting of intestinal contents, infection, renal failure
E. Metabolic alkalosis as a result of failure of mechanism
   1. Excess base bicarbonate in the body
   2. Signs of metabolic alkalosis include muscle hypertonicity, tetany, confusion, shallow slow respirations, convulsions, coma
   3. Common causes include vomiting of stomach contents or prolonged gastric suction, excessive ingestion of alkaline drugs, potent diuretics
F. Metabolic compensation for respiratory imbalance
   1. In respiratory acidosis the urinary system excretes increased hydrogen ions to compensate for the respiratory system's inability to blow off CO_2
   2. In respiratory alkalosis the urinary system may decrease excretion of hydrogen ions to compensate and maintain the body's pH in the normal range

CHEMICAL PRINCIPLES RELATED TO FLUIDS, ELECTROLYTES, ACIDS, BASES, AND SALTS

Water
General Information
A. Chemical combination of oxygen and hydrogen
B. Most abundant compound
C. Essential to life
D. Sixty percent of the average adult human body weight is water; may be as high as 80% in infants and as low as 40% to 50% in the elderly

Physical Properties
A. Colorless, tasteless, odorless liquid
B. Exists chiefly as ice at low temperatures, liquid at moderate temperatures, and gas at elevated temperatures
   1. Water changes from liquid to solid at the freezing point 0° C
   2. Water changes from liquid to gas at the boiling point 100° C
   3. These transition points in the physical states of water are the basis of the Celsius temperature scale
   4. Conversion from one temperature scale to the other is accomplished by using the formula

$$(°F - 32) \, {}^5/_9 = °C$$

Chemical Properties
A. Water molecule is a dipolar structure; because of this molecular shape, it is an excellent solvent for ionic or slightly ionic substances
B. Water is a stable compound; it dissociates very slightly to H^+ and OH^- under normal conditions
C. Electrolysis can dissociate water into its components, hydrogen and oxygen
D. Many chemical reactions need water as a solvent before they can occur
E. Process of splitting a substance with the addition of water is called hydrolysis, which is the basis for the digestion of food
F. Crystals formed with water in their molecule are called hydrates

Importance of Water
A. Necessary for life; universal solvent
B. Essential for many chemical reactions
C. Needed for digestion (hydrolysis) of food
D. Forms large percentage of plant and animal tissue
E. Necessary for circulation of blood; plasma is a water solution
F. Necessary for elimination; urine, sweat, feces contain water
G. Lubricating fluid at joints (synovial fluid) contains water
H. Water has a great capacity for absorbing heat or

giving off absorbed heat; useful in ice packs, hydrotherapy, and hot compresses

Water as a Standard

A. Thermometer scales: the freezing and boiling points of water are used to standardize Celsius scale
B. Specific gravity: compares the density of a volume of water to the density of the same volume of another substance
C. Weight: 1 g is the mass of 1 ml of water at 4° C
D. Calorie: the heat needed to raise 1 g of water 1° C
E. pH: water acts as neutrality point on acid-base scale

Proteins

A. Polymers of alpha amino acids connected by peptide bonds
B. Characteristics of proteins
   1. Protein molecules are very large
   2. Proteins form colloid particles in solution
   3. Synthesis of proteins occurs in ribosomes of cell according to specific genetic patterns under direction of the nucleic acids DNA and RNA
   4. Structure patterns of proteins are extremely specific; proteins differ from species to species, individual to individual, and organ to organ; this presents a problem in transplant operations
   5. Proteins are the tissue builders of the body
C. Classification of proteins
   1. Simple proteins: give amino acids on hydrolysis
      a. Albumins: water soluble, coagulated by heat (e.g., lactalbumin [milk], serum albumin [blood], egg white); albumin is most important in the development of the plasma colloid osmotic pressure, which helps control (through osmosis) the flow of water between the plasma and interstitial fluid; during a condition such as starvation, a fall in the albumin level of the blood results in a fall in the plasma colloid osmotic pressure; this leads to edema because less fluid is being drawn by osmosis into the capillaries from the interstitial spaces
      b. Globulins: insoluble in water, soluble in dilute salt solutions, coagulated by heat (e.g., lactoglobulin [milk], serum globulin [blood], gamma serum globulin [forms antibodies of blood])

Solutions

Basic Concepts

A. Substances that dissolve in other substances form solutions
B. A solution can be classified as a homogeneous mixture
C. Solids, liquids, and gases can be dissolved in other solids, liquids, and gases
   1. Substance dissolved is called the solute
   2. Substance in which the solute is dissolved is called the solvent
   3. Common solution is one in which a solid, liquid, or gas is dissolved in a liquid (e.g., blood, a colloid, is mainly a liquid [water] containing dissolved ions, sugars, amino acids, and respiratory gases)

Factors Affecting Solubility

A. Chemical and physical nature of the solvent
B. Chemical and physical nature of the solute
C. Amount of solvent versus amount of solute
D. Temperature: warming aids some solutes (solids) to dissolve; cooling aids others (gases) to dissolve
E. Presence or absence of mixing; mixing usually speeds solution reaction
F. Pressure: especially when one of the components is a gas

Types of Solutions

A. Dilute: small amount of solute in a relatively large amount of solvent
B. Concentrated: large amount of solute in a relatively small amount of solvent
C. Unsaturated: holding less solute than is possible for it to dissolve at a certain temperature and pressure
D. Saturated: holding all the solute it can dissolve at a certain temperature and pressure
E. Supersaturated: unique case of a solution holding more solute than it normally should for a particular temperature and pressure
   1. Very unstable condition
   2. Excess solute easily precipitates from solution
F. Percent solution: grams of solute per gram of solution
G. Molar solution (M): number of gram-molecular weights of solute per liter of solution
H. Normal solution (N): number of gram-equivalent weights of solute per liter of solution
I. Molar solution: gram-molecular weight of solute in 1000 g of solvent

Osmosis

A. Process of selective diffusion
B. More concentrated solution is separated from a less concentrated solution by a membrane that is permeable only to the solvent
C. Solvent moves more rapidly from the dilute solution into the concentrated solution than in the reverse direction
D. Pressure forcing the solvent across the membrane is called osmotic pressure
E. Isotonic solutions: when the osmotic pressures of two liquids are equal, the flow of solvent is equalized and the two solutions are said to be isotonic to each other
   1. Physiologic saline—0.89% NaCl in distilled water—is isotonic to blood and body tissues
   2. Five-percent dextrose in water is isotonic to blood and body tissues

3. When isotonic solutions are administered intravenously, the blood cells remain intact

F. Hypertonic solutions: when one solution has less osmotic pressure (is more concentrated) than another, it draws fluid from the other and is said to be hypertonic to it

G. Hypotonic solutions: when one solution has more osmotic pressure (is more dilute) than another, it forces fluid into the other and is said to be hypotonic to it

H. Both hypertonic and hypotonic types of solution may be destructive to body cells and should be used with caution in intravenous infusions

I. Osmosis constantly occurs as part of the normal physiology of human beings
   1. Capillary membrane: the colloid osmotic pressure of the plasma draws fluid from the tissue spaces back into the capillaries; edema results when disease states upset the normal colloid osmotic pressure (e.g., starvation, kidney disease)
   2. Plasma membranes: water freely flows from interstitial fluid into intracellular fluid and vice versa, depending on the relative concentration of water in these two fluid compartments

Kind of Solution Determined by Size of Solute Particles

A. Atomic, ionic, and most molecular-sized particles are extremely small: submicroscopic
   1. Particles are freely dispersed by solvent
   2. Particles are kept in solution by movement and attraction of solvent molecules
   3. Substances of this class are called crystalloids
   4. Crystalloids form true solutions
      a. Clear in appearance: particles cannot be seen
      b. Solute stays in solution as long as the solvent is not removed by evaporation or other means
      c. Solute accompanies solvent as it passes through filters and most membranes (e.g., the ions Na^+, K^+, Cl^-, HCO_3^- dissolved in plasma are in true solution)

B. Large particles of matter do not form solutions in the real sense of the term
   1. Solute particles easily settle out of solvent
   2. Solute particles can be seen by the naked eye or with a microscope when suspended in solvent
   3. Solutes can be removed by ordinary filtration
   4. Substances of this class are called coarse suspensions (e.g., the erythrocytes are suspended in plasma and can be seen microscopically and removed by fine filters or centrifugation)

C. The colloid particle
   1. Intermediate in size between the crystalloid and the coarse suspensoid
   2. Particle much larger than the crystalloid particle although smaller than particle of coarse

suspensoid; diameter of colloid around 0.0000001 to 0.00001 mm

3. Solutions of colloids
   a. Solute particles dispersed by solvent
   b. Solution: clear, cloudy, or opalescent
   c. Show bright path of reflected light passed through the solution: Tyndall effect
   d. More stable than coarse suspensoids, less stable than true solutions
   e. With time, colloid particles will settle out
   f. Affect osmotic pressure less than do crystalloids
   g. Most of the proteins in plasma are dispersed as colloid particles
   h. Blood is classified as a colloid and a suspension

4. Colloid particles will pass through ordinary filters but will be held back by most membranes

5. Colloid particles carry electric charges on their surfaces: not to be confused with ionic charges

6. Importance of colloid suspensions
   a. Proteins, fats, and many carbohydrates form molecules in the colloid size range
   b. These form colloid solutions in the cells and body fluids
   c. Protoplasm of cell itself is a colloid

Ionization

Ion

A. When an atom loses or gains an electron (electrons), it is no longer a neutral atom but a charged particle: an ion

B. The charge on this particle depends on whether electrons are lost (+) or gained (−) and the number of electrons lost or gained

C. An electron is a negative particle; the loss of 1 electron makes the ion positive (less negative) by 1; with loss of 2 electrons, the ion is 2+, etc.

D. The gain of 1 electron makes ion negative by 1; with 2 electrons gained, the ion is 2−, etc.

Ionization and Water

A. When certain compounds are placed in water, the polar water molecules dissociate the molecules of the compound into ions: a process called ionization

B. A substance that will ionize when placed in water is called an electrolyte

C. A substance that will ionize in water (an electrolyte) will allow the passage of an electric current through its solution

D. Acids, bases, and salts ionize in water and conduct an electric current

Factors Affecting Strength of Electrolytes

A. Amount of electrolyte present in solution

B. How well the electrolyte dissociates in solution: degree of ionization

1. Weak electrolytes are substances that dissociate into ions to only a slight degree
2. Strong electrolytes are substances that dissociate into ions to a larger degree

Bases, Acids, and Salts
Bases
A. Definition: a base is a substance that usually adds a hydroxyl ion (OH⁻) to any solution in which it is placed

$$\text{NaOH} \xrightarrow{\text{in water}} \text{Na}^+ + \text{OH}^-$$

B. Properties of a base
1. Bitter taste
2. Slippery feeling
3. Electrolyte in water
4. Reacts with indicators, giving a base color
a. Methyl orange: yellow
b. Litmus: blue
c. Phenolphthalein: red
5. Reacts with acids to form water and a salt (neutralization)
6. Reacts with certain metals to release hydrogen gas
7. Combines with organic acids (fatty acids) to form soaps
8. In high concentration destroys organic material; corrosive
C. Names and formulas of common bases
1. Calcium hydroxide (Ca[OH]$_2$): water solution, called lime water
2. Sodium hydroxide (NaOH): caustic soda
3. Potassium hydroxide (KOH): soap making
4. Ammonium hydroxide (NH$_4$OH): household cleaner
5. Magnesium hydroxide (Mg[OH]$_2$): water solution marketed under trade name Milk of Magnesia; antacid, mild laxative
6. Aluminum hydroxide (Al[OH]$_3$): component of antacid pills

Acids
A. Definition: an acid is ordinarily thought of as a substance that liberates an H$^+$ (hydrogen ion) to a solution in which it is placed

$$\text{H}_2\text{CO}_3 \xrightarrow{\text{in water}} \text{H}^+ + \text{HCO}_3^-$$

B. Properties of an acid
1. Sour taste
2. Reacts with indicators giving an acid color
a. Methyl orange: red
b. Litmus: red
c. Phenolphthalein: colorless
3. Combines with certain metals, releasing hydrogen gas
4. Reacts with bases to form water and a salt (neutralization)
5. Reacts with carbonates to give carbon dioxide gas
6. Acts as an electrolyte in water
7. In high concentration destroys organic materials: corrosive
C. Names and formulas of common acids
1. Hydrochloric acid (HCl): secreted by the parietal cells of the stomach; transforms pepsinogen into pepsin, which is a protein-digesting enzyme of gastric juice
2. Nitric acid (HNO$_3$): used in test for proteins
3. Sulfuric acid (H$_2$SO$_4$): in storage batteries
4. Carbonic acid (H$_2$CO$_3$)
a. One form in which CO$_2$ is transported in the blood
b. Part of the bicarbonate buffer system, which is the most important buffer system regulating the pH of body fluids
5. Boric acid (H$_3$BO$_3$): mild antiseptic
6. Acetic acid (CH$_3$COOH): vinegar
7. Lactic acid (CH$_3$CHOHCOOH): builds up in muscle tissue during exercise; most lactic acid is then transported to the liver via the circulatory system, where it is completely oxidized into CO$_2$, water, and energy (as adenosine triphosphate [ATP])

General Considerations Concerning Acids and Bases
A. Weak acids produce few hydrogen ions in solution, whereas strong acids produce many
B. Weak bases produce few hydroxyl ions in solution, whereas strong bases produce many
C. Strong acids and bases can cause serious damage to human tissue
D. Acids and bases can be used to neutralize each other: therefore, in the event of acid or base burn, flood with water and add the opposite chemical in weak, diluted form

Salts
A. Definition: the compound (besides water) formed when an acid is neutralized by a base is a salt; e.g.,

$$\underset{\textbf{Acid}}{\text{HCl}} + \underset{\textbf{Base}}{\text{KOH}} \longrightarrow \underset{\textbf{Water}}{\text{H}_2\text{O}} + \underset{\textbf{Salt}}{\text{KCl}}$$

B. Properties of a salt
1. Crystalline in nature
2. Ionic even in the dry crystal
3. Electrolyte in solution
4. "Salty" taste
C. Names and formulas of common salts
1. Sodium chloride (NaCl): salt of intercellular and extracellular spaces
2. Calcium phosphate (Ca$_3$[PO$_4$]$_2$): bone and tooth formation

3. Potassium chloride (KCl): salt of intracellular spaces
4. Calcium carbonate ($CaCO_3$): limestone
5. Barium sulfate ($BaSO_4$): when taken internally, outlines internal structures for x-ray studies
6. Silver nitrate ($AgNO_3$): antiseptic
7. Iron sulfate ($FeSO_4$): treatment of anemia
8. Sodium bicarbonate ($NaHCO_3$): antacid
9. Calcium sulfate ($CaSO_4$): hydrated form is plaster of paris (casts for broken bones)
10. Magnesium sulfate ($MgSO_4$): Epsom salt

Hydrogen Ion Concentration (pH)

A. The p in pH comes from the French word puissance, meaning power
B. The H in pH stands for hydrogen
C. Thus pH denotes the power or strength of hydrogen (ions) in a solution
D. A neutral solution has the same amount of acid-reacting ions, H^+ (actually H_3O^+), as basic-reacting ions, OH^-
E. An acid-reacting solution has more H^+ than OH^-
F. A basic-reacting solution has more OH^- than H^+
G. pH is used to represent these conditions
1. A neutral solution has a pH of 7.00
2. An acid solution would have a pH in the range from 0 to 6.99; the lower the pH, the more acid the solution
3. A basic solution would have a pH in the range from 7.01 to 14.00; the higher the pH, the more basic the solution
4. The pH of the extracellular (vascular and interstitial) fluid is in the narrow range of 7.35 to 7.45; fluctuations in pH of 0.4 unit above or below this range can result in body distress; a prolonged blood pH of 7 or less or 7.8 or more can result in death
5. Certain body fluids have a pH different from 7.4; gastric juice has a pH of 1 or 2 caused by the presence of hydrochloric acid; bile is basic; urine may be acidic or basic

GENERAL NURSING CARE OF CLIENTS WITH FLUID AND ELECTROLYTE PROBLEMS

A. DATA COLLECTION

1. Obtain history to identify risk factors affecting fluid and electrolyte status (Table 6-3)
2. Monitor vital signs
3. Evaluate skin turgor, hydration, and temperature
4. Auscultate breath sounds
5. Weigh client daily
6. Monitor intake and output
7. Evaluate changes in behavior and energy level
8. Review laboratory tests
   a. Urinary specific gravity
   b. Serum pH and serum electrolytes
   c. Hematocrit
   d. Blood urea nitrogen (BUN)
   e. Creatinine clearance

B. ANALYSIS AND INTERPRETATION

1. Activity intolerance related to muscle weakness
2. Decreased cardiac output related to cardiac dysrhythmias
3. Fluid volume deficit related to:
   a. Diarrhea
   b. Loss of gastric contents (vomiting, nasogastric intubation)
   c. Diaphoresis
   d. Polyuria
4. Fluid volume excess related to:
   a. Anuria
   b. Decreased cardiac output
   c. Altered regulatory mechanisms
   d. Trapping of fluid in third space; where extracellular fluid accumulates and is physiologically unavailable to the body
5. Impaired gas exchange related to excessive secretions
6. Risk for injury related to sensory and perceptual alterations
7. Altered nutrition: less than body requirements related to:
   a. Anorexia
   b. Nausea
   c. Vomiting
8. Risk for impaired skin integrity related to poor skin turgor

C. PLANNING/IMPLEMENTATION

1. Manage fluid and electrolyte intake
   a. Fluids may be encouraged to correct deficit (usually 3000 ml/day; may be restricted to prevent excess)
   b. Nutritional intake can be increased or restricted to correct electrolyte disturbances
      (1) Sodium: table salt, dairy products, processed meats, soup, canned foods
      (2) Potassium: bananas, oranges, nuts, dark leafy greens, dried fruit
      (3) Calcium: milk, cheese, yogurt
2. Administer intravenous therapy
   a. Fluids
      (1) Dextrose in water
         (a) Provides fluid and limited calories (1 L of 5% dextrose provides 170 calories)
         (b) Used to correct dehydration, ketosis, and hypernatremia
      (2) Dextrose in sodium chloride (NaCl): used to correct fluid loss from excessive perspiration or vomiting and to prevent alkalosis

TABLE 6-3 Etiology, manifestations, and treatment of major fluid and electrolyte distributions

Fluid/electrolyte imbalance	Etiology	Signs and symptoms	Treatment
Extracellular fluid deficit	Decreased fluid intake Prolonged fever Vomiting Excessive use of diuretics	Increased thirst Dry skin and mucous membranes Increased temperature Flushed skin Rapid, thready pulse Increased Hct, Na$^+$, and specific gravity	Administration of hypotonic or isotonic fluids
Extracellular fluid excess	Congestive heart failure Liver disease Malnutrition (decreased plasma protein) Renal disease Excessive parenteral fluids	Weight gain Crackles Edema Ascites Confusion Weakness Decreased Hct	Administration of diuretics Fluid restriction
Hypokalemia	Diarrhea Vomiting Diabetic acidosis Diuretics Inadequate intake	Loss of muscle tone Cardiac dysrhythmias Abdominal distension Vomiting Decreased serum K$^+$	Parenteral/oral administration of potassium supplement Increased dietary intake of potassium
Hyperkalemia	Advanced kidney disease Severe burns or tissue trauma Excessive dosages of potassium	Cardiac irregularities Weakness Diarrhea Nausea Irritability Increased serum K$^+$	Administration of potassium-free fluids Dialysis Potassium-removing resin
Hyponatremia	Diuretics Electrolyte-free IV fluids Diarrhea GI suction Excessive perspiration followed by increased water intake	Abdominal cramps Convulsions Oliguria Decreased serum Na$^+$ and specific gravity	Administration of IV solutions containing NaCl Administration of NaCl tablets
Hypernatremia	Diabetes insipidus Excess NaCl IV fluid intake	Dry, sticky mucous membranes Oliguria Firm tissue turgor Dry tongue Increased serum Na$^+$ and specific gravity	Low Na$^+$ diet Increased Na$^+$-free fluid intake
Hypocalcemia	Removal of parathyroid glands Administration of electrolyte-free solutions	Tingling of extremities Tetany Cramps Convulsions	Oral/parenteral calcium replacement
Hypercalcemia	Hyperparathyroidism Prolonged immobility Excessive intake of Ca$^+$ or vitamin D	Flank pain (renal calculi) Deep bone pain Relaxed muscles	Correction of primary problem Increased fluid intake

(3) NaCl: used to manage alkalosis, fluid loss, and adrenal cortical insufficiency
(4) Ringer's solution
    (a) Contains Na$^+$, Cl$^-$, K$^+$, Ca^{++}
    (b) Used to correct dehydration from vomiting, diarrhea, or inadequate intake

(5) Lactated Ringer's solution
    (a) Contains Na$^+$, Cl$^-$, K$^+$, Ca^{++}, and lactate
    (b) Lactate is metabolized by liver and forms bicarbonate (HCO$_3^-$)
    (c) Used to correct extracellular fluid shifts and moderate metabolic acidosis

(6) Plasma expanders
  (a) Examples include dextran and albumin
  (b) Used to increase blood volume in trauma or burn victims

b. Regulation of flow rate
  (1) Manual regulation of gravity flow with clamp

Per minute drop rate =

$$\frac{\text{Milliliters to be infused} \times \text{drop factor (drops per 1 ml)}}{\text{Number of hours} \times 60 \text{ minutes}}$$

  (2) Use of infusion pump or controller
    (a) Drop control: usually drops per minute (follow manufacturer's instructions when setting desired rate of flow)
    (b) Volume control: usually milliliters per hour (follow manufacturer's instructions when setting desired rate of flow)

c. Monitor client for complications
  (1) Infiltration
    (a) Catheter is displaced, allowing fluid to leak into tissues
    (b) Insertion site is pale, cool, and edematous; flow rate decreases
    (c) IV must be removed and restarted in a new site
  (2) Phlebitis
    (a) Vein is irritated by catheter or medications
    (b) Insertion site is red, painful, and warm; flow rate is decreased
    (c) IV must be removed and restarted in a new site; warm compresses are applied to inflammation
  (3) Circulatory overload
    (a) Flow rate exceeds cardiovascular system's capability to adjust to the increased fluid volume
    (b) Client exhibits dyspnea, crackles, distended neck veins, and increased blood pressure
    (c) Rate is decreased to keep the vein open; physician is notified and diuretics, if prescribed, are administered

3. Administer pharmacologic agents
  a. Diuretics (thiazide, potassium-sparing, loop, or osmotic diuretics)
  b. Electrolyte replacement (e.g., potassium chloride, calcium gluconate)
  c. Potassium-removing resin: sodium polystyrene sulfonate (Kayexalate)

4. Provide care based on specific clinical findings (e.g., skin care, safe environment)

D. EVALUATION/OUTCOMES
1. Maintains fluid balance
2. Serum electrolyte levels are within normal limits
3. Vital signs are within normal limits

PERIOPERATIVE CARE

REVIEW OF PHARMACOLOGY RELATED TO PERIOPERATIVE CARE

General Anesthetics

A. Description
1. Used in a "balanced" combination to facilitate the surgical experience by producing varying types of loss of consciousness, pain control, and skeletal muscle relaxation
2. Act by depressing the CNS through the following progressive sequence
  a. Stage I: euphoria; gradual loss of consciousness
  b. Stage II: hyperexcitement; hyperactive reflexes; pupil dilation
  c. Stage III: depression of corneal reflex and pupillary response to light; absence of voluntary control; decreased muscle tone; stage of surgical anesthesia
  d. Stage IV: medullary paralysis (respiratory/cardiac failure); death
3. General anesthetics are available in parenteral (IM, IV) and inhalation preparations; ultrashort-acting IV barbiturates are useful in the induction of anesthesia because of their ability to quickly penetrate the blood-brain barrier; IV and IM nonbarbiturates produce a special type of anesthesia in which the client appears to be awake but dissociated from the environment, resulting in amnesia for the surgical experience (neuroleptanalgesia)

B. Examples
1. Inhalation anesthetics
  a. Cyclopropane
  b. Enflurane (Ethrane)
  c. Ether
  d. Halothane (Fluothane)
  e. Methoxyflurane (Penthrane)
  f. Nitrous oxide
2. IV barbiturates: high lipoid affinity provides prompt effect on cerebral tissue
  a. Methohexital sodium (Brevital)
  b. Thiamylal sodium (Surital)
  c. Thiopental sodium (Pentothal)
3. IV and IM nonbarbiturates: induce a cataleptic state and produce amnesia for the procedure
  a. Ketamine HCl (Ketaject)
  b. Midazolam HCl (Versed)
  c. Combination product: fentanyl and droperidol (Innovar)

C. Major side effects
1. Inhalation anesthetics
   a. Excitement and restlessness (initial CNS stimulation)
   b. Nausea and vomiting (stimulation of chemoreceptor trigger zone in medullary vomiting center)
   c. Respiratory distress (depression of medullary respiratory center)
2. IV barbiturates
   a. Respiratory depression (depression of medullary respiratory center)
   b. Hypotension and tachycardia (depression of cardiovascular system)
   c. Laryngospasm (depression of laryngeal reflex)
3. IV and IM nonbarbiturates
   a. Respiratory failure (depression of medullary respiratory center)
   b. Changes in blood pressure: hypertension; hypotension (alterations in cardiovascular system)
   c. Rigidity (enhancement of muscle tone)
   d. Psychic disturbances (emergence reaction-recovery period)

D. Nursing care
1. Assess for allergies and other medical problems that could alter the client's response to the anesthetic agents
2. Have O_2 and emergency resuscitative equipment available
3. Assess vital signs before, during, and after anesthetic administration
4. Maintain a calm environment during induction of anesthesia
5. Use safety precautions with flammable agents
6. Protect client during postanesthetic period because of decreased sensory awareness
7. Judiciously administer narcotics in the initial postanesthetic period
8. Evaluate client's response to medications

Local Anesthetics

A. Description
1. Used to produce pain control without rendering the client unconscious; useful for obstetric, dental, and minor surgical procedures
2. Act in a reversible manner to block nerve impulse conduction in sensory, motor, and autonomic nerve cells by decreasing nerve membrane permeability to sodium ion influx
3. Available in topical, spinal, and nerve block preparations; epinephrine may be added to these preparations to enhance the duration of the local anesthetic effect

B. Examples
1. Topical: local infiltration of tissue
   a. Benzocaine
   b. Cocaine
   c. Dibucaine (Nupercainal)
   d. Lidocaine HCl (Xylocaine); also used for nerve block
   e. Piperocaine HCl (Metycaine)
   f. Tetracaine HCl (Pontocaine); also used for spinal anesthesia and nerve block
2. Spinal: injected into the spinal subarachnoid space
   a. Lidocaine HCl (Xylocaine)
   b. Procaine HCl (Novocain); also used for nerve block
3. Epidural: injected into the epidural space of the spinal column
   a. Bupivacaine HCl (Sensorcaine)
   b. Lidocaine HCl (Xylocaine)
   c. Mepivacaine HCl (Carbocaine)
4. Nerve block: injected at perineural site distant from desired anesthesia site
   a. Bupivacaine HCl (Marcaine)
   b. Chloroprocaine HCl (Nesacaine)
   c. Mepivacaine HCl (Carbocaine)

C. Major side effects
1. Allergic reactions; anaphylaxis (hypersensitivity)
2. Respiratory arrest (depression of medullary respiratory center)
3. Dysrhythmias; cardiac arrest (depression of cardiovascular system)
4. Convulsions (depression of central nervous system)
5. Hypotension (depression of cardiovascular system)

D. Nursing care
1. Assess for allergies and other medical problems that could alter the client's response to the anesthetic agent
2. Have O_2 and emergency resuscitative equipment available
3. Assess vital signs before, during, and after anesthetic administration
4. Protect anesthetized body parts from mechanical and/or thermal injury
5. Maintain a calm environment while the client is anesthetized
6. Keep client flat for a specified period (usually 6 to 12 hours) after spinal anesthesia to prevent severe headache; avoid pillows
7. Use safety precautions (side rails up) and maintain bed rest until sensation returns to lower extremities after spinal anesthesia
8. Maintain side-lying position to prevent aspiration after general anesthesia

9. Restrict oral intake after client has had general anesthesia until ability to swallow has returned
10. Evaluate client's response to medications and understanding of teaching

Sedatives/Hypnotics

A. Description
   1. Produce sedation in small doses and sleep in larger doses
   2. Used for clients experiencing anxiety-related situations and insomnia
   3. Act by depressing the CNS
   4. Available in oral, parenteral (IV, IM), and rectal preparations

B. Examples
   1. Barbiturates: depress CNS starting with diencephalon
     a. Amobarbital (Amytal)
     b. Butabarbital sodium (Butisol)
     c. Pentobarbital sodium (Nembutal)
     d. Phenobarbital (Luminal)
     e. Secobarbital (Seconal)
   2. Nonbarbiturates: depress CNS and relax skeletal muscles
     a. Chloral hydrate
     b. Ethchlorvynol (Placidyl)
     c. Flurazepam HCl (Dalmane)
     d. Glutethimide

C. Major side effects
   1. Drowsiness (depression of CNS)
   2. Hypotension (depression of cardiovascular system)
   3. Dizziness (hypotension)
   4. Gastrointestinal irritation (local oral effect)
   5. Skin rash (hypersensitivity)
   6. Blood disorders (hematologic alterations)
   7. Drug dependence
   8. Barbiturates
     a. Hangover (persistence of low barbiturate concentration in body caused by decreased metabolism)
     b. Photosensitivity (hypersensitivity)
     c. Excitement in children and elderly (paradoxic reaction)

D. Nursing care
   1. Avoid administration with other CNS depressants
   2. Caution client to avoid engaging in hazardous activity; avoid concurrent use of alcohol
   3. Assess for signs of dependence
   4. Use safety precautions at night for hospitalized clients (side rails up)
   5. Implement supportive measures to promote sleep (back rub; warm milk)
   6. Instruct client to avoid placing medication within reach to prevent possible overdose while drowsy

7. Monitor blood work during long-term therapy
8. Administer controlled substances according to appropriate schedule restrictions
9. Evaluate client's response to medication and understanding of teaching

Analgesics

A. Description
   1. Used to relieve pain
   2. Divided into two classes
     a. Nonnarcotic analgesics relieve mild to moderate pain
     b. Narcotic analgesics relieve moderate to severe pain
   3. Nonnarcotic analgesics
     a. Act by a peripheral mechanism at the level of the damaged tissue by inhibiting prostaglandin and other chemical mediator synthesis involved in the pain phenomenon
     b. Exert antipyretic activity by action on the hypothalamic heat-regulating center to reduce fever
     c. Salicylates, which belong to this class, also exert antiinflammatory, uricosuric, and antiplatelet-aggregating effects
     d. Nonsalicylates, such as acetaminophen, are nonirritating to the gastrointestinal mucosa
   4. Narcotic analgesics act by blocking opioid receptors in the CNS, thereby altering awareness of pain
     a. Depress CNS and also produce effects on multiple body systems
     b. Produce euphoria and are addicting
   5. Available in oral, parenteral (IV, SC, IM), and rectal preparations; many combination products exist that contain both a narcotic and nonnarcotic analgesic component

B. Examples
   1. Nonnarcotic (salicylates)
     a. Aspirin (ASA; Ecotrin)
     b. Magnesium salicylate
   2. Nonnarcotic (nonsalicylates)
     a. Acetaminophen (Tylenol)
     b. Diflunisal (Dolobid)
   3. Narcotic
     a. Codeine sulfate
     b. Meperidine HCl (Demerol)
     c. Morphine sulfate
     d. Oxycodone HCl (Percodan)
     e. Pentazocine HCl (Talwin)
     f. Propoxyphene HCl (Darvon)

C. Major side effects
   1. Nonnarcotic (salicylates)
     a. Gastric irritation (local effect)
     b. Visual disturbances (salicylism)

c. Prolonged bleeding time (suppression of platelet aggregation)

d. Tinnitus (early toxicity-salicylism)

2. Nonnarcotic (nonsalicylates)

a. Sore throat, fever (depression of WBCs)

b. Skin rash (hypersensitivity)

c. Hepatotoxicity (direct liver toxic effect)

3. Narcotic

a. Respiratory depression (depression of medullary respiratory center)

b. Hypotension (depression of cardiovascular system)

c. Constipation (decreased peristalsis)

d. Euphoria (central nervous system effect)

e. Urinary retention (increased smooth muscle tone of sphincter)

f. Miosis (stimulation of sphincter muscle of iris)

D. Nursing care

1. Assess for covert signs of pain

a. Monitor vital signs

b. Evaluate nonverbal communication (grimacing; protective motions)

2. Administer medication before pain becomes severe

3. Administer narcotics as ordered

a. Do not administer if respirations are less than 12 per minute

b. Have narcotic antagonist available (naloxone [Narcan])

c. Observe for overdosage triad: respiratory depression, pinpoint pupils, and coma

d. Avoid administration with CNS depressants

e. Avoid use in clients with head injuries

f. Assess for signs of dependence

g. Use safety precautions with hospitalized clients; supervise ambulation; side rails up, especially at night

h. Note automatic stop orders

i. Controlled substances: administer according to appropriate schedule restrictions

4. Evaluate client's response to medications and understanding of teaching

CLASSIFICATION OF SURGERY

A. Ambulatory surgery: useful in offering clients early ambulation, an active role in an individual's recovery process, and cost containment

1. Hospital-based outpatient settings

a. Client has diagnostic workup in hospital several days before surgery

b. Client is admitted directly to the ambulatory surgical section by the perioperative nurse

c. Client is discharged from the postanesthesia or clinical unit generally the same day as the surgery is performed; when complica-

tions occur, the physician must admit the client to the hospital

2. Hospital satellite settings

a. Client has diagnostic workup in hospital or physician's office before surgery

b. Client is admitted to satellite unit and discharged from same when recovery is satisfactory

3. Private surgical offices

a. Surgical procedures are performed by the surgeon in a private office, which has a surgical suite and surgical staff (technicians and nurses)

b. Preoperative workup is performed by hospital, physician, or clinic before surgery

B. Inpatient surgical care

1. Client is admitted to the hospital setting for surgical care

2. Surgery may be classified as:

a. Elective

b. Diagnostic

c. Urgent or emergency surgery

d. Ablative

e. Palliative

f. Curative

GENERAL NURSING CARE OF CLIENTS DURING THE PREOPERATIVE PERIOD

A. DATA COLLECTION

1. Obtain history of current health problems and factors that would influence recovery

2. Perform physical assessment to identify potential health problems

3. Determine client's understanding of disease and treatment plan

4. Identify client's emotional state and coping skills

B. ANALYSIS AND INTERPRETATION

1. Fear related to:

a. Surgical procedure

b. Prognosis

2. Knowledge deficit related to unfamiliarity with hospital procedures/personnel/ environment

3. Sleep-pattern disturbance related to anxiety

C. PLANNING/IMPLEMENTATION

1. Allow the client time to ask questions about procedures and surgery

2. Explain all procedures to the client and give reasons for them

3. Determine the client's level of understanding of operative procedure to ascertain whether signature on permit represents informed consent

4. Allow and encourage the client to ventilate feelings about diagnosis and surgery

5. Tell the client what to expect in the operating room, recovery, and/or intensive care units, including use of anticipated equipment
6. Inform the client if the plan is to return him or her to other than the present room
7. Encourage nutritional assessment so that any nutrient deficiencies can be corrected
8. Provide a spiritual counselor if desired by the client or family
9. Consider needs of the family when discussing surgery
10. Teach the client the activities that will be instituted after surgery related to ventilatory function
    a. Diaphragmatic breathing
    b. Controlled coughing
    c. Deep breathing
    d. Incentive spirometry
    e. Splinting
    f. Turning
11. Teach the client physical exercises that will be used to promote circulation after surgery
    a. Leg exercises including dorsiflexion
    b. Ambulation routines
    c. Isometric exercises
12. Inform the client to expect some discomfort after surgery and teach the importance of requesting medication for pain
13. Make certain that history, physical examination results, recent laboratory tests, and chest x-ray report are entered on the chart
14. Inform all members of the medical team, especially the anesthetist, of the client's allergies and other health problems and prominently mark the chart
15. Minimize the risk of postoperative infection by proper skin preparation
    a. Cleanse the skin thoroughly with antimicrobial preparation as ordered
    b. Shampoo hair when procedure involves head, neck, or upper chest area
    c. Shave skin if ordered, however, hair removal recommended only if necessary and then only immediately prior to surgery
16. Carry out ordered preoperative preparation
    a. Enemas (often until clear returns)
    b. Douches
    c. Irrigations
17. Remove nail polish from fingers and toes
18. Administer prescribed sleeping medications
    a. Sedative-hypnotics
    b. Antianxiety agents
19. Inform the client not to take anything by mouth after midnight the night before surgery, remove fluid, and place obvious signs at bedside

20. Provide care for the client on the day of surgery
    a. In the morning, check the client's vital signs and assess overall physical status; record and report any deviations to physician
    b. Check the client's medical chart to ensure that pertinent test results are present
    c. Complete the preoperative checklist
    d. Provide hygiene and assist client into hospital gown
    e. Have the client void
    f. Remove any prosthetics such as dentures and wigs
    g. Apply antiembolic stockings as ordered
    h. Arrange for insertion of any tubes as ordered
       (1) Nasogastric tube
       (2) Indwelling urinary catheter
    i. Arrange for insertion of intravenous line as ordered
    j. Store any client valuables according to hospital policy
    k. Make sure identification band is on client's wrist
    l. Administer prescribed preoperative medications as ordered
       (1) Antianxiety agents (e.g., diazepam HCl [Valium])
       (2) Sedatives (e.g., lorazepam [Ativan])
       (3) Narcotic analgesics (e.g., meperidine HCl [Demerol])
       (4) Anticholinergics (e.g., glycopyrrolate [Robinul], atropine sulfate)
    m. Put side rails up after administering medications
    n. Transfer the client to a stretcher when operating room calls; fasten the stretcher strap in place before transporting
    o. Consider the emotional needs of both the client and family on the day of surgery
21. Provide care for the client in the operative suite
    a. Take client to a holding area outside of the operating room
    b. Insert an intravenous catheter (if not already in place); usually done by the nurse or anesthetist
    c. Transfer client to the operating room by stretcher
    d. Complete checklist
    e. Apply monitoring devices as needed
    f. Allay client's anxiety; ambulatory surgical clients remain aware during most of their stay in the operating room because local anesthetics are frequently used
    g. Anesthesia is introduced by anesthetist to produce four stages of anesthesia

(1) Stage 1: Client becomes drowsy and loses consciousness

(2) Stage 2: Stage of excitement; muscles are tense, breathing may be irregular

(3) Stage 3: Depression of vital signs and reflexes; operation begins during this phase

(4) Stage 4: Complete respiratory depression

h. Anesthetist inserts an endotracheal tube or airway after the administration of an intravenous anesthetic

i. Position client for surgery

j. Operating room nurse assumes role of client advocate during the intraoperative phase

(1) The scrub nurse hands the surgeon sterile instruments and supplies; counts sponges, needles, and instruments; and disposes of used instruments

(2) The circulating nurse positions the client on the table, drapes the client, and assists the surgeon and scrub nurse to don sterile attire

D. EVALUATION/OUTCOMES

1. Verbalizes fears concerning operative process
2. Controls long-standing health problems
3. Demonstrates an understanding of preoperative teaching
4. Remains free from injury

GENERAL NURSING CARE OF CLIENTS DURING THE POSTOPERATIVE PERIOD

A. DATA COLLECTION

1. Verify patency of airway
2. Establish baseline vital signs, breath sounds
3. Determine level of consciousness
4. Observe tubes for patency and placement and drainage for characteristics
5. Inspect dressing if present
6. Determine if client has sufficient urinary output
7. Assess for signs of normal wound healing after initial postoperative period

B. ANALYSIS AND INTERPRETATION

1. Ineffective airway clearance related to prolonged sedation
2. Risk for aspiration related to reduced level of consciousness
3. Ineffective breathing pattern related to incisional pain
4. Constipation related to decreased peristalsis
5. Fear related to surgical procedure and prognosis
6. Risk for fluid volume deficit related to:
   a. Inadequate intake
   b. Wound drainage
7. Hyperthermia related to inflammatory process
8. Risk for infection related to surgical wound

9. Risk for injury related to anesthesia and sedation
10. Impaired physical mobility related to pain and/or dressing
11. Pain related to surgical incision
12. Sleep pattern disturbance related to:
    a. Anxiety and pain
    b. Environmental stimuli
13. Altered urinary elimination related to:
    a. Effects of anesthesia
    b. Decreased intake
14. Inability to sustain spontaneous ventilation related to effects of anesthesia

C. PLANNING/IMPLEMENTATION

1. Provide immediate care
   a. Respiratory needs: anesthesia may result in depression of respiratory function
      (1) Maintain a patent airway by keeping the artificial airway in place until gag reflex returns
      (2) Position client on one side with neck slightly extended to prevent aspiration and accumulation of mucus secretions
      (3) Monitor the rate, rhythm, symmetry of chest movement, breath sounds, pulse oximeter, and color of mucous membranes
      (4) Suction artificial airway and the oral cavity as needed to remove secretions
      (5) Administer oxygen as ordered
      (6) Remove airway when the gag reflex has returned, suctioning prior to removal to clear mucous plugs and secretions as needed
      (7) Encourage coughing and deep breathing as soon as the client is able to cooperate
   b. Circulatory needs: anesthesia and immobilization during surgery may result in circulatory compromise
      (1) Monitor the heart rate and rhythm as well as the blood pressure at frequent intervals, approximately every 15 minutes
      (2) Monitor peripheral circulation by noting the color, temperature, capillary refill, and presence of pulses to ensure tissue perfusion
      (3) Monitor for hemorrhage by measuring blood pressure for hypotension and observing and measuring wound drainage
      (4) Report signs of hemorrhage to the surgeon immediately
   c. Neurologic needs: preoperative and anesthetic agents depress the central nervous system
      (1) Monitor the client's level of consciousness and responses to stimuli

(2) Monitor pupillary blink and gag reflexes

(3) Monitor for loss or return of sensation or movement when specific areas have been surgically treated

(4) Reorient the client to time, place, and situation

(5) Call the client by name

(6) Answer questions as honestly and simply as possible and avoid complicated, involved explanations

(7) Expect and accept repetitious questions and give the client necessary reassurance

d. Wound care

(1) Note the location of the wound and the color, odor, amount, and consistency of drainage

(2) Circle drainage on the dressing to allow for more objective assessment of drainage

(3) Reinforce postoperative dressings because surgeons generally perform the first dressing change

e. Care of drains and tubes

(1) Maintain patency of tubing

(2) Attach tubing to appropriate collection containers; maintain negative pressure in portable wound drainage systems

(3) Monitor output of drains to assess for hemorrhage

f. Fluid and electrolyte needs

(1) Maintain intravenous therapy as ordered

(2) Record intake and output accurately

g. Comfort needs

(1) Assess the client's level of pain

(2) Medicate as ordered to reduce pain and increase postoperative compliance with breathing, coughing, and activity regimens

(3) Teach client how to use patient-controlled analgesia (PCA)

2. Provide care for the ambulatory surgical client

a. All care included under immediate postoperative care applies to the ambulatory surgical client

b. Recovery time is generally less for this client because outpatient anesthesia is intended to provide for a quick recovery time and few side effects

c. When the client is responsive, encourage sips of water and ambulate to chair

d. Provide a light meal when tolerated

e. When the client is stable, has retained foods, and has voided, reinforce postoperative teaching and discharge planning with client and family members; evaluate understanding of teaching

3. Provide care for the inpatient surgical client

a. Protect the client from injury by keeping under close observation, keeping side rails in place, positioning to prevent excessive pressure on body parts or on tubing, controlling restlessness and preventing the client from pulling on tubes or dressing, and making certain that all equipment is in safe working condition and properly used

b. Turn frequently; encourage deep breathing and coughing and use of incentive spirometer to prevent the development of atelectasis or hypostatic pneumonia

c. Perform or encourage range of motion and isometric exercises and early ambulation to prevent phlebitis, paralytic ileus, and circulatory stasis

d. Maintain patency of tubing (e.g., catheter, gastric tubes, T-tube, chest tubes, incisional drains) to promote drainage and maintain decompression to reduce pressure on suture line

e. Use surgical aseptic technique when changing dressings or as necessary when irrigating tubing or emptying portable wound drainage systems to prevent infection

f. Monitor intake and output to prevent dehydration, fluid and electrolyte imbalance, and urinary suppression or retention

g. Observe for abdominal distention to prevent discomfort and intestinal obstruction

h. Give medication for pain as ordered to prevent discomfort and restlessness

i. Regulate IV therapy to prevent overload or circulatory collapse

j. Encourage the client to support and splint the incisional site when coughing, moving, or turning to prevent tension on the suture line

k. Position the client as required by type of surgery to prevent misalignment and prevent accumulation of fluid or blocking the drainage tubes

l. Provide emotional support; assist client to cope with changes in body image

4. Provide for nutritional needs

a. Maintain IV therapy to provide water and electrolytes (oral intake needed as soon as possible for adequate nutrition)

b. Monitor parenteral nutrition (total parenteral nutrition [TPN] and peripheral parenteral nutrition [PPN]); parenteral nutrition is of high nutrient density; solutions of amino acids, glucose, electrolytes, minerals, vitamins; fat emulsions (intralipids); TPN usually inserted into larger veins (inferior or superior vena cava) to avoid thrombosis in peripheral veins; used in clients with major tissue trauma, injury, or extensive surgery

   c. Gradually increase oral intake as permitted
     (1) Liquid diets
       (a) Clear liquid: clear broth, bouillon, juices, plain gelatin, fruit-flavored water, ices, ginger ale, coffee, tea
       (b) Full liquid: may add milk and items made with milk, such as cream soups, milk drinks, sherbet, ice cream, puddings, custard
     (2) Soft diet: may add all soft, cooked foods, such as refined cereals; pasta; rice, white bread and crackers; eggs; cheese; meat; potatoes; cooked, whole vegetables; cooked fruits; few soft, ripe, plain fruits without membranes or skins; simple desserts
     (3) Light diet: same as soft with few additional whole, cooked foods; light, raw foods such as fruit; mainly avoid heavily seasoned or fried foods
     (4) Full diet: full, well-balanced diet of all foods as desired and tolerated, including a wide variety for interest and flavor

   d. Provide for special nutritional needs
     (1) Protein: increased need caused by protein losses and the anabolism of recovery and tissue healing; approximate requirement for adult is 1.2 to 2 g/kg/day
     (2) Calories: adequate amount to supply energy and spare protein for tissue building
     (3) Water: adequate fluid therapy to prevent dehydration caused by large fluid losses
     (4) Vitamins and minerals: need for most will be increased following surgery and the nutrition program must be designed to ensure that individual requirements are met; special attention to mineral adequacy to maintain electrolyte balance is essential
       (a) Zinc
         [1] Increases the tensile strength (force needed to separate edges) of the healing wound
         [2] Supplemental dosages of 4 to 6 mg/day orally are recommended
       (b) Vitamin C
         [1] Required for collagen formation
         [2] Supplemental dosages of 500 to 1000 mg/day should be administered to promote optimal wound healing

D. EVALUATION/OUTCOMES
   1. Avoids respiratory complications
   2. Remains free of infection
   3. Experiences relief of pain
   4. Verbalizes understanding of postoperative limitations
   5. Demonstrates ability to care for self
   6. Maintains fluid balance
   7. Reestablishes urinary function
   8. Reestablishes bowel function
   9. Effectively copes with changes resulting from surgery

NEOPLASTIC DISORDERS

(See related body system for specific diseases.)

CLASSIFICATION OF NEOPLASMS

A. Benign neoplasia
   1. Cells adhere to each other and the growth remains circumscribed
   2. Generally not life threatening unless they occur in a restricted area (e.g., skull)
   3. Classified according to the tissue involved
     a. Adenoma—glandular tissue
     b. Leiomyoma—smooth muscle
     c. Chondroma—cartilaginous tissue
     d. Osteoma—bone osteoblast
     e. Hemangioma—blood vessels
     f. Lymphangioma—lymphatics
     g. Neuroma—nerve cells
     h. Lipoma—adipose tissue
     i. Papilloma—epithelial tissue
     j. Rhabdomyoma—skeletal tissue
     k. Fibroma—fibrous tissue

B. Malignant neoplasia
   1. Cells infiltrate surrounding tissue
   2. Cells invade other tissues and produce secondary lesions
   3. May spread (metastasize) by direct extension, lymphatic permeation and embolization, and diffusion of cancer cells by mechanical means
   4. Tumors are classified according to the tissue involved
     a. Adenocarcinoma—glandular epithelial tissue
     b. Carcinoma—epithelial surface tissue
     c. Sarcoma—connective tissue
     d. Osteosarcoma—bone osteoblasts
     e. Hemangiosarcoma—blood vessels
     f. Lymphangiosarcoma—lymphatics
     g. Neurofibrosarcoma (neurilemic sarcoma)—nerve sheath
     h. Liposarcoma—adipose tissue
     i. Melanoma—melanocytes

5. Tumors are often classified by a universal system of staging classification, the TNM system
   a. T designates a primary tumor
   b. N designates lymph node involvement
   c. M designates metastasis
   d. Numbers 0 to 4 designate degree of involvement
   e. TIS designates carcinoma in situ, or one which is noninfiltrating

PHARMACOLOGY RELATED TO NEOPLASTIC DISORDERS

Basic Concepts

A. Used to destroy malignant cells by interfering with reproduction of the cancer cell
B. Act at specific points in the cycle of cell division (cell-cycle specific) or at any phase of the cycle of cell division (cell-cycle nonspecific)
C. Affect any rapidly dividing cell within the body, thus having the potential for toxicity development in healthy, functional tissue (bone marrow, hair follicles, GI mucosa); to reduce the possibility of toxicity, combination therapy is often used
D. Available in oral, parenteral (IM, SC, IV), intraarterial, intrathecal, and topical preparations

Antineoplastic Drugs

Alkylating Agents

A. Cell-cycle nonspecific; attack the DNA of rapidly dividing cells
B. Examples
   1. Busulfan (Myleran)
   2. Chlorambucil (Leukeran)
   3. Cisplatin (Platinol)
   4. Cyclophosphamide (Cytoxan)
   5. Lomustine (CeeNU)
   6. Melphalan (Alkeran)

Antibiotics

A. Cell-cycle specific; inhibit RNA and protein synthesis of rapidly dividing tissue
B. Examples
   1. Dactinomycin (Cosmegen)
   2. Daunorubicin (Cerubidine)
   3. Doxorubicin hydrochloride (Adriamycin)
   4. Mithramycin (Mithracin)
   5. Mitomycin (Mutamycin)
   6. Procarbazine hydrochloride (Matulane)

Antimetabolites

A. Cell-cycle specific; inhibit protein synthesis in rapidly dividing cells during "S" phase
B. Examples
   1. Azathioprine (Imuran)
   2. Cytarabine (Cytosar-U)
   3. Floxuridine (FUDR)
   4. Fluorouracil (5-FU)
   5. Hydroxyurea (Hydrea)
   6. Mercaptopurine (6-MP, Purinethol)
   7. Methotrexate

Hormones

A. Tissue specific; inhibit RNA and protein synthesis in tissues that are dependent on the opposite (sex) hormone for development
B. Examples
   1. Androgens
   2. Estrogens (estramustine phosphate sodium [Emcyt])
   3. Progestins
   4. Steroids (prednisone [Meticorten])
   5. Other
      a. Mitotane (Lysodren) cortisol antagonist
      b. Tamoxifen citrate (Nolvadex) estrogen antagonist

Immune Agents

A. Involves introduction of noncancerous antigens or other agents into the body to stimulate production of lymphocytes and antibodies
B. Examples
   1. Bacillus of Calmette-Guérin (BCG) vaccine: provides active immunity
   2. Interferon alfa-2a (Roferon-A); interferon alfa-2b (Intron A)

Miscellaneous Agents

A. Leucovorin calcium
   1. A reduced form of folic acid
   2. Antidote to folic acid antagonists
B. Paclitaxel (Taxol)
   1. Inhibits the reorganization of the microtubule network that is needed for interphase and mitotic cellular functions
   2. Causes abnormal bundles of microtubules during cell cycle and multiple esters of microtubules during mitosis
C. Vinblastine (Velban)
   1. An alkaloid extracted from periwinkle
   2. Arrests mitosis during metaphase, blocking cell division

Common Combinations of Neoplastic Agents

A. ABVD
   1. Doxorubicin hydrochloride (Adriamycin)
   2. Bleomycin sulfate (Blenoxane)
   3. Vinblastine sulfate (Velban)
   4. Dacarbazine (DTIC-Dome)
B. CHOP
   1. Cyclophosphamide (Cytoxan)
   2. Doxorubicin hydrochloride (Adriamycin)
   3. Vincristine sulfate (Oncovin)
   4. Prednisone
C. CMF (may be referred to as CMFP when prednisone is included)
   1. Cyclophosphamide (Cytoxan)

    2. Methotrexate (Mexate)

    3. Fluorouracil (5-FU)

D. COPP (may be referred to as A-COPP when doxorubicin hydrochloride [Adriamycin] is included)

    1. Cyclophosphamide (Cytoxan)

    2. Vincristine sulfate (Oncovin)

    3. Procarbazine hydrochloride (Matulane)

    4. Prednisone

E. CVP

    1. Cyclophosphamide (Cytoxan)

    2. Vincristine sulfate (Oncovin)

    3. Prednisone

F. FAC

    1. Fluorouracil (5-FU)

    2. Doxorubicin hydrochloride (Adriamycin)

    3. Cyclophosphamide (Cytoxan)

G. MOPP

    1. Mechlorethamine hydrochloride (Nitrogen mustard, Mustargen)

    2. Vincristine sulfate (Oncovin)

    3. Procarbazine hydrochloride (Matulane)

    4. Prednisone

H. VAC

    1. Vincristine sulfate (Oncovin)

    2. Dactinomycin (Actinomycin D)

    3. Cyclophosphamide (Cytoxan)

Major Side Effects

A. Anorexia, nausea, vomiting (irritation of GI tract; quick uptake by rapidly dividing alimentary tract tissue)

B. Diarrhea (irritation of GI tract; quick uptake by rapidly dividing alimentary tract tissue)

C. Bone marrow depression (quick uptake by rapidly dividing myeloid tissue)

D. Stomatitis (irritation of GI tract; quick uptake by rapidly dividing alimentary tract tissue)

E. Blood dyscrasias (bone marrow depression)

F. Alopecia (rapid uptake by rapidly dividing hair follicle cells)

G. CNS disturbances (neurotoxicity)

H. Hepatic disturbances (hepatotoxicity)

I. Hyperuricemia (release of large quantities of breakdown products—uric acid)

J. Kidney failure (direct kidney toxic effect)

K. Doxorubicin: cardiac toxicity (direct cardiac toxic effect)

L. BCG: allergic reactions, anaphylaxis

RADIATION

Purpose

A. Diagnosis

B. Treatment

    1. Curative: destroys neoplasm by irradiation

    2. Palliative: shrinks neoplasm by irradiation

    3. Adjuvant: used in conjunction with chemotherapy or surgery to shrink or destroy neoplasm

Examples

A. Alpha particle: fast-moving helium nucleus

    1. Weight: 4 atomic weight units (awu)

    2. Charge: 2^+

    3. Penetration: slight

B. Beta particle: fast-moving electron

    1. Weight: practically 0 awu

    2. Charge: 1^-

    3. Penetration: moderate

C. Gamma ray: penetrating ray, similar to light ray

    1. Weight: none

    2. Charge: none

    3. Penetration: high

D. Gold (^{198}Au): ascites; pleural effusions

E. Sodium iodide (^{131}I): thyroid gland

F. Sodium phosphate (^{32}P): erythrocytes

Major Side Effects

A. Localized skin irritation

B. Varies based on site

    1. Gastrointestinal tract

        a. Nausea

        b. Vomiting

        c. Diarrhea

    2. Gonads

        a. Temporary sterility

        b. Permanent sterility

    3. Bone marrow

        a. Leukopenia

        b. Thrombocytopenia

    4. Respiratory tract—pneumonitis

    5. Genitourinary tract—cystitis

Methods Of Delivery

A. External beam radiotherapy or teletherapy delivers radiation to a tumor by means of an external machine (cobalt or linear accelerator) at a predetermined distance

B. Internal radiation therapy or brachytherapy delivers radiation by systemic, interstitial, or intracavity means

    1. Systemic (metabolized) involves administration by intravenous or oral routes

    2. Interstitial involves implantation of needles, wires, or seeds into the tissue

    3. Intracavity radiation involves placing an implant into a body cavity and may require a surgical procedure

Influencing Factors

A. Type of tumor

B. Location of the tumor

C. Tolerance of adjacent tissue

D. Extent of the disease process
E. Health status of the client
F. Age of the client

GENERAL NURSING CARE OF CLIENTS WITH NEOPLASTIC DISORDERS RECEIVING EITHER CHEMOTHERAPY OR RADIATION THERAPY

A. DATA COLLECTION
   1. Obtain a description of onset and progression of symptoms
   2. Perform physical assessment to determine general state of health and nutrition
   3. Determine client's understanding of disease and treatment plan

B. ANALYSIS AND INTERPRETATION
   1. Decisional conflict (choices regarding health or death) related to:
      a. Choice or continuation of treatment modality
      b. Religious, moral, or ethical beliefs
   2. Fatigue related to depletion of body reserve
   3. Fear related to:
      a. Diagnosis
      b. Death
      c. Intractable pain
   4. Risk for infection related to altered immune response
   5. Risk for injury related to disease process/therapeutic modalities (radiation, chemotherapy)
   6. Altered nutrition: less than body requirements related to:
      a Disease process
      b. Therapeutic modalities
   7. Altered oral mucous membrane related to:
      a Disease process
      b. Therapeutic modalities
   8. Pain related to:
      a. Disease process
      b. Therapeutic modalities
   9. Powerlessness related to diagnosis/prognosis
   10. Impaired tissue integrity related to treatment modalities

C. PLANNING/IMPLEMENTATION
   1. Review infection control guidelines with client
   2. Teach client to report temperature higher than 37.7° C to physician
   3. Instruct client regarding special measures to limit infection and injury (e.g., gentle oral hygiene, prevention of pathologic fractures)
   4. Explain side effects that influence appearance and encourage positive adaptations (e.g., purchase of wigs, scarves, hats)
   5. Implement measures to reduce or eliminate nausea such as antiemetics, hypnosis, relaxation modalities, small frequent feedings, adjustment of meal times in relation to therapy, avoidance of spicy foods
   6. Monitor blood work during therapy
      a. White blood cells
      b. Red blood cells
      c. Platelets
      d. Tumor markers
         (1) Alpha-fetoprotein—liver, testes
         (2) CA-125—ovaries, gastrointestinal
         (3) Carcinoembryonic antigen (CEA)—breast, colon, lung
         (4) Prostatic specific antigen (PSA)—prostate
   7. Offer emotional support to client and family; answer questions and encourage verbalization of fears
   8. Encourage conservation of client's decreasing energy
   9. Encourage client to follow the Canadian Cancer Society's "Chemotherapy and You : A Guide to Self Help" during treatment
   10. Support natural defense mechanisms of client; encourage intake of foods rich in the immune-stimulating nutrients, especially vitamins A, C, and E, and the mineral selenium (whole grains and seeds)
   11. Encourage optimal intake of high nutrient density foods; bland or mechanical soft diet may be indicated if stomatitis exists; routinely monitor weight
   12. Encourage women of childbearing age to use birth control measures while receiving therapy because of mutagenic/teratogenic effects; avoid use of birth control pill
   13. Counsel male clients regarding use of sperm bank if permanent infertility may result
   14. Keep client well hydrated (3000 ml/24 hr); monitor intake and output
   15. Assess client for pain; administer analgesics as needed; provide for client comfort
   16. Encourage client to become involved in decision making; support client's decisions whenever possible, even if they differ from the nurse's philosophy
   17. Specific care for clients receiving chemotherapy
      a. Monitor intravenous infusion site for infiltration to prevent local tissue necrosis
      b. Follow established protocols for handling chemotherapeutic agents and equipment to minimize exposure
      c. Institute protective isolation if WBCs are low
      d. Wear double gloves when handling urine and other excretions
      e. Observe for signs of bleeding; avoid anticoagulants because of decreased platelets
      f. Avoid skin contact with drugs during preparation for administration; wear gloves; if contact occurs, rinse area well with water

g. Avoid use of rectal thermometers, enemas, IM injections, and razor blades because of increased bleeding tendency

h. Monitor renal function for nephrotoxicity

i. Monitor vital signs; monitor for cardiac toxicity

j. Encourage client to check with physician before consuming over-the-counter (OTC) drugs, such as aspirin or alcohol

18. Specific care for clients receiving external radiation

a. Avoid washing off the marks placed by the radiologist

b. Instruct client to avoid creams, soaps, powders, and deodorants in the area during the treatment periods

c. Assess skin for erythema, dryness, burning

d. Instruct client to wear cotton, loose-fitting clothing

e. Protect skin from sunlight

f. Apply a nonadherent dressing to areas of skin breakdown

g. Reassure others that the client will not be a source of radiation

19. Specific care for clients receiving internal radiation

a. Avoid overexposure to the client and use the principles of time, distance, and shielding

b. Postpone routine hygiene while implant is in place

c. Ascertain if body excreta has to be placed in lead containers for disposal when systemic (metabolized) radiation is used

D. EVALUATION/OUTCOMES

1. Remains free from infection

2. Verbalizes feelings about disease and treatment

3. Maintains skin integrity

4. Consumes nutritionally adequate diet

5. Verbalizes details concerning self-care related to treatment regimen

EMERGENCY SITUATIONS

FIRST AID

A. Maintain or establish:
1. Airway
2. Breathing
3. Circulation

B. Provide for physical safety
1. Remove client from immediate danger
2. Control bleeding
3. Avoid unnecessary movement of spinal column or extremities

4. Control pain
5. Monitor level of consciousness

C. Establish priority for care
1. Triage: system of client evaluation to establish priorities and assign appropriate treatment or personnel
2. Determination of priority
   a. Emergency situations: greatest risk receives priority
   b. Major disasters: classification based on principles to benefit the largest number; those requiring highly specialized care may be given minimal or no care

D. Offering psychologic support
1. Establish and maintain open communication with the client and family to mediate feelings of "loss of control"
2. Allow contact between the client and family as soon as feasible

SPECIFIC EMERGENCIES

A. Circulatory
1. See specific disease: myocardial infarction, hypertensive crisis, shock, asystole
2. Uncontrolled hemorrhaging
   a. Stop the bleeding by direct pressure, application of a pressure dressing or ice to constrict vessels, elevation of the involved extremity, or (rarely) tourniquet application
   b. Treat for shock

B. Respiratory
1. See specific disease: pneumothorax, pulmonary edema, pulmonary embolism, carbon monoxide poisoning, chronic obstructive pulmonary disease (COPD), acute respiratory distress syndrome (ARDS)
2. Near drowning
   a. Assessment
      (1) Possible airway obstruction from bronchospasm
      (2) Adventitious or absent breath sounds
      (3) Hypoxia, hypercarbia, and acidosis
      (4) Possible pulmonary edema
         (a) Salt water: high osmotic pressure of aspirated water draws additional fluid into alveolar spaces from the vascular bed
         (b) Fresh water: removes surfactant, leading to alveolar collapse
   b. Treatment and nursing care
      (1) Establish an airway and ventilate with 100% oxygen and positive pressure
      (2) Correct the acidosis
      (3) Insert a nasogastric tube to prevent aspiration of gastric contents

(4) Treat pulmonary edema and hypothermia if present
C. Gastrointestinal (see specific diseases: perforated peptic ulcer, appendicitis, intestinal obstruction, bleeding esophageal varices associated with cirrhosis)
D. Genitourinary (see specific disease: bladder trauma)
E. Endocrine (see specific diseases: hypoglycemia, ketoacidosis, thyroid storm)
F. Neuromusculoskeletal (see specific diseases: fractures, spinal cord injury, head injury, cerebral vascular accident, myasthenic crisis)
G. Integumentary (see specific disease: burns)
H. Poisoning (see Pediatric Nursing: Poisoning)
I. Thermal trauma
   1. Heatstroke
      a. Risk factors: advanced age, strenuous exercise in heat, medications such as anticholinergics that interfere with sweating
      b. Signs and symptoms
         (1) Hot, dry, flushed skin progressing to pallor in the late stages of circulatory collapse
         (2) Elevation of body temperature above 40.5° C
         (3) Complaints of dizziness, nausea, and headaches
         (4) Convulsions
         (5) Altered level of consciousness
      c. Treatment and nursing care
         (1) Rapidly reduce temperature: hypothermia blanket, cold-water baths, and cool enemas
         (2) Administer oxygen to meet increased metabolic demands
         (3) Institute seizure precautions
   2. Hypothermia
      a. Risk factors: exposure to cold; submersion in cold water; age (elderly and very young)
      b. Signs and symptoms
         (1) Local (frostbite): pallor, paresthesia, pain to absence of sensation of involved body part
         (2) Systemic: core temperature less than 34.4° C, weak and irregular pulse, decreased level of consciousness
      c. Treatment and nursing care
         (1) Monitor core temperature
         (2) Continually assess cardiac status, arterial blood gases, electrolytes, glucose, and blood urea nitrogen (BUN)
         (3) Rewarm: to prevent cardiovascular collapse, core rewarming with heated oxygen and/or irrigations must precede surface rewarming
         (4) Correct fluid and electrolyte imbalances

CIRCULATORY SYSTEM

REVIEW OF ANATOMY AND PHYSIOLOGY OF THE CIRCULATORY SYSTEM

Functions of the Circulatory System

A. Primary function: provides communication between widely separated body parts through transportation of hormones, nutrients, wastes, respiratory gases, vitamins, minerals, enzymes, water, leukocytes, antibodies, and buffers
B. Secondary functions: contributes directly or indirectly to all the body's metabolic functions: tissue perfusion with oxygen and nutrients, water balance, immunity, enzymatic reactions, and pH and temperature regulation

Structures of the Circulatory System

Blood

A. Blood components
   1. Serum: plasma with fewer or no coagulating proteins
   2. Plasma (Table 6-4)
      a. Water: 3 L in average adult; constitutes 90% of plasma
      b. Ions: see fluid and electrolytes
      c. Proteins: all act as buffers; fractionated and separated from each other by electrophoretic and ultracentrifugation techniques
         (1) Albumin
            (a) Largest component of plasma proteins
            (b) Principally responsible for plasma colloid osmotic pressure (COP)
            (c) Reversibly combines with and transports certain lipids, bilirubin, thyroxin, and certain drugs, such as barbiturates
         (2) Alpha and beta globulins
            (a) Help establish COP
            (b) Transport certain vitamins, iron, copper, and cortisol
            (c) Hemostasis (prothrombin and fibrinogen are in this blood fraction)
         (3) Gamma globulins: antibodies
      d. Glucose: prime oxidative metabolite of body cells
   3. Formed elements
      a. Erythrocytes
         (1) Shape: pliable biconcave disc that maximizes surface area proportional to volume for ease of diffusion of respiratory gases
         (2) Number: males: 4.2 to 5.4 × 10^{12}/L; females: 3.6 to 5.0 × 10^{12}/L

(3) Formation: erythropoiesis
　(a) Location: red marrow of vertebrae, sternum, ribs, iliac crests, clavicles, scapulae, and skull
　(b) Maturation process: mature ery-

TABLE 6-4 Plasma Constituents

Constituent	Normal concentration range
Ions	
Sodium (Na^+)	135 to 147 mmol/L
Potassium (K^+)	3.5 to 5.3 mmol/L
Calcium (Ca^{++})	2.1 to 2.6 mmol/L
Magnesium (Mg^{++})	0.65 to 1.05 mmol/L
Chloride (Cl^-)	98 to 108 mmol/L
Bicarbonate (HCO_3^-)	22 to 30 mmol/L
Phosphate ($H_2PO_4^-$, $HPO_4^=$)	0.87 to 1.45 mmol/L
Plasma proteins	
Albumin	0 to 222 mmol/L
Ig G	8 to 18 g/L
Ig A	0.9 to 4.5 g/L
Ig M male	0.6 to 2.5 g/L
female	0.7 to 2.8 g/L
Glucose	3.6 to 6.1 mmol
HgA_{1c}	3.4% to 6.0%
Nitrogenous substances	
Blood urea nitrogen (BUN)	2.8 to 7.1 mmol/L
Uric acid male	180 to 420 μmol/L
female	120 to 360 μmol/L
Creatinine	70 to 110 μmol/L
Amino acids	Variable concentrations
Bilirubin	0 to 4 μmol/L
Lipids	
Cholesterol	
18 to 30 yrs	3.2 to 4.6 mmol/L
31 to 49 yrs	3.8 to 5.1 mmol/L
50 to 64 yrs	4.2 to 5.1 mmol/L
65+ yrs	4.2 to 6.2 mmol/L
HDL	
male	
18 to 49 yrs	0.9 to 1.6 mmol/L
50 to 64 yrs	0.9 to 1.8 mmol/L
65+ yrs	0.9 to 2.0 mmol/L
female	
18 to 49 yrs	0.9 to 2.0 mmol/L
50 to 64 yrs	0.9 to 2.2 mmol/L
65+ yrs	0.9 to 2.4 mmol/L
LDL	
18 to 30 yrs	1.7 to 3.0 mmol/L
31 to 49 yrs	2.0 to 3.4 mmol/L
50 to 64 yrs	2.2 to 3.4 mmol/L
65+ yrs	2.4 to 4.1 mmol/L
Triglycerides	0.6 to 2.3 mmol/L
INR	0.8 to 1.4 mmol/L
Other constituents	
Respiratory gases (O_2 and CO_2)	Variable concentrations
Hormones	Variable concentrations
Vitamins	Variable concentrations

throcytes are mainly sacs of hemoglobin without a nucleus, mitochondria, ribosomes, endoplasmic reticula, or Golgi bodies; process requires folic acid and vitamin B_{12}; vitamin B_{12} plus intrinsic factor from the parietal cells of the stomach form hemopoietic factor, which stimulates erythrocyte formation (see Pernicious Anemia)
　(c) Under conditions of low O_2 tension, liver and kidneys secrete proteins into blood that combine to form erythropoietin, which stimulates erythrocyte production
(4) Principal component is hemoglobin
　(a) Conjugated protein: globulin plus 4 molecules of heme
　(b) Formed within the erythrocyte utilizing copper, cobalt, iron, nickel, and vitamin B_6
　(c) Functions to bind O_2 through iron in heme and CO_2 through globulin portion; can carry both simultaneously
(5) Erythrocytes live for about 120 days; old or deteriorated ones are removed by reticuloendothelial cells of the liver, spleen, and bone marrow; 3.5×10^{12} die and are replaced daily; heme is converted to bilirubin, which is excreted from the liver as part of the bile

b. Leukocytes
(1) Types
　(a) Granulocytes (polymorphonuclear): originate in red marrow and consist of neutrophils (50% to 70% of total), eosinophils (1% to 4% of the total), and basophils (0% to 1% of the total)
　(b) Agranulocytes (mononuclear): originate in red marrow and lymphatic tissue and consist of monocytes (3% to 8% of the total), which become macrophages in tissue spaces, and lymphocytes (25% to 40% of the total)
(2) Functions
　(a) Phagocytosis of bacteria by neutrophils and macrophages; phagocytosis of antibody-antigen complexes by eosinophils
　(b) Antibody synthesis: B lymphocytes produce antibodies; they also become plasma cells, which produce most circulatory antibodies
　(c) Destruction of transplanted tissues

and cancer cells by T lymphocytes, which form in lymphoid tissue and mature in the thymus

(3) Leukocytes live for a few hours or days; some T lymphocytes live for many years and provide long-term immunity

c. Thrombocytes: anucleate cellular fragments associated with hemostasis

(1) Origin: fragmentation of megakaryocytes in bone marrow

(2) Number: 150 to 500 $\times$ 10^9/L

(3) Function in blood coagulation

(a) Adhere to each other and to damaged areas of circulatory system to limit or prevent blood loss

(b) Release chemicals that constrict damaged blood vessels

B. Physical properties of blood

1. Volume

a. Male: 5 to 6 L; female: 4.5 to 5.5 L

b. Hematocrit: percent blood volume occupied by red cells (normal range: 36% to 45%)

2. Specific gravity (sp gr): normal range: 1.05 to 1.06

3. Viscosity: about 5.5 times as viscous as pure water

C. Blood groups

1. Names: indicate type antigens on or in red blood cell membrane (e.g., type A blood means that red blood cells have A antigens, type O that red blood cells have no antigens)

2. Every person's blood belongs to one of the 4 blood groups: type A, type B, type AB, or type O—and is either Rh positive or Rh negative

3. Plasma: normally contains no antibodies against antigens present on its own red blood cells, but does contain antibodies against other A or B antigens not present on its red blood cells (e.g., type A plasma does not contain antibodies against A antigen, but does contain antibodies against B antigen)

4. Blood does not normally contain anti-Rh antibodies; Rh-positive blood never contains them; Rh-negative blood will contain anti-Rh antibodies if the individual has been transfused with Rh-positive blood or has carried an Rh-positive fetus

5. The potential danger in transfusing blood is that the donor's blood may be agglutinated (clumped) by the recipient's antibodies

D. Hemostasis: arrest of bleeding

1. Vasoconstriction: reflex spasm in cut or ruptured vessel's smooth muscles

2. Aggregation of platelets: adhere to damaged blood vessel walls forming plugs

3. Blood coagulation (clotting): blood becomes gel as soluble fibrinogen is converted to insoluble fibrin; process brought about by at least a dozen different chemical clotting factors operating in sequence after mechanism is triggered

a. Extrinsic clotting mechanism: trigger for mechanism is blood contacting damaged tissue

b. Intrinsic clotting mechanism: trigger for mechanism is release of chemicals (platelet factors) from platelets aggregated either at the site of a wound or at a rough spot on the blood vessel wall

4. Some facts about the blood proteins essential for clotting

a. Liver cells synthesize prothrombin, fibrinogen, and other clotting factors; adequate amounts of vitamin K must be present in blood for the liver to make normal amounts of prothrombin, Stuart factor (X), factor VIII, and Christmas factor (IX) (a plasma thromboplastin component [PTC])

b. Normal blood prothrombin content: 0.1 to 0.15 g/L of plasma

c. Normal blood fibrinogen content: 350 mg/100 ml of plasma

d. Both prothrombin and fibrinogen are soluble proteins normally present in blood in adequate amounts for clotting to occur at the normal rapid rate

e. Fibrin is an insoluble protein formed from the soluble protein fibrinogen, in the presence of the enzyme thrombin; fibrin appears as a tangled mass of threads having a jellylike texture; blood cells become enmeshed in these threads, and red blood cells give the clot its red color

f. INR 0.8 to 1.4 mmol/L

5. Clinical applications

a. Hemophilia: hereditary sex-linked disease characterized by defect in clotting ability of blood caused by lack of a blood protein essential for clotting (factor VIII, or less frequently factor IX)

b. Thrombosis: partial or complete occlusion of a blood vessel, caused by presence of a stationary clot (thrombus)

c. Embolism: partial or complete occlusion of a blood vessel by a moving clot (embolus)

d. Atherosclerosis: plaques of lipoid material deposited in endothelium act as rough spots, causing platelet disintegration and thrombus formation

Heart

A. Location: in pericardial cavity within the mediastinum with apex on diaphragm and pointing to left (apical beat may be counted by placing stethoscope in fifth intercostal space on line with left midclavicular point); two thirds of bulk of heart lies to left of midline of body, one third to right

B. Covering: pericardium
   1. Structure
      a. Fibrous pericardium: loose-fitting, inextensible sac around heart
      b. Serous pericardium: consists of two layers
         (1) Parietal layer: lines inner surface of fibrous pericardium
         (2) Visceral layer (epicardium): adheres to outer surface of the heart; pericardial space, lying between the parietal and visceral layers, contains a few drops of lubricating pericardial fluid
   2. Function: protects heart against friction and erosion by providing well-lubricated, smooth sac in which the heart beats
C. Structure of heart
   1. Heart wall
      a. Myocardium: composed of cardiac muscle cells
      b. Endocardium: delicate endothelial lining of myocardium
      c. Cardiac skeleton: continuous dense connective tissue regions at the heart's base and in the interventricular septum serving as points of origin and insertion for cardiac muscle fibers and as supports for the heart's valves
   2. Cavities
      a. Upper two called atria
      b. Lower two called ventricles
   3. Valves and openings
      a. Openings between atria and ventricles known as atrioventricular orifices
         (1) Guarded by cuspid valves
            (a) Tricuspid on right
            (b) Mitral (bicuspid) on left
         (2) Valves consist of three parts
            (a) Flaps or cusps
            (b) Chordae tendineae
            (c) Papillary muscles
      b. Opening from right ventricle into pulmonary artery guarded by the pulmonary semilunar valve
      c. Opening from left ventricle into the aorta guarded by the aortic semilunar valve
   4. Blood supply to myocardium (heart muscle)
      a. Two vessels: the right and left coronary arteries, the first branches of the aorta
      b. Both coronary arteries send branches to both sides of the heart
      c. Right coronary branches supply right side of

heart mainly but also carry some blood to the left ventricle
      d. Left coronary branches supply left side of heart mainly but also carry some blood to the right ventricle
      e. Most abundant blood supply goes to the myocardium of the left ventricle
      f. Greatest flow of blood into myocardium occurs when heart relaxes as a result of decreased arterial compression
      g. Relatively few anastomoses (branches from one artery to another artery) exist between the larger branches of the coronary arteries (poor collateral circulation); hence, if one of these vessels becomes occluded, little or no blood can reach the myocardial cells supplied by that vessel; deprived of an adequate blood supply, the cells soon die (myocardial infarction)
   5. Nerve supply to heart
      a. Sympathetic fibers (in cardiac nerves) and parasympathetic fibers (in the vagus nerve) form the cardiac plexuses
      b. Fibers from the cardiac plexuses terminate mainly in the sinoatrial node
      c. Sympathetic impulses tend to accelerate and strengthen heartbeat
      d. Parasympathetic (vagal) impulses slow the heartbeat
   6. Conduction system of heart
      a. Sinoatrial (SA) node: a cluster of cells located in the right atrial wall near the opening of the superior vena cava
      b. Atrioventricular (AV) node: a small mass of special conducting cells located in the base of the right atrium at the top of the interventricular septum
      c. AV bundle of His: special conducting fibers that originate in the AV node and extend by two branches down the two sides of the interventricular septum (right and left bundle branches)
      d. Purkinje's fibers: special conducting fibers that extend from the AV bundles throughout the wall of the ventricles
      e. Normally a nerve impulse begins its course through the heart in the heart's own pacemaker, the SA node; it quickly spreads through both atria, via special conducting fibers, to the AV node; after a short delay at this node, the impulse is conducted by two branches of the AV bundle of His down both sides of the interventricular septum; from there, the impulse travels over Purkinje's fibers to the lateral walls of the ventricles
      f. Impulse conduction through the heart generates electric currents that spread through

surrounding tissues to the skin, from which visible records of conduction can be made with the electrocardiograph or oscillograph; conduction from the SA node through the atria causes atrial contraction and gives rise to the so-called P wave of the electrocardiogram; conduction from the AV node down the bundle of His and out the Purkinje's fibers causes ventricular contraction and gives rise to the QRS wave; ventricular repolarization is associated with the T wave

    g. Refractory period: particularly long ($^1/_4$ second) to ensure against extra beats arising as electrical energy flows around the surface of the heart; only SA node depolarizations, occurring after a refractory period, produce the next beat

D. Physiology of heart
1. Function: to pump varying amounts of blood through the vessels as the needs of cells change
2. Cardiac cycle
   a. Consists of systole (contraction) and diastole (relaxation) of atria and of ventricles; atria contract, and as they relax ventricles contract
   b. Time required: about $^4/_5$ second for one cardiac cycle; so there are 70 to 80 cycles or heartbeats per minute
3. Auscultatory events (heart sounds): first sound (S_1), "lub," occurs at the beginning of ventricular systole due to closing of the atrioventricular valves (tricuspid and mitral); second sound (S_2), "dub," occurs at the end of ventricular systole as a result of closing of the semilunar valves

Blood Vessels

A. Kinds
1. Arteries: vessels that carry blood away from the heart (all arteries except pulmonary artery carry oxygenated blood); arteries branch into smaller and smaller vessels called arterioles, which branch into microscopic vessels, the capillaries
2. Veins: vessels that carry blood toward the heart (all veins except the pulmonary veins carry deoxygenated blood); veins branch into venules, which collect blood from capillaries; veins in cranial cavity formed by dura mater are called sinuses
3. Capillaries: microscopic vessels that carry blood from arterioles to venules; capillaries unite to form small veins or venules, which, in turn, unite to form veins; exchange of substances between blood and interstitial fluid occurs in capillaries

B. Structure of blood vessels
1. Arteries
   a. Lining (tunica intima) of endothelium
   b. Middle coat (tunica media) of smooth muscle, elastic, and fibrous tissues; this coat permits constriction and dilation
   c. Outer coat (tunica adventitia or externa) of fibrous tissue; its firmness makes arteries stand open instead of collapsing when cut
2. Veins
   a. Same three coats, but thinner and fewer elastic fibers
   b. Veins collapse when cut
   c. Semilunar valves present in most veins over 2 mm in diameter
3. Capillaries
   a. Only lining coat present (intima)
   b. Wall only one cell thick

C. Fetal circulation: structures that are essential for fetal circulation but that normally cease to exist after birth
1. Umbilical arteries: two extensions of hypogastric arteries (internal iliacs) carry fetal blood to placenta
2. Placenta: attached to uterine wall
3. Umbilical vein: extends from placenta back to fetus' body; returns oxygenated blood from placental to fetal circulation; two umbilical arteries and one umbilical vein constitute umbilical cord
4. Ductus venosus: small vessel that connects umbilical vein with inferior vena cava in fetus
5. Foramen ovale: opening in fetal heart septum between right and left atria
6. Ductus arteriosus: small vessel connecting pulmonary artery with descending thoracic aorta
7. Only two fetal blood vessels carry oxygenated blood: umbilical vein and ductus venosus; as soon as blood enters inferior vena cava from ductus venosus, it becomes mixed with venous blood

Physiology of Circulation

A. Definitions
1. Circulation: blood flow through circuit of vessels
2. Systemic circulation: blood flow from left ventricle into aorta, other arteries, arterioles, capillaries, venules, and veins to right atrium of heart
3. Pulmonary circulation: blood flow from right ventricle to pulmonary artery to lung arterioles, capillaries, and venules, to pulmonary veins, to left atrium
4. Hepatic portal circulation: blood flow from capillaries, venules, and veins of stomach, intestines, spleen, pancreas, and gallbladder into portal vein, liver sinusoids, to hepatic veins, to inferior vena cava

5. Cardiac output (CO): volume of blood pumped per minute by the ventricles; average for adult at rest is approximately 3 to 5 L per minute; cardiac output is the stroke volume (systolic discharge) times heart rate; CO increases if heart rate increases or if stroke volume increases, as by sympathetic stimulation
   a. Preload: the extent to which the left ventricle stretches at the height of diastole
   b. Afterload: force required to overcome arterial resistance and eject contents of the left ventricle during systole
B. Regulation of cardiac output
   1. Starling's law of the heart: within physiologic limits, the heart, when stretched by an increased returning volume of blood, contracts more strongly and pumps out the extra returned blood; the heart pumps in proportion to peripheral demand
   2. Autoregulation: volume of blood returning to the heart and subsequently pumped by the heart is determined by the tissues; precapillary sphincters, which precede every capillary bed of the body, relax and permit more blood flow when O_2 tension falls; they constrict and restrict flow when O_2 tension rises
   3. Venous return: sum of all volumes of blood flowing through all capillary beds of the body; initiates Starling's law of the heart
   4. Nervous and hormonal influences on heart: physiologic limit on heart's ability to increase output as venous return increases; maximum at about 15 L/minute; sympathetic stimulation and epinephrine raise upper limit of cardiac output to 25 to 30 L/minute in normal individuals and to 35 L/minute in athletes; parasympathetic stimulation decreases heart rate and stroke volume
   5. Neural influence on veins: venous constriction due to sympathetic stimulation milks blood toward heart, increasing venous return and cardiac output
C. Principles of circulation
   1. Blood circulates because a blood pressure gradient exists in the vessels; similar to all fluids, blood moves from regions where its pressure is greater to regions where the pressure is less; because blood pressure is highest in the left ventricle and aorta, successively lower in arteries, arterioles, capillaries, venules, veins, and lowest in the central veins (venae cavae and right atrium), blood flows through the circulatory system in this order
   2. Normal range of systolic blood pressure is 100 to 139 mm Hg; consistent readings in 140s and 150s are borderline high; readings 160 and

above are high; difference between systolic and diastolic pressures is the pulse pressure, normally between 30 and 40 mm Hg
3. Blood pressure normally remains relatively constant over a wide range of activities as a result of:
   a. Neural regulation: maintains blood pressure on a minute-by-minute basis; increase in arterial pressure stimulates baroreceptors in aorta and carotid sinus, which leads to increased parasympathetic impulses to the heart via the vagus nerve, which slow the heart rate; a decrease in arterial pressure inhibits baroreceptors in the aorta and carotid sinus and thereby leads to decreased parasympathetic impulses and increased sympathetic impulses to the heart, which in turn cause a faster heart rate
   b. Intrinsic circulatory regulation: maintains blood pressure on an hour-to-hour basis; increased blood pressure raises the hydrostatic pressure of plasma, leading to increased filtration of plasma from circulatory system to interstitial spaces; this results in reduced venous return, decreased cardiac output, and decreased blood pressure
   c. Kidney regulation: provides long-term day-to-day regulation of blood pressure; increased blood pressure drives more blood through the kidneys, which in turn make and excrete more urine; as a result venous return, cardiac output, and blood pressure all decrease
4. Blood flow through the capillary bed: plasma filters through capillary wall at arterial end of capillary bed and becomes interstitial fluid; fluid flows over cells in capillary bed, and diffusion of nutrients and wastes occurs between fluid and cells; about half the interstitial fluid filters back into venous end of capillary bed, becoming plasma again; remaining half of interstitial fluid enters lymphatic channels, along with leaked plasma proteins, and returns to venous system
5. Regulation of blood flow in the circulatory system: rate of flow in liters per minute is directly proportional to blood pressure gradient and diameter of blood vessels; as pressure gradient and vessel diameter increase, flow rate increases; rate of flow is inversely proportional to blood vessel length and blood viscosity; as vessel length and blood viscosity increase, flow rate decreases; peripheral resistance refers to the combined effects of blood vessel radius and length and blood viscosity
6. Under nonpathologic conditions, blood pressure remains relatively constant; because ves-

sel length and blood viscosity are constant, the rate of flow depends almost entirely on blood vessel radius (constriction and dilation)

  a. Sympathetic discharge constricts muscular arteries and arterioles leading to the viscera, kidneys, and skin and dilates those leading to skeletal muscles

  b. Postural reflexes (baroreceptor system): arterioles are constricted when one suddenly stands after sitting or lying down; this raises blood pressure and ensures adequate perfusion of brain cells with oxygen and nutrients

  c. Sympathetic discharge constricts blood reservoirs, such as the veins, and propels blood toward the heart

D. Pulse

  1. Definition: alternate expansion and elastic recoil of blood vessel

  2. Cause: variations in pressure within vessel caused by intermittent injections of blood from heart into aorta with each ventricular contraction; pulse can be felt because of elasticity of arterial walls

  3. Pulse can be felt wherever artery lies near surface and over firm background such as bone; some of those most easily palpated are:

    a. Radial artery: at wrist

    b. Temporal artery: in front of ear, or above and to outer side of eye

    c. Common carotid artery: along anterior edge of sternocleidomastoid muscle, at level of lower margin of thyroid cartilage

    d. Facial artery: at lower margin of lower jaw bone, on line with corners of mouth, in groove in mandible about one third of way forward from angle of bone

    e. Brachial artery: at bend of the elbow, along the inner margin of the biceps muscle

    f. Posterior tibial artery: behind the medial malleolus (inner "ankle bone")

    g. Dorsalis pedis: on anterior surface of the foot, just below the bend of the ankle

  4. Venous pulse: in large veins only; produced by changes in venous pressure brought about by alternate contraction and relaxation of the atria rather than the ventricles, as in arterial pulse

Lymphatic System

Lymph Vessels

A. Structure: lymph capillaries similar to blood capillaries in structure; larger lymphatics similar to veins but are thinner walled, have more valves, and have lymph nodes in certain places along their course

B. Names: largest lymphatic known as thoracic duct; drains lymph from entire body, except upper right quadrant, into the left subclavian vein (where it joins the internal jugular); right lymphatic ducts drain lymph from the upper right quadrant into the right subclavian vein

C. Functions

  1. Lymphatics return fluid and proteins to blood from interstitial fluid; about 60% of fluid filtered out of blood capillaries returns to circulation via lymphatics rather than by osmosis into venous ends of capillaries; about 50% of total blood proteins leak out of capillaries per day; the only way these large molecules can return to blood is via lymphatics

  2. Adequate lymph return is essential for maintaining homeostasis of blood proteins and therefore of blood volume

  3. Interference with the return of proteins to the blood results in edema caused by the loss of protein and changes in colloid osmotic pressure

Lymph Nodes

A. Structure: lymphatic tissue, separated into compartments by fibrous partitions; afferent lymphatic vessels enter each node; one (usually) efferent vessel drains lymph out of node

B. Location: usually in clusters, some of the more important groups, from nursing viewpoint, are:

  1. Submental and submaxillary groups in floor of mouth; lymph from nose, lips, and teeth drains through these nodes

  2. Superficial cervical nodes in neck, along sternocleidomastoid muscle; lymph from head and neck drains through these nodes

  3. Superficial cubital nodes at bend of elbow; lymph from hand and forearm drains through these nodes

  4. Axillary nodes in armpit; lymph from arm and upper part of the chest wall, including the breast, drains through these nodes (may be removed during mastectomy for carcinoma)

  5. Inguinal nodes in groin; lymph from the leg and external genitals drains through these nodes

C. Functions

  1. Help defend the body against injurious substances (notably, bacteria and tumor cells) by filtering them out of lymph and thereby preventing their entrance into bloodstream; leukocytes in lymph nodes destroy many of these substances by phagocytosis and antibody action

  2. Lymphatic tissue of lymph nodes carries on the process of hemopoiesis; specifically, it forms T and B lymphocytes

Lymph

A. Definition: fluid in lymphatics

B. Source: interstitial fluid that has entered the lymphatic capillaries

1. Interstitial fluid is the fluid in the microscopic tissue spaces
2. Interstitial fluid is formed by plasma filtering out of the blood capillaries into the tissue spaces

Spleen
A. Location: left hypochondrium, above and behind cardiac portion of the stomach
B. Structure: lymphatic tissue, similar to lymph nodes; size varies, contains numerous spaces filled with venous blood
C. Functions
   1. Defense: phagocytosis of particles such as microbes, red blood cell fragments, and platelets by reticuloendothelial cells of spleen (reticuloendothelial system—phagocytic cells, located mainly in the liver; spleen; bone marrow; and lymph nodes; also, macrophages of connective tissue and microglia in the brain and cord); antibody formation by plasma cells of spleen
   2. Hemopoiesis: lymphatic tissue of the spleen, similar to that of the lymph nodes, forms lymphocytes and possibly monocytes
   3. Spleen serves as blood reservoir; sympathetic stimulation causes constriction of its capsule, squeezing out an estimated 200 ml of blood into general circulation within 1 minute

REVIEW OF PHYSICAL PRINCIPLES RELATED TO THE CIRCULATORY SYSTEM

Principles of Mechanics
Newton's Laws of Motion

A. First law: a body remains at rest or in uniform motion in a straight line unless forces act on it to make it change its state of rest or uniform motion; in other words, bodies continue to do whatever they are doing unless some force acts on them
   EXAMPLE: The heart produces the force that propels the blood through the vessels; without such a force the blood would come to rest as a result of friction between the blood and the blood vessels
B. Second law: if a body is accelerated, the greater the force applied to it, the greater the acceleration; the greater the mass of the body, the more force needed to produce a desired acceleration
   EXAMPLE: In polycythemia the greater cell mass of each unit volume of blood requires greater force of cardiac contraction to produce a desired rate of blood flow
C. Third law: for every action there is an equal and opposite reaction

EXAMPLE: As blood flows through an artery, it exerts an action force on the walls of the artery; the walls of the artery exert a reaction force on the blood, which helps to provide the pressure to keep the blood flowing

Law of Gravitation
Any two objects in the universe are attracted to each other with a force equal to the product of the masses of the two objects divided by the square of the distance between them (e.g., the greater the mass of the bodies, the greater the gravitational force; the closer they are together, the greater the gravitational force)
EXAMPLE: When a person is standing, blood tends to pool in the lower extremities, resulting in bulging of veins in lower parts of the body and requiring greater pumping force from the heart to overcome such pooling; orthostatic hypotension and recovery by the baroreceptor reflex are a direct result of gravitational forces; the evolutionary development of valves in the venous system (particularly in the legs) is due to gravitational forces

Momentum
A. Basic concept: an object's momentum depends on its mass and the velocity at which it is moving
   EXAMPLE: A 112-kg person in a heavy motorized wheelchair moving down a corridor at 5 km/h has greater momentum than a 45-kg person in a light wheelchair rolling along at 8 km/h
B. Changes in momentum: an object's momentum can be changed by applying a force to the object for a certain length of time; the greater the force applied and/or the longer the time that the force is applied, the greater is the change in momentum of the object
   EXAMPLE: During exercise, the contracting heart imparts great momentum to the blood because the force of contraction of the myocardium is great, and the duration of contraction of the myocardium is relatively long

Energy
A. Basic concept: a property that enables a body to perform work
   EXAMPLE: The heart possesses energy because it is capable of doing the work of circulating the blood
B. Work: the product of the force exerted and the distance through which the force moves
   EXAMPLE: The heart exerts a force that moves the blood a certain distance
C. Laws concerning energy
   1. First law of thermodynamics (law of conservation of energy): energy cannot be created or destroyed but may be transformed from one form into another
   EXAMPLE: The potential energy of the ATP molecule is transformed into the kinetic energy of the cardiac muscle contraction during the cardiac cycle

2. Second law of thermodynamics: all systems in the universe have a natural tendency to become disorderly or randomized; the energy of the system continually becomes more spread out and dilute
   a. Molecules tend to move from areas where they are in high concentration to areas where they are in low concentration; this is usually stated as the law of diffusion
      EXAMPLES
      (1) The diffusion of oxygen and carbon dioxide between the air sacs and capillaries of the lungs
      (2) The diffusion of water through the membrane systems of cells (osmosis)
   b. Heat always flows from a hot body into a colder one
      EXAMPLES
      (1) Some of the chemical energy stored in muscles is transformed into heat when muscles contract; this heat flows from the hot body (the muscles) into cooler bodies (the surrounding tissues, including blood) and helps to maintain the human body temperature of 37° C
      (2) When the human body is too hot, vasodilation occurs in the skin and heat radiates from the body into the cooler surrounding air

Efficiency

Efficiency: never total, since friction that occurs when two surfaces rub together produces resistance and heat; the greater the efficiency, the less heat produced; friction causes mechanical devices eventually to be worn away

EXAMPLE: If friction did not operate, the human heart would only have to beat once in a lifetime because the initial force would propel the blood indefinitely through the blood vessels; friction continuously slows blood flow, and consequently the adult heart beats an average of 72 times each minute

Principles of Physical Properties of Matter

Solids

Concept of elasticity: because of external or internal stresses, solids may change their shape or size

EXAMPLE: Heart and blood vessels constantly change shape as blood pressure and degree of neural stimulation undergo change

Liquids

A. Hydrostatic pressure: force per unit area caused by the weight of the fluid on matter submerged in the fluid
   EXAMPLE: The weight of blood in a capillary exerts a hydrostatic force that helps to filter the blood

plasma through the capillary wall, forming interstitial fluid

B. Pascal's principle: when pressure is applied to a fluid in a closed, nonflexible container, it is transmitted undiminished throughout all parts of the fluid and acts in all directions
   EXAMPLES: In the circulatory system the pressure exerted as a result of the contracting ventricles is transmitted throughout the blood vessels of the circulatory system; this pressure is responsible for blood flow
   1. Pressure: fluid always flows from regions of higher pressure to those of lower pressure; the pressure in the human circulatory system is highest in the ventricles during systole, decreases throughout the length of the circulatory system, and is lowest in the atria; the normal pressure of blood in the circulatory system varies with age and disease
   2. Lumen of the tube: the flow of fluid through a tube is larger when the radius of the tube is larger (e.g., the degree of constriction of the arterioles for the most part determines the quantity of blood entering the capillary beds and returning to the heart)
   3. Length of the tube: the longer the tube, the less fluid flow there is through it in a unit of time; when blood circulation to the skin is greatly increased, the heart must increase its output to maintain normal circulation, since many more miles of tubing (capillaries) have been added to the system
   4. Viscosity: the molecular components of a fluid exert forces of attraction on each other; as the fluid flows along, an internal friction, caused by the molecular attractions of the fluid's components, tends to impede it; viscosity is a measure of this internal resistance to fluid flow
      a. Anemia: because of a reduced number of erythrocytes, the viscosity of the blood is decreased; therefore blood returns to the heart more rapidly, increasing cardiac output, which may overwork the heart during periods of increased exercise
      b. Polycythemia: an increased number of erythrocytes in the blood increases its viscosity; blood flows more sluggishly and the blood pressure increases to compensate

C. Capillarity: when a small-diameter tube is dipped into water or other fluid, the water will rise in the tube because of adhesion of the water molecules to the components of the glass; surface tension then causes the film of water to contract and pull itself up the tube; the water continues to rise until its weight balances the adhesive force; this rise of the fluid level in a tube is called capillarity or capillary action

EXAMPLE: Capillarity draws blood into a capillary tube when a technician takes a small blood sample for various analyses

Gases

Gases are carried in the circulatory system by adhering to other molecules

Principles of Acoustics

Basic concept: sound is a wave caused by mechanical vibration that cannot occur in a vacuum; it is propagated best through solids and through liquids better than gases; it travels in waves from a vibrating source such as human vocal cords, a loudspeaker, or a dropped object

EXAMPLES

1. A very faint heartbeat can be heard only with a stethoscope or by placing the ear on the chest; even strong heartbeats cannot be heard distinctly with just the ears
2. The sound vibrations (waves) pass readily through the tissue of the human body to the surface of the skin where the stethoscope can pick them up
3. Ultrasonic fetal heart monitors can detect the fetal heartbeat as early as the twelfth week of gestation
4. Echocardiography: a sound wave–constructed picture of the heart helps in the identification of cardiac diseases

Principles of Electricity

Electric Force

A. The atoms composing all matter represent an almost perfect balance of protons and electrons; the attraction of a positive proton for a negative electron (opposite charges attracting) is the electric force that also makes like charges repel each other
B. Electric forces hold atoms and molecules together and thus hold solid matter together; electric forces also provide the source for all chemical energy; the molecular rearrangements associated with cellular metabolism derive their energy from electric forces between enzymes, substrates, and cofactors

Conductors and Insulators

A. Conductors are good transferrers of electric charges and the energy they contain; copper and aluminum are good conductors and are commonly used for all electric wiring, including the electrodes for cardiac monitoring
B. Insulators: rubber and most nonmetals are good insulators, as is the connective tissue that separates the atria and ventricles of the heart and electrically insulates these regions; consequently the only way electrical energy can flow from the AV node to the ventricles is through the heart's specialized conducting system (bundle of His) in the interventricular septum
C. Water as a conductor: distilled water is a poor conductor, although tap water contains enough charged particles (ions) to make it a fairly good electric conductor; the ions (electrolytes) of body fluids make them excellent conductors of electrical energy

Application of Electricity

A. Electronic devices used in health care
   1. Electronic cardiac pacemakers: battery-operated devices supplement or replace defective electric stimulation in the human heart and thus help maintain the individual's heartbeat at a selected rate
   2. Defibrillator: electronic device that delivers electrical energy through electrodes strategically placed on an individual whose heart is in atrial or ventricular fibrillation; the use of such a device is based on the premise that the sustaining mechanism of the fibrillation process is different from the initiating mechanism; thus, if the initiating mechanism is no longer present and the sustaining mechanism is terminated by the defibrillating electric current, sinus rhythm will ensue
B. Applications to the human body: the contraction of all types of muscle is preceded by depolarization of the muscle fibers; ions carry the electric charges

   EXAMPLE: Electrocardiograms measure and record the electric activity of the heart as this activity is carried to the surface of the body by the ions of the body fluids; this information provides an electric picture of the heart's activity

REVIEW OF CHEMICAL PRINCIPLES RELATED TO THE CIRCULATORY SYSTEM

A. Organic catalysts enter into reactions and are reformed at end of reaction
B. Needed in minute amounts
C. Protein in nature and inactivated by all factors that denature proteins (e.g., high temperature, changes in pH)
D. Substrate is the substance acted on by an enzyme (e.g., carbon dioxide and water are the substrate for the enzyme carbonic anhydrase, found in the erythrocyte, which catalyzes the conversion of CO_2 and H_2O into carbonic acid)
E. Enzymes usually have ending "-ase" added on to name of substrate or to action of enzyme (e.g., sucrase: enzyme hydrolyzing sucrose; lactic acid dehydrogenase: enzyme removing hydrogen from lactic acid)

F. Enzymes, being proteins, are usually quite specific in action
   1. One enzyme will usually catalyze only one reaction: substrate specificity
   2. Enzyme activity will be high at temperature specific for the enzyme and low at other temperatures: temperature specificity
   3. Enzyme activity will be high at the pH specific for the enzyme and low at other pH values: pH specificity
G. Certain inorganic ions act to speed up or slow down enzyme activity: enzyme activators and enzyme inhibitors
H. Enzymes acting within cells are called intracellular enzymes (e.g., the enzymes that bring about the breakdown of glucose and other sugars and the synthesis of carbohydrates, proteins, and nucleic acids all function within cells and are intracellular enzymes)
I. Enzymes acting outside cells are called extracellular enzymes (e.g., the digestive enzymes that are found in the mouth, stomach, and small intestine all function outside cells and are extracellular enzymes)
J. Some enzymes exist in two parts
   1. Apoenzyme: protein part of enzyme (inactive)
   2. Coenzyme: nonprotein part of enzyme (inactive)
   3. Holoenzyme: the apoenzyme and the coenzyme together (active molecule)

REVIEW OF MICROORGANISMS RELATED TO THE CIRCULATORY SYSTEM

A. *Streptococcus pyogenes*: gram-positive streptococcus; the most virulent strain (group A beta hemolytic) causes scarlet fever, septic sore throat, tonsillitis, cellulitis, puerperal fever, erysipelas, rheumatic fever, and glomerulonephritis
B. *Streptococcus viridans*: gram-positive streptococcus; distinguishable from *S. pyogenes* by its alpha hemolysis (rather than beta) of red blood cells; the most common cause of subacute bacterial endocarditis

PHARMACOLOGY RELATED TO CIRCULATORY SYSTEM DISORDERS

Cardiac Glycosides

A. Description
   1. Used to improve the pumping ability of the heart, thus increasing cardiac output
   2. Produce a positive inotropic effect (increased force of contraction) by increasing permeability of cardiac muscle membranes to the calcium and sodium ions required for contraction of muscle fibrils
   3. Produce a negative chronotropic effect (decreased rate of contraction) by an action mediated through the vagus nerve, which slows firing of the SA node and impulse transmission by the AV node
   4. Responsible for a diuretic effect caused by increased renal blood flow
   5. Effective in the treatment of congestive heart failure and atrial flutter and fibrillation
   6. Available in oral and parenteral (IM, IV) preparations
   7. Initially, loading dose is administered to digitalize the client; after the desired effect is achieved, the dosage is lowered to a maintenance level, which replaces the amount of drug metabolized and excreted each day
B. Examples
   1. Digitalis
   2. Digitoxin (Digitaline)
   3. Digoxin (Lanoxin)
   4. Lanatoside C (Cedilanid)
C. Major side effects
   1. Nausea, vomiting, diarrhea (local oral effect—stimulates chemoreceptor zone in medulla)
   2. Anorexia (nausea and vomiting caused by chemoreceptor zone stimulation)
   3. Malabsorption of all nutrients (nausea, vomiting, diarrhea)
   4. Bradycardia (increased vagal tone at AV node)
   5. Toxicity
      a. Dysrhythmias (premature ventricular beats [PVBs]) (increased spontaneous rate of ventricular depolarization)
      b. Xanthopsia (yellow vision) (effect on visual cones)
      c. Muscle weakness (CNS effect, neurotoxicity, hypokalemia)
D. Nursing care
   1. Check apical pulse prior to administration
      a. In the adult, if pulse is below 60 withhold dose and notify the physician
      b. In adults, if pulse increases to >120 it may indicate toxicity—notify the physician
   2. Administer oral preparations with meals to reduce GI irritation
   3. Encourage intake of high nutrient density foods
   4. Assess client for signs of impending toxicity (anorexia, nausea, vomiting, palpitations, xanthopsia)
   5. Monitor the client for hypokalemia, which potentiates the effects of digitalis
   6. Instruct the client to:
      a. Count radial pulse and record before each administration
      b. Notify physician of occurrence of any side effects

c. Report any changes in heart rate to physician (irregular heartbeats; increased or decreased rate)

7. Digoxin—monitor blood level during therapy (normal serum: 0.6 to 2.6 mmol/L)

8. Evaluate client's response to medication and understanding of teaching

Antidysrhythmics

A. Description
  1. Used to treat abnormal variations in cardiac rate and rhythm; also used to prevent the occurrence of dysrhythmias in clients with the potential for their occurrence
  2. Available in oral and parenteral (IM, IV) preparations
B. Examples
  1. Calcium ion antagonists: control atrial dysrhythmias by decreasing cardiac automaticity and impulse conduction (diltiazem, nifedipine, verapamil)
  2. Disopyramide phosphate: controls ventricular dysrhythmias by decreasing the rate of diastolic depolarization
  3. Lidocaine HCl: controls ventricular irritability by shortening the refractory period and suppressing ectopic foci
  4. Phenytoin (Dilantin): controls atrial or ventricular dysrhythmias by reducing automaticity without decreasing conduction
  5. Procainamide HCl (Pronestyl): controls ventricular and atrial dysrhythmias by prolonging the refractory period of the heart and slowing the conduction of cardiac impulses
  6. Propranolol (Inderal): controls supraventricular dysrhythmias by decreasing cardiac impulse conduction through a beta-adrenergic blocking action
  7. Quinidine preparations: control atrial dysrhythmias by prolonging the effective refractory period and slowing depolarization
C. Major side effects
  1. Hypotension (decreased cardiac output caused by vasodilation)
  2. Dizziness (hypotension)
  3. Nausea, vomiting (irritation of gastric mucosa)
  4. Heart block (direct cardiac toxic effect; cardiac depressant)
  5. Anticholinergic effect (decreased parasympathetic stimulation)
  6. Blood dyscrasias (decreased RBCs, WBCs, platelet synthesis)
  7. Toxicity
    a. Diarrhea (GI irritation)
    b. CNS disturbances (neurotoxicity)
    c. Sensory disturbances (neurotoxicity)

D. Nursing care
  1. Assess vital signs during course of therapy
  2. Use cardiac monitoring during IV administration
  3. Instruct client to:
    a. Notify physician of occurrence of any side effects
    b. Report any changes in heart rate or rhythm to physician (irregular beats; increased or decreased rate)
  4. Monitor blood levels during therapy; heart block occurs at 8 > mg/L
    a. Quinidine (varies considerably)
    b. Procainamide (17 to 42 mmol/L)
    c. Lidocaine (6.4 to 25.6 μmol/L)
    d. Phenytoin (40 to 80 μmol/L)
  5. Monitor blood work during long-term therapy
  6. Administer oral preparations with meals to reduce GI irritation
  7. Monitor electrocardiograms (ECGs) during course of therapy
  8. Use infusion-control device for continuous IV administration
  9. Use safety precautions (supervise ambulation, side rails up) when CNS effects are manifested
  10. Evaluate client's response to medication and understanding of teaching

Cardiac Stimulants

A. Description
  1. Used to increase the heart rate
  2. Act by either indirect or direct mechanisms affecting the autonomic nervous system
  3. Available in parenteral (IM, IV), intracardiac, and intrathecal preparations
B. Examples
  1. Atropine sulfate: suppresses parasympathetic nervous system control at SA and AV nodes, thus allowing heart rate to increase
  2. Epinephrine HCl (Adrenalin): stimulates the rate and force of cardiac contraction via the sympathetic nervous system
  3. Isoproterenol HCl (Isuprel): stimulates beta-adrenergic receptors of the sympathetic nervous system, thus increasing heart rate
C. Major side effects
  1. Tachycardia (sympathetic stimulation)
  2. Headache (dilation of cerebral vessels)
  3. CNS stimulation (sympathetic stimulation)
  4. Cardiac dysrhythmias (cardiovascular system stimulation)
  5. Atropine: anticholinergic effects (dry mouth, blurred vision, urinary retention as a result of decreased parasympathetic stimulation)
D. Nursing care
  1. Assess vital signs during course of therapy
  2. Use cardiac monitoring during IV administration
  3. Monitor ECG during course of therapy

4. Utilize safety precautions (side rails up) during administration
5. Evaluate client's response to medication and understanding of teaching

Coronary Vasodilators

A. Description
1. Used to decrease cardiac work and myocardial oxygen requirements by their vasodilatory action to decrease preload and decrease afterload
2. Nitrates act directly at "nitrate" receptors in smooth muscles causing relaxation of the smooth muscle (vasodilation); produces marked venodilation, which decreases the preload, thus decreasing cardiac workload
3. Calcium ion antagonists inhibit the influx of the calcium ion across the cell membrane during depolarization of the cardiac and vascular smooth muscle
4. Effective in the treatment of angina pectoris
5. Available in oral, sublingual, buccal, and topical, including transdermal, preparations
B. Examples
1. Nitrates (sublingual)
   a. Erythrityl tetranitrate (Cardilate)
   b. Isosorbide dinitrate (Isordil)
   c. Nitroglycerin
2. Nitrates (oral)
   a. Erythrityl tetranitrate (Cardilate)
   b. Isosorbide dinitrate (Isordil)
3. Nitrates (topical)
   a. Nitroglycerin ointment
      (1) Nitro-Bid
      (2) Nitrol
   b. Nitroglycerin transdermal
      (1) Nitrodisc
      (2) Nitro-Dur
      (3) Transderm-Nitro
4. Calcium-ion antagonists (calcium channel blockers)
   a. Diltiazem (Cardizem)
   b. Felodipine (Plendil)
   c. Nifedipine (Adalat)
   d. Verapamil hydrochloride (Isoptin)
C. Major side effects
1. Headache (dilation of cerebral vessels)
2. Flushing (peripheral vasodilation)
3. Orthostatic hypotension (loss of compensatory vasoconstriction with position change)
4. Tachycardia (reflex reaction to severe hypotension)
5. Dizziness (orthostatic hypotension)
D. Nursing care
1. Assess for signs and symptoms of hypotension before administering; if present, withhold drug
2. Encourage client to change positions slowly

3. Use safety precautions (supervise ambulation; side rails up)
4. Nitroglycerin: instruct client to:
   a. Take sublingual preparations before angina-producing activities
   b. Note slight stinging, burning, tingling under the tongue; indicates potency of drug
   c. Avoid placing the drug in heat, light, moisture, or plastic; store in original amber, glass container
   d. Take sublingual preparations every 5 minutes, not to exceed 3 tablets in 15 minutes for chest pain; if pain persists, get emergency care
5. Evaluate client's response to medication and understanding of teaching

Antihypertensives

A. Description
1. Used to promote dilation of peripheral blood vessels, thus decreasing blood pressure and afterload
2. Available in oral, parenteral (IM, IV), and transdermal preparations
B. Examples
1. Captopril (Capoten): angiotensin-converting enzyme (ACE) inhibitor
2. Clonidine (Catapres): sympatholytic; centrally acting
3. Diltazem (Cardizen): calcium-entry blocker
4. Enalapril maleate (Vasotec): angiotensin converting enzyme (ACE) inhibitor
5. Hydralazine HCl (Apresoline): direct smooth muscle relaxation; increases excretion of vitamin B_6 (vasodilator)
6. Hydrochlorothiazide (HydroDiuril): thiazide diuretic
7. Hydrochlorthiazide/amiloride (Moduret): combination thiazide and potassium-sparing diuretic
8. Methyldopa (Aldomet): sympatholytic
9. Nifedipine (Adalat): calcium entry blocker; vasodilator
10. Prazosin HCl (Minipress): direct smooth muscle relaxation (alpha blocker)
11. Propranolol (Inderal): beta-adrenergic blocker (sympatholytic)
12. Reserpine (Serpasil): peripheral norepinephrine depletion; centrally acting
C. Major side effects
1. Orthostatic hypotension (loss of compensatory vasoconstriction with position change)
2. Dizziness (orthostatic hypotension)
3. Cardiac rate alteration
   a. Bradycardia (sympatholytics) (decreased sympathetic stimulation to the heart)
   b. Tachycardia (direct relaxers) (reflex reaction to severe hypotension)

4. Sexual disturbances (failure of erection or ejaculation due to loss of vascular tone)
5. Blood dyscrasias (decreased RBCs, WBCs, platelet synthesis)
6. Drowsiness (cerebral hypoxia)

D. Nursing care
1. Monitor blood pressure in standing and supine positions during therapy
2. Instruct client to:
   a. Follow a low-sodium diet
   b. Change positions slowly
   c. Continue to take medication as prescribed; therapy is usually for life
   d. Report occurrence of any side effects to physician
   e. Avoid engaging in hazardous activities when initially placed on antihypertensive drug therapy
3. Reserpine: assess client for mental depression; implement suicide precautions
4. Nitroprusside: protect IV solution from light; discard unused portions according to manufacturer's schedule
5. Assess vital signs, especially pulse, during the course of therapy
6. Encourage intake of foods high in B-complex vitamins
7. Evaluate client's response to medication and understanding of teaching

Diuretics

A. Description
1. Used to increase urine output, which reduces hypervolemia; decreases preload and afterload
2. Interferes with sodium reabsorption in the kidney
3. Available in oral and parenteral (IM, SC, IV) preparations

B. Examples
1. Thiazides: interfere with sodium ion transport at loop of Henle and inhibit carbonic anhydrase activity at distal tubule sites
   a. Chlorthalidone (Hygroton)
   b. Hydrochlorothiazide (HydroDiuril)
   c. Indapamide (Lozide)
   d. Methyclothiazide (Enduron)
2. Potassium-sparers: interfere with aldosterone-induced reabsorption of sodium ions at distal nephron sites to increase sodium chloride excretion and decrease potassium ion loss
   a. Spironolactone (Aldactone)
   b. Triamterine (Dyrenium)
3. Loop diuretics: interfere with active transport of sodium ions in loop of Henle and inhibit sodium chloride and water reabsorption at proximal tubule sites

   a. Ethacrynic acid
   b. Furosemide (Lasix)

C. Major side effects
1. GI irritation (local effect)
2. Hyponatremia (inhibition of sodium reabsorption at the kidney tubule)
3. Orthostatic hypotension (reduced blood volume)
4. Hyperuricemia (partial blockage of uric acid excretion)
5. Dehydration (excessive sodium and water loss)
6. All diuretics except potassium-sparers
   a. Hypokalemia (increased potassium excretion)
   b. Increased urinary excretion of magnesium
   c. Increased urinary excretion of zinc
7. Potassium-sparers
   a. Hyperkalemia (reabsorption of potassium at the kidney tubule)
   b. Hypomagnesemia (increased excretion of magnesium at kidney tubule)
   c. Increased urinary excretion of calcium

D. Nursing care
1. Maintain intake and output records
2. Weigh daily (same time, same scale, same clothing)
3. Administer the drug in the morning so that the maximal effect will occur during the waking hours
4. Assess vital signs, especially pulse and blood pressure, during course of therapy
5. Encourage intake of foods high in calcium, magnesium, zinc, and potassium (except for potassium-sparers)
6. Assess client for signs of fluid-electrolyte imbalance
7. Instruct client to change positions slowly
8. Thiazides and loop diuretics: monitor blood sugar in diabetics; may cause hyperglycemia
9. Be alert for signs of hypokalemia except for potassium sparers (muscle weakness, cramps)
10. Evaluate client's response to medication and understanding of teaching

Peripheral Vasoconstrictors

A. Description
1. Used to elevate the blood pressure
2. Act by constriction of peripheral blood vessels through alpha-adrenergic stimulation
3. Available in parenteral (IV) preparations

B. Examples
1. Levarterenol bitartrate
2. Mephentermine sulfate
3. Metaraminol bitartrate
4. Phenylephrine HCl

C. Major side effects
1. Hypertension (compression of cerebral blood vessels)

2. Headache (increase in blood pressure)
3. Gastrointestinal disturbance (autonomic dysfunction)
D. Nursing care
1. Assess vital signs during course of therapy
2. Monitor blood pressure at frequent intervals
3. Assess for IV infiltration; may lead to tissue necrosis
4. Titrate IV depending on blood pressure readings to prevent hypertension
5. Do not leave client unattended
6. Encourage intake of high-fiber foods to reduce the potential of constipation
7. Evaluate client's response to medication and understanding of teaching

Anticoagulants

A. Description
1. Used to prevent clot formation and clot extension
2. Act to prevent fibrin formation by interfering with the production of various clotting factors in the coagulation process
3. Anticoagulants available in oral and parenteral (SC, IV) preparations
B. Examples
1. Heparin sodium: must be administered parenterally
2. Oral anticoagulants
   a. Dicumarol
   b. Warfarin sodium (Coumadin)
C. Major side effects
1. Fever, chills (hypersensitivity)
2. Skin rash (hypersensitivity)
3. Hemorrhage (interference with clotting mechanisms)
4. Diarrhea (GI irritation)
D. Nursing care
1. Monitor blood work during course of therapy, especially coagulation studies
2. Assess client for signs of bleeding
3. Have appropriate antidote available
   a. Vitamin K for warfarin
   b. Protamine sulfate for heparin
4. Avoid administration of salicylates during anticoagulant therapy
5. Avoid IM injections of other drugs if possible
6. Instruct client to:
   a. Report any signs of bleeding to the physician immediately
   b. Carry a medical alert card
   c. Avoid use of alcohol during therapy
   d. Use an electric razor and soft toothbrush
   e. Avoid taking OTC medications containing aspirin
   f. Keep appointments for laboratory tests (coagulation studies)

g. Eat a consistent diet of vitamin K–containing foods (leafy green vegetables)
7. Evaluate client's response to medication and understanding of teaching

Antianemics

A. Description
1. Used to promote RBC production
2. Include iron-containing compounds and vitamin replacements necessary for erythrocyte formation
3. Effective in the treatment of iron-deficiency and nutritional anemias
4. Available in oral and parenteral (IM, SC, IV) preparations
B. Examples
1. Iron compounds (oral)
   a. Ferrous gluconate
   b. Ferrous sulfate
2. Iron compounds (parenteral)
   a. Iron dextran
   b. Iron sorbitex
3. Vitamin replacements
   a. Cyanocobalamin: Vitamin B_{12}
   b. Folic acid: Vitamin B_9
C. Major side effects
1. Iron replacements
   a. Nausea, vomiting (irritation of gastric mucosa)
   b. Constipation (delayed passage of iron and stool in GI tract)
   c. Black stools (presence of unabsorbed iron in stool)
   d. Stained teeth (liquid preparations) (contact of liquid iron with enamel)
   e. Tissue staining (injectable preparations) (leakage of iron into tissue)
2. Vitamin replacements
   a. Local irritation (local tissue effect)
   b. Allergic reactions, anaphylaxis (hypersensitivity)
   c. Diarrhea (GI irritation)
D. Nursing care
1. Iron replacements
   a. Inform client about side effects of therapy
   b. Use Z-track procedure for IM administration
   c. Administer liquid preparations through a straw after diluting with water or fruit juice; encourage good oral hygiene
   d. Administer oral preparations on an empty stomach if possible for optimum absorption; ascorbic acid (vitamin C) increases absorption
   e. Encourage intake of foods high in iron, vitamin B_{12}, and folic acid
   f. Encourage intake of high-fiber foods to reduce the potential of constipation

    g. Deferoxamine mesylate (Desferal) is the antidote for iron toxicity
2. Vitamin replacements
    a. Vitamin B_{12}: inform client that this drug cannot be administered orally; therapy is for life
    b. Folic acid: instruct client on dietary sources of folic acid (fresh fruits, vegetables, and meats)
3. Evaluate client's response to medication and understanding of teaching

Antilipemics

A. Description
  1. Used to lower serum lipid levels by reducing cholesterol or triglyceride synthesis or both
  2. Available in oral preparations
B. Examples
  1. Cholestyramine (Questran)
  2. Clofibrate
  3. Colestipol hydrochloride
  4. Dextrothyroxine
  5. Gemfibrozil
  6. Lovastatin
  7. Niacin
  8. Probucol
C. Major side effects
  1. Nausea, vomiting (irritation to gastric mucosa)
  2. Diarrhea (GI irritation)
  3. Musculoskeletal disturbances (direct musculoskeletal tissue effect)
  4. Hepatic disturbances (hepatic toxicity)
  5. Skin rash (hypersensitivity)
  6. Reduced absorption of fat and fat-soluble vitamins (A, D, E, K) as well as vitamin B_{12} and iron (except for Nicobid)
  7. Niacin: flushing (transient) (vasodilation)
  8. Lovastatin and gemfibrozil: visual disturbances (ocular alterations)
D. Nursing care
  1. Encourage the following dietary program:
    a. Low cholesterol, low fat (especially saturated)
    b. Replace vegetable oils high in polyunsaturated fatty acid (PUFA) with those high in monounsaturated fatty acid (MUFA) such as olive, avocado
    c. Eat fish that are high in omega-3 fatty acids several times per week (salmon, tuna)
    d. Increase intake of high-fiber foods such as fruits, vegetables, cereal grains, and legumes; soluble fiber is particularly effective in reducing blood lipids (oat bran, legumes)
  2. Offer emotional support to client; long-term therapy may be necessary
  3. Administer medications with meals to reduce GI irritation
  4. Monitor serum cholesterol and triglyceride levels during therapy

  5. Monitor hemoglobin and RBC levels during therapy
  6. Monitor blood levels of fat-soluble vitamins during therapy
  7. Monitor liver function tests during therapy
  8. Cholestyramine: mix with full glass of liquid
  9. Clofibrate: assess for potentiation of anticoagulant effect
  10. Lovastatin and gemfibrozil: assess for visual disturbances with prolonged use
  11. Evaluate client's response to medication and understanding of teaching

Thrombolytics

A. Description
  1. Used to dissolve occluding thrombi in the coronary arteries
  2. Act by converting plasminogen to plasmin, which initiates local fibrinolysis
  3. Administered intravenously or intraarterially (via cardiac catheterization)
  4. Initially, loading dose is administered; lower doses may be continued for 24 to 72 hours
  5. Therapy must be instituted within 4 to 6 hours of the onset of the myocardial infarction
B. Examples
  1. Streptokinase
  2. Tissue plasminogen activator
  3. Urokinase
C. Major side effects
  1. Bleeding (increased fibrinolytic activity)
  2. Allergic reactions (introduction of a foreign protein)
  3. Low-grade fever (resulting from absorption of infarcted tissue)
D. Nursing care
  1. Observe for signs of bleeding
  2. Monitor partial thromboplastin time (PTT) and fibrinogen concentration
  3. Monitor vital signs
  4. Assess for signs of allergic reactions such as chills, urticaria, pruritis, rash, and malaise
  5. Keep aminocaproic acid, a fibrinolysis inhibitor, available on nursing unit
  6. Evaluate client's response to medication and understanding of teaching

PROCEDURES RELATED TO THE CIRCULATORY SYSTEM

Angiography

A. Definition: an x-ray examination using contrast dye to visualize the patency of an artery
B. Nursing care
  1. Inform the client of the risks involved in this procedure (allergic reaction, embolus, cardiac dysrhythmia)

2. Administer mild sedative as ordered before procedure
3. Observe the client for complications
4. Postprocedure care involves checking the injection site for bleeding and inflammation, assessing circulatory status of the extremities, and enforcing bed rest
5. Evaluate client's response to procedure

Angioplasty

A. Definition: Percutaneous transluminal coronary angioplasty (PTCA) is the introduction of a balloon-tipped catheter into the coronary artery to the point of stenosis to reduce or eliminate the occlusion; may be used with laser angioplasty that vaporizes the plaque
  1. Procedure is performed in a coronary catheterization laboratory using fluoroscopy
  2. Heparin infusion is used during the procedure to prevent thrombus formation
  3. Thrombolytic therapy may be combined with PTCA in some situations
  4. Intracoronary stents may be left in place following balloon angioplasty to maintain patency; clients would require long-term anticoagulation therapy
  5. If lesions are calcified and cannot be removed by PTCA, an atherectomy can be performed; this procedure mechanically removes the plaque by shaving and retrieving it from the vessel's lumen

B. Nursing care
  1. See care for Cardiac Catheterization
  2. Transfer client to an institution with equipment for this procedure, if necessary
  3. Administer vasoactive drugs such as calcium-channel blockers and nitroglycerin before, during, and after this procedure, as ordered
  4. Monitor client for angina and dysrhythmias
  5. Evaluate client's response to procedure

Blood Transfusion

A. Purpose
  1. Restore blood volume after hemorrhage
  2. Maintain hemoglobin levels in severe anemias
  3. Replace specific blood components

B. Nursing care
  1. Check that blood or blood components have been typed and cross-matched, indicating that the blood of the donor and recipient are compatible
  2. Blood must never be administered straight from the refrigerator
  3. A baseline of the client's temperature, blood pressure, pulse, and respirations should be determined before administration
  4. An IV with normal saline infusing through a large bore angiocath and a blood administration set containing a filter are used to start the infusion; solutions containing glucose may cause the blood to clot in the tubing and should not be used
  5. Maintain standard (universal) precautions when handling blood or IV equipment
  6. Before starting the infusion, it is advisable for two nurses to verify the blood type, Rh factor, client and blood numbers, and expiration date
  7. The container should be inverted gently to suspend the red blood cells within the plasma
  8. Observe for signs of hemolytic reaction, which generally occur early in the transfusion (within the first 10 to 15 minutes)
    a. Shivering
    b. Headache
    c. Lower back pain
    d. Increased pulse and respiratory rate
    e. Hemoglobinuria
    f. Oliguria
    g. Hypotension
  9. Observe for signs of febrile reaction, which usually occur within 30 minutes
    a. Shaking
    b. Headache
    c. Elevated temperature
    d. Back pain
    e. Confusion
    f. Hematemesis
  10. Observe for allergic reaction
    a. Hives
    b. Wheezing
    c. Pruritus
    d. Joint pain
  11. If any reaction occurs:
    a. Stop infusion immediately
    b. Notify the physician
    c. Maintain patency of the IV with normal saline
    d. Send blood to the laboratory
    e. Monitor vital signs frequently
    f. Send a urine specimen to the laboratory if a hemolytic reaction is suspected
  12. Evaluate client's response to procedure

Bone Marrow Aspiration

A. Definition: puncture to collect tissue from the bone marrow
  1. Sites used include the sternum, vertebral body, iliac crest, or the tibia in infants
  2. Performed to study the cells involved in blood production

B. Nursing care
  1. Obtain informed consent
  2. Attempt to allay anxiety of the client
  3. Assist the physician in maintaining a sterile field and positioning the client

4. Send the specimen to the laboratory in a proper container with appropriate label
5. Evaluate client's response to procedure

Cardiac Catheterization

A. Definition: introduction of a catheter into the heart via a peripheral vessel
   1. Injection of contrast material for visualization of chambers, coronary circulation, and great vessels
   2. Withdrawal of blood samples to evaluate cardiac function
   3. Measurement of pressures within chambers and blood vessels (e.g., pulmonary wedge pressure)
B. Nursing care
   1. Obtain an informed consent; the client should be aware of the procedure's purpose, its possible complications, and the sensations it causes (e.g., urge to cough, nausea, heat)
   2. Allow time for verbalization of fears
   3. Keep the client NPO for 6 to 8 hours before the procedure
   4. Determine the presence of allergies, particularly to iodine
   5. Administer sedatives as ordered prior to the procedure
   6. After catheterization
      a. Monitor vital signs frequently; cardiac dysrhythmias are more common during the procedure but may occur afterward
      b. Assess the puncture site for bleeding (sandbags or ice packs may be ordered if the femoral artery is used)
      c. Assess the involved extremity for signs of ischemia (e.g., absence of peripheral pulses, changes in sensation, color, and temperature)
      d. Maintain bed rest for the prescribed number of hours
   7. Evaluate client's response to procedure

Cardiac Monitoring

A. Definition
   1. Electric observation of the conductivity patterns of the heart by the use of skin electrodes and a monitoring device; the heart's electric activity is conducted to the surface of the skin by the salty fluids bathing the cells and tissues
   2. Used in heart disease, during surgery and intrusive procedures, or when danger of dysrhythmias (cardiac irregularities in rhythm) is apparent
   3. P, Q, R, S, and T segments are parts of the normal electrocardiogram (ECG); P wave represents atrial depolarization, QRS waves (QRS complex) ventricular depolarization, and T wave ventricular repolarization (Fig. 6-4)

B. Nursing care
   1. Explain the procedure to client and attempt to allay anxiety
   2. Prepare the skin on the chest for electrode attachment
      a. Cleanse area with alcohol swab to remove dirt and oils
      b. Shave the area to improve skin-electrode contact if appropriate
   3. Place electrodes on the skin and attach to the monitor cable as indicated
      a. RA (attach to right upper chest)
      b. LA (attach to left upper chest)
      c. RL (attach to right lower chest [ground])
      d. LL (attach to left lower chest)
   4. Turn on the monitor scope and set the machine's sensitivity when a clear picture is obtained
   5. Observe the monitor for changes in rate and rhythm
   6. Set the alarm and readout attachment (if available) so an electric printout will be made if there is a change in cardiac activity
   7. If dysrhythmia occurs, act appropriately
      a. Emergency dysrhythmias require immediate intervention
      b. If the dysrhythmia is a nonemergency, document its occurrence with a rhythm strip and notify the physician
   8. Intervene immediately when life-threatening dysrhythmias occur
      a. Ventricular fibrillation (Fig. 6-5): repetitive rapid stimulation from ectopic ventricular foci to which the ventricles are unable to respond; ventricular contraction is replaced by uncoordinated twitching; circulation ceases, and death ensues
         (1) Defibrillate immediately
         (2) Inject medications per protocol
         (3) Institute cardiopulmonary resuscitation
         (4) Document the dysrhythmia and notify the physician
      b. Ventricular tachycardia (Fig. 6-6): series of 3 or more bizarre premature ventricular beats that occur in a regular rhythm; this electric activity results in decreased cardiac output and may rapidly convert to ventricular fibrillation
         (1) Administer medications per protocol
         (2) Be prepared to administer defibrillation and cardiopulmonary resuscitation
         (3) Document the dysrhythmia and notify the physician
      c. Premature ventricular beats (PVBs) (Fig. 6-7) originate in the ventricles and occur before the next expected sinus beat; they can be life threatening when they occur

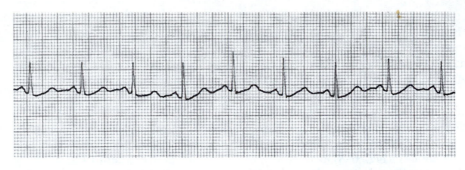

FIGURE 6-4 Regular sinus rhythm. (From Sheehy SB: *Emergency nursing*, ed 3, St. Louis, 1992, Mosby.)

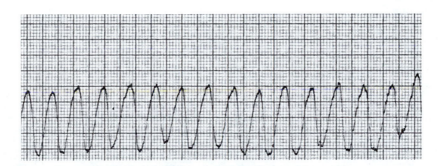

FIGURE 6-5 Ventricular fibrillation. (From Sheehy SB: *Emergency nursing*, ed 3, St. Louis, 1992, Mosby.)

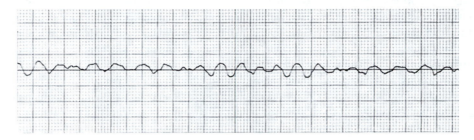

FIGURE 6-6 Ventricular tachycardia. (From Sheehy SB: *Emergency nursing*, ed 3, St. Louis, 1992, Mosby.)

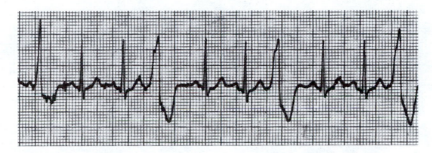

FIGURE 6-7 Premature ventricular beats. (From Sheehy SB: *Emergency nursing*, ed 3, St. Louis, 1992, Mosby.)

close to the T wave because cardiac repolarization is interfered with and ventricular fibrillation may ensue
(1) Administer medications per protocol
(2) Document the dysrhythmia and notify the physician
(3) Long-term institution of oral antiarrhythmics may be indicated
d. Third-degree atrioventricular block (complete heart block) (Fig. 6-8) occurs when there is no electric communication between the atria and ventricles and each beats independently; this activity will not provide long-term adequate circulation, and syncope, congestive failure, or cardiac arrest may ensue
(1) Document the dysrhythmia and notify the physician
(2) Administer medications per protocol
(3) Prepare for pacemaker insertion (see procedure)
e. Cardiac standstill (asystole) (Fig. 6-9) occurs when there is no cardiac activity, demonstrated on the ECG tracing as a flat line; this terminates in death unless intervention is begun immediately
(1) Institute cardiopulmonary resuscitation
(2) Document the dysrhythmia and notify the physician

(3) Cardiac stimulants may be given via IV or intracardiac route
(4) Pacemaker insertion may be indicated (see procedure)
9. Evaluate client's response to procedure

Cardiac Pacemaker Insertion
A. Definition: artificial pacemakers replace natural electric stimulation of the heart and are indicated in the treatment of:
1. Third-degree atrioventricular block: impulses generated from the SA node of the heart do not reach the ventricles; the atria and ventricles beat independently of each other
2. Second-degree atrioventricular block: intermittent failure of impulse to reach the ventricles
3. Adams-Stokes syndrome: a sudden drop in ventricular rate that causes syncope and temporary loss of consciousness
B. Pacemakers: involve the insertion of an electrode catheter into the heart, which transmits the impulses generated by the pacing unit
1. Demand pacemakers are most frequently used; the pacemaker will stimulate the ventricles to contract only if the client's ventricular rate falls below the rate set on the pacemaker
2. Fixed-rate pacemakers stimulate the heart a specific number of times per minute regardless of the client's rhythm

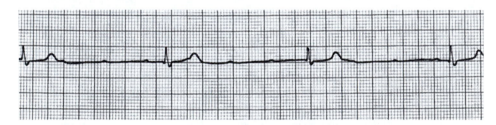

FIGURE 6-8 Third-degree atrioventricular block (complete heart block). (From Sheehy SB: *Emergency nursing*, ed 3, St. Louis, 1992, Mosby.)

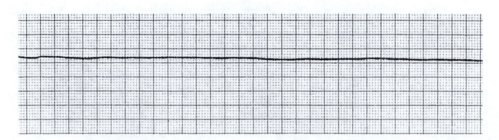

FIGURE 6-9 Ventricular standstill (asystole). (From Sheehy SB: *Emergency nursing*, ed 3, St. Louis, 1992, Mosby.)

3. Pacemakers may be temporary and worn externally or permanent and surgically placed under the skin
C. Nursing care
   1. Explain the procedure to the client
   2. Observe the cardiac monitor before, during, and after the procedure to verify pacemaker capture (QRS following pacemaker spike), and observe for dysrhythmias
   3. Have emergency medications (e.g., lidocaine, atropine sulfate, isoproterenol) available, as well as a defibrillator
   4. Teach the client how to take pulse, to keep a diary of pulse, and to notify the physician immediately if the rate falls below that set on the pacemaker
   5. Teach the client to remain under a physician's supervision, since batteries must be replaced periodically; pacemaker function may be checked by special telephone devices
   6. Encourage the client to wear a bracelet or carry a medical alert card
   7. Teach client to avoid high magnetic fields such as airport security devices, high-tension wires, and magnetic resonance imaging (MRI); when in doubt consult physician
   8. Evaluate client's response to procedure

Cardiopulmonary Resuscitation (CPR)

A. Definition: institution of artificial ventilation and circulation with rescue breathing and external cardiac compression
B. Nursing care
   1. Assess level of consciousness
      a. Shake victim's shoulder and shout, "Are you OK?"
      b. If no response, call for help or activate the EMS system
   2. Establish an airway
      a. Use head tilt or chin lift maneuver
      b. Determine if air is being exchanged
         (1) Look: is the chest moving
         (2) Listen: can air be heard escaping during exhalation
         (3) Feel: can air be felt escaping during exhalation
      c. If not breathing, proceed to step 3
   3. Initiate rescue breathing
      a. Maintain the head-tilt or chin-lift maneuver and pinch the victim's nostrils
      b. Give two full mouth-to-mouth breaths
   4. Assess circulation
      a. Palpate carotid pulse
      b. If carotid pulse is not palpable, proceed to step 5
   5. Deliver external cardiac compressions

a. Ensure that the victim is on a firm surface and in the supine position
b. Place heel of hand over lower half of body of sternum, interlock hands and compress the chest 3.8 to 5 cm for an adult
c. Maintain the ventilation/compression ratio
   (1) One rescuer: two breaths after every 15 compressions (rate, 80 to 100 per minute)
   (2) Two rescuers: one breath after every five compressions (rate, 80 to 100 per minute)
   (3) Reassess carotid pulse after first 4 cycles and then every few minutes
6. Terminate CPR as indicated
   a. Return of cardiac rhythm and spontaneous respirations
   b. Rescuer exhaustion
   c. Physician orders cessation
7. Evaluate client's response to procedure

Central Venous Pressure (CVP) Monitoring

A. Definition
   1. CVP is the right atrial pressure, which is normally 2 to 6 mm Hg or 3 to 10 cm H_2O
   2. A catheter is passed from the subclavian vein into the superior vena cava or right atrium
B. Nursing care
   1. Obtain informed consent
   2. Assist the physician with insertion of the catheter using surgical aseptic technique
   3. Obtain chest x-ray film after insertion to ascertain the position of the catheter
   4. Take readings as ordered
      a. Place the client in a supine position
      b. Place the stopcock of the manometer at the midaxillary line (which is approximately the level of the right atrium) and fill with fluid from primary line; if a transducer and pressure monitor are used, the transducer is fixed at the midaxillary line
      c. Allow fluid to enter the catheter by placing the stopcock in such a position as to interfere with the flow of fluid between the IV solution and the client
      d. If the client is on a ventilator, remove it during readings
   5. Record and report changes in CVP readings; often these readings are used to regulate the rate of administration of IVs (high readings are present in congestive heart failure, low readings in hypovolemia)
   6. Evaluate client's response to procedure

Exercise Stress Testing

A. Definition: assessment of cardiac function by ECG,

blood pressure, and pulse rate during sustained exercise

1. Common aerobic activities involved include walking on a treadmill or riding a stationary bicycle
2. Cardiac workload is increased either by constant level of activity or by graduating levels of difficulty to evaluate ability of the coronary circulation to supply adequate amounts of oxygen to the heart muscle when maximum heart rates are approached (depression of ST segment of ECG is one indication of myocardial hypoxia)

B. Nursing care

1. Obtain an informed consent
2. Attempt to allay anxiety of the client
3. Instruct the client to have only a light meal several hours prior to the test and to avoid stimulants and depressants
4. Ensure that the client does not smoke (nicotine causes peripheral vasoconstriction)
5. Ask the client to report dizziness, chest pain, dyspnea, fatigue, or nausea if experienced during the test
6. Continually observe the client, the vital signs, and the ECG during the test
7. Ensure ready access to emergency cardiac drugs and equipment (e.g., defibrillator)
8. Observe the client after the test and reinforce any medical instructions as required
9. Evaluate client's response to procedure

Nuclear Medicine Procedures

A. Multiple gated angiographic radioisotope (MUGA) scan

1. Involves intravenous injection of a radioisotope, which has an affinity for red blood cells
2. Volume of blood pumped during one ventricular contraction is compared with the total volume in the left ventricle, which yields an ejection fraction
3. The ejection fraction gives important information on ventricular size and wall motion abnormalities

B. Thallium stress testing or imaging

1. Intravenous injection of a radioisotope, which is taken up by the heart muscle
2. Damaged myocardial tissue takes up the isotope more slowly and retains it for a longer period
3. The isotope can be injected during and after exercise to determine myocardial perfusion

C. Pyrophosphate scan or technetium 99m pyrophosphate imaging

1. This radioisotope binds with free calcium in damaged myocardial tissue after intravenous injection

2. Injured myocardium binds as much as 20 times more than normal tissue
3. Test may be performed from 16 hours to 7 days after onset of symptoms

D. Positron emission tomography (PET) scan

1. A positron-emitting isotope is administered intravenously
2. Provides detailed information about cardiac circulation
3. Clients should be encouraged to drink fluids after the test to facilitate excretion of the isotope

E. Nursing care

1. Explain procedure to client
2. Monitor client's vital signs prior to and after test
3. Determine history of allergies and notify radiology prior to test
4. Offer emotional support to client who may be apprehensive about test and results; allay client's fears about the use of radioactive substances
5. Evaluate client's response to procedures

Pulmonary Artery Catheter Procedure

A. Definition: catheter used to measure pulmonary capillary wedge pressure, pulmonary artery pressure, and right atrial pressure

1. The double-lumen catheter with a balloon tip is inserted into a vein and advanced through the superior vena cava, into the right atrium and ventricle, and into the pulmonary artery; the catheter is guided further until, when the balloon is inflated, it is wedged in the distal arterial branch
2. This catheter functions to yield information on the client's circulatory status, left ventricular pumping action, and vascular tone

B. Nursing care

1. Obtain informed consent for procedure
2. Assist the physician in inserting the catheter using surgical aseptic technique
3. Observe the insertion site for inflammation
4. Observe the line for patency and air bubbles
5. Take readings with transducer at the level of the client's sternal notch
6. Change the dressing as ordered using surgical asepsis
7. Notify the physician if the waveform changes or pressure readings are altered
8. Ensure that balloon does not remain inflated after wedge pressure determination
9. Normal readings
   a. Pulmonary capillary wedge pressure: 5 to 13 mm Hg
   b. Pulmonary artery pressure
      (1) Systolic: 16 to 30 mm Hg
      (2) Diastolic: 0 to 7 mm Hg
   c. Right atrial pressure: 5 mm Hg

d. Cardiac output is determined by injecting iced or room-temperature saline through the proximal lumen of the pulmonary artery catheter; a thermistor unit can detect temperature changes in the right atrium that allows the computer to calculate cardiac output

10. Keep emergency medications and a defibrillator available

GENERAL NURSING DIAGNOSES FOR CLIENTS WITH CIRCULATORY SYSTEM DISORDERS

A. Risk for activity intolerance related to:
   1. Decreased cardiac output
   2. Decreased tissue perfusion
   3. Decreased oxygen-carrying capacity of the blood
   4. Pain
B. Ineffective breathing pattern related to trauma of chest surgery
C. Decreased cardiac output related to:
   1. Excessive cardiac workload
   2. Decreased tissue perfusion
   3. Blood loss
   4. Decreased venous return
D. Ineffective individual coping related to type A personality
E. Ineffective coping related to denial of prognosis and disease process
F. Fatigue related to:
   1. Decreased cardiac output
   2. Decreased oxygen-carrying capacity of the blood
G. Fear related to questionable prognosis and potential disability/death
H. Fluid volume deficit related to blood loss
I. Fluid volume excess related to decreased cardiac output
J. Risk for infection related to disease process or treatment modalities
K. Risk for injury related to diagnostic and therapeutic modalities
L. Noncompliance (with therapeutic regimen) related to denial of diagnosis
M. Altered nutrition, less than body requirements, related to inadequate dietary intake
N. Pain related to:
   1. Impaired tissue perfusion
   2. Operative trauma
O. Personal identity disturbance related to sick role
P. Self-care deficit (total) related to imposed restrictions
Q. Sexual dysfunction related to fear, medication, and disease process
R. Risk for impaired skin integrity related to altered peripheral tissue perfusion
S. Altered thought processes related to decreased cerebral perfusion

T. Altered tissue perfusion related to:
   1. Decreased cardiac output
   2. Peripheral vasoconstriction or obstruction
   3. Inadequate, excessive, or inappropriate nutrition
   4. Venous stasis

MAJOR DISORDERS OF THE CIRCULATORY SYSTEM

▼ HYPERTENSION

Data Base

A. Etiology and pathophysiology
   1. Hypertension increases the risk of coronary artery disease, heart failure, myocardial infarction, cerebral vascular accidents (CVAs), and renal failure
   2. Often asymptomatic; diagnosis requires three assessments of elevated blood pressure on separate occasions
   3. Blood pressure is now divided into seven categories: normal, high normal, hypertension stage one, hypertension stage two, hypertension stage three, hypertension stage four, and isolated systolic hypertension
   4. Stages of hypertension
      a. Stage 1: systolic 140 to 159 and diastolic 90 to 99
      b. Stage 2: systolic 160 to 179 and diastolic 100 to 109
      c. Stage 3: systolic 180 to 209 and diastolic 110 to 119
      d. Stage 4: systolic equal to or greater than 210 and diastolic equal to or greater than 120
   5. Essential hypertension
      a. Anxiety and other stresses are believed to play a role in releasing a pressor from kidneys that causes chronic vasoconstriction, thereby raising blood pressure
      b. Individuals with essential hypertension have difficulty handling hostile feelings, are less assertive, and have more obsessive-compulsive traits than do nonhypertensive individuals
      c. Onset is generally between 25 and 55 years of age
   6. Renal hypertension
      a. Narrowing of the lumen of a renal artery as a result of atherosclerosis causes release of renin
      b. Renin sets off series of reactions, which cause sodium retention and subsequent rise in blood pressure
      c. Onset is generally after 50 years of age

7. Malignant hypertension results from sustained hypertension of any form, which causes necrosis of the arterioles and proliferative changes of the renal arteries leading to renal failure, CVA, and heart failure, if untreated

8. Hypertensive crisis may also be caused by endocrine disorders (pheochromocytoma), increased intracranial pressure, and encephalopathy

B. Clinical findings
   1. Subjective
      a. Headache (occipital area)
      b. Lightheadedness
      c. Tinnitus
      d. Easy fatigue
      e. Visual disturbances
      f. Palpitations
      g. Brief lapses in memory
   2. Objective
      a. Blood pressure greater than 140/90 mm Hg that has been obtained on three separate occasions
      b. Retinal changes
      c. Possible hematuria
      d. Epistaxis
      e. Cardiac hypertrophy

C. Therapeutic interventions
   1. Life-style modifications:
      a. Sodium restriction (1 to 3 g daily)
      b. Weight control or reduction
      c. Alcohol restriction
      d. Cessation of smoking
      e. Regular exercise program
   2. Pharmacologic treatment
      Selection of drug therapy can be guided by concomitant medical conditions (e.g., diabetes, abnormal lipids, CHF, asthma, COPD, renal disease) and blood pressure response as recommended by the Canadian Hypertension Society. The goal of therapy is reducing diastolic blood pressure to less than 90 mm hg
      If there are no coexisting medical conditions or target-organ damage, pharmacologic treatment of essential hypertension includes an incremental approach:
      a. Initial therapy: monotherapy with either a low-dose thiazide diuretic or beta-blocker
      b. If response is inadequate or there are adverse effects, substitute the alternate drug
      c. If there is a partial response, consider a combination of a diuretic and beta-blocker or monotherapy with an alpha-blocker, ACE inhibitor, calcium-entry blocker, or centrally acting drug
      d. If blood pressure is still not controlled, consider combinations such as a low-dose diuretic with an ACE inhibitor, a calcium-entry blocker, a centrally acting drug, or beta-blocker

e. Resistant hypertension may require combinations of three or more drug groups
      For hypertensive clients with coexisting medical conditions or target-organ damage, drug treatment should be individualized to obtain maximum benefit with minimum risk
      Elderly people are more heterogenous than younger ones in mood, life satisfaction, intellectual performance, physiologic reserve, and mobility. Even more than chronologic age, factors such as coexisting disease and concurrent drug therapy (especially NSAIDs) must be considered in treating hypertension in the older client
      a. Prepared initial therapy is thiazide diuretics
      b. When diuretics are contraindicated or not preferred, initial treatment with beta-blockers in small doses is recommended and should be used as a second choice because of their lower efficacy, more frequent adverse effects, and less clear benifits
      c. Third choice monotherapy: calcium-entry blockers should be considered when diuretics or beta-blockers are contraindicated or not tolerated
   3. Relaxation modalities such as biofeedback and imagery

Nursing Care of Clients with Hypertension

A. DATA COLLECTION
   1. Vital signs with client in both upright and recumbent positions
   2. Baseline weight
   3. Headaches, tinnitus, fatigability, memory loss, palpitations

B. ANALYSIS AND INTERPRETATION
   Refer to General Nursing Diagnoses for Clients with Circulatory System Disorders for the following diagnoses: D, E, L, T 1, T 2

C. PLANNING/IMPLEMENTATION
   1. Monitor vital signs with client in both upright and recumbent positions
   2. Weigh client daily when there is a threat of congestive heart failure
   3. Pay particular attention to calcium and potassium intake because hypertension has been associated with deficiencies of these minerals; monitor blood work
   4. Reassure and support any expression of emotions
   5. If epistaxis occurs, place an ice pack on the back of the neck, which may alleviate it; packing is sometimes required
   6. Educate the client regarding drugs, follow-up care, activity restrictions, and diet; note that many salt substitutes contain potassium chloride rather than sodium chloride and may be

permitted by the physician if client has no renal impairment (see Antihypertensives and Diuretics for additional dietary information)

7. Teach information related to specific medications

D. EVALUATION/OUTCOMES
1. Reduces blood pressure to an acceptable level
2. Understands and adheres to medical regimen
3. Verbalizes need for stress reduction

▼ ARTERIOATHEROSCLEROSIS

Data Base

A. Etiology and pathophysiology
1. Deposition of fatty plaques along inner wall of the artery; most often affects the peripheral arteries, aorta, coronary arteries, and arteries supplying the brain
2. Considered to be a loss of elasticity, or "hardening," of the arteries
3. May be limited by eating a diet low in fat and cholesterol and high in dietary fiber, exercising regularly, controlling weight, and not smoking

B. Clinical findings
1. Subjective
   a. Intermittent claudication of the lower extremities
   b. Pain, depending on location and degree to which circulation is impaired
   c. Forgetfulness
2. Objective
   a. Decreased skin temperature
   b. Pallor
   c. Diminished pulsations
   d. Decreased hair growth
   e. May lead to ulcerations and gangrene
   f. Elevated serum cholesterol and lipids
   g. Objective memory loss on testing

C. Therapeutic interventions
1. Drugs that cause vasodilation
2. Weight loss
3. Dietary restriction of cholesterol and fat along with increased dietary fiber
4. Smoking cessation
5. Avoidance of constrictive garments
6. Coronary artery bypass graft surgery (CABG) if the coronary arteries are affected

Nursing Care of Clients with Arterioatherosclerosis

A. DATA COLLECTION
1. Peripheral pulses
2. Color and temperature of extremities
3. History relative to causative factors such as smoking and high-fat diet

B. ANALYSIS AND INTERPRETATION
Refer to General Nursing Diagnoses for Clients with Circulatory System Disorders for the following diagnoses: A 2, C 2, N 1, N 2, T 2, and T 3

C. PLANNING/IMPLEMENTATION
1. Discourage positions that hamper circulation (e.g., sitting cross-legged)
2. Teach the client the hazards of smoking (nicotine causes peripheral vasoconstriction)
3. Encourage the following dietary program:
   a. Low cholesterol, low fat (especially saturated)
   b. Replace vegetable oils high in PUFA with those high in MUFA, such as olive and avocado
   c. Eat fish that are high in omega-3 fatty acids several times per week (salmon, tuna)
   d. Increase intake of high-fiber foods such as fruits, vegetables, cereal grains, and legumes; soluble fiber is particularly effective in reducing blood lipids (oat bran, legumes)
4. Teach importance of warm clothing
5. Teach importance of not vigorously massaging involved area

D. EVALUATION/OUTCOMES
1. Maintains adequate peripheral circulation
2. Adheres to prescribed diet

▼ANGINA PECTORIS

Data Base

A. Etiology and pathophysiology
1. Commonly caused by narrowed coronary arteries (coronary artery disease); may be caused by coronary artery spasms
2. Clients with aortic stenosis or extremely low blood pressure may also have impaired coronary artery blood flow
3. Increased metabolic demands due to strenuous exercise, emotional stress, hyperthyroidism, or severe anemia may also precipitate angina pectoris
4. When oxygen supplied by the blood cannot meet the metabolic demands of the muscle, hypoxia occurs
5. Pain is thought to be a result of anaerobic metabolic end products

B. Classification
1. Unstable preinfarction
2. Chronic stable
3. Nocturnal
4. Resting (Prinzmetal)

C. Clinical findings
1. Subjective
   a. Chest pain associated with activity; generally subsides after a few minutes of rest
   b. Pain is usually substernal and can be described as "crushing" or "pressure"

   c. Pain may radiate to the left shoulder and arm, jaw, epigastric area, or right shoulder

   d. Palpitations

   e. Faintness

   f. Dyspnea

   g. Levine's sign—client clenches fist over sternum when describing discomfort

  2. Objective

   a. Diaphoresis

   b. Blood pressure may be elevated

   c. Signs of underlying disease may be evident (cardiac enlargement, valvular disease, dysrhythmias)

   d. ECG recordings, which vary at rest and during exercise

   e. ECG often indicates a previous infarction

D. Therapeutic interventions

  1. Restricted activity

  2. Pharmacologic management

   a. Nitrates

   b. Beta-blocking agents

   c. Calcium channel–blocking agent

   d. Antilipidemics

   e. Thrombolytics

  3. Weight loss

  4. Restriction of cholesterol and fat in diet

  5. Oxygen therapy during attack

  6. Percutaneous transluminal coronary angioplasty (PTCA)

  7. Coronary artery bypass surgery if medical regimen not successful

Nursing Care of Clients with Angina Pectoris

A. DATA COLLECTION

  1. Vital signs

  2. Activity tolerance

  3. History of precipitating factors

B. ANALYSIS AND INTERPRETATION

  Refer to General Nursing Diagnoses for Clients with Circulatory System Disorders for the following diagnoses: A 2, C 1, G, N 1, and O

C. PLANNING/IMPLEMENTATION

  1. Provide physical and mental rest

  2. Relieve pain by administration of vasodilators

  3. Discourage smoking

  4. Educate the client regarding diet, medication, and activity

  5. Provide necessary emotional support to client regarding required alterations in life-style

D. EVALUATION/OUTCOMES

  1. Describes the use of therapeutic medications

  2. Assumes life-style that contributes to improvement in disease process

  3. Episodes of pain are decreased in frequency, intensity, and duration

▼ MYOCARDIAL INFARCTION

Data Base

A. Etiology and pathophysiology

  1. Acute necrosis of part of the heart muscle caused by interruption of oxygen supply to the area, resulting in altered function and reduced cardiac output

  2. Possible causes include atherosclerosis, thrombus formation, decreased blood flow, which can be influenced by the client's history of smoking, obesity, high-cholesterol/low-density lipoprotein diet, and physical/emotional stress

  3. Risk can be decreased by:

   a. Maintaining serum lipoprotein ratio

    (1) Low-density lipoprotein (LDL) carries cholesterol through the blood and deposits it in the arteries, which forms plaque

    (2) Very low-density lipoprotein (VLDL) is a substance used by the liver to manufacture LDL; it is the precursor of LDL

    (3) High-density lipoprotein (HDL): protective fraction of cholesterol which draws cholesterol away from the arteries

    (4) The ratio between LDL and HDL is important as an indicator of heart disease; the higher the ratio, the greater the risk

   b. Eating a diet low in fat and cholesterol and high in dietary fiber, exercising regularly, controlling weight, and not smoking

B. Clinical findings

  1. Subjective

   a. Sudden, severe, crushing, or viselike pain in the substernal region; may radiate to the arms, neck, and back

   b. Nausea

   c. Severe anxiety and dyspnea

  2. Objective

   a. Vomiting

   b. Slight elevation of temperature

   c. Changes in ECG

   d. Changes in blood serum enzyme and isoenzyme levels

    (1) Creatine kinase or creatine phosphokinase (CK or CPK): elevated 3 to 6 hours after infarction, peaking at 24 hours, and returning to normal within 72 to 96 hours

    (2) CK isoenzymes or CPK isoenzymes (CK-MB or CPK-MB): elevated 4 to 6 hours after pain, peaking within 24 hours, and returning to normal within 72 hours; specific for myocardial damage

(3) Lactic dehydrogenase (LDH): elevated on first day, reaching its peak on third to fourth day, and then gradually subsiding

(4) LDH_1 and LDH_2: elevate in 4 hours and peak 48 hours after infarction

(5) LDH isoenzymes: following a myocardial infarction (MI) LDH_1 is greater than LDH_2

(6) Aspartate aminotransferase (AST) (formerly SGOT); elevated on days 2 to 4

e. Complete blood studies, particularly white blood cells and sedimentation rate, to determine presence of inflammatory process

f. Coagulation studies: prothrombin time (PT) and partial thromboplastin time (PTT)

g. Signs of shock: cold, clammy skin; profuse diaphoresis; decreased blood pressure; rapid, thready pulse

C. Therapeutic interventions
1. Admit the client to the coronary care unit
2. Morphine sulfate IV or SC to relieve pain and reduce apprehension
3. Bed rest with cardiac precautions to reduce demand for oxygen
4. Oxygen as necessary
5. Cardiac monitoring for continued surveillance of the heart's electrical activity
6. Frequent monitoring of vital signs, including temperature, pulse (apical and radial), respirations, blood pressure, intake and output
7. Pharmacologic management to stabilize client and prevent complications
   a. Thrombolytic agents
   b. Anticoagulants
   c. Antidysrhythmics
   d. Narcotic analgesics
   e. Nitrates
   f. Beta-blocking agents
   g. Calcium antagonists
   h. Diuretics
   i. Potassium salts
   j. Sedatives
   k. Hypnotics
   l. Laxatives
8. IV fluids at slow rate to keep vein open for administration of medications
9. Thrombolytic therapy (streptokinase, urokinase, TPA) may be employed to dissolve thrombi in the coronary arteries immediately after onset of infarction
10. Pulmonary artery catheter is used to monitor pressure in pulmonary artery, which reflects function of left ventricle
11. Intraaortic balloon pump that inflates during diastole and deflates during systole may be used to decrease cardiac workload by decreasing afterload
12. Clear liquid diet is prescribed initially to decrease oxygen consumption and then advanced to low sodium

Nursing Care of Clients with Myocardial Infarction

A. DATA COLLECTION
1. Changes in rate, rhythm, and conduction of heart function evident on electrocardiogram
2. Life-threatening dysrhythmias (ventricular fibrillation and ventricular standstill)
3. Dysrhythmias such as PVBs close to a T wave, ventricular tachycardia, and atrial fibrillation; if they occur, administer prescribed medications and document the rhythm
4. Vital signs every 15 minutes until stable
5. Intake and output
6. Pulmonary congestion and dependent edema
7. Occurrence of pain and restlessness
8. Cyanosis and dyspnea

B. ANALYSIS AND INTERPRETATION
Refer to General Nursing Diagnoses for Clients with Circulatory System Disorders for the following diagnoses: A 1, A 2, C 2, D, E, N 1, and T 1

C. PLANNING/IMPLEMENTATION
1. Respond to dysrhythmias with medications per protocol, defibrillation, or cardiac massage
2. Administer analgesics and other medications as ordered
3. Administer oxygen as necessary
4. Recognize that the client is subject to sensory overload
   a. Orient to the unit and machinery
   b. Allow the client time to express feelings and fears
5. Provide gradual increase in activity
6. Apply antiembolism stockings
7. Provide emotional support to client and family
8. Reduce anxiety and accept client's fears

D. EVALUATION/OUTCOMES
1. Remains pain free or pain is reduced
2. Maintains adequate tissue perfusion
3. Verbalizes a reduction in anxiety and fear
4. Adheres to prescribed regimen (dietary, pharmacologic, and exercise)

▼ INFLAMMATORY DISEASES OF THE HEART (PERICARDITIS, MYOCARDITIS, INFECTIVE SUBACUTE BACTERIAL ENDOCARDITIS)

Data Base

A. Etiology and pathophysiology

1. Pericarditis
   a. Acute or chronic inflammation of the pericardium (membranous sac around the heart)
   b. May be idiopathic or result from:
      (1) Bacterial infection (*Streptococcus, Staphylococcus, Gonococcus, Meningococcus* organisms)
      (2) Viral infection (coxsackievirus, influenza)
      (3) Mycotic (fungal) infection
      (4) Rickettsial and parasitic infestation
      (5) Trauma
      (6) Collagen disease
      (7) Rheumatic fever
      (8) Neoplastic disease
   c. Sequelae
      (1) Loss of pericardial elasticity or an accumulation of fluid within the sac
      (2) Heart failure or cardiac tamponade (compression of the heart caused by a collection of fluid within the pericardial sac)
2. Myocarditis
   a. Inflammation of the myocardium (heart muscle)
   b. May result from:
      (1) Viral, bacterial, mycotic, parasitic, protozoal, or spirochetal infections or infestations
      (2) Rheumatic fever
      (3) Endocarditis
   c. Sequelae
      (1) Impaired contractility of the heart caused by the inflammatory process
      (2) Myocardial ischemia and necrosis
3. Infective subacute bacterial endocarditis
   a. Inflammation of the inner lining of the heart and valves
   b. May result from:
      (1) Rheumatic heart disease
      (2) Prosthetic valve surgery
      (3) Mitral prolapse
      (4) Infected teeth, gums, or tonsils
      (5) *Streptococcus viridans*, bacterial, fungal, or rickettsiae infections
   c. Sequelae
      (1) Structural damage to the valves
      (2) Pump failure
B. Clinical findings
   1. Subjective
      a. Precordial or substernal pain
      b. Dyspnea
      c. Chills
      d. Fatigue and malaise
   2. Objective
      a. Dysrhythmias
      b. Increased cardiac enzymes
      c. Fever

   d. Positive blood cultures
   e. Friction rubs evident on auscultation
C. Therapeutic interventions
   1. Oxygen therapy
   2. Bed rest
   3. Antibiotics to relieve underlying infection
   4. Corticosteroids
   5. Antidysrhythmics
   6. Pericardectomy (surgical removal of scar tissue and the pericardium), if indicated
   7. Salicylates to suppress rheumatic activity
   8. Cardiac monitoring when dysrhythmias occur

Nursing Care of Clients with Inflammatory Disease of the Heart

A. DATA COLLECTION
   1. Signs of shock, heart failure, and dysrhythmias
   2. Temperature to obtain baseline data
   3. Distention of neck veins
   4. Friction rub and murmur
   5. Overt and covert indicators of pain

B. ANALYSIS AND INTERPRETATION
   Refer to General Nursing Diagnoses for Clients with Circulatory System Disorders for the following diagnoses: A, C 1, F, G, J, and T

C. PLANNING/IMPLEMENTATION
   1. Maintain a tranquil environment and help the client achieve maximum rest
   2. Medicate for discomfort as needed
   3. Allow for expression of concerns
   4. Explain posthospitalization therapy to improve compliance (lifelong doses of penicillin prophylactically when undergoing invasive procedures)
   5. Administer IV antibiotics as ordered
   6. Monitor temperature and blood cultures to determine the effect of antibiotic therapy
   7. If surgical intervention is undertaken, care for chest tubes and follow the postoperative chest surgery routine (see Cardiac Surgery)

D. EVALUATION/OUTCOMES
   1. Verbalizes pain is relieved
   2. Achieves afebrile state
   3. Maintains vital signs within normal limits
   4. Adheres to therapeutic regimen

▼ CONGESTIVE HEART FAILURE (CHF)

Data Base

A. Etiology and pathophysiology
   1. Inability of the heart to meet the demands of the body
   2. Pump failure may be caused by cardiac abnormalities or conditions that place increased demands on the heart

a. Myocardial infarctions
b. Valvular defects
c. Hypertension
d. Anemia
e. Hyperthyroidism
f. Obesity
g. Circulatory overload

3. When one side of the heart "fails," there is essentially a buildup of pressure in the vascular system feeding into that side: signs of right-ventricular failure will be evident in the systemic circulation, those of left-ventricular failure in the pulmonary system

B. Clinical findings
1. Right-ventricular failure
a. Subjective
(1) Abdominal pain
(2) Fatigue
(3) Bloating
(4) Nausea
b. Objective
(1) Dependent, pitting edema; ankle edema is frequently the first sign of CHF; often subsides at night when legs are elevated
(2) Ascites from increased pressure within the portal system
(3) Hepatomegaly
(4) Respiratory distress
(5) Increased CVP
(6) Diminished urinary output
2. Left-ventricular heart failure
a. Subjective
(1) Dyspnea from fluid within the lungs
(2) Orthopnea
(3) Fatigue
(4) Paroxysmal nocturnal dyspnea
b. Objective
(1) Crackles
(2) Peripheral cyanosis
(3) Cheyne-Stokes respirations
(4) Frothy, blood-tinged sputum

C. Therapeutic interventions
1. Rest to reduce cardiac workload
2. Morphine sulfate therapy to reduce anxiety and dyspnea
3. Oxygen by mask or cannula; however, if acute ventricular failure exists, the client may require endotracheal intubation and placement on a ventilator
4. Cardiac glycosides to increase the efficiency of the heart's pumping action
5. Diuretics such as furosemide (Lasix) to remove excess fluid, thereby decreasing cardiac workload
6. Vasodilators to allow for more efficient ventricular emptying and increased venous capacity
7. Potassium supplements to prevent digitalis toxicity and hypokalemia

8. Rotating tourniquets (dry phlebotomy) to decrease venous return; generally tourniquets are applied to three of the extremities, and every 15 minutes a tourniquet is removed and rotated in a clockwise direction; when the client is stable, tourniquets are removed one at a time in 15-minute intervals
9. A paracentesis if ascites exists and is causing respiratory distress
10. Sodium-restricted diet
11. Hemodynamic monitoring through a multilumen pulmonary artery catheter

Nursing Care of Clients with Congestive Heart Failure

A. DATA COLLECTION
1. Baseline vital signs
2. Body weight
3. Baseline CVP and pulmonary wedge pressure, when indicated
4. Electrolyte levels (sodium, chloride, potassium)
5. Intake and output

B. ANALYSIS AND INTERPRETATION
Refer to General Nursing Diagnoses for Clients with Circulatory System Disorders for the following diagnoses: A 1, C 1, F, G, I, P, and T 2

C. PLANNING/IMPLEMENTATION
1. Maintain the client in high-Fowler's position
2. Elevate extremities except when the client is in acute distress
3. Frequently monitor vital signs
4. Change position frequently
5. Monitor intake and output and daily weight
6. Restrict fluids as ordered
7. Monitor invasive lines
8. Teach the client and family and provide emotional support
9. Refer to glycoside and diuretic medications for additional nursing actions
10. Use aseptic procedures when caring for invasive lines

D. EVALUATION/OUTCOMES
1. Maintains adequate tissue perfusion
2. Reduces peripheral edema/ascites
3. Verbalizes understanding of pharmacologic and diet therapy

▼ CARDIAC SURGERY

Data Base
A. May be used to:
1. Correct abnormalities
a. Mitral stenosis or regurgitation
b. Aortic stenosis or insufficiency
c. Coronary occlusion
d. Ventricular aneurysm

2. Replace failing heart (cardiac transplantation)
   a. Terminal heart disease with life expectancy of less than 1 year
   b. Viral myocarditis
   c. Toxic injury to the myocardium
   d. Severe coronary artery disease
B. Types of procedures: open or closed heart surgery (when extracorporeal circulation or the heart-lung machine is used, it is called open heart surgery; hypothermia may be used in either open or closed heart surgery to decrease the metabolic demands of the body)
   1. Mitral commissurotomy or valvotomy involves splitting the joined portions of the mitral valve that are present in mitral stenosis
   2. Mitral valve replacement is done for mitral insufficiency, which occurs when the mitral valve does not close properly to block the reflux of blood from the ventricle into the atrium during systole (regurgitation)
   3. Aortic valve replacement is performed for aortic stenosis or insufficiency; aortic stenosis results in left ventricular hypertrophy and diminished function; insufficiency results in regurgitation of blood into the left ventricle with a wide pulse pressure, bounding pulse, and dyspnea
   4. Tricuspid valve repair or replacement is indicated for tricuspid insufficiency or stenosis; both these conditions result in dilation of the right atrium and right-ventricular heart failure
   5. Aneurysmectomy is done to correct a ventricular aneurysm (which occurs in approximately 10% to 30% of clients with myocardial infarction; i.e., a weakened ventricular wall balloons out, causing decreased cardiac efficiency)
   6. Cardiac transplantation involves replacement of the client's diseased heart with one from a compatible donor
   7. Surgical removal (ablation) of foci and pathways of dysrhythmias; involves mapping cardiac electrophysiologic function to locate the source of the dysrhythmic foci; surgical resection of the focus is made through a sternotomy; indicated in Wolf-Parkinson-White syndrome and atrial and ventricular dysrhythmias
   8. Percutaneous transluminal coronary angioplasty (PTCA) is indicated for individuals with single-vessel disease; procedure involves inserting a balloon-tipped catheter into the diseased vessel and inflating it to reduce stenosis
   9. Coronary artery bypass graft (CABG) surgery is done when severe arteriosclerotic disease causes angina pectoris; involves anastomosis of a graft or a segment of a vessel (often the internal mammary artery and the saphenous vein), bypassing the diseased portion of a coronary artery; one or more vessels may be bypassed

Nursing Care of Clients Undergoing Cardiac Surgery

A. DATA COLLECTION
   1. Vital signs
   2. Airway patency
   3. Tubes to ensure patency and to assess drainage
   4. Incision for signs of hemorrhage or infection
B. ANALYSIS AND INTERPRETATION
   Refer to General Nursing Diagnoses for Clients with Circulatory System Disorders for the following diagnoses: B, C 3, J, N 2, P, and T 4
C. PLANNING/IMPLEMENTATION
   1. Monitor cardiac functioning
   2. Evaluate vital signs, including peripheral pulses and neurologic signs
   3. Monitor temperature closely
   4. Maintain airway; the client will have an endotracheal tube in place postoperatively and require mechanical ventilation; suction as necessary
   5. Monitor intake and output; weigh regularly
   6. Assess state of hydration by frequent checks of pulmonary artery pressure (PAP), pulmonary wedge pressure (PWP), and central venous pressure (CVP) readings, electrolytes, and observation of the client
   7. Assess pain (nature, site, duration, type) and provide relief
   8. Monitor arterial blood gases
   9. Maintain a Foley catheter in place; in addition to output, monitor specific gravity
   10. Care for chest tubes
       a. Maintain patency of tubes
       b. Avoid kinked tubing
       c. Drainage should not be more than 200 ml/hour
   11. Encourage coughing and deep breathing; change position frequently
   12. Administer parenteral therapy, including electrolytes and blood
   13. Plan with the client and family for meeting both short- and long-term goals
   14. Provide relief of anxiety and fear by staying with the client and explaining procedures; encourage verbalization of feelings; provide emotional support
   15. If saphenous vein has been used, assess the site for signs of impaired circulation or infection
   16. Administer cardiac medications as ordered
   17. Monitor client for signs of complications
       a. Hemorrhage that can lead to hypovolemia
          (1) Decreased blood pressure, increased pulse rate

(2) Restlessness, apprehension
(3) Lowered CVP readings
(4) Pallor
b. Cardiac tamponade caused by collection of fluid or blood within pericardium
  (1) Decreased arterial pressure
  (2) Elevated CVP
  (3) Rapid, thready pulse
  (4) Diminished output
c. Congestive heart failure
  (1) Dyspnea
  (2) Elevated CVP
  (3) Tachycardia
  (4) Edema
d. Transplant rejection
  (1) Fever
  (2) Malaise, fatigue
  (3) Signs of congestive heart failure
e. Myocardial infarction
f. Renal failure
g. Embolism
h. Psychosis resulting from an inability to cope with anxiety associated with cardiac surgery
18. Specific care for the client with a cardiac transplant
a. Maintain protective isolation when immunosuppressants (cyclosporine and azathioprine) are used
b. Teach client not to strain for defecation and to avoid lifting or pulling for at least 8 weeks after surgery
c. Teach client and family the importance of adhering to a sodium- and cholesterol-restricted diet (usually 2 g sodium and 300 mg cholesterol)
d. Provide emotional support during periods of euphoria or fear
e. Instruct client to avoid temperature extremes
f. Tell client to report signs of respiratory infection and urinary tract infection to the physician
g. Stress the importance of foot care and oral care
h. Encourage client to take temperature daily and report elevations to the physician immediately
i. Instruct client to take immunosuppressive drugs before meals diluted 1:10 in milk
j. Inform client that frequent nodal biopsies will be performed to identify rejection
k. Teach client that when rejection is found to be moderate to severe, hospitalization will be necessary for intensive immunosuppressive therapy
l. Explain that chest x-ray examination will be required every 2 to 6 weeks following surgery

m. Alert the client and family to signs of rejection and the need to notify the physician
  (1) Increased temperature
  (2) Increased pulse
  (3) Dependent edema
  (4) Weight gain
  (5) Malaise
  (6) Dyspnea
  (7) Confusion
D. EVALUATION/OUTCOMES
  1. Achieves adequate cardiac output
  2. Maintains painless state
  3. Performs self-care activities
  4. Maintains cardiac/peripheral tissue perfusion
  5. Achieves and maintains afebrile state
  6. Verbalizes understanding of and adheres to therapeutic regimen (diet, exercise, and medications)

▼ THROMBOPHLEBITIS

Data Base
A. Etiology and pathophysiology
  1. Thrombophlebitis is the inflammation of a vein and is associated with clot formation (thrombus)
  2. An embolus is a clot or solid particle carried by the bloodstream that may interfere with circulation to vital organs
  3. Risk factors thought to contribute to this disorder include immobilization, venous stasis, trauma to vessels, pregnancy, obesity, and contraceptive therapy
  4. Surgical procedures involving the pelvic area increase the risk of phlebitis because of the vascularity of the area and subsequent vascular impairment
B. Clinical findings
  1. Subjective
    a. Pain on dorsiflexion of affected extremity (Homans' sign)
    b. Sometimes no signs are present until embolus is released and lodges in a vessel supplying a vital organ (e.g., pulmonary embolus)
  2. Objective
    a. Swollen limb with hard veins that are sensitive to pressure
    b. Redness and warmth of area along the vein
C. Therapeutic interventions
  1. Bed rest with antiembolytic stockings to promote venous return
  2. Warm moist heat to promote vasodilation; however, some believe this may dislodge the clot, and ice packs are ordered
  3. Elevation of extremity to reduce edema

4. Anticoagulants to prevent recurrence of deep vein involvement
5. Vasodilators to prevent vascular spasm
6. Thrombolytic therapy (e.g., streptokinase) may be used to dissolve clot
7. Transvenous filter or thrombectomy

Nursing Care of Clients with Thrombophlebitis

A. DATA COLLECTION
1. Increased temperature of affected leg
2. Calf circumference
3. History of leg pain
4. Presence of leg edema

B. ANALYSIS AND INTERPRETATION
Refer to General Nursing Diagnoses for Clients with Circulatory System Disorders for the following diagnoses: A 2, K, N 1, N 2, and T 2

C. PLANNING/IMPLEMENTATION
1. Observe frequently for signs of vascular impairment (e.g., pallor, cyanosis, coolness)
2. Assist in understanding the rationale for prolonged bed rest and minimal activity
3. Apply antiembolism stockings; remove and replace as ordered
4. Observe and record vital signs, including peripheral pulses
5. Instruct the client to avoid tight and constricting clothing, cigarette smoking, or maintaining one position for long periods
6. Observe for signs of pulmonary embolism (e.g., sudden pain, cyanosis, hemoptysis, shock)
7. Provide specific care for the client undergoing surgery after the acute phase of thrombophlebitis
   a. Monitor for hemorrhage; notify physician if bleeding suspected
   b. Assess circulatory status of extremity
   c. Keep extremity elevated
   d. Allow out of bed as ordered; avoid prolonged hip flexion
   e. Administer ordered analgesics and anticoagulants

D. EVALUATION/OUTCOMES
1. Decreases edema of extremity
2. Maintains adequate peripheral/pulmonary tissue perfusion
3. Verbalizes understanding of precautions associated with anticoagulant therapy

▼ VARICOSE VEINS

Data Base

A. Etiology and pathophysiology
   1. The veins in the lower trunk and extremities become dilated, congested, and tortuous
   2. Results from weakness of valves or loss of elasticity of vessel walls
   3. Risk factors include family history, prolonged standing, pregnancies, leg trauma, or thrombophlebitis

B. Clinical findings
   1. Subjective
      a. Heaviness or fullness in legs
      b. Leg fatigue
      c. Leg cramping that intensifies at night
   2. Objective
      a. Positive venogram
      b. A positive Trendelenburg test result is diagnostic of varicose veins: the client lies down with legs elevated until veins empty completely; the client then stands, and observation of filling of veins is made; a normal vein fills from below, whereas a varicose vein fills from above
      c. Skin discoloration, usually brown
      d. Stasis ulcer formation
      e. Distended protruding veins

C. Therapeutic interventions
   1. Weight loss
   2. Avoidance of standing for prolonged periods or sitting with legs crossed
   3. Support or antiembolism stockings
   4. Sclerotherapy involves the injection of a chemical irritant into the vein
   5. Surgical intervention involves ligation of the vein above the varicosity and removal of the involved vein; the great saphenous vein may be ligated near the femoral junction
   6. Postoperative early ambulation is essential to prevent formation of thrombi by compression

Nursing Care of Clients with Varicose Veins

A. DATA COLLECTION
1. Contributing risk factors such as prolonged standing and leg crossing
2. Extremities for color and pulses
3. Family history of varicosities
4. Vital signs

B. ANALYSIS AND INTERPRETATION
Refer to General Nursing Diagnoses for Clients with Circulatory System Disorders for the following diagnoses: A 4, N1, N 2, and T 4

C. PLANNING/IMPLEMENTATION
1. Instruct client about the importance of weight loss and exercise
2. Administer analgesics as ordered
3. Have client use support stockings as ordered
4. Provide specific care for the client following a vein ligation
   a. Elevate the foot of the bed for first 24 hours

b. Observe vital signs and incisions for indications of hemorrhage

c. Maintain compression with dressings

d. Assist the client with ambulation

D. EVALUATION/OUTCOMES

1. Maintains reduction in pain or discomfort
2. Maintains adequate peripheral tissue perfusion
3. Verbalizes details of weight-loss program

▼ PERIPHERAL VASCULAR DISORDERS (PVDS)

Data Base

A. Etiology and pathophysiology

1. Reduced or occluded arterial blood flow due to atherosclerosis, thrombus, or embolus
2. Buerger's disease (thromboangiitis obliterans)
   a. Peripheral circulation impaired by inflammatory occlusions of the peripheral arteries
   b. Thromboses of arteries or veins may occur
   c. Incidence is highest in young adult males who smoke
3. Raynaud's disease
   a. Spasms of digital arteries thought to be caused by abnormal response of the sympathetic nervous system to cold or emotional stress; usually bilateral
   b. Primarily occurs in young females
   c. Rarely leads to gangrene
4. Raynaud's phenomenon
   a. Episodic arterial spasms of the extremities
   b. Secondary to another disease or abnormality

B. Clinical findings

1. Subjective
   a. Paresthesia
   b. Aching to severe pain
2. Objective
   a. Pallor or cyanosis
   b. Gangrenous ulcers (more common in Buerger's disease)
   c. Diminished pulses in Buerger's disease

C. Therapeutic interventions

1. Vasodilators may be given
2. Sympathectomy to sever the sympathetic ganglia supplying the area; there is local vasodilation with improved circulation
   a. Lumbar sympathectomy deprives the leg and foot of innervation
   b. Cervicothoracic sympathectomy relieves vasospasm in the arms and hands
3. Femoropopliteal bypass grafting
   a. Saphenous vein grafting from femoral artery to the area below the obstruction
   b. Polyester fiber grafts in aortic iliac obstructions
4. Amputation if vascular supply is severely impaired
   a. Below-the-knee amputation provides the client with a more natural gait because knee movement is maintained
   b. Above-the-knee amputation limits the client's movement because prosthesis contains knee joint
   c. A guillotine amputation, in which the wound is left open and skin traction is applied, is performed when the area is infected, gangrenous, or extensively traumatized or if the client is a poor surgical risk
   d. A flap-type amputation is less prone to infection because the skin covers the area and healing occurs within 2 weeks; may be above or below the knee

Nursing Care of Clients with Peripheral Vascular Disorders

A. DATA COLLECTION

1. Vital signs
2. Color, temperature, pulses, sensation, and movement of involved extremities

B. ANALYSIS AND INTERPRETATION

Refer to General Nursing Diagnoses for Clients with Circulatory System Disorders for the following diagnoses: A 4, N 1, N 2, T 2, and T 4

C. PLANNING/IMPLEMENTATION

1. Associated with medical management
   a. Instruct the client not to smoke or wear constrictive garments
   b. Keep extremities warm; instruct the client to wear gloves when exposed to cold
   c. Protect from injury because of decreased wound-healing ability; lubricants may be applied to keep skin supple
   d. Assess color, temperature, pulses, and sensation of involved extremities
2. Associated with sympathectomy
   a. Monitor vital signs frequently because shock can occur
   b. Change position gradually because dizziness may be a problem
   c. Apply elastic bandages if ordered
3. Associated with femoropopliteal bypass grafting
   a. Assess circulation of involved extremity by checking pulses, color, temperature, and neurologic function
   b. Observe blood pressure frequently, since hypotension increases the possibility of thrombus formation
   c. Observe for signs of hemorrhage, including pain, change in skin color, and alteration of vital signs

d. Ambulate as ordered; sitting should be avoided in femoropopliteal bypass surgery

4. Associated with amputation (see Amputation in Neuromusculoskeletal System)

D. EVALUATIONS/OUTCOMES

1. Maintains adequate peripheral perfusion
2. Verbalizes a reduction in pain

▼ ANEURYSMS

Data Base

A. Etiology and pathophysiology
   1. Distention at the site of a weakness in the arterial wall
      a. Saccular aneurysm: pouchlike projection at one side of the artery
      b. Fusiform aneurysm: entire circumference of the artery wall is dilated
      c. Mycotic aneurysm: tiny weaknesses in the arterial wall that result from infection
      d. Dissecting aneurysm: tear in the inner lining of an arteriosclerotic aortic wall causes blood to form a hematoma between layers of the artery, which compresses the lumen of the artery
   2. Causes
      a. Congenital weakness such as Ehlers-Danlos syndrome
      b. Atherosclerosis (most common cause of both thoracic and abdominal aortic aneurysms)
      c. Syphilis
      d. Trauma
   3. Represent surgical emergency if ruptured
   4. Occur most frequently in middle-aged white males
   5. Risk factors include history of hypertension, obesity, stress, hypercholesterolemia, cigarette smoking

B. Clinical findings
   1. Thoracic aortic aneurysm
      a. Subjective
         (1) May be asymptomatic
         (2) Pain resulting from pressure against the nerves or vertebrae
         (3) Dyspnea
         (4) Dysphagia
      b. Objective
         (1) Hoarseness, aphonia from impingement on laryngeal nerve
         (2) Cough
         (3) Unequal pulses and arterial pressure in upper extremities
         (4) Trachea may be displaced from midline because of adhesions between trachea and aneurysm

   2. Abdominal aortic aneurysm
      a. Subjective
         (1) May be asymptomatic
         (2) Lower back or abdominal pain (severe if aneurysm is leaking)
         (3) Sensory changes in the lower extremities if aneurysm ruptures
      b. Objective
         (1) Hypertension
         (2) Pulsating abdominal mass
         (3) Mottling of the lower extremities if aneurysm ruptures
         (4) Increased abdominal girth if aneurysm ruptures
   3. Dissecting aortic aneurysm
      a. Subjective
         (1) Restlessness and anxiety
         (2) Severe pain
      b. Objective
         (1) Diminished pulses
         (2) Signs of shock

C. Therapeutic interventions
   1. Resection of the aneurysm and use of a Teflon or Dacron graft
   2. Surgical procedures involving the aorta would necessitate use of a heart-lung device (cardiopulmonary bypass)
   3. Medical treatment is aimed at decreasing cardiac output and blood pressure through the use of drugs

Nursing Care of Clients with Aneurysms

A. DATA COLLECTION

1. History including age, sex, race, cigarette usage, and familial occurrence
2. Pulsation in abdomen (palpate gently)
3. History of pain

B. ANALYSIS AND INTERPRETATION

Refer to General Nursing Diagnoses for Clients with Circulatory System Disorders for the following diagnoses: A 4, O, and R

C. PLANNING/IMPLEMENTATION

1. Monitor the vital signs and pulses of all extremities, including the posterior tibial and dorsalis pedis
2. Monitor central venous pressure (CVP) frequently
3. Record intake and output, since renal failure may occur after surgery
4. Administer narcotics as ordered to alleviate pain
5. Apply abdominal binders to provide support when the client is coughing, deep breathing, and ambulating
6. Prevent flexion of hip and knees to eliminate pressure on the arterial wall

7. Apply elastic stockings and encourage dorsi-flexion of the foot to decrease the risk of thrombophlebitis
8. Maintain patency of the nasogastric tube if present
9. Provide emotional support to client and family

D. EVALUATION/OUTCOMES
1. Maintains adequate peripheral circulation
2. Identifies ways to modify risk factors

▼ SHOCK

Data Base

A. Etiology and pathophysiology
   1. Hypovolemic: occurs when there is a loss of fluid resulting in inadequate tissue perfusion; caused by:
      a. Excessive bleeding
      b. Excessive diarrhea or vomiting
      c. Fluid loss from fistulas or burns
   2. Cardiogenic: occurs when pump failure causes inadequate tissue perfusion; caused by:
      a. Congestive heart failure
      b. Myocardial infarction
      c. Cardiac tamponade
   3. Neurogenic: caused by rapid vasodilation and subsequent pooling of blood within the peripheral vessels; caused by:
      a. Spinal anesthesia
      b. Emotional tension
      c. Drugs that inhibit the sympathetic nervous system
   4. Anaphylactic: caused by an allergic reaction that causes a release of histamine and subsequent vasodilation
   5. Septic: similar to anaphylaxis and is the body's reaction to bacterial toxins (generally gram-negative infections), which results in the leakage of plasma into tissues
B. Clinical findings
   1. Subjective
      a. Apprehension
      b. Restlessness
      c. Paresis of extremities
   2. Objective
      a. Weak, rapid, thready pulse
      b. Diaphoresis
      c. Cold, clammy skin
      d. Decreased blood pressure
      e. Decreased urine output
      f. Pallor
      g. Progressive loss of consciousness
      h. Lowered CVP readings
C. Therapeutic interventions
   1. Aimed at correcting the underlying cause
   2. Fluid and blood replacement
   3. Oxygen therapy
   4. Vasoconstricting drugs to increase blood pressure
   5. Cardiac monitoring
   6. Cardiotonics, such as digitalis preparations, for cardiogenic shock
   7. Antihistamines for anaphylactic shock
   8. Antibiotics for septic shock based on blood cultures
   9. Elevation of lower extremities to ensure circulation to vital organs
   10. Intraaortic balloon pump may be used to aid the failing heart

Nursing Care of Clients in Shock

A. DATA COLLECTION
1. History of causative and risk factors from client
2. Fluid intake and output over the previous 24 hours
3. Signs of covert bleeding
   a. Weak, thready pulse
   b. Hypotension
   c. Increased respirations
   d. Pain
4. Cold clammy skin
5. Mental status

B. ANALYSIS AND INTERPRETATION
Refer to General Nursing Diagnoses for Clients with Circulatory System Disorders for the following diagnoses: C 3, C 4, H, and S

C. PLANNING/IMPLEMENTATION
1. Keep the client warm
2. Check vital signs and monitor hemodynamic functioning
3. Monitor urine output and specific gravity
4. Allay client's anxiety
5. Carefully observe all responses to therapy
6. Administer intravenous fluids as ordered
7. Monitor oxygen saturation and provide oxygen therapy as indicated

D. EVALUATION/OUTCOMES
1. Reduces blood/fluid loss
2. Restores normal circulating volume
3. Maintains a urine output of 30 ml or more per hour
4. Remains oriented to time, place, and person
5. Maintains adequate cardiac output

▼ IRON DEFICIENCY ANEMIA

Data Base

A. Etiology and pathophysiology
   1. Poor dietary habits leading to inadequate intake of iron, vitamin B_{12}, and/or folacin

2. Iron is essential for the formation of hemoglobin and the erythrocytes needed to carry oxygen to cells; B_{12} and folacin are essential to erythrocyte synthesis

B. Clinical findings
   1. Subjective
      a. Fatigue
      b. Headache
      c. Paresthesias
   2. Objective
      a. Ankle edema
      b. Dry, pale mucous membranes
      c. Pearly white sclera
      d. Decreased hemoglobin, erythrocytes, and ferritin (most sensitive indicator)
      e. Increased iron-binding capacity
      f. Megaloblastic condition of blood

C. Therapeutic interventions
   1. Improve diet; include ascorbic acid, which stimulates iron uptake
   2. Appropriate supplements of iron, vitamin B_{12}, and/or folic acid

Nursing Care of Clients with Iron Deficiency Anemia

A. DATA COLLECTION
1. History of dietary habits
2. Status of skin, mucous membranes, and sclera
3. Fatigue, headache, and parasthesias

B. ANALYSIS AND INTERPRETATION
Refer to General Nursing Diagnoses for Clients with Circulatory System Disorders for the following diagnoses: A 3 and M

C. PLANNING/IMPLEMENTATION
1. Teach client about foods high in iron, folic acid, and vitamin B_{12}
2. Teach about the side effects of medications
3. Assist client with activities of daily living (ADL) as needed

D. EVALUATION/OUTCOMES
1. States dietary sources of iron, folic acid, and B_{12}
2. States no fatigue noted when performing ADL

▼ PERNICIOUS ANEMIA

Data Base

A. Etiology and pathophysiology
   1. Lack of intrinsic factor in the stomach prevents the absorption of vitamin B_{12} in the lower portion of the ileum
   2. Subsequent reduced number of erythrocytes formed, leading to anemia

B. Clinical findings
   1. Subjective
      a. Weakness

b. Sore mouth
c. Paresthesias
d. Dyspnea
   2. Objective
      a. Pallor
      b. Beefy red tongue
      c. Positive Romberg test (loss of balance when eyes closed)
      d. Gastric analysis: no intrinsic factor
      e. Schilling test: urine test for B_{12} absorption

C. Therapeutic intervention: lifelong injections of cyanocobalamin (B_{12})

Nursing Care of Clients with Pernicious Anemia

A. DATA COLLECTION
1. Presence of pallor
2. Presence of beefy tongue
3. Presence of paresthesias

B. ANALYSIS AND INTERPRETATION
Refer to General Nursing Diagnoses for Clients with Circulatory System Disorders for the following diagnoses: A 3 and M

C. PLANNING/IMPLEMENTATION
1. Explain disease process and the need for continued treatment
2. Teach family member(s) how to give IM injections or make referral to visiting nurse

D. EVALUATION/OUTCOMES
1. Verbalizes an understanding of need for long-term therapy
2. Administers IM injection to self correctly

▼ APLASTIC ANEMIA (HYPOPLASTIC ANEMIA)

Data Base

A. Etiology and pathophysiology
   1. Bone marrow is depressed or destroyed by a chemical or drug
   2. Leukopenia, thrombocytopenia, and decreased erythrocytes, agranulocytosis

B. Clinical findings
   1. Subjective
      a. Headache
      b. Weakness
      c. Anorexia
      d. Dyspnea
   2. Objective
      a. Fever
      b. Bleeding from mucous membranes
      c. Decreased leukocytes, erythrocytes, and platelets

C. Therapeutic interventions
   1. Identify and eliminate causative agent
   2. Blood transfusions

3. Maintenance of fluid and electrolyte balance
4. Corticosteroids and androgens to stimulate bone marrow function
5. Splenectomy when enlarged organ destroys normal RBCs
6. Bone marrow transplant if suitable donor is available

Nursing Care of Clients with Aplastic Anemia

A. DATA COLLECTION
1. Detailed history to determine causative agents
2. Baseline temperature
3. Bleeding from mucous membranes

B. ANALYSIS AND INTERPRETATION
Refer to General Nursing Diagnoses for Clients with Circulatory System Disorders for the following diagnoses: A 3, F, and J

C. PLANNING/IMPLEMENTATION
1. Support the client and family in understanding illness
2. Prevent infection by protective isolation
3. Provide blood transfusion therapy as ordered

D. EVALUATION/OUTCOMES
1. Remains afebrile
2. Performs ADL

▼ AUTOIMMUNE THROMBOCYTOPENIC PURPURA

Data Base
A. Etiology and pathophysiology
 1. Appears to result from the production of an antiplatelet antibody, which coats the surface of platelets
 2. Coated platelets are then easily destroyed by phagocytic leukocytes
B. Clinical findings
 1. Subjective
  a. History of epistaxis
  b. History of gum bleeding
 2. Objective
  a. Low platelet count
  b. Ecchymotic areas
  c. Hemorrhagic petechiae
C. Medical interventions
 1. Corticosteroids
 2. Immunosuppressive agents
 3. Splenectomy
 4. Platelet transfusions

Nursing Care of Clients with Autoimmune Thrombocytopenic Purpura

A. DATA COLLECTION
1. History of bleeding and tendency to bruise easily
2. Low energy level and unexplained fatigue

B. ANALYSIS AND INTERPRETATION
Refer to General Nursing Diagnoses for Clients with Circulatory System Disorders for the following diagnoses: G and H

C. PLANNING/IMPLEMENTATION
1. Prevent injury and bruises
2. Encourage client to adhere to medical regimen
3. Teach the side effects of medications, particularly proneness to infection
4. Provide postoperative care related to splenectomy

D. EVALUATION/OUTCOMES
1. Remains injury free
2. Complies with drug regimen
3. Describes signs of bleeding

▼ POLYCYTHEMIA VERA

Data Base
A. Etiology and pathophysiology
 1. A sustained increase in the number of erythrocytes, leukocytes, and platelets
 2. Thought to be associated with a form of malignancy similar to leukemia
B. Clinical findings
 1. Subjective
  a. Headache
  b. Weakness
  c. Itching
 2. Objective
  a. Increased hemoglobin
  b. Purple-red complexion
  c. Dyspnea
C. Therapeutic interventions
 1. Phlebotomy several times yearly
 2. Diet low in iron
 3. Radioactive phosphorus; busulfan (Myleran)

Nursing Care of Clients with Polycythemia Vera

A. DATA COLLECTION
1. History of:
  a. Weakness
  b. Dyspnea
  c. Bleeding from mucous membranes
2. Stasis in lower extremities
3. Presence or absence of pulses in lower extremities

B. ANALYSIS AND INTERPRETATION
Refer to General Nursing Diagnoses for Clients with Circulatory System Disorders for the following diagnoses: R and T 4

C. PLANNING/IMPLEMENTATION
1. Discuss diet with the client and family
2. Provide supportive care and prevent hemorrhage

3. Assist with phlebotomy
4. Instruct client to elevate legs while sitting

D. EVALUATION/OUTCOMES
1. Remains injury free
2. Complies with dietary restrictions
3. Remains under medical supervision
4. Performs activities that support peripheral circulation

▼ AGRANULOCYTOSIS

Data Base

A. Etiology and pathophysiology
1. Results in a decreased number of leukocytes
2. Thought to arise from physical agents (e.g., heavy metals) and cytotoxic drugs
B. Clinical findings
1. Subjective
a. Fatigue
b. Malaise
2. Objective
a. High fever
b. Necrotic ulcers of mucosa
c. Rapid weak pulse
C. Therapeutic interventions
1. Removal of causative agent
2. Transfusions
3. Antibiotics

Nursing Care of Clients with Agranulocytosis

A. DATA COLLECTION
1. Baseline temperature
2. History to determine causative agent
3. Presence of mucosal ulcers
B. ANALYSIS AND INTERPRETATION
Refer to General Nursing Diagnoses for Clients with Circulatory System Disorders for the following diagnoses: J and R
C. PLANNING/IMPLEMENTATION
1. Prevent infection and observe for signs of infection
2. Provide careful oral hygiene
3. Provide for bed rest
4. Encourage diet consisting of high nutrient density foods that are rich in vitamins and minerals
D. EVALUATION/OUTCOMES
1. Remains afebrile
2. Lists warning signs of infection
3. Verbalizes understanding of dietary plan
4. Demonstrates oral hygiene activities

▼ DISSEMINATED INTRAVASCULAR COAGULATION (DIC)

Data Base

A. Etiology and pathophysiology
1. Body's response to injury or disease in which microthrombi obstruct the blood supply of organs
2. Complicated by hemorrhage at various sites throughout the body
B. Clinical findings
1. Subjective
a. Restlessness
b. Anxiety
2. Objective
a. Laboratory tests indicate low fibrinogen and prolonged prothrombin and partial thromboplastin times
b. Hemorrhage, both subcutaneous and internal
C. Therapeutic interventions
1. Goal is to relieve the underlying cause
2. Heparin to prevent the formation of thrombi
3. Transfusion of blood products
4. Antifibrinolytic therapy to prevent bleeding may be necessary

Nursing Care of Clients with Disseminated Intravascular Coagulation

A. DATA COLLECTION
1. History of causative factors (generally septicemia and septic shock)
2. Subcutaneous hemorrhages
B. ANALYSIS AND INTERPRETATION
Refer to General Nursing Diagnoses for Clients with Circulatory System Disorders for the following diagnoses: A 2, C 3, G, and T 2
C. PLANNING/IMPLEMENTATION
1. Observe for bleeding
2. Minimize skin punctures
3. Prevent injury
4. Provide emotional support
D. EVALUATION/OUTCOMES
1. Maintains circulation to all tissues
2. Verbalizes a decrease in fears
3. Maintains adequate cardiac output

▼ LEUKEMIA
See Leukemia in Pediatric Nursing (Chapter 5)

Data Base

A. Etiology and pathophysiology
1. Incidence highest in children ages 3 to 4; declines until age 35, at which point there is a steady increase

2. Etiology unknown, although exposure to certain toxic substances such as radiation seems to increase the incidence
3. In general, an uncontrolled proliferation of white blood cells
4. Classified according to the type of white blood cell affected
   a. Acute lymphocytic leukemia (ALL)
      (1) Primarily occurs in children
      (2) Most favorable prognosis with chemotherapy
      (3) Results from abnormal leukocytes in blood-forming tissue
   b. Acute myelogenous leukemia (AML)
      (1) Occurs throughout life cycle
      (2) Prognosis is poor with or without chemotherapy
      (3) Results from inability of leukocytes to mature; those that do are abnormal
   c. Chronic myelogenous leukemia (CML)
      (1) Occurs after the second decade
      (2) Prognosis is poor
      (3) Results from abnormal production of granulocytic cells
   d. Chronic lymphocytic leukemia (CLL)
      (1) Occurs after age 35 years
      (2) Life expectancy: 4 to 5 years
      (3) Results from increased production of leukocytes and lymphocytes and proliferation of cells within the bone marrow, spleen, and liver
B. Clinical findings
   1. Subjective
      a. Malaise
      b. Bone pain
   2. Objective
      a. Anemia
      b. Thrombocytopenia
      c. Elevated leukocytes
      d. Decreased platelets
      e. Petechiae
      f. Gingival bleeding
C. Therapeutic interventions
   1. Chemotherapy
   2. Transfusions of whole blood or blood fractions
   3. Analgesics
   4. Bone marrow transplant
   5. Radiation to areas of lymphocytic infiltration

Nursing Care of Clients with Leukemia

A. DATA COLLECTION
1. Frequency and severity of the infectious processes
2. Overt and covert bleeding
3. Skin, gums, and urine for bleeding
4. Baseline vital signs observing for signs of anemia, such as increased pulse and respiratory rates and decreased blood pressure

B. ANALYSIS AND INTERPRETATION
Refer to General Nursing Diagnoses for Clients with Circulatory System Disorders for the following diagnoses: F, J, and K

C. PLANNING/IMPLEMENTATION
1. Discuss the importance of follow-up care with the client and family
2. Provide emotional support for the client and family
3. Provide specific nursing care related to particular chemotherapeutic therapy, transfusion, or diagnostic tests
4. Provide a safe injury-free environment
5. Use appropriate infection control techniques
6. Pace care to avoid fatigue and assist client as necessary

D. EVALUATION/OUTCOMES
1. States signs of infection
2. Remains free from bleeding episodes
3. Verbalizes positive feelings about self
4. Verbalizes a decrease in fears
5. Limits activity when fatigued
6. Plans strategies to avoid excess energy expenditure
7. Continues medical supervision

▼ INFECTIOUS MONONUCLEOSIS

Data Base
A. Etiology and pathophysiology
   1. Acute infectious disease of the lymphatic system due to Epstein-Barr (EB) herpesvirus
   2. Transmitted by respiratory droplets
   3. Incubation period is uncertain; probably 28 to 42 days
   4. Incidence highest between ages 15 and 35
   5. Complications include hepatitis, ruptured spleen, pericarditis, and meningoencephalitis
B. Clinical findings
   1. Subjective
      a. Sore throat
      b. Malaise
      c. Stiff neck
      d. Nausea
   2. Objective
      a. Elevated temperature
      b. Enlarged, tender lymph nodes (generally, posterior cervical nodes involved first)
      c. Splenomegaly in approximately 50% of clients
      d. Elevated lymphocyte and monocyte counts
      e. Positive heterophile antibody agglutination test

C. Therapeutic interventions
1. Generally directed toward symptoms (recovery is approximately 3 weeks)
2. ASA; steroids if severely ill
3. If spleen ruptures, splenectomy and blood transfusions

Nursing Care of Clients with Infectious Mononucleosis

A. DATA COLLECTION
1. Temperature for baseline data
2. History of lethargy and fatigue
3. Cervical lymphadenopathy
4. Hepatomegaly
5. Splenomegaly
6. Inflammation of throat—swelling, grayish white exudate on tonsils

B. ANALYSIS AND INTERPRETATION
Refer to General Nursing Diagnoses for Clients with Circulatory System Disorders for the following diagnoses: F and J

C. PLANNING/IMPLEMENTATION
1. Provide rest
2. Administer aspirin as ordered
3. Assess for signs of complications; the spleen should not be palpated once the diagnosis is made
4. Increase fluid intake
5. Support natural defense mechanisms; encourage intake of foods rich in the immune-stimulating nutrients, especially vitamins A, C, and E, and the minerals selenium and zinc

D. EVALUATION/OUTCOMES
1. Reduces fatigue
2. Maintains afebrile state

▼ HODGKIN'S DISEASE

Data Base

A. Etiology and pathophysiology
1. Cause unknown
2. Higher incidence in males and young adults
3. Proliferation of malignant cells (Reed-Sternberg cells) within lymph nodes
4. All tissues may eventually be involved, but chiefly lymph nodes, spleen, liver, tonsils, and bone marrow
5. Classification by staging and the presence or absence of systemic symptoms

B. Clinical findings
1. Subjective
   a. Dyspnea and dysphagia caused by pressure from enlarged nodes
   b. Pruritus
   c. Anorexia

2. Objective
   a. Enlarged lymph nodes (generally cervical nodes are involved first)
   b. Diagnosis confirmed by histologic examination of a lymph node
   c. Progressive anemia
   d. Elevated temperature
   e. Enlarged spleen and liver may occur
   f. Pressure from enlarged lymph nodes may cause symptoms of edema and obstructive jaundice
   g. Thrombocytopenia if spleen and bone marrow involved

C. Therapeutic interventions
1. Staging procedures include: CBC; liver function studies; CT of thorax and abdomen; bone marrow and lymph node biopsies; lymphangiography
2. Radiotherapy
   a. Vital organs must be shielded
   b. Potential side effects
      (1) Nausea
      (2) Skin rashes
      (3) Dry mouth
      (4) Dysphagia
3. Surgical intervention includes excision of masses to relieve pressure on other organs
4. Chemotherapy
   a. MOPP and ABVD protocols
   b. Nitrogen mustard
   c. Thiophosphoramide
   d. Chlorambucil
   e. Vincristine
   f. Doxorubicin (Adriamycin)
   g. Prednisone
   h. Procarbazine hydrochloride
   i. Bleomycin (Blenoxane)
   j. Vinblastine sulfate (Velban)
   k. Dacarbazine

Nursing Care of Clients with Hodgkin's Disease

A. DATA COLLECTION
1. Lymph nodes to determine enlargement
2. Temperature for baseline data
3. Liver and spleen to determine enlargement

B. ANALYSIS AND INTERPRETATION
Refer to General Nursing Diagnoses for Clients with Circulatory System Disorders for the following diagnoses: F, G, J, and M

C. PLANNING/IMPLEMENTATION
1. Provide emotional support for the client and family
2. Protect from infection
3. Monitor temperature

4. Observe for signs of anemia; provide adequate rest
5. Examine sclera and skin for signs of jaundice
6. Encourage high nutrient density foods; observe for anorexia and nausea

D. EVALUATION/OUTCOMES
1. Remains afebrile
2. Conserves energy
3. Verbalizes feelings related to therapy and prognosis
4. Continues medical supervision

▼ LYMPHOSARCOMA

See Hodgkin's Disease for Data Base and Nursing Care

RESPIRATORY SYSTEM

REVIEW OF ANATOMY AND PHYSIOLOGY OF THE RESPIRATORY SYSTEM

Functions of the Respiratory System
A. The upper portion of the respiratory system filters, moistens, and warms air during inspiration
B. The lower portion of the respiratory system enables the exchange of gases between blood and air to regulate serum PO_2, PCO_2, and pH

Structures of the Respiratory System

Nose
A. Structure
  1. Portions
    a. Internal: in skull, above roof of mouth
    b. External: protruding from face
  2. Cavities
    a. Divisions: right and left
    b. Meati: superior, middle, and lower; named for turbinates located above each meatus
    c. Openings
      (1) To exterior: anterior nares
      (2) To nasopharynx: posterior nares
    d. Conchae (turbinates)
      (1) Superior and middle processes of ethmoid bone; interior conchae, separate bones
      (2) Conchae partition each nasal cavity into three passageways or meati
    e. Floor: formed by palatine bones and maxillae; these also act as roof of mouth
  3. Lining: ciliated mucosa
  4. Sinuses draining into the nose (paranasal sinuses)
    a. Frontal

  b. Maxillary (antrum of Highmore)
  c. Sphenoidal
  d. Ethmoidal
B. Functions
  1. Serves as passageway for incoming and outgoing air, filtering, warming, moistening, and chemically examining it
  2. Organ of smell (olfactory receptors located in the nasal mucosa)
  3. Aids in phonation

Pharynx
A. Structure: composed of muscle with mucous lining
  1. Divisions
    a. Nasopharynx: behind the nose
    b. Oropharynx: behind the mouth
    c. Laryngopharynx: behind the larynx
  2. Openings
    a. Nasopharynx has four openings: two auditory (eustachian) tubes and two posterior nares
    b. Oropharynx has one opening: fauces, archway into mouth
    c. Laryngopharynx has two openings: into esophagus and into larynx
  3. Organs in the pharynx
    a. Nasopharynx: nasopharyngeal tonsils (adenoids) and eustachian tubes
    b. Oropharynx: palatine and lingual tonsils
B. Functions
  1. Serves as a passageway and entrance to the respiratory and digestive tracts
  2. Aids in phonation
  3. Tonsils function to destroy incoming bacteria and detoxify certain foreign proteins

Larynx
A. Location: at upper end of the trachea, just below the pharynx
B. Structure
  1. Cartilages: nine pieces arranged in a boxlike formation; thyroid cartilage is the largest (called the Adam's apple); epiglottis (the lid cartilage); cricoid (the signet ring cartilage)
  2. Vocal cords
    a. False cords: folds of mucous lining
    b. True cords: fibroelastic bands stretched across the hollow interior of the larynx; the paired vocal cords (folds) and the posterior arytenoid cartilages make up the glottis; the slit between the vocal cords, through which air enters and leaves the lower respiratory passages, is the rima glottidis
  3. Lining: ciliated mucosa
C. Functions
  1. Voice production: during expiration, air passing through the larynx causes the vocal cords

to vibrate; short, tense cords produce a high pitch; long, relaxed cords, a low pitch
2. Serves as part of the passageway for air and as the entrance to the lower respiratory tract

Trachea

A. Structure
   1. Walls: smooth muscle; contain C-shaped rings of cartilage at intervals; these keep the tube open at all times but do not constrict the esophagus, which is directly behind the trachea
   2. Lining: ciliated mucosa
   3. Extent: from the larynx to the bronchi; 10 to 11 cm long
B. Function: furnishes open passageway for air going to and from lungs

Lungs

A. Structure
   1. Size: large enough to fill pleural divisions of thoracic cavity
   2. Shape: cone, base downward
   3. Location: in pleural divisions of thorax; extend from slightly above clavicle to diaphragm; base of each lung rests on diaphragm
   4. Divisions
      a. Lobes: three in the right lung, two in the left
      b. Root: consists of the primary bronchus and pulmonary artery and veins bound together by connective tissue
      c. Hilum: vertical slit on medial surface of the lung, through which root structures enter the lung
      d. Apex: pointed upper part of the lung
      e. Base: broad, inferior surface of the lung
   5. Bronchial tree: consists of the following:
      a. Bronchi: right and left, formed by branching of the trachea; right bronchus slightly larger and more vertical than left; each primary bronchus branches, on entering the lung, into 10 segmental bronchi in each lung; primary and segmental bronchi all contain C-shaped cartilage
      b. Bronchioles: small branches off the secondary bronchi; distinguished by lack of C-shaped cartilage and a duct diameter of about 1 mm
      c. Terminal bronchioles: last ones possess a ciliated mucosa
      d. Respiratory bronchioles: composed of cuboidal nonciliated cells
      e. Alveolar ducts: microscopic branches off bronchioles composed of a thin squamous epithelium
      f. Alveoli: microscopic sacs composed of a single layer of extremely thin squamous epithelial cells; each alveolar duct termi-

nates in a cluster of alveoli, often likened to a bunch of grapes; each alveolus enveloped by a network of lung capillaries
      6. Covering of lung: visceral layer of pleura
B. Function: place where air and blood can come in close enough contact for rapid diffusion of gases to occur
   1. Bronchi, bronchioles, alveolar ducts: lower part of airway through which air moves into and out of alveoli
   2. Alveoli: microscopic sacs in which gases are exchanged rapidly between the air and blood; membranous walls of the millions of alveoli provide a surface area large enough and thin enough to make possible rapid gas exchange
   3. Alveolar surfaces coated with group of substances called surfactant; effect is to lower alveolar surface tension to facilitate breathing, since sacs have less tendency to collapse with their walls adhering to each other

Physiology of Respiration

A. Mechanism of inspiration
   1. Respiratory muscles contract
   2. Thorax increases in size
   3. Intrathoracic pressure decreases
   4. Lungs increase in size
   5. Intrapulmonic pressure decreases
   6. Air rushes from positive pressure in the atmosphere to negative pressure in the alveoli
   7. Inspiration is completed
B. Mechanism of expiration
   1. Respiratory muscles relax
   2. Thorax decreases in size
   3. Intrathoracic pressure increases
   4. Lungs decrease in size
   5. Intrapulmonic pressure increases
   6. Air expelled from higher pressure in the lung to lower pressure in the atmosphere
   7. Expiration is completed
C. Neural control
   1. Alveolar stretch receptors respond to inspiration (lung inflation) by sending inhibitory impulses to inspiratory neurons in brainstem; this is the Hering-Breuer inflation reflex, and it prevents lung overdistention
   2. During expiration (lung deflation) the stretch receptors no longer inhibit inspiratory neurons, and inspiration may begin again; this is the Hering-Breuer deflation reflex
D. Chemical control
   1. Blood pH: decrease in pH stimulates respiration by direct stimulation of neurons of respiratory center and indirectly by stimulation of carotid and aortic chemoreceptors

2. Blood PCO_2: increase in arterial PCO_2 results in decrease in pH and mimics effects in no.1 above

3. Blood PO_2: decrease in arterial PO_2 produces effects similar to decreased blood pH

4. Stimulation of respiratory center neurons or chemoreceptors results in hyperventilation; hypoventilation occurs when the arterial pH rises or the arterial PCO_2 falls

E. Amount of air exchanged in breathing
   1. Directly related to gas pressure gradient between atmosphere and alveoli and inversely related to resistance opposing air flow; the greater the difference between atmospheric pressure and alveolar pressure, the greater the amount of air exchanged in breathing; the greater the resistance opposing air flow to or from the lungs, the less air exchanged
   2. Measured by apparatus called a spirometer
   3. Tidal volume: average amount expired after normal inspiration; approximately 500 ml
   4. Expiratory reserve volume (ERV): largest additional volume of air that can be forcibly expired after a normal inspiration and expiration; normal ERV 1000 to 1200 ml
   5. Inspiratory reserve volume (IRV): largest additional volume of air that can be forcibly inspired after a normal inspiration; normal IRV 3000 to 3300 ml
   6. Residual volume: air that cannot be forcibly expired from lungs; about 1200 ml
   7. Minimal air: air that can never be removed from alveoli if they have been inflated even once, even though lungs are subjected to atmospheric pressure that squeezes part of residual air out
   8. Vital capacity: approximate capacity of lungs as measured by amount of air that can be forcibly expired after forcible inspiration; varies with size of thoracic cavity, which is determined by various factors (e.g., size of rib cage, posture, volume of blood and interstitial fluid in the lungs, size of the heart)
   9. Forced expiratory flow rate: an individual should be able to exhale 70% of vital capacity in the first second and empty more than 90% in 3 seconds; asthma and emphysema prevent such normal, forced expiratory rates; measurable with a spirometer; the forced expiratory volume (FEV) can also be measured for a specified time

F. Diffusion of gases between air and blood occurs across alveolar-capillary membranes (i.e., in lungs between air in alveoli and venous blood in lung capillaries)
   1. Direction of diffusion
      a. Oxygen: net diffusion toward lower oxygen pressure gradient (i.e., from alveolar air to blood)

      b. Carbon dioxide: net diffusion toward lower carbon dioxide pressure gradient (i.e., from blood to alveolar air)
   2. Mechanism of oxygen diffusion (Fig. 6-10)
   3. Mechanism of carbon dioxide diffusion (Fig. 6-11)

G. How blood transports oxygen
   1. As solute: about 0.5 ml of oxygen is dissolved in 100 ml of blood; produces the blood PO_2 (pressure of oxygen in the blood)

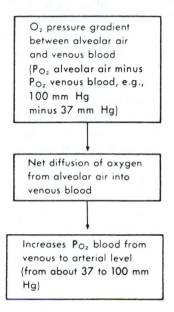

FIGURE 6-10 Mechanism of oxygen diffusion.

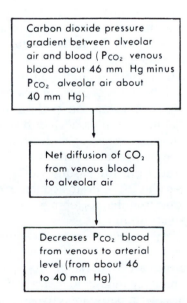

FIGURE 6-11 Mechanism of carbon dioxide diffusion.

2. As oxyhemoglobin: each gram of hemoglobin can combine with 1.34 ml of oxygen; hence, with normal hemoglobin content (e.g., 15 g/100 ml of blood) and 100% oxygen saturation, about 20 ml (15×1.34) of oxygen is transported as oxyhemoglobin

3. Various factors influence rate at which oxygen associates with hemoglobin to form oxyhemoglobin, including:
   a. Increasing pressure of oxygen in the blood
   b. Decreasing pressure of carbon dioxide in the blood

4. Various factors influence the rate at which oxygen dissociates from hemoglobin, including:
   a. Decreasing pressure of oxygen in the blood
   b. Increasing pressure of carbon dioxide in the blood
   c. Increased blood temperature

H. How blood transports carbon dioxide
   1. As solute: small amount dissolves in plasma
   2. As bicarbonate ion: more than half of carbon dioxide in blood is present in the plasma as bicarbonate ion (HCO_3^-) formed by ionization of carbonic acid
   3. As carbhemoglobin: less than one third of carbon dioxide is transported in combination with hemoglobin

I. Diffusion of gases between arterial blood and tissues occurs in tissue capillaries
   1. Oxygen: net diffusion of dissolved oxygen out of the blood into the tissues because of lower PO_2 there (perhaps 30 mm Hg, compared to arterial PO_2 of 100 mm Hg); diffusion of dissolved oxygen out of the blood lowers blood PO_2 from arterial to venous level (from 100 to 40 mm Hg); decreasing PO_2 as the blood moves through tissue capillaries causes oxygen to dissociate from hemoglobin, thereby releasing more oxygen for diffusion out of the blood to the tissue cells
   2. Carbon dioxide: net diffusion of carbon dioxide into the blood because of lower PCO_2 there (40 mm Hg compared with probably more than 50 mm Hg in tissues); diffusion of carbon dioxide into tissue capillaries increases blood PCO_2 from arterial to venous level (from 40 to 46 mm Hg); increasing PCO_2, similar to decreasing PO_2, tends to accelerate oxygen dissociation from hemoglobin

J. Normal breath sounds
   1. Bronchial sounds (over trachea, bronchi)
      a. Result of air passing through larger airways
      b. Sounds are loud, harsh, high pitched
      c. Expiratory phase longer than inspiratory phase with pause in between

2. Vesicular sounds (over entire lung field except large airways)
   a. Result of air moving in and out of alveoli; may reflect sound of air in larger passages that is transmitted through lung tissue
   b. Sounds are quiet, low pitched
   c. Inspiratory phase much longer than expiratory phase

3. Bronchovesicular sounds (near main stem bronchi)
   a. Result of air moving through smaller air passages
   b. Sounds are moderately pitched, breezy
   c. Inspiratory and expiratory phases equal

K. Adventitious breath sounds
   1. Crackles (rales)
      a. Result of air passing through fluid in small airways and alveoli
      b. Sound may be simulated by rubbing a few strands of hair between fingers next to ear
      c. Most common during inspiratory phase
      d. Associated with conditions such as COPD and pulmonary edema
   2. Wheezes
      a. Result of air passing through narrowed small airways
      b. Sounds are high pitched, musical, or rumbling (sonorous rhonchi)
      c. Most common on expiration
      d. Associated with conditions causing narrowing of airways, such as asthma, and with conditions that involve partial obstruction of airway by mucus, foreign body, or tumor
   3. Pleural friction rub
      a. Result of roughened pleural surfaces rubbing across each other
      b. Sounds are crackling, grating
      c. Associated with conditions causing inflammation of the pleura

REVIEW OF PHYSICAL PRINCIPLES RELATED TO THE RESPIRATORY SYSTEM

Principles of Mechanics
Law of Gravitation
EXAMPLES

1. Postural drainage: positioning the client so the throat is below the level of the lungs to help drain fluid from the lungs
2. Rocking beds: abdominal viscera alternately push against and then away from the diaphragm, thus aiding in respiration
3. Position of the head postoperatively: head is placed on one side; thus, the force of gravity pulls the tongue down, breathing remains unobstructed and allows for drainage in case of vomiting

4. Use of chest tubes without suction to restore negative pressure to intrapleural space

Momentum
EXAMPLES
1. During a cough or a sneeze, the abdominal and intercostal muscles apply a large force on the air in the lungs; the sudden opening of the vocal cords and epiglottis results in the explosive propulsion of air from the lungs; in this case momentum of the air stream is great, not because of the mass of the particles (since the molecules of gases in air are light), but because of their high velocity
2. When a person speaks, the vocal cords vibrate and in turn produce vibrations in the air molecules surrounding them; the momentum in these vibrating molecules is transferred from air molecule to air molecule all the way to the ear of the listener, where the vibrations are converted into nerve impulses that the brain interprets as sound

Energy
EXAMPLES
1. Epithelial cells of the human respiratory tract possess energy because their cilia beat back and forth and thus do the work of pushing mucus and foreign matter up toward the throat
2. Every living cell in the body possesses energy because it does work to maintain certain water and electrolyte concentrations within itself
3. The cilia exert a force that moves them through a certain distance in the fluid surrounding them
4. The cell membranes exert a force that moves ions a certain distance through the membrane
5. First law of thermodynamics

Principles of Physical Properties of Matter
Solids
Concept of elasticity

EXAMPLE: The elastic recoil of the lungs during quiet respiration provides the entire force necessary to affect expiration

Liquids
Surface tension: molecules of a liquid exert forces of attraction on one another; at the surface of the liquid the molecules are attracted by other molecules at the bottom and sides, but not at the top since air is there; this results in a force of contraction at the liquid surface called surface tension

EXAMPLE: The alveoli and respiratory passages of the human lungs have a mixture of surface tension–reducing substances collectively called surfactant that reduce surface tension and the pull that the water molecules would ordinarily have on each other if these surface active agents were absent; breathing is therefore much easier because of this agent

Gases
The molecules composing gases are so far apart that they do not exert any cohesive forces on each other; consequently, the gas will expand to fill any container and will exert pressure on the container because of elastic rebound of the gas molecules with the walls of the container

A. Boyle's law: at constant temperature the pressure exerted by a gas is inversely proportional to its volume; as the volume of a gas is decreased, its pressure increases, and as the volume is increased, the pressure decreases
   1. Respiration: contraction and downward movements of the dome-shaped diaphragm increase the volume of the thoracic cavity containing the lungs; since the volume of air in the lungs is increased, the pressure exerted by the air is decreased; air now flows from the area of higher pressure outside body to the area of lower pressure inside lungs; conversely, during expiration, the upward movement of the diaphragm and the elastic recoil of the lungs themselves decrease the volume of air in the thoracic cavity and lungs as air flows out
   2. Pneumothorax: opening that connects the outside air with the intrapleural space; result is that air flows into the intrapleural space; this eliminates the pressure gradient between the thoracic cavity and the atmosphere, and the lungs cannot inflate
   3. Intermittent positive pressure breathing (IPPB) apparatus: special valve is operated by the individual's own respirations; on inspiration, one part of the valve opens and oxygen or a mixture of gases is forcefully pushed under greater-than-atmospheric pressure (positive pressure) into the lungs through a special mouthpiece or face mask
B. Dalton's law: pressure exerted (in millimeters of mercury [mm Hg]) by a gas in a mixture of gases is proportional to its percentage in the mixture; e.g., partial pressure of oxygen (O_2) in alveoli is 104 mm Hg; partial pressure of O_2 in pulmonary artery and alveolar capillaries is 40 mm Hg; therefore O_2 diffuses from alveoli air sacs into capillaries
C. Henry's law: quantity of gas dissolving in a liquid is proportional to the partial pressure of the gas at a given temperature; that is, a person overcome by smoke inhalation or who has some obstruction to normal breathing can benefit from inhalation of either pure O_2 or a mixture of gases having a higher partial pressure of O_2 than is found in air
D. Bernoulli's principle: moving air exerts less pressure than motionless air

Principles of Light

A. X-rays use high-frequency electromagnetic waves
    EXAMPLE: The chest x-ray examination permits observation of a variety of lung disorders, such as pneumonia, tumors, and tuberculosis

B. Total internal reflection: at a certain critical angle, light between two media is not refracted (bent) through the media but is reflected back into the first medium, provided the first medium is more dense than the second medium
    EXAMPLE: Fiberoptics allow illumination and visualization of trachea and bronchi (bronchoscopy); the image picked up by the lens internally reflects along fiberoptic tubing (even if bent) until it reaches the eye of the observer

REVIEW OF CHEMICAL PRINCIPLES RELATED TO THE RESPIRATORY SYSTEM

(See Fluid, Electrolyte, and Acid-Base Balance)

REVIEW OF MICROORGANISMS RELATED TO THE RESPIRATORY SYSTEM

A. Bacterial pathogens
   1. *Bordetella pertussis*: small, gram-negative coccobacillus; causes pertussis or whooping cough
   2. *Streptococcus pneumoniae*: gram-positive, encapsulated diplococcus; on the basis of the antigenic nature of the capsule, there are about 100 types, the most important being types I, II, and III; causes pneumococcal pneumonia (most commonly lobar) and often responsible for sinusitis, otitis media, and meningitis
   3. *Haemophilus influenzae*: small, gram-negative, highly pleomorphic bacillus; causes acute meningitis and upper respiratory tract infections
   4. *Klebsiella pneumoniae* (Friedlander's bacillus): gram–negative, encapsulated, nonspore-forming bacillus; causes pneumonia and urinary tract infections
   5. *Mycobacterium tuberculosis* (tubercle bacillus): acid-fast actinomycete (thin, waxy rods, often bent, nonmotile, nonspore-forming); causes tuberculosis
   6. *Pseudomonas aeruginosa*: gram-negative, non–spore-forming bacillus; important cause of hospital-acquired infections; respiratory equipment can be source; causes pneumonia, urinary tract infections, and the sepsis that complicates severe burns

B. Rickettsial pathogen: *Coxiella burnetii*: only Rickettsiae species not associated with a vector; causes Q fever, an infection clinically similar to primary atypical pneumonia

C. Viral pathogens
   1. DNA viruses
      Adenoviruses: spheric, 70 to 80 nm in diameter; cause acute respiratory tract disease, adenitis, pharyngitis, and other respiratory tract infections, as well as conjunctivitis
   2. RNA viruses
      a. Coronaviruses: enveloped pleomorphic viruses; frequently associated with a mild upper respiratory tract infection
      b. Picornaviruses: spheric and 20 to 30 nm in diameter; cause poliomyelitis, coxsackie disease, common cold, and various diseases of animals
      c. Reoviruses: double-stranded RNA virus involved in mild respiratory tract infections of humans

D. Fungal pathogen: *Histoplasma capsulatum*: dimorphic fungus producing characteristic spores (chlamydospores) in infected tissue; causes histoplasmosis (a primary lung infection)

E. Protozoan pathogen: *Pneumocystis carinii*: a unicellular protozoan thought to be transmitted by airborne droplets

PHARMACOLOGY RELATED TO RESPIRATORY SYSTEM DISORDERS

Bronchodilators

A. Description
   1. Used to reverse bronchoconstriction, thus opening air passages in the lungs
   2. Act by:
      a. Stimulating beta-adrenergic sympathetic nervous system receptors
      b. Directly relaxing bronchial smooth muscle
   3. Available in oral, parenteral (IM, SC, IV), rectal, and inhalation preparations

B. Examples
   1. Adrenergics: act at beta-adrenergic receptors in bronchus to relax smooth muscle and increase respiratory volume
      a. Albuterol
      b. Epinephrine HCl (Adrenalin)
      c. Ephedrine sulfate (Neorespin)
      d. Isoproterenol HCl (Isuprel)
      e. Metaproterenol sulfate
      f. Pseudoephedrine HCl (Sudafed)
      g. Terbutaline sulfate (Brethine)
   2. Xanthines: act directly on bronchial smooth muscle, decreasing spasm and relaxing smooth muscle of the vasculature
      a. Aminophylline
      b. Oxtriphylline (Choledyl)
      c. Theophylline (Theo-Dur)

3. Combination products
   a. Actifed
   b. Dristan
   c. Marax
   d. Sinutab
   e. Tedral
   f. Triaminic

C. Major side effects
   1. Dizziness (decrease in blood pressure)
   2. CNS stimulation (sympathetic stimulation)
   3. Palpitations (beta-adrenergic stimulation)
   4. Gastric irritation (local effect)

D. Nursing care
   1. Avoid administration to clients with hypertension, hyperthyroidism, and cardiovascular dysfunction
   2. Avoid concurrent administration of CNS stimulants (adrenergics) and bronchoconstricting agents (beta blockers)
   3. Administer during waking hours
   4. Encourage clients to avoid smoking
   5. Assess vital signs, especially respirations
   6. Assess intake and output
   7. Administer with food
   8. Evaluate client's response to medication and understanding of teaching

Mucolytic Agents and Expectorants

A. Description
   1. Used to liquify secretions in the respiratory tract, thus promoting a productive cough
   2. Mucolytics act directly to break up mucous plugs in the tracheobronchial passages
   3. Expectorants act indirectly to liquify mucus by increasing respiratory tract secretions via oral absorption
   4. Mucolytic agents are available in inhalation preparations; expectorants are available in oral preparations

B. Examples
   1. Mucolytic: acetylcysteine (Mucomyst)
   2. Expectorants
      a. Ammonium chloride
      b. Guaifenesin (Robitussin)
      c. Potassium iodide (SSKI)

C. Major side effects
   1. Gastrointestinal irritation (local effect)
   2. Skin rash (hypersensitivity)
   3. Oropharyngeal irritation (mucolytics)
   4. Bronchospasm (mucolytics) (hypersensitivity)

D. Nursing care
   1. Promote adequate fluid intake
   2. Encourage coughing and deep breathing
   3. Avoid administering fluids immediately after taking expectorants

4. Assess respiratory status
5. Have suction apparatus available
6. Evaluate client's response to medication and understanding of teaching

Antitussives

A. Description
   1. Used to suppress the cough reflex
   2. Act by inhibiting the cough reflex either by direct action on the medullary cough center or by indirect action peripherally on sensory nerve endings
   3. Available in oral preparations

B. Examples
   1. Narcotic
      a. Codeine
      b. Hydrocodone bitartrate (Hycodan)
      c. Hydromorphone HCl (Dilaudid cough syrup)
   2. Nonnarcotic
      a. Benzonatate (Tessalon)
      b. Dextromethorphan hydrobromide
      c. Diphenhydramine HCl (Benadryl)

C. Major side effects
   1. Drowsiness (CNS depression)
   2. Nausea (GI irritation)
   3. Dry mouth (anticholinergic effect of antihistamine in combination products)

D. Nursing care
   1. Provide adequate fluid intake
   2. Avoid administering fluids immediately after liquid preparations
   3. Encourage high-Fowler's position
   4. Avoid use postoperatively and in clients with head injury
   5. Administer narcotics cautiously
      a. Avoid administration with CNS depressants
      b. Caution client to avoid engaging in hazardous activity
      c. Assess for signs of dependence
   6. Evaluate client's response to medication and understanding of teaching

Narcotic Antagonists

See Substance-Related Disorders in Psychiatric/Mental Health Nursing (Chapter 4)

A. Description
   1. Used to reverse respiratory depression caused by narcotic overdosage
   2. Act to displace narcotics at respiratory receptor sites via competitive antagonism
   3. Available in parenteral (IV, SC, IM) preparations

B. Examples
   1. Levallorphan tartrate (Lorfan)
   2. Naloxone HCl (Narcan)

C. Major side effects
   1. CNS depression (acts on opioid receptors in CNS)

2. Nausea, vomiting
3. Pupillary constriction
D. Nursing care
   1. Assess vital signs, especially respirations
   2. Have O_2 and emergency resuscitative equipment available
   3. Avoid use in cases of nonnarcotic respiratory depression
   4. Evaluate client's response to medication and understanding of teaching

Antihistamines

A. Description
   1. Used to relieve symptoms of the common cold and allergies, which are mediated by the chemical histamine
   2. Act by blocking the action of histamine at receptor sites via competitive inhibition; they also exert antiemetic, anticholinergic, and CNS depressant effects
   3. Available in oral and parenteral (IM, IV, SC) preparations
B. Examples
   1. Brompheniramine maleate (Dimetane)
   2. Chlorpheniramine maleate (Chlor-Trimeton)
   3. Diphenhydramine HCl (Benadryl)
   4. Promethazine HCl (Phenergan)
   5. Combination products
      a. Allerest
      b. Drixoral
      c. Ornade
      d. Triaminic
C. Major side effects
   1. Drowsiness (CNS depression)
   2. Dizziness (CNS depression)
   3. Gastrointestinal irritation (local effect)
   4. Dry mouth (anticholinergic effect of decreased salivation)
   5. Excitement (in children) (paradoxic effect)
D. Nursing care
   1. Avoid administration with CNS depressants
   2. Caution client to avoid engaging in hazardous activities
   3. Administer with food or milk to avoid GI irritation
   4. Offer gum or hard candy to promote salivation
   5. Evaluate client's response to medication and understanding of teaching

PROCEDURES RELATED TO THE RESPIRATORY SYSTEM

Abdominal Thrust (Heimlich Maneuver)

A. Definition: short, abrupt pressure against the abdomen (halfway between the umbilicus and xiphoid) to raise intrarespiratory pressure, which

will dislodge an obstruction such as a bolus of food or a foreign body
B. Symptoms of obstruction
   1. Partial: noisy respiration, dyspnea, lightheadedness, dizziness, flushing of face, bulging of eyes, repeated coughing
   2. Total: cessation of breathing, inability to speak or cough, extension of head, facial cyanosis, bulging of eyes, panic, unconsciousness
C. Nursing care
   1. Assess client no longer than 3 to 5 seconds
      a. Ask if client is choking
      b. Determine if victim can speak or cough
      c. Observe for universal choking sign (thumb and forefinger encircling throat under chin)
      d. Assess for respirations (particularly in unconscious victim)
         (1) Observe for rise and fall of chest
         (2) Listen for escape of air from nose and mouth on expiration
         (3) Feel for flow of air from nose and mouth on expiration
   2. Initiate intervention in the presence of a partial obstruction
      a. Allow the individual's expulsive cough to dislodge the obstruction
      b. Assess for signs of total obstruction
      c. Remove foreign bodies coughed up into the mouth
   3. Initiate intervention in the presence of a total obstruction
      a. Open the individual's mouth and remove the obstruction if possible
      b. Standing behind the conscious victim, encircle the hypochondrium and thrust upward and inward against the diaphragm with intertwined clenched fists
      c. Straddling the hips of the unconscious supine victim, place the heel of one hand on the other and thrust upward and inward against the diaphragm; activate emergency medical service (EMS) system
      d. Repeat abdominal thrust several times (may require 6 to 10 thrusts) until foreign body is dislodged or until help arrives
      e. Determine patency of airway; remove foreign objects from mouth; attempt rescue breathing
      f. Continue pattern of abdominal thrusts if breathing is not reestablished
      g. If an airway cannot be established, an emergency cricothyrotomy may be necessary
      h. Assess for signs of injury to liver or spleen; there is a higher risk when abdominal thrusts are performed with the victim in recumbent position
   4. Evaluate client's response to procedure

Administration of Oxygen

A. Definition
1. Administration of supplemental oxygen when the client's respiratory system is compromised and tissue hypoxia is threatened
2. May be accomplished via a catheter, cannula, mask, or tent

B. Nursing care
1. Explain the procedure to the client and family
2. Attach "oxygen in use" signs to door of room and instruct the client and visitors not to smoke
3. Assess the client's color (nail beds, general appearance) and vital signs before and during therapy
4. Ascertain that client does not have chronic lung disease before administering high concentrations of oxygen
5. Attach appropriate apparatus to the oxygen source and fill the humidification canister prn with water to prevent drying of mucous membranes
6. Evaluate client's response to procedure

Arterial Blood Gases

A. Definition: measurement of arterial pH, partial pressures of oxygen and carbon dioxide, bicarbonate ion, and oxygen saturation (see Acid-Base Balance)

B. Nursing care
1. Explain procedure to the client
2. Obtain a heparinized syringe or vacuum container tube
3. Notify the laboratory to calibrate equipment
4. Aseptically obtain approximately 3 ml of arterial blood; most common sites include the radial, brachial, and femoral arteries
5. Avoid introducing room air into the syringe, for this can alter results
6. Apply pressure over the arterial site for 5 minutes after the needle is removed to prevent bleeding
7. Place the specimen in ice to decrease the metabolic rate of blood cells and subsequent alteration of values; transport promptly to the laboratory
8. Evaluate client's response to procedure

Bronchoscopy

A. Definition
1. Visualization of the tracheobronchial tree via a scope advanced through the mouth or nose into the bronchi
2. Procedure may be performed to remove foreign body, to remove secretions, or to obtain specimens of tissue or mucus for further study

B. Nursing care
1. Obtain an informed consent
2. Maintain the client NPO before procedure and remove dentures and jewelry
3. Administer ordered preprocedure medications to produce sedation and decrease anxiety
4. Inform client to expect some hemoptysis after the procedure
5. Advise client to avoid coughing or clearing throat
6. Observe the client for signs of hemorrhage and/or respiratory distress
7. Monitor vital signs until stable
8. Do not allow the client to drink until the gag reflex returns
9. Evaluate client's response to procedure

Chest Tubes

A. Definition
1. Use of tubes and suction to return negative pressure to the intrapleural space
2. To drain air from the intrapleural space, the chest tube is placed in the second or third intercostal space; to drain blood or fluid, the catheter would be placed at a lower site, usually the eighth or ninth intercostal space

B. Types of drainage systems
1. One-chamber underwater system: allows air or fluid to drain from the pleural cavity by gravity; a glass rod, which extends approximately 2 cm below the surface of the water within the collection bottle, provides the water seal
2. Two-chamber drainage system: involves one bottle that acts as a collection chamber and provides the water seal while a second bottle can be connected to a suction apparatus; the bubbling of water within the second bottle indicates that the desired suction is maintained
3. Three-chamber system: includes one bottle that serves to collect drainage, one that acts as the water-seal chamber, and one that controls suction
4. Commercially prepared plastic unit designed for closed chest suction: combines the features of the other systems and may or may not be attached to suction (e.g., PleurEvac)

C. Nursing care
1. Ensure that the tubing is not kinked; tape all connections to prevent separation
2. Gently milk the tubing, if ordered, in the direction of the drainage system to maintain patency; milking can cause a pneumothorax
3. Maintain the drainage system below the level of the chest
4. Turn the client frequently, making sure the chest tubes are not compressed
5. Report drainage on dressing immediately, because this is not a normal occurrence

6. Observe for fluctuation of fluid in tube; the level will rise on inhalation and fall on exhalation; if there are no fluctuations, either the lung has expanded fully or the chest tube is clogged

7. Palpate the area around the chest tube insertion site for subcutaneous emphysema or crepitus, which indicates that air is leaking into the subcutaneous tissue

8. Situate the drainage system to avoid breakage

9. Place two clamps at the bedside for use if the underwater–seal bottle is broken; clamp the chest tube immediately to prevent air from entering the intrapleural space, which would cause pneumothorax to occur or extend; clamps are used judiciously and only in emergency situations

10. Encourage coughing and deep breathing every 2 hours, splinting the area as needed

11. Instruct the client to exhale or strain (Valsalva's maneuver) as the tube is withdrawn by the physician; apply a gauze dressing immediately and firmly secure with tape to make an airtight dressing

12. Encourage movement of the arm on the affected side

13. Evaluate client's response to procedure

Incentive Spirometry

A. Purpose
   1. Mechanical device used to maximize inspiration
   2. Prevents atelectasis
   3. Mobilizes secretions
B. Nursing care
   1. Verify predetermined volume; set at 500 ml and progressively increase
   2. Instruct client to use lips to form a seal around the mouthpiece
   3. Have client inspire deeply and hold the inspiration a few seconds before completely expelling the air
   4. Explain that the machine provides feedback only when preset volume is reached; feedback may be a light or a rising ball depending on the specific device
   5. Avoid spirometry at mealtime to prevent nausea
   6. Evaluate client's response to procedure

Mechanical Ventilation

A. Definition: use of a mechanical device to instill a mixture of air and oxygen into the lungs using positive pressure
B. Types of ventilators
   1. Volume control: delivers a preset tidal volume at various pressures

2. Pressure control: delivers preset pressure at various volumes
C. Modes of ventilation
   1. Controlled mandatory ventilation (CMV): the client receives a specified volume at a specific pressure with no triggering of the machine by the client; the nurse may have to administer drugs such as pancuronium bromide (Pavulon) or morphine to decrease the client's own respiratory response; rarely used
   2. Assist control ventilation (ACV): the client triggers the machine so that the rate may vary; however, if the client has periods of apnea, the machine will take over initiation of respirations at a preset tidal volume
   3. Intermittent mandatory ventilation (IMV): the client receives a predetermined number of breaths per minute with a specified tidal volume; the rate is low so that the client controls the respiratory rate and depth between mechanical ventilations; can be gradually reduced as a client is weaned from the ventilator
   4. Synchronized intermittent mandatory ventilation (SIMV): same as IMV but the ventilator-triggered breaths are synchronized with the client's own breaths; often used for weaning
   5. Pressure support ventilation (PSV): the client initiates all breaths, which are then supplemented by positive pressure, improving the tidal volume and reducing respiratory efforts; may be used alone or with IMV/SIMV
   6. Positive end expiratory pressure (PEEP): maintains positive pressure at the end of expiration to keep alveoli open, increasing the functional residual capacity (FRC)
   7. Continuous positive airway pressure (CPAP): similar to PEEP but exerts positive pressure throughout the respiratory cycle; the client must be breathing spontaneously; may be used without intubation or mechanical ventilation
D. Nursing care
   1. Keep the respirator at settings as ordered and notify the respiratory therapy department and the physician if distress occurs
   2. Maintain a sealed system between the respirator and the client so that volume to be delivered is kept constant and air is not lost around the tubing; this is accomplished by inflating the cuff of the endotracheal tube or tracheostomy tube to the minimum occlusive volume
   3. Perform suction as necessary, because humidified oxygen helps to liquefy secretions that must be removed
   4. Observe for signs of respiratory insufficiency, such as tachypnea, cyanosis, and changes in sensorium

5. Ascertain blood gases as ordered to determine effectiveness of ventilation
6. Establish a means of communication because client will be unable to speak while on a ventilator
7. Evaluate client's response to procedure; revise plan as necessary

Pulmonary Function Tests

A. Definition
   1. Series of tests used to detect problems in the performance capabilities of the pulmonary system
   2. A spirometer is used to measure amounts of gas exchanged between the client and the atmosphere; nose clips are used to allow only mouth breathing and prevent air leakage
   3. Measurement studies include:
      a. Tidal volume: amount of air inhaled or exhaled during one respiration
      b. Vital capacity: volume of air that can be forcefully exhaled after a maximum inspiration
      c. Total lung capacity: volume of air in the lungs following a maximum inspiration
      d. Forced expiratory volume (FEV): volume of air that can be forcefully exhaled within a specific amount of time, usually 1, 2, or 3 seconds
B. Nursing care
   1. Explain procedure to the client to allay anxiety and promote compliance at time of test
   2. Notify the respiratory therapist of all medications the client is receiving that affect respiratory function
   3. Evaluate client's response to procedure

Pulse Oximetry

A. Definition: noninvasive, continuous monitoring of arterial oxygen saturation by use of red and infrared light beams and a photodetector to determine relative light absorption
B. Nursing care
   1. Explain procedure to the client
   2. Select the appropriate transducer or sensor (adult finger or nasal transducer, neonatal foot or infant toe transducer, or pediatric finger transducer)
   3. Apply transducer to extremity and maintain at heart level; do not select an extremity that has any impediment to blood flow (blood pressure cuff or arterial line)
   4. Check the preset alarm for oxygen saturation and pulse rate
   5. Evaluate client's response to procedure

Sputum Studies

A. Definition: analysis of sputum for pathogenic bacteria or tumor cells
   1. Culture and sensitivity: identification of bacteria and appropriate antibiotic therapy; the specimen should be obtained before institution of antibiotic therapy
   2. Acid-fast bacillus (AFB): staining technique to identify bacilli as acid fast, generally indicative of *Mycobacterium tuberculosis*
   3. Cytology: microscopic examination of pulmonary epithelial cells that have sloughed off into the sputum; performed when malignancy is suspected
B. Nursing care
   1. Collect specimen in the early morning before client has food or fluid; can also be obtained after an aerosol treatment
   2. Have client rinse mouth with water to decrease contamination of specimen with oropharyngeal microorganisms
   3. Instruct client to take several deep breaths and cough deeply to raise sputum and expectorate into a sterile specimen container; care must be taken to avoid touching the inside of the container
   4. Transport specimen to laboratory promptly
   5. Offer oral hygiene after collection to eliminate unpleasant taste of sputum
   6. Evaluate client's response

Suctioning of Airway

A. Definition
   1. Mechanical aspiration of mucous secretions from the tracheobronchial tree by application of negative pressure
   2. Used to maintain a patent airway, obtain a sputum specimen, or stimulate coughing
   3. May be nasotracheal, oropharyngeal, or through an endotracheal or tracheostomy tube
B. Nursing care
   1. Maintain surgical asepsis
   2. Assess proper functioning of the equipment
   3. Hyperoxygenate client by increasing flow rate; encourage deep breathing
   4. Lubricate the suction catheter with sterile water
   5. Insert the catheter
      a. If tracheal suction is being used, insert to the end of the tube (approximately 4 inches)
      b. If nasotracheal suction is being used, insert until the cough reflex is induced
   6. Apply no suction while the catheter is being inserted
   7. Rotate and withdraw the catheter while suction is applied; do not exceed 10 to 15 seconds

8. Clear the catheter with sterile solution and encourage the client to breathe deeply
9. If deeper suction is required, the client's head should be turned to the side to permit entry of a smaller catheter into the opposite bronchus
10. Evaluate client's response to procedure; revise plan as necessary

Thoracentesis

A. Definition
1. Surgical aseptic procedure in which the chest wall is punctured with a trocar to remove fluid or air; this is done for diagnostic purposes or to alleviate respiratory embarrassment
2. No more than 1000 ml of fluid should be removed at a time; fluid withdrawn should be sent to the laboratory for culture and sensitivity tests
3. Complications include pneumothorax from trauma to the lung and pulmonary edema resulting from sudden fluid shifts
B. Nursing care
1. Obtain an informed consent
2. Explain procedure to the client
3. Ensure that chest x-ray examination is done before and after the procedure
4. Assist and support the client in the sitting position
5. Set up a sterile field for the physician
6. Assess pulse and respirations before, during, and after the procedure
7. Inform the client not to cough during the procedure to prevent trauma to the lungs
8. After the procedure, label and send specimens for laboratory tests
9. Note and record the amount, color, and clarity of the fluid withdrawn
10. Place the client on opposite side for approximately 1 hour to prevent leakage of fluid through the thoracentesis site
11. Observe the client for coughing, bloody sputum, and rapid pulse rate and report their occurrence immediately
12. Evaluate client's response to procedure

Tracheostomy Care

A. Definition: removal of dried secretions from the cannula to maintain a patent airway, prevent infection, and prevent irritation
B. Nursing care
1. Provide tracheostomy care at least every 8 hours
2. Suction to remove secretions from the lumen of the tube (see procedure for suctioning of airways)
3. If an inner cannula is present
   a. Remove disposable inner cannula and replace with new one
   b. Care for nondisposable inner cannula

(1) Remove and place in peroxide; rinse with normal saline, using surgical aseptic technique
(2) Remove secretions within the cannula with a sterile brush
(3) Drain excess saline before reinserting the tube, which is then locked in place
4. Clean around the stoma with saline, using aseptic technique; apply antiseptic ointment if ordered
5. Change the tracheostomy tape, being careful not to dislodge the cannula; tie with a double knot
6. Place a tracheostomy dressing or fenestrated 10×10 cm (unfilled) dressing below the stoma to absorb expelled secretions
7. Humidify inhaled air mechanically or by the use of a moistened 10×10 cm dressing over the tracheostomy because air is bypassing normal humidification process in the nasopharynx
8. Evaluate client's response to procedure

GENERAL NURSING DIAGNOSES FOR CLIENTS WITH RESPIRATORY SYSTEM DISORDERS

A. Risk for activity intolerance related to oxygen deprivation
B. Ineffective airway clearance related to:
1. Improper positioning
2. Mechanical obstruction
3. Excessive secretions
4. Tumor growth
C. Anxiety related to:
1. Oxygen deprivation
2. Pain
D. Body image disturbance related to disfiguring head and neck surgery
E. Ineffective breathing patterns related to:
1. Chemical toxicity
2. Anxiety
3. Pain
4. CNS damage
5. Tachypnea
F. Impaired verbal communication related to an alteration in structures necessary for speech
G. Fatigue related to:
1. Oxygen deprivation
2. Coughing
H. Fear related to:
1. Air hunger
2. Pain
3. Mechanical ventilation
I. Impaired gas exchange related to:
1. Excessive secretions
2. Loss of functioning lung tissue

3. Insufficient oxygen supply
4. Inadequate ventilation/perfusion ratio
5. Respiratory muscle fatigue
J. Risk for infection related to microbial invasion
K. Altered nutrition: less than body requirements related to:
   1. Excessive secretions
   2. Easy fatigability
L. Knowledge deficit related to disease treatment
M. Pain related to:
   1. Inflammation of lung tissue
   2. Pressure of tumor
   3. Medical or surgical therapy
N. Inability to sustain spontaneous ventilation related to disease process
O. Altered thought processes related to decreased cerebral oxygenation
P. Dysfunctional ventilatory weaning response (DVWR) related to prolonged mechanical ventilation

MAJOR DISORDERS OF THE RESPIRATORY SYSTEM

▼ PULMONARY EMBOLISM AND INFARCTION

Data Base
A. Etiology and pathophysiology
   1. Postoperative clients, as well as those confined to bed, are prone to venous stasis, which causes peripheral thrombus formation
   2. When an embolus lodges in the pulmonary artery causing hemorrhage and necrosis of lung tissue it is called a pulmonary infarction
B. Clinical findings
   1. Subjective
      a. Severe dyspnea that occurs suddenly
      b. Anxiety
      c. Restlessness
      d. Sharp upper abdominal or thoracic pain
   2. Objective
      a. Violent coughing with hemoptysis
      b. On auscultation, dullness over area of infarction
      c. Increased temperature
C. Therapeutic interventions
   1. Anticoagulant therapy
   2. Thrombolytic therapy
   3. Angiography; if the condition is severe, an embolectomy may be indicated
   4. Vena caval interruption; a filter may be implanted in the inferior vena cava preventing the passage of large thrombi

Nursing Care of Clients with Pulmonary Embolism and Infarction
A. **DATA COLLECTION**
   1. Data related to causative factors
   2. Pleural pain
   3. Sputum for presence of blood
   4. Crackles on auscultation
   5. Vital signs for baseline data
B. **ANALYSIS AND INTERPRETATION**
   Refer to General Nursing Diagnoses for Clients with Respiratory System Disorders for the following diagnoses: C 2, E 2, and I 2
C. **PLANNING/IMPLEMENTATION**
   1. Place in the high-Fowler's position to aid respirations
   2. Monitor vital signs
   3. Administer thrombolytics, anticoagulants, and oxygen as ordered
   4. Maintain safe environment to decrease fear
D. **EVALUATION/OUTCOMES**
   1. Maintains normal breathing patterns
   2. Exchanges adequate gases to maintain tissue perfusion
   3. Verbalizes feelings of control over situation

▼ PULMONARY EDEMA

Data Base
A. Etiology and pathophysiology
   1. An acute emergency condition characterized by a rapid accumulation of fluid in the alveolar spaces resulting from increased pressure within the pulmonary system
   2. Possible causes include valvular disease, left-ventricular failure, circulatory overload, or congestive heart disease
B. Clinical findings
   1. Subjective
      a. History of premonitory symptoms such as shortness of breath, paroxysmal nocturnal dyspnea, wheezing, and orthopnea
      b. Acute anxiety, apprehension, restlessness
   2. Objective
      a. Rapid, thready pulse
      b. Pink, frothy sputum
      c. Elevated central venous pressure (CVP)
      d. Elevated pulmonary capillary wedge pressure (PCWP)
      e. Cyanosis
      f. Wheezing; crackles
      g. Stertorous respirations
C. Therapeutic interventions
   1. Medications aimed at decreasing cardiac workload and improving cardiac output, such as

morphine sulfate, digitalis, diuretics, bronchodilators
2. Oxygen in high concentration or by PEEP as necessary
3. Phlebotomy to remove approximately 500 ml of blood or the application of rotating tourniquets to reduce the volume of circulating blood
4. Cardiac monitoring

Nursing Care of Clients with Pulmonary Edema

A. DATA COLLECTION

1. Vital signs
2. Activity level
3. Mental status
4. Rate, depth, and quality of respirations
5. Frothy sputum
6. Crackles on auscultation of lungs
7. Assumption of orthopneic position

B. ANALYSIS AND INTERPRETATION

Refer to General Nursing Diagnoses for Clients with Respiratory System Disorders for the following diagnoses: A, H 1, and I 4

C. PLANNING/IMPLEMENTATION

1. Support client in a high-Fowler's or semi-Fowler's position
2. Observe and record vital signs and monitor cardiac activity and intake and output
3. Provide a reassuring environment to allay anxiety
4. Suction as needed to maintain a patent airway
5. Apply rotating tourniquets when ordered
   a. Tourniquets are placed around three extremities without completely obliterating the pulse
   b. One tourniquet is released in a clockwise direction every 15 minutes; may be done manually or by an automated machine
   c. Assess arterial pulses of all extremities every 15 minutes
   d. When client is no longer in distress, remove tourniquets one at a time, at 15-minute intervals, to prevent sudden cardiac overload; legs are rotated off last

D. EVALUATION/OUTCOMES

1. Demonstrates activity tolerance within level of cardiac function
2. Maintains adequate gas exchange
3. Verbalizes decreased fear

▼ PLEURAL EFFUSION

Data Base

A. Etiology and pathophysiology
   1. Collection of fluid in the pleural space
   2. Generally occurs secondary to diseases such as cancer of the lung, tuberculosis, and congestive heart failure

B. Clinical findings
   1. Subjective
      a. Pleuritic pain that is sharp and increases on inspiration
      b. Dyspnea
      c. Malaise
   2. Objective
      a. Tachycardia
      b. Elevated temperature
      c. Cough (may be productive or nonproductive, depending on cause)
      d. Decreased breath sounds
      e. Chest x-ray examination shows obliteration of the angle between the ribs and diaphragm; may also reveal a mediastinal shift away from the fluid

C. Therapeutic interventions
   1. Thoracentesis (see procedure)
   2. Treatment of underlying cause

Nursing Care of Clients with Pleural Effusion

A. DATA COLLECTION

1. Temperature for baseline data
2. Respiratory status
3. Diminished lung sounds on auscultation

B. ANALYSIS AND INTERPRETATION

Refer to General Nursing Diagnoses for Clients with Respiratory System Disorders for the following diagnoses: A, C 1, and I 2

C. PLANNING/IMPLEMENTATION

1. Encourage coughing and deep breathing
2. Increase fluid intake
3. Place the client in a high-Fowler's position for maximum air exchange
4. In addition to standard precautions, use airborne and/or droplet precautions if indicated

D. EVALUATION/OUTCOMES

1. Maintains adequate air exchange
2. Verbalizes a decrease in anxiety
3. Performs ADL without respiratory difficulty

▼ PLEURISY

Data Base

A. Etiology and pathophysiology
   1. Inflammation of the visceral and parietal membranes, which rub together during respiration and cause pain
   2. Caused by chest trauma, tuberculosis, pneumonia, or chest surgery

B. Clinical findings
   1. Subjective
      a. Knifelike pain on inspiration

b. Apprehension

c. Dyspnea

2. Objective

a. Decreased excursion of the involved chest wall

b. Pleural friction rub discernible on auscultation of chest wall

C. Therapeutic interventions

1. Treat the underlying condition

2. Analgesics for pain

3. Applications of heat or cold to thoracic area

Nursing Care of Clients with Pleurisy

A. DATA COLLECTION

1. Lung sounds to determine extent of inflammation (pleural friction rub)

2. Pain at height of inspiration

3. Vital signs, particularly respirations

B. ANALYSIS AND INTERPRETATION

Refer to General Nursing Diagnoses for Clients with Respiratory System Disorders for the following diagnoses: C 2, E 2, and E 3

C. PLANNING/IMPLEMENTATION

1. Instruct the client to lie on the affected side to splint the chest wall and lessen pain on inspiration

2. Administer medications as ordered

3. Allay anxiety by checking at frequent intervals

4. Observe for signs of shock or pulmonary emboli

5. In addition to standard precautions, use airborne and/or droplet precautions if indicated

D. EVALUATION/OUTCOMES

1. Maintains optimal gas exchange

2. Remains pain free

3. Verbalizes reduction in anxiety

▼ EMPYEMA

Data Base

A. Etiology and pathophysiology

1. Collection of pus within the pleural cavity

2. May occur following staphylococcal pneumonia, tuberculosis, chest trauma, or surgery

B. Clinical findings

1. Subjective

a. Unilateral chest pain

b. Malaise

c. Anorexia

d. Dyspnea

2. Objective

a. Chest x-ray examination shows pleural exudate

b. Elevated temperature

c. Cough

d. Unequal chest expansion

C. Therapeutic interventions

1. Thoracentesis to obtain a specimen of exudate to culture

2. Chest tubes inserted to drain pleural cavity

3. Antibiotics may be instilled through the chest tube or given systemically

4. If condition is long-standing, the area of inflammation is surgically removed; this is known as decortication

Nursing Care of Clients with Empyema

A. DATA COLLECTION

1. Temperature for baseline data

2. Chest expansion for diminished motion and inequality of expansion

3. Decreased breath sounds on auscultation

4. Flat note on percussion

5. Decreased or absent fremitus on palpation

B. ANALYSIS AND INTERPRETATION

Refer to General Nursing Diagnoses for Clients with Respiratory System Disorders for the following diagnoses: A, C 1, I 1, and J

C. PLANNING/IMPLEMENTATION

1. Monitor chest tube (see procedure)

2. Provide emotional support

3. Administer antibiotics as ordered

4. Monitor vital signs, particularly temperature and character of respirations

5. In addition to standard precautions, use airborne and/or droplet precautions as indicated

D. EVALUATION/OUTCOMES

1. Maintains maximum gas exchange

2. Verbalizes reduction in anxiety

3. Performs ADL without respiratory distress

4. Remains afebrile

▼ PNEUMONIA

Data Base

A. Etiology and pathophysiology

1. Inflammatory disease usually caused by an infectious agent (bacterial, viral, protozoan, or fungal) but may also be caused by inhalation of chemicals and aspiration of gastric contents

2. Pneumonia is commonly spread by respiratory droplets

3. Pneumococcal pneumonia, the most common type of bacterial pneumonia, occurs in winter and spring; other bacterial pneumonias include *Klebsiella pneumoniae*, *Haemophilus influenzae*, *Pseudomonas*, *Proteus*, and *Streptococcus* species, and *Staphylococcus aureus*

4. Aspiration pneumonia occurs when gastric contents and the normal flora of the upper respiratory tract are aspirated into the lung

5. *Pneumocystis carinii* pneumonia, a rare protozoan infection, is seen in clients with impaired immune function (e.g., AIDS)
6. Viral pneumonias include influenza virus type A and cytomegalovirus

B. Clinical findings
1. Subjective
   a. Lassitude
   b. Chest pain that increases on inspiration
   c. Dyspnea
2. Objective
   a. Elevated temperature
   b. Increased WBC
   c. Cough
   d. Chest x-ray examination shows pulmonary infiltration
   e. Sputum production
      (1) Pneumococcal: purulent, rusty sputum
      (2) Staphylococcal: yellow, blood-streaked sputum
      (3) *Klebsiella*: red, gelatinous sputum
      (4) Mycoplasmal: nonproductive that advances to mucoid sputum

C. Therapeutic interventions
1. If bacterial pneumonia, culture and sensitivity tests will be done on blood and sputum to determine appropriate antibiotic therapy
2. Oxygen therapy usually via nasal cannula
3. Inhalation therapy and the use of incentive spirometer

Nursing Care of Clients with Pneumonia

A. DATA COLLECTION
1. Breathing pattern
2. Color, amount, and consistency of sputum
3. Adventitious sounds on auscultation of lung
4. Mental status
5. Skin for rashes that occur with mycoplasma, cytomegalovirus, or Rocky Mountain spotted fever infections

B. ANALYSIS AND INTERPRETATION
Refer to General Nursing Diagnoses for Clients with Respiratory System Disorders for the following diagnoses: A, B 3, E 5, I 1, and I 2

C. PLANNING/IMPLEMENTATION
1. Encourage coughing and deep breathing, splinting the chest as necessary
2. Collect sputum specimen for culture and sensitivity tests in sterile container; notify the physician if organism is resistant to the antibiotic being given
3. Increase fluid intake
4. Monitor vital signs
5. Observe for signs of respiratory distress, such as labored respirations, cool clammy skin, and cyanosis

6. Plan rest periods
7. Instruct client to cover nose and mouth when coughing
8. Administer antibiotics as ordered
9. In addition to standard precautions, use airborne and/or droplet precautions as indicated

D. EVALUATION/OUTCOMES
1. Maintains patent airway
2. Performs ADL without assistance
3. Remains afebrile
4. Breathes without difficulty

▼ ATELECTASIS

Data Base
A. Etiology and pathophysiology
1. Respirations shallow and ineffective, as in postoperative clients
2. Bronchioles obstructed by secretions, and alveoli distal to the bronchioles collapse; many small bronchioles or a stem of the bronchus may be involved
3. Causes include compression resulting from large pleural effusion, empyema, or pneumothorax, obstruction of a bronchus by a tumor, and deficiency of surfactant in an infant

B. Clinical findings
1. Subjective
   a. Restlessness
   b. Anxiety
2. Objective
   a. Rapid, shallow respirations
   b. Diminished breath sounds in lower lobes
   c. Productive cough
   d. Temperature elevation

C. Therapeutic interventions
1. Oxygen therapy
2. Prophylactic antibiotics

Nursing Care of Clients with Atelectasis

A. DATA COLLECTION
1. Lungs for evidence of decreased ventilation
2. Baseline temperature

B. ANALYSIS AND INTERPRETATION
Refer to General Nursing Diagnoses for Clients with Respiratory System Disorders for the following diagnoses: C 1 and I 2

C. PLANNING/IMPLEMENTATION
1. Encourage coughing and deep breathing
2. Monitor respirations closely
3. Place in a high-Fowler's position; turn every 2 hours
4. Encourage use of incentive spirometer

D. EVALUATION/OUTCOMES
1. Maintains adequate gas exchange
2. Verbalizes reduced feelings of anxiety

▼ SARCOIDOSIS

Data Base

A. Etiology and pathophysiology
1. Characterized by epithelioid cell tubercles, most commonly in the lung
2. Cause unknown, although 80% have high titers of Epstein-Barr virus
3. Incidence is highest in blacks and young adults

B. Clinical findings
1. Subjective
   a. Fatigue
   b. Malaise
   c. Dyspnea
2. Objective
   a. Night sweats
   b. Fever
   c. Weight loss
   d. Cough
   e. Nodules of face
   f. Polyarthritis
   g. Mild anemia
   h. Elevated serum calcium
   i. Kveim test: sarcoid node antigen is injected intradermally and causes local nodular lesion in approximately 1 month
   j. Biopsy of skin, lymph node, or liver
   k. X-ray findings include bilateral hilar and paratracheal adenopathy
   l. Pulmonary function studies reveal decreased lung compliance

C. Therapeutic interventions
1. No specific treatment
2. Corticosteroids to control symptoms

Nursing Care of Clients with Sarcoidosis

A. DATA COLLECTION
1. Baseline temperature
2. Lungs to determine extent of lung involvement

B. ANALYSIS AND INTERPRETATION
Refer to General Nursing Diagnoses for Clients with Respiratory System Disorders for the following diagnoses: A, G 2, I 4, and K 2

C. PLANNING/IMPLEMENTATION
1. Increase fluid intake
2. Provide frequent periods of rest
3. Provide small, nutritious meals, taking into consideration the client's preferences

D. EVALUATION/OUTCOMES
1. Performs ADL with minimal fatigue

2. Maintains normal body weight
3. Maintains adequate oxygenation

▼ PULMONARY TUBERCULOSIS

Data Base

A. Etiology and pathophysiology
1. Infection of lungs caused by *Mycobacterium tuberculosis*, an acid-fast bacterium
2. Causes tubercles, fibrosis, and calcification within the lungs
3. Tubercle bacillus may be communicated to others by means of droplet formation (inhalation), ingestion, or inoculation
4. Predisposing factors include debilitating diseases such as alcoholism, cardiovascular disease, HIV infection, diabetes mellitus, and cirrhosis, as well as poor nutrition and crowded living conditions
5. The emergence of multi–drug-resistant tuberculosis has complicated management of the disease
6. Chronic, progressive, and reinfection phase is most frequently encountered in adults and involves progression or reactivation of primary lesions after months or years of latency
7. Swallowing infected sputum may lead to laryngeal, oropharyngeal, and intestinal tuberculosis

B. Clinical findings
1. Subjective
   a. Malaise
   b. Pleuritic pain
   c. Easily fatigued
2. Objective
   a. Fever
   b. Night sweats
   c. Cough that progressively becomes worse
   d. Hemoptysis
   e. Weight loss
   f. Chest x-ray examination to determine presence of active or calcified lesions
   g. Analysis of sputum and gastric contents for the presence of acid-fast bacilli
   h. Tuberculin testing
      (1) Examples
         (a) Tine
         (b) Heaf
         (c) Mantoux, which frequently involves the use of purified protein derivative (PPD)
      (2) Determines antibody response to the tubercle bacillus
      (3) Indicates prior exposure to bacillus, which may or may not indicate active

disease state (a sudden change from negative to positive requires follow-up testing)

(4) In each test, either old tuberculin (OT) or PPD is injected intradermally; an induration of 8 mm or greater present 48 to 72 hours later indicates a positive finding

C. Therapeutic interventions
1. Program of combined antituberculin drugs such as isoniazid, paraminosalicylic acid, streptomycin, pyrazinamide, rifampin, and ethambutol hydrochloride for 9 to 24 months
2. Bed rest until symptoms abate or therapeutic regimen is established
3. Determine whether surgical resection of the involved lobe is necessary if symptoms such as hemorrhage develop or chemotherapy is unsatisfactory
4. Provide prophylactic therapy to immediate contacts (all cases and follow-up of contacts must be reported to public health agency)
5. Have the client begin a high-carbohydrate, high-protein, high-vitamin diet with supplemental vitamin B_6

Nursing Care of Clients with Pulmonary Tuberculosis

A. DATA COLLECTION
1. Detailed history related to exposure, travel, or BCG inoculation
2. Fatigue, anorexia, low-grade fever, and night sweats
3. Sputum for color, amount, and consistency

B. ANALYSIS AND INTERPRETATION
Refer to General Nursing Diagnoses for Clients with Respiratory System Disorders for the following diagnoses: G 2, I 2, J, K 2, and L

C. PLANNING/IMPLEMENTATION
1. Teach client to provide for scheduled rest periods
2. Teach which foods to include in the diet and which are nutritious between-meal supplements
3. Teach the importance of adhering, without variation, to the drug program that has been established
4. Teach the proper techniques to prevent spread of infection
   a. Frequent hand washing
   b. Cover the mouth when coughing
   c. Proper use and disposal of tissues
   d. Proper cleansing of eating utensils and disposal of food wastes
   e. In addition to standard precautions, use airborne precautions with high filtration masks when sputum is positive for the organism

5. Encourage client to participate in developing a schedule of activities and therapy and follow the schedule once established
6. Instruct client to be alert to the early symptoms of hemorrhage, such as hemoptysis, and to contact the physician immediately if any occur
7. Instruct client to be alert to the early symptoms of adverse drug reactions (e.g., neuritis, ringing in the ears, ataxia, dermatitis) and to contact the physician immediately if any occur
8. Encourage client to follow prescribed program for productive coughing and deep breathing
9. Instruct client to avoid any medications such as cough syrups without physician's approval
10. Explain the need and instruct client to continue follow-up care and supervision
11. Encourage client to express feelings about disease and the many ramifications (stigma, isolation, fear) it creates
12. Expect and accept client's expression of feelings related to the disease
13. Encourage client to limit activities until the physician gives approval for gradual increase
14. Help client plan a realistic schedule for taking the large number of necessary medications
15. Monitor client's compliance with therapeutic regimen

D. EVALUATION/OUTCOMES
1. Complies with treatment regimen
2. Maintains adequate body weight
3. Remains afebrile

▼ CHRONIC OBSTRUCTIVE PULMONARY DISEASE (COPD)

Data Base
A. Etiology and pathophysiology
1. Group of diseases that result in an obstruction of airflow; causes include air pollution, smoking, chronic respiratory infections, exposure to molds and fungi, and allergic reactions
2. Types
   a. Asthma: obstruction of the bronchioles characterized by attacks that occur suddenly and last from 30 to 60 minutes; an asthmatic attack that is difficult to control is referred to as status asthmaticus
   b. Bronchitis: inflammation of the bronchial walls with hypertrophy of the mucous goblet cells; characterized by a chronic cough
   c. Emphysema: characterized by distended, inelastic, or destroyed alveoli with bronchiolar obstruction and collapse; these alterations greatly impair the diffusion of gases through the alveolar capillary membrane

d. Bronchiectasis: chronic dilation of the bronchi and bronchioles as a result of infection or obstruction

3. Clients with COPD become accustomed to an elevated residual carbon dioxide level and do not respond to high CO_2 concentrations as the normal respiratory stimulant; they respond instead to a drop in oxygen concentration in the blood

B. Clinical findings
   1. Subjective
      a. Fatigue and weakness
      b. Headache, impaired sensorium
      c. Dyspnea
   2. Objective
      a. Orthopnea, expiratory wheezing, stertorous breathing sounds, cough
      b. Barrel chest, cyanosis, clubbing of fingers
      c. Distention of neck veins
      d. Edema of extremities
      e. Increased PCO_2 and decreased PO_2 of arterial blood gases
      f. Polycythemia

C. Therapeutic interventions
   1. Antibiotics and cortisone to prevent and reduce inflammation
   2. Bronchodilators to reduce muscular spasm
   3. Mucolytics and expectorants to liquify secretions and to facilitate their removal
   4. Oxygen at 1 to 2 L even if hypoxia is severe
   5. Respiratory therapy program to include nebulizer therapy, postural drainage, and exercise
   6. High-protein, soft diet in small, frequent feedings is most easily tolerated

Nursing Care of Clients with Chronic Obstructive Pulmonary Disease

A. DATA COLLECTION
1. History of increased symptoms: during early morning, in cold weather, when sleeping, and when smoking
2. Breathing patterns: abdominal, paradoxical, pursed lip, asynchronous
3. Frequency of respiratory infections
4. Chest measurement to determine presence of barrel chest
5. Chest auscultation to assess depth of inspiration and presence of adventitious sounds

B. ANALYSIS AND INTERPRETATION
Refer to General Nursing Diagnoses for Clients with Respiratory System Disorders for the following diagnoses: A, B 3, C 1, G 1, H 1, I 1, I 4, I 5, J, L, and N

C. PLANNING/IMPLEMENTATION
1. Advise the elimination of smoking and other external irritants, such as dust, as much as possible

2. Supervise client's respiratory exercises, such as pursed lip or diaphragmatic breathing
3. Teach proper use of nebulizer and other special equipment
4. Carefully observe for symptoms of carbon dioxide intoxication (CO_2 narcosis) if oxygen is being administered
5. Teach client to adjust activities to avoid overexertion
6. Teach client to avoid people with respiratory infections
7. Teach the client to avoid the use of sedatives or hypnotics, which could compromise respirations
8. Teach client to maintain the highest resistance possible by getting adequate rest, eating nutritious food, dressing properly for weather conditions
9. Teach client to be alert to early symptoms of infection, hypoxia, hypercapnea, or adverse response to medications
10. Encourage client to continue with close medical supervision
11. Encourage client to express feelings about disease and therapy
12. Accept feelings about life-long restrictions in activity
13. Encourage client to take an active role in planning therapy
14. Encourage client to take medications as ordered
15. Support efforts to give up smoking by providing diversional activities such as eating hard candies
16. Encourage the family to support client's efforts to give up smoking
17. Monitor client's compliance with therapeutic regimen

D. EVALUATION/OUTCOMES
1. Demonstrates pursed lip breathing and diaphragmatic breathing
2. Describes and complies with treatment regimen
3. States methods for reducing/controlling feelings of anxiety/fear

▼ OCCUPATIONAL LUNG DISEASE: SILICOSIS (BLACK LUNG), ASBESTOSIS, AND PNEUMOCONIOSIS

Data Base
A. Etiology and pathophysiology
   1. Fibrotic disease of lungs caused by inhalation of inorganic dusts over long periods
   2. Common in people whose professions expose them to free silica, such as miners and sandblasters

3. Tuberculosis a frequent complication
B. Clinical findings
   1. Subjective
      a. Exertional dyspnea
      b. Anxiety
   2. Objective
      a. Frequent respiratory infections
      b. Sputum may be blood streaked
      c. Cough
      d. Chest x-ray examination reveals nodular lesions and enlarged hilar nodes
      e. Biopsy to establish diagnosis
      f. Pulmonary function studies reveal decreased volume and forced vital capacity
C. Therapeutic interventions
   1. Relieve cough with antitussives
   2. Prescribe medications for complications such as tuberculosis
   3. Eliminate toxic substances from the environment
   4. Administer oxygen therapy

Nursing Care of Clients with Occupational Lung Diseases

A. DATA COLLECTION
   1. Onset of acute or chronic symptoms
   2. Sputum for amount, color, and consistency
   3. Lung auscultation for presence of adventitious sounds and extent of involvement

B. ANALYSIS AND INTERPRETATION
   Refer to General Nursing Diagnoses for Clients with Respiratory System Disorders for the following diagnoses: A, C 1, H 1, I 2, I 4, and J

C. PLANNING/IMPLEMENTATION
   1. Teach self-administration of oxygen
   2. Encourage coughing and deep breathing
   3. Involve the client and family in programs aimed at improved occupational health and safety
   4. Teach how to balance rest and activity

D. EVALUATION/OUTCOMES
   1. Maintains adequate oxygenation
   2. Verbalizes a reduction in anxiety and fear
   3. Reduces frequency and severity of episodes of shortness of breath
   4. Administers oxygen to self safely

▼ PNEUMOTHORAX

Data Base
A. Etiology and pathophysiology
   1. Collapse of a lung resulting from disruption of the negative pressure that normally exists within the intrapleural space caused by the presence of air in the pleural cavity

   2. Reduces the surface area for gaseous exchange and leads to hypoxia and retention of carbon dioxide (hypercarbia)
   3. Types
      a. Spontaneous: thought to occur when a weakened area of the lung (bleb) ruptures; air then moves from the lung to the intrapleural space causing collapse; highest incidence is in men 20 to 40 years of age
      b. Open: laceration (e.g., a stab wound) through the chest wall into the intrapleural space
      c. Hemothorax: collection of blood within the pleural cavity
      d. Hydrothorax: accumulation of fluid in the pleural cavity
      e. Tension: buildup of pressure as air accumulates within the pleural space; the pressure increase likely to induce a mediastinal shift
   4. Mediastinal shift may occur toward the uninvolved side as a result of increased pressure within the pleural space; this involves the trachea, esophagus, heart, and great vessels
B. Clinical findings
   1. Subjective
      a. Chest pain, usually described as sharp and increasing on exertion
      b. Dyspnea
   2. Objective
      a. Rapid, shallow respirations (nonsymmetric)
      b. Breath sounds on the affected side will be diminished or absent
      c. Chest x-ray examination will reveal extent of the pneumothorax
      d. Tachycardia
      e. Hypotension
C. Therapeutic interventions
   1. Bed rest initially
   2. Analgesics
   3. Negative pressure is returned to the intrapleural space by the insertion of chest tubes attached to underwater drainage

Nursing Care of Clients with Pneumothorax
A. DATA COLLECTION
   1. Auscultation of lung fields for diminished or absent breath sounds
   2. Chest percussion for hyperresonance
   3. Chest motion during inhalation for inequality
   4. Baseline vital signs
   5. Skin for changes in color

B. ANALYSIS AND INTERPRETATION
   Refer to General Nursing Diagnoses for Clients with Respiratory System Disorders for the following diagnoses: C 1, C 2, H 1, H 2, and I 2

C. PLANNING/IMPLEMENTATION
   1. Maintain constant supervision until stable

2. Maintain patency of chest tubes (see Chest Tubes Procedure)
3. Place in high-Fowler's position
4. Offer fluids frequently
5. Monitor vital signs, particularly respirations
6. Monitor respiratory status

D. EVALUATION/OUTCOMES
1. Maintains adequate gas exchange
2. Verbalizes reduction in anxiety and fear
3. Verifies reduction or absence of chest pain

▼ CHEST INJURIES

Data Base
A. Etiology and pathophysiology
   1. Penetrating or crushing wounds of the chest wall generally caused by acts of violence (stabbing, gunshot wounds) or motor vehicle accidents
   2. Flail chest: occurs when ribs are fractured in more than one area; the chest wall on the involved side becomes unstable; the portion of lung below the injury moves in the opposite direction to the remainder of the lung, which results in hypoxia
B. Clinical findings
   1. Subjective
      a. Dyspnea
      b. Anxiety
   2. Objective
      a. Presence of a wound with a sucking sound on inspiration
      b. Presence of cyanosis and symptoms of mild to profound shock, depending on wound
      c. Mediastinal shift may occur toward the unaffected side caused by the pressure exerted by a pneumothorax or hemothorax, causing a change in the site of the apical pulse and paradoxical respirations
      d. Absence of breath sounds on the affected side
C. Therapeutic interventions
   1. Pressure dressing over the wound
   2. Aspiration of the pleural cavity to promote lung expansion
   3. Water-seal suction drainage
   4. Bed rest and limitation of activity
   5. Oxygen as necessary
   6. Restoration of blood volume and treatment of shock
   7. Antibiotics and mild analgesics
   8. Respiratory therapy to promote lung expansion
   9. Volume-controlled ventilation in cases of severe chest trauma

Nursing Care of Clients with Chest Injuries
A. DATA COLLECTION
1. Presence of paradoxic chest movement
2. Respirations for dyspnea
3. Pulse for tachycardia
4. Skin for changes in color

B. ANALYSIS AND INTERPRETATION
Refer to General Nursing Diagnoses for Clients with Respiratory System Disorders for the following diagnoses: A, C 1, E 2, E 3, G 1, H 1, H 2, and I 2

C. PLANNING/IMPLEMENTATION
1. Maintain chest tubes if present (see procedure)
2. Observe client's respiratory status
3. Encourage client to move and cough and use an incentive spirometer
4. Teach client to self-splint with hands and arms
5. Explain the purpose and functioning of chest tubes and water-seal drainage
6. Administer oxygen and analgesics as ordered and as necessary

D. EVALUATION/OUTCOMES
1. Verbalizes feelings of decreased anxiety
2. Breathes without difficulty
3. Performs ADL without difficulty

▼ BRONCHOGENIC CARCINOMA

Data Base
A. Etiology and pathophysiology
   1. Carcinoma of the lungs may be primary or metastatic
   2. Smoking is the most significant risk factor
   3. Leading type of cancer that causes death
   4. Incidence highest in men over the age of 40
   5. Symptoms may occur after metastasis to other organs such as the ribs, liver, adrenal glands, mediastinal organs, kidneys, and brain
   6. Classification of lung cancers
      a. Large cell (undifferentiated)
      b. Small cell (oat cell carcinoma)
      c. Epidermoid (squamous cell)
      d. Adenocarcinoma
B. Clinical findings
   1. Subjective
      a. Dyspnea
      b. Chills
      c. Fatigue
      d. Chest pain
   2. Objective
      a. Persistent cough
      b. Hemoptysis
      c. Unilateral wheeze detected by auscultation
      d. Weight loss
      e. Clubbing of fingers
      f. Pleural effusion

g. "Coin" lesions detected by x-ray examination of the chest

h. Results of cytologic test of sputum positive

C. Therapeutic interventions

1. Surgical

a. Lobectomy: removal of one lobe of the lung when the lesion is limited to one area

b. Wedge section: removal of a small confined lesion; may also be done for biopsy

c. Pneumonectomy: removal of an entire lung

d. Exploratory thoracotomy: opening of the thoracic cavity to determine extent and further therapy

e. Thoracoplasty: removal of ribs to reduce the size of the pleural cavity; may be done to prevent complications after resection of lung

f. Laser surgery: removal of tumor via endoscope inserted between the ribs

2. Radiation therapy may be used as an adjunct therapy or to alleviate symptoms of pain, dyspnea, and hemoptysis

3. Chemotherapy (e.g., cyclophosphamide, methotrexate, vincristine)

Nursing Care of Clients with Bronchogenic Carcinoma

A. DATA COLLECTION

1. Sputum quantity and characteristics

2. Lung auscultation for areas of absent breath sounds

3. Chest percussion for dullness over tumors

4. Respirations for shallowness, stridor, and use of accessory muscles

5. Persistent cough

B. ANALYSIS AND INTERPRETATION

Refer to General Nursing Diagnoses for Clients with Respiratory System Disorders for the following diagnoses: B 4, C 2, G 2, I 2, L, and M 2

C. PLANNING/IMPLEMENTATION

1. Maintain open communication between self, the client, and the family; refer to community agencies and mental health practitioner as necessary

2. Monitor temperature and vital signs

3. Encourage coughing and deep breathing

4. Change client's position frequently; semi-Fowler's or high-Fowler's promotes greater lung expansion

5. Provide specific care based on therapy being used

a. Care of client with chest tubes (see Procedure)

b. Radiation therapy (see Nursing Care for Clients with Neoplastic Disorders Receiving Either Chemotherapy or Radiation)

c. Chemotherapy (see Nursing Care for Clients with Neoplastic Disorders Receiving Either Chemotherapy or Radiation)

6. Provide high-protein, high-calorie diet, and supplements

7. Use interventions to manage pain: analgesics, distraction, relaxation, imagery

D. EVALUATION/OUTCOMES

1. Verbalizes a reduction of pain

2. Maintains patent airway

3. States understanding of treatment

4. Breathes with minimal effort

▼ CANCER OF THE LARYNX

Data Base

A. Etiology and pathophysiology

1. Most tumors of the larynx (vocal cords, epiglottis, laryngeal cartilages, and ventricle) are squamous cell carcinoma

2. Cigarette smoking and heavy alcohol consumption appear to be related to increased incidence

3. More common in men 50 to 65 years of age

B. Clinical findings

1. Subjective

a. Sore throat

b. Dyspnea

c. Dysphagia

d. Weakness

2. Objective

a. Increasing hoarseness

b. Weight loss

c. Enlarged cervical lymph nodes

d. Foul breath

C. Therapeutic interventions

1. Radiation therapy

2. Chemotherapy (e.g., methotrexate, bleomycin, fluorouracil)

3. Surgical intervention

a. Thyrotomy: removal of tumor from the larynx via an incision through the thyroid cartilage

b. Total laryngectomy: removal of total larynx with construction of a permanent tracheal stoma

c. Radical neck dissection (used when the tumor has metastasized into surrounding tissue and lymph nodes): removal of larynx, surrounding tissue and muscle, lymph nodes, and glands with a permanent tracheal stoma

Nursing Care of Clients with a Total Laryngectomy

A. DATA COLLECTION

1. Voice for hoarseness

2. Oropharyngeal inspection for masses

3. Neck palpation for masses and nodal enlargement

B. ANALYSIS AND INTERPRETATION

Refer to General Nursing Diagnoses for Clients with Respiratory System Disorders for the following diagnoses: B 4, D, F, H 2, and L

C. PLANNING/IMPLEMENTATION

1. Provide time to discuss the diagnosis and the ramifications of surgery
2. Assist and encourage the client to express feelings
3. Answer questions as thoroughly and honestly as possible
4. Arrange for individuals with laryngectomies to visit and discuss the rehabilitative process
5. Instruct the client as to the method of communication that will be used after surgery (e.g., slate board and chalk, pencil and paper, sign language; electronic voice)
6. Observe for obstruction of airway by mucous plugs, edema, or blood (e.g., air hunger, dyspnea, cyanosis, gurgling)
7. Observe for signs of hemorrhage (e.g., increased pulse rate, drop in blood pressure, cold clammy skin, appearance of blood on dressing)
8. Stay with the client but provide a bell or other system for the client to signal for help
9. Provide, at the bedside, suction apparatus and catheters (additional laryngectomy tube and a surgical instrument set with additional hemostats should be immediately available in case tube becomes dislodged or blocked)
10. Suction the laryngectomy tube that is left in place for approximately 3 days (see Suctioning of Airway Procedure)
11. Provide humidity to compensate for loss of normal humidification of air in the nasopharynx; later the stoma may be covered with a moistened, unfilled gauze pad
12. Prevent cross-infection and contamination of the wound by providing special oral hygiene, cleanliness at tracheal site, avoidance of people with respiratory tract infections, use of sterile equipment
13. With clients receiving radiation or chemotherapy, observe for signs of adverse reactions
14. Expect and accept a period of mourning, but prevent withdrawal from reality by:
    a. Involving the client in laryngectomy care
    b. Keeping channels of communication open
    c. Supporting the client's strengths
    d. Encouraging a return to activities of daily living
    e. Allowing the client time to write responses or use sign language

15. Encourage the client to become involved in speech therapy and realistically support efforts and gains
16. Teach the skills necessary to handle altered body functioning
    a. Method of tracheobronchial suctioning to maintain patency of airway, emphasizing pressure, depth, frequency, and safety
    b. Method of changing, cleaning, and securing the laryngectomy tube
    c. Care of skin around the opening (stoma)
    d. Importance of providing humidified air for inspiration to prevent drying of secretions (can be achieved by use of moist dressing or cloth bib)
17. Teach the client to avoid activities that may permit water or irritating substances to enter the trachea, because the usual defensive mechanisms (glottis and cilia) are absent; the client should avoid showers (unless wearing a protective cover), swimming, dust, hair spray, and other volatile substances
18. Teach the client to avoid wearing clothes with tight collars or constricting necklines
19. Teach the client that certain other activities will be interrupted (e.g., sipping through a straw, whistling, blowing the nose)

D. EVALUATION/OUTCOMES

1. States a reduction in feelings of fear
2. Maintains patent airway
3. States acceptance of body image
4. Verbalizes understanding of laryngeal cancer and treatment
5. Uses an alternate form of communication

▼ ADULT RESPIRATORY DISTRESS SYNDROME (ARDS)

Data Base

A. Etiology and pathophysiology
1. Respiratory failure in clients with previously healthy lungs as a complication of conditions such as trauma, aspiration, prolonged mechanical ventilation, severe infection, or open heart surgery
2. Involves:
    a. Pulmonary capillary damage with loss of fluid and interstitial edema
    b. Impaired alveolar gas exchange and tissue hypoxia due to pulmonary edema
    c. Alteration in surfactant production; collapse of alveoli
    d. Atelectasis resulting in labored and inefficient respiration

B. Clinical findings
1. Subjective
   a. Restlessness
   b. Anxiety
   c. Dyspnea
2. Objective
   a. PCO_2 initially decreased and later increased, and decreased PO_2 arterial blood gases
   b. Tachycardia
   c. Cyanosis
   d. Grunting respirations
   e. Intercostal retractions
   f. Chest x-ray examination reveals pulmonary edema
C. Therapeutic interventions
1. Relieve the underlying cause
2. Mechanical ventilation
3. Positive end expiratory pressure (PEEP): this setting on a mechanical ventilator maintains positive pressure within the lungs at the end of expiration, which increases the residual capacity, reducing hypoxia
4. Monitoring arterial blood gases
5. Corticosteroids may be used

Nursing Care of Clients with Adult Respiratory Distress Syndrome

A. DATA COLLECTION
1. Respirations for dyspnea
2. Pain that increases on inspiration
3. Sputum for quantity and characteristics
4. Chest percussion for hyperresonance
5. Baseline vital signs

B. ANALYSIS AND INTERPRETATION
Refer to General Nursing Diagnoses for Clients with Respiratory System Disorders for the following diagnoses: C 1, F, G 1, H 1, H 3, I 2, I 4, J, N, and P

C. PLANNING/IMPLEMENTATION
1. Allow frequent rest periods between therapeutic interventions
2. Provide tranquil, supportive environment; sedation is contraindicated because of its depressant effect on respirations
3. Observe behavioral changes and vital signs because confusion and hypertension may indicate cerebral hypoxia
4. Auscultate breath sounds to observe for signs of pneumothorax when the client is on PEEP (lung tissue that is frail may not withstand increased intrathoracic pressure, and pneumothorax occurs)
5. Monitor arterial blood gases, as ordered; use a heparinized syringe to obtain specimen
6. Maintain a patent airway
7. Care for the client on mechanical ventilation (see Procedure)

8. Measure central venous or pulmonary artery pressures

D. EVALUATION/OUTCOMES
1. Maintains adequate gas exchange
2. Communicates reduction in anxiety
3. Performs activities without respiratory distress or fatigue
4. Demonstrates an absence of infection
5. Uses alternate form of communication when on ventilator

▼ CARBON MONOXIDE POISONING

Data Base
A. Etiology and pathophysiology
1. Caused by inadequately vented combustion devices
2. Carbon monoxide combines with hemoglobin more readily than does oxygen, causing tissue anoxia
B. Clinical findings
1. Subjective
   a. Headache
   b. Faintness
   c. Vertigo
   d. Tinnitus
2. Objective
   a. Color may be normal, cyanotic, or flushed, but is usually cherry pink
   b. Paralysis
   c. Loss of consciousness
   d. ECG changes
C. Therapeutic interventions
1. Mechanical ventilation
2. 100% oxygen until carboxyhemoglobin is reduced to less than 5% and respirations are normal
3. Hyperbaric pressure chamber to accelerate elimination of carbon dioxide

Nursing Care of Clients with Carbon Monoxide Poisoning

A. DATA COLLECTION
1. History to determine extent of exposure
2. Color of skin
3. Baseline vital signs
4. Level of consciousness

B. ANALYSIS AND INTERPRETATION
Refer to General Nursing Diagnoses for Clients with Respiratory System Disorders for the following diagnoses: I 3 and O

C. PLANNING/IMPLEMENTATION
1. Remove the individual from the immediate area of poisoning
2. Evaluate for cardiopulmonary function

3. Institute cardiopulmonary resuscitation if necessary and maintain until additional help arrives
4. Administer oxygen if available
5. Maintain respirations with assistance if needed
6. Maintain body temperature
7. Monitor vital signs, with special concern for respirations
8. Maintain oxygen flow at prescribed levels

D. EVALUATION/OUTCOMES
1. Maintains adequate oxygen levels
2. Remains conscious and alert

ENDOCRINE SYSTEM

REVIEW OF ANATOMY AND PHYSIOLOGY OF THE ENDOCRINE SYSTEM

Functions of the Endocrine System

Endocrine glands secrete products called hormones, which are chemical messengers that deliver stimulatory or inhibitory signals to target cells (Table 6-5)

Structures of the Endocrine System

Thyroid Gland

A. Anatomy
1. Soft, red-brown mass having right and left pear-shaped lobes joined by a narrow isthmus
2. Extends from sides of cricoid and thyroid cartilages to sixth tracheal cartilage
3. Half of glands observed have a pyramidal lobe extending upward from the isthmus
B. Actions of thyroid hormones (Table 6-6)
1. Accelerate cellular reactions in most body cells
   a. Increase basal metabolic rate (BMR)
   b. Accelerate growth
   c. Alter the metabolic rate of more than 100 enzyme systems by profound stimulatory effect on cellular protein synthesis
2. Bind to nuclear and cytoplasmic receptor sites
   a. Intranuclear chromatin protein binds thyroid hormones; this stimulates cellular protein synthesis and influences growth, development, and cell differentiation
   b. Mitochondrial membranes bind thyroid hormones, which regulate energy metabolism
C. Metabolism (inactivation) of thyroid hormones
1. Liver the principal organ regulating blood concentration of thyroid hormones; thyroxine and triiodothyronine deaminated, deiodinated, and conjugated; conjugates excreted in the bile
2. Skeletal muscle, kidney, liver, and heart tissues deiodinate thyroid hormones; this mechanism of hormone inactivation not as important as conjugation in liver

D. Calcitonin (thyrocalcitonin)
1. Decreases loss of calcium from bone through inhibition of osteocytic and osteoclastic osteolysis (cAMP mechanism)
   a. Action opposite that of parathormone
   b. Some bone cells respond specifically to calcitonin; others to parathormone
2. Decreases loss of calcium from bone and promotes hypocalcemia; this effect offsets postprandial hypercalcemia

Parathyroid Glands

A. Anatomy: generally four small, yellow glands (but may be two to twelve); 0.6 cm (in diameter at their widest part; usually embedded in the capsule of the posterior part of the thyroid (but may be behind the pharynx or in the thorax with the thymus)
B. Actions of parathyroid hormones (Table 6-6)
1. Parathormone: major sites of action are skeleton, kidneys, and intestine
   a. Bone tissue releases calcium into blood (requires active form of vitamin D)
      (1) Osteoclastic osteolysis stimulated
      (2) Osteocytic osteolysis stimulated
      (3) Enhanced rate of maturation of precursor cells into osteoclasts and osteoblasts
      (4) Inhibition of osteoblastic collagen synthesis
   b. Kidney tubule reabsorption of calcium and magnesium is enhanced, which helps prevent further decreases in serum calcium levels; excretion of potassium, phosphorus, and bicarbonate also is enhanced; that of hydrogen and ammonia is decreased
   c. Parathormone, through adenylate cyclase activation, stimulates kidney's production of the enzyme that converts dihydroxycholecalciferol into hydroxycholecalciferol, which is the active form of vitamin D that works with parathormone in bone to mobilize calcium
   d. The intestinal mucosa increases its absorption of calcium and phosphorus, with subsequent release into the blood

Testes

A. Anatomy (see Genitourinary System)
B. Actions of testicular (androgenic) hormones (Table 6-7)
1. Major androgenic action in target tissues is stimulation of protein synthesis through enhancement of nuclear DNA and RNA
2. Increased protein synthesis manifests itself as increased tissue growth, particularly in younger individuals; at puberty, rise in androgen level induces growth of long bones, muscular development, enlargement of the exter-

TABLE 6-5 Location and hormones of endocrine glands

Endocrine gland	Location	Hormones
Pituitary Anterior (adenohypophysis)	Cranial cavity, in sella turcica of sphenoid bone	Growth hormone (GH, somatotropin, somatropic hormone, STH)* Thyrotropin (thyroid-stimulating hormone, or TSH) Adrenocorticotropic hormone (ACTH, corticotropin)* Follicle-stimulating hormone (FSH) Luteinizing hormone (LH) in female; interstitial cell-stimulating hormone (ICSH) in male Prolactin (PRL, lactogenic hormone, luteotropin) Melanocyte-stimulating hormone (MSH) Alpha and beta lipotropins
Posterior (neurohypophysis)	In sella turcica of sphenoid bone	Antidiuretic hormone (ADH, vasopressin)† Oxytocin†
Pineal	Midbrain	Melatonin
Thyroid	Overlies thyroid cartilage below the larynx	Thyroid hormones (thyroxine and triiodothyronine), calcitonin
Parathyroids	Usually four beads on posterior wall of the thyroid	Parathormone
Thymus	Root of neck and anterior thorax	Thymosin‡
Adrenals	Situated on medial anterior surface of each kidney	
Cortex		Glucocorticoids (mainly cortisol and corticosterone) Mineralocorticoids (mainly aldosterone) Sex hormones (small amounts of androgens and estrogens)
Medulla		Epinephrine (mainly) Norepinephrine
Pancreas (islets of Langerhans)	Retroperitoneal in abdominal cavity	Insulin (secreted by beta cells) Glucagon (secreted by alpha cells) Somatostatin Pancreatic polypeptide
Ovaries Graafian follicles Corpus luteum	Pelvic cavity (female)	Estrogens (estradiol, estrone) Progesterone
Testes Interstitial cells of testes	Scrotum (male)	Testosterone

*Also present in placenta along with estrogens and progesterone.
†ADH and oxytocin are synthesized in the hypothalamus but are secreted by the posterior pituitary gland. Synthesis occurs in cell bodies of neurons of the supraoptic and paraventricular nuclei. From here they migrate down the neurons' axons into the posterior pituitary gland, which secretes them into the blood.
‡ One of several active thymic hormones.

nal genitalia, increased sex drive, laryngeal growth, and growth of body hair

3. Androgens influence fetal brain development through contributing to establishment of neural pathways that help to regulate adult brain functions and behavior

C. Metabolism of androgens

1. Liver the major site for androgen metabolism; testosterone and other androgenic steroids are enzymatically converted into other less androgenic steroids and then conjugated with glucuronic acid or sulfate
2. The generally biologically inactive conjugates are excreted in bile and urine

TABLE 6-6 Functions of thyroid and parathyroid hormones

Hormones	Functions	Hypofunction effects	Hyperfunction effects
Thyroid hormones			
Thyroxine	Stimulates metabolic rate; therefore essential for normal physical and mental development	Cretinism, if occurs early in life; myxedema, if occurs in older children or adults	Hyperthyroidism
Triiodothyronine	Inhibits anterior pituitary secretion of TSH		
Thyrocalcitonin (calcitonin)	Quickly decreases blood calcium concentration if Ca^{++} increases about 20% above normal level; presumably accelerates calcium movement from blood into bone		
Parathyroid hormone (parathormone)	Increases blood calcium concentration by accelerating following three processes: 1. Breakdown of bone with release of calcium into blood 2. Calcium absorption from intestine into blood 3. Kidney tubule reabsorption of calcium from tubular urine into blood, thereby decreasing calcium loss in urine	Decreased blood calcium (hypocalcemia), which causes increased neural excitability and tetany	Increased blood calcium (hypercalcemia), which causes decreased neural excitability and muscle weakness Bone "softening"–decalcification
	Decreases blood phosphate concentration by slowing its reabsorption by kidney tubules and thereby increasing phosphate loss in urine	Increased blood phosphorus (hyperphosphatemia)	Hypophosphatemia

TABLE 6-7 Sex hormones (ovarian and testicular)

Hormones	Functions
Estrogens (secreted by graafian follicle and corpus luteum) Estradiol Estrone Estriol	Stimulate proliferation of epithelial cells of female reproductive organs (e.g., thickening of endometrium, breast development) Stimulate uterine contractions Accelerate protein anabolism (including bone matrix synthesis) to promote growth; but also promote epiphyseal closure to limit height Mildly accelerate sodium and water reabsorption by kidney tubules; increase water content of uterus High blood estrogen concentration inhibits anterior pituitary secretion of FSH and prolactin but stimulates its secretion of LH Low blood estrogen concentration after delivery of baby stimulates anterior pituitary secretion of prolactin
Progesterone (secreted by corpus luteum and placenta)	Name "progesterone" indicates hormone's general function, "favoring pregnancy": Stimulates secretion by endometrial glands, thereby preparing endometrium for implantation of fertilized ovum Inhibits uterine contractions, thereby favoring retention of implanted embryo Promotes development of alveoli (secreting cells) of estrogen-primed breasts; necessary for lactation Protein-catabolic and salt and water-retaining effects similar to those of corticoids but milder; increases water content of endometrium
Testosterone (secreted by interstitial cells of testes)	Growth and development of male reproductive organs; promotes "maleness" Marked stimulating effect on protein anabolism, including synthesis of bone matrix and muscular development, hence, promotes growth; however, it also tends to limit height by promoting epiphyseal closure Mild acceleration of kidney tubule reabsorption of sodium chloride and water Inhibits secretion of ICSH by anterior pituitary

Ovaries

A. Anatomy

See Structures of the Female Reproductive System in Childbearing and Women's Health (Chapter 3)

B. Actions of ovarian hormones (Table 6-7)

1. Estrogens
   a. Enter target cells, bind cytoplasmic receptors, and enter nucleus; estrogen receptor complex regulates mRNA synthesis with overall effect of stimulating cellular RNA and protein synthesis
   b. Stimulate uterine and liver lipid metabolism
   c. Stimulate long-bone calcification
   d. Play a major role in the ovulatory-menstrual cycle
   e. Increased protein and lipid synthesis are manifested in the reproductive system as uterine growth
   f. Participate also in growth of pubic and axillary hair, pelvic enlargement, subcutaneous lipid distribution, growth of mammary glands, and maturation of skin (increased glandular activity)

2. Progesterone
   a. Increases mucous secretory activity of endometrium; such action required for implantation of young embryo
   b. Promotes growth of breasts
   c. Keeps uterine smooth muscle quiescent during pregnancy
   d. Inhibits oxytocin release by neurohypophysis (otherwise released in response to vaginal distention)

C. Metabolism of estrogens and progesterone

1. Liver conjugates estrogens with glucuronic and sulfuric acids; the conjugates are excreted chiefly in urine
2. Conversion of estradiol to the less active estrone in the liver; placenta also carries out this conversion
3. Liver converts progesterone, synthesized from cholesterol in corpus luteum, placenta, and adrenals, to pregnanediol, which is then conjugated with glucuronic acid or sulfate; conjugates are excreted in urine

Adrenal Glands

A. Anatomy

1. Wedge-shaped, flattened, yellowish structure positioned like a cap at the kidney's superior border
2. Actually two closely associated structures: inner adrenal medulla and outer adrenal cortex; medulla and cortex each produce hormones with distinct effects on distant target structures

3. Medulla produces two catecholamines, D-epinephrine and D-norepinephrine, in approximate ratio of 80% to 20%, respectively
4. Cortex secretes three steroid hormones in relatively large amounts: aldosterone (a mineralocorticoid), cortisol (known as hydrocortisone), and corticosterone (both glucocorticoids); also small amounts of several androgenic steroids; adrenocortical secretion is circadian, with higher levels produced during daytime; aldosterone secretion increases as sodium ions decrease or potassium ions increase

B. Actions of adrenal hormones

1. Epinephrine and norepinephrine
   a. Stimulate liver and skeletal muscle to break down glycogen
   b. Increase oxygen use and increase carbon dioxide production
   c. Increase blood concentration of free fatty acids through stimulation of lipolysis in adipose tissue
   d. Cause constriction of nearly all blood vessels of body, thereby greatly increasing total peripheral resistance and arterial pressure
   e. Increase heart rate and force of contraction and thereby raise cardiac output
   f. Epinephrine significantly dilates bronchial smooth muscle
   g. Inhibit contractions of gastrointestinal and uterine smooth muscle

2. Glucocorticoids and mineralocorticoids (Table 6-8)

C. Metabolism of adrenocortical steroids

1. Liver the major organ metabolizing adrenal steroids
2. Conjugation of steroids with glucuronic acid or sulfate produces inactive products primarily excreted in urine
3. In liver disease, adrenal steroids increase in the blood as a result of decreased inactivation

Pancreas

A. Anatomy (see Gastrointestinal System)

B. Actions of pancreatic hormones

1. Regulate glucose homeostasis through action of insulin and glucagon; also secrete somatostatin and pancreatic polypeptide
2. Insulin stimulates intracellular macromolecular syntheses, such as glycogen synthesis, protein synthesis, and lipogenesis
3. Insulin stimulates cellular uptake of sodium and potassium (latter is significant in the treatment of diabetic coma with insulin); glucose also requires potassium supplement to offset hypokalemia
4. Glucagon induces liver glycogenolysis similar to that produced by epinephrine, but glucagon functions at lower concentration and also does

TABLE 6-8 Functions of adrenal cortex hormones

Functions	Hypofunction effects (e.g., in Addison's disease)	Hyperfunction effects (e.g., in Cushing's syndrome)
Glucocorticoids (mainly cortisol [hydrocortisone] and corticosterone)		
In general, a normal blood concentration of glucocorticoids promotes normal metabolism of all three kinds of foods and a high blood concentration produces various stress responses		
Accelerates mobilization and catabolism of fats; i.e., causes shift from usual use of carbohydrates for energy to fat use		
Accelerates tissue protein mobilization and catabolism (tissue proteins hydrolyzed to amino acids, which enter blood and are carried to liver for deamination and gluconeogenesis)		Muscle atrophy and weakness; osteoporosis
Accelerates liver gluconeogenesis (i.e., formation of glucose from mobilized proteins [hyperglycemic effect])	Hypoglycemia	Hyperglycemia
Causes atrophy of lymphatic tissues, notably thymus and lymph nodes		Lymphocytopenia
Decreases antibody formation (immunosuppressive, antiallergic effect)		Decreased immunity Decreased allergy Spread of infections; slower wound healing
Slows the proliferation of fibroblasts characteristic of inflammation (antiinflammatory effect)		
Mild acceleration of sodium and water reabsorption and potassium excretion by kidney tubules		High blood sodium (hypernatremia); sodium retention; also water retention; low blood potassium (hypokalemia)
Decreases ACTH secretion		
Mineralocorticoids (mainly aldosterone)		
Marked acceleration of sodium and water reabsorption by kidney tubules	Low blood sodium (hyponatremia); dehydration, hypovolemia High blood potassium (hyperkalemia)	High blood sodium (hypernatremia); water retention; edema Low blood potassium (hypokalemia)
Marked acceleration of potassium excretion by kidney tubules		

not raise blood pressure; antagonizes the glycogen synthesis stimulated by insulin

5. Glucagon inhibits hepatic protein synthesis; this makes amino acids available for gluconeogenesis and also increases urea production

6. Glucagon stimulates hepatic ketogenesis and release of glycerol and fatty acids from adipose tissue

7. Primary target organs are muscle, liver, and adipose cells, but other tissues also affected

8. Somatostatin inhibits release of both insulin and glucagon

9. Pancreatic polypeptide increases pancreatic and gastric secretions; secreted into blood after a protein-rich meal; secretion inhibited by somatostatin

TABLE 6-9 Functions of anterior pituitary hormones

Functions	Hyposecretion effects	Hypersecretion effects
GROWTH HORMONE (GH) Promotes protein anabolism (hence, essential for normal growth) Promotes fat mobilization and catabolism (i.e., causes shift from carbohydrate catabolism to fat catabolism) Slows carbohydrate metabolism; has antiinsulin, hyperglycemic, diabetogenic effect (promotes glucagon secretion)	Dwarfism (well-formed type) if it occurs before skeletal growth is completed Simmonds' disease after skeletal maturity	Giantism if it occurs before skeletal growth is completed Acromegaly if it occurs after skeletal maturity Hyperglycemia, chronic excess GH may cause diabetes mellitus
THYROID-STIMULATING HORMONE (TSH) Stimulates synthesis and secretion of thyroid hormones	Hypothyroidism: cretinism in early life, myxedema in adults	Hyperthyroidism (exophthalmic goiter, various other names)
ADRENOCORTICOTROPIC HORMONE (ACTH) Stimulates adrenal cortex growth and secretion of glucocorticoids; slight mineralocorticoid stimulation	Atrophy of adrenal cortex and hyposecretion (e.g., Addison's disease) Increased skin pigmentation	Hypertrophy of adrenal cortex and hypersecretion (Cushing's syndrome)
FOLLICLE-STIMULATING HORMONE (FSH) Stimulates primary graafian follicle to start growing and to develop to maturity Stimulates follicle cells to secrete estrogens In male, FSH stimulates development of seminiferous tubules and spermatogenesis by them	Failure of follicle and ovum to grow and mature; sterility	
LUTEINIZING HORMONE (LH) Essential for bringing about complete maturation of follicle and ovum Required for ovulation Causes formation of corpus luteum in reptured follicle following ovulation; hence the name luteinizing hormone Stimulates corpus luteum to secrete progesterone In males LH is called interstitial–cell-stimulating hormone (ICSH) because it stimulates interstitial cells of testes to secrete testosterone		
PROLACTIN Promotes breast development during pregnancy Initiates milk secretion after delivery of fetus Stimulates progesterone secretion by corpus luteum	Failure to lactate	
ALPHA AND BETA LIPOPROTEINS Cause release of lipid from adipose cells		

Thymus

A. Anatomy
1. Soft, pink mass extending from lower border of thyroid to the fourth costal cartilages; great variation in size; two asymmetric lobes
2. Large at birth; decreases in size after puberty; hardly visible beyond middle age

B. Actions of thymic hormones
1. Regulate immunologic processes, possibly through regulation of the numbers and types of lymphoid cells; decrease in immune response with aging; parallels thymus involution and decreasing blood concentrations of thymic hormones
2. Just after birth the thymus produces T-lymphocytes that migrate to peripheral regions (e.g., lymph nodes, spleen) to provide immunologic potential
3. Thymus synthesizes hormones that regulate the rate of development of lymphoid cells, particularly T cells

Pineal Gland

A. Anatomy
1. A firm, reddish, conical structure lying in the midbrain between the superior colliculi and attached by a short stalk to the roof of the third ventricle
2. Composed of cords of pinealocytes (or chief cells) separated by connective tissue; septa continuous with the pia mater covering the organ; cells accumulate calcareous granules (brain sand) by age 18 years, clearly visible with x-ray examination

B. Actions of pineal hormone
1. Secretes melatonin

2. Melatonin may regulate diurnal fluctuations of hypothalamic-hypophyseal hormones

Pituitary Gland

A. Anatomy
1. Rounded body 1.2 cm in diameter extending downward from the floor of the brain's third ventricle by a stalk (infundibulum); supported and protected by the sella turcica of the sphenoid bone; located near the optic chiasm
2. Composed of an anterior lobe (adenohypophysis) and a posterior lobe (neurohypophysis)

B. Actions of pituitary hormones (Tables 6-9 and 6-10)

PHARMACOLOGY RELATED TO ENDOCRINE SYSTEM DISORDERS

Antidiabetic Agents

A. Description
1. Used to treat diabetes mellitus
2. Classified into two types: insulin for parenteral use and oral hypoglycemics
3. Insulin acts to facilitate the transport of glucose across the cell membrane and to promote glycogenesis
4. Insulin is available in three forms: beef, pork, and human; human and purified pork insulins are less antigenic than the other forms
5. Insulin is available in rapid-acting, intermediate-acting, and long-acting forms; rapid-acting and intermediate-acting forms are available in mixed preparations (e.g., Humulin 70/30, which contains 70% NPH and 30% regular insulin)
6. Oral hypoglycemics stimulate pancreatic beta

TABLE 6-10 Functions of posterior hormones		
Functions	**Hyposecretion effects**	**Hypersecretion effects**
ANTIDIURETIC HORMONE (ADH) VASOPRESSIN Increased water reabsorption by kidney's distal and collecting tubules, thereby producing antidiuresis (less urine volume; name based on this effect) Stimulates vasoconstriction; raises blood pressure	Diuresis (polyuria); diabetes insipidus	Antidiuresis (oliguria)
OXYTOCIN Stimulates powerful contractions by pregnant uterus Stimulates milk ejection from alveoli (milk-secreting cells) of lactating breasts into ducts; essential before milk can be removed by suckling		
COHERIN Regulates peristaltic rhythmicity in intestinal smooth muscle		
MELANOCYTE-STIMULATING HORMONE (MSH) Stimulates synthesis and dispersion of melanin in skin, causing darkening		

cells to produce insulin in clients with residual functioning cells

B. Examples
1. Insulin: exogenous replacement of insulin hormone; parenteral administration only (Table 6-11)
2. Oral hypoglycemics are medications capable of decreasing blood glucose. There are two categories of medications with differing mechanisms of action, sulphonylureas and biguanides
    a. Sulphonylureas lower blood glucose by stimulating release of insulin from pancreatic beta cells. Other potential actions are to decrease insulin resistance and decrease hepatic glucose production
        (1) Glyburide (Diabeta/Euglucon)
        (2) Gliclazide (Diamicron)
        (3) Tolbutamide (Orinase)
        (4) Chlorpropamide (Diabinese)
        (5) Acetohexamide (Dimelor)
    b. Biguanides: primary mechanism of action is to enhance glucose utilization by skeletal muscle. Metformin is the only marketed biguanide in Canada: may also enhance insulin binding

Drug	Onset (hours)	Duration (hours)
Glyburide	1.5	10-14
Gliclazide		24
Tolbutamide	1	6-12
Chlorpropamide	1	72
Acetohexamide	1	10-14

of the cell. Positive effects include changes in triglycerides and cholesterol with weight loss. Metformin is useful for the obese patient with type II diabetes and hyperinsulinemia

C. Major side effects
1. Important side effects of sulphonylureas
    a. Hypoglycemia (give oral glucose in some form)
    b. Nausea (give with meals)
    c. Dyspepsia (give with meals)
    d. Dizziness (rule out hypoglycemia)
    e. Headache (rule out hypoglycemia)
    f. Rash, maculopapular, erythematous, or pruritis (discontinue or change sulphonylureas)
2. Adverse effects of metformin (a biguanide)
    a. Hypoglycemia (give oral glucose in some form)
    b. Diarrhea (give with meals)
    c. Abdominal discomfort (give with meals)
    d. Nausea (give with meals)
    e. Anorexia (give with meals)
    f. Metallic taste (give with meals)
    g. Hyperventilation (rapid onset) and drowsiness with abdominal pain (may be a sign of lactic acidosis, rare but potentially severe reaction; more common in clients with renal impairment and hepatic disease)

D. Nursing care
1. Assess client for signs of hypoglycemia
2. Instruct client to:
    a. Use proper medication administration procedure

TABLE 6-11 Types of insulin

Insulin	Action in hours		
	Onset	Peak	Duration
RAPID ACTING*			
Insulin human (Humulin R)	½ to 1	2 to 3	5 to 7
Insulin injection (regular insulin)	1 to 3	2 to 3	5 to 7
Prompt insulin zinc suspension (Semilente)	1 to 3	2 to 8	12 to 16
INTERMEDIATE ACTING*			
Globin zinc insulin injection	2 to 3	8 to 16	18 to 24
Human insulin zinc suspension (Humulin L)	1 to 2	8 to 12	18 to 24
Insulin zinc suspension (Lente)	1 to 2	8 to 12	18 to 24
Isophane insulin human (Humulin N, Insulatard NPH human)	1 to 2	8 to 12	18 to 24
Isophane insulin suspension (NPH)	1 to 2	8 to 12	18 to 24
LONG ACTING			
Extended insulin zinc suspension (Ultralente)	4 to 6	18 to 24	34 to 36
Protamine zinc insulin suspension (PZI)	4 to 6	14 to 24	30 to 36

*Rapid-acting and intermediate-acting insulins are available in mixed preparations (e.g., Humulin 70/30, which contains 70% NPH and 30% regular insulin)

b. Comply with dietary program

c. Avoid alcohol, especially when taking chlorpropamide; severe nausea, vomiting, and malaise can result

d. Use proper procedure for urine and/or blood testing

e. Carry medical alert card

f. Be prepared for hypoglycemic incidents (rapid-acting glucose solution, hard candy, orange juice)

3. Administer insulin
   a. Administer all forms of insulin subcutaneously
   b. Only regular insulin may be given intravenously
   c. When mixing insulins, draw regular insulin (clear) into the syringe first
   d. Rotate sites of administration
   e. Slight dosage adjustment may be necessary when switching from one form of insulin to another because of differing pharmacokinetics

4. Offer emotional support to client; therapy is lifelong

5. Evaluate client's response to medication and understanding of teaching

Thyroid Enhancers

A. Description
   1. Used to replace thyroid hormone in clients experiencing a reduction in or absence of thyroid gland function
   2. Thyroid hormone regulates the metabolic rate of body cells; aids in growth and development of bones and teeth; and affects protein, fat, and carbohydrate metabolism
   3. Available in oral and parenteral (IV) preparations
B. Examples
   1. Levothyroxine sodium (Eltroxin)
   2. Liotrix (Euthroid, Thyrolar)
   3. Thyroglobulin (Proloid)
   4. Thyroid desiccated (Thyrar)
   5. Thyrotropin (thytropar)
C. Major side effects
   1. Increased metabolism (increased serum T_3, T_4)
   2. Hyperactivity (increased metabolic rate)
   3. Cardiac stimulation (increased cardiac metabolism)
D. Nursing care
   1. Instruct client to:
      a. Report the occurrence of any side effects to the physician immediately
      b. Take medication as scheduled at the same time each day; do not stop abruptly
      c. Take radial pulse; notify physician if greater than 100 beats/minute

d. Carry medical alert card

e. Keep all scheduled appointments with physician; medical supervision is necessary

2. Assess client for potentiation of anticoagulant effect

3. Offer emotional support to client; therapy may be lifelong

4. Assess client for signs of hyperthyroidism

5. Evaluate client's response to medication and understanding of teaching

Thyroid Inhibitors

A. Description
   1. Used to treat hyperthyroidism
   2. Act by interfering with the synthesis and release of thyroid hormone; inhibit oxidation of iodides to prevent their combination with tyrosine in formation of thyroxine
   3. Available in oral and parenteral (IV) preparations
B. Examples
   1. Iodine (Lugol's solution)
   2. Methimazole (Tapazole)
   3. Propylthiouracil (Thyracil)
C. Major side effects
   1. Agranulocytosis (decreased WBCs)
   2. Skin disturbances (hypersensitivity)
   3. Nausea, vomiting (irritation of gastric mucosa)
   4. Decreased metabolism (decreased production of serum T_3, T_4)
   5. Iodine: bitter taste; stains teeth (local oral effect on mucosa and teeth)
D. Nursing care
   1. Instruct client to:
      a. Report the occurrence of any side effects to physician, especially sore throat and fever
      b. Avoid crowded places and potentially infectious situations
   2. Administer liquid iodine preparations diluted in beverage of choice through a straw
   3. Assess client for signs of hypothyroidism
   4. Evaluate client's response to medication and understanding of teaching

Adrenocorticosteroids

A. Description
   1. Interfere with the release of factors important in producing the normal inflammatory and immune responses
   2. Increase glucose and fat formation and promote protein breakdown
   3. Available in oral, parenteral (IM, IV), inhalation, intraarticular, and topical, including ophthalmic, preparations
B. Examples
   1. Betamethasone preparations

2. Dexamethasone (Decadron)
3. Hydrocortisone (Cortef)
4. Hydrocortisone succinate (Solu-Cortef)
5. Methylprednisolone sodium succinate (Solu-Medrol)
6. Prednisone (Deltasone)

C. Major side effects
1. Cushing-like symptoms (increased glucocorticoid activity)
2. Hypertension (promotion of sodium and water retention)
3. Hyperglycemia (increased carbohydrate catabolism; gluconeogenesis)
4. CNS stimulation (CNS effect)
5. Euphoria (CNS effect)
6. GI irritation and ulcer formation (local GI effect)
7. Cataracts (hyperglycemia)
8. Hypokalemia (promotion of potassium excretion)

D. Nursing care
1. Administer oral preparations with food, milk, or antacid
2. Monitor client's weight, blood pressure, and serum electrolytes during therapy
3. Avoid placing client in potentially infectious situations
4. Assess for GI bleeding; monitor blood glucose in diabetics
5. Instruct client to:
   a. Avoid exposure to infections; notify physician if fever or sore throat occurs
   b. Avoid using salt; encourage foods high in potassium
   c. Avoid immunizations during therapy
   d. Carry medical alert card
   e. Avoid missing, changing, or withdrawing drug suddenly
6. Withdraw drug therapy gradually to permit adrenal recovery
7. Evaluate client's response to medication and understanding of teaching

Antidiuretic Hormone

A. Description
1. Used in the treatment of diabetes insipidus
2. Acts to:
   a. Promote water reabsorption by the distal renal tubules
   b. Cause vasoconstriction and increased muscle tone of the bladder, GI tract, uterus, and blood vessels
3. Available in parenteral (IM, SC) or nasal preparation

B. Examples
1. Desmopressin acetate (DDAVP): intranasal administration
2. Vasopressin (Pitressin)

C. Major side effects
1. Increased intestinal activity (direct peristaltic stimulant)
2. Hyponatremia (promotion of water reabsorption)
3. Pallor (hemodilution)
4. Water intoxication (promotion of water reabsorption)
5. Cardiac disturbances (fluid/electrolyte imbalance)
6. Nasal irritation (lypressin has local effect on nasal mucosa)

D. Nursing care
1. Assess client for signs of dehydration during therapy
2. Monitor intake and output
3. If drug is administered to improve bladder or bowel tone, assess for continence or passage of flatus
4. Assess vital signs, especially blood pressure, during course of therapy
5. Evaluate client's response to medication and understanding of teaching

PROCEDURES RELATED TO THE ENDOCRINE SYSTEM

Capillary Blood Glucose Monitoring

A. Definition: capillary blood is analyzed as direct measure of blood glucose (being replaced by noninvasive techniques)
B. Nursing care
1. Cleanse skin with soap and water (usually sufficient)
2. Prick fingertip or earlobe with sterile needle or lancet to obtain blood specimen
3. Apply free-flowing drop of blood to glucose-sensitive reagent strip
4. Blot or wipe strip after specified interval according to manufacturer's instructions
5. Visually compare color of reagent to manufacturer's chart or use computerized blood glucose monitoring system; adhere to specific time frames
6. Chart results
7. Administer usual insulin coverage as ordered
8. Instruct client about individual method of self monitoring of blood glucose (SMBG)
9. Evaluate client's response to procedure

Sugar and Acetone (Fractional Urine Tests)

A. Definition
1. Sugar refers to the percentage of glucose in the urine as indirect measure of blood glucose
2. Acetone refers to the amount of ketones, a

byproduct of fat metabolism, present in the urine
B. Nursing care
1. Obtain a recently voided specimen approximately half an hour before meals and at bedtime; a double-voided specimen would produce most accurate results (client empties bladder and half an hour later is asked to void again)
2. Test urine with appropriate reagent (Clinitest, Acetest)
3. Chart results
4. Administer usual insulin coverage as ordered
5. Evaluate client's response to procedure

GENERAL NURSING DIAGNOSES FOR CLIENTS WITH ENDOCRINE SYSTEM DISORDERS

A. Activity intolerance related to altered metabolic rate
B. Body image disturbance related to hormonal changes
C. Constipation related to decreased metabolic rate
D. Ineffective individual coping related to chronic nature of disability
E. Diarrhea related to increased metabolic rate
F. Fatigue related to altered metabolic processes
G. Fluid volume deficit related to increased urinary output
H. Fluid volume excess related to:
1. Chronic nature of disability
2. Hormonal imbalance
I. Risk for infection related to:
1. Impaired immune response caused by disease process
2. Trauma to extremities
3. Decreased peripheral tissue perfusion
J. Risk for injury related to:
1. Hormonal imbalance
2. Peripheral neuropathy
K. Noncompliance related to:
1. Inability to accept chronic disease
2. Difficulty in carrying out treatment modalities
L. Altered nutrition: less than body requirements related to:
1. Increased metabolic rate
2. Altered use of nutrients
M. Sensory/perceptual alteration related to metabolic dysfunction
N. Sexual dysfunction related to:
1. Hormonal changes
2. Results of disease process
O. Sleep pattern disturbance related to increased metabolic rate

MAJOR DISORDERS OF THE ENDOCRINE SYSTEM

▼ HYPERPITUITARISM
Data Base

A. Etiology and pathophysiology
1. May be due to overactivity of gland or the result of an adenoma
2. Characterized by an excessive concentration of pituitary hormones (GH, ACTH, PRL) in the blood, overactivity, and changes in the anterior lobe of the pituitary gland
3. Two classifications of GH overproduction
   a. Giantism: generalized increase in size, especially in children; involves the long bones
   b. Acromegaly: occurs after epiphyseal closing, with subsequent enlargement of cartilage, bone, and soft tissues of body
4. ACTH overproduction leads to Cushing's disease
B. Clinical findings
1. Subjective
   a. Headaches
   b. Depression
   c. Weakness
2. Objective
   a. Increased soft tissue and bone thickness
   b. Facial features become coarse and heavy, with enlargement of lower jaw, lips, and tongue
   c. Enlarged hands and feet
   d. Increased growth hormone (GH), corticotrophic (ACTH), or prolactin (PRL)
   e. X-ray examination of long bones, skull (sella turcica area), and jaw demonstrates change in structure
   f. Amenorrhea
   g. Glycosuria
   h. Diabetes and hyperthyroidism may also occur
C. Therapeutic interventions
1. Medications to relieve symptoms of other endocrine imbalances resulting from pituitary hyperfunctioning
2. Surgical intervention (hypophysectomy) or irradiation of the pituitary

Nursing Care of Clients with Hyperpituitarism
A. DATA COLLECTION
1. Changes in energy level; sexual function; menstrual patterns; and sizes of hat, gloves, or rings
2. Face, hands, and feet for thickening and enlargement

3. Presence of dysphagia or voice changes
4. Presence of hypogonadism as a result of hyperprolactinemia
5. Reaction to changes in physical appearance and sexual function

B. ANALYSIS AND INTERPRETATION

Refer to General Nursing Diagnoses for Clients with Endocrine System Disorders for the following diagnoses: B, F, I 1, N 1, and N 2

C. PLANNING/IMPLEMENTATION

1. Help the client accept the altered body image that is irreversible
2. Assist family to understand what the client is experiencing
3. Help the client recognize that medical supervision will be required for life
4. Help the client understand the basis for the change in sexual functioning
5. Assist the client in expressing feelings
6. Care for the client following a hypophysectomy
   a. Encourage following an established medical regimen
   b. Protect from stress situations
   c. Protect from infection
   d. Follow and maintain an established schedule for hormone replacement
   e. Refer to nursing care for the client undergoing intracranial surgery
      (1) Perform neurologic assessments
      (2) Measure specific gravity of urine, monitor intake and output, and check daily weight to identify complication of diabetes insipidus
      (3) Check clear nasal drainage for glucose to determine presence of CSF
      (4) Encourage deep breathing, but not coughing
      (5) Institute measures to prevent constipation because straining increases intracranial pressure

D. EVALUATION/OUTCOMES

1. Verbalizes an improved body image
2. Reports satisfying sexual relationship
3. Continues medical supervision

▼ HYPOPITUITARISM

Data Base

A. Etiology and pathophysiology
   1. Deficiency of one or more anterior pituitary hormones
   2. Total absence of pituitary hormones referred to as panhypopituitarism (Simmonds' disease)
   3. Occurs when there is destruction of the ante-

rior lobe of the gland by trauma, tumor, or hemorrhage
   4. Clinical findings vary with target organs affected

B. Clinical findings
   1. Subjective
      a. Lethargy
      b. Loss of strength and libido
      c. Decreased tolerance for cold
   2. Objective
      a. Decreased temperature
      b. Postural hypotension
      c. Hypoglycemia
      d. Diminished axillary and pubic hair
      e. Sterility
      f. Loss of secondary sexual characteristics
      g. Visual disturbances if tumor impinges on optic nerve

C. Therapeutic interventions
   1. Replace hormones
   2. If tumor is present, surgical intervention is indicated

Nursing Care of Clients with Hypopituitarism

A. DATA COLLECTION

1. Baseline vital signs
2. Sexual patterns
   a. Loss of libido
   b. Painful intercourse
   c. Inability to maintain an erection
3. Past and present menstrual patterns
4. Visual acuity
5. Loss of secondary sexual characteristics
6. Activity tolerance

B. ANALYSIS AND INTERPRETATION

Refer to General Nursing Diagnoses for Clients with Endocrine System Disorders for the following diagnoses: B, F, K 1, K 2, N 1, and N 2

C. PLANNING/IMPLEMENTATION

1. Monitor effects of hormone replacement
2. Discuss the importance of adhering to medical regimen on a long-term basis
3. Allow the client ample time to verbalize feelings regarding the long-term nature of the disease and impact on daily life
4. Provide adequate rest periods

D. EVALUATION/OUTCOMES

1. Complies with medical regimen
2. Expresses positive feelings of body image
3. Establishes satisfying sexual relationship

▼ DIABETES INSIPIDUS

Data Base

A. Etiology and pathophysiology

1. A deficient production or secretion of the antidiuretic hormone (ADH); may be familial, idiopathic, secondary to trauma, surgery, tumors, infections, or autoimmune disorders
2. Neurogenic diabetes insipidus, a renal tubular defect resulting in decreased water absorption, may be familial or result from renal disorders, primary aldosteronism, or excessive water intake (primary polydipsia); results in impaired renal concentrating ability

B. Clinical findings
   1. Subjective
      a. Polydipsia
      b. Craving for cold water
   2. Objective
      a. Polyuria (5 to 25 L/24 hr)
      b. Dilute urine; specific gravity 1.001 to 1.005; osmolarity 50 to 200 mOsm/kg
      c. Signs of dehydration (poor skin turgor, dry mucous membranes, elevated temperature)

C. Therapeutic interventions
   1. Antidiuretic hormone replacement: vasopressin (Pitressin), lypressin (Diapid), desmopressin (DDAVP)
   2. Treatment of underlying cause

Nursing Care of Clients with Diabetes Insipidus

A. DATA COLLECTION
   1. Intake and output, weight, and specific gravity of urine to establish baseline data
   2. Results of serum electrolyte evaluation
   3. Dryness of skin and mucous membranes

B. ANALYSIS AND INTERPRETATION

Refer to General Nursing Diagnoses for Clients with Endocrine System Disorders for the following diagnoses: D, G, and H 2

C. PLANNING/IMPLEMENTATION
   1. Continue monitoring of fluid and electrolyte status: intake and output, daily weight, skin turgor, electrolyte levels
   2. Replace fluid by mouth or parenterally
   3. Monitor response to ADH replacement
   4. Teach client on long-term vasopressin therapy the need for daily weight records, recognition of polyuria, and wearing a medical alert bracelet; overdosage may cause syndrome of inappropriate antidiuretic hormone (SIADH), leading to water retention and hyponatremia
   5. Advise client to avoid alcohol because it suppresses ADH secretion

D. EVALUATION/OUTCOMES
   1. Maintains fluid balance
   2. States signs of overmedication and undermedication with ADH replacement

▼ HYPERTHYROIDISM (GRAVES' DISEASE, THYROTOXICOSIS)

Data Base

A. Etiology and pathophysiology
   1. Etiology is believed to be involved with an autoimmune process of impaired regulation; secondary to other autoimmune disorders
   2. Excessive concentration of thyroid hormones in the blood as a result of thyroid disease or increased TSH
   3. Overactivity and changes in the thyroid gland may be present
   4. May occur at periods of high physiologic and psychologic stress, although considered by some to be an autoimmune reaction
   5. The gland may also enlarge (goiter) as a result of decreased iodine intake; no increase in secretion of thyroid is present

B. Clinical findings
   1. Subjective
      a. Polyphagia
      b. Emotional lability and apprehension
      c. Heat intolerance
   2. Objective
      a. Weight loss
      b. Increased systolic blood pressure, temperature, pulse, and respiration
      c. Tremors, hyperactive reflexes
      d. Diaphoresis
      e. Insomnia
      f. Exophthalmos, corneal ulceration
      g. Increased BMR
      h. Decreased TSH levels if thyroid disorder; increased TSH levels if secondary to a pituitary disorder
      i. Increased triiodothyronine (T_3), thyroxine (T_4), protein-bound iodine (PBI), long-acting thyroid stimulator (LATS), and radioactive iodine uptake
      j. Loose stools
      k. Thyrotoxic crisis (thyroid storm): a state of hypermetabolism that may lead to heart failure; usually precipitated by a period of severe physiologic or psychologic stress, thyroid surgery, or radioactive iodine therapy

C. Therapeutic interventions
   1. Antithyroid medications such as propylthiouracil (Thyracil) and methimazole (Tapazole) to block the synthesis of thyroid hormone
   2. Antithyroid medications such as iodine (Lugol's solution or SSKI) to reduce the vascularity of the thyroid gland
   3. Radioactive iodine to destroy thyroid gland

cells, thereby decreasing the production of thyroid hormone (atomic cocktail)

4. Medications to relieve the symptoms related to the increased metabolic rate (e.g., digitalis, propranolol [Inderal], phenobarbital)

5. Well-balanced, high-calorie diet with vitamin and mineral supplements

6. Surgical intervention involves a subtotal or total thyroidectomy

Nursing Care of Clients with Hyperthyroidism

A. DATA COLLECTION

1. History of weight loss, diarrhea, insomnia, emotional lability, palpitations, and heat intolerance
2. Eyes for exophthalmos, tearing, and sensitivity to light
3. Neck palpation for enlarged thyroid gland
4. Weight and vital signs to establish baseline

B. ANALYSIS AND INTERPRETATION

Refer to General Nursing Diagnoses for Clients with Endocrine System Disorders for the following diagnoses: B, D, E, F, J 1, L 1, and O

C. PLANNING/IMPLEMENTATION

1. Assign the client a private room with the means for temperature control when possible; clients usually prefer a cool room
2. Monitor vital signs regularly
3. Provide for periods of uninterrupted rest
4. Administer medications to promote sleep as prescribed
5. Use nursing measures such as warm milk, warm bath, and back rub to establish a climate for rest
6. Protect the client from stress-producing visitors
7. Provide diet high in calories, proteins, and carbohydrates with supplemental feedings between meals and at bedtime; vitamin and mineral supplements should be given as prescribed
8. Understand that the client is upset by lability of mood and exaggerated response to environmental stimuli; take time to explain disease processes involved
9. Provide eye care; eye drops and eye patches may be needed
10. Care for the client before a thyroidectomy
    a. Administer prescribed antithyroid medications to achieve euthyroid state
    b. Teach deep breathing exercises and use of hands to support neck and to avoid strain on suture line
11. Care for the client following a thyroidectomy
    a. Observe for signs of respiratory distress and laryngeal stridor caused by tracheal edema (keep tracheotomy set available)
    b. Provide humidity with cold steam nebulizer to keep secretions moist when at home
    c. Keep the bed in a semi-Fowler's position without pillows and teach client to support head
    d. Use a soft cervical collar if ordered to prevent unnecessary neck movement
    e. Observe dressings at the operative site and back of the neck and shoulders for signs of hemorrhage
    f. Observe for signs of thyroid storm; may result from manipulation of the gland during surgery, which releases thyroid hormone into bloodstream
       (1) High fever
       (2) Tachycardia
       (3) Irritability, delirium
       (4) Coma
    g. Notify the physician immediately if signs of thyroid storm occur; administer propanolol (Inderal), iodides, propylthiouracil and steroids as ordered
    h. Observe for signs of tetany, which can occur after accidental trauma or removal of the parathyroid glands
       (1) Numbness or twitching of extremities
       (2) Spasm of the glottis
    i. If tetany occurs, give calcium gluconate or calcium chloride (IV) as prescribed
    j. Assess for hoarseness; may result from endotracheal intubation or laryngeal nerve damage
12. Teach client signs and symptoms of:
    a. Hypothyroidism that may result from inadequate thyroid hormones
    b. Hyperthyroidism that may result from thyroid storm or overmedication with thyroid hormone–replacement therapy
13. Teach the importance of taking antithyroid medications regularly and to observe for adverse effects

D. EVALUATION/OUTCOMES

1. Establishes regular routine of activity and rest
2. Establishes effective communication with family
3. States adverse effects of therapy
4. Maintains vital signs within normal range
5. Maintains ideal body weight
6. Maintains visual acuity

▼ HYPOTHYROIDISM

Data Base

A. Etiology and pathophysiology
1. Absence or decreased production of thyroid

hormone because of primary thyroid disease, response to decreased TSH, or effect of thyroid surgery or radioactive iodine (RAI) treatment; most common cause is Hashimoto's thyroiditis, an autoimmune disorder

2. Classified according to the time of life in which it occurs
   a. Cretinism: hypothyroidism in infants and young children
   b. Hypothyroidism without myxedema: mild degree of thyroid failure in older children and adults
   c. Hypothyroidism with myxedema: severe degree of thyroid failure in older individuals
3. Myxedema coma is the most severe degree of hypothyroidism, representing a potentially fatal endocrine emergency; precipitated by a severe physiologic stress, myxedema coma involves hypothermia, bradycardia, hypoventilation and progressive loss of consciousness
4. Decreased levels of thyroid hormones may interfere with erythropoiesis and lipid metabolism

B. Clinical findings
1. Subjective
   a. Dull mental processes
   b. Apathy
   c. Lethargy
   d. Intolerance to cold
   e. Anorexia
2. Objective
   a. Lack of facial expression
   b. Increase in weight
   c. Constipation
   d. Subnormal temperature and pulse
   e. Dry, brittle hair
   f. Pale, dry, coarse skin
   g. Enlarged tongue; drooling
   h. Decreased BMR
   i. Decreased thyroxine (T_4), triiodothyronine (T_3), T_3 resin uptake (T_3RU), and radioactive iodine uptake; delayed or poor response to TSH stimulation test in secondary hypothyroidism, increased TSH in primary hypothyroidism
   j. Hoarseness
   k. Thinning of lateral eyebrows
   l. Scalp, axilla, and pubic hair loss
   m. Diminished hearing
   n. Anemia
   o. Decreased libido
   p. Periorbital edema

C. Therapeutic interventions
1. Administer thyroid hormones
2. Maintain vital functions

Nursing Care of Clients with Hypothyroidism

A. DATA COLLECTION
1. History of therapeutic interventions that may have contributed to condition
2. Activity tolerance, bowel elimination, sleeping patterns, sexual function, and intolerance to cold
3. Skin and hair for characteristic changes
4. Weight and vital signs to establish baseline
5. Signs of anemia or atherosclerosis

B. ANALYSIS AND INTERPRETATION
Refer to General Nursing Diagnoses for Clients with Endocrine System Disorders for the following diagnoses: A, B, C, D, F, K 1, M, N1, and N 2

C. PLANNING/IMPLEMENTATION
1. Have patience with a lethargic client; activity tolerance and mental functioning will improve with therapy
2. Teach the client and family to be alert for signs of complications
   a. Angina pectoris: chest pain, feeling of indigestion
   b. Cardiac failure: dyspnea, palpitations
   c. Myxedema coma: weakness, syncope, slow pulse rate, subnormal temperature, slow respirations, lethargy
3. Teach the client to seek medical supervision on a regular basis and when any signs of illness develop
4. Explain the importance of continued hormone replacement through life
5. Review the signs of hypothyroidism and hyperthyroidism to help client recognize signs of undermedication or overmedication
6. Explain that increased sensitivity to narcotic analgesics and tranquilizers necessitates dosage adjustment; OTC drugs should be avoided unless approved by physician
7. Help the client and family recognize that client's inability to adapt to cold temperature requires additional protection and modification of outdoor activity in cold weather
8. Teach the client to avoid constipation by the use of adequate hydration and roughage in the diet
9. Apply moisturizers to skin
10. Teach the need to restrict calories, cholesterol, and fat in the diet

D. EVALUATION/OUTCOMES
1. Completes ADL without fatigue
2. Complies with dietary, exercise, and medication regimen
3. Establishes regular pattern of bowel elimination
4. Communicates concerns to family or significant others
5. Maintains vital signs within normal range

▼ HYPERPARATHYROIDISM

Data Base

A. Etiology and pathophysiology
   1. Hyperfunction of the parathyroid glands; usually caused by adenoma; hypertrophy and hyperplasia of the glands may also be responsible
   2. As a result the absorption of calcium and excretion of phosphorus by the kidneys is increased
   3. If dietary intake is not enough to meet calcium levels demanded by high levels of parathormone, demineralization of the bone occurs
B. Clinical findings
   1. Subjective
      a. Apathy
      b. Fatigue
      c. Muscular weakness
      d. Anorexia, nausea
      e. Emotional irritability
      f. Deep bone pain (if demineralization occurs)
      g. Constipation
   2. Objective
      a. Bone cysts, pathologic fractures
      b. Renal calculi composed of calcium
      c. Pyelonephritis, renal damage, uremia, polyuria
      d. Vomiting
      e. Elevated serum calcium and parathormone levels
      f. Decreased serum phosphorus
      g. Cardiac dysrhythmias
C. Therapeutic interventions
   1. Surgical excision of a parathyroid tumor
   2. Increased fluid intake
   3. Activity encouraged
   4. Calcium intake restricted
   5. Administration of furosemide (Lasix) to increase renal excretion of calcium
   6. Administration of calcitonin or plicamycin with glucocorticoid or mithramycin to lower calcium level in acute situations

Nursing Care of Clients with Hyperparathyroidism

A. DATA COLLECTION
   1. Presence of GI disturbance or bone pain
   2. History of renal calculi or fractures
   3. Signs of renal calculi such as hematuria or flank pain
   4. History of use of thiazide diuretics or vitamin D, which can also increase serum calcium
   5. Serum calcium and phosphorus levels
   6. Baseline vital signs, particularly heart rate and rhythm

B. ANALYSIS AND INTERPRETATION
Refer to General Nursing Diagnoses for Clients with Endocrine System Disorders for the following diagnoses: D, F, and J 1

C. PLANNING/IMPLEMENTATION
   1. Strain the urine, observing for calculi
   2. Encourage fluid intake
   3. Assist the client with ambulating to help prevent demineralization; avoid high-impact activities
   4. Monitor intake and output
   5. Encourage foods such as prune juice and roughage to combat constipation
   6. Instruct the client to limit intake of foods high in calcium, especially milk products
   7. Provide cardiac monitoring if hypercalcemia is severe
   8. If surgery is performed, provide postoperative care the same as for clients undergoing thyroidectomy (see Hyperthyroidism)

D. EVALUATION/OUTCOMES
   1. Reports fewer incidents of irritability or depression
   2. Maintains skeletal integrity
   3. Remains free of urinary complications

▼ HYPOPARATHYROIDISM

Data Base

A. Etiology and pathophysiology
   1. Parathyroid glands may not secrete a sufficient amount of parathormone after thyroid surgery, parathyroid surgery, or radiation therapy of the neck; idiopathic hypoparathyroidism rare
   2. As levels of parathormone drop, the serum calcium also drops, causing signs of tetany; a concomitant rise in serum phosphate occurs
B. Clinical findings
   1. Subjective
      a. Photophobia
      b. Diplopia
      c. Muscle cramps
      d. Irritability
      e. Dyspnea
      f. Tingling of extremities
   2. Objective
      a. Trousseau's sign (carpopedal spasm)
      b. Chvostek's sign (contraction of the facial muscle in response to tapping near the angle of the jaw)
      c. Decreased serum calcium
      d. Elevated serum phosphate
      e. Stridor, wheezing from laryngeal spasm
      f. Convulsions
      g. Cataracts if the disease is chronic

h. X-ray examination reveals increased bone density
i. Cardiac dysrhythmias
j. Alkalosis

C. Therapeutic interventions
1. Calcium chloride or calcium gluconate given IV for emergency treatment
2. Calcium salts administered orally (calcium carbonate, calcium gluconate)
3. Vitamin D (dihydrotachysterol, ergocalciferol) to increase absorption of calcium from the GI tract
4. Parathormone injections
5. High-calcium, low-phosphate diet
6. Aluminum hydroxide to decrease absorption of phosphorus from the GI tract

Nursing Care of Clients with Hypoparathyroidism

A. DATA COLLECTION
1. History of muscle spasms, numbness or tingling of extremities, visual disturbances, or convulsions
2. Presence of neuromuscular irritability
3. Status of respiratory functioning
4. Heart rate and rhythm
5. Serum calcium and phosphate levels

B. ANALYSIS AND INTERPRETATION
Refer to General Nursing Diagnoses for Clients with Endocrine System Disorders for the following diagnoses: J 1, L 2, and M

C. PLANNING/IMPLEMENTATION
1. Observe for respiratory distress and have emergency equipment available to perform a tracheostomy
2. Maintain seizure precautions
3. Monitor serum calcium and phosphate levels
4. Check vital signs frequently if a history of cardiac problems is present; place on a monitor
5. Provide a calm environment free of harsh stimuli
6. Provide drug and dietary instruction including elimination of milk, cheese, and egg yolks because of high phosphorus content
7. Teach symptoms of hypocalcemia and hypercalcemia; instruct client to contact physician immediately if either should occur

D. EVALUATION/OUTCOMES
1. Adheres to high-calcium, low-phosphate diet
2. Remains free from neuromuscular irritability
3. Maintains respiratory functioning within normal limits

▼ DIABETES MELLITUS

Data Base

A. Etiology and pathophysiology
1. Occurs when there is insufficient supply of insulin and/or cells become insulin resistant; may be due to:
   a. Failure in body's production
   b. Blockage of insulin supply
   c. Autoimmune response wherein the insulin may bind to an immune serum globulin fraction, preventing use
   d. Excess body fat, which alters glucose metabolism
2. Incidence increases with obesity, aging, and familial predisposition
3. Type I: insulin-dependent diabetes mellitus (IDDM), formerly called juvenile type; has a rapid onset and requires insulin administration because of minimal or absence of beta cell function
4. Type II: non–insulin dependent diabetes mellitus (NIDDM), formerly called adult-onset type; more than 90% of all diabetes is of this type; has a gradual onset and often can be controlled with diet and exercise; caused by decreased sensitivity of insulin receptors (insulin resistance) and decreased insulin secretion; often associated with obesity
5. Diabetes may occur as a result of pancreatectomy, Cushing's syndrome, and certain drugs
6. Body does not have enough insulin to drive glucose into cells or to convert glucose into glycogen; cells become insensitive to insulin
   a. Glucose level in the blood remains high
   b. Body attempts to rid itself of excess glucose by excreting some via the kidneys
   c. Osmotic force is created within the kidneys due to glucose excretion, and body fluid is lost
   d. Body is unable to use carbohydrates properly, and fat is oxidized as a compensatory mechanism; oxidation of fats gives off ketone bodies (see Diabetic Ketoacidosis)
7. Long-term complications of diabetes include retinopathy, renal failure, peripheral neuropathy, cardiovascular and peripheral vascular diseases

B. Clinical findings
1. Subjective
   a. Polydipsia
   b. Polyphagia
   c. Fatigue
   d. Blurred vision from retinopathy
   e. Peripheral neuropathy

2. Objective
   a. Polyuria
   b. Weight loss
   c. Hyperglycemia: detected by fasting blood sugar, glucose tolerance test, 2-hour post-prandial glucose, and glycosylated hemo-globin (provides measure of average glucose level over preceding 2 to 3 months) [HbA$_{1C}$]
   d. Glycosuria
   e. Peripheral vascular changes and gangrene

C. Therapeutic interventions
   1. Attempt to manage with life-style changes
      a. Weight control: if overweight or obese, client should lose excess body fat, which alters glucose metabolism (obesity leads to insulin resistance); this can be reversed by weight loss
      b. Exercise: increases insulin sensitivity but must be regular; vigorous but not jarring exercise, such as brisk walking, swimming, and bicycling, is recommended
      c. Diet: current recommendations include:
         (1) Calories controlled to maintain ideal body weight
         (2) 50% to 60% of caloric intake should be from carbohydrates; emphasis should be on complex carbohydrates, high-fiber foods rich in water-soluble fiber (oat bran, peas, all forms of beans, pectin-rich fruits and vegetables); particular attention should be paid to the glycemic effect of foods, those with a high glycemic index should be avoided; Glycemic index refers to the effect of particular foods on blood glucose (e.g., water-insoluble fiber has little effect on blood glucose)
         (3) Protein: intake should be consistent with the Canadian Dietary Guidelines, usually between 60 and 85 g depending on calorie intake; should be 12% to 20% of daily calories
         (4) Moderate fat intake: should not exceed 30% of daily calories (70 to 90 g/day); keep saturated fat intake low; emphasize monounsaturated and polyunsaturated fats
         (5) Dietary ratio: carbohydrate to protein to fat usually about 5:1:2
         (6) Distribute food fairly evenly throughout the day in three or four meals, with snacks added between and at bedtime

as needed in accordance with total food allowance and therapy (insulin or oral hypoglycemics)
         (7) Basic tools for planning diet: food exchange groups, using the exchange system of dietary control; food composition tables showing amount and type of fiber in foods; glycemic index of foods

2. Insulin administration
   a. Adjusted after considering the client's physical and emotional stresses, selecting a specific type of insulin, depending on the condition and needs of the client (see pharmacology section for discussion of insulin)
   b. Somogyi effect: insulin-induced hypoglycemia that rebounds to hyperglycemia
      (1) Epinephrine is released and the blood glucose level is low
      (2) Glucagon is released by alpha cells of the pancreas
      (3) These reactions cause mobilization of the liver's stored glucose and iatrogenically induce hyperglycemia
      (4) Somogyi phenomenon is treated by gradually lowering insulin dosage while monitoring blood glucose, particularly during the night (when hypoglycemia is most likely to occur)
   c. Mixing insulin: "order of insulin in the process of mixing is generally cloudy, clear, clear, cloudy" (i.e., air into cloudy vial, then clear, invert clear vial and draw up insulin, then draw up cloudy;) the clear insulin is generally drawn up first because it is fast acting, and this eliminates the possibility that a slow-acting insulin will enter the multidose vial
   d. Insulin pump
      (1) Battery-operated device worn on a belt or harness that delivers insulin through a needle inserted into subcutaneous tissue
      (2) Small (basal) doses of regular insulin are delivered every few minutes; bolus doses (extra preset amounts) are delivered before meals
      (3) Improves glucose control for clients with wide variations in insulin requirements as a result of irregular schedules, pregnancy, or growth requirements
      (4) Insulin concentration and basal and bolus doses are programmed into computer of pump
      (5) Appropriate amount of insulin for 24 hours plus priming is drawn into syringe

(6) The administration set is primed and needle inserted aseptically, usually into abdomen

3. Oral hypoglycemics for certain clients; however, these clients must have some functioning beta cells in the islets of Langerhans; more commonly prescribed for adults with late-developing mild diabetes (see Pharmacology Related to Endocrine System Disorders)

4. Other therapies include pancreas islet cell grafts, pancreas transplants, implantable insulin pumps that continually monitor blood glucose and release insulin accordingly, cyclosporine therapy to prevent beta-cell destruction in insulin-dependent (type I) diabetes

5. Monitoring glucose control
   a. Self-monitoring of blood glucose; may be done before meals and at bedtime
   b. Glycosylated hemoglobin; reflects long-term serum glucose control and is done at routine medical evaluations (HbA_{1C})

Nursing Care of Clients with Diabetes Mellitus

A. DATA COLLECTION

1. Familial history of diabetes mellitus
2. Cardinal signs of polyuria, polydipsia, and polyphagia
3. History of fatigue, visual changes, impaired wound healing, urinary tract infections, fungal infections, and altered sensation
4. Blood glucose levels
5. Visual acuity and retinal changes
6. Vital signs and weight for baseline data
7. Renal function
8. Dietary and exercise patterns

B. ANALYSIS AND INTERPRETATION

Refer to General Nursing Diagnoses for Clients with Endocrine System Disorders for the following diagnoses: A, D, F, G, I 1, I 2, I 3, J 1, J 2, K 1, K 2, L 2, M, N 1, and N 2

C. PLANNING/IMPLEMENTATION

1. Assist the client to accept the diagnosis
2. Encourage the client to express feelings about illness and the necessary changes in life-style and self-image
3. Assist the client and family in understanding the disease process
4. Help the client with the administration of medication until self-administration is both physically and psychologically possible
5. Assist the client to recognize the need for continuing health supervision
6. Assist the client in recognizing the need for activities and diet that promote and maintain normal body weight

7. Teach client to:
   a. Use blood-glucose–monitoring system to test blood sugar
   b. Test urine for ketones when blood glucose is high
   c. Avoid infection
   d. Care for the legs, feet, and toenails properly; inspect, bathe, dry, and lubricate except between toes; avoid exposure of feet to heat sources
   e. Administer insulin by using sterile technique; rotating injection sites; measuring dosage; noting types, strengths of insulin, and peak action periods; need to carry carbohydrate source
   f. Use dietary chart and make proper substitutions
   g. Avoid tight shoes and smoking, which will constrict circulation
8. Encourage the client to continue medical supervision and follow-up care, including visits to an eye care specialist and podiatrist
9. Teach the client and the family the signs of impending hypoglycemia (headache; nervousness; diaphoresis; rapid, thready pulse; slurred speech)
10. Teach the client and family the signs of impending diabetic coma (restlessness; hot, dry, flushed skin; thirst; rapid pulse; nausea; fruity odor to breath)
11. Teach client how to use the insulin pump
    a. How to insert the needle and fill the syringe; use of aseptic methods
    b. When to remove the pump (e.g., before showering or sexual relations)
    c. How to test capillary blood-glucose levels to monitor insulin dosage at home
12. Encourage follow-up nutritional counseling
13. Teach client and family about Somogyi effect and the associated signs and symptoms

D. EVALUATION/OUTCOMES

1. Complies with medical regimen of diet, exercise, and medications
2. Verbalizes an increased sense of well-being
3. Maintains ideal body weight
4. Remains free from infection
5. Establishes a satisfying sexual relationship
6. Maintains skin integrity
7. Maintains visual acuity
8. Maintains blood glucose levels within an acceptable range

▼ DIABETIC KETOACIDOSIS (DKA; DIABETIC COMA)

Data Base

A. Etiology and pathophysiology
   1. Occurs in insulin-dependent (type I) diabetes when there is insufficient insulin available, a systemic infection, diarrhea and vomiting, overindulgence in eating, emotional stress, injury, surgery, or pregnancy
   2. Lack of insulin results in alterations of metabolism; proteins and fats are used; dehydration and electrolyte imbalance occur; and ketone bodies appear in the urine
B. Clinical findings
   1. Subjective
      a. Thirst
      b. Anorexia
      c. Drowsiness
      d. Headache
   2. Objective
      a. Vomiting
      b. Flushed appearance
      c. Lowered blood pressure
      d. Coma
      e. Sweet odor to breath
      f. Kussmaul breathing due to acidosis: very deep respirations as the body attempts to blow off carbon dioxide
      g. Hyperglycemia
      h. Glycosuria and ketonuria
C. Therapeutic interventions
   1. IV to provide fluid replacement and direct access to the circulatory system, and a Foley catheter to monitor urine output
   2. Rapid-acting insulin based on serum glucose levels
   3. Replacement of lost electrolytes, using blood studies to determine dosage
   4. Cardiac monitoring if circulatory collapse is imminent or dysrhythmias associated with electrolyte imbalance occur
   5. Establish cause of acidosis and treat appropriately

Nursing Care of Clients with Diabetic Ketoacidosis

A. DATA COLLECTION
1. Blood glucose and vital signs
2. Urine for ketones
3. Precipitating factors from history: increased food intake, stress, infection
4. Fluid and electrolyte balance
5. Classic signs of DKA: anorexia, nausea, vomiting; thirst; headache, drowsiness, coma; flushed appearance; sweet odor to breath; deep, rapid breathing; hypotension

B. ANALYSIS AND INTERPRETATION
Refer to General Nursing Diagnoses for Clients with Endocrine System Disorders for the following diagnoses: A, D, F, G, J 1, K 1, K 2, L 2, and M

C. PLANNING/IMPLEMENTATION
1. Administer regular insulin as ordered
2. Maintain IV for replacement of fluid and electrolytes as ordered
3. Keep accurate records of urine and blood tests, vital signs, and fluid balance
4. Teach the client about diet, prevention of infection, and signs of ketoacidosis
5. Monitor cardiac rhythm

D. EVALUATION/OUTCOMES
1. Returns serum glucose to within acceptable range
2. Exhibits increased level of consciousness
3. Maintains stable vital signs
4. Identifies precipitating factors
5. States signs and symptoms of impending DKA

▼ HYPERGLYCEMIC HYPEROSMOLAR NONKETOTIC COMA (HHNK COMA)

Data Base

A. Etiology and pathophysiology
   1. Similar to ketoacidosis, but occurs in non-insulin–dependent (type II) diabetes and does not involve ketosis
   2. Precipitating factors include infection, diarrhea, and vomiting; failure to comply with dietary/medication regimen; prolonged exposure to drugs that induce hyperglycemia (e.g., steroids)
   3. High serum glucose level increases osmotic pressure, leading to polyuria and cellular dehydration
B. Clinical findings
   1. Subjective
      a. Thirst
      b. Drowsiness
      c. Confusion
      d. History of polyuria
   2. Objective
      a. Flushed appearance
      b. Dry, hot skin
      c. Hyperglycemia
      d. Glycosuria
      e. Hypotension
C. Therapeutic interventions (see Diabetic Ketoacidosis)

Nursing Care of Clients with Hyperglycemic Hyperosmolar Nonketotic Coma

See Nursing Care of Clients with Diabetic Ketoacidosis

HYPOGLYCEMIA

Regardless of the cause, the end result is an imbalance between the blood glucose concentration and the body's need for glucose

▼ EXOGENOUSLY INDUCED HYPOGLYCEMIA (INSULIN COMA, SHOCK, OR REACTION)

Data Base
A. Etiology and pathophysiology
   1. Occurs when blood glucose levels fall below 60 mg/dl or less
   2. Occurs as a side effect of insulin therapy or oral hypoglycemics
   3. May result when a diabetic client omits a meal, takes excessive insulin, vomits a meal, or over-exercises
   4. Signs and symptoms occur as a result of sympathetic nervous system stimulation or reduced glucose supply to the brain
B. Clinical findings
   1. Subjective
      a. Muscular weakness
      b. Diplopia
      c. Faintness
      d. Numbness and tingling in fingers, tongue, lips
   2. Objective
      a. Diaphoresis
      b. Trembling
      c. Tachycardia
      d. Disorientation
C. Therapeutic interventions
   1. Oral glucose administration if the client is alert
   2. Administration of glucagon parenterally to stimulate glucogenolysis
   3. Insertion of an IV line for access to a vein in an emergency
   4. Administration of 50% dextrose

Nursing Care of Clients with Exogenously Induced Hypoglycemia
A. **DATA COLLECTION**
   1. Precipitating factors from history
   2. Neurologic status
   3. Vital signs and blood glucose levels to establish a baseline
B. **ANALYSIS AND INTERPRETATION**
   Refer to General Nursing Diagnoses for Clients with Endocrine System Disorders for the following diagnoses: D, J 1, L 1, L 2, and M
C. **PLANNING/IMPLEMENTATION**
   1. Supply 10 to 15 g of a simple sugar (glucose tablets, orange juice, soda, candy) if client is alert; follow with a complex carbohydrate
   2. Administer medications as ordered
   3. Keep accurate record of intake and output, vital signs, and finger-stick test results
   4. If ordered, give client protein or fat after an easily absorbed carbohydrate meal is given
   5. Teach signs and symptoms of hypoglycemia and need to carry glucose source
D. **EVALUATION/OUTCOMES**
   1. Experiences a reduction in symptoms
   2. Carries a glucose source when out of the home
   3. Identifies signs and symptoms of hypoglycemia

▼ ENDOGENOUSLY INDUCED HYPOGLYCEMIA (REACTIVE HYPOGLYCEMIA)

Data Base
A. Etiology and pathophysiology
   1. Occurs when blood glucose levels fall below 60 mg/dl
   2. Precipitated by the overproduction of insulin or insulin-like substances
      a. Insulin-producing tumors
      b. Autoimmune disease
   3. Precipitated by the underproduction of glucose
      a. Hormonal deficiencies (ACTH, catecholamines, glucagon)
      b. Acquired liver disease
      c. Drugs (alcohol, propranolol, salicylates)
B. Clinical findings
   See Exogenously Induced Hypoglycemia
C. Therapeutic interventions
   1. Surgery to remove insulin-producing tumors
   2. Diazoxide therapy to suppress insulin secretion
   3. Correction of hormonal deficiency
   4. Discontinuance of drugs that cause hypoglycemia
   5. Correction of hepatic disease
   6. Low-carbohydrate, high-protein diet with avoidance of simple sugars and fasting

Nursing Care of Clients with Endogenously Induced Hypoglycemia
A. **DATA COLLECTION**
   1. Precipitating events from history
   2. Dietary intake
   3. Vital signs for a baseline
   4. Serum glucose level
B. **ANALYSIS AND INTERPRETATION**
   Refer to General Nursing Diagnoses for Clients with Endocrine System Disorders for the following diagnoses: F, J 1, L 1, L 2, and M

C. PLANNING/IMPLEMENTATION

1. Help client distinguish between symptoms that are hypoglycemia induced and those that are not
2. Instruct client regarding dietary intake of protein, complex carbohydrates, and fiber
3. Teach client to eat small, frequent meals rather than three large meals a day

D. EVALUATION/OUTCOMES

1. Avoids simple sugars in diet
2. Maintains normal blood glucose levels through appropriate dietary and exercise patterns

▼ REACTIVE (FUNCTIONAL) HYPOGLYCEMIA

Data Base

A. Etiology and pathophysiology

1. True reactive hypoglycemia occurs with rapid gastric emptying (a frequent complication following gastric surgery) that stimulates the production of excessive insulin and results in a lowered blood glucose level
2. Idiopathic postprandial syndrome is a condition in which symptoms of hypoglycemia occur without a documented decrease in blood glucose; a decrease in blood glucose may be found after a 5-hour glucose tolerance test

B. Clinical findings

1. Subjective
   a. Anxiety
   b. Irritability
   c. Weakness
   d. Fatigue
2. Objective
   a. Hypoglycemia
   b. Pallor
   c. Diaphoresis

C. Therapeutic interventions

1. Avoidance of rapidly absorbed simple sugars
2. Frequent meals
3. Increased emphasis on intake of protein, complex carbohydrates, and fiber, which delay gastric emptying and slow glucose absorption

Nursing Care of Clients with Reactive Hypoglycemia

See Nursing Care of Clients with Endogenously Induced Hypoglycemia

▼ PRIMARY ALDOSTERONISM (CONN'S SYNDROME)

Data Base

A. Etiology and pathophysiology

1. Aldosterone, a mineralocorticoid secreted in response to the renin-angiotensin system and ACTH, causes the kidneys to retain sodium and excrete potassium
2. Hypersecretion of aldosterone is usually caused by an adenoma of the adrenal cortex, but may also be caused by hyperplasia or carcinoma
3. The disease is more common in females

B. Clinical findings

1. Subjective
   a. Muscle weakness
   b. Polydipsia, polyuria
   c. Paresthesia
2. Objective
   a. Hypertension
   b. Hypokalemia
   c. Hypernatremia
   d. Alkalosis
   e. Elevated urinary aldosterone levels
   f. Renal damage
      (1) Proteinuria
      (2) Decreased specific gravity of urine
      (3) Pyelonephritis

C. Therapeutic interventions

1. Surgical removal of the tumor
2. Temporary management with spironolactone
3. Occasionally a bilateral adrenalectomy involving lifelong corticosteroid therapy is necessary

Nursing Care of Clients with Primary Aldosteronism

A. DATA COLLECTION

1. Vital signs for a baseline
2. Electrolyte levels
3. Motor and sensory functions for alterations
4. Cardiac dysrhythmias as a result of hypokalemia

B. ANALYSIS AND INTERPRETATION

Refer to General Nursing Diagnoses for Clients with Endocrine System Disorders for the following diagnoses: F, L 2, and M

C. PLANNING/IMPLEMENTATION

1. Monitor vital signs
2. Observe for signs of electrolyte imbalance
3. Provide fluids to meet excessive thirst
4. Encourage continued medical supervision
5. Monitor intake and output and specific gravity of urine
6. Care for the client following a bilateral adrenalectomy
   a. Monitor vital signs, hemodynamic state, and blood glucose level
   b. Administer steroids with milk or antacid

c. Protect the client from infection and stressful situations

d. Explain drug and side effects to client

e. Instruct the client to carry medical alert identification card

7. Provide dietary instruction; include foods high in potassium, such as orange juice and bananas, and avoid or limit intake of foods that contain sodium

D. EVALUATION/OUTCOMES

1. Maintains blood pressure at an acceptable level

2. Selects foods low in sodium and high in potassium

3. Performs routine ADL without fatigue

▼ CUSHING'S SYNDROME

Data Base

A. Etiology and pathophysiology

1. Results from excess secretion of adrenocortical hormones

2. Caused by hyperplasia or by a tumor of the adrenal cortex; however, the primary lesion may occur in the pituitary gland, causing excess production of ACTH

3. Administration of excess glucocorticoids or ACTH will also cause Cushing's syndrome

B. Clinical findings

1. Subjective

   a. Weakness

   b. Decreased libido

   c. Mood swings to psychosis

2. Objective

   a. Obese trunk with relatively thin arms and legs

   b. Hypertension

   c. Moon face

   d. Buffalo hump

   e. Acne

   f. Increased susceptibility to infections

   g. Hirsutism

   h. Ecchymotic areas

   i. Purple striae on the breast and abdomen

   j. Amenorrhea

   k. Hyperglycemia

   l. Hypokalemia

   m. Elevated plasma cortisol level

   n. Elevated 17-hydroxycorticosteroids and 17-ketosteroids in urine

   o. Osteoporosis may be evident on x-ray examination

C. Therapeutic interventions

1. Reduce dosage of externally administered corticoids

2. If lesion on pituitary is causing hypersecretion of ACTH, a hypophysectomy or irradiation of the pituitary may be done

3. Surgical excision of adrenal tumors (adrenalectomy)

4. Administration of cyproheptedine (Periactin), which inhibits ACTH secretion

5. Potassium supplements

6. High-protein diet with sodium restriction

Nursing Care of Clients with Cushing's Syndrome

A. DATA COLLECTION

1. Vital signs, weight, and blood glucose level to establish a baseline

2. Electrolyte levels

3. Urine specimens for diagnostic purposes

4. Physical appearance

5. Changes in coping from history

6. Changes in sexuality from history

B. ANALYSIS AND INTERPRETATION

Refer to General Nursing Diagnoses for Clients with Endocrine System Disorders for the following diagnoses: B, D, F, H 1, H 2, I 1, J 1, N 1, and N 2

C. PLANNING/IMPLEMENTATION

1. Monitor vital signs, daily weight, intake and output, blood glucose, and electrolytes

2. Protect the client from exposure to infections

3. Encourage ventilation of feelings by the client and spouse, since changes in body image and sex drives can alter marital support

4. Attempt to minimize stress in the environment by measures such as limiting visitors and explaining procedures carefully

5. Instruct client regarding diet and supplementation; encourage diet rich in nutrient-dense foods such as fruits, vegetables, whole grains, and legumes to improve and maintain nutritional status and prevent any possible drug-induced nutrient deficiencies

6. Care for the client following a bilateral adrenalectomy (see Primary Aldosteronism)

7. Care for the client following a hypophysectomy (see Hyperpituitarism)

D EVALUATION/OUTCOMES

1. Participates in care without fatigue

2. Maintains fluid balance

3. Remains free of infection

4. Maintains integrity of skeletal system

5. Discusses feelings regarding physical changes

▼ ADDISON'S DISEASE

Data Base

A. Etiology and pathophysiology

1. Hyposecretion of adrenocortical hormones
2. Generally caused by destruction of the cortex or by idiopathic atrophy

B. Clinical findings
   1. Subjective
      a. Weakness
      b. Easy fatigue
      c. Nausea
      d. Anorexia
   2. Objective
      a. Increased bronze pigmentation of skin
      b. Vomiting
      c. Diarrhea
      d. Hypotension
      e. Hypoglycemia
      f. Small heart
      g. Decreased serum cortisol level
      h. Increased plasma ACTH
      i. Decreased 17-ketosteroids and 17-hydroxysteroids in 24-hour urine studies
      j. Hyponatremia
      k. Hyperkalemia

C. Therapeutic interventions
   1. Replacement of hormones
      a. Glucocorticoids to correct metabolic imbalance
      b. Mineralocorticoids to correct electrolyte imbalance and hypotension
   2. Correction of fluid and electrolyte losses
   3. High-carbohydrate, high-protein diet

Nursing Care of Clients with Addison's Disease
A. DATA COLLECTION

1. Vital signs, weight, and serum glucose level for baseline data
2. 24-hour urine specimens for diagnostic purposes (17-hydroxycorticosteroids and 17-ketosteroids)
3. Electrolyte levels
4. Appearance of skin
5. Changes in energy or activity from history

B. ANALYSIS AND INTERPRETATION

Refer to General Nursing Diagnoses for Clients with Endocrine System Disorders for the following diagnoses: F, G, I 1, J 1, K 1, K 2, and L 2

C. PLANNING/IMPLEMENTATION

1. Monitor vital signs four times a day; be alert for elevation in temperature (infection, dehydration), alterations in pulse rate and rhythm (hyperkalemia), and alterations in blood pressure
2. Observe for signs of sodium and potassium imbalance
3. Monitor intake and output and weigh daily
4. Administer steroids as ordered
5. Administer steroids with milk or an antacid to limit ulcerogenic factor of the drug
6. Put the client in a private room to prevent contact with clients having infectious diseases
7. Limit the number of visitors
8. Teach client need for lifelong hormone replacement with increased dosage during stress
9. Review signs of adrenal hypofunction or hyperfunction so client can recognize need for adjustment of steroid dose
10. Instruct client to wear medical alert band
11. Encourage diet consistent with Canada's Food Guide, with emphasis on diet high in nutrient-dense foods
12. Administer antiemetics to prevent fluid and electrolyte loss by vomiting

D. EVALUATION/OUTCOMES

1. Completes ADL without fatigue
2. Maintains fluid balance
3. Remains free from infection
4. Complies with medical regimen
5. Lists adverse effects of steroid therapy

▼ PHEOCHROMOCYTOMA

Data Base

A. Etiology and pathophysiology
   1. Tumor of the adrenal medulla; usually benign
   2. Causes increased secretion of epinephrine and norepinephrine
   3. Heredity believed to be involved in the development of the tumor

B. Clinical findings
   1. Subjective
      a. Headache
      b. Visual disturbances
      c. Nausea
      d. Anxiety
   2. Objective
      a. Hypertension and orthostatic hypotension
      b. Tachycardia
      c. Diaphoresis
      d. Increased BMR
      e. Increased urinary catecholamines and vanillymandelic acid (VMA), a product of catecholamine breakdown
      f. Hyperglycemia

C. Therapeutic interventions
   1. Surgical removal of the tumor
   2. Antihypertensive and antidysrhythmic drugs such as nitroprusside (Nipride) and propranolol (Inderal)

Nursing Care of Clients with Pheochromocytoma

A. DATA COLLECTION

1. Blood pressures, taken with client in both upright and horizontal positions
2. Symptoms associated with episodic hypertension
3. 24-hour urine specimens for VMA and catecholamine studies; instruct client to avoid coffee, chocolate, beer, wine, citrus fruit, bananas, and vanilla before the test for VMA

B. ANALYSIS AND INTERPRETATION

Refer to General Nursing Diagnoses for Clients with Endocrine System Disorders for the following diagnoses: F, G, J 1, and O

C. PLANNING/IMPLEMENTATION

1. Monitor blood pressure frequently in both upright and horizontal positions (orthostatic blood pressures)
2. Administer parenteral fluids and blood as ordered before and after surgery to maintain blood volume
3. Decrease environmental stimulation
4. If bilateral adrenalectomy is performed, instruct the client regarding maintenance doses of steroids (see Care for the Client Following a Bilateral Adrenalectomy under Primary Aldosteronism)
5. Emphasize the importance of continued medical supervision and screening for other family members

D. EVALUATION/OUTCOMES

1. Maintains blood pressure at an acceptable level
2. Remains free of complications of hypertension (such as strokes and renal failure)

INTEGUMENTARY SYSTEM

REVIEW OF ANATOMY AND PHYSIOLOGY OF THE INTEGUMENTARY SYSTEM

Functions of the Integumentary System

A. Prevents loss of body fluids
B. Protects deeper tissues from pathogenic organisms, noxious chemicals, and short-wavelength ultraviolet radiation
C. Helps regulate body temperature
D. Provides location for sensory reception of touch, pressure, temperature, pain, wetness, tickle, etc.
E. Assists in vitamin-D synthesis
F. Plays a minor excretory role

Structures of the Integumentary System

A. Epidermis: contains no blood or lymphatic vessels; cells nourished by diffusion from underlying dermal papillae
   1. Layers from the dermis outward
      a. Stratum germinativum: cell layers undergoing mitosis; gradually pushed to surface to replace those exfoliated
      b. Stratum granulosum: granule-filled cells in several layers; contain keratohyalin, intermediate in keratin formation; most free nerve endings of epidermis are here; contains epidermal pigment
      c. Stratum lucidum: translucent layers; nails are outgrowths of this layer
      d. Stratum corneum: upper horny layer of flat, dead cells that exfoliate rapidly, taking bacterial flora with them; responsible for variations in skin thickness
   2. Melanocytes of the lower epidermis produce melanin, which colors skin
   3. Exceptional epidermal regions
      a. Conjunctiva: epidermis so thin it is transparent
      b. Lips: epidermis very thin and highly vascular, which accounts for redness
B. Dermis
   1. Extremely vascular fabric of collagen and elastic fibers woven to provide strength and flexibility
   2. Upper papillary layer joined to epidermis by upward projecting papillae; vascular loops in papillae nourish overlying epidermis; contain abundant touch receptors; double-row papillae in finger pads and palms and soles give great strength against shearing stress, provide fingerprint pattern as unique arrangement of ridges projected to epidermal surface, and allow hands and feet to grip surfaces
   3. Deeper reticular layer contains loose arrangement of connective tissue gradually merging with subcutaneous fatty layer (superficial fascia)
   4. Skin stretched beyond certain limits (e.g., during pregnancy) may rupture dermal collagen and elastic fibers; consequent scar tissue repair produces striae gravidarum
C. Glands
   1. Eccrine: tubular coiled glands deep in dermis; duct rises straight through dermis and spirals through epidermis, opening in sweat pore on crest of skin ridges; secretes clear fluid
   2. Apocrine: scent glands; very large branched tubular glands found in the axillary, mammary, and genital areas that produce an originally odorless secretion rapidly metabolized by bacteria to produce typical body odors

3. Ceruminous: wax glands in external auditory canal; large branched glands frequently opening into hair sheaths along with sebaceous glands

4. Sebaceous: small, saclike glands lacking innervation, usually forming close to hairs and opening into upper portion of hair follicle; form independently of hairs at corners of mouth and in eyelids as meibomian glands; absent on palms and soles, accounting for wrinkling of these areas after lengthy immersion in water

5. Mammary: milk-secreting, compound tubular alveolar glands developing to full extent only during pregnancy

D. Hair
1. Long strands of tightly compacted and cemented, dead and keratinized cells sheathed in hair follicles (tubes of epidermal cells plunged obliquely into dermis surrounded by dermal connective tissue sheath)

2. About the same number of follicles in males and females; hormones stimulate differential growth

3. Shape determines appearance; round (straight hair); ribbon shaped (kinky hair); alternately round and oval (wavy hair)

4. Arrector pili (smooth muscle) attached at one end to connective sheath in middle of the hair follicle and at other end to the dermal papillary region of the dermis; on contraction, elevates hair and surrounding skin but depresses skin overlying the dermal papillary attachment point; result is "goose-flesh"; such contraction also stimulates sebaceous gland secretion

Tissue Repair

A. Inflammation
1. Vascular changes: initially there is vasoconstriction (5 to 10 minutes); vessel walls lined with leukocytes (margination); then vasodilation with increased blood flow and increased vessel permeability (effects of histamine from mast cells, kinins, and prostaglandins); lymphatics become plugged with fibrin to wall off damaged area

2. Polymorphonuclear and mononuclear leukocytes leave the vessels (diapedesis) and phagocytize foreign substances

3. Chronic inflammation: longer-lived mononuclear leukocytes (macrophages) predominate, and fibroblasts deposit a wall of collagen around each group of macrophages and foreign substances; stage of granuloma formation

B. Fibroplasia
1. Epithelization: epithelial cells of the epidermis begin to cover tissue defect through migration of basal cells across wound defect with continued mitosis in intact epithelium

2. Deep in the wound, fibroblasts synthesize collagen and ground substance; process begins about fourth or fifth day and continues for 2 to 4 weeks

3. Capillaries regenerate by endothelial budding; tissue becomes red

4. Fibrin plugs are lysed

C. Scar maturation
1. Collagen fibers rearranged into a stronger, more organized pattern

2. Scar remodels, sometimes for months and years as a result of collagen turnover; if collagen synthesis exceeds breakdown, a hypertrophic scar or keloid forms; if collagen breakdown exceeds synthesis, scar gradually softens and fades

3. Wound contracture: contraction of wound margins begins about 5 days after injury; caused by fibroblast migration into the wound along the lines of fibrin strands initially deposited in the wound; assists in closing the defect but may also result in contractures that can be debilitating

REVIEW OF PHYSICAL PRINCIPLES RELATED TO THE INTEGUMENTARY SYSTEM

Principle of Mechanics

Friction: epidermal ridges resulting from upthrusting dermal papillae provide palms of hands, fingers, and soles of feet with friction surfaces for grasping and walking

Principles of Physical Properties of Matter

Elasticity: molecular structure of elastin, a protein, permits stretching of skin under tension and the ability to snap back to its original shape when tension is relieved; less elastic properties of collagen give skin its strength to resist tearing and shearing forces

Principles of Heat

A. Conduction: heat brought to the dermis by blood passes through the epidermis; allows for elimination of excess heat

B. Evaporation: sweat evaporating cools the body surface and acts to drain heat from the body interior

Principle of Light

Radiation absorption: ultraviolet absorption by melanin protects the skin and underlying structures from damage; quantity and degree of dispersed melanin, which absorbs visible light wavelengths differently, produces different skin colors

REVIEW OF CHEMICAL PRINCIPLES RELATED TO THE INTEGUMENTARY SYSTEM

Solutions (Solubility)

A. Fat-soluble substances have a greater tendency to penetrate skin than do water-soluble substances

EXAMPLE: Oleoresins of poison ivy, fat-soluble vitamins (A,D,E), and insecticides are absorbed, whereas water is repelled

B. Fat-soluble (oily) substances secreted by the meibomian glands (modified sebaceous glands) of the eyelids, which are not capable of mixing with water; act as barriers to prevent tears from constantly flooding over lower eyelid

Water

Dehydration of epidermal cells leaves water-insoluble keratin impregnated in surface and corneum providing a water-resistant protective barrier

PHARMACOLOGY RELATED TO INTEGUMENTARY SYSTEM DISORDERS

Antibiotics and Antifungals

See Pharmacology Related to Infection

Pediculocides/Scabicides/Ovicides

A. Description
1. Used to destroy parasitic arthropods
2. Act at the parasite's nerve cell membrane to produce death of the organism
3. Available in topical preparations

B. Examples
1. Crotamiton (Eurax): antipruritic/scabicide
2. Esdepallethrin piperonyl butoxide (Scabene): scabicide
3. Gamma benzene hexachloride (Kwellada, Lindane): scabicide
4. Permethrin (Nix cream rinse): topical pediculocide/ovicide
5. Permethrin (Nix dermal cream): topical scabicide
6. Pyrethrins/piperonyl butoxide (Lice-Enz): pediculocide

C. Major side effects
1. Skin irritation (hypersensitivity)
2. Contact dermatitis (local irritation)

D. Nursing care
1. Inspect skin, particularly the scalp, for scabies and pediculosis before and after treatment
2. Use gown, gloves, and cap to prevent spread of parasitic arthropods
3. Keep linen of an infected client separate to prevent reinfection

4. Assess for skin irritation during therapy
5. Assess source of infection; provide client and family education
6. Avoid drug contact with the eyes and mucous membranes
7. Evaluate client's response to medication and understanding of teaching

Antiinfectives

A. Description
1. Agents that act on the bacterial cell wall or alter cellular function to produce bactericidal effects
2. Available in topical preparations

B. Examples
1. Silver nitrate 0.5% solution
2. Silver sulfadiazine (Flamazine, Silvadene)

C. Major side effects
1. Silver sulfadiazine: skin irritation; hemolysis in clients with G-6-PD deficiency
2. Mafenide acetate: metabolic acidosis; burning sensation when first applied
3. Silver nitrate: electrolyte imbalance; brownish-black discoloration produced on contact

D. Nursing care
1. Adhere to strict surgical asepsis
2. Assess burns and the client's general condition during therapy
3. Provide comprehensive nursing burn care; offer emotional support
4. Cleanse and debride before application
5. Apply prescribed medications
   a. Silver sulfadiazine
      (1) Apply to a thickness of 1.6 mm
      (2) Monitor G-6-PD level before initiation of treatment
   b. Mafenide acetate: assess client for signs of acidosis during course of therapy
   c. Silver nitrate
      (1) Apply dressings soaked in silver nitrate
      (2) Avoid contact with the drug
      (3) Assess for signs of electrolyte imbalance during course of therapy
6. Evaluate client's response to medication and understanding of teaching

Antipruritics

A. Description
1. Used to relieve itching and promote comfort
2. Act by inhibiting sensory nerve impulse conduction at the local site and by exerting a local anesthetic effect
3. Available in topical preparations

B. Examples
1. Benzocaine (Anbesol, Solarcaine)
2. Lidocaine HCl (Xylocaine)

3. Phenol
4. Pramoxine HCl/Hydrocortisone acetate (Pramox H.C.)
5. Tars
6. Tetracaine HCl (Pontocaine)

C. Major side effects
   1. Skin irritation (hypersensitivity)
   2. Contact dermatitis (local irritation)
D. Nursing care
   1. Assess the lesion, including location and size
   2. Assess for local irritation during course of therapy
   3. Question client regarding relief obtained from treatment
   4. Discourage client from scratching; keep nails well trimmed
   5. Advise medical follow-up, since these medications provide only temporary relief of symptoms
   6. Evaluate client's response to medication and understanding of teaching

Antiinflammatory Agents

A. Description
   1. Reduce signs of inflammation
   2. Produce vasoconstriction, which decreases swelling and pruritis
   3. Available in topical preparations
B. Examples
   1. Betamethasone benzoate (Bepen): topical
   2. Betamethasone valerate (Betacart)
   3. Dexamethasone (Dexazone)
   4. Fluocinonide (Lyderm)
   5. Hydrocortisone (Emocort)
   6. Triamcinolone acetonide (Kenacort)
C. Major side effects
   1. Skin irritation (hypersensitivity)
   2. Contact dermatitis (local irritation)
   3. Adrenal insufficiency if absorbed systemically (suppression of hypothalamic-pituitary-adrenal axis)
D. Nursing care
   1. Assess lesions for color, location, and size
   2. Protect skin from scratching or rubbing
   3. Use appropriate topical agent
      a. Lotions: axillae; groin
      b. Creams: draining lesions
      c. Ointments: dry lesions
   4. Avoid contact with eyes
   5. Cleanse skin before application
   6. Utilize occlusive dressings if ordered
   7. Assess client for signs of sensitivity during therapy
   8. Evaluate client's response to medication and understanding of teaching

Dermal Agents

A. Description
   1. Inhibits keratinization and sebaceous gland function to improve cystic acne and reduce sebum excretion
   2. Available preparation: oral
B. Examples
   1. Isotretinoin (Accutane)
   2. Vitamin A acid (Retin-A)
C. Major side effects
   1. Visual disturbances (corneal opacities)
   2. Decreased night vision (vitamin A toxicity—effect on visual rods)
   3. Papilledema, headache (pseudotumor cerebri)
   4. Hepatic dysfunction (hepatotoxicity)
   5. Cheilitis (vitamin A toxicity)
   6. Pruritis, skin fragility (dryness)
   7. Hypertriglyceridemia (increased plasma triglycerides)
D. Nursing care
   1. Assess visual and hepatic status before administration
   2. Monitor blood lipids before and during therapy
   3. Instruct client to:
      a. Avoid pregnancy during and for 1 month after therapy; use contraception if sexually active to avoid pregnancy
      b. Avoid vitamin A supplements
      c. Side effects are reversible when therapy is discontinued
   4. Evaluate client's response to medication and understanding of teaching

PROCEDURES RELATED TO THE INTEGUMENTARY SYSTEM

Biopsy

A. Definition: a sample of tissue generally 3 mm or more is removed by use of a sharp, circular punch; when more tissue is needed, a wedge is excised through an incision
B. Nursing care
   1. Offer emotional support to client
   2. Assist the physician and help to maintain strict surgical aseptic technique
   3. Place specimen in appropriate container and send to pathology laboratory for analysis
   4. Use surgically aseptic technique when dressing wound at biopsy site
   5. Evaluate client's response to procedure

Cultures of the Skin

A. Definition
   1. To determine the presence of fungi on the skin, the skin is covered with a 10% potassium

hydroxide solution before scraping for microscopic examination

2. To determine bacterial infection of the skin, adequate tissue sampling is obtained using a sterile applicator or swab
3. Organisms obtained from the skin are observed in the laboratory so that identification may be made

B. Nursing care
1. Explain procedure to client
2. Allay anxiety and offer reassurance
3. Obtain samples using surgically aseptic technique prior to instituting antibiotic therapy
4. Notify physician of results so that appropriate therapy may be instituted
5. Evaluate client's response to procedure

Skin Grafts

A. Definition
1. Covering of denuded tissue with skin to prevent infection and loss of body fluids, promote healing, and prevent contractures
2. When used for burn sites, it is applied between the fifth and twenty-first day, depending on extent of the burn
3. May be partial or split thickness, involving the epidermis and part of the dermis, or full thickness, involving the entire epidermis and dermis
4. Types of skin grafts
   a. Xenografts: skin from animals, usually pigs (porcine xenograft)
   b. Homografts: skin from another person
   c. Autografts: skin from another part of the client's body
      (1) Mesh graft: machine used to mesh skin obtained from a donor site so it can be stretched to cover a larger area of burn
      (2) Postage stamp graft: earlier method of accomplishing the same goal as a mesh graft; a small amount of skin is used to cover a larger area; the donor skin is cut into small pieces and applied to the burn
      (3) Sheet grafting: large strips of skin placed over the burn as close together as possible

B. Nursing care
1. Explain procedure; obtain a written consent
2. Prepare the donor site carefully
3. After surgery, keep donor sites (which are covered with a nonadherent dressing and wrapped in an absorbent gauze) dry; remove absorbent gauze as ordered; nonadherent dressing will separate as healing occurs
4. Monitor the grafts, which are generally left with a light pressure dressing for approximate-

ly 3 days; after the graft has "taken," roll cotton-tipped applicators gently over the graft to remove underlying exudate; allowed to remain, exudate could promote infection, which could prevent the graft from adhering; instruct client to restrict mobility of the affected part
5. Observe for foul-smelling drainage, temperature elevation, and other signs of infection
6. Instruct the client to avoid exposure of the graft and donor sites to the sun
7. Evaluate client's response to procedure

Wood's Light Examination

A. Definition: the skin is viewed under ultraviolet light through special glass (Wood's glass) to identify superficial infections of the skin
B. Nursing care
1. Explain procedure to client
2. Reassure client that procedure is noninvasive and painless
3. Evaluate client's response to procedure

GENERAL NURSING DIAGNOSES FOR CLIENTS WITH INTEGUMENTARY SYSTEM DISORDERS

A. Anxiety related to fear of death
B. Body image disturbance related to altered appearance
C. Fluid volume deficit related to:
1. Excess loss via skin or kidney
2. Fluid shift into interstitial spaces
D. Fluid volume excess related to:
1. Response to stress
2. Disease process
3. Therapeutic modalities
E. Impaired gas exchange related to damaged mucous membranes
F. Risk for infection related to disruption of the skin surface
G. Risk for injury related to:
1. Altered mobility
2. Pain
H. Pain related to irritation/exposure of nerve endings
I. Impaired physical mobility related to:
1. Pain
2. Contractures
3. Scar tissue
J. Impaired skin integrity related to disruption of the skin surface
K. Ineffective thermoregulation related to interrupted skin integrity

MAJOR DISORDERS OF THE INTEGUMENTARY SYSTEM

PRIMARY SKIN LESIONS

A. Macule: flat circumscribed area from 1 to several centimeters in size, without elevation (freckle, flat pigmented moles)

B. Papule: raised circumscribed area less than 1 cm in size (acne)

C. Nodule: raised solid mass that extends into the dermis and is 1 to 2 cm in size (pigmented nevi)

D. Tumor: solid raised mass that extends into the dermis and is over 2 cm in size (dermatofibroma)

E. Wheal: flattened collection of fluid 1 mm to several centimeters in size (mosquito bites)

F. Vesicle: raised collection of fluid less than 1 cm in size (chickenpox, herpes simplex)

G. Bulla: fluid-filled vesicle over 1 cm in size (second-degree burn, pemphigus)

H. Pustule: vesicle or bulla filled with pus, over 1 cm in size (acne vulgaris)

I. Cyst: mass of fluid-filled tissue that extends to the subcutaneous tissues or dermis, over 1 cm in size (epidermoid cyst)

SECONDARY SKIN LESIONS

A. Fissure: a linear crack in the skin (athlete's foot)

B. Erosion: nonbleeding loss of superficial dermis (chickenpox rupture)

C. Ulcer: deep loss of skin surface that may bleed (stasis ulcer)

D. Crust: dried residue from blood or pus (impetigo)

E. Scale: flake of exfoliated epidermis (dandruff)

▼ PRESSURE ULCERS (DECUBITUS ULCERS)

Data Base

A. Etiology and pathophysiology
1. Caused by interruption of circulation when pressure on the skin exceeds capillary pressure of 32 mm Hg
2. Most ulcers commonly occur over bony prominences: sacrum, greater trochanter, heels, scapulae, elbows, malleoli, occiput, ears, and ischeal tuberosities
3. Contributing factors
   a. Immobility—results in prolonged pressure
   b. Aging—decreased epidermal thickness, elasticity, and secretion by sebaceous glands
   c. Moisture—causes skin maceration
   d. Inadequate nutrition—loss of subcutaneous tissue reduces padding; inadequate protein intake leads to negative nitrogen balance
   e. Pyrexia—causes increased cellular demand for oxygen
   f. Inadequate tissue oxygenation—anemia and circulatory disturbances result in less oxygen delivered to tissues
   g. Incontinence—substances in urine and feces irritate the skin
   h. Dryness—skin less supple
   i. Shearing force or friction—exerts excessive tension on skin
   j. Sensory deficits—client not aware of discomfort and does not take protective precautions
   k. Equipment—causes pressure, tension, or shearing forces on skin
4. Staging determined by depth of tissue damage
   a. Stage I: nonblanchable area of erythema; skin is intact
   b. Stage II: superficial ulceration of epidermis and/or dermis
   c. Stage III: full-thickness ulceration involving the epidermis and dermis, as well as subcutaneous tissue
   d. Stage IV: extensive tissue damage involving full-thickness skin loss, as well as damage to muscle, bone, and/or supporting structures

B. Clinical findings
1. Subjective
   a. Pain
   b. Loss of sensation if sensory nerve damage is present
2. Objective
   a. Erythema
   b. Tissue damage (see Staging under Etiology and Pathophysiology of Pressure Ulcers)
   c. Exudate
   d. Pyrexia and leukocytosis if systemic infection is present

C. Therapeutic interventions
1. Elimination of pressure on the ulcer through positioning and supportive devices (e.g., air-fluidized beds, low–air-loss beds, or kinetic beds)
2. Administration of protein supplements to prevent negative nitrogen balance state
3. Administration of vitamin and mineral supplements to promote wound healing, particularly vitamin C and zinc
4. Debridement of necrotic tissue, which interferes with healing and promotes bacterial growth
   a. Mechanical irrigation
   b. Chemical debridement with enzyme preparations
   c. Surgical debridement
   d. Wet to damp/dry dressings

5. Dressings to promote wound healing
   a. Moist gauze: maintains wound humidity that promotes epithelial cell growth
   b. Polyurethane film: provides barrier to bacteria and external fluid, promotes a moist environment, and permits viewing of the wound
   c. Hydrocolloid dressing: absorbs drainage, maintains wound humidity, liquifies necrotic debris, and provides a protective cushion
   d. Absorptive dressing: absorbs drainage
6. Antibiotic therapy
7. Skin grafts

Nursing Care of Clients with Pressure Ulcers

A. DATA COLLECTION
1. Stage, size, and location
2. Type and amount of exudate
3. Risk factors
   a. Degree of immobility
   b. Age
   c. Nutritional state (e.g., albumin, transferrin)
   d. Skin turgor
   e. Incontinence
   f. History of anemia or cardiovascular disease

B. ANALYSIS/NURSING DIAGNOSIS
Refer to General Nursing Diagnoses for Clients with Integumentary System Disorders for the following diagnoses: F and J

C. PLANNING/IMPLEMENTATION
1. Emphasize preventive care as soon as risk factors are identified
2. Change client's position at least every 1 to 2 hours
3. Use supportive devices (e.g., pillows, heel and elbow pads, cushions, special mattresses or bed) to reduce pressure on bony prominences
4. Encourage activity to enhance circulation
5. Bathe the skin to remove irritants and stimulate circulation
6. Massage around bony prominences, but avoid massaging reddened areas which are already damaged
7. Ensure adequate fluid intake
8. Provide well-balanced diet; emphasize importance of protein, zinc, and vitamins C, A, and B
9. Avoid shearing force by lifting, not dragging, the client during position changes
10. Administer wound care as prescribed
11. Instruct client about the importance of regular skin assessment, position changes, hygiene, and diet

D. EVALUATION/OUTCOMES
1. Maintains intact skin
2. Consumes diet high in protein, zinc, and vitamins C, A, and B

3. Changes position every hour
4. Inspects skin routinely

▼ BURNS

Data Base
A. Etiology and pathophysiology
1. Thermal, radiation, electrical, and chemical burns: cause cell destruction and result in depletion of fluid and electrolytes
2. Extent of the fluid and electrolyte loss directly related to extent and degree of the burn
   a. Superficial partial-thickness (first-degree) burn affects epidermis causing erythema, edema, and pain; fluid loss slight, especially if less than 15% of body surface is involved
   b. Deep partial-thickness (second-degree) burn affects epidermis and dermis causing erythema, pain, vesicles with oozing; fluid loss slight to moderate, especially if less than 15% of the body surface is involved
   c. Full-thickness (third-degree) burn affects entire dermis and at times the subcutaneous tissue, resulting in charred or pearly white, dry skin and absence of pain; fluid loss usually severe, especially if more than 2% of the body surface is involved
3. Classification of burns
   a. Minor burns: no involvement of hands, face, or genitalia; total partial-thickness burn area does not exceed 15%
   b. Moderate burns: partial-thickness involvement of 15% to 25% of body; but full-thickness burns do not exceed 10% of body area
   c. Major burns: involvement exceeds 25% (if partial-thickness) or 10% (if full-thickness) of body surface; involvement of hands, face, genitalia, or feet; this classification is also used if the client has a preexisting chronic health problem, is under 18 months or over 50 years of age, or has additional injuries
4. Pulmonary injury should be suspected if two of the following factors are present, and expected if three or all four are present:
   a. Hair in nostrils singed
   b. The client was trapped in a closed space
   c. Face, nose, and lips burned
   d. Initial blood sample contains carboxyhemoglobin
5. Percentage of body-surface involvement can be estimated by rule of nines or other burn area chart

6. Curling's ulcer may occur after a burn
   a. The client may complain of gastric discomfort, or there may be profuse bleeding
   b. Usually occurs by end of the first week after a burn
   c. Treatment essentially the same as for a gastric ulcer; however, mortality following surgical repair is high because of the client's debilitated state

B. Clinical findings
   1. Subjective
      a. Extreme anxiety
      b. Restlessness
      c. Pain, severity depending on the type of burn
      d. Paresthesia
      e. Disorientation
   2. Objective
      a. Changes in appearance of skin indicate degree of burn (see Etiology and Pathophysiology)
      b. Hematuria; blood hemolysis with subsequent rise in plasma hemoglobin may occur with full-thickness burns
      c. Elevated hematocrit as a result of fluid loss
      d. Electrolyte imbalance: cellular destruction results initially in hyperkalemia and hyperuricemia
      e. Presence of symptoms of hypovolemic shock caused by circulatory failure resulting from seepage of water, plasma, proteins, and electrolytes into burned area
      f. Presence of symptoms of neurogenic shock (symptoms similar to hypovolemic shock) caused by the fright, terror, hysteria, and pain involved in the situation
      g. Evidence of renal impairment (e.g., increased BUN and creatinine levels) if acute tubular necrosis occurs as a result of circulatory collapse

C. Therapeutic interventions
   1. Establishment of airway and administration of oxygen; mechanical ventilation as needed
   2. IV replacement (electrolyte solutions and colloids such as blood and plasma) to maintain circulation
      a. Volume of fluid replacement is based on percentage of body surface area involved and client's weight (e.g., Parkland/Baxter formula, Evans formula)
      b. Half of fluid is administered in first 8 hours; second half is administered over next 16 hours
   3. Reduction of total IV solutions during second 24 hours depends on the urinary output, blood work, and hemodynamic pressures

4. Foley catheter; monitor the urinary output and specific gravity hourly to observe kidney functioning and determine fluid replacement
5. Insertion of central line to monitor hemodynamic pressures (e.g., CVP, PCWP)
6. Vital signs monitored every 15 minutes
7. Serum electrolytes and blood gases to observe for levels and assist in deciding replacement therapy
8. Tetanus toxoid administration
9. Nothing by mouth except mineral water for first 24 to 48 hours; clear liquids as tolerated after 2 days; then high-protein, high-carbohydrate, high-fat, high-vitamin diet as tolerated
10. Maintenance of surgical asepsis
11. Daily Hubbard tank baths after the fifth day; use of antibiotic ointment and Kling dressing
12. Surgical debridement and skin grafting (see Procedures) to promote healing and limit contractures
13. Mechanical debridement (e.g., wet to damp/dry dressings) or enzymatic debridement may be used
14. IV and topical antibiotics to limit infection (Keflin and penicillin intravenously; mafenide acetate ointment; gentamicin; silver nitrate solution; and silver sulfadiazine)
15. Narcotics to reduce pain and sedatives to decrease anxiety, given IV or orally because of decreased muscle absorption

Nursing Care of Clients with Burns
A. DATA COLLECTION
   1. Signs of airway involvement: burns of face, neck, or chest; sooty sputum; or hoarseness
   2. Vital signs, arterial blood gases, and breath sounds to establish a baseline for respiratory function
   3. Central venous pressure (CVP) or pulmonary capillary wedge pressure (PCWP), urine output, and specific gravity to establish baseline for assessment of circulation
   4. Estimated body surface area involvement and severity of burns

B. ANALYSIS AND INTERPRETATION
Refer to General Nursing Diagnoses for Clients with Integumentary System Disorders for the following diagnoses: A, D 1, D 2, D 3, E, F, H, I 1, I 2, I 3, J, and K

C. PLANNING/IMPLEMENTATION
   1. Monitor vital signs, CVP or PCWP, intake and output (hourly urine output), and specific gravity as ordered; notify the physician if deviations occur or if output falls below 30 ml or rises above 50 ml per hour

2. Maintain patency of the Foley catheter to ascertain the correct information regarding fluid balance
3. Observe for signs of electrolyte imbalance (calcium, potassium, and sodium) and metabolic acidosis
4. Administer fluid and electrolytes as ordered
5. Monitor respiratory function: characteristics of respirations, breath sounds, and arterial blood gases
6. Administer oxygen as ordered
7. Elevate head of the bed
8. Encourage client to cough, deep breathe, and use incentive spirometer
9. Observe for signs of infection (rising temperature and white blood cell count, odor)
10. Follow principles of infection control (gown, gloves, mask, hair covering) during contact because the client's ability to resist infection is compromised
11. Administer tetanus toxoid as ordered
12. Administer IV and topical antibiotics as ordered
13. Use sterile technique for wound care
14. Apply pressure dressings as ordered to reduce contractures and scarring
15. Support the joints and extremities in a functional position and perform range-of-motion exercises
16. Support the client physically and emotionally while turning
17. Keep room temperature warm and humidity high
18. Observe for symptoms of stress ulcer; give ordered drugs to decrease or neutralize HCl
19. Provide small, frequent feedings; diet should be high in protein, carbohydrates, vitamins, and minerals; moderate in fat, with adequate calories for protein sparing
20. Give medication for pain as ordered and particularly before dressing change
21. Expect the client to express negative feelings about burns, and accept it
22. Explain need for staff wearing gowns and masks
23. Give realistic reassurance
24. Encourage participation in self-care
25. Refer client and family to support groups and rehabilitative services

D. EVALUATION/OUTCOMES
1. Maintains respiratory function
2. Maintains vital signs within normal limits
3. Maintains fluid balance
4. Remains free of infection
5. Participates in decision making and care
6. Expresses feelings about altered body image
7. Establishes effective communication with support system

▼ ACNE VULGARIS

Data Base
A. Etiology and pathophysiology
1. Hormonal activity produces hyperkeratosis of the follicular orifices, leading to blockage of secretions and the subsequent formation of fatty plugs known as blackheads (comedones) and whiteheads
2. When a blackhead (comedo) forms, the sebaceous gland involved becomes hypertrophic and infected
3. Cysts and nodules form, leaving scars
4. Most common among adolescents
B. Clinical findings
1. Subjective
   a. Pain when sebaceous glands become infected
   b. Depression
2. Objective
   a. Blackheads
   b. Whiteheads
   c. Pustules
   d. Nodules or cysts
C. Therapeutic interventions
1. Mechanical removal with a comedo extractor
2. Abrasive cleaners, astringents, and bacteriostatic creams
3. Topical administration of vitamin A acid, retinoic acid
4. Cryotherapy to produce desquamation of skin
5. Oral administration of antibiotics such as tetracycline
6. Intralesional injections of corticosteroids
7. Dermabrasion to improve the scars but not to cure the condition
   a. Instrument that functions at a high speed with a cylinder of wire or sandpaper at its end
   b. Epidermis and some dermis are removed at high points of the scars so they do not appear as deep
   c. Local anesthesia for treatment of small areas; general is indicated for large areas

Nursing Care of Clients with Acne Vulgaris
A. DATA COLLECTION
1. Client's personal hygiene and nutritional habits
2. Type and extent of lesions
3. Location and degree of inflammation
4. Client's perception of skin changes
B. ANALYSIS AND INTERPRETATION
Refer to General Nursing Diagnoses for Clients with Integumentary System Disorders for the following diagnoses: B and F

C. PLANNING/IMPLEMENTATION

1. Promote hygienic care when instructing how to wash areas and apply topical medications
2. Discuss the use of water-based cosmetics to prevent clogging of pores
3. Instruct the client how to take medications and to observe for side effects (see Pharmacology)
4. Emphasize importance of diet, which should be high in fruits, vegetables, whole grains, and legumes, and low in fats and animal foods; vitamin A is essential to promote proper epidermal function and status
5. Provide postoperative care following dermabrasion
   a. Apply ointment to lubricate skin and remove crust from area
   b. Observe serum draining from the area and report copious amounts of drainage to the surgeon
   c. Explain that the feeling of being sunburned is normal after dermabrasion

D. EVALUATION/OUTCOMES

1. Establishes and maintains skin-cleansing routine
2. Reduces incidence of infected lesions
3. Verbalizes improved self-esteem and body image

▼ CONTACT DERMATITIS

Data Base

A. Etiology and pathophysiology
   1. Results from contact with a substance that reacts with the protein in the skin to form an antigen in a sensitized client
   2. Antigen causes proliferation of lymphocytes, and the interaction of these factors causes eczematous changes
   3. Common causes: poison ivy, hair dye containing paraphenylenediamine, benzocaine, soaps, cements, insecticides, rubber compounds
B. Clinical findings
   1. Subjective
      a. Discomfort
      b. Pruritus
   2. Objective
      a. Erythema at the point of contact
      b. Vesicles and papules
      c. Edema
      d. Thickening of the skin and scaling
C. Therapeutic interventions
   1. Identification of the allergen through patch testing; a suspected allergen is applied to the unbroken skin; the skin is observed for erythe-

ma, papules, and vesicles in 24 to 48 hours
   2. Antihistamines, antipruritics, corticosteroids
   3. Topical corticosteroids

Nursing Care of Clients with Contact Dermatitis

A. DATA COLLECTION

1. History of onset and progression of symptoms
2. Allergies and potential exposure to irritants
3. Lesions, noting type, location, size, distribution, color, and drainage
4. Results of patch tests to identify allergens

B. ANALYSIS AND INTERPRETATION

Refer to General Nursing Diagnoses for Clients with Integumentary System Disorders for the following diagnoses: B, F, H, and J

C. PLANNING/IMPLEMENTATION

1. Instruct the client to avoid situations or substances that involve the identified allergen
2. Maintain cool environment
3. Provide tepid baths, adding colloidal preparations, oils, or cornstarch as indicated to alleviate pruritis
4. Trim fingernails to help control injury from scratching
5. Provide diversional activities
6. If topical corticosteroids are ordered, apply occlusive plastic dressing (Saran Wrap) over the ointment or lotion as ordered
7. Explain side effects of and related precautions for corticosteroids and antihistamines (see Pharmacology)

D. EVALUATION/OUTCOMES

1. Reports alleviation of pruritis
2. Verbalizes perceived improvement in appearance
3. Avoids exposure to known allergens
4. Maintains skin integrity

▼ CELLULITIS

Data Base

A. Etiology and pathophysiology
   1. Infection of upper layers of the dermis and subcutaneous tissue
   2. Usually caused by streptococcal or staphylococcal organisms
   3. Spreads along connective tissue planes
B. Clinical findings
   1. Subjective
      a. Pain
      b. Itching
   2. Objective
      a. Swelling
      b. Redness

c. Warmth

d. Leukocytosis

C. Therapeutic interventions

1. IV, IM, or oral antibiotic therapy following cultures of the area

2. Rest with elevation of extremity

3. Hot compresses

Nursing Care of Clients with Cellulitis

A. DATA COLLECTION

1. Description of onset and progression of symptoms

2. Signs of inflammation

3. Evidence of trauma

4. Evidence of impaired immune response from history

5. Vital signs and white blood cell count for database

B. ANALYSIS AND INTERPRETATION

Refer to General Nursing Diagnoses for Clients with Integumentary System Disorders for the following diagnoses: B, F, H, and I 1

C. PLANNING/IMPLEMENTATION

1. Monitor vital signs and white blood cell count for evidence of systemic involvement

2. Use appropriate aseptic technique when cleaning area

3. Use isolation precautions if necessary; see Infection for additional information

4. Administer analgesics and antibiotics as ordered

5. Elevate extremity

6. Apply warm compresses as ordered; protect from thermal trauma

D. EVALUATION/OUTCOMES

1. Experiences resolution of inflammatory process

2. Reports relief of pain

3. Explains the need to complete course of antibiotic therapy

▼ PSORIASIS

Data Base

A. Etiology and pathophysiology

1. Inflammatory disease involving epidermal proliferation that may be acute or chronic

2. Genetic predisposition is thought to be a factor

3. Uncommon in blacks

4. Exacerbations precipitated by climatic changes, trauma, infection, and psychologic stress

5. Exposure to sunlight in warm climates seems to reduce symptoms

B. Clinical findings

1. Subjective

a. Mild pruritus (severe if in skin folds)

b. If psoriatic arthritis is present, joint pain and stiffness

2. Objective

a. Bright-red, well-demarcated plaque covered with silvery scales, usually on knees, elbows, and scalp

b. Stippling of the nails and separation from nail bed

C. Therapeutic interventions

1. Exposure to solar or ultraviolet irradiation

2. Application of coal-tar ointment or antiinflammatory topical agents

3. Exposure to long-wave ultraviolet light (UVA) after oral administration of a psoralen derivative to increase photosensitivity; useful in treatment of intractable cases; also known as PUVA therapy

4. Systemic corticosteroid therapy may be used in severe cases

5. Methotrexate may also be used for severe psoriasis

Nursing Care of Clients with Psoriasis

A. DATA COLLECTION

1. History of onset and progression of symptoms

2. Factors contributing to the development of lesions

3. Presence of lesions noting type, color, location, size, and distribution

B. ANALYSIS AND INTERPRETATION

Refer to General Nursing Diagnoses for Clients with Integumentary System Disorders for the following diagnoses: B, F, H, and J

C. PLANNING/IMPLEMENTATION

1. Encourage ventilation of feelings about changes in body image; show acceptance

2. Assess lesions and the response to therapy

3. Determine factors linked to flare-ups; the client may need help coping with stressful situations

4. Instruct the client to use a soft brush to remove scales when bathing

5. If occlusive dressings are ordered with topical ointment, use plastic wrap, plastic bags, or gloves

6. Encourage diet rich in nutrient-dense foods such as fruits, vegetables, whole grains, and legumes to improve and maintain nutritional status and prevent possible drug-induced nutrient deficiencies; vitamin A is essential to promote improved epidermal status

7. Caution client to wear dark glasses during exposure to ultraviolet light

8. Review short-term and long-term effects of therapies with client

D. EVALUATION/OUTCOMES
1. Complies with medical regimen to improve skin integrity
2. Experiences alleviation of pruritis
3. Reports improvement in self-perception and self-esteem

▼ PEMPHIGUS VULGARIS

Data Base

A. Etiology and pathophysiology
1. Potentially fatal skin disease
2. Occurs only in adults
3. Associated with an autoimmune response
B. Clinical findings
1. Subjective
a. Debilitation
b. Malaise
c. Pain associated with lesions
d. Dysphagia
2. Objective
a. Bullae on normal skin and mucosa
b. Separation of epidermis caused by rubbing skin (Nikolsky's sign)
c. Acantholysis (changes in intercellular connections of the epidermis) evident on microscopic examination
d. Leukocytosis, eosinophilia
e. Foul-smelling discharge
C. Therapeutic interventions
1. Oral corticosteroids and immunosuppressive agents
2. Antibiotics for secondary infections
3. Topical treatment for relief of symptoms
a. Potassium permanganate baths
b. Oatmeal baths
c. Viscous xylocaine for oral lesions

Nursing Care of Clients with Pemphigus Vulgaris

A. DATA COLLECTION
1. History of onset and progression of symptoms
2. Presence of lesions noting location, size, distribution, and drainage
3. Degree to which lesions have compromised client's ADL
4. Vital signs for baseline

B. ANALYSIS AND INTERPRETATION
Refer to General Nursing Diagnoses for Clients with Integumentary System Disorders for the following diagnoses: B, C 2, D 1, D 2, F, H, I 1, J, and K

C. PLANNING/IMPLEMENTATION
1. Obtain lesion discharge for culture
2. Protect from infection
3. Watch for signs of infection such as elevated temperature and WBCs
4. Provide oral hygiene and increased fluid intake to soothe oral lesions
5. Provide skin care: therapeutic baths, gentle drying, avoidance of use of tape when applying protective dressings
6. Monitor intake and output (NaCl and fluid are lost through the skin)
7. Monitor serum protein and albumin levels (protein is lost through the skin)
8. Administer prescribed steroids with antacid or milk to prevent gastric irritation
9. Explain the need to observe for adverse effects of steroid therapy
10. Encourage ventilation of feelings; clients are often discouraged and depressed
11. Encourage diet rich in nutrient-dense foods such as fruits, vegetables, whole grains, and legumes to improve and maintain nutritional status and compensate for nutrient interactions of corticosteroid and other treatment medications; vitamin A is essential to promote improved epidermal status

D. EVALUATION/OUTCOMES
1. Maintains adequate oral intake
2. Experiences an improvement in skin integrity
3. Remains free from infection
4. Reports that pain is reduced
5. Identifies adverse effects of steroid therapy
6. Participates in personally fulfilling activities

▼ CANCER OF THE SKIN

Data Base

A. Etiology and pathophysiology
1. Most common cancer; however, early detection and slow progression make the cure rate high
2. Exposure to the sun, irritating chemicals, and chronic friction implicated; more common in persons with fair complexions
3. Types
a. Basal cell carcinoma: generally located on the face and appears as a waxy nodule that may have telangiectasias visible; the most common type of skin cancer, but metastasis is rare
b. Squamous cell carcinoma: develops rapidly and may metastasize through local lymph nodes; may develop secondarily to precancerous lesions such as keratosis and leukoplakia and is found most frequently on upper extremities and face, which are exposed to the sun; it appears as a small, red, nodular lesion

c. Malignant melanoma: most serious type and arises from the pigment-producing melanocytes; the color of the lesion may vary greatly (white, flesh, gray, brown, blue, black); changes in size, color, sensation, or characteristics of a mole suggest the possibility of malignant melanoma; metastasis via blood can be extensive

B. Clinical findings
   1. Subjective
      a. Pruritus may or may not be present
      b. Localized soreness
   2. Objective
      a. Change in color, size, or shape of preexisting lesion
      b. Oozing, bleeding, or crusting
      c. Biopsy of tumor reveals type of cancer
      d. Lymphadenopathy if metastasis has occurred

C. Therapeutic interventions
   1. Surgical excision of the lesion and surrounding tissue
   2. Chemosurgery, which involves the use of zinc chloride to fix the cells before they are dissected by layers
   3. Cryosurgery utilizing liquid nitrogen to destroy the tumor cells by freezing
   4. Radiation (malignant melanoma does not respond well to this mode of treatment)
   5. Chemotherapy
   6. Nonspecific immunostimulants such as BCG vaccine

Nursing Care of Clients with Cancer of the Skin

A. DATA COLLECTION
   1. History of changes in size, color, shape, sensation, or unusual bleeding of lesions
   2. Risk factors from history
   3. Skin for presence of suspicious lesions, documenting objective and subjective characteristics

B. ANALYSIS AND INTERPRETATION
   Refer to General Nursing Diagnoses for Clients with Integumentary System Disorders for the following diagnoses: B, F, and J

C. PLANNING/IMPLEMENTATION
   1. Monitor appearance of skin lesions
   2. Instruct the client to examine moles for changes and have those subject to chronic irritation (bra or belt line) removed
   3. Encourage to avoid exposure to the sun; use sunscreens with a rating higher than 15 SPF (solar protection factor); wear protective clothing
   4. Emphasize continued medical supervision
   5. Use surgical aseptic technique when caring for surgical site

   6. Encourage verbalization; maintain a therapeutic environment
   7. Provide care to the client receiving radiation
      a. Observe skin for local reaction
      b. Avoid use of ointments or powders containing metals
   8. Provide care related to specific chemotherapeutic agents (see Pharmacology Related to Neoplastic Disorders)
   9. Support natural defense mechanisms of client; encourage intake of nutrient-dense foods with emphasis on fruits, vegetables, whole grains, and legumes, especially those high in the immune-stimulating nutrients selenium and vitamins A, C, and E; beta-carotene has been associated with prevention of skin cancer
   10. Encourage client to verbalize fears
   11. Answer client's questions honestly

D. EVALUATION/OUTCOMES
   1. Avoids exposure to the sun and known irritants
   2. Examines skin lesions regularly and reports changes to physician
   3. Expresses concerns and feelings to health care provider
   4. Verbalizes acceptance of physical appearance after surgical excision of lesions

▼ HERPES ZOSTER (SHINGLES)

Data Base
A. Etiology and pathophysiology
   1. Acute viral infection of nerve structures caused by the varicella-zoster virus
   2. Inflammation occurs along the pathway of one or more peripheral sensory nerves
   3. Occurs in clients who have not had chickenpox and are exposed to an affected individual
   4. Occurs in immunosuppressed clients who have previously had chickenpox (e.g., leukemia, lymphoma)
   5. May involve the eye, leading to keratitis, uveitis, and blindness

B. Clinical findings
   1. Subjective
      a. Malaise
      b. Headache
      c. Pain
      d. Paresthesias
      e. Pruritis
   2. Objective
      a. Painful, pruritic vesicles arranged along the pathway of the involved nerves
      b. Stains made from lesion exudate isolate the organism

C. Therapeutic interventions
1. Administration of acyclovir (Zovirax)
2. Medications for pain, relaxation, itching, and preventing secondary infection
3. Control of pain by blocking the nerve through injection of drugs such as lidocaine or applying medication such as triamcinolone (Kenalog)
4. Antiinflammatory drugs such as systemic or topical steroids

Nursing Care of Clients with Herpes Zoster

A. DATA COLLECTION
1. Description of onset and progression of symptoms from history
2. Factors in history that can compromise the immune response (e.g., age, disease, chemotherapy)
3. Presence of characteristic lesion

B. ANALYSIS AND INTERPRETATION
Refer to General Nursing Diagnoses for Clients with Integumentary System Disorders for the following diagnoses: F, H, I 1, and J

C. PLANNING/IMPLEMENTATION
1. Administer analgesics and other medications as ordered
2. Reduce itching and protect lesions from air by the application of salves, ointments, lotions, and sterile dressings as ordered
3. Protect from pressure by use of air mattress; bed cradle; and light, loose clothing (avoid synthetic and woolen materials and use cotton fabrics)
4. In addition to standard precautions, use airborne and/or contact precautions as indicated
5. Administer antibiotics as ordered
6. Encourage client to avoid scratching and to use gloves at night to limit the possibility of accidental scratching
7. Assist the client to understand the basis for the rash and the itch
8. Allay fears that may be based on old wives' tales about shingles
9. Encourage the client to express feelings
10. Encourage diet rich in nutrient-dense foods such as fruits, vegetables, whole grains, and legumes to improve and maintain nutritional status and prevent possible drug-induced nutrient deficiencies; encourage intake of vitamin C because it has been reported to stimulate the immune response to viral infection by increasing interferon, which limits viral reproduction in early stages
11. Teach proper hand washing to help prevent spreading of the virus; individuals who have not had chickenpox should not be assigned to provide care

D. EVALUATION/OUTCOMES
1. Experiences an improvement in skin integrity
2. Reports that pain and pruritis have subsided
3. Performs ADL

▼ SYSTEMIC LUPUS ERYTHEMATOSUS (SLE)

Data Base
A. Etiology and pathophysiology
1. Origin unknown; affects the connective tissue and is thought to be due to a defect in the body's immunologic mechanisms, genetic predisposition, or to environmental stimuli
2. Immune complex deposits in blood vessels, among collagen fibers, and on organs
3. Necrosis of the glomerular capillaries, inflammation of cerebral and ocular blood vessels, necrosis of lymph nodes, vasculitis of the GI tract and pleura, and degeneration of the basal layer of skin
4. More common in females, ages 13 to 40
B. Clinical findings
1. Subjective
a. Malaise
b. Photosensitivity
c. Joint pain
2. Objective
a. Fever
b. Butterfly erythema on the face
c. Erythema of palms
d. Positive lupus erythematosus preparation (LE prep); increased antinuclear antibodies (ANA) in blood
e. Raynaud's phenomenon
f. Weight loss
g. Evidence of impaired renal (nephritis), gastrointestinal (esophagitis), cardiac (pericarditis), respiratory (pneumonitis), and neurologic functions
C. Therapeutic interventions
1. Corticosteroids and analgesics to reduce pain and inflammation
2. Supportive therapy as major organs become affected (heart, kidneys, CNS, GI tract)

Nursing Care of Clients with Systemic Lupus Erythematosus

A. DATA COLLECTION
1. Description of onset and progression of symptoms from the history
2. Presence of skin lesions
3. Sensitivity to light (photosensitivity)
4. Vital signs for baseline data
5. Heart and lung sounds

6. Abdomen for enlargement of liver and spleen
7. Neurologic status
8. Renal function (review BUN and creatinine analysis results)

B. ANALYSIS AND INTERPRETATION

Refer to General Nursing Diagnoses for Clients with Integumentary System Disorders for the following diagnoses: A, B, D 2, D 3, E, G 1, H, I 1, I 2, I 3, and J

C. PLANNING/IMPLEMENTATION

1. Administer corticosteroids and observe for side effects, teaching client to do the same (see Pharmacology Related to Integumentary System Disorders)
2. Help the client and family cope with severity of the disease, as well as its poor prognosis
3. Explain the importance of protecting skin
   a. Use of mild soap
   b. Avoidance of exposure to sunlight
   c. Use of sun-blocking agents
4. Assist client to establish regular program of exercise balanced by rest periods to avoid fatigue
5. Instruct client to alter the consistency and frequency of meals if dysphagia and anorexia exist
6. Encourage diet rich in nutrient-dense foods such as fruits, vegetables, whole grains, and legumes to improve and maintain nutritional status and compensate for nutrient interactions of corticosteroid and other treatment medications; emphasize vitamin C because it is essential in the biosynthesis of collagen, and large doses have been found to increase total collagen synthesis
7. Emphasize the need for continued medical follow-up

D. EVALUATION/OUTCOMES

1. Demonstrates a reduction in skin lesions
2. Establishes a schedule of exercise and rest periods
3. States that pain is reduced
4. Verbalizes fears with family and health care providers
5. Participates in decisions about care
6. Remains active in activities that provide satisfaction
7. Continues medical supervision

▼ POLYARTERITIS NODOSA

Data Base

A. Etiology and pathophysiology
1. Cause unknown
2. Collagen disease that causes inflammation and necrosis of small and medium-sized arteries

3. When healing of the arteries occurs, there is a thickening of the walls with subsequent circulatory impairment
4. Common areas involved are the kidneys, heart, liver, and GI tract

B. Clinical findings
1. Subjective
   a. Malaise
   b. Weakness
   c. Severe abdominal pain, muscle aches
2. Objective
   a. Weight loss
   b. Low-grade fever
   c. Bloody diarrhea
   d. Proteinuria if kidneys are affected
   e. Positive rheumatoid factor (RF) and elevated sedimentation rate

C. Therapeutic interventions
1. Corticosteroids and analgesics to control pain and inflammation
2. Balanced diet to combat weight loss

Nursing Care of Clients with Polyarteritis Nodosa

See Nursing Care of Clients with Systemic Lupus Erythematosus

▼ SCLERODERMA (PROGRESSIVE SYSTEMIC SCLEROSIS)

Data Base

A. Etiology and pathophysiology
1. Thought to be caused by an autoimmune defect; occurs in women more frequently than in men
2. Systemic disease that causes fibrotic changes in connective tissue throughout the body
3. May involve the skin, blood vessels, synovial membranes, esophagus, heart, lungs, kidneys, or GI tract
4. CREST syndrome refers to a group of symptoms associated with a poor prognosis
   a. Calcium deposits in organs
   b. Raynaud's phenomenon
   c. Esophageal dysfunction
   d. Sclerodactyly (scleroderma of the digits)
   e. Telangiectasia

B. Clinical findings
1. Subjective
   a. Articular pain
   b. Muscle weakness
2. Objective
   a. Hard skin that eventually adheres to underlying structures; face becomes mask-like

b. Telangiectases on the lips, fingers, face, and tongue
c. Dysphagia
d. Restriction of body motion as the disease progresses
e. Raynaud's phenomenon
f. Positive LE prep, elevated gamma-globulin levels, presence of antinuclear antibodies

C. Therapeutic interventions
1. Corticosteroids
2. Salicylates or analgesics for joint pain
3. Vasodilators for symptoms of Raynaud's phenomenon
4. Physical therapy

Nursing Care of Clients with Scleroderma

A. DATA COLLECTION
1. Onset and progression of symptoms from history
2. Skin, particularly of the hands and face
3. Joints for inflammation
4. Vital signs for baseline data

B. ANALYSIS AND INTERPRETATION
Refer to General Nursing Diagnoses for Clients with Integumentary System Disorders for the following diagnoses: A, B, D 2, D 3, E, G 1, G 2, H, I 2, and J

C. PLANNING/IMPLEMENTATION
1. Ensure that vital capacity and renal function studies are performed
2. Support the client and family emotionally; there is no cure at present
3. Use mild soaps and lotions for skin care
4. Provide small, frequent meals
5. Instruct client to avoid smoking and exposure to cold
6. Encourage deep-breathing exercises
7. Teach the client the importance of observing for side effects of corticosteroids or other immunosuppressive drugs
8. Emphasize the need for continued medical follow-up
9. Monitor function of all vital organs (e.g., cardiac, respiratory, and renal status)

D. EVALUATION/OUTCOMES
1. Maintains skin integrity
2. Participates in self-care activities with minimal discomfort
3. Verbalizes acceptance of changes in appearance and disease
4. Reports symptoms of vital organ involvement
5. Lists side effects of corticosteroid therapy

▼ KAPOSI'S SARCOMA

Data Base
A. Etiology and pathophysiology
1. Cause is unknown: occurs primarily in individuals with a compromised immune system; often occurs in individuals with AIDS
2. Lesions generally begin in the epidermis and extend into the dermis, but may develop as extracutaneous lesions
3. There are four classifications of lesions
   a. Nodular: found on the extremities and slow growing
   b. Florid: very rapid growing and ulcerated
   c. Infiltrate: penetrating deeper structures, including bone
   d. Lymphadenopathic: disseminated type, rare, generally found in children
4. Involvement of GI organs, bone, and lung are common

B. Clinical findings
1. Subjective
   a. Pain may or may not be present
   b. Depend on organ involved
2. Objective
   a. Purplish lesions on skin and mucous membranes
   b. Positive identification obtained through biopsy

C. Therapeutic interventions
1. Radiation may be used alone or in conjunction with chemotherapy
2. Chemotherapeutic treatment may be administered intravenously, intraarterially, or intralesionally
3. Immunotherapy may be employed to stabilize the immune system
4. Cryotherapy

Nursing Care of Clients with Kaposi's Sarcoma

A. DATA COLLECTION
1. Onset and progression of symptoms from history
2. Skin and oral mucosa for lesions, noting location, size, color, and number
3. Other manifestations of immunosuppressive disorders (see Acquired Immunodeficiency Syndrome)

B. ANALYSIS AND INTERPRETATION
Refer to General Nursing Diagnoses for Clients with Integumentary System Disorders for the following diagnoses: A, B, F, H, I 1, and J

C. PLANNING/IMPLEMENTATION
1. Provide emotional support as an individual and by appropriate referrals
2. Provide for pain relief

3. Use precautions to maximize skin integrity including a diet high in vitamin A and foods that are of high nutrient density
4. Use aseptic technique when applying dressings over open lesions
5. Use appropriate aseptic techniques if client is severely immune depressed; use standard (universal) precautions
6. Provide care for the client receiving radiation therapy or chemotherapy (see Nursing Care of Clients with Neoplastic Disorders Receiving Chemotherapy or Radiation)

D. **EVALUATION/OUTCOMES**
1. Remains free from infection
2. Verbalizes acceptance of disease
3. Copes with altered body image
4. Continues to seek medical follow-up

INFECTIOUS DISEASES

See discussion of Infection for additional information

GENERAL NURSING DIAGNOSES FOR CLIENTS WITH INFECTIOUS DISEASES

A. Body image disturbance related to altered body appearance
B. Diarrhea related to increased peristalsis and altered gastrointestinal flora
C. Fatigue related to increased metabolic rate and decreased oxygen-carrying capacity of blood
D. Fluid volume deficit related to:
   1. Diaphoresis/fever
   2. Diarrhea
E. Hyperthermia related to pyrogenic activity
F. Knowledge deficit related to misinformation about transmission
G. Altered nutrition: less than body requirements related to:
   1. Decreased intake
   2. Increased metabolic needs
H. Pain related to inflammatory response
I. Disturbance in self-esteem related to contagious nature of illness
J. Impaired skin integrity related to disease process
K. Social isolation related to imposed isolation precautions
L. Altered peripheral tissue perfusion related to interrupted skin integrity

MAJOR INFECTIOUS DISEASES

▼ GAS GANGRENE

Data Base

A. Etiology and pathophysiology
   1. Caused by an anaerobic gram-positive clostridium (*Clostridium perfringens*, *C. welchii*, *C. novyi*) that enters through a deep wound
   2. Usually occurs 2 to 5 days after injury
   3. Bacilli colonize in muscle tissue surrounding the wound
B. Clinical findings
   1. Subjective
      a. Pain
      b. Apprehension
      c. Anorexia
      d. Chills
   2. Objective
      a. Bronzed or blackened wound tissue
      b. Crepitus
      c. Sweetish-smelling exudate
      d. Necrosis of muscle tissues
      e. Presence of clostridia on culture
      f. Pallor
      g. Diarrhea
      h. Vomiting
      i. Temperature elevation (may be slight)
      j. Anemia
C. Therapeutic interventions
   1. Multiple incisions for decompression and drainage
   2. Extirpation and debridement of involved tissue with copious irrigations
   3. Penicillin G, tetracycline, chloramphenicol, or erythromycin, depending on drug sensitivity
   4. Amputation
   5. Hyperbaric oxygenation
   6. Whole blood, packed erythrocytes, or plasma transfusions to combat hemolysis and profound anemia
   7. Antitoxin therapy may be started

Nursing Care of Clients with Gas Gangrene

A. Refer to General Nursing Care of Clients at Risk for Infection
B. Refer to General Nursing Diagnoses for Clients with Infectious Diseases
C. Prevent infection whenever the wound is near the rectum because the organism is found in feces
D. Use standard precautions
E. Monitor fluid and electrolyte balance
F. Check cardiovascular status frequently to determine complications

G. Instruct client regarding side effects of medications and importance of diet to support immune system (see Pharmacologic Control of Infection)

▼ HANSEN'S DISEASE (LEPROSY)

Data Base
A. Etiology and pathophysiology
   1. Thought to be transmitted by direct contact with the acid-fast bacillus *Mycobacterium leprae*
   2. Bacillus causes lesions of the peripheral nervous system that extend to and destroy nearby skin tissues
B. Clinical findings
   1. Subjective: loss of sensation
   2. Objective: painless, colorless, or red-brown macules and papules, nodules, sores, and ulcers
C. Therapeutic interventions
   1. Sulfone drugs (e.g., dapsone)
   2. Reconstructive surgery

Nursing Care of Clients with Hansen's Disease
A. Refer to General Nursing Care of Clients at Risk for Infection
B. Refer to General Nursing Diagnoses for Clients with Infectious Diseases
C. Provide emotional support for the client and the family, allowing ample time for verbalization of feelings
D. Maintain mobility of the client with decreased use of painful extremities
E. Use standard precautions
F. Encourage case-finding examinations of all family members and friends; assure them that the disease has a very low incidence of communicability

▼ TOXOPLASMOSIS

Data Base
A. Etiology and pathophysiology
   1. Caused by protozoan (*Toxoplasma gondii*), a parasite of warm-blooded animals
   2. Contracted by eating raw meat containing cysts or by exposure to contaminated cat feces
   3. Disease can be transmitted to fetus through placental circulation causing death or congenital anomalies, even though mother may be asymptomatic
   4. Leading cause of encephalitis in immunosuppressed clients
B. Clinical findings
   1. Subjective
      a. Malaise
      b. Fatigue

   2. Objective
      a. Fever
      b. Lymphadenopathy
C. Therapeutic interventions
   1. Usually no treatment required for adults
   2. Pregnant women and immunosuppressed clients may be treated with pyrimethamine, trisulfapyrimidine, sulfadiazene, and folic acid

Nursing Care of Clients with Toxoplasmosis
A. Refer to General Nursing Care of Clients at Risk for Infection
B. Refer to General Nursing Diagnoses for Clients with Infectious Diseases
C. Provide emotional support to pregnant clients
D. Caution pregnant clients to avoid cleaning cat litter pans or gardening where they may be exposed to cat feces
E. Teach client about proper handling, preparation, and storage of meat, washing fruits and vegetables, and care of cat litter
F. Encourage a diet rich in nutrient-dense foods
G. Use standard precautions

▼ MALARIA

Data Base
A. Etiology and pathophysiology
   1. Caused by a protozoan (*Plasmodium falciparum, P. vivax, P. ovale, P. malariae*) that enters during a bite by an infected Anopheles mosquito, through the use of dirty needles, or by a transfusion from an infected donor
   2. When the parasite enters the bloodstream, it invades the red blood cells; destruction of red blood cells, blockage of capillaries, and irreversible damage to the spleen and liver may follow
   3. Rare complication is "blackwater fever"; name derived from the fact that there is intravascular hemolysis and hemoglobinuria
   4. Individuals with the sickle cell trait have natural resistance to malaria
B. Clinical findings
   1. Subjective
      a. Malaise
      b. Headache
      c. Muscle aches
      d. Chills
      e. Thirst
   2. Objective
      a. High fever
      b. Anemia
      c. Enlarged spleen
      d. Dehydration

e. Renal failure

C. Therapeutic interventions
   1. Antimalarial drugs (see Chemoprophylaxis under Nursing Care)
   2. Aspirin

Nursing Care of Clients with Malaria

A. Refer to General Nursing Care of Clients at Risk for Infection
B. Refer to General Nursing Diagnoses for Clients with Infectious Diseases
C. Monitor fluid and electrolyte balance
D. Use standard precautions
E. Use sprays and wear protective clothing to prevent mosquito bites
F. Use therapeutic measures such as sponges to decrease the fever; maintain hydration
G. Maintain bed rest until the fever and other symptoms have ceased
H. Assist with dialysis and monitor blood transfusions as needed when blackwater fever is present
I. Teach preventive measures
   1. Avoid stagnant pools
   2. Initiate chemoprophylaxis 1 week before visiting endemic areas and regularly while in the area: pyrimethamine, proguanil hydrochloride, chloroquine phosphate, or amodiaquine hydrochloride
J. Support natural defense mechanisms of client; encourage intake of nutrient-dense foods with emphasis on fruits, vegetables, whole grains, and legumes, especially those high in the immune-stimulating nutrients selenium and vitamins A, C, and E

▼ RABIES (HYDROPHOBIA)

Data Base

A. Etiology and pathophysiology
   1. Caused by a virus found in the saliva of an infected animal and usually spread by bite; the animal can be a carrier and not be ill with the disease
   2. Incubation period is 10 to 50 days in bites of the upper parts of the body, 4 months in bites of the lower parts
   3. Bites are usually unprovoked; suspected animals are observed for 10 days
   4. Negri bodies (round objects) found in the brain tissue of infected animals
   5. Virus spreads from the soft tissue surrounding the wound to the peripheral nerves and ultimately affects the CNS; may cause punctate hemorrhages and neuronal destruction

B. Clinical findings
   1. Subjective
      a. Anxiety
      b. Depression, malaise, lethargy
      c. Irritability
      d. Headaches
      e. Stiff neck
      f. Anorexia, nausea
      g. Photophobia
      h. Respiratory difficulty such as wheezing, hyperventilation, and dyspnea
      i. Thirst
      j. Paresthesia or pain near the bite or in the bitten extremity
   2. Objective
      a. Severe difficulty swallowing
      b. Excessive salivation
      c. Choking
      d. Aerophobia
      e. Apnea
      f. Paralysis
      g. Coma
      h. Cardiac dysrhythmias
C. Therapeutic interventions
   1. Cleansing of the wound with soap and water
   2. Tracheostomy if severe respiratory embarrassment develops
   3. Human rabies immune globulin for passive immunity; dose given in the buttock; wound is bathed with the drug
   4. Human diploid cell vaccine is used to induce active immunity; treatment consists of five doses over 4 weeks followed by a sixth dose after 2 months; duck embryo rabies vaccine (DEV) was formerly used requiring a total of 23 doses administered subcutaneously
   5. Sedative or anesthetics as necessary; phenytoin used for seizures

Nursing Care of Clients with Rabies

A. Refer to General Nursing Care of Clients at Risk for Infection
B. Refer to General Nursing Diagnoses for Clients with Infectious Diseases
C. Maintain standard precautions to avoid contact with saliva of infected client
D. Monitor blood gases, fluid and electrolyte balance, and electrocardiograms
E. Keep the room dark and quiet to prevent agitation
F. Monitor the tracheostomy and the need for suctioning
G. Prevent drafts, which may result in spasms
H. Allow the family and client to verbalize their feelings

▼ ROCKY MOUNTAIN SPOTTED FEVER

Data Base

A. Etiology and pathophysiology
 1. Contamination of an individual by a tick infected with *Rickettsia rickettsii* (through bite or contamination by a crushed tick on the fingers or in the eye); there may or may not be a history of a tick bite
 2. Sudden onset, with an incubation period of 3 to 17 days
 3. Organism attacks endothelial cells and extends into the vessel walls, causing thrombi, inflammation, and necrosis
B. Clinical findings
 1. Subjective
  a. Malaise
  b. Insomnia
  c. Headache
  d. Anorexia
  e. Photophobia
  f. Joint and muscle discomfort
 2. Objective
  a. Fever
  b. Rash (rose-colored macules)
  c. Edema
  d. Subcutaneous hemorrhage
  e. Necrosis
  f. Enlarged spleen
  g. Hearing loss
  h. Hypotension
  i. Circulatory collapse
C. Therapeutic interventions
 1. Prompt recognition and treatment vital
 2. Tetracycline or chloramphenicol therapy continued until the client is afebrile for 3 to 5 days
 3. Treatment of symptoms and complications as they develop

Nursing Care of Clients with Rocky Mountain Spotted Fever

A. Refer to General Nursing Care of Clients at Risk for Infection
B. Refer to General Nursing Diagnoses for Clients with Infectious Diseases
C. Assure the family that the client's disturbed emotional responses are associated with the disease
D. Monitor symptoms to determine progression of the disease
E. Assess the cardiovascular status to determine developing circulatory collapse
F. Use standard precautions
G. Reassure that hearing loss will last only several weeks
H. Teach prevention such as wearing tick repellents, checking pants legs and animals for the presence of ticks, and removal of ticks
I. Teach all individuals to kill ticks with a tweezer to prevent contamination of fingers

▼ LYME DISEASE

Data Base

A. Etiology and pathophysiology
 1. Caused by spirochete bacteria, *Borrelia burgdorferi*
 2. Disease is most often carried by mice, deer, or raccoons; cats, dogs, and horses may also be carriers
 3. Transmitted by carrier tick that acquired bacterium from infected host (deer tick, Western black-legged tick, or lone star tick)
 4. Most common in coastal areas during June and July, but tick is active from April to October
 5. Infectious organism can survive in host 10 years or more
 6. Initial rash and flulike symptoms; later neuromusculoskeletal symptoms
 7. Named for mysterious 1972 outbreak of arthritis in Lyme, Connecticut
B. Clinical findings
 1. Subjective
  a. Chills
  b. Muscle aches
  c. Joint pain
  d. Headache
  e. Dizziness
  f. Stiff neck
 2. Objective
  a. Fever
  b. Red-ringed, circular rash
  c. Blood work positive for causative bacterium
  d. Swollen joints
  e. Lack of coordination
  f. Facial palsy
  g. Paralysis
  h. Dementia
C. Therapeutic interventions
 1. Antibiotics such as penicillin, tetracycline, ceftriaxone sodium
 2. Symptomatic treatment

Nursing Care of Clients with Lyme Disease

A. Refer to General Nursing Care of Clients at Risk for Infection
B. Refer to General Nursing Diagnoses for Clients with Infectious Diseases

C. Question clients with arthritic symptoms about possible exposure
D. Use standard precautions
E. Teach clients to:
1. Avoid tall grass
2. Use chemical repellents
3. Wear light colors to enhance tick identification
4. Wear long sleeves and pants tucked in high boots when walking in areas with tick infestation
5. Shower and inspect skin
6. Remove ticks with tweezers, grasping close to skin to avoid breaking mouth parts

▼ TETANUS (LOCKJAW)

Data Base
A. Etiology and pathophysiology
1. Caused by the anaerobic bacillus *Clostridium tetani*, which is transmitted through an open wound
2. Symptoms from 2 days to 3 weeks after exposure to the bacillus
3. Toxins from the bacillus invade the nervous tissue, and the motor and sensory nerves become hypersensitive, resulting in prolonged contractions and respiratory failure
B. Clinical findings
1. Subjective
a. Irritability
b. Restlessness
c. Pain from muscle spasms
2. Objective
a. Muscle rigidity
b. Local or general spastic contractions of the voluntary muscles
c. Trismus (spasm of the masticatory muscles)
d. Spasms of the respiratory tract
e. Convulsions
C. Therapeutic interventions
1. Tetanus immune globulin (TIG) to provide temporary passive immunity; tetanus toxoid may also be given in a different site
2. Maintenance of adequate pulmonary ventilation
3. Debridement of the wound to allow exposure to air
4. Control of muscle spasms
5. Penicillin G to limit secondary infection
6. Maintenance of fluid balance and nutrition
7. Diazepam and barbiturates to sedate the client and limit spasms

8. Once symptoms develop, specific therapy is ineffective; therefore institution of supportive therapy is necessary until toxins are reduced by time

Nursing Care of Clients with Tetanus
A. Refer to General Nursing Care of Clients at Risk for Infection
B. Refer to General Nursing Diagnoses for Clients with Infectious Diseases
C. Prevent the disease through immunization with tetanus toxoid to provide active immunity; prophylaxis in suspect injuries
D. Maintain a quiet environment to decrease excessive stimuli, which may result in convulsions
E. Frequently assess respiratory status; administer oxygen as needed; client may require mechanical ventilation
F. Frequently suction the airway to maintain patency and promote ventilation; keep an endotracheal tube and tracheostomy set at the bedside
G. Use standard precautions
H. Allow the client and family to verbalize fears and feelings

▼ TYPHOID FEVER

Data Base
A. Etiology and pathophysiology
1. Caused by the bacterium *Salmonella typhi*, which can be carried in human feces and transmitted through sewage, flies, and shellfish
2. Incubation period 3 to 20 days
3. Bacterium invades the GI tract and localizes in lymph tissue of the intestinal wall (Peyer's patches); these areas may become thrombosed and tissue sloughs off, leaving ulcers
4. Hemorrhage, peritonitis, perforation, and hepatitis are serious complications
B. Clinical findings
1. Subjective
a. Headaches
b. Drowsiness
2. Objective
a. Fever
b. Bradycardia
c. Rose-colored papules on the abdomen
d. Enlarged spleen
e. Enlarged liver
f. Delirium
g. Constipation during the early stage; diarrhea during the late stage
C. Therapeutic interventions
1. Chloramphenicol, ampicillin, or trimethoprim and sulfamethoxazole
2. Corticosteroids the first 4 to 5 days of treatment

Nursing Care of Clients with Typhoid Fever

A. Refer to General Nursing Care of Clients at Risk for Infection
B. Refer to General Nursing Diagnoses for Clients with Infectious Diseases
C. Maintain safety if delirium is present
D. Encourage a diet rich in high nutrient density foods and high-calorie foods
E. Employ methods to decrease the fever
F. Monitor fluid and electrolytes to prevent imbalance
G. Monitor for urinary retention
H. In addition to standard precautions, use contact precautions if the client is incontinent of feces
I. Use soft diet to prevent perforation and stool softeners as ordered to limit constipation
J. Educate the public to prevent disease through proper sewage treatment
K. Encourage vaccination programs with booster injections every 3 years in endemic areas
L. Allow the client and family ample time to verbalize emotional reactions and concerns resulting from the illness

URINARY/REPRODUCTIVE SYSTEMS

REVIEW OF ANATOMY AND PHYSIOLOGY OF THE URINARY SYSTEM

Functions of the Urinary System

A. Secrete urine
B. Eliminate urine from body (urination, micturition, or voiding) to:
   1. Excrete various normal and abnormal metabolic wastes
   2. Regulate the composition and volume of blood and regulate blood pressure; especially important in maintenance of fluid and electrolyte balance and acid-base balance (see Maintenance of Fluid, Electrolyte, and Acid-Base Balance)

Structures of the Urinary System

Kidneys

A. Gross anatomy
   1. Size, shape, and location: about $10 \times 5 \times 2.5$ cm; shaped like lima beans; lie against the posterior abdominal wall, behind the peritoneum at the level of the last thoracic and first three lumbar vertebrae; right kidney slightly lower than the left
   2. External structure
      a. Hilum: concave notch on the mesial surface; blood vessels, nerves, lymphatics, and ureter enter through this notch
      b. Renal capsule: protective fibrous tissue that envelops the kidney
   3. Internal structure
      a. Cortex: outer layer of the kidney substance; composed of renal corpuscles, convoluted tubules, and adjacent parts of loops of Henle
      b. Medulla: inner portion of the kidney; composed of loops of Henle and collecting tubules
      c. Pyramids: triangular wedges of medullary substance that have a striped appearance and are composed of collecting tubules
      d. Columns: inward extensions of cortex between the pyramids
      e. Papillae: apices of the pyramids; collecting tubules drain into minor calyces here
      f. Calyces: bell-mouthed cups that drain the papillae; 8 to 12 minor calyces open into 2 or 3 major calyces that form the pelvis
      g. Pelvis: a small funnel tapering into the ureter and formed by union of several calyces
B. Blood flow in the kidney
   1. Kidneys receive 20% of cardiac output during rest; reduced to 2% to 4% during physical or emotional stress
   2. Abdominal aorta gives rise to the renal artery, which enters the hilum of each kidney; renal artery branches into interlobar arteries that fan out into kidney cortex; smaller arterial branches form afferent arterioles, which enter glomerular capillary beds
   3. Efferent arterioles leave the glomerular capillary bed forming the peritubular capillary network, which then converges into progressively larger veins until the renal vein leaves the kidney
C. Nephron: anatomic and functional unit of the kidney; approximately 1 million per kidney
   1. Anatomy
      a. Glomerulus: cluster of capillaries invaginated into Bowman's capsule
      b. Bowman's capsule: the funnel-shaped upper end of the urinary tubules
      c. Renal corpuscle: composed of Bowman's capsule and the glomerulus invaginated into it
      d. Proximal convoluted tubule: first portion of kidney tubules
      e. Henle's loop: second portion of kidney tubules
      f. Distal convoluted tubule: third portion of kidney tubules
   2. Physiology: nephron functions via principles of filtration, reabsorption, and secretion (Fig. 6-12)
      a. Glomerulus: urine formation starts with process of filtration; water and solutes

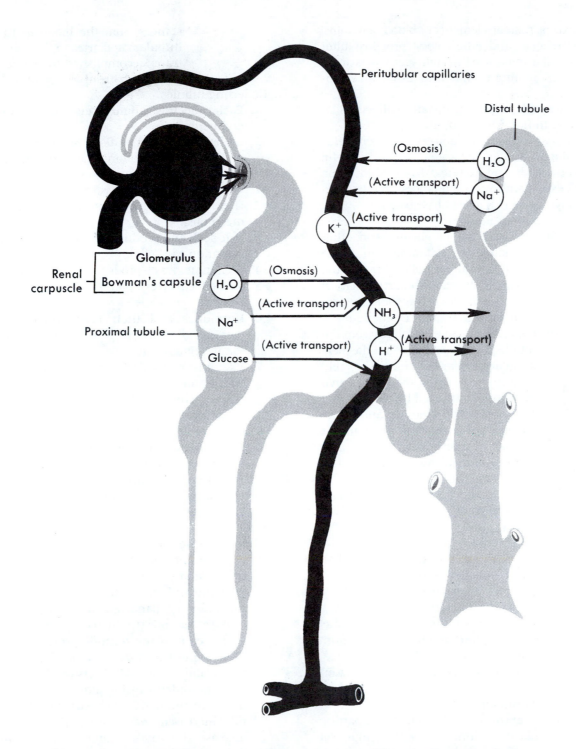

FIGURE 6-12 Diagram showing glomerular filtration, tubular reabsorption, and tubular secretion—the three processes by which the kidneys secrete urine. In the proximal tubule, note that water is reabsorbed from the tubular filtrate and moves into the blood by osmosis (a passive transport mechanism) but that sodium and glucose are reabsorbed mainly by active transport mechanisms. Note also that water and sodium are reabsorbed from the distal tubule. Potassium and hydrogen ions (K^+ and H^+) and ammonia (NH_3), by contrast, are secreted into the tubule from the blood. (From Thibodeau GA, Patton KT: *Anatomy and physiology*, ed 2, St. Louis, 1993, Mosby.)

(except cellular elements of blood, albumins, fibrinogen, and other blood proteins) filter out of capillaries through glomerular-capsular membrane and into Bowman's capsule

b. Bowman's capsule: filtrate collects here prior to flow to the tubules

c. Tubular reabsorption and secretion: epithelial lining of tubules reabsorbs substances useful to the body and excretes, dissolved in water, all excess and waste substances; secretes electrolytes essential to acid-base balance

(1) Proximal tubule

(a) Reabsorption of glucose and other nutrients (e.g., vitamins and amino acids) from the tubular filtrate to the blood in the peritubular capillaries; mainly by active transport mechanisms in the tubular epithelium

(b) Reabsorption of electrolytes from the tubule filtrate to blood in the peritubular capillaries; cations (notably sodium) are reabsorbed by active transport, stimulated by aldosterone; anions (notably chloride and bicarbonate) are reabsorbed by diffusion following cation transport

(c) Reabsorption of about 80% of the water from the tubular filtrate to the blood in the peritubular capillaries by osmosis as a result of electrolyte reabsorption

(2) Loop of Henle

(a) Establishes osmotic conditions that promote water reabsorption

(b) Actively transports chloride ions from the filtrate, thus passively removing sodium ions with the chloride; sodium chloride excretion results in increased osmotic force and promotes reabsorption of water in the collecting tubules

(3) Distal tubule

(a) Reabsorption of electrolytes, particularly sodium, under the influence of the mineralocorticoid aldosterone

(b) Reabsorption of water into the blood by osmosis; ADH controls the amount of water osmosing out of the distal tubule, whereas amount of electrolytes reabsorbed controls the amount of osmosis out of the proximal tubule

(c) Secretion of hydrogen, potassium, ammonia, and some other substances from the blood in the peritubular capillaries to the tubular filtrate; accomplished by active transport mechanism

D. Collecting tubules

1. Each collecting tubule receives urine from several nephrons

2. Under ADH influence, final osmotic reabsorption of most of the remaining water in urine occurs

E. Urine composition

1. Water: 1.5 L per day average

2. Urea: waste product of protein and amino acid metabolism

3. Uric acid: end product of purine metabolism or oxidation in the body

4. Creatinine: waste product of muscle metabolism

5. Ions (electrolytes): potassium, sodium, calcium, chloride

6. Hormones and their breakdown products: presence of chorionic gonadotropin is the basis for a pregnancy test

7. Vitamins: particularly the water-soluble B vitamins and C

8. Drugs secreted in the urine (e.g., aspirin, penicillin, sulfa)

9. Other molecules, in low concentrations

10. Abnormal constituents: glucose, albumin, red blood cells, calculi

F. Urine volume is controlled normally by mechanisms that regulate the amount of water reabsorbed by the kidney tubules; only under abnormal conditions does the glomerular filtration rate influence urine volume

1. ADH mechanism: neurons in the hypothalamus (mainly in the supraoptic nucleus) produce the antidiuretic hormone, and the posterior pituitary gland secretes it into the blood; ADH secretion is stimulated by two conditions, an increase in the osmotic pressure of extracellular fluid or a decrease in the volume of extracellular fluid; ADH acts on distal and collecting tubules, causing more water to osmose from the tubular filtrate back into the blood; this increased water reabsorption tends to increase the total volume of body fluid by decreasing the urine volume; ADH has both a water-retaining and an antidiuretic effect

2. Aldosterone mechanism: an increase in aldosterone secretion tends to decrease urine volume by stimulating kidney tubules to reabsorb primarily more sodium and secondarily more water; thus aldosterone tends to produce sodium retention, water retention, and a low urine volume

3. Control by the amount of solutes in tubular filtrate; in general, an increase in tubular solutes

causes decreased osmosis of water from proximal tubule back into blood and therefore an increase in urine volume (e.g., in diabetes, excess glucose in the tubular filtrate leads to increased urine volume [polyuria, diuresis])

  4. Glomerular filtration rate normally is quite constant at about 125 ml per minute; it does not vary enough to alter volume of urine produced, but in certain pathologic conditions glomerular filtration rate may change markedly and alter urine volume (e.g., in shock the glomerular filtration decreases or even ceases, causing decreased urine volume [oliguria] or urinary suppression [anuria])

G. Control of amount of blood flow through kidneys
  1. Reduced renal blood flow results in renal excretion of the hormone renin
  2. Renin chemically interacts with blood proteins, producing angiotensin II
  3. Angiotensin II causes vasoconstriction and aldosterone secretion, resulting in an increase in blood pressure and renal blood flow

Ureters

A. Location: behind the parietal peritoneum; extend from the kidneys to posterior part of the bladder floor
B. Structure: ureter expands as it enters the kidney to form the renal pelvis; subdivided into calyces, each of which contains renal papillae; ureter walls composed of smooth muscle with mucosa lining and fibrous outer coat
C. Function: collect urine secreted by the kidney cells and propel it to the bladder by peristaltic waves

Urinary Bladder

A. Location: behind symphysis pubis, below parietal peritoneum
B. Structure: collapsible bag of smooth muscle lined with mucosa arranged in rugae, three openings—two from ureters and one into the urethra
C. Functions
  1. Reservoir for urine until sufficient amount accumulated for elimination
  2. Expulsion of urine from body by way of urethra

Urethra

A. Location
  1. Female: behind the symphysis pubis, anterior to the vagina
  2. Male: extends through the prostate gland, fibrous sheet, and penis
B. Structure: musculomembranous tube lined with mucosa; opening to exterior called urinary meatus
C. Functions
  1. Female: passageway for expulsion of urine
  2. Male: passageway for expulsion of both urine and semen

REVIEW OF ANATOMY AND PHYSIOLOGY OF THE REPRODUCTIVE SYSTEM

Functions of the Male Reproductive System

A. Procreation of species
B. Contribution to development of secondary sexual characteristics
C. Pleasure

Structures of the Male Reproductive System

Glands

A. Main male sex glands (gonads) are the testes
  1. Structure: fibrous capsule covers each testis and sends partitions into interior of gland, dividing it into lobules composed of tiny tubules called seminiferous tubules, embedded in connective tissue containing interstitial cells; ducts emerge from top of gland to enter head of epididymis
  2. Location: in the scrotum, one testis in each compartment (two compartments)
  3. Functions
    a. Seminiferous tubules carry on spermatogenesis; that is, they form spermatozoa, the male sex cells, or gametes
    b. Interstitial cells secrete testosterone, the main androgen, or male hormone
  4. Structure of spermatozoon: consists of a head, middle piece, and whiplike tail that propels sperm; microscopic
B. Accessory glands
  1. Seminal vesicles
    a. Location: on posterior surface of the bladder
    b. Structure: convoluted pouches, mucous lining
    c. Function: secrete nutrient-rich fluid estimated to constitute about 30% of semen
  2. Prostate gland
    a. Location: encircles urethra just below bladder
    b. Structure: walnut-sized gland with ducts opening into urethra
    c. Function: secretes estimated 60% of semen; prostatic secretion is alkaline, which increases sperm motility; prostatic secretion contains abundance of enzyme, acid phosphatase; therefore blood level of this enzyme increases in metastasizing cancer of prostate
  3. Bulbourethral glands (Cowper's)
    a. Location: just below prostate gland
    b. Structure: small, pea-shaped structures with duct leading into urethra
    c. Function: secrete alkaline fluid that lubricates urethra prior to ejaculation

Ducts

A. Epididymis
1. Location: lies along top and side of each testis
2. Structure: each epididymis consists of single, tightly coiled tube enclosed in fibrous casing
3. Function: conducts seminal fluid (semen) from testes to vas deferens; secretes small part of semen; stores semen prior to ejaculation, sperm mature during this period

B. Vas deferens (seminal ducts)
1. Location: extend through inguinal canal into abdominal cavity, over top and down posterior surface of bladder to join ducts from seminal vesicles
2. Structure: pair of tubes or ducts
3. Function: conduct sperm and small amount of fluid from each epididymis to an ejaculatory duct
4. Clinical application: vasectomy is the surgical procedure in which a short section of each vas is cut out and its separated ends tied off; as a result, sperm cannot enter the ejaculatory ducts and be ejaculated; semen from a vasectomized male contains no sperm; hence vasectomy sterilizes a man (infertile); it does not render him impotent; it does, however, slightly decrease the amount of semen ejaculated

C. Ejaculatory ducts: formed by union of each vas with duct from seminal vesicle; pass through prostate gland to terminate in urethra; function is to ejaculate semen into urethra

D. Urethra: described under Urinary System

Supporting Structures

A. External: scrotum and penis
1. Scrotum: skin-covered pouch suspended from perineal region; divided into two compartments, each containing testis, epididymis, and first part of seminal duct; allows sperm to develop at 2° to 3° below the temperature of rest of body, which is ideal for sperm development
2. Penis: made up of three cylindric masses of erectile tissue that contain large vascular spaces; filling of these with blood causes erection of penis; two larger upper cylinders (corpora cavernosa) and one smaller lower cylinder (corpus cavernosum); the lower cylinder surrounds the urethra; glans penis: a bulging structure at distal end of the penis, over which a double fold of skin, the prepuce or foreskin, fits loosely (removed in circumcision)

B. Internal: spermatic cords are fibrous tubes located in each inguinal canal; serve as casing around each vas deferens and its accompanying blood vessels, lymphatics, and nerves

Functions of the Female Reproductive System

See Structures of the Female Reproductive System in Childbearing and Women's Health (Chapter 3) and Ovaries in Review of Anatomy and Physiology of the Endocrine System in this chapter

Structures of the Female Reproductive System

See Structures of the Female Reproductive System in Childbearing and Women's Health (Chapter 3) and Ovaries in Review of Anatomy and Physiology of the Endocrine System in this chapter

REVIEW OF PHYSICAL PRINCIPLES RELATED TO THE URINARY/REPRODUCTIVE SYSTEMS

Principles of Mechanics

Newton's Laws of Motion

EXAMPLES
1. Pumping action of the heart supplies hydrostatic force to filter blood in the glomerular capillary bed
2. Contraction of muscle is responsible for the force of propulsion of semen along and out of the male reproductive tract

Momentum

EXAMPLE: During micturition, the walls of the urinary bladder exert a force of prolonged duration that imparts great momentum to the urine being expelled from the body

Energy

EXAMPLE: Chemical energy of ATP is used to actively transport nutrients and electrolytes from glomerular filtrate into the tubular epithelium

Principles of Physical Properties of Matter

Elasticity

EXAMPLES
1. Elastic properties of the bladder permit it to hold several hundred milliliters of urine before micturition
2. Elastic properties of uterine connective tissue partly account for the tremendous increase in size of the uterus during pregnancy

Surface Area

EXAMPLE: The proximal convoluted tubules of the nephron have a brush border consisting of numerous microvilli that have a very high surface-to-volume ratio; these tiny cellular extensions greatly increase the surface area of the tubule for reabsorption of materials from the glomerular filtrate

Liquids: Pascal's principle

EXAMPLE: In conditions causing a lack of the micturition reflex, manual pressure over the bladder region will be transmitted to the urine, which results in the opening of the sphincters and the expulsion of urine from the bladder

REVIEW OF CHEMICAL PRINCIPLES RELATED TO THE URINARY/REPRODUCTIVE SYSTEMS

Urine

A. Water solution of inorganic salts and organic compounds
B. Important in excretion of wastes
C. Analysis yields information of physical condition in health and disease
D. Normal urine
   1. Amount: 800 to 1800 ml/24 hours
   2. Color: light yellow to dark brown, resulting from pigments (urobilin, urochrome, etc.)
   3. Odor: aromatic (fresh); food and drugs alter odor
   4. Sediment: varies; caused by diet and other normal changes
      a. Few blood cells
      b. Few epithelial cells
      c. Phosphates
      d. Urates
      e. Uric acid crystals
      f. Calcium oxalate
   5. Specific gravity (1.005 to 1.025) varies greatly, depending on fluid intake and the quantity of solutes dissolved in the urine; the individual having diabetes insipidus may excrete 5 to 15 L of urine daily; this urine has a very low specific gravity (close to that of pure water); a person with diabetes mellitus may excrete urine of high specific gravity caused by excessive quantities of glucose dissolved in the urine
   6. Reaction: usually acid (pH 4.5 to 7.5 is the normal range); alkaline immediately after a meal
   7. Proteins: none; protein in the urine is usually associated with a pathologic condition, although albumin traces will occasionally appear after heavy exercise or cold showers (these are of no consequence)
   8. Sugar: trace to none; the presence of urinary carbohydrate is usually indicative of a pathologic condition
   9. Ketone bodies: none; ketone bodies in the urine appear in metabolic disorders
   10. Indican: none; positive results indicate intestinal obstruction
   11. Bile: none; positive results indicate liver or gallbladder dysfunction
   12. Blood: trace to none; positive results indicate bleeding in organs of urinary system

Hormones

See Review of Anatomy and Physiology of the Endocrine System in this chapter

REVIEW OF MICROORGANISMS RELATED TO THE URINARY/REPRODUCTIVE SYSTEMS

Bacterial Pathogens

A. *Enterobacter aerogenes*: small, gram-negative bacillus (morphologically indistinguishable from *Escherichia coli*); causes urinary tract infections
B. *Haemophilus ducreyi*: morphologically indistinguishable from *H. influenzae* and *H. aegyptius*; causes the venereal ulcer called chancroid (soft chancre)
C. *Neisseria gonorrhoeae*: gram-negative diplococcus; causes gonorrhea (transmitted sexually)
D. *Pseudomonas aeruginosa*: gram-negative, motile bacillus; a common secondary invader of wounds, burns, outer ear, and urinary tract; the infection characterized by blue-green pus; may be transmitted by catheters and other hospital instruments
E. *Treponema pallidum*: long, slender, highly motile spirochete; causes syphilis (transmitted sexually)

Protozoal Pathogen

Trichomonas vaginalis, a flagellated protozoan, causes trichomonas vaginitis (transmitted sexually)

Viral Pathogens

A. Human immunodeficiency virus (HIV); causes acquired immunodeficiency syndrome (AIDS) (transmitted sexually and by blood)
B. *Herpesvirus hominis*; transmitted via genital or oral-genital route; causes herpes genitalis

PHARMACOLOGY RELATED TO URINARY SYSTEM DISORDERS

Kidney-Specific Antiinfectives

A. Description
   1. Used to treat local urinary tract infections
   2. Exert an antibacterial effect on renal tissue, including the ureters and bladder
   3. Available in oral and parenteral (IV) preparations
B. Examples
   1. Methenamines
   2. Nalidixic acid
   3. Nitrofurantoin
C. Major side effects
   1. Nausea, vomiting (irritation of gastric mucosa)
   2. Skin rash (hypersensitivity)
   3. CNS disturbances (neurotoxicity)
   4. Blood dyscrasias (decreased RBCs, WBCs, and platelet synthesis)

D. Nursing care
  1. Administer with meals to reduce GI irritation
  2. Monitor blood work, cultures, and urinary output during therapy
  3. Encourage increased fluid intake to promote drug excretion and prevent toxicity
  4. Nalidixic acid
     a. Assess for potentiation of anticoagulant effect
     b. Utilize Clinistix for urine testing, because false positives are obtained with Clinitest tablets, Fehling's, and Benedict's solutions
  5. Nitrofurantoin
     a. Dilute oral suspensions in milk or juice to prevent staining of teeth
     b. Instruct client that the urine will appear brown in color
  6. Evaluate client's response to medication and understanding of teaching

Sulfonamides

See Pharmacologic Control of Infection in this chapter

Urinary Spasmolytics

A. Description
  1. Used for symptomatic relief of incontinence
  2. Directly affects the smooth muscle of the urinary tract
B. Examples
  1. Flavoxate HCl (Urispas)
  2. Oxybutynin Cl (Ditropan)
C. Major side effects
  1. Tachycardia, palpitations
  2. Dry mouth
  3. Constipation
  4. Drowsiness
  5. Blurred vision
  6. Urinary retention
D. Nursing care
  1. Do not administer if GI obstruction is present
  2. Administer cautiously to clients with glaucoma
  3. Advise client to avoid driving and other hazardous activities
  4. Monitor urinary output
  5. Evaluate client's response to medication and understanding of teaching

Androgens

A. Description
  1. Hormones that aid in the development of secondary sex characteristics in men and have anabolic properties, which stimulate the building and repair of body tissue
  2. Used in debilitating conditions, inoperable breast cancer, and to restore hormone levels in males; also effective for treatment of fibrocystic breast disease, dysmenorrhea, and severe postpartum breast engorgement in nonnursing mothers
  3. Available in oral, parenteral (IM, SC), and buccal preparations
B. Examples
  1. Danazol (Cyclomen)
  2. Ethylestrenol
  3. Fluoxymesterone
  4. Nandrolone phenpropionate
  5. Norethandrolone
  6. Testosterone preparations
C. Major side effects
  1. Weight gain, edema (sodium and water retention)
  2. Acne (androgen effect)
  3. Changes in libido (androgen effect)
  4. Hoarseness, deep voice (virilism—androgen effect)
  5. Nausea, vomiting (irritation of gastric mucosa; hypercalcemia)
D. Nursing care
  1. Assess for signs of virilization in females
  2. Encourage a diet high in calories and proteins to aid in building body tissues
  3. Encourage clients to restrict sodium intake to control edema
  4. Administer with meals to reduce GI irritation
  5. Monitor blood pressure during course of therapy
  6. Assess for potentiation of anticoagulant effect
  7. Evaluate client's response to medication and understanding of teaching

Estrogens

See Pharmacology Related to Female Reproductive System Disorders in Childbearing and Women's Health (Chapter 3)

Progestins

See Pharmacology Related to Female Reproductive System Disorders in Childbearing and Women's Health (Chapter 3)

PROCEDURES RELATED TO THE URINARY SYSTEM

Common Urine Tests

A. Definition
  1. Urinalysis: microscopic examination of urine for cells, as well as chemical study for pH and specific gravity
  2. Culture and sensitivity tests of urine: microscopic examination of urine for bacterial growth and determination of antibiotic appropriate to control growth

3. Specific gravity: estimation of the concentration of urine relative to water; reflects concentrating ability of the kidneys; normal value of 1.005 to 1.025 depends on fluid intake and loss

B. Nursing care
1. Explain procedure to the client
2. Obtain container for the specimen
   a. For urinalysis a urine container is used
   b. For culture and sensitivity a sterile specimen container is used
3. For urinalysis obtain a freshly voided specimen and place in the container
4. For culture and sensitivity obtain a clean-catch or midstream specimen
   a. Cleanse the outer urinary meatus with a bacteriostatic solution
   b. Instruct the client to void a small amount into a bedpan, urinal, or toilet, and then to stop the stream
   c. Instruct the client to continue voiding into a container without contaminating the lid or inside of the container
   d. Seal the container
5. Send the specimen to the laboratory with label indicating contents, client's name, and date
6. For specific gravity
   a. Obtain freshly voided specimen
   b. Fill specific gravity container one-half to two-thirds full with urine
   c. Place hydrometer (urinometer) in urine and spin gently
   d. Read scale at level of meniscus
7. Evaluate client's response to procedure

Cystoscopy

A. Definition
1. The visualization of the bladder wall through a tube with a fiberoptic end
2. Indicated as a diagnostic measure or as a means to enter the bladder for therapy
B. Nursing care
1. Obtain an informed consent
2. Maintain the client NPO before the procedure (which may be done with or without general anesthesia)
3. Provide care following the procedure
   a. Maintain the client in a comfortable state
   b. Observe the client's urine for blood and clots
   c. Ascertain that the client has voided through observation and palpation of the bladder
4. Evaluate client's response to procedure

Intravenous Pyelogram (IVP)

A. Definition: x-ray examination of the kidneys, ureters, and bladder after the injection of a contrast medium into an antecubital vein

B. Nursing care
1. Explain procedure to the client
2. Obtain an informed consent
3. Administer a cathartic as ordered the evening before the test to remove feces and flatus
4. Provide a light supper before the procedure and maintain the client NPO for 6 to 8 hours prior to the test
5. Evaluate client's response to procedure

Urinary (Retention) Catheter Care

A. Definition: special care to the urinary meatus and catheter to reduce the likelihood of infection
B. Nursing care
1. Explain procedure to the client
2. Provide privacy
3. Gather equipment, wash hands, and don gloves
4. Perform catheter care at least twice daily
5. Wash the genital area well with soap and warm water and dry; uncircumcised males should have foreskin retracted to remove sebaceous secretions
6. Use soap and water to wash encrustations from catheter (may harbor microorganisms)
7. Check drainage tubing at frequent intervals to assess for kinks or clogs
8. Fasten catheter to the client's thigh to prevent tension
9. Keep the drainage bag below bladder level without loops or kinks to ensure gravity drainage
10. Use a syringe to remove urine if a specimen is needed; use the port site and surgical aseptic technique
11. Empty the drainage bag at least every 8 hours and record the amount, odor, color, and consistency
12. Change the drainage bag and catheter according to institutional policy
13. Evaluate client's response to procedure

Urinary Catheterization

A. Definitions
1. Sterile introduction of a catheter through the urethra to the bladder for the purpose of urine collection
2. Intermittent catheterization is performed with a one-lumen catheter, which is removed after the bladder is drained (clients with neurogenic bladder dysfunction may be taught this procedure)
3. Retention catheterization involves use of a catheter with an inflatable balloon around its tip to hold it in place in the bladder (Foley catheter); once inserted, it is attached to a collecting bag, and thus the bladder is continually emptied by gravity

4. Catheterization for residual urine involves the use of a straight catheter that is inserted after a client voids; the bladder should normally be empty at this time

B. Nursing care
1. Explain procedure to the client
2. Provide privacy
3. Obtain equipment, including a bright light
4. Position the female client supine with the knees flexed and abducted and the male client supine with the knees slightly abducted
5. Wash hands, open catheterization tray, and put on sterile gloves
6. Place the sterile fenestrated drape over the external genitalia, exposing the meatus
7. Lubricate tip of the catheter and leave catheter on the sterile tray
8. Saturate cotton pledgets with a suitable cleaning solution
9. Cleanse the urinary meatus
   a. For female clients separate the labia minora with thumb and forefinger and cleanse from anterior to posterior using one pledget for each stroke (keep labia separated)
   b. For male clients hold the penis between thumb and forefinger and cleanse from meatus to shaft using one pledget for each stroke (retract foreskin during this procedure)
10. Insert lubricated catheter into the bladder
    a. For female clients insert approximately 7.5 cm or slightly past the point at which urine returns
    b. For male clients, hold the penis perpendicular to the body and insert catheter 17 to 25 cm or slightly past the point at which urine returns
11. Drain urine slowly
    a. Intermittent catheterization: remove catheter when bladder is empty
    b. Retention catheterization: inflate the balloon with sterile solution after the bladder is emptied and the catheter is attached to a sterile closed collection system (to reduce chance of infection)
12. Assist the client to a comfortable position, remove equipment, and record data on appropriate records
13. Evaluate client's response to procedure

Mammography

See Procedures Related to the Female Reproductive System in Childbearing and Women's Health (Chapter 3)

Breast Biopsy

See Procedures Related to the Female Reproductive System in Childbearing and Women's Health (Chapter 3)

Infertility and Sterility Testing

See Diagnostic Measures Associated with Infertility and Sterility in Childbearing and Women's Health (Chapter 3)

GENERAL NURSING DIAGNOSES FOR CLIENTS WITH URINARY/ REPRODUCTIVE SYSTEMS DISORDERS

A. Anxiety related to reduced urine output
B. Body image disturbance related to:
   1. Dependency on technology
   2. Alterations in structure
   3. Loss of function
C. Constipation related to pressure on colon
D. Fluid volume excess related to inability to secrete urine
E. Anticipatory grieving related to:
   1. Loss of independence
   2. Concerns about dying
   3. Loss of body part
   4. Infertility
F. Incontinence (functional, reflex, stress, total, urge) related to disease process
G. Risk for infection related to:
   1. Altered immune response
   2. Knowledge deficit
H. Knowledge deficit related to prevention/treatment protocols
I. Altered nutrition: less than body requirements related to anorexia
J. Pain related to:
   1. Inflammation
   2. Obstruction of urine
   3. Pressure
K. Impaired physical mobility related to:
   1. Pain
   2. Inflammation
L. Altered role performance related to:
   1. Interference with sexual functioning
   2. Chronic debilitation
M. Self-esteem disturbance related to chronic debilitation
N. Sensory-perceptual alteration related to chemical toxins
O. Sexual dysfunction related to:
   1. Altered body image
   2. Inadequate tissue perfusion
   3. Surgery
   4. Imposed restrictions
P. Altered sexuality patterns related to:
   1. Fear of transmission of infection
   2. Loss of function
Q. Impaired skin integrity related to:
   1. Presence of irritants
   2. Presence of lesions

R. Social isolation related to social stigma

S. Altered thought processes related to chemical toxins

T Altered urinary elimination related to:
1. Microbiologic irritants
2. Physical obstruction
3. Trauma

U. Urinary retention related to physical obstruction

MAJOR DISORDERS OF THE URINARY/REPRODUCTIVE SYSTEMS

See Childbearing and Women's Health (Chapter 3) for additional disorders of the urinary/reproductive systems in women

▼ CYSTITIS

Data Base

A. Etiology and pathophysiology
1. Inflammation of the bladder wall usually caused by an ascending bacterial infection (*Escherichia coli* most common)
2. More common in females due to:
   a. Shorter urethra
   b. Childbirth
   c. Anatomic proximity of the urethra to the rectum

B. Clinical findings
1. Subjective
   a. Urgency, frequency, burning, and pain on urination
   b. Nocturia
   c. Bearing down on urination
2. Objective
   a. Pyuria and hematuria
   b. Bacterial growth evident on culture of urine

C. Therapeutic interventions
1. Chemotherapeutic and antibiotic agents such as sulfonamides, penicillin, tetracycline
2. Antispasmodics to soothe the irritable bladder such as flavoxate (Urispas, oxybutynin (Ditropan)
3. Urinary antiseptics such as nitrofurantoin, trimethoprim
4. Diet directed toward altering the properties of urine (e.g., cranberry juice)
5. Intake of additional fluids to dilute the urine
6. Sitz baths to provide comfort

Nursing Care of Clients with Cystitis

A. DATA COLLECTION
1. History to obtain baseline data
2. Urine for color, clarity, odor, blood, or mucus
3. Lower abdomen for bladder distention
4. In males, rectal examination for prostate tenderness or enlargement

B. ANALYSIS AND INTERPRETATION
Refer to General Nursing Diagnoses for Clients with Urinary/Reproductive System Disorders for the following diagnoses: H, J 1, and T 1

C. PLANNING/IMPLEMENTATION
1. Teach the client to seek medical attention at the first sign of symptoms
2. Teach the client to take medications as directed
3. Encourage the client to drink additional fluids
4. Promote physical comfort
5. Teach the client preventive measures such as perineal care, avoiding tub baths, voiding after intercourse, and wearing cotton underwear

D. EVALUATION/OUTCOMES
1. Expresses relief of pain on urination
2. Resumes normal urinary patterns
3. Describes methods to prevent recurrence of infection

▼ UROLITHIASIS AND NEPHROLITHIASIS

Data Base

A. Etiology and pathophysiology: formation of stones in the urinary tract; stones may be composed of calcium phosphate, uric acid, or oxalate; they tend to recur and may cause obstruction, infection, and/or hydronephrosis

B. Clinical findings
1. Subjective
   a. Severe pain in kidney area radiating down the flank to the pubic area (renal colic)
   b. Frequency and urgency of urination
   c. History of prior or associated health problems (e.g., gout, parathyroidism, immobility, dehydration, urinary tract infections)
   d. Nausea
2. Objective
   a. Diaphoresis, pallor, nausea, vomiting
   b. Hematuria; pyuria may occur if infection is present

C. Therapeutic interventions
1. Narcotics for pain
2. Antispasmodics to reduce the renal colic
3. Allopurinal or sulfinpyrazone to reduce uric acid excretion
4. Antibiotics to reduce infection
5. Monitor intake and output; strain urine
6. Diet therapy
   a. Large fluid intake to produce dilute urine
   b. Diet altered according to type of stone

(1) Calcium stones: low-calcium diet of about 400 mg daily, achieved mainly by eliminating dairy products; if phosphate involvement, limit high-phosphorus foods—dairy products, meat; if oxalate involvement, avoid oxalate-rich foods—tea, almonds, cashews, chocolate, cocoa, beans, spinach, and rhubarb; since calcium stones have an alkaline chemistry, an acid ash diet can be used to create an acidic urinary tract, which is less conducive to their formation; stress whole grains, eggs, and cranberry juice, and limit milk, vegetables, and fruit

(2) Uric acid stones: low purine (uric acid is a metabolic product of purines in the body), controlling purine foods such as meat, especially organ meats, meat extractives, and to a lesser extent plant sources (e.g., whole grains and legumes); alkaline ash, since the stone composition is acid

(3) Cystine stones (rare): low methionine, since methionine is the essential amino acid from which the nonessential amino acid cystine is formed; controlling protein foods such as meat, milk, eggs, cheese; alkaline ash, since the stone is an acid composition

7. Surgical intervention if stone is not passed or complications are present (e.g., nephrolithotomy, ureterolithotomy, cystotomy)
8. Percutaneous ultrasonic lithotripsy (PUL)
    a. Nephroscope is inserted through skin into kidney
    b. Ultrasonic waves disintegrate stones
    c. Stone fragments are removed by suction and irrigation
    d. Less traumatic alternative to conventional surgery
9. Extracorporeal shock-wave lithotripsy (ESWL): Client is immersed in water and exposed to shock waves that disintegrate stones so that they can be passed with urine; procedure is noninvasive

Nursing Care of Clients with Urolithiasis and Nephrolithiasis

A. DATA COLLECTION
1. History of causative factors and progression of symptoms
2. Vital signs, particularly temperature for baseline data
3. Urine for color, clarity, pH, and odor
4. Intake and output
5. Urine for presence of stones (strain all urine)

B. ANALYSIS AND INTERPRETATION
Refer to General Nursing Diagnoses for Clients with Urinary/Reproductive System Disorders for the following diagnoses: H, J 3, and U

C. PLANNING/IMPLEMENTATION
1. Administer analgesics as ordered
2. Permit the client to set own pattern of activity
3. Plan care to provide the client with periods of undisturbed rest
4. Encourage fluid intake of 3000 to 4000 ml daily
5. Administer antibiotics as ordered to prevent infection
6. Encourage the client to accept medication for pain
7. Provide as much privacy as possible
8. Encourage client to remain on diet; those on calcium-restricted diets will need daily riboflavin supplements; those on an acid ash diet will need daily supplementation of vitamins C and A and folic acid
9. Teach the client to read labels on food preparations for the presence of contraindicated additives such as calcium or phosphate
10. Whenever possible, encourage daily weight-bearing exercise to prevent hypercalciuria caused by release of calcium from the bones
11. Provide care following a nephrolithotomy or percutaneous ultrasonic lithotripsy
    a. Change dressings frequently during the first 24 hours after a nephrolithotomy
    b. Maintain patency of ureteral catheter as well as urethral catheter to prevent hydronephrosis
    c. Encourage use of incentive spirometry and coughing and deep breathing to prevent atelectasis

D. EVALUATION/OUTCOMES
1. Expresses relief of pain
2. Establishes normal urine flow
3. Describes strategies for prevention of stone formation

▼ HYDRONEPHROSIS

Data Base
A. Etiology and pathophysiology
1. Obstruction at any point in the urinary system leading to pressure that can damage renal tissue
2. Caused by tumors, trauma, calculi, polycystic disease, congenital abnormalities, lymph enlargement, or nephrotosis (floating kidney)
B. Clinical findings
1. Subjective
    a. Pain, local tenderness

b. Dull pain in flank region or colicky pain
2. Objective
   a. Nausea and vomiting
   b. Nocturia
C. Therapeutic interventions
   1. Treat the underlying cause
   2. Promote urinary drainage with a catheter
   3. Urinary antiseptics
   4. Antispasmodics for colicky spasm

Nursing Care of Clients with Hydronephrosis

A. DATA COLLECTION
   1. Flank areas for asymmetry
   2. Abdomen for bladder distention
   3. Urinary leakage associated with application of gentle pressure over bladder

B. ANALYSIS AND INTERPRETATION
   Refer to General Nursing Diagnoses for Clients with Urinary/Reproductive System Disorders for the following diagnoses: A, J 2, and U

C. PLANNING/IMPLEMENTATION
   1. Observe for signs of uremia
   2. Medicate as ordered
   3. Maintain patency of drainage tubes

D. EVALUATION/OUTCOMES
   1. Establishes normal urine flow
   2. Describes reduction of pain

▼ ACUTE RENAL FAILURE

Data Base

A. Etiology and pathophysiology
   1. Usually follows direct trauma to the kidneys or overwhelming physiologic stress (e.g., burns, septicemia, nephrotoxic drugs and chemicals, hemolytic blood transfusion reaction, severe shock, renal vascular occlusion) that decreases blood flow to the glomeruli or to the nephrons
   2. Sudden and almost complete loss of glomerular and/or tubular function
   3. Acute renal failure may result in death from acidosis, potassium intoxication, pulmonary edema, or infection
   4. May progress from the anuric or oliguric phase through the diuretic phase to the convalescent phase (which can take 6 to 12 months) to recovery of function
   5. May progress to chronic renal failure; chronic renal failure may develop as a separate entity and does not have to be a sequela of acute failure
B. Clinical findings
   1. Subjective
      a. Lethargy and drowsiness that can progress from stupor to coma
      b. Irritability and headache
      c. Circumoral numbness
      d. Tingling extremities
      e. Anorexia
   2. Objective
      a. Sudden dramatic drop in urinary output appearing a few hours after the causative event
      b. Oliguria: urinary output less than 400 ml but more than 100 ml/24 hours; anuria: urinary output less than 100 ml/24 hours
      c. Restlessness, twitching, convulsions
      d. Nausea and vomiting
      e. Skin pallor, anemia, and increased bleeding time, which can progress to epistaxis and internal hemorrhage
      f. Ammonia (urine) odor to breath and perspiration, which can progress to uremic frost on skin and pruritus
      g. Generalized edema, hypervolemia, hypertension, and increased venous pressure, which can progress to pulmonary edema and congestive heart failure
      h. In addition, respirations are deep and rapid as a compensatory response to the developing metabolic acidosis
      i. Elevated serum levels of
         (1) BUN
         (2) Creatinine
         (3) Potassium
      j. Decreased serum levels of:
         (1) Calcium
         (2) Sodium
         (3) pH
         (4) Carbon dioxide combining power
      k. Anemia
      l. Albumin in urine
      m. Decreased specific gravity
C. Therapeutic interventions
   1. Direct treatment toward correcting the underlying cause of renal failure (e.g., treat shock, eliminate drugs and toxins, treat transfusion reactions, restore integrity of urinary tract)
   2. Maintain client on complete bed rest
   3. Diet therapy
      a. Protein low to moderate according to tolerance: 30 to 50 g
      b. Carbohydrate relatively high for energy: 300 to 400 g
      c. Fat relatively moderate: 70 to 90 g
      d. Calories adequate for maintenance and to prevent tissue breakdown: 2000 to 2500 daily
      e. Sodium controlled according to serum levels and excretion tolerance: varying from 400 to 2000 mg daily

f. Potassium controlled according to serum levels and excretion capacities: varying from 1300 to 1900 mg

g. Water controlled according to excretion: about 800 to 1000 ml; careful intake and output records vital

h. Calcium intake of 1000 mg/day is needed to prevent or delay progression of renal osteodystrophy, or demineralization of bone, which can result from chronic acidosis and altered vitamin A metabolism; because of dietary restrictions, supplementation may be prescribed; calcium supplements, however, should not be given unless serum phosphate is under control because of risk of precipitation of calcium phosphate in the kidney

i. Phosphorus intakes of less than 600 mg/day have been shown to delay progression of renal insufficiency; this level is usually achieved by restricting milk intake to 1 cup or less per day, avoiding soft drinks and beer, and restriction of meats, poultry, fish, eggs, and cereal grain products

j. Renal diet is low in water-soluble vitamins, iron, and zinc, necessitating daily supplements; dialyzed clients will need daily supplements of vitamins B_6 (5 to 10 mg), C (70 to 100 mg), and folic acid (1 mg) administered following dialysis

k. Total parenteral nutrition (TPN) and parenteral intralipid therapy may be used

4. Frequent monitoring of vital signs and intake and output

5. Packed cells, electrolytes, and glucose IV as necessary

6. Exchange resins to decrease serum potassium

7. Antibiotics to reduce possibility of infection

8. Peritoneal dialysis or hemodialysis

9. Surgical intervention if kidney transplant is a viable alternative

Nursing Care of Clients with Acute Renal Failure

A. DATA COLLECTION

1. Daily weight
2. Signs of hyperkalemia and hyponatremia
3. History of clinical symptoms and potential causative factors

B. ANALYSIS AND INTERPRETATION

Refer to General Nursing Diagnoses for Clients with Urinary/Reproductive System Disorders for the following diagnoses: A, B 1, B 3, D, H, I, N, and S

C. PLANNING/IMPLEMENTATION

1. Monitor intake and output at frequent intervals
2. Limit fluid intake as ordered

3. Observe for signs of overhydration (e.g., dependent, pitting, sacral, or periorbital edema; crackles or dyspnea; headache, distended neck veins, and hypertension)

4. Continue to monitor for hyperkalemia and hyponatremia

5. Administer electrolytes as ordered

6. Provide periods of undisturbed rest to conserve energy and oxygen

7. Protect client from injury caused by bleeding tendency, the possibility of convulsions, and a clouded sensorium

8. Protect client from cross-infection

9. Observe for early signs and symptoms of complications (e.g., hemorrhage, convulsions, cardiac problems, pulmonary edema)

10. Provide special skin care frequently to prevent breakdown and remove uremic frost

11. Monitor vital signs and physical status at frequent intervals; record and report any deviations immediately

12. Administer antibiotics as ordered

13. Encourage intake of diet as ordered and record amount consumed

14. Allow the client as much choice as possible in the selection of food while recognizing that little variation is possible

15. Provide mouth care before, after, and between meals

16. Administer dietary and electrolyte supplements as ordered

17. Administer antiemetics to control nausea and sodium-free antacids to reduce GI irritation

D. EVALUATION/OUTCOMES

1. Maintains adequate dietary intake
2. Remains free of infection
3. Remains free from injury
4. Describes treatment protocols and plans for compliance
5. Maintains fluid and electrolyte balance within acceptable limits

▼ CHRONIC RENAL FAILURE

Data Base

A. Etiology and pathophysiology
   1. Chronic renal failure can occur as the result of chronic kidney infections, developmental abnormalities, vascular disorders, and destruction of kidney tubules
   2. The ongoing deterioration in renal function results in uremia

B. Clinical findings
   1. Subjective
      a. Lethargy or drowsiness

b. Headache

c. Nausea

d. Pruritis

2. Objective

a. Vomiting

b. Mental clouding

c. Anemia (decreased red blood cells, hemoglobin and hematocrit)

d. Decreased serum pH (metabolic acidosis)

e. Hypertension

f. Increased serum phosphate, decreased serum calcium

g. Renal osteodystrophy

h. Kussmaul respirations

i. Uremic frost (powdery substance on the skin from urate wastes)

j. Convulsions, coma, death

C. Therapeutic interventions

1. Fluid and salt restrictions

2. Antihypertensive medications

3. Recombinant human erythropoietin to manage the anemia

4. Peritoneal dialysis: warmed dialyzing solution is introduced via a catheter inserted in the peritoneal cavity; the peritoneal membrane is used as a dialyzing membrane to remove toxic substances, metabolic wastes, and excess fluid

a. Intermittent: involves 6 to 48 hours several times a week

b. Continuous ambulatory peritoneal dialysis (CAPD): involves approximately four exchanges a day, 7 days a week, and can be administered by the client at home

5. Hemodialysis: the client is attached (via a surgically created arteriovenous fistula or graft) directly to a machine that pumps the blood along a semipermeable membrane; dialyzing solution is on the other side of the membrane, and osmosis and/or diffusion of wastes, toxins, and fluid from the client occurs

6. Continuous arteriovenous hemofiltration (CAVH); hemofiltration of micromolecules is based on the principle of convection, which is that some elements in plasma water are conveyed across a semipermeable membrane as a result of differences in hydrostatic pressure in the system; can use previously established fistulas or externally placed access points without the need for external pumps or dialysis machines; the client's blood pressure is the driving force

7. Diet management

a. General protein and electrolyte control

b. The low-protein, essential-amino-acid diet (modified Giordano-Giovannetti regimen) to sustain clients with uremia and alleviate their difficult symptoms

(1) Very low protein (20 g); minimal essential amino acids

(2) Controlled potassium (1500 mg); feed only essential amino acids, causing the body to use its own excess urea nitrogen to synthesize the nonessential amino acids needed for tissue protein production; foods used include 1 egg, 6 oz milk, low-protein bread, 2 to 4 fruits, and 2 to 4 vegetables from special lists to control protein and potassium

c. See Acute Renal Failure for additional diet therapy information

8. Kidney transplant from donor with compatible ABO and HLA antigens

Nursing Care of Clients with Chronic Renal Failure

A. DATA COLLECTION

1. Detailed history of signs, symptoms, and causative factors

2. Data related to urinary elimination patterns

3. Neurologic status including attention span, weakness, and neuropathies

4. Client's breath for an ammonia odor

5. Oral cavity for stomatitis

6. Urine for consistency, odor, and amount

7. Skin for urochromatic pigmentation (bronze pigmentation of the skin)

B. ANALYSIS AND INTERPRETATION

Refer to General Nursing Diagnoses for Clients with Urinary/Reproductive System Disorders for the following diagnoses: A, B 1, B 3, D, E 2, H, J 1, J 2, L 1, M, N, P 2, and Q 1

C. PLANNING/IMPLEMENTATION

1. Monitor intake and output

2. Provide skin care as needed

3. Monitor vital signs

4. Provide care for the client undergoing dialysis

a. Explain the procedure and answer questions related to it

b. Take vital signs and weigh the client before the procedure is begun

c. Use surgical asepsis in preparation of the site (abdomen or area of fistula)

d. Assure the client that a staff member will be available at all times

e. If an abdominal catheter is not in place for peritoneal dialysis, have the client void before procedure is started

f. Once the procedure is instituted by the physician, monitor the client's response and add dialysate as prescribed

g. Take vital signs every 15 minutes; assess for hypotension

h. During peritoneal dialysis keep an accurate flow chart and monitor for signs of peritonitis

i. During hemodialysis watch the site for clotting; check clotting time and administer heparin as prescribed by the physician; monitor for patency of an internal fistula between treatments by palpating for a thrill and auscultating for a bruit

j. During both procedures check tubes for patency

k. Since both procedures are long, provide back care to promote comfort and diversional activities to help pass the time

l. Encourage client and family to seek nutritional counseling; stress importance of lifelong dietary modifications

D. EVALUATION/OUTCOMES

1. Maintains fluid and electrolyte balance within acceptable limits
2. Follows diet/fluid restrictions
3. Discusses plans for long-term treatment program
4. Verbalizes feelings related to altered functioning and potential prognosis
5. Remains free from infection
6. Remains free from injury

▼ KIDNEY TRANSPLANTATION

Data Base

A. Etiology and pathophysiology
  1. Clients with chronic renal failure who have no kidney function are candidates for transplantation
  2. Human leukocyte antigen (HLA) tests are done to decrease risk of rejection; least risk of rejection of the new kidney occurs if donor and recipient are identical twins
  3. At the time of surgery, the client's own kidney is not removed unless it is infected or enlarged
  4. New kidney is placed generally in the iliac fossa retroperitoneally, and the donor's ureter is attached to the bladder to prevent reflux of urine

B. Clinical findings
  See Clinical findings under Chronic Renal Failure

C. Therapeutic interventions
  1. Human leukocyte antigen studies
  2. Tissue typing
  3. Blood typing
  4. Surgical replacement of kidney

Nursing Care of Clients Undergoing Kidney Transplantation

A. DATA COLLECTION
  1. Complete body assessment

2. Emotional status of client and support group

B. ANALYSIS AND INTERPRETATION
Refer to General Nursing Diagnoses for Clients with Urinary/Reproductive System Disorders for the following diagnoses: A, E 2, G 1, H, J 1, and K

C. PLANNING/IMPLEMENTATION

1. Preoperative nursing care
  a. Prepare the client and family emotionally for the possible outcomes of surgery
  b. Explain that, postoperatively, immunosuppressive drugs and dialysis may be indicated, as well as isolation to prevent infection
  c. Explain routine preoperative and postoperative procedures

2. Postoperative nursing care
  a. Maintain patency of the drainage tubes, including the Foley catheter; gross hematuria or clots are not expected postoperatively
  b. Monitor fluid and electrolyte balance carefully; initial output increased because of sodium diuresis; sharp decrease may signal rejection
  c. Monitor vital signs, weight, and temperature
  d. Observe for and teach the client signs of rejection
    (1) Increased serum creatinine
    (2) Decreasing urinary output
    (3) Malaise
    (4) Fever
    (5) Flank pain or tenderness
  e. Administer steroids and immunosuppressives, such as azathioprine (Imuran) and cyclosporine, as ordered to prevent rejection
  f. Teach the client the need for lifelong immunosuppressive therapy
  g. Observe client for signs of opportunistic infections such as candidiasis, cytomegalovirus, virus, and *Pneumocystis carinii* pneumonia
  h. Emphasize need to prevent infection by avoiding crowds and utilizing aseptic techniques

D. EVALUATION/OUTCOMES

1. Verbalizes decrease in incisional pain
2. Maintains appropriate dietary intake
3. Maintains adequate urinary output
4. Discusses concerns about prognosis
5. Remains free from infection
6. Describes signs and symptoms of rejection
7. Continues medical supervision

▼ ADENOCARCINOMA OF THE KIDNEY

Data Base

A. Etiology and pathophysiology

1. Most common cancer affecting the kidneys
2. Common sites of metastasis include lungs, liver, and long bones
3. Incidence higher in males

B. Clinical findings
1. Subjective
   a. There may be none until metastasis
   b. Dull back pain
   c. Weakness
2. Objective
   a. Painless hematuria
   b. Enlarged kidney palpable during physical examination
   c. Elevated temperature
   d. Weight loss
   e. Anemia

C. Therapeutic interventions
1. Nephrectomy
2. Radiation therapy if tumor is sensitive
3. Chemotherapy
4. Hormonal therapy with medroxyprogesterone (Provera)

Nursing Care of Clients with Adenocarcinoma of the Kidney

A. DATA COLLECTION
1. History of signs and symptoms including presence of hematuria
2. Flank regions for asymmetry
3. History of pain

B. ANALYSIS AND INTERPRETATION
Refer to General Nursing Diagnoses for Clients with Urinary/Reproductive System Disorders for the following diagnoses: A, E 2, E 3, J 1, and J 3

C. PLANNING/IMPLEMENTATION
1. Monitor intake and output
2. Increase oral fluid intake
3. Administer analgesics as ordered to alleviate postoperative pain
4. Encourage coughing and deep breathing while splinting the incision
5. Examine dressing and linen under the client for drainage; a small amount of serosanguinous drainage is expected
6. Maintain integrity of the urinary drainage system; avoid kinking of tubes
7. Observe urine for color, amount, and any abnormal components
8. Support natural defense mechanisms of client; encourage intake of foods rich in the immune-stimulating nutrients, especially vitamins A, C, and E, and the mineral selenium

D. EVALUATION/OUTCOMES
1. Expresses reduction in pain
2. Discusses feelings related to prognosis
3. Maintains adequate urine output

▼ GLOMERULONEPHRITIS

Data Base
A. Etiology and pathophysiology
1. Involves damage to both kidneys resulting from filtration and trapping of antibody-antigen complexes within the glomeruli
2. As a result, inflammatory and degenerative changes affect all renal tissue
3. Often follows some form of streptococcal infection such as tonsillitis
4. May be acute or chronic in nature; decreases life expectancy if progressive renal damage occurs
5. Complications include hypertensive encephalopathy, heart failure, and infection

B. Clinical findings
1. Subjective
   a. Flank pain, costovertebral tenderness
   b. Headache
   c. Malaise
   d. Dyspnea due to salt and fluid retention
   e. Weakness
   f. Visual disturbances
2. Objective
   a. Hematuria
   b. Periorbital and facial edema
   c. Oliguria
   d. Fever
   e. Tachycardia
   f. Urinalysis reveals protein and casts
   g. Elevated plasma BUN and creatinine
   h. Anemia

C. Therapeutic interventions
1. Antibiotics such as penicillin to treat underlying infection
2. Dietary restriction of sodium, fluids, and protein based on clinical status
3. Diuretics and antihypertensives to control blood pressure

Nursing Care of Clients with Glomerulonephritis

A. DATA COLLECTION
1. History of recent upper respiratory or skin infections or invasive procedures
2. Blood pressure for baseline data
3. Urine for color
4. History of dyspnea and edema
5. Neck veins for engorgement

B. ANALYSIS AND INTERPRETATION
Refer to General Nursing Diagnoses for Clients with Urinary/Reproductive System Disorders for the following diagnoses: A, H, and I

C. PLANNING/IMPLEMENTATION
1. Monitor intake and output

2. Assess specific gravity of urine
3. Weigh the client daily
4. Monitor vital signs and temperature
5. Special prophylactic skin care (these clients are prone to skin breakdown)
6. Protect the client from infection
7. Observe for complications such as renal failure, cardiac failure, and hypertensive encephalopathy
8. Evaluate laboratory results (BUN, creatinine, urinalysis)
9. Encourage continued medical supervision
10. Refer to social service as needed; the long-term nature of the illness may create economic problems for the family

D. EVALUATION/OUTCOMES
1. Complies with medical regimen, particularly dietary and fluid restrictions
2. Stabilizes fluid volume to within acceptable limits
3. Maintains adequate nutritional status
4. Identifies signs of complications

▼ BLADDER TUMORS

Data Base

A. Etiology and pathophysiology
1. Occur most frequently in men over 50 years of age
2. Smoking, exposure to radiation, schistosomiasis, and exposure over prolonged periods to certain chemicals increase the risk of development of tumor
3. Common sites of metastasis include lymph nodes, bone, liver, and lungs
B. Clinical findings
1. Subjective
a. Frequency and urgency of urination
b. Dysuria
2. Objective
a. Direct visualization by cystoscopic examination
b. Painless hematuria
C. Therapeutic interventions
1. Surgical intervention
a. Resection of tumor
b. Cystectomy (removal of the bladder); requires urinary diversion
(1) Ureterosigmoidostomy: ureters are attached to the sigmoid colon, and urine is excreted through the rectum; these clients have constant drainage and are usually troubled by recurrent infection of the urinary tract

(2) Ileal conduit: section of the ileum is resected and attached to the ureters; one end of this ileal segment is sutured closed and the other is brought to the skin as an ileostomy to drain urine; technique most widely used to divert urine
(3) Continent ileal urinary reservoir (Koch's pouch): similar to an ileal conduit, but involves the surgical creation of a nipplelike valve that can be drained by insertion of a catheter
(4) Nephrostomy: catheter is inserted into the kidney through an incision
(5) Ureterostomy: ureters are implanted in the abdominal wall to drain urine
2. Radiation therapy
3. Chemotherapy

Nursing Care of Clients with Bladder Tumors

A. DATA COLLECTION
1. History of signs and symptoms and causative factors
2. Abdomen for signs of bladder distention
3. Urine for hematuria
B. ANALYSIS AND INTERPRETATION
Refer to General Nursing Diagnoses for Clients with Urinary/Reproductive System Disorders for the following diagnoses: B 2, E 3, G 2, H, J 1, and Q1
C. PLANNING/IMPLEMENTATION
1. Allow time for the client to verbalize fears of surgery, cancer, death, and body-image alterations
2. Preoperatively, in addition to routine care and explanations, prepare the bowel by cleansing with laxatives, antibiotics, and enemas as ordered
3. Assess the color and amount of urine frequently; maintain patency of drainage system
4. Care for the client following a ureterosigmoidostomy
a. Monitor the drainage tube, which may be in the rectum for several days
b. After the tube in the rectum is removed, encourage the client to void frequently via the rectum to prevent complications such as reflux and absorption of urine through the intestinal wall
5. Care for the client with an ileal conduit
a. Maintain the urinary drainage bag, which will be cemented around the stoma to collect urine
b. After equipment is collected, remove the collection bag; use water or a commercial solvent to loosen the adhesive

c. Hold a rolled gauze pad against the stoma to absorb urine during the procedure

d. Cleanse the skin around the stoma and under the drainage bag with soap and water; inspect for excoriation

e. After the skin is dry, apply skin adhesive to the area around the stoma and to the appliance

f. Place the appliance over the stoma and secure in place by an adjustable belt

g. Encourage self-care; teach the client to change the appliance by using a mirror

6. Care for the client with a continent ileal urinary reservoir (Koch pouch): teach client to insert catheter through nipple valve to drain urine at prescribed times, thus preventing absorption of metabolic wastes from the urine as well as urine reflux into the ureters

7. Expect a variety of psychologic manifestations, such as anger or depression, postoperatively

8. Arrange visit from a member of an ostomy club

9. Set realistic goals

10. Encourage fluids such as cranberry juice to help prevent infection

11. Support natural defense mechanisms of client; encourage intake of foods rich in the immune-stimulating nutrients, especially vitamins A, C, and E, and the mineral selenium

D. EVALUATION/OUTCOMES

1. Discusses feelings related to prognosis

2. Demonstrates correct care of stoma and appliance

3. Remains free from infection

▼ BLADDER TRAUMA (RUPTURE)

Data Base

A. Etiology and pathophysiology

1. Traumatic rupture of the bladder occurs following external crushing injury to the area, as in automobile accidents

2. An overdistended bladder at time of trauma increases the risk of this occurrence

B. Clinical findings

1. Subjective

a. Pain

b. Anxiety

2. Objective

a. Oliguria or anuria

b. Hematuria

C. Therapeutic interventions

1. Exploration of the bladder to aid in diagnosing rupture

2. Surgical repair of laceration

3. Insertion of a suprapubic catheter to aid in urinary drainage (a tube inserted directly through the peritoneal cavity into the bladder to drain urine)

Nursing Care of Clients with Bladder Trauma

A. DATA COLLECTION

1. Vital signs for baseline data

2. Urine for amount and color

3. Routine preoperative history

B. ANALYSIS AND INTERPRETATION

Refer to General Nursing Diagnoses for Clients with Urinary/Reproductive System Disorders for the following diagnoses: G 2, H, J 1, J 2, J 3, K, and T 3

C. PLANNING/IMPLEMENTATION

1. Observe vital signs for changes indicative of shock or hemorrhage

2. Observe urine for amount and color

3. Promote rest and analgesia

4. Maintain patency of catheters

D. EVALUATION/OUTCOMES

1. Describes decrease in pain

2. Remains free from infection

3. Reestablishes regular pattern of urinary elimination

▼ URETHRITIS

Data Base

A. Etiology and pathophysiology

1. Inflammation of the urethra caused by staphylococci, *Escherichia coli*, *Pseudomonas* species, and streptococci

2. Although inflammatory symptoms are similar to gonorrheal urethritis, sexual contact is not the cause

B. Clinical findings

1. Subjective

a. Burning on urination

b. Urgency

c. Frequency

2. Objective

a. Purulent drainage

b. Bacteria in urine

C. Therapeutic interventions

1. Identification of the causative organism through a culture of urine

2. Antibiotics

3. Warm sitz baths

4. Dilation of the urethra and subsequent instillation of antiseptic solution

Nursing Care of Clients with Urethritis

A. DATA COLLECTION

1. History of dysuria, burning, discharge, or frequency

2. Urine for pyuria

B. ANALYSIS AND INTERPRETATION

Refer to General Nursing Diagnoses for Clients with Urinary/Reproductive System Disorders for the following diagnoses: G 2, H, J 1, P 1, and T 1

C. PLANNING/IMPLEMENTATION

1. Promote rest and comfort
2. Encourage fluid intake
3. Observe urine for clarity and hemorrhage
4. Teach preventive measures such as adequate fluid intake daily, wearing cotton underwear, perineal hygiene particularly after a bowel movement

D. EVALUATION/OUTCOMES

1. Verbalizes a decrease in pain on urination
2. Demonstrates an absence of microorganisms in the urine
3. Describes measures to avoid reinfection

▼ PROSTATITIS

Data Base

A. Etiology and pathophysiology
   1. Generally the result of urethritis
   2. Prostate gland becomes swollen and tender
B. Clinical findings
   1. Subjective
      a. Difficult urination
      b. Pain, backache
   2. Objective
      a. Fever
      b. Hematuria
C. Therapeutic interventions
   1. Antibiotics or chemotherapeutics
   2. Application of heat

Nursing Care of Clients with Prostatitis

A. DATA COLLECTION

1. History of signs and symptoms and their progression
2. Prostate for irregularity, enlargement, and/or tenderness

B. ANALYSIS AND INTERPRETATION

Refer to General Nursing Diagnoses for Clients with Urinary/Reproductive System Disorders for the following diagnoses: A, G 2, H, J 1, T 1, and U

C. PLANNING/IMPLEMENTATION

1. Teach importance of increasing fluid intake
2. Administer antibiotics as ordered
3. Apply heat as ordered
   a. Sitz baths
   b. Rectal irrigations
4. Instruct client regarding activities that drain the prostate (e.g., masturbation, intercourse, massage of the prostate)

D. EVALUATION/OUTCOMES

1. Maintains urinary output
2. Describes decrease in pain
3. Discusses activities in treatment protocol and prevention

▼ BENIGN PROSTATIC HYPERTROPHY (BPH)

Data Base

A. Etiology and pathophysiology
   1. Slow enlargement of the prostate gland common in men over 40 years of age
   2. Constriction of urethra and subsequent interference in urination
B. Clinical findings
   1. Subjective
      a. Frequency and urgency
      b. Difficulty initiating stream
      c. Feeling of incomplete emptying of bladder after urination
   2. Objective
      a. Decreased force of stream
      b. Nocturia
      c. Hematuria
      d. Urinary retention
C. Therapeutic interventions
   1. Relief of acute obstruction by insertion of indwelling catheter or cystostomy tube
   2. Urinary antiseptics to prevent infection from stasis of urine
   3. Pharmacologic management
      a. Finasteride; inhibits the enzyme 5-alpha reductase thus blocking the uptake and utilization of androgens by the prostate reducing glandular hyperplasia and prostatic size
      b. Alpha-1-adrenergic receptor blocking agents such as Terazosin (Hytrin)
   4. Surgical removal of the prostate
      a. Transurethral (TURP)—requires no surgical incision; resectoscope or laser is inserted through the urethra
      b. Suprapubic—requires incision of abdomen and bladder
      c. Retropubic—requires abdominal incision
      d. Perineal—requires perineal incision; associated with highest risk for incontinence, impotence, and wound contamination
   5. Reduction of prostatic obstruction of urethra via balloon catheter technique; procedure is called transurethral dilatation of the prostate (TUDP)
   6. Intermittent or continuous bladder irrigation (CBI) after surgery to promote hemostasis and limit clots that block the catheter

Nursing Care of Clients with Benign Prostatic Hypertrophy

A. DATA COLLECTION

1. Description of onset and progression of symptoms
2. Rectal examination for enlarged prostate
3. Abdomen for bladder distention
4. Signs indicating impaired renal function as a result of prolonged obstruction

B. ANALYSIS AND INTERPRETATION

Refer to General Nursing Diagnoses for Clients with Urinary/Reproductive System Disorders for the following diagnoses: A, B 2, B 3, F, J 1, J 2, J 3, O 3, T 1, T 2, and U

C. PLANNING/IMPLEMENTATION

1. Encourage increased fluid intake (2400 to 3000 ml/day)
2. Administer antiseptics and antibiotics as ordered to prevent or treat urinary tract infections after urine for culture is obtained
3. Instruct the client to avoid anticholinergics and antihistamines because they can cause urinary retention
4. Assist the hospitalized client to a standing position to void
5. Care for the client after a prostatectomy
   a. Observe for signs of hemorrhage (e.g., change in vital signs, nature of drainage, pain, symptoms of shock, frank bleeding)
   b. Observe for or initiate measures to maintain patency of the catheter
      (1) Maintaining unobstructed gravity flow
      (2) Increasing fluid intake
      (3) Providing continuous bladder irrigation (CBI)
      (4) Irrigating catheter with a 60-ml irrigating syringe as prescribed
   c. Maintain integrity of the closed drainage systems
   d. Monitor output; volume of irrigant must be subtracted from drainage for clients with CBI
   e. Administer prescribed stool softeners to prevent straining and pressure on the operative site
   f. Maintain suprapubic catheter after suprapubic prostatectomy; change dressings frequently after removal of the catheter because of urine leakage
   g. Encourage client to express concerns about sexual functioning (a prostatectomy, except when radical, does not usually cause impotence)
   h. Provide as much privacy as possible
   i. Instruct client to perform perineal exercises to regain urinary control; dribbling is common after surgery

D. EVALUATION/OUTCOMES

1. Maintains appropriate urine output
2. Remains free of urinary tract infection
3. Verbalizes concerns about urinary and sexual functioning
4. Performs perineal exercises to improve urinary control

▼ CANCER OF THE PROSTATE

Data Base

A. Etiology and pathophysiology
   1. Slow, malignant change in the prostate gland
   2. Tends to spread by direct invasion of surrounding tissues and metastases to the bony pelvis and spine
   3. Incidence increases with age
B. Clinical findings
   1. Subjective
      a. Frequency and urgency
      b. Difficulty initiating stream
   2. Objective
      a. Decreased force of stream
      b. Urinary retention
      c. Elevated serum acid phosphatase and carcinoembryonic antigen (CEA); increased prostate-specific antigen (PSA); alkaline phosphatase rises with bone metastasis
      d. Enlarged hardened prostate on palpation
      e. Positive diagnosis made by biopsy
C. Therapeutic interventions
   1. Type of surgical intervention depends on the extent of the lesion, the physical condition of the client, and the client's full awareness of the outcome (impotency follows radical prostatectomy)
   2. Radical prostatectomy, done by perineal or retropubic approach, removing the seminal vesicles and a portion of the bladder neck
   3. Radiation therapy alone or in conjunction with surgery may be ordered preoperatively or postoperatively to reduce the lesion and limit metastases; high doses of external-beam radiotherapy and/or ^{125}I seed therapy may be used
   4. Diethylstilbestrol (estrogen) may be ordered to reduce the size of an inoperable lesion or postoperatively to limit metastases
   5. Orchiectomy may be done to limit production of testosterone and thus slow the spread of the disease

Nursing Care of Clients with Cancer of the Prostate

A. DATA COLLECTION

1. History of onset and progression of symptoms of urinary obstruction

2. Presence of back pain
3. Rectal examination to palpate prostate for enlargement
4. Possible presence of metastasis to bone, lungs, liver, or kidneys

B. ANALYSIS AND INTERPRETATION

Refer to General Nursing Diagnoses for Clients with Urinary/Reproductive System Disorders for the following diagnoses: A, B 2, B 3, E 2, E 3, J 2, M, O 3, T 2, and U

C. PLANNING/IMPLEMENTATION

1. Provide care similar to the client who has undergone a prostatectomy for benign prostatic hypertrophy (see Benign Prostatic Hypertrophy)
2. Explain to the client that development of secondary female characteristics will occur as a result of estrogen therapy and not the surgery
3. Allow time and opportunity for the client to express concerns about impotence
4. Support the client's male image
5. Assist the client and family in dealing with the diagnosis of cancer
6. Monitor for evidence of metastasis
7. Provide care for the client receiving radiation (see Nursing Care of Clients with Neoplastic Disorders Receiving Either Chemotherapy or Radiation in this chapter)

D. EVALUATION/OUTCOMES

1. Maintains normal urine output
2. Remains free of pain
3. Maintains satisfying sexual expression
4. Verbalizes concerns regarding sexuality and prognosis

▼ CANCER OF THE TESTES

Data Base

A. Etiology and pathophysiology
  1. Etiology unknown; contributing factors include infection, cryptorchidism, genetics, and hormone levels
  2. Leading cause of death due to cancer in men 20 to 35 years old
  3. Most are germ cell tumors (seminomas, embryonal carcinomas, teratomas, and choriosarcomas)
  4. Metastasizes to the retroperitoneal nodes, lungs, and CNS
B. Clinical findings
  1. Subjective
    a. Heaviness or dull ache in scrotal area
    b. Backache or abdominal pain
  2. Objective
    a. Enlarged testes

b. Hydrocele
c. Palpable mass
d. Elevated tumor markers: alpha-fetoprotein, beta–human chorionic gonadotropin
e. Weight loss
f. CT scan of chest and abdomen may reveal metastasis

C. Therapeutic interventions
  1. Orchiectomy (removal of the testis)
  2. Retroperitoneal lymph node dissection (RPLND)
  3. Radiation
  4. Chemotherapy
    a. Cysplatin
    b. Dactinomycin
    c. Vinblastine

Nursing Care of Clients with Cancer of the Testes

A. DATA COLLECTION

1. Palpation of the testes for enlargement
2. Evidence of metastasis
   a. Back pain
   b. Dyspnea, cough
   c. Dysphagia
   d. Altered mental state
   e. Visual changes

B. ANALYSIS AND INTERPRETATION

Refer to General Nursing Diagnoses for Clients with Urinary/Reproductive System Disorders for the following diagnoses: B 1, B 2, B 3, E 2, E 3, E 4, J 1, J 2, J 3, L 1, L 2, O 1, O 2, O 3, O 4, and P 2

C. PLANNING/IMPLEMENTATION

1. Discuss the possibility of banking sperm prior to treatment because of risk of infertility
2. Encourage discussion of feelings
3. See Nursing Care of Clients with Neoplastic Disorders Receiving Either Chemotherapy or Radiation

D. EVALUATION/OUTCOMES

1. Demonstrates ability to perform testicular self-examination
2. Verbalizes feelings about sexuality and treatment
3. Maintains satisfying sexual expression

▼ EPIDIDYMITIS

Data Base

A. Etiology and pathophysiology
  1. Acute or chronic inflammation of the epididymis
  2. Occurs as a sequela of urinary tract infections, sexually transmitted disease (STD), prostatitis
B. Clinical findings
  1. Subjective

a. Chills
b. Scrotal pain
c. Groin pain
2. Objective
a. Fever
b. Edema
c. Elevated WBCs
d. Pyuria and bacteriuria

C. Therapeutic interventions
1. Medications to control pain, fever, and infection
2. Scrotal support to facilitate drainage
3. Notification of the State Department of Health if a reportable sexually transmitted disease (STD) is present

Nursing Care of Clients with Epididymitis

A. DATA COLLECTION

1. Description of onset and progression of symptoms
2. Vital signs and white blood cell count for baseline data
3. History of causative factors
   a. Gonorrhea or chlamydia exposure
   b. Urinary tract infection
   c. Prostatic surgery

B. ANALYSIS AND INTERPRETATION

Refer to General Nursing Diagnoses for Clients with Urinary/Reproductive System Disorders for the following diagnoses: G 2, H, J 1, L 1, O 4, P 1, and T 1

C. PLANNING/IMPLEMENTATION

1. Obtain urethral and/or urine specimens for culture
2. Maintain the client in a restful state
3. Explain the importance of good hygiene practices
4. Encourage fluid intake
5. Apply cold compresses or administer sitz baths as ordered
6. Advise client to avoid heavy lifting, straining, or sexual activity until infection subsides
7. Ascertain contacts if due to STD
8. Teach the client to protect himself from contracting most STDs by use of a condom

D. EVALUATION/OUTCOMES

1. Experiences a reduction in pain
2. Demonstrates an absence of microorganisms in cultures
3. Describes safer sexual practices

▼ SYPHILIS

Data Base

A. Etiology and pathophysiology
1. Caused by the spirochete *Treponema pallidum*

2. Incubation is 10 to 90 days for primary syphilis
3. If untreated, organism enters blood stream 6 to 8 weeks after infection (usually sexually transmitted)
4. Secondary syphilis is a systemic response to the infection occurring up to 6 months after exposure
5. Latent phase begins after the secondary stage and may last several months to years; client is asymptomatic
6. Tertiary syphilis may occur 18 to 20 years later
   a. Gummas (granulomas) attack any organ and cause cardiovascular syphilis (aortitis and thoracic aortic aneurysms) and neurosyphilis
   b. During this stage it is rare for an individual to infect another; however, a fetus can be infected

B. Clinical findings
1. Primary syphilis
   a. Chancre on genitalia, mouth, or anus
   b. Serous drainage from chancre
   c. Enlarged lymph nodes
   d. Positive test for syphilis: Venereal Disease Research Laboratory (VDRL), rapid plasma reagin circle card test (RPR-CT), automated reagin test (ART), fluorescent treponemal antibody absorption test (FTA-ABS)
2. Secondary syphilis
   a. Skin rash on palms and soles of feet
   b. Erosions of oral mucous membrane
   c. Alopecia
   d. Enlarged lymph nodes
   e. Fever
3. Tertiary syphilis
   a. Cardiovascular changes
   b. Personality changes
   c. Ataxia
   d. Stroke
   e. Blindness

C. Therapeutic interventions
1. Penicillin
2. Probenecid to delay excretion of penicillin
3. Tetracycline or erythromycin if client is allergic to penicillin

Nursing Care of Clients with Syphilis

A. DATA COLLECTION

1. Description of onset and progression of symptoms
2. Potential source of infection and date of exposure
3. Client's sexual partners so that they can be notified and treated
4. Genitalia, rectum, and oropharynx for inflammation, lesions, or drainage

5. Regional lymph nodes for enlargement
6. History of allergies, particularly to penicillin

B. ANALYSIS AND INTERPRETATION

Refer to General Nursing Diagnoses for Clients with Urinary/Reproductive System Disorders for the following diagnoses: G 2, H, P 1, Q 2, and R

C. PLANNING/IMPLEMENTATION

1. Provide a supportive, nonjudgmental environment
2. Encourage the use of early screening and educational programs such as STD clinics, hot lines, and workshops
3. Explain that careful cleansing of the genitals, as well as the use of condoms, helps prevent transmission of most STDs
4. Teach about the disease and its transmission
5. Continue to encourage client to identify prior contacts so they can be treated
6. Inform client that the disease must be reported to the health department, but that confidentiality will be maintained
7. Explain need to complete course of antibiotic therapy
8. Tell client to avoid any sexual activity until tests are negative
9. If client is sexually active, encourage monogamous relationship and advise not to have sexual contact with multiple partners, unknown individuals, individuals with known sexually transmitted diseases, or individuals who have multiple sexual partners themselves

D. EVALUATION/OUTCOMES

1. Skin integrity is restored
2. Identifies "safer sex" practices to reduce risk of reinfection
3. Avoids sexual contact until follow-up testing indicates that transmission will not occur
4. Maintains satisfying interpersonal relationships while abstaining from sexual contact

▼ GONORRHEA

Data Base

A. Etiology and pathophysiology
   1. Caused by *Neisseria gonorrhoeae*, a gram-negative diplococcus
   2. Penicillinase-producing *N. gonorrhoeae* is a newer strain resistant to penicillin
   3. Symptoms depend on nature of sexual contact and may appear within a few days after exposure
   4. Client may remain asymptomatic
   5. Untreated, inflammation subsides in 2 to 4 weeks, but client may become a carrier

B. Clinical findings
   1. Subjective
      a. Lower abdominal discomfort
      b. Dysuria
      c. Urgency
      d. Joint pain
      e. Anal pruritis
      f. Painful defecation
   2. Objective
      a. Purulent penile or vaginal discharge
      b. Fever
      c. Urethral or endocervical smear positive for gonococcus; cultures should be obtained from the urethra, endocervix, anal canal, and pharynx
      d. If untreated, complications such as sterility, urethral stricture, prostatitis, epididymitis, proctitis, and pharyngitis can occur

C. Therapeutic interventions
   1. Penicillin, drug of choice
   2. Tetracycline
   3. Doxycycline
   4. Ceftriaxone sodium
   5. Amoxicillin

Nursing Care of Clients with Gonorrhea

A. DATA COLLECTION

See Assessment under Nursing Care of Clients with Syphilis

B. ANALYSIS AND INTERPRETATION

Refer to General Nursing Diagnoses for Clients with Urinary/Reproductive System Disorders for the following diagnoses: E 4, G 2, H, J 1, J 2, J 3, K, P 1, P 2, R, and T 1

C. PLANNING/IMPLEMENTATION

1. Instruct client to wash hands to prevent conjunctivitis
2. Make arrangements for follow-up culture 2 weeks after therapy is initiated
3. Monitor urinary and bowel elimination
4. Allow time for client to verbalize concerns about potential infertility
5. See Nursing Care of Clients with Syphilis for additional information

D. EVALUATION/OUTCOMES

1. Voids without pain
2. Defecates without pain
3. Maintains reproductive functions
4. Identifies "safer sex" practices to reduce risk of reinfection
5. Maintains satisfying interpersonal relationships while abstaining from sexual contact

▼ HERPES GENITALIS

Data Base
A. Etiology and pathophysiology
   1. Most commonly caused by herpes simplex type II (herpesvirus hominus type II): may also be caused by type I, which is most often associated with lesions (cold sores) of the mouth
   2. Lesions occur 3 to 7 days after infection (usually by sexual contact) and may last several weeks
   3. When symptoms resolve, virus lies dormant in spinal root ganglia and is capable of repeatedly causing lesions
   4. May cause aseptic meningitis, proctitis, and prostititis
   5. Newborn may be infected during vaginal delivery
   6. Associated with higher rate of cervical cancer
   7. Transmitted only when active lesions are present
B. Clinical findings
   1. Subjective
      a. Anorexia
      b. Genital pain
      c. Dysuria
      d. Tingling sensation before vesicles appear
   2. Objective
      a. Vesicles and papules on genitalia
      b. Leukorrhea
      c. Vaginal bleeding
      d. Urinary retention
      e. Cultures reveal herpesvirus type II
C. Therapeutic interventions
   1. No cure; acyclovir sodium reduces healing time and severity of symptoms; not as effective in subsequent episodes
   2. Sedation for severe pain
   3. Alcohol may be used to dry lesions

Nursing Care of Clients with Herpes Genitalis
A. DATA COLLECTION

See Assessment under Nursing Care of Clients with Syphilis

B. ANALYSIS AND INTERPRETATION

Refer to General Nursing Diagnoses for Clients with Urinary/Reproductive System Disorders for the following diagnoses: G 2, H, J 1, O 4, P 1, Q 1, Q 2, R, and T 1

C. PLANNING/IMPLEMENTATION
1. Provide emotional support to deal with incurable nature of disease
2. Assist client to develop stress-reduction strategies; stress precipitates recurrences
3. Encourage increased fluid intake
4. Relieve local discomfort as ordered
   a. Prescribed analgesics
   b. Topical anesthetic agents
   c. Sitz baths
   d. Application of heat or cold
5. Stress the need to avoid sexual contact when lesions exist
6. Advise female client to have annual Papanicolaou smears
7. See Planning/Implementation under Nursing Care of Clients with Syphilis

D. EVALUATION/OUTCOMES
1. Reports relief of dysuria
2. Experiences a reduction in pain
3. Avoids stressful situations
4. Exhibits intact skin without lesions
5. Abstains from sexual contact when lesions are present
6. Identifies "safer sex" practices
7. Maintains satisfying interpersonal relationships while abstaining from sexual contact

▼ CHLAMYDIA

Data Base
A. Etiology and pathophysiology
   1. Caused by *Chlamydia trachomatis*
   2. Most prevalent sexually transmitted disease
   3. Causes epididymitis, urethritis, cervical inflammation, pelvic inflammatory disease
B. Clinical findings
   1. Subjective
      a. Urgency
      b. Dysuria
      c. Pelvic discomfort
   2. Objective
      a. Positive culture
      b. Frequency
      c. Thin, white, vaginal or urethral discharge
      d. Inflammation of cervix
C. Therapeutic interventions
   1. Doxycycline (Doxycin)
   2. Erythromycin

Nursing Care of Clients with Chlamydia
See Syphilis, Epididymitis, and Pelvic Inflammatory Disease in this chapter for nursing care associated with these disorders

▼ ACQUIRED IMMUNODEFICIENCY SYNDROME (AIDS)

Data Base
A. Etiology and pathophysiology
   1. Caused by the human immunodeficiency virus (HIV); a retrovirus

2. HIV infects helper T-lymphocytes (T_4/CD_4 cells), B-lymphocytes, macrophages, promyelocytes, fibroblasts, and epidermal Langerhans cells

3. When the normal number of T_4/CD_4 cells (600 to 1200/microliter) fall below 200/microliter the risk of opportunistic infections is greatest because the immune system is severely depressed

4. Protozoal (*Pneumocystis carinii* pneumonia, toxoplasmosis, cryptosporidiosis), fungal (candidiasis, cryptococcosis, histoplasmosis), bacterial (*Mycobacterium avium-intracellulare* complex, *Mycobacterium tuberculosis* [MTB]), and viral (herpes simplex virus, varicella-zoster virus, cytomegalovirus) infections, and malignancies (Kaposi's sarcoma, lymphoma) frequently occur with AIDS

5. Classification system for HIV infection
   a. T_4/CD_4 categories
      (1) Category 1: less than or equal to 500 cells/microliter
      (2) Category 2: 200 to 499 cells/microliter
      (3) Category 3: less than 200 cells/microliter
   b. Clinical categories
      (1) Category A: categories B and C have not occurred; asymptomatic HIV infection; persistent generalized lymphadenopathy; acute (primary) HIV infection
      (2) Category B: category C has not occurred; presence of conditions attributed to HIV infection; conditions considered to have a clinical course or require management that is complicated by HIV infection
      (3) All clinical conditions listed as advanced HIV disease or AIDS; once a person is in category C, the person remains in this category

6. The HIV is present in blood, semen, vaginal secretions, saliva, tears, breast milk, and cerebrospinal fluid; transmission occurs through contact with infected blood, semen, and vaginal secretions; oral secretions and breast milk have been implicated

7. The adult is considered HIV positive when blood tests reveal the presence of HIV or antibodies to the HIV

8. Once individuals are infected with HIV, they are capable of transmitting the virus

9. Incubation period estimates range from 6 months to 10 years and may be even longer; the antibodies produced by the body can generally first be detected in the blood from 2 weeks to 3 months or longer after infection; a test that detects the virus can determine its presence within 24 hours of infection

B. Clinical findings
   1. Subjective
      a. Anorexia
      b. Fatigue
      c. Dyspnea
      d. Chills
      e. Sore throat
   2. Objective
      a. Positive test for HIV antibody
         (1) ELISA (enzyme-linked immunosorbent assay)
         (2) Western blot
      b. Positive test for presence of HIV itself; polymerase chain reaction (PCR)
      c. Decreased T_4/CD_4 cells to less than 200/microliter
      d. Decreased T_4 cell (helper cell) : T_8 cell (suppressor cell) ratio
      e. Night sweats
      f. Fever
      g. Diarrhea
      h. Enlarged lymph nodes
      i. Weight loss and emaciation
      j. HIV encephalopathy: memory loss, lack of coordination, partial paralysis, mental deterioration
      k. Opportunistic infections such as:
         (1) *Pneumocystis carinii* pneumonia (PCP) (see Pneumonia)
         (2) Cytomegalovirus infection of retina, intestines, liver, lungs, or CNS
         (3) *Candida albicans* infection of mouth, esophagus, or airways
         (4) *Mycobacterium avium-intracellulare* (MAI), *M. kansasii*, or *M. tuberculosis* (MTB)
         (5) Toxoplasmosis of the brain
      l. Malignancies
         (1) Kaposi's sarcoma, normally a rare skin cancer, manifested by dark purplish lesions (for additional information see Kaposi's sarcoma in Integumentary System)
         (2) Non-Hodgkin's lymphoma

C. Therapeutic interventions
   1. There is no cure; prevention is the key to control
   2. Zidovudine (AZT)
   3. Didanosine or dideoxyinosine
   4. Zalcitabine
   5. Specific treatment of opportunistic infections
      a. *Pneumocystis carinii*: trimethoprim sulfamethoxazole (Bactrim), pentamidine

b. Tuberculosis: isoniazid (INH), rifampin, ethambutal

c. Fungal infections: nystatin (Mycostatin), amphotericin B, ketoconazole

d. Viral infections: acyclovir

6. Management of symptoms

7. Research to control the disease involves genetic manipulation and vaccines to prevent HIV infection in uninfected individuals

Nursing Care of Clients with Acquired Immunodeficiency Syndrome

A. DATA COLLECTION

1. Identify risk factors from history
   a. Sexual practices
      (1) Multiple partners
      (2) Anal intercourse
      (3) Sexual intercourse without the use of condoms
   b. IV drug abuse
   c. Blood transfusions
   d. Other exposure to HIV-infected blood and/or body fluids
2. Weight and vital signs for baseline
3. Description of onset and progression of symptoms
4. Presence of lymphadenopathy
5. Skin and mucous membranes for evidence of Kaposi's sarcoma or opportunistic infections
6. Respiratory function (e.g., characteristics of respiration, arterial blood gases, breath sounds)

B. ANALYSIS AND INTERPRETATION

1. Refer to General Nursing Diagnoses for Clients with Urinary/Reproductive System Disorders for the following diagnoses: B 3, E 1, E 2, G 2, H, I, M, O 1, O 4, P 1, P 2, Q 1, Q 2, and R
2. Where appropriate, see Analysis/Nursing Diagnoses under associated diseases such as Pneumonia, Pulmonary Tuberculosis, Kaposi's Sarcoma, and Toxoplasmosis

C. PLANNING/IMPLEMENTATION

1. Use standard (universal) precautions for all clients, regardless of diagnosis, because the virus can be transmitted before the client shows signs of the disease
2. Refer client and significant others to counselor or support group
3. Provide emotional support; client and family must deal with social rejection and death
4. Protect the client from secondary infection; carefully assess for early signs
5. Monitor client receiving zidovudine for blood dyscrasias
6. Provide frequent rest periods
7. Encourage verbalization of feelings

8. Teach client the importance of:
   a. Informing sexual contacts of diagnosis
   b. Avoiding sexual intercourse unless using a condom
   c. Not sharing needles with other individuals
   d. Continuing medical supervision
9. Provide high-calorie, high-protein diet to prevent weight loss
10. Support natural defense mechanisms of client; encourage intake of foods rich in the immune-stimulating nutrients, especially vitamins A, C, and E, and the mineral selenium
11. Provide skin care
12. See Planning/Implementation under Pneumonia, Pulmonary Tuberculosis, Kaposi's Sarcoma, and Toxoplasmosis for additional nursing care

D. EVALUATION/OUTCOMES

1. Avoids opportunistic infections
2. Maintains body weight
3. Completes self-care activities without fatigue
4. Maintains skin integrity
5. Experiences decreased frequency of loose stools
6. Shares feelings with family and health care providers
7. Is aware of community support groups

GASTROINTESTINAL SYSTEM

REVIEW OF ANATOMY AND PHYSIOLOGY OF THE GASTROINTESTINAL SYSTEM

Functions of Gastrointestinal System

A. Digestion of food, essential preparation for absorption and metabolism

B. Absorption of digested food

C. Elimination of wastes of digestion

Digestion

A. Definition: all changes that food undergoes in the alimentary canal

B. Purpose: conversion of foods into chemical and physical forms that can be absorbed and metabolized

C. Kinds
   1. Mechanical digestion: all movements of the alimentary tract that:
      a. Change physical state of foods from comparatively large solid pieces into minute dissolved particles
      b. Propel food forward along the alimentary tract, finally eliminating digestive wastes from the body
         (1) Deglutition: swallowing
         (2) Peristalsis: wavelike movements that

squeeze food downward in the tract
(3) Mass peristalsis: moving of entire intestinal contents into the sigmoid colon and rectum; usually occurs after a meal
(4) Defecation: emptying of the rectum (bowel movement)
c. Churn intestinal contents so all become well mixed with digestive juices and all parts of contents come in contact with the intestinal mucosa to facilitate absorption
2. Chemical digestion: series of hydrolytic processes dependent on specific enzymes; hydrolysis, decomposition of complex compound into two or more simple compounds by means of chemical reaction with water
D. Control of digestive gland secretion
1. Secretion of saliva: neural control of this reflex results from parasympathetic impulses to glands, initiated by taste, smell, and sight of food (cephalic phase of digestion)
2. Gastric juice
a. Neural control similar to that of salivary glands
b. Hormonal control: partially digested proteins cause gastric mucosa to release hormone (gastrin) into blood; gastrin stimulates gastric mucosa to secrete juice with high pepsin and hydrochloric acid content
3. Pancreatic juice
a. Hormonal control: hydrochloric acid in chyme entering the duodenum from the stomach causes intestinal mucosa to release a hormone, secretin, into the blood; secretin stimulates pancreatic cells to secrete a juice high in sodium bicarbonate to neutralize hydrochloric acid but low in enzymes; products of protein digestion (e.g., proteoses, peptones, and amino acids) cause the intestinal mucosa to release another hormone, pancreozymin, that stimulates the pancreatic cells to secrete enzymes
b. Neural control: reflex secretion of pancreatic juice results from parasympathetic impulses via the vagus nerve
4. Bile
a. Although bile is secreted continuously, secretin increases amount of bile secreted
b. Presence of fats in the intestine causes the intestinal mucosa to release a hormone, cholecystokinin, into the blood; cholecystokinin stimulates the smooth muscle of the gallbladder to contract, ejecting bile into the duodenum
5. Intestinal juice: control obscure, but believed to be both reflexive and hormonal; food in the small intestine causes the mucosa to release hormone (enterocrinin) into blood; enterocrinin stimulates intestinal glands to secrete

Absorption
A. Definition: passage of substances through the intestinal mucosa into the blood or lymph
B. Accomplished mainly through active transport by the intestinal cells; makes it possible for both water and solutes to move through the intestinal mucosa in a direction opposite that expected in osmosis and diffusion
C. Absorption occurs in the duodenum and jejunum of the small intestine; however, absorption of alcohol, certain drugs, and some water occurs in the stomach; most water is absorbed from the large intestine
D. Absorption of protein, carbohydrate, and fat (Table 6-12)

Metabolism
A. Definition: sum of all the chemical reactions in the body
B. Catabolism
1. Consists of a complex series of chemical reactions that take place inside the cells and yield energy, carbon dioxide, and water; about half the energy released from food molecules by catabolism is put back in storage as unstable, high-energy bonds of ATP molecules; the rest is transformed to heat; the energy in high-energy bonds of ATP can be released as rapidly as needed for cellular work
2. Two processes involved; glycolysis and the Krebs' cycle with the electron transport chain
3. Purpose: to provide cells continually with utilizable energy
C. Anabolism
1. Synthesis of various compounds from simpler compounds
2. Cellular work that uses some of the energy made available by catabolism
D. Metabolism of carbohydrates
Consists of the following processes:
1. Glucose transport through cell membranes and phosphorylation
a. Insulin promotes this transport through cell membranes
b. Glucose phosphorylation: conversion of glucose to glucose-6-phosphate, catalyzed by the enzyme hexokinase; insulin increases the activity of glucokinase and promotes glucose phosphorylation, which is essential prior to both glycogenesis and glucose catabolism
2. Glycogenesis: conversion of glucose to glycogen for storage; occurs mainly in the liver and muscle cells

TABLE 6-12 Absorption of nutrients

Substance	Structures into which absorbed	Circulation
Protein—amino acids	Into blood in intestinal capillaries	Portal vein, liver, hepatic vein, inferior vena cava to heart, etc.
Carbohydrate—monosaccharides (glucose and fructose)	Same as amino acids	Same as amino acids
Fat—glycerol and fatty acids; fatty acids are insoluble and must first combine with bile salts to form water-soluble units called micelles	Chiefly into lymph in intestinal lacteals; some into blood	During absorption while in epithelial cells of intestinal mucosa, glycerol and fatty acids recombine and complex with protein to form microscopic particles called chylomicrons (a type of lipoprotein); lymphatics carry them by way of thoracic duct to left subclavian vein, superior vena cava, heart, etc.
Vitamins		
Fat-soluble	Same as fat	Same as fat
Water-soluble	Same as amino acid	Same as amino acid
Minerals	Same as amino acid	Same as amino acid

3. Glycogenolysis
   a. In muscle cells glycogen is changed back to glucose-6-phosphate, which is then catabolized in the muscle cells
   b. In liver cells glycogen is changed back to glucose; an enzyme, glucose phosphatase, is present in the liver cells and catalyzes the final step of glycogenolysis, the changing of glucose-6-phosphate to glucose; glucagon and epinephrine accelerate liver glycogenolysis
4. Glucose catabolism
   a. Glycolysis: series of anaerobic reactions that break one glucose molecule down into two pyruvic acid molecules, with conversion of about 5% of energy stored in glucose to heat and ATP molecules
   b. Krebs' citric acid cycle with the electron transport chain: series of aerobic chemical reactions by which two pyruvic acid molecules (from one glucose molecule) are broken down to six carbon dioxide and six water molecules, with the release of some energy as heat and some stored again in ATP; the aerobic reactions release about 95% of the energy stored in glucose, while the anaerobic reactions release only about 5%; the aerobic reactions occur in the mitochondria of cells
5. Gluconeogenesis: sequence of chemical reactions carried on in liver cells; process converts protein or fat compounds into glucose
6. Principles of normal carbohydrate metabolism
   a. Principle of preferred energy fuel: most cells first catabolize glucose, sparing fats and proteins (muscle cells prefer fatty acids as long as adequate oxygen is available); when the glucose supply becomes inadequate, most cells (not nerve cells) next catabolize fats; nerve cells require glucose, thus causing proteins to be sacrificed to provide the amino acids needed to produce more glucose (gluconeogenesis); also small amounts of glucose can be made from the glycerol portion of fats
   b. Principle of glycogenesis: glucose in excess of about 6.7 to 7.8 mmol/L blood brought to the liver by the portal veins enters the liver cells, where it undergoes glycogenesis and is stored as glycogen
   c. Principle of glycogenolysis: when blood glucose decreases below the midpoint of normal, liver glycogenolysis accelerates and tends to raise the blood glucose concentration back toward the midpoint of normal
   d. Principle of gluconeogenesis: when blood glucose decreases below normal or when the amount of glucose entering the cells is inadequate, liver gluconeogenesis accelerates and raises blood glucose levels
   e. Principle of glucose storage as fat: when the blood insulin content is adequate, glucose in excess of the amount used for catabolism and glycogenesis is converted to fat and stored in fat depots
E. Control of metabolism: primarily by hormones
   1. Pancreatic hormones
      a. Insulin: exerts predominant control over carbohydrate metabolism but also affects protein and fat metabolism; in general, it

accelerates carbohydrate metabolism by the cells, thereby decreasing blood glucose

   b. Glucagon: primarily accelerates liver glycogenolysis but also promotes gluconeogenesis and lipolysis when blood insulin levels are low

   c. Somatostatin: inhibits the release of insulin and glucagon

2. Anterior pituitary hormones

   a. Growth hormone tends to:

      (1) Accelerate protein anabolism; hence promotes growth of skeleton and soft tissues

      (2) Accelerate fat mobilization from adipose cells, which tends to bring about a shift from the use of glucose to the use of fats for catabolism

      (3) Accelerate liver gluconeogenesis from fats, which tends to increase blood glucose

      (4) Stimulate glucagon secretion, which in turn stimulates liver glycogenolysis and glucose release into the blood

   b. ACTH (the adrenocorticotropic hormone): stimulates the secretion of glucocorticoids by the adrenal cortex

3. Adrenal cortex hormones (glucocorticoids) mainly cortisol and corticosterone, tend to:

   a. Accelerate fat mobilization and catabolism, thereby promoting shift to fat catabolism from glucose catabolism whenever the latter is inadequate for energy needs

   b. Accelerate tissue protein mobilization (catabolism)

   c. Accelerate liver gluconeogenesis that becomes necessary to maintain blood glucose for nerve cells when carbohydrate availability is limited

4. Adrenal medulla hormones: epinephrine and norepinephrine (catecholamines) tend to accelerate both liver and muscle glycogenolysis, with release of glucose from the liver into the circulation; therefore tend to increase blood sugar

5. Male sex gland hormone: testosterone, secreted by interstitial cells of testes, tends to accelerate protein anabolism

F. Metabolic rate: calories of heat energy produced and expended per hour or per day

1. Basal metabolic rate (BMR): calories of heat produced when an individual is awake but resting in a comfortably warm environment 12 to 18 hours after the last meal

   a. Factors determining basal metabolic rates

      (1) Size: BMR is directly related to square meters of surface area of the body; the larger the surface area, the higher the BMR

      (2) Sex: 5% to 7% higher in males than in females of the same size and age

      (3) Age: BMR inversely related to age; as age increases, BMR decreases

      (4) Amount of thyroid hormones secreted; thyroid hormones accelerate BMR

      (5) Body temperature: BMR directly related to body temperature; 1° C increase in body temperature above normal is accompanied by about a 13% increase in BMR

      (6) Miscellaneous factors such as sleep (decreases BMR), pregnancy, and emotions (increase BMR)

   b. Measurement

      (1) Determined by measuring the amount of oxygen inspired in a given time

      (2) Reported as normal or as a definite percentage above or below normal

2. Total metabolic rate: calories of heat energy expended per day; equal to basal metabolic rate plus number of calories of energy used for muscular work, eating and digesting food, and adjusting to cool temperatures

3. Some principles about the metabolic rate and its relation to body weight

   a. For body weight to remain constant (except for variations in water content) the energy balance must be maintained; body weight remains constant when energy input equals energy output

   b. Whenever the energy input (food intake) is greater than the energy output (total metabolic rate), body weight increases

   c. Whenever energy input (food intake) is less than the energy output (total metabolic rate), body weight decreases

Structures of Gastrointestinal System

Mouth (Buccal Cavity)

A. Lips

B. Cheeks

C. Hard palate: formed by two palatine bones and palatine processes of maxillae

D. Soft palate: formed of muscle in shape of an arch that forms a partition between the mouth and nasopharynx; fauces (archway) or opening from mouth into oropharynx; uvula, conical dependent process; possesses numerous mucus-secreting glands

E. Gums (gingivae)

F. Teeth

1. Deciduous or "baby teeth": 10 in each jaw (20 in set)

2. Permanent: 16 per jaw (32 in set)
3. Eruption
    a. Deciduous: first one erupts usually at 6 months of age; rest follow at intervals of 1 or more months; however, great individual variation in time of eruption of teeth; deciduous teeth are shed between 6 and 13 years of age
    b. Permanent: usually between 6 years and about 17 years; third molars (wisdom teeth) last to erupt
G. Tongue
    1. Papillae: many rough elevations on surface
    2. Taste buds: specialized receptors of cranial nerves VII (facial) and IX (glossopharyngeal); located in papillae
    3. Frenum (or frenulum): fold of mucous membrane that helps anchor tongue to floor of mouth
H. Tonsils: lymphatic tissue connected to the surface epithelium by a channel (crypt); produces lymphocytes; defense against infection
I. Salivary glands: produce saliva, a mixture of water, mucin, salts, enzyme (salivary amylase)
    1. Parotid: below and in front of the ear
    2. Submandibular: posterior part of floor of mouth
    3. Sublingual: anterior part of floor of mouth, under tongue

Pharynx

See Anatomy and Physiology of the Respiratory System in this chapter

Esophagus

A. Location and extent
    1. Posterior to trachea; anterior to the vertebral column
    2. Extends from the pharynx through an opening in the diaphragm (hiatus) to the stomach
B. Structure: collapsible muscular tube; about 25 cm long
C. Secretions and functions: secretes mucus; facilitates movement of food

Stomach

A. Size, shape, position
    1. Size: varies in different persons and according to degree of distention
    2. Shape: elongated pouch, with greater curve forming the lower left border
    3. Position: in epigastric and left hypochondriac portions of the abdominal cavity
B. Divisions
    1. Fundus: the uppermost portion of the stomach; the bulge adjacent to and extending above the esophageal opening
    2. Body: central portion
    3. Pylorus: constricted lower portion
C. Curves
    1. Lesser: upper right border

2. Greater: lower left border
D. Sphincters
    1. Cardiac: guarding opening of the esophagus into the stomach
    2. Pyloric: guarding opening of the pylorus into the duodenum
E. Glands of the stomach: secrete gastric juice composed of mucus, hydrochloric acid, and enzymes
    1. Simple columnar epithelial cells form the surface of the gastric mucosa; goblet cells secrete mucus
    2. Millions of microscopic gastric glands embedded in gastric mucosa composed of different types of cells; mainly chief cells (zymogenic cells) that secrete gastric juice enzymes, and parietal cells that secrete hydrochloric acid and intrinsic factor
F. Functions: food storage and liquefaction (chyme)

Small Intestine

A. Size: approximately 2.5 cm in diameter, 6.0 m in length when relaxed
B. Divisions
    1. Duodenum: joins pylorus of the stomach; about 25 cm in length; C-shaped
    2. Jejunum: middle section about 2.4 m in length
    3. Ileum: lower section, about 3.6 m in length; no clear boundary between jejunum and ileum
C. Functions: digestion and absorption
D. Process: mixing movements; peristalsis; secretion of water, ions, and mucus; receives secretions from the liver, gallbladder, and pancreas

Large Intestine

A. Size: approximately 6.3 cm in diameter, but only 1.5 to 1.8 m long when relaxed
B. Divisions
    1. Cecum: first 5 to 7.6 cm
    2. Colon
        a. Ascending: extends vertically along the right border of the abdomen up to level of the liver
        b. Transverse: extends horizontally across the abdomen, below liver and stomach, and above the small intestine
        c. Descending: extends vertically down the left side of the abdomen to level of the iliac crest
        d. Sigmoid: S-shaped part of large intestine curving downward below the iliac crest to join the rectum; lower part of the sigmoid curve that joins rectum bends toward the left
    3. Rectum: last 17.7 or 20.3 cm of intestines
    4. Anus: terminal opening of the alimentary tract
C. Functions: water and sodium ion absorption; temporary storage of fecal matter; defecation

D. Process: weak mixing movements, mass movements, and peristalsis

Vermiform Appendix

A. Size, shape, location: about size and shape of a large angleworm; blind-end tube off the cecum just beyond the ileocecal valve; 7.5 to 10 cm long; 0.6 cm in diameter

B. Structure: same coats as compose the intestinal wall

C. Function: part of the immune system; submucosa unique in the large size of its lymphatic nodules

Liver

A. Location and size: occupies most of the right hypochondrium and part of the epigastrium; largest gland in the body

B. Lobes: divided into thousands of lobules by blood vessels and fibrous partitions
   1. Right lobe: subdivided into two smaller lobes (caudate and quadrate) and right lobe proper
   2. Left lobe: single lobe

C. Ducts
   1. Hepatic duct: from liver
   2. Cystic duct: from gallbladder
   3. Common bile duct: formed by union of the hepatic and cystic ducts in a Y formation; drains bile into the duodenum at the hepatopancreatic papilla, surrounded by the sphincter of Oddi

D. Functions: liver is one of the most vital organs because of its role in metabolism of proteins, carbohydrates, and fats
   1. Carbohydrate metabolism by liver cells
      a. Glycogenesis: conversion of glucose to glycogen for storage
      b. Glycogenolysis: conversion of glycogen to glucose and release of glucose into the blood; epinephrine and glucagon accelerate glycogenolysis
      c. Gluconeogenesis: formation of glucose from proteins or fats; glucocorticoids (hydrocortisone, corticosterone) have an accelerating effect on gluconeogenesis
   2. Fat metabolism by liver cells
      a. Ketogenesis: occurs during accelerated fat catabolism; occurs mainly in liver cells; consists of a series of reactions by which fatty acids are broken down into molecules of acetyl CoA (beta oxidation), which are then combined (two at a time) to form ketone bodies (acetoacetic acid, acetone, beta-hydroxybutyric acid)
      b. Fat storage
      c. Synthesis of triglycerides, phospholipids, cholesterol, and the B complex factor choline
   3. Protein metabolism by liver cells
      a. Anabolism: synthesis of various proteins, notably blood proteins (e.g., prothrombin, fibrinogen, albumins, alpha and beta globulins, and clotting factors V, VII, IX, and X)
      b. Deamination: first step in protein catabolism; chemical reaction by which amino group is split off from amino acid to form ammonia and a keto acid
      c. Urea formation: liver cells convert most of the ammonia formed by deamination to urea
   4. Secretes bile, substance important for emulsifying fats prior to digestion and as a vehicle for excretion of cholesterol and bile pigments
   5. Detoxifies various substances (e.g., drugs, hormones)
   6. Vitamin metabolism: stores vitamins A, D, K, and B_{12}; synthesizes B_3 from tryptophan

Gallbladder

A. Size, shape, location: approximately the size and shape of a small pear; lies on the undersurface of the liver

B. Structure: sac made of smooth muscle, lined with mucosa arranged in rugae (expandable longitudinal folds)

C. Functions: concentrates and stores bile

Pancreas

A. Size, shape, location: larger in men than in women, but considerable individual variation; fish shaped, with body, head, and tail; extends from the duodenal curve to the spleen

B. Structure: that of both a duct gland and a ductless gland
   1. Pancreatic cells: pour secretion (pancreatic juice) into the duct that runs length of the gland and empties into the duodenum at the hepatopancreatic papilla
   2. Islets of Langerhans: clusters of cells not connected with pancreatic ducts (two main types of cells compose islets, namely, alpha and beta cells); constitute the endocrine gland

C. Functions
   1. Pancreatic cells connected with pancreatic ducts secrete pancreatic juice, enzymes of which help digest all three kinds of foods
   2. Islet cells constitute endocrine gland
      a. Alpha cells secrete the hormone glucagon, which accelerates liver glycogenolysis and initiates gluconeogenesis; hence, tends to increase blood glucose level
      b. Beta cells secrete insulin, one of the most important metabolic hormones, which exerts a profound influence on the metabolism of carbohydrates, proteins, and fats (Fig. 6-13)
         (1) Insulin accelerates the active transport of glucose (along with potassium and phosphate ions) through cell mem-

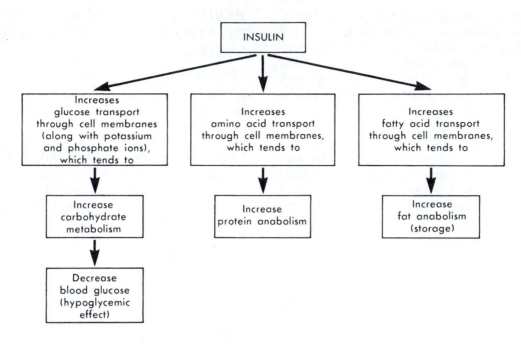

FIGURE 6-13 Major insulin effects.

branes; therefore it tends to decrease blood glucose (hypoglycemic effect) and to increase glucose utilization by the cells for either catabolism or anabolism

(2) Insulin stimulates the production of liver cell glucokinase; therefore it promotes liver glycogenesis, another effect that tends to lower blood glucose

(3) Insulin inhibits liver cell phosphatase and therefore inhibits liver glycogenolysis

(4) Insulin accelerates the rate of amino acid transfer into cells, so it promotes anabolism of proteins within the cells

(5) Insulin accelerates the rate of fatty acid transfer into cells, promotes fat anabolism (also called fat deposition or lipogenesis), and inhibits fat catabolism

REVIEW OF PHYSICAL PRINCIPLES RELATED TO THE GASTROINTESTINAL SYSTEM

Principles of Mechanics
Law of Motion
EXAMPLE: The greater the force of contraction of the intestinal wall and the more frequent the contractions, the more rapid the propulsion of food and fecal matter through the digestive tract; under irritating conditions, rapid powerful peristalsis leads to abdominal cramps and diarrhea

Gravity
EXAMPLES: Colostomy irrigations and enemas
Energy
A. Potential and kinetic energy
EXAMPLE: The potential energy in glucose (food) molecules is captured in the bonds of the high-energy molecule ATP; such potential energy is released as kinetic energy when ATP powers the contraction of muscle and the beating of cilia and flagella

B. First law of thermodynamics
EXAMPLE: The energy stored in an ATP molecule exactly equals the work (of muscles, cilia, etc.) and heat energy liberated during the process
C. Second law of thermodynamics
EXAMPLE: The diffusion of nutrients and enzymes in the various digestive juices results in their collisions and chemical interactions because it is the natural tendency of molecules and systems to become more randomized

Principles of Physical Properties of Matter
Solids
EXAMPLE: The elastic properties of the connective and muscular tissues of the stomach permit distention during a meal and the consequent storage and slow digestion and absorption of food over the next several hours
Liquids
A. Pascal's principle
EXAMPLE: The voluntary contraction of muscles of

the abdominal wall, such as the external and internal oblique, applies pressure on the fluids of the abdominal cavity, which is transmitted undiminished throughout the abdominopelvic cavity and aids in defecation; chronic constipation with chronic straining during defecation may predispose to hemorrhoids

B. Surface tension

EXAMPLE: Bile salts partly combine with fats and with water; this dual combination lowers the surface tension of the water molecules surrounding large fat droplets, which disperse into thousands of smaller droplets whose greater total surface area promotes more rapid hydrolysis (digestion) by pancreatic lipase

Gases:

Boyle's law

EXAMPLES:

1. During gastric analysis, the volume of gas in the tube is increased as the barrel of the syringe attached to the tube is pulled out; the result is a flow of gastric contents from the stomach due to the decreased pressure exerted by the gas in the tube as compared with gas pressure in the stomach
2. The same applies during paracentesis
3. During gastric gavage the process is reversed

Heat

A. Body temperature maintained by heat produced as a byproduct of biochemical reactions; basal metabolic rate is a measure of heat production under specified conditions

B. The normal metabolism in each of the cells of the human body produces heat; in addition, heat is a byproduct of muscular contraction

Light

A. Refraction

EXAMPLE: Total internal reflection in fiberoptics permits viewing of interior walls of stomach and intestines for diagnostic purposes such as endoscopic procedures, gastroscopy, sigmoidoscopy, and proctoscopy

B. X-rays

EXAMPLES

1. GI series and barium enemas allow visualization of the soft tissues of the upper and lower gastrointestinal tract; the barium salts coat the inner walls of the alimentary tube and absorb the x-rays striking them; as a result, the organ surfaces are outlined
2. Fluoroscopy can be considered the observation of "live" x-ray images; after the x-rays pass through the individual, they strike a fluorescent screen that absorbs them and emits visible light; with x-ray-opaque (radiopaque) chemicals the intestinal and biliary tracts can be observed

REVIEW OF CHEMICAL PRINCIPLES RELATED TO THE GASTROINTESTINAL SYSTEM

Oxidation and Reduction

A. Uniting oxygen with a substance results in oxidation

B. Uniting hydrogen with a substance results in reduction

Oxidation-Reduction Reactions in the Body

A. Important in body chemistry as a source of energy through cellular oxidation of foods in cytoplasm and mitochondria; oxidation of nutrients like glucose results in the formation of high-energy ATP molecules and heat—both useful to the body

B. Oxygen is the usual oxidizing agent in cells

C. Some forms of life (anaerobes) can use substances other than oxygen for cellular oxidation (e.g., *Clostridium perfringens* found in gangrenous tissue)

Diffusion and Osmosis

EXAMPLES

1. Diffusion of nutrients and enzymes results in the collisions necessary to promote chemical (metabolic) reactions
2. Absorption of water by osmosis occurs through the mucosa of the GI tract

Active Transport

The movement of molecules against a concentration gradient due to energy (ATP) expenditure

EXAMPLE: The absorption of most simple sugars and amino acids in the small intestine involves active transport processes

Buffers

Pairs of chemical substances that resist changes in pH

EXAMPLE: The sodium bicarbonate part of the bicarbonate buffer system secreted from the pancreas into the duodenum acts as a buffer to prevent acidification of intestinal juices due to the presence of hydrochloric acid from gastric juice

Types of Compounds

Organic Acids

All organic acids contain the carboxyl group

EXAMPLES

1. Lactic acid: end product of anaerobic muscle metabolism; converted to pyruvic acid and oxidized completely to carbon dioxide and water aerobically
2. Citric acid: one intermediate in the Krebs citric acid cycle; cycle occurs in mitochondria as a major oxidation-reduction pathway for the generation of ATP (potential chemical energy)
3. Salicylic acid: synthesis of aspirin

Amino Acids

A. Amino acids possess two functional groups: an amine group and an acid or carboxyl group

B. Amino acids are amphoteric: act as both acids or bases; therefore proteins act as buffers in body fluids

C. Reactions of amino acids
1. Amino acids are able to act as an acid and as a base (amphoteric character)
2. Condense via peptide bond to form proteins

D. Essential amino acids cannot be synthesized well enough in the body to maintain health and growth and must be supplied in the food

Carbohydrates

A. Aldehyde or ketone derivatives of single oxidation of polyhydric alcohols, or compounds yielding aldehyde or ketone derivatives on hydrolysis

B. Include simple sugars, starches, celluloses, gums, and resins

C. Widespread in plant and animal tissue

D. Contain carbon, hydrogen, and oxygen; the hydrogen and oxygen are present in approximately the ratio of 2 to 1

E. Synthesis: plants synthesize carbohydrates from carbon dioxide and water with the aid of the green pigment chlorophyll (which acts as an enzyme) and solar energy

F. Classification
1. By functional group
a. Carbohydrates having the aldehyde group are called aldoses (e.g., glucose)
b. Carbohydrates having the ketone group are called ketoses (e.g., fructose)
2. By complexity of the molecule
a. Carbohydrate having a single ketose or aldose molecule is called a monosaccharide: a simple sugar (e.g., glucose, fructose)
b. Carbohydrate formed by combining two aldose molecules or an aldose and a ketose molecule is called a disaccharide (e.g., sucrose, lactose, maltose)
c. Carbohydrate having more than two simple sugars joined in a molecule is called a polysaccharide (e.g., starch, glycogen)

G. Tests for glucose in urine
1. Benedict's test and Clinitest tablets use copper ions in basic medium: show presence of sugar in urine by change in color
2. Positive reaction gives colors from green (very little glucose) to brick red (111.0 mmol/L)
3. Iron ions and silver ions can be used instead of copper to give a test for glucose
4. Most monosaccharides and disaccharides except sucrose are reducing sugars; therefore sucrose put into urine will not produce a reaction

H. Important carbohydrates
1. Glycerose and dihydroxyacetone: triose intermediates in cellular metabolism of carbohydrates
2. Ribose and deoxyribose: pentose constituents in nucleic acids
3. Glucose (dextrose) hexose monosaccharide; a sugar found abundantly in body fluids, fruits, and vegetables; the pancreatic hormones insulin and glucagon regulate the blood glucose concentration in the normal range of 3.9 to 6.1 mmol/L blood; glucose is the basic food molecule that is broken down first in glycolysis (in the cytoplasm of cells) and then in the Krebs' cycle (in mitochondria); the breakdown of each molecule of glucose results in the release of 38 molecules of ATP, which can be used in almost all cellular energy-requiring functions
4. Fructose (levulose): ketose monosaccharide; found in fruits and honey, sweetest sugar known; important intermediate in cellular metabolism of carbohydrates
5. Galactose: hexose monosaccharide; present in brain and nervous tissue
6. Lactose (milk sugar): disaccharide of glucose and galactose molecules; bacterial fermentation of lactose to lactic acid causes milk to sour
7. Sucrose (cane sugar): disaccharide of glucose and fructose molecules; nonreducing sugar, common table sugar used in sweetening and baking
8. Maltose: disaccharide of two glucose molecules; found in grains and malt
9. Starch: mixed polysaccharide of glucose molecules found in plants
a. Amylose: straight-chained glucose polymer
b. Amylopectin: branched-chain glucose polymer
c. Chief food carbohydrate in human nutrition
d. Starch polymers react with iodine to form a blue complex; used as a test for starch
(1) Test becomes colorless as starch is hydrolyzed
(2) Starch (blue) → amylodextrin (purple) → erythrodextrin (red) → achromdextrin (colorless) → maltose (colorless) → glucose (colorless)
10. Glycogen: polysaccharide polymer of glucose molecules found in human and animal tissue; storage compound in the body; hydrolyzes to glucose, maintaining blood glucose levels
11. Cellulose: polysaccharide polymer of glucose found in plants; not digestible by humans; important in the manufacture of cotton cloth, paper, and cellulose acetate synthetics

12. Inulin: polysaccharide polymer of fructose, used in kidney function test (insulin clearance test)
13. Agar-agar: polysaccharide polymer of galactose used as a solid medium for bacteriologic studies
14. Hemicellulose, gums and pectin: polysaccharide polymers of glucose with high water-binding capacity; have been found to be important dietary components of disease prevention and treatment programs

Lipids
A. Organic substances essentially insoluble in water but soluble in organic solvents (ether, chloroform, acetone, etc.)
B. Fatty acids: important constituents of all lipids (except sterols)
   1. Usually straight-chain carboxylic acids
   2. Naturally-occurring fatty acids contain even numbers of carbon atoms
   3. Saturated fatty acids: have no double bonds (points of unsaturation) between their carbon atoms
   4. Unsaturated fatty acids: have one or more points of unsaturation between their carbon atoms
   5. Essential fatty acids: cannot be synthesized by the body; must be taken in by diet
C. Classification of lipids
   1. Simple lipids: esters of fatty acids and alcohols
      a. Fats: the alcohol of fats is the trihydric alcohol glycerol
         (1) Solid fats: fats that are solid at room temperature contain long-chain saturated fatty acids
         (2) Liquid fats (oils): fats that are liquid at room temperature contain short-chain unsaturated fatty acids
      b. Waxes: esters of long-chained fatty acids and an alcohol other than glycerol; lanolin, a mixed wax from wool, is used in creams and salves
      c. Reactions of simple lipids
         (1) Hydrolysis: splitting into fatty acid(s) and alcohol by breaking the ester bond is affected by acid, base, or enzyme action
         (2) Saponification: basic hydrolysis; soap is formed from organic salts of a fatty acid and metal ion of base
         (3) Addition: fats containing unsaturated fatty acids will form additional products at points of unsaturation
            (a) Addition of oxygen will cause fat to become rancid; antioxidants slow this reaction in packaged foods

            (b) Unsaturated oils used in paints add oxygen, and oils become hard and glossy
            (c) Hydrogenation: liquid fats can form solid fats by adding in hydrogen at double bonds
   2. Compound lipids: fats containing chemical substances other than fatty acids and alcohols
      a. Phospholipids: contain alcohol, fatty acids, phosphoric acid, and a nitrogenous base (or inositol)
         (1) Lecithins: contain the alcohol glycerol, fatty acids, phosphoric acid, and the nitrogenous base choline; are found in brain and nervous tissue; in blood, lecithin serves to render fats soluble in plasma (a lipotropic agent)
         (2) Cephalins: similar in structure to lecithin except base is ethanolamine; important in brain and nerve tissue; help blood-clotting mechanism
         (3) Sphingomyelins: made from amino alcohol (sphingosinol), a fatty acid; phosphoric acid, and choline; important in brain and nerve tissue
      b. Cardiolipids: made from unsaturated fatty acids, glycerol, and phosphoric acid; found in heart tissue
      c. Glycolipids (cerebrosides): structure contains the monosaccharide galactose, amino alcohol (sphingosine), and a fatty acid; found in brain tissue and the myelin sheaths of nerves
   3. Steroids: complex monohydroxy alcohols found in plant and animal tissues—basic structure, the phenanthrene structure plus a cyclopentane ring; characteristic side chains determine specific steroids
      a. Cholesterol: a sterol found in human and animal tissue, chiefly in brain and nerve tissue; an important, normal component of membranes; found in blood within a normal range of 3.88 to 5.15 mmol/L; high blood cholesterol seems associated with coronary thrombosis
      b. Ergosterol: a plant sterol that can be converted to vitamin D by ultraviolet light
      c. Bile acids: sterols that aid in digestion and absorption of fats
      d. Steroid hormones: sex and adrenal gland hormones (glucocorticoids, mineralocorticoids)
      e. Vitamin D: steroid helping to control calcium metabolism by regulating calcium uptake from the gastrointestinal tract

Proteins

A. Classification of proteins

  1. Simple proteins: give amino acids on hydrolysis

     a. Albumins: water soluble, coagulated by heat (e.g., lactalbumin [milk], serum albumin [blood], egg white); albumin is most important in the development of the plasma colloid osmotic pressure (oncotic pressure), which helps control (through osmosis) the flow of water between the plasma and interstitial fluid; during a condition such as starvation, a fall in the albumin level of the blood leads to a fall in the plasma colloid osmotic pressure; this results in edema because less fluid is drawn by osmosis into the capillaries from the interstitial spaces

     b. Globulins: insoluble in water, soluble in dilute salt solutions, coagulated by heat (e.g., lactoglobulin [milk], serum globulin [blood], gamma serum globulin—forms antibodies of blood)

     c. Glutenins: soluble in dilute bases or acids, insoluble in neutral solutions; coagulated by heat (e.g., glutenin [wheat])

     d. Albuminoids: soluble in water (e.g., collagen [connective tissue], elastin [ligaments])

     e. Histone: water soluble (e.g., globin [hemoglobin])

     f. Prolamines: insoluble in water, soluble in 70% to 80% alcohol (e.g., gliadin [wheat], zein [corn])

     g. Protamines: water soluble (e.g., protamine [fish spermatozoa])

  2. Compound proteins: contain molecules other than amino acids

     a. Chromoproteins: proteins containing a colored molecule (e.g., hemoglobin, flavoproteins)

     b. Glycoproteins: proteins containing carbohydrate molecule(s) (e.g., mucopolysaccharide of synovial fluid)

     c. Lipoproteins: simple proteins combined with lipid substances

        (1) Low-density lipoproteins (beta lipoproteins)

           (a) VLDL: very low-density lipoproteins that contain a high proportion of triglycerides and a small amount of protein

           (b) LDL: low-density lipoproteins that are chief carriers of cholesterol and are low in triglycerides

           (c) Contribute to atherosclerotic plaque formation

        (2) High-density lipoproteins (HDL) (alpha lipoproteins)

           (a) Consist of 50% protein and 20% cholesterol

           (b) Inversely associated with coronary artery disease

     d. Nucleoproteins: proteins complexed with nucleic acids (e.g., the DNA found in chromosomes is complexed with proteins); chromosomes are sometimes referred to as nucleoprotein structures

     e. Metalloproteins: proteins containing metal ions (e.g., ferritin [iron transport compound of plasma])

     f. Phosphoproteins: proteins containing the phosphoric acid radical (e.g., casein of milk)

  3. Derived proteins: also called denatured proteins; treatment with acids, bases, heat, x-radiation, ultraviolet rays, etc., causes proteins to alter their molecular arrangements

B. Reactions of proteins

  1. Amphoteric properties: like the amino acids forming them, proteins can act as an acid or a base in solution; can act as buffers

  2. Hydrolysis: acid, base, or enzyme hydrolysis splits the peptide bond; yields proteose → peptones → peptides → amino acids

  3. Denaturation: change in structure renders the protein less soluble, leads to coagulation of the protein

     a. Heat: protein and heat → coagulated protein (e.g., cooked egg white, cooked meat)

     b. Salts of heavy metals: silver, lead, mercury, etc.; taken internally, they are poison, because they denature the enzymes of the cells, which are protein in nature

     c. Acetone and alcohol: both harden skin proteins

     d. Inorganic acids and bases: coagulate and hydrolyze proteins

     e. Alkaloids and organic acids: tanning of hides, precipitation of blood proteins for clinical tests

     f. Rays: x-rays, infrared rays, ultraviolet rays; long exposure can cause cataracts (precipitation of lens protein in the eye)

  4. Salting out: concentrated salt solutions render soluble proteins insoluble

Nucleoproteins

A. Specific proteins found in cells, made of large and complex molecules having important functions

B. Composition of nucleoproteins

  1. Hydrolysis of nucleoproteins results in nucleic acids and protein

  2. Hydrolysis of nucleic acid yields

a. Phosphoric acid: H_3PO_4
b. Pentose sugars: ribose or deoxyribose
c. Purine or pyrimidine bases
   (1) Purine bases: adenine, guanine
   (2) Pyrimidine bases: cytosine, uracil, thymine
3. Combination of a purine or pyrimidine base with either ribose or deoxyribose forms a nucleoside
4. Addition of phosphoric acid to a nucleoside forms a nucleotide
5. Polymerization of nucleotide molecules via ester bonds yields a nucleic acid: the shape of DNA is that of a double helix

C. Two main forms of nucleic acid: RNA and DNA (ribonucleic acid and deoxyribonucleic acid)
   1. RNA yields the following on hydrolysis: adenine, guanine, cytosine, uracil, ribose, phosphoric acid
   2. DNA yields the following on hydrolysis: adenine, guanine, cytosine, thymine, deoxyribose, phosphoric acid

D. Role of DNA and RNA in protein synthesis
   1. DNA is found chiefly in the chromatin material of interphase cells and in the chromosomes of cells in mitosis
      a. Portions of DNA molecules are the genes of classic genetics; the genetic code consists of sequences of bases (adenine, guanine, cytosine, and thymine) linearly arranged along the DNA molecule; every three bases represent a code for one amino acid (a triplet code)
      b. One enormous DNA molecule represents thousands of genes separated from each other by specific triplets (codons) representing periods or commas; i.e., the linear triplet code is punctuated so it can eventually be translated correctly on the ribosome
      c. DNA is also found in mitochondria, chloroplasts, and certain other cellular organelles (like centrioles) and is thought to play some role in their replication and metabolism
   2. RNA is found both inside the nucleus and in the cytoplasm of cells
   3. RNA occurs in three forms: messenger RNA (mRNA), transfer RNA (tRNA), and ribosomal RNA (rRNA)
      a. DNA transcribes its coded message of how to make proteins into mRNA; the function of mRNA is to carry this coded genetic information from the DNA in the nucleus to the ribosome in the cytoplasm where proteins can be synthesized
      b. The transcribed genetic code being carried by mRNA is translated into the synthesis of

proteins on the ribosomes; these proteins then serve both structurally and enzymatically in the cell
      c. tRNA molecules each carry an amino acid to the ribosome where protein synthesis is occurring; there is a specific tRNA molecule for each amino acid
      d. rRNA is part of the structure of the ribosome
   4. The protein difference between individuals is ultimately determined by differences in the genetic code carried by DNA; the DNA and RNA molecules are presently the only known molecules that store information and can result in the accurate transmission of genetic information from one generation of cell or organism to the next; the cellular mitotic and meiotic processes are elaborate and precise mechanisms for partitioning the genetic material appropriately between daughter cells

E. Other important related compounds
   1. ATP and ADP (adenosine triphosphate and adenosine diphosphate) are energy-storing compounds in cells
   2. NAD (nicotinamide adenine dinucleotide) and NADP (nicotinamide adenine dinucleotide phosphate) are important in hydrogen transport in the metabolism of foods

Enzymes

Hormones involved in regulating the GI tract
A. Gastrin: stimulates flow of gastric juices
B. Enterogastrone: inhibits flow of gastric juices
C. Secretin: stimulates flow of sodium bicarbonate from the pancreas to the duodenum
D. Pancreozymin: stimulates the flow of pancreatic enzymes from the pancreas to the duodenum
E. Cholecystokinin: stimulates contraction of the gallbladder
F. Enterocrinin: stimulates flow of intestinal juice

REVIEW OF MICROORGANISMS RELATED TO THE GASTROINTESTINAL SYSTEM

Bacterial Pathogens

A. Brucella: three species (*B. abortus*, *B. suis*, and *B. melitensis*); small, gram-negative, somewhat pleomorphic (variable shape) bacilli, cause brucellosis, an infection primarily of domestic animals (cattle, goats, swine, sheep); humans can acquire it by drinking infected milk
B. *Escherichia coli*: small, gram-negative bacillus composing the major portion of the normal flora of the large intestine; certain strains are the most common cause of urinary tract infections and infantile diarrhea

C. *Clostridium difficile*: anaerobic, spore-forming bacterial pathogen; produces toxins that affect bowel mucosa; major cause of nosocomial diarrhea

D. *Leptospira icterohaemorrhagiae*: long, tightly coiled spirochete similar in appearance to *Treponema pallidum*; causes infectious jaundice (Weil's disease)

E. Shigella: gram-negative bacillus, similar to Salmonella; *Shigella dysenteriae* and a number of other species cause an illness known as bacillary dysentery or shigellosis

F. *Vibrio cholerae* (formerly *V. comma*): curved, gram-negative bacillus with a single polar flagellum; causes Asiatic cholera

Protozoal Pathogens

A. *Balantidium coli*: ciliated protozoan; causes enteritis
B. *Entamoeba histolytica*: an amoeba; causes amebiasis (amebic dysentery)
C. *Giardia lamblia*: flagellated protozoan; causes enteritis

Parasitic Pathogens

A. Nematodes (roundworms)
   1. *Ancylostoma duodenale* (hookworm): intestinal parasite similar to *Necator americanus*
   2. *Ascaris lumbricoides* (roundworm): intestinal parasite resembling the earthworm
   3. *Enterobius vermicularis* (pinworm, seatworm): small, white, parasitic worm found in upper part of the large intestine; the female lays eggs in perianal area, causing irritation
   4. *Necator americanus* (the American hookworm): intestinal parasite about 1.2 cm long
   5. *Trichuris trichiura* (whipworm): intestinal parasite about 5 cm long
B. Cestodes (tapeworm)
   1. *Diphyllobothrium latum* (fish tapeworm): large tapeworm 6 m long found in adult form in the intestine of cats, dogs, and humans (vertebrate and aquatic hosts in sequence)
   2. *Echinococcus granulosa* (dog tapeworm): small tapeworm of dogs; larval stage (hydatid) may develop in humans forming hydatid tumors or cysts in the liver, lungs, kidneys, and other organs
   3. *Hymenolepsis nana* (dwarf tapeworm): a species about 2.5 cm long, found in adult form in the intestine
   4. *Taenia marginata* (beef tapeworm): the common tapeworm of humans, a species 3.6 to 7.6 m long, found in adult form in the human intestine
   5. *Taenia solium* (pork tapeworm): a species 0.9 to 1.8 m long, found in the adult form in the intestines of humans

C. Trematodes (flukes)
   1. *Clonorchis sinensis*: one of the most common liver flukes, especially in China and Japan
   2. *Fasciola hepatica*: common liver fluke of herbivorous animals; occasionally found in the human liver
   3. *Fasciolopsis buski*: largest of the intestinal flukes
   4. *Paragonimus westermani*: lung fluke; found in cysts in the lungs, liver, abdominal cavity, and elsewhere

PHARMACOLOGY RELATED TO GASTROINTESTINAL SYSTEM DISORDERS

Antiemetics

A. Description
   1. Used to alleviate nausea and vomiting
   2. Act by:
      a. Diminishing the sensitivity of the chemoreceptor trigger zone (CTZ) to irritants or
      b. Decreasing labyrinthine excitability
   3. Effective in the prevention and control of emesis and motion sickness
   4. Available in oral, parenteral (IM, IV), rectal, and transdermal preparations
B. Examples
   1. Centrally acting agents
      a. Benzquinamide
      b. Ondansetron HCl
      c. Prochlorperazine (Stemetil)
      d. Trimethobenzamide HCl
   2. Agents for motion sickness control
      a. Dimenhydrinate (Gravol)
      b. Meclizine HCl
      c. Promethazine HCl (Phenergan)
      d. Thiethylperazine maleate
   3. Agents that promote gastric emptying
      a. Cisapride (Propulsid)
      b. Metoclopramide (Maxeran)
C. Major side effects
   1. Drowsiness (CNS depression)
   2. Hypotension (vasodilation via central mechanism)
   3. Dry mouth (decreased salivation from anticholinergic effect)
   4. Blurred vision (pupillary dilation from anticholinergic effect)
   5. Incoordination (an extrapyramidal symptom due to dopamine antagonism)
D. Nursing care
   1. Observe occurrence and characteristics of vomitus
   2. Eliminate noxious substances from the diet and environment
   3. Provide good oral hygiene

4. Caution client to avoid engaging in hazardous activities during therapy
5. Offer sugar-free chewing gum or hard candy to promote salivation
6. Instruct client to change positions slowly
7. Evaluate client's response to medication and understanding of teaching

Anorexiants

A. Description
   1. Used to suppress the appetite
   2. Act at the hypothalamic appetite centers to suppress the desire for food; they generally produce CNS stimulation
   3. Available in oral preparations
B. Examples
   1. Amphetamine sulfate
   2. Benzphetamine HCl
   3. Dextroamphetamine sulfate
   4. Fenfluramine HCl
   5. Phenmetrazine HCl
C. Major side effects
   1. Nausea, vomiting (irritation of gastric mucosa)
   2. Constipation (delayed passage of stool in GI tract)
   3. Tachycardia (sympathetic stimulation)
   4. CNS stimulation (sympathetic activation)
   5. Fenfluramine: CNS depression (direct effect)
D. Nursing care
   1. Educate client regarding:
      a. Drug misuse (controlled substances)
      b. Concurrent exercise and diet therapy
      c. Need for medical supervision during therapy
      d. Possibility of affecting ability to engage in hazardous activities
   2. Fenfluramine: assess for history of depression, alcohol abuse, or suicidal tendencies; avoid administration in these situations
   3. Evaluate client's response to medication and understanding of teaching

Antacids

A. Description
   1. Used to neutralize gastric acid
   2. Act by providing a protective coating on the stomach lining and lowering the gastric acid level, which allows more rapid movement of stomach contents into the duodenum
   3. Effective in the treatment of ulcers
   4. Available in oral preparations
B. Examples
   1. Aluminum carbonate gel
   2. Aluminum hydroxide gel (Amphojel)
   3. Aluminum hydroxide with magnesium trisilicate (Gelusil)
   4. Aluminum and magnesium hydroxides (Maalox)
   5. Aluminum phosphate gel
   6. Magaldrate (Riopan)
   7. Sodium bicarbonate: systemic antacid; may cause alkalosis
C. Major side effects
   1. Constipation (aluminum compounds) (aluminum delays passage of stool in GI tract)
   2. Diarrhea (magnesium compounds) (magnesium stimulates peristalsis in GI tract)
   3. Alkalosis (systemic antacids) (absorption of alkaline compound into the circulation)
   4. Reduced absorption of calcium and iron (increase in gastric pH)
D. Nursing care
   1. Instruct the client regarding:
      a. Prevention of overuse of antacids
      b. Need for continued supervision
      c. Dietary restrictions related to gastric distress
      d. Encouraging foods high in calcium and iron
   2. Caution client on a sodium-restricted diet that many antacids contain sodium
   3. Shake oral suspensions well prior to administration
   4. Administer with small amount of water to ensure passage to stomach
   5. Evaluate client's response to medication and understanding of teaching

Gastrointestinal Anticholinergics

A. Description
   1. Used to alleviate pain associated with peptic ulcer
   2. Act by inhibiting smooth muscle contraction in the GI tract
   3. Available in oral and parenteral (IM, SC, IV) preparations
B. Examples
   1. Atropine sulfate
   2. Belladonna leaf, tincture
   3. Dicyclomine HCl
   4. Glycopyrrolate
   5. Methantheline bromide
   6. Propantheline bromide (Pro-Banthine)
C. Major side effects (all related to decreased parasympathetic stimulation)
   1. Abdominal distention (decreased peristalsis)
   2. Constipation (decreased peristalsis)
   3. Dry mouth (decreased salivation)
   4. Urinary retention (decreased parasympathetic stimulation)
   5. CNS disturbances (direct CNS toxic effect)
D. Nursing care
   1. Provide dietary counseling with emphasis on bland foods

2. Offer sugar-free chewing gum or hard candy to promote salivation
3. Evaluate client's response to medication and understanding of teaching

Gastrointestinal Antihistamines

A. Description
1. Used to inhibit gastric acid secretion
2. Act at the H_2 receptors of the stomach parietal cells
3. Effective in the short-term therapy of peptic ulcer
4. Available in oral and parenteral (IM, IV) preparations
B. Examples
1. Cimetidine (Tagamet)
2. Famotidine (Pepcid)
3. Nizatidine (Axid)
4. Omeprazole (Prilosec)
5. Ranitidine (Zantac)
C. Major side effects
1. CNS disturbances (decreased metabolism of drug because of liver or kidney impairment)
2. Blood dyscrasias (decreased RBCs, WBCs, platelet synthesis)
3. Skin rash (hypersensitivity)
4. Reduced calcium and iron absorption (increase in gastric pH)
D. Nursing care
1. Do not administer at same time as antacids; allow 1 to 2 hours between drugs
2. Administer oral preparations with meals
3. Assess for potentiation of oral anticoagulant effect
4. Instruct client regarding dietary restrictions; also encourage foods high in calcium and iron (see Peptic Ulcer for more dietary information)
5. Instruct client to follow prescription exactly; Prilosec administration should not exceed 8 weeks
6. Evaluate client's response to medication and understanding of teaching

Antidiarrheals

A. Description
1. Used to alleviate diarrhea
2. Act by various mechanisms to promote the formation of a formed stool
3. Available in oral and parenteral (IM) preparations
B. Examples
1. Fluid adsorbents: decrease the fluid content of stool
   a. Bismuth subcarbonate
   b. Kaolin and pectin (Kaopectate)

2. Enteric bacteria replacements: enhance production of lactic acid from carbohydrates in the intestinal lumen; acidity suppresses pathogenic bacterial overgrowth
   a. *Lactobacillus acidophilus*
   b. *Lactobacillus bulgaricus*
3. Motility suppressants: decrease GI tract motility so that more water will be absorbed from the large intestine
   a. Diphenoxylate HCl (Lomotil)
   b. Tincture of opium (paregoric)
   c. Loperamide HCl (Imodium)
C. Major side effects
1. Fluid adsorbents
   a. GI disturbances (local effect)
   b. CNS disturbances (direct CNS toxic effect)
2. Enteric bacteria replacements
   a. Excessive flatulence (increased microbial gas production)
   b. Abdominal cramps (increased microbial gas production)
3. Motility suppressants
   a. Urinary retention (decreased parasympathetic stimulation)
   b. Tachycardia (vagolytic effect on cardiac conduction)
   c. Dry mouth (decreased salivation from anticholinergic effect)
   d. Sedation (CNS depression)
   e. Paralytic ileus (decreased peristalsis)
   f. Respiratory depression (depression of medullary respiratory center)
D. Nursing care
1. Monitor bowel movements (BMs) for color, characteristics, and frequency
2. Assess for fluid/electrolyte imbalance
3. Assess and eliminate cause of diarrhea
4. Motility suppressants
   a. Warn client of risk of physical dependence with long-term use
   b. Offer sugar-free chewing gum and hard candy to promote salivation
   c. May interfere with ability to perform hazardous activities
5. Evaluate client's response to medication and understanding of teaching

Cathartics/Laxatives

A. Description
1. Used to alleviate or prevent constipation
2. Act by various mechanisms to promote evacuation of a normal stool
3. Available in oral and rectal preparations
B. Examples
1. Intestinal lubricants: decrease dehydration of feces; lubricate intestinal tract

a. Mineral oil
b. Olive oil
2. Fecal softeners: lower surface tension of feces in colon; allow water and fats to penetrate feces
   Dioctyl sodium sulfosuccinate (Colace)
3. Bulk-forming laxatives: increase bulk in intestinal lumen, which stimulates propulsive movements by pressure on mucosal lining
   a. Methylcellulose
   b. Psyllium hydrophilic mucilloid (Metamucil)
4. Colon irritants: stimulate peristalsis by reflexive response to irritation of intestinal lumen
   a. Bisacodyl (Dulcolax)
   b. Cascara sagrada
   c. Castor oil
   d. Senna (Senokot)
5. Saline cathartics: increase osmotic pressure within intestine, drawing fluid from blood and bowel wall, thus increasing bulk and stimulating peristalsis
   a. Effervescent sodium phosphate (Fleet Phospho-Soda)
   b. Magnesium citrate solution
   c. Magnesium sulfate (Epsom salts)
   d. Milk of magnesia
C. Major side effects
1. Laxative dependence with long-term use (loss of normal defecation mechanism)
2. GI disturbances (local effect)
3. Intestinal lubricants
   a. Inhibited absorption of fat-soluble vitamins (coat the GI mucosa prohibiting absorption of vitamins A, D, E, K)
   b. Anal leaking of oil (accumulation of lubricant near rectal sphincter)
4. Saline cathartics
   a. Dehydration (fluid volume depletion due to hypertonic state in GI tract)
   b. Hypernatremia (increased sodium absorption into circulation; loss of some fluid from vasculature)
D. Nursing care
1. Instruct the client regarding:
   a. Overuse of cathartics and intestinal lubricants
   b. Increasing intake of fluids and dietary fiber
   c. Increasing activity level
   d. Compliance with bowel-retraining program
2. Monitor BMs for consistency and frequency of stool
3. Intestinal lubricants: utilize peripad to protect clothing
4. Bulk-forming laxatives: mix thoroughly in 240 ml of fluid and follow with another 240 ml of fluid to prevent obstruction

5. Administer at bedtime to promote defecation in the morning
6. Evaluate client's response to medication and understanding of teaching

Intestinal Antibiotics

See Aminoglycosides in Pharmacologic Control of Infection

Pancreatic Enzymes

A. Description
1. Used to promote the digestion of proteins, fats, and starches
2. Act as replacements for natural endogenous pancreatic enzymes (protease, lipase, amylase)
3. Available in oral preparations
B. Examples
1. Pancreatin (Viokase)
2. Pancrelipase (Cotazym)
C. Major side effects
1. Nausea (GI irritation)
2. Diarrhea (GI irritation)
D. Nursing care
1. Administer with meals; teach client to take with meals
2. Avoid crushing preparations that are enteric coated
3. Provide a balanced diet to prevent indigestion
4. Evaluate client's response to medication and understanding of teaching

PROCEDURES RELATED TO THE GASTROINTESTINAL SYSTEM

Barium Enema

A. Definition: introduction of barium, an opaque medium, into the intestines for the purpose of x-ray visualization for pathologic changes
B. Nursing care
1. Explain procedure to the client
2. Prepare the client for the procedure by:
   a. Administering cathartics and/or enemas as ordered to evacuate the bowel
   b. Maintaining the client NPO for 8 to 10 hours prior to the test
3. Inspect stool after the procedure for the presence of barium
4. Administer enemas and/or cathartics as ordered if the stool does not return to normal
5. Encourage fluid intake
6. Evaluate client's response to procedure

Colostomy Irrigation and Care

A. Definition
1. Instillation of fluid into the lower colon via a stoma on the abdominal wall to stimulate peristalsis and facilitate the expulsion of feces

2. Cleansing the colostomy stoma and collection of feces (stool consistency will depend on location of the ostomy: a colostomy of the sigmoid colon will tend to produce formed stools; a transverse or ascending colostomy will produce less formed stools)
B. Nursing care
1. Secure a physician's order
2. Irrigate the stoma at the same time each day to approximate normal bowel habits
3. Insert a well-lubricated catheter tip into the stoma approximately 7 cm in the direction of the remaining bowel (anatomy of ascending, transverse, and descending colon should be considered); as the solution is allowed to flow, the catheter may be advanced
4. Hold the irrigating container 30 to 45 cm above the colostomy; irrigating solution should be 40.5° C
5. Clamp tubing or temporarily lower the container if the client complains of cramping
6. Provide privacy while waiting for fecal returns or permit the client to ambulate with the collection bag in place to further stimulate peristalsis
7. Cleanse the stoma; if excoriation occurs, a soothing ointment may be ordered
8. Apply a colostomy bag or gauze dressing (if the colostomy is well regulated)
9. Teach the client to control odor when necessary by placing two aspirin tablets (or commercially available deodorizers) in the colostomy bag or by taking bismuth subcarbonate tablets orally to control odor
10. Evaluate client's response to procedure

Endoscopy

A. Definition: visualization of the esophagus, stomach, colon, or rectum using a hollow tube with a lighted end
1. Gastroscopy: stomach
2. Esophagoscopy: esophagus
3. Sigmoidoscopy: sigmoid colon
4. Proctoscopy: rectum
B. Nursing care
1. Obtain an informed consent for the procedure
2. If rectal examination is indicated, administer cleansing enemas prior to the test
3. Restrict diet (NPO) prior to procedure
4. Following the procedure, observe for bleeding, changes in vital signs, or nausea
5. If the throat is anesthetized (as for a gastroscopy or esophagoscopy), check for the return of gag reflex before offering oral fluids
6. Evaluate client's response to procedure

Enemas

A. Definitions
1. Tap-water enema (TWE): introduction of water into the colon to stimulate evacuation
2. Soapsuds enema (SSE): introduction of soapy water into the colon to stimulate peristalsis by bowel irritation; contraindicated as a preparation for an endoscopic procedure because it may alter the appearance of the mucosa
3. Hypertonic enema: commercially prepared small-volume enema that works on the principle of osmosis
4. Harris flush or drip: introduction of water into the colon as tolerated and subsequent repeated drainage of that water through the same tubing to facilitate passage of flatus
5. High colonic irrigation: introduction of water into the upper portion of the colon to facilitate complete fecal evacuation
6. Instillation: introduction of a liquid (usually mineral oil) into the colon to facilitate fecal activity through lubricating effect
B. Nursing care
1. Explain procedure to client
2. Provide privacy
3. Obtain the correct solution
4. Lubricate the tip of a rectal catheter with water-soluble jelly
5. Insert the catheter 10 to 15 cm into the rectum
6. Allow the solution to enter slowly; keep it no more than 30 to 45 cm above the rectum
7. Allow ample time for the client to expel the enema
8. Observe and record the amount and consistency of returns
9. Evaluate client's response to procedure

Gastric Analysis

A. Definition
1. Analysis of stomach contents for the presence of abnormal constituents or lack of normal constituents such as hydrochloric acid, blood, acid-fast bacteria, and lactic acid
2. Acid content is elevated in ulcers, decreased in malignant conditions of the stomach, and absent in pernicious anemia
B. Nursing care
1. Explain procedure to client
2. Maintain the client NPO prior to the test and have a nasogastric tube passed at time of procedure
3. Administer histamine or caffeine to stimulate hydrochloric acid secretion prior to the procedure if ordered

4. Obtain stomach contents, secure in an appropriate container, and send to laboratory
5. Evaluate client's response to procedure

Gastrointestinal (GI) Series

A. Definition: introduction of barium, an opaque medium, into the upper GI tract via the mouth, gastrostomy tube, or nasogastric tube to visualize the area by x-ray methods
B. Nursing care
   1. Explain procedure to client
   2. Maintain the client NPO after midnight
   3. Inform client that the stool will be white or pink for 24 to 72 hours after procedure
   4. Encourage fluids and administer cathartics as ordered
   5. Evaluate client's response to procedure

Gavage (Tube Feeding)

A. Definitions
   1. Nasogastric
      a. Placement of a tube through the nose into the stomach, securing it in place with tape
      b. Prepared nutritional supplements are introduced through this tube
   2. Intestinal
      a. Placement of a tube through the nose into the small intestine, securing it in place with tape
      b. There is less likelihood of aspiration because the pyloric sphincter inhibits backflow
   3. Surgically placed feeding tubes
      a. Cervical esophagostomy: tube is sutured directly into the esophagus for clients who have had head and neck surgery
      b. Gastrostomy: tube is placed directly into stomach through the abdominal wall and sutured in place; used for clients who require tube feeding on a long-term basis
      c. Jejunostomy: tube is inserted directly into the jejunum for clients with pathologic conditions of the upper GI tract
   4. Percutaneous endoscopic gastrostomy (PEG)
      a. Stomach is punctured during endoscopy procedure
      b. Does not require general anesthesia or laparotomy
      c. Dressing should be changed daily
      d. Although associated with reduced risks, accidental removal and aspiration still may occur
B. Nursing care
   1. Verify placement of tube prior to feeding
      a. Inject a small amount of air into the tube and, with a stethoscope placed over the epigastric area, listen for the passage of air into the stomach
      b. Aspirate for presence of stomach contents; reinstill to avoid electrolyte imbalance
      c. Test aspirate for acid pH
      d. Small-bore tube placement must be verified by x-ray examination
   2. Aspirate contents of stomach prior to feeding to determine residual; reinstill to avoid electrolyte imbalance; withhold feeding if the residual is greater than 150 ml
   3. Intermittent feeding
      a. Position the client so that the head is elevated during and for 1 hour after the feeding
      b. Appropriately verify placement of tube
      c. Introduce a small amount of water (30 ml) first to verify the patency of the tube; the tube should not be allowed to empty during feeding so that excess air is not forced into the stomach
      d. Slowly administer the feeding at room or body temperature; observe and question the client to determine tolerance; the higher the feeding container and the larger the lumen of the feeding tube, the more rapid the flow
      e. Administer a small amount of water to clear the tube at the completion of the feeding
      f. Clamp the tubing and clean the equipment
      g. Place client in sitting position for 1 hour after feeding
   4. Continuous feeding
      a. Place prescribed feeding in gavage bag and prime tubing to prevent excess air from entering stomach
      b. Set rate of flow; rate of flow can be manually regulated by setting drops per minute or mechanically regulated by using an electric pump
      c. Position the client to keep the head elevated throughout the feeding
      d. Appropriately verify placement of tube when adding additional fluid to a continuous feeding
      e. Flush tube intermittently with water to prevent occlusion of tube with feeding
      f. Monitor for gastric distention and aspiration; since smaller amounts of feeding are generally administered within a given period, gastric distention and subsequent aspiration are less frequent
      g. Discard unused fluid that has been in gavage administration bag at room temperature for longer than 4 hours
   5. Care common for all clients receiving tube feedings
      a. Monitor for abdominal distention; changes in bowel sounds

b. Discontinue feeding if nausea and/or vomiting occur

c. Provide oral hygiene

d. When appropriate, encourage the client to chew foods that will stimulate gastric secretions while providing psychologic comfort; chewed food may not be swallowed

e. Provide special skin care; if the client has a gastrostomy tube sutured in place, the skin may become irritated from gastrointestinal enzymes; if the client has a nasogastric tube, the skin may become excoriated at point of entry because of irritation

f. Evaluate client's response to the procedure

Ileostomy Care

A. Definition: physical care of the ileostomy stoma and surrounding skin

B. Nursing care

1. Protect the skin from irritation, since the feces will be liquid because of the anatomic location of the stoma

2. Explain procedure to the client and family and encourage self-care

3. Do not irrigate the stoma

4. Affix an appliance with an adequate seal (e.g., karaya) to prevent accidental leakage around the stoma; the appliance is generally changed every 2 to 4 days but emptied every 6 hours

5. Evaluate client's response to procedure

Irrigation of Nasogastric (Levin) Tube

A. Definition

1. The Levin tube is commonly used for gastric decompression

2. Purposes of insertion of a nasogastric tube include emptying the stomach, obtaining a specimen for diagnostic purposes, or providing a means for nourishment

3. Irrigation is the insertion and then removal of fluid (usually normal saline) to maintain patency

B. Nursing care

1. Check that the order for irrigations has been written by the physician

2. Ascertain the patency of the Levin tube attached to intermittent suction by observing for drainage; nausea or abdominal discomfort may indicate that the tube is occluded

3. Assemble equipment: 30-ml syringe or bulb syringe, irrigating solution, and basin for returning fluid

4. Verify placement (see gavage)

5. Instill approximately 30 ml of fluid into the tube

6. Gently withdraw the same volume of fluid as was instilled; if the client has undergone gastric surgery, the physician will generally order instillations; in this case, irrigation fluid is instilled but not withdrawn; the amount instilled must be subtracted from total gastric output

7. Chart the amount, color, and consistency of drainage

8. Evaluate client's response to procedure

Paracentesis

A. Definition: surgical puncture of the peritoneal membrane of the abdominal cavity for the purpose of removing fluid

B. Nursing care

1. Explain the procedure; obtain consent

2. Have the client void prior to procedure to avoid accidental trauma to the bladder

3. Assist the client to a sitting position

4. Observe for signs of shock; sudden fluid shifts can result in hypotension

5. Chart the amount and characteristics of fluid withdrawn

6. Apply a dry sterile dressing to the puncture site

7. Properly label the specimen if required and send to the laboratory

8. Evaluate client's response to the procedure

Parenteral Replacement Therapy

A. Definitions

1. Peripheral parenteral nutrition (PPN)

a. Administration of isotonic lipid and amino acid solutions through a peripheral vein

b. Amino acid content should not exceed 4%; dextrose content should not be greater than 10%

c. Assists in maintaining a positive nitrogen balance

2. Total parenteral nutrition (TPN)

a. Administration of carbohydrates, amino acids, vitamins, and minerals via a central vein (usually the superior vena cava)

b. High osmolality solutions (25% dextrose) are administered in conjunction with 5% to 10% amino acids, electrolytes, minerals, and vitamins

c. Assists in maintaining a positive nitrogen balance

3. Intralipid therapy

a. Infusion of 10% to 20% fat emulsion that provides essential fatty acids

b. Provides increased caloric intake to maintain positive nitrogen balance

4. Total nutrient admixture (TNA or "3 in 1")

a. Combination of dextrose, amino acids and lipids in one container; vitamins and minerals may be added

b. Administered through a central line over 24 hours

B. Nursing care
1. Infuse fluid through a large vein such as the subclavian because of the high osmolarity of the solution used in TPN
2. Ensure proper placement of the tube by chest x-ray examination after insertion of a catheter; accidental pneumothorax can occur during insertion
3. Precisely regulate the fluid infusion rate; an intravenous pump should be used if available
   a. Rapid infusion may result in movement of the fluid into the intravascular compartment; dehydration, circulatory overload, and hyperglycemia can occur
   b. Slow infusion may result in hypoglycemia, since the body adapts to the high osmolarity of this fluid by secreting more insulin; for this reason, therapy is never terminated abruptly but is gradually discontinued
4. Use aseptic technique when handling the infusion or changing the dressing (in many institutions, only nurses specially prepared are allowed to change the dressing because of the high risk of infection)
5. Consult manufacturer's instructions about tubing when administering lipids
6. Utilize a filter for TPN; filters cannot be used for lipids
7. Use surgically aseptic technique when changing tubing
8. Record daily weights, and monitor urinary sugar and acetone or blood glucose levels frequently
9. Check laboratory reports daily, especially glucose, creatine, BUN, and electrolytes; serum lipids and liver function studies if lipids are administered
10. Monitor temperature every four hours since infection is the most common complication of TPN; if the client has a temperature elevation, order cultures of blood, urine, and sputum to rule out other sources of infection
11. Evaluate client's response to procedure

Stool Specimens

A. Definitions
1. Stool for guaiac (occult blood): specimen or smear of stool on a commercially prepared card is analyzed for the presence of blood; positive results indicate the presence of blood in the stool and may suggest diverse diseases such as peptic ulcer, gastritis, gastric or colonic carcinoma, colitis, or diverticulitis

2. Stools for O and P (ova and parasites): must be sent to the laboratory while still warm for microscopic examination unless a preservative is available
3. Stool culture: specimen or swab of stool is sent in a sterile container for identification of abnormal bacterial growth

B. Nursing care
1. Explain procedure to the client
2. Collect specimen in an appropriate container
3. Label the container with the client's name, identification number, physician, and room number
4. Chart that the specimen was sent and any unusual assessment of the stool

GENERAL NURSING DIAGNOSES FOR CLIENTS WITH GASTROINTESTINAL SYSTEM DISORDERS

A. Activity intolerance related to malaise
B. Anxiety related to:
1. Prognosis
2. Pain
C. Risk for aspiration related to:
1. Interference with swallowing
2. Wired jaws
3. Gastrointestinal tube feedings
D. Body image disturbance related to:
1. Disease process (fluid retention or malnutrition)
2. Alterations in structure or function because of surgical intervention
E. Bowel incontinence related to impaired sphincter control
F. Colonic constipation related to less than adequate fiber/fluid intake
G. Constipation related to:
1. Dietary habits
2. Inadequate intake of fluids
3. Inactivity
4. Obstruction
5. Fear of pain when defecating
6. Absence of motility
H. Diarrhea related to:
1. Local inflammatory process
2. Anxiety
3. Food intolerance
4. Contaminated foods
I. Risk for fluid volume deficit related to:
1. Hypovolemia
2. Increased intestinal motility
J. Fluid volume excess related to ascites
K. Risk for infection related to altered mucous membranes
L. Risk for injury related to:

1. Hemorrhage
2. Metastasis
3. Strangulation
4. Sensory/perceptual alterations
M. Ineffective management of therapeutic regimen (families) related to:
 1. Complexity of therapeutic regimen
 2. Feelings concerning secretions and/or excretions
N. Ineffective management of therapeutic regimen (individual) related to:
 1. Complexity of therapeutic regimen
 2. Feelings concerning secretions and/or excretions
O. Altered nutrition: less than body requirements related to:
 1. Anorexia
 2. Inability to ingest
 3. Malabsorption
 4. Changes in metabolism
 5. Therapeutic nothing-by-mouth status
 6. Nausea
P. Altered nutrition: risk for more than body requirements related to excess ingestion
Q. Altered oral mucous membrane related to chemical and/or microbiologic irritants
R. Pain related to:
 1. Pathologic processes
 2. Diagnostic procedures
 3. Therapeutic modalities
S. Impaired skin integrity related to:
 1. Pruritis
 2. Irritation by intestinal drainage
T. Social isolation related to:
 1. Disfiguring surgery
 2. Risk of transmission
U. Impaired swallowing related to obstruction in oropharyngeal and/or esophageal structures
V. Risk for trauma related to mechanical devices used for irrigation

MAJOR DISORDERS OF THE GASTROINTESTINAL SYSTEM

▼ STOMATITIS

Data Base
A. Etiology and pathophysiology
 1. Inflammation of the buccal mucosa because of disease, trauma, irritants, nutritional deficiencies, or medications
 2. Categories
  a. Aphthous stomatitis: canker sore that can result from chronic cheek biting
  b. Herpes simplex: virus that causes vesicle formation in mouth, on lips, or on nose
  c. Vincent's angina: ulceration of the buccal membrane due to *Borrelia vincentii* (trench mouth)
  d. Thrush: fungal invasion of the mouth by *Candida albicans*, characterized by white patches
B. Clinical findings
 1. Subjective
  a. Foul taste in the mouth
  b. Pain in the mouth
 2. Objective
  a. Erythema of the mucous membranes
  b. Changes in salivation
  c. Unpleasant odor to the breath
  d. Bleeding gums in Vincent's angina
  e. White patches in thrush
C. Therapeutic interventions
 1. Adequate nutrition and hydration
 2. Alkaline mouthwashes
 3. Antifungal agents for thrush
 4. Antibiotics for Vincent's angina
 5. Viscous xylocaine

Nursing Care of Clients with Stomatitis
A. DATA COLLECTION
 1. Size and shape of, and color and amount of, drainage from oral lesions
 2. Presence of fever, malaise, nausea, and vomiting
B. ANALYSIS AND INTERPRETATION
 Refer to General Nursing Diagnoses for Clients with Gastrointestinal System Disorders for the following diagnoses: K, O 2, Q, and R 1
C. PLANNING/IMPLEMENTATION
 1. Administer medications as ordered
 2. Provide mouthwashes every 2 hours
 3. Encourage foods that can be tolerated, such as soft foods, cool drinks, eggnogs; utilize nutritional supplements
 4. Promote oral hygiene; use soft toothbrush or padded tongue blade
D. EVALUATION/OUTCOMES
 1. Adheres to oral hygiene regimen
 2. States pain is relieved
 3. Maintains nutritional status through balanced diet

▼ FRACTURE OF THE JAW

Data Base
A. Etiology and pathophysiology: generally the result of trauma such as motor vehicle accidents or physical combat
B. Clinical findings
 1. Subjective

a. History of trauma to the face
b. Pain in the face and jaw
2. Objective
a. Bloody discharge from the mouth
b. Swelling of face on the affected side
c. Difficulty opening or closing the mouth
C. Therapeutic interventions
1. Separated fragments of the broken bone are reunited and immobilized by wires and rubber bands; usually placed without surgical incision
2. Open reduction of the jaw is indicated for severely fractured or displaced bones; interosseous wiring is done

Nursing Care of Clients with Fracture of the Jaw

A. DATA COLLECTION

1. Respiratory status for presence of distress
2. Presence of nausea and potential for vomiting
3. Structures of the face and neck for signs of edema

B. ANALYSIS AND INTERPRETATION

Refer to General Nursing Diagnoses for Clients with Gastrointestinal System Disorders for the following diagnoses: C 2, K, and O 2

C. PLANNING/IMPLEMENTATION

1. Postoperatively control vomiting and reduce the chance of aspiration pneumonia by positioning client on abdomen or side
2. Keep wire cutters at the bedside to release the wires and rubber bands if emesis occurs and aspiration cannot be prevented by suctioning
3. Explain diet to the client and family; no solid foods are permitted; encourage high-protein liquids or blenderized soft foods
4. Stress the importance of regular oral hygiene and institute it early in the postoperative period

D. EVALUATION/OUTCOMES

1. Remains free from nausea and vomiting
2. Adheres to nutritionally balanced safe diet
3. Demonstrates oral hygiene techniques
4. Describes technique for releasing wires and rubber bands if emesis occurs

▼ CANCER OF THE ORAL CAVITY

Data Base

A. Etiology and pathophysiology
1. Primarily in clients who smoke and drink alcohol in large quantities
2. Cancer of the lip, easily diagnosed; prognosis is very good; incidence highest in pipe smokers
3. Cancer of the tongue, usually occurs with cancer of the floor of the mouth; metastasis to the neck common

4. Cancer of the submaxillary glands, highly malignant and grows rapidly
B. Clinical findings
1. Subjective
a. Pain (not an early symptom)
b. Alterations of taste sensation
2. Objective
a. Leukoplakia (white patches on mucosa), which is considered precancerous
b. Ulcerated, bleeding areas in the involved structure
C. Therapeutic interventions
1. Reconstructive surgery if indicated
2. Radiation or implantation of radioactive material may arrest growth of tumor

Nursing Care of Clients with Cancer of the Oral Cavity

A. DATA COLLECTION

1. History of hemoptysis and pain
2. Baseline nutritional data including weight, dietary intake, and ability to chew
3. Characteristics of lesions in oral cavity

B. ANALYSIS AND INTERPRETATION

Refer to General Nursing Diagnoses for Clients with Gastrointestinal System Disorders for the following diagnoses: B 1, B 2, C 1, D 2, K, L 2, O 2, R 1, T 1, and U

C. PLANNING/IMPLEMENTATION

1. Maintain fluid and electrolyte balance
2. Provide for a means of communication
3. If radiation therapy is indicated, relieve dryness of the mouth by frequent saline mouthwashes and ample fluids
4. Consider time and distance in relation to the radioactive material when giving nursing care

D. EVALUATION/IMPLEMENTATION

1. States pain is relieved
2. Maintains adequate nutrition
3. Discusses feelings of changes in body image
4. Remains free from infection
5. Maintains airway patency

▼ CANCER OF THE ESOPHAGUS

Data Base

A. Etiology and pathophysiology
1. Etiology unknown: occurs predominantly in persons with a history of alcohol abuse or hiatus hernia
2. Tumor may develop anywhere in the esophagus, but most commonly in the middle and lower third
B. Clinical findings
1. Subjective

a. Dysphagia

b. Substernal pain

c. Substernal burning after drinking hot liquids

2. Objective

a. Regurgitation

b. X-ray examination of esophagus reveals irregularities of the lumen

c. Cytologic examination of cells, obtained after esophageal lavage, reveals malignant cells

C. Therapeutic interventions

1. Surgical removal of the esophagus is the treatment of choice

a. Esophagogastrostomy: resection of a portion of the esophagus; a portion of the bowel may be grafted between the esophagus and stomach, or the stomach may be brought up to the proximal end of the esophagus

b. Esophagectomy: removal of part or all of the esophagus, which is replaced by a Dacron graft

c. Gastrostomy: opening directly into the stomach in which a feeding tube is usually inserted to bypass the esophagus

2. Radiation and/or chemotherapy may be used prior to or instead of surgery as a palliative measure

Nursing Care of Clients with Cancer of the Esophagus

A. DATA COLLECTION

1. History of nutritional status and weight loss

2. Presence of pain and dysphagia

3. History of foul breath, eructation, nausea, and vomiting

B. ANALYSIS AND INTERPRETATION

Refer to General Nursing Diagnoses for Clients with Gastrointestinal System Disorders for the following diagnoses: B 1, B 2, L 2, O 2, R 1, T 1, and U

C. PLANNING/IMPLEMENTATION

1. Support the client and family emotionally

2. Formulate realistic goals in planning client care

3. Observe for respiratory distress caused by pressure of tumor on the trachea; place in a semi-Fowler's or high-Fowler's position to facilitate respirations

4. Monitor vital signs, especially respirations

5. Provide oral care, since dysphagia may result in increased accumulation of saliva in mouth

6. Maintain nutritional status by providing high-protein liquids along with vitamin and mineral replacements

D. EVALUATION/OUTCOMES

1. Maintains adequate nutrition

2. Maintains airway

3. States relief from pain

4. Discusses emotional impact of disease

▼ HIATAL HERNIA

Data Base

A. Etiology and pathophysiology

1. Portion of the stomach protruding through a hiatus (opening) in the diaphragm into the thoracic cavity

2. May result from a congenital weakness of the diaphragm or from injury, pregnancy, or obesity

3. Function of the cardiac sphincter is lost, gastric juices enter the esophagus, and edema and hyperemia may result

B. Clinical findings

1. Subjective

a. Substernal burning pain or fullness

b. Heartburn after eating, which increases in the recumbent position

c. Nocturnal dyspnea

2. Objective

a. GI series and endoscopy show protrusion of the stomach through the diaphragm

b. Regurgitation

C. Therapeutic interventions

1. Small, frequent, bland feedings

2. Pharmacologic management

a. Antacids

b. Gastrointestinal antihistamines

c. Antiemetics, especially those that promote gastric emptying

3. Surgical repair (done infrequently)

Nursing Care of Clients with Hiatal Hernia

A. DATA COLLECTION

1. History of heartburn, pain, and reflux

2. Relationship of body position to presence of symptoms

3. Respiratory status

B. ANALYSIS AND INTERPRETATION

Refer to General Nursing Diagnoses for Clients with Gastrointestinal System Disorders for the following diagnoses: Q and R 1

C. PLANNING/IMPLEMENTATION

1. Teach the client and family about the dietary regimen

2. Encourage attempts at weight loss

3. Avoid constricting clothing

4. Elevate head of the bed after meals

5. Encourage the client to eat slowly

6. Encourage the client to avoid drinking fluids with meals to limit the volume in the stomach; drink fluids between meals

D. EVALUATION/OUTCOMES
1. States symptoms of reflux are absent or greatly reduced
2. Remains free from respiratory complications

▼ GASTRITIS

Data Base
A. Etiology and pathophysiology
  1. Inflammation of the stomach; either acute or chronic
  2. May be caused by:
     a. Ingestion of irritating chemicals such as salicylates, steroids, indomethacin, and alcohol
     b. Bacterial or viral infections; *Helicobacter pylori* and *Campylobacter pylori*
     c. Allergic reactions
     d. Chronic uremia, which often leads to chronic gastritis
B. Clinical findings
  1. Subjective
     a. Anorexia
     b. Nausea and vomiting
     c. Epigastric fullness
  2. Objective
     a. Diarrhea and cramps if caused by an infection
     b. Dehydration
     c. Hemorrhage if aspirin or other chemicals are involved
C. Therapeutic interventions
  1. Early treatment aimed at correcting the fluid and electrolyte imbalance; the client is kept NPO during the acute phase of illness and then progresses to a bland diet
  2. If caused by microorganisms, appropriate antibiotics may be given
  3. Other medications that may be prescribed include antispasmodics, anticholinergics, antiemetics, gastrointestinal antihistamines, and antacids

Nursing Care of Clients with Gastritis
A. DATA COLLECTION
1. Characteristics of pain and relationship to types of food ingested and time food is consumed
2. Abdomen for epigastric tenderness, increased bowel sounds, and guarding
3. History of dietary patterns, foods ingested, and alcohol consumption

B. ANALYSIS AND INTERPRETATION
Refer to General Nursing Diagnoses for Clients with Gastrointestinal System Disorders for the following diagnoses: B 2, O 1, and R 1

C. PLANNING/IMPLEMENTATION
1. Observe for signs of dehydration and electrolyte imbalance
2. Provide adequate fluid intake
3. Alert the client to possible causes
4. Teach the client the necessary dietary alterations, such as maintaining a bland diet and the omission of coffee, alcohol, and spices

D. EVALUATION/OUTCOMES
1. States pain is reduced or absent
2. Maintains adequate weight, nutritional status, and fluid volume
3. Describes and complies with treatment plan

▼ PEPTIC ULCER DISEASE (PUD)

Data Base
A. Etiology and pathophysiology
  1. Ulcerations of the gastrointestinal mucosa and underlying tissues caused by gastric secretions that have a low pH (acid)
  2. Causes include conditions that increase the secretion of hydrochloric acid by the gastric mucosa or that decrease that tissue's resistance to the acid
     a. Infection of the gastric and/or duodenal mucosa by *Campylobacter pylori* or *Helicobacter pylori*
     b. Zollinger-Ellison syndrome: tumors secreting gastrin, which will stimulate the production of excessive hydrochloric acid
     c. Certain drugs such as aspirin, steroids, and indomethacin will decrease tissue resistance
     d. Smoking is a risk factor
     e. Although very controversial, some still believe that emotional factors are related to peptic ulcers; a person who is considered a perfectionist may have an increased risk of developing a peptic ulcer
  3. Peptic ulcers may be present in the esophagus, stomach, or duodenum (the most common site)
  4. Complications include pyloric or duodenal obstruction, hemorrhage, and perforation
B. Clinical findings
  1. Subjective
     a. Gnawing or burning epigastric pain that occurs 1 to 2 hours after eating and may be relieved by eructation, vomiting, food, or antacids
     b. Nausea

2. Objective
   a. If bleeding occurs, signs of anemia will be evident; passage of tarry stools (melena) may occur
   b. Vomiting (the color of coffee grounds to port wine if bleeding has occurred)
C. Therapeutic interventions
   1. Institute measures to neutralize or buffer hydrochloric acid, inhibit acid secretion, and decrease the activity of pepsin and hydrochloric acid, such as:
      a. Radiation and gastric hypothermia to suppress gastric secretions
      b. Antacids to reduce acidity
      c. Diet regulation through the use of bland foods, and restriction of irritating substances such as nicotine, caffeine, alcohol, spices, and gassy foods
   2. Type and cross-match so that blood will be available if gastric hemorrhage occurs
   3. Sedatives, tranquilizers, anticholinergics, and analgesics for pain and restlessness
   4. Histamine H_2 receptor antagonist to limit gastric acid secretion
   5. Antiemetics for nausea and vomiting
   6. Antibiotic therapy if microorganism is identified; tetracycline, metronidazole, and bismuth
   7. Bed rest to reduce physical activity
   8. Counseling or psychotherapy to explore the emotional components of the illness
   9. If hemorrhage occurs, a nasogastric tube is inserted and saline lavages may be ordered; irrigations with medications that cause vasoconstriction to control bleeding are also used
   10. Surgical intervention
       a. Vagotomy: cutting the vagus nerve (X), which innervates the stomach, to decrease the secretion of hydrochloric acid
       b. Billroth I: removal of the lower portion of the stomach and attachment of the remaining portion to the duodenum
       c. Billroth II: removal of the antrum and distal portion of the stomach and subsequent anastomosis of remaining section to the jejunum
       d. Antrectomy: removal of the antral portion of the stomach
       e. Gastrectomy: removal of 60% to 80% of the stomach
       f. Common complications of partial or total gastric resection
          (1) Dumping syndrome: involves the rapid passage of food from the stomach to the jejunum; the food, being hypertonic (especially if high in carbohydrates), will draw fluid from the circulating blood into the jejunum causing diaphoresis, faintness, and palpitations
          (2) Hemorrhage
          (3) Pneumonia
          (4) Pernicious anemia

Nursing Care of Clients with Peptic Ulcer Disease

A. DATA COLLECTION

See Assessment under Nursing Care of Clients with Gastritis

B. ANALYSIS AND INTERPRETATION

Refer to General Nursing Diagnoses for Clients with Gastrointestinal System Disorders for the following diagnoses: B 2, I 1, L 1, O 1, and R 1

C. PLANNING/IMPLEMENTATION

1. Allow ample time for the client to express feelings and concerns
2. Administer and assess effects of sedatives, antacids, anticholinergics, H_2 receptor antagonists, antibiotics, and dietary modifications
3. Encourage hydration to reduce anticholinergic side effects and dilute the hydrochloric acid in the stomach
4. Instruct client to:
   a. Eat small to medium-sized meals because this helps prevent gastric distention; encourage between-meal snacks to achieve adequate calories when necessary
   b. Avoid foods that increase gastric acid secretion or irritate gastric mucosa, such as alcohol, caffeine-containing foods and beverages, decaffeinated coffee, red or black pepper; replace with decaffeinated soft drinks and teas; use seasonings like thyme, basil, sage, etc., to replace pepper
   c. Avoid foods that cause distress; varies for individuals but common offenders are the gas producers (legumes, carbonated beverages, the cruciferous vegetables)
   d. Eat meals in pleasant, relaxing surroundings to reduce acid secretion
   e. Administer calcium and iron supplements as ordered if client's medication increases gastric pH
5. Refrain from administering drugs such as salicylates, phenylbutazone, steroids, and ACTH, which are normally contraindicated
6. Observe for complications such as gastric hemorrhage, perforation, and drug toxicity
7. Provide postoperative care after gastric resection
   a. Monitor vital signs; assess the dressing for drainage
   b. Maintain a patent nasogastric tube to the suction apparatus to prevent stress on the suture line

c. Observe the color and amount of nasogastric drainage; excessive bleeding or the presence of bright red blood after 12 hours should be reported immediately
d. Have the client cough, deep breathe, and change position frequently to prevent the occurrence of pulmonary complications
e. Monitor intake and output
f. Apply antiembolism stockings; have the client ambulate early to prevent vascular complications
g. To prevent dumping syndrome, instruct the client to:
   (1) Eat smaller meals at more frequent intervals
   (2) Avoid high-carbohydrate intake
   (3) Consume liquids only between meals (at least 1 hour before or after meals)
   (4) Lie down or rest after eating
   (5) In severe cases, pectin or guar gum (5-g dose) may be prescribed with meals; these water-soluble fibers delay gastric emptying and absorption of carbohydrates
8. Teach drug regimen and signs and symptoms of recurrence
9. Prevent recurrence by teaching client to modify dietary, working, and living patterns; maintain regularity in activities of daily living; continue medical supervision

D. EVALUATION/OUTCOMES
1. States pain is reduced or relieved
2. Identifies signs of hemorrhage and need for immediate medical care
3. Follows a nutritionally sound diet
4. Discusses feelings
5. Identifies strategies to cope with stress

▼ CANCER OF THE STOMACH

Data Base
A. Etiology and pathophysiology
   1. Often not diagnosed until metastasis occurs; the stomach is able to accommodate to the growth of a tumor, and pain occurs late in the disease
   2. May metastasize by direct extension, lymphatics, or blood to the esophagus, spleen, pancreas, liver, or bone
   3. Heredity apparently a factor in the development of carcinoma of the stomach, as is the presence of precursors such as ulcerative disease and pernicious anemia
   4. Incidence higher in men more than 40 years of age; Japan has a 4 times greater rate of cancer of the stomach than does the United States

B. Clinical findings
   1. Subjective
      a. Anorexia
      b. Nausea
      c. Belching (eructation)
      d. Heartburn
   2. Objective
      a. Weight loss
      b. Anemia
      c. Positive stools for guaiac (occult blood)
      d. Achlorhydria (absence of hydrochloric acid, determined by gastric analysis)
C. Therapeutic interventions
   1. Subtotal or total gastrectomy
   2. Radiation
   3. Chemotherapy (fluorouracil is often used)

Nursing Care of Clients with Cancer of the Stomach
A. DATA COLLECTION
1. History of causative factors, pain, and weight loss
2. Axillary lymph nodes and left supraclavicular nodes for hard nodes, indicative of metastasis
3. Skin for pallor and acanthosis nigricans, symmetrically distributed hard and soft papillary growths with hyperpigmentation and hyperkeratosis

B. ANALYSIS AND INTERPRETATION
Refer to General Nursing Diagnoses for Clients with Gastrointestinal System Disorders for the following diagnoses: B 1, B 2, I 1, L 1, L 2, O 1, O 3, O 4, and R1

C. PLANNING/IMPLEMENTATION
1. Offer the client every opportunity to verbalize fears (i.e., cancer, death, family problems, self-image)
2. Postoperative care the same as nursing care after a gastric resection (see Peptic Ulcer); in addition, if a total gastrectomy is performed, the chest cavity is usually entered, so the client will have chest tubes (see Pneumothorax for related nursing care)
3. Modify diet to include smaller, more frequent meals (see Peptic Ulcer for more dietary information)
4. If total gastrectomy has been performed, the client will have a vitamin B_{12} deficiency (see Pernicious Anemia)
5. Client may require gavage feedings via nasogastric tube or gastrostomy tube (see Gavage procedure)

D. EVALUATION/OUTCOMES
1. States relief from discomfort and pain
2. Maintains adequate nutritional status
3. Follows medical regimen
4. Verbalizes feelings related to prognosis

▼ CHOLELITHIASIS/CHOLECYSTITIS

Data Base

A. Etiology and pathophysiology
1. Inflammation of the gallbladder; usually caused by the presence of stones (cholelithiasis), which are composed of cholesterol, bile pigments, and calcium
2. Diseased gallbladder is unable to contract in response to fatty foods entering the duodenum because of obstruction by calculi or edema
3. When the common bile duct is completely obstructed, the bile is unable to pass into the duodenum and is absorbed into the blood
4. Incidence is highest in obese women in the fourth decade

B. Clinical findings
1. Subjective
   a. Indigestion after eating fatty or fried foods
   b. Pain, usually in the right upper quadrant of the abdomen, which may radiate to the back
   c. Nausea
2. Objective
   a. Vomiting
   b. Elevated temperature and WBC
   c. Jaundice
   d. Diagnostic tests
      (1) Serum bilirubin will be elevated
      (2) Ultrasonography to determine the presence of gallstones
      (3) Gallbladder series; approximately six radiopaque tablets such as Telepaque or Bilopaque are taken with water the evening before so that the gallbladder will be visible on x-ray examination; this test may be done if the ultrasonography is inconclusive
      (4) Intravenous cholangiogram; clients who are allergic to the dye will complain of sensation of warmth, urticaria, nausea, and vomiting

C. Therapeutic interventions
1. Medical management
   a. Rest
   b. Nasogastric suctioning to reduce nausea and eliminate vomiting
   c. Narcotics to decrease pain
   d. Antispasmodics and anticholinergics to reduce spasms and contractions of the gallbladder
   e. Antibiotic therapy if infection is suspected
   f. In cases where clients are poor surgical risks, ursodeoxycholic acid (Ursofalk) is taken orally over a period of 6- 12 months to dissolve radiolucent cholesterol stones, particularly if they are small

   g. Lithotripsy: ultrasonic soundwaves fragment stones to enable their passage without surgical intervention
   h. Low-fat diet to avoid stimulating the gallbladder, which constricts to excrete bile with subsequent pain; calories principally from carbohydrate foods in acute phases; if weight loss is indicated, calories may be reduced to 1000 to 1200; postoperatively clients may take fat-restricted diets initially but progress to regular diets
2. Surgical intervention
   a. Cholecystotomy: incision into the gallbladder for the purpose of drainage
   b. Abdominal cholecystectomy: removal of the gallbladder through an abdominal incision
   c. Laparoscopic cholecystectomy: removal of the gallbladder through an endoscope inserted through the abdominal wall; also called endoscopic laser cholecystectomy (not used if infection is present)
   d. Choledochotomy: incision into the common bile duct for removal of stones

Nursing Care of Clients with Cholelithiasis/Cholecystitis

A. DATA COLLECTION

1. Characteristics of pain
2. Presence of pain in relation to ingestion of foods high in fat
3. Abdomen for rebound tenderness that increases on inspiration (peritoneal inflammation)
4. Stools for color (clay colored) and fat (steatorrhea)

B. ANALYSIS AND INTERPRETATION

Refer to General Nursing Diagnoses for Clients with Gastrointestinal System Disorders for the following diagnoses: B 2, O 6, and R 1

C. PLANNING/IMPLEMENTATION

1. Teach dietary modification to achieve a low-fat intake (about 25% of the kcal), because reduced bile flow will reduce fat absorption; supplementation with water-miscible forms of vitamins A and E may be prescribed
2. Relieve pain both preoperatively and postoperatively
3. Observe for signs of bleeding (vitamin K is fat soluble and is not absorbed in the absence of bile); administer vitamin K preparations as ordered
4. Teach the client receiving ursodeoxycholic acid (Ursofalk) that:
   a. Effects will be monitored every 6 to 12 months by cholecystogram or ultrasonogram
   b. Side effects include hepatotoxicity and diarrhea

5. Provide care following a cholecystectomy
   a. Monitor nasogastric tube attached to suction to prevent distention
      (1) Maintain patency of the tube
      (2) Assess and measure drainage
   b. Provide fluids and electrolytes via intravenous route
      (1) Monitor intake and output
      (2) Check IV site for redness, swelling, heat, or pain
   c. Keep the client in a low-Fowler's position
   d. Have the client cough and deep breathe; splint the incision (incision is high and midline, making coughing extremely uncomfortable)
   e. Provide care for the client with a T-tube (if the common bile duct has been explored, a T-tube is inserted to maintain patency)
      (1) Secure the drainage bag; avoid kinking of the tube
      (2) Measure drainage at least every shift; drainage during the first day may reach 500 to 1000 ml and then gradually decline
      (3) Apply ordered protective ointments around tube to prevent excoriation
      (4) When the tube is removed, usually in 7 days, observe stool for normal brown color, which indicates bile is again entering the duodenum

D. EVALUATION/OUTCOMES
1. Verbalizes decrease in discomfort
2. Maintains adequate fluid volume
3. Discusses feelings

▼ ACUTE PANCREATITIS

Data Base
A. Etiology and pathophysiology
   1. Inflammation of pancreas caused by pancreatic enzymes, primarily trypsin
   2. May result from gallstones, alcoholism, carcinoma, or acute trauma to the pancreas or abdomen
   3. Inflammation with or without edema of pancreatic tissues, suppuration, abscess formation, hemorrhage, or necrosis, depending on the severity of the disease and the cause
B. Clinical findings
   1. Subjective
      a. Abrupt onset of pain in the central epigastric area that may radiate to shoulder, chest, and back described as aching, burning, stabbing, or pressing
      b. Abdominal tenderness
      c. Nausea
      d. Pruritis associated with jaundice
   2. Objective
      a. Elevated temperature
      b. Vomiting
      c. Tachycardia
      d. Changes in character of stools
      e. Abdominal distention
      f. Hypotension
      g. Shock
      h. Jaundice
      i. Grossly elevated serum amylase and lipase
      j. Decreased serum calcium
   3. Severity of symptoms depends on the cause of the problem, the amount of fibrous replacement of normal duct tissue, the degree of autodigestion of the organ, the type of associated biliary disease if present, and the amount of interference in blood supply to the pancreas
   4. Symptoms may be exaggerated by the development of complications such as pseudocysts, abscesses, and pancreatic fistulas that may be assessed by endoscopic retrograde cholangiopancreatography (ERCP)
C. Therapeutic interventions
   1. Antacids to neutralize gastric secretions
   2. Barbiturates and tranquilizers to reduce emotional tension
   3. Narcotics to control pain; morphine is contraindicated because it causes spasms of the sphincter of Oddi
   4. Cardiotonics to lessen strain on the heart caused by increased metabolic demands and altered circulatory volume
   5. Bed rest to decrease metabolic demands and promote healing
   6. Nothing by mouth and nasogastric decompression to control nausea, reduce stimulation of the pancreas to secrete enzymes, and remove gastric hydrochloric acid
   7. Anticholinergics to suppress vagal stimulation and decrease gastric motility and duodenal spasm
   8. Antibiotics to prevent secondary infections and abscess formation
   9. Pancreatic enzymes and bile salts if necessary
   10. Diet regulated according to the client's condition: nothing by mouth; parenteral administration of fluids and electrolytes, total or peripheral parenteral nutrition; diet low in fats and proteins, with restriction of stimulants such as caffeine and alcohol
   11. Surgical intervention if the client fails to respond to medical management, exhibits persistent jaundice, develops a pseudocyst or bleeds; type of surgery is determined by the cause (e.g., biliary tract surgery, removal of gallstones, drainage of cysts)

Nursing Care of Clients with Acute Pancreatitis

A. **DATA COLLECTION**
1. History of causative factors, pain, and recent weight loss
2. Presence of jaundice
3. Abdomen for rigidity and guarding
4. Changes in behavior and sensorium

B. **ANALYSIS AND INTERPRETATION**

Refer to General Nursing Diagnoses for Clients with Gastrointestinal System Disorders for the following diagnoses: B 2, I 1, O 1, O 5, O 6, R 1, and S 1

C. **PLANNING/IMPLEMENTATION**
1. Provide care for a client with a nasogastric tube
   a. Administer frequent, thorough mouth care
   b. Apply lubricant to the external nares to prevent irritation and eventual breakdown of mucous membranes
   c. Observe for electrolyte imbalances (manifested by symptoms such as tetany, irritability, jerking, muscular twitching, mental changes, and psychotic behavior)
   d. Observe for signs of adynamic ileus (e.g., nausea and vomiting, abdominal distention)
2. Be alert for hyperglycemic states
3. Monitor vital signs
4. Administer prescribed analgesics
5. Maintain NPO during the acute stage of illness
6. Use the semi-Fowler's position and encourage deep breathing and coughing to promote deeper respiration and prevent respiratory problems
7. Closely monitor IV feedings until oral feedings can be tolerated
8. Teach dietary modifications as required by the client's condition, usually starting with small feedings of low-fat, non–gas-producing liquids and progressing to a more liberalized diet that is low in fat but high in protein and carbohydrates; if fat malabsorption is severe, vitamins A and E may be necessary; daily supplements of calcium and zinc may also be needed; if insulin secretion is impaired, a Canadian Diabetes Association (CDA) diet is indicated (see Diabetes Mellitus for details)
9. Teach importance of taking medication containing pancreatic enzymes (amylase, lipase, trypsin, etc.) with each meal to improve digestion of food if the disease becomes chronic
10. Encourage the adoption of a life-style that allows for emotional stability, rest, follow-up medical care
11. Teach the client and family the importance of dietary discretion, especially the avoidance of alcohol, coffee, spicy foods, and heavy meals, while recognizing religious and cultural factors
12. Help the client set realistic goals for convalescent period
13. Teach the client and family about prevention of recurrences and/or control of symptoms (e.g., diet therapy, drug therapy, avoiding foods and substances such as alcohol and caffeine, regular medical supervision, rest requirements)

D. **EVALUATION/OUTCOMES**
1. Reports decrease in discomfort
2. Maintains adequate nutritional status
3. Lists the treatment strategies and need for follow-up care
4. Identifies and avoids precipitating foods and liquids

▼ CANCER OF THE PANCREAS

Data Base

A. Etiology and pathophysiology
1. Malignant growth from the epithelium of the ductal system producing cells that block the ducts of the pancreas
2. Fibrosis, pancreatitis, and obstruction of the pancreas
3. Lesion tends to metastasize by direct extension to the duodenal wall, splenic flexure of the colon, posterior stomach wall, and common bile duct
4. Cause unknown; heredity, environmental toxins, alcohol, a high-fat diet, and smoking are associated with increased incidence
5. History of chronic pancreatitis, diabetes mellitus, and alcoholism is common
6. More common in middle-aged men than women

B. Clinical findings
1. Subjective
   a. Anxiety, depression, anorexia, and nausea
   b. Severe pain present in most clients
   c. Pruritis associated with jaundice
2. Objective
   a. Jaundice
   b. Weight loss
   c. Diarrhea and steatorrhea, along with clay-colored stools and dark urine
   d. In later stages usually demonstrates presence of a right upper quadrant mass
   e. Decreased serum amylase and lipase levels due to decreased secretion of enzymes
   f. Increased serum bilirubin and alkaline phosphatase levels when biliary ducts are obstructed
   g. Ascites may develop

C. Therapeutic interventions
1. Preparation for surgical intervention by ordering red blood cell and blood volume replacement and medications to correct coagulation problems and nutritional deficiencies
2. Chemotherapy and radiation when surgery is not possible or desired to provide comfort, or in conjunction with surgery to limit metastasis
3. Medications to control diabetes if present
4. Drug therapy such as pancreatic enzymes, bile salts, and vitamin K to correct deficiencies
5. Analgesics and tranquilizers for pain
6. Surgery (the treatment of choice, although the postsurgical prognosis is grim): Whipple's procedure (removal of the head of the pancreas, the duodenum, a portion of the stomach, and the common bile duct) or a cholecystojejunostomy (creation of an opening between the gallbladder and jejunum)

Nursing Care of Clients with Cancer of the Pancreas

A. DATA COLLECTION

1. Presence of jaundice
2. Stool for clay-color
3. Urine for characteristics of dark-amber color and frothy appearance
4. Abdomen for enlargement of liver and gallbladder
5. Characteristics of pain
6. History of anorexia, nausea, and weight loss
7. Abdominal dullness on percussion indicating early ascites

B. ANALYSIS AND INTERPRETATION

Refer to General Nursing Diagnoses for Clients with Gastrointestinal System Disorders for the following diagnoses: A, B 1, B 2, I 1, J, L 1, L 2, O 1, O 3, O 6, R 1, and S 1

C. PLANNING/IMPLEMENTATION

1. Provide emotional support for the client and family, and set realistic goals in planning care
2. Administer analgesics as ordered, and as soon as needed, to promote rest and comfort
3. Use soapless bathing and antipruritic agents to relieve pruritus
4. Observe for complications such as peritonitis, gastrointestinal obstruction, jaundice, hyperglycemia, and hypotension
5. Observe the stools for undigested fat
6. Frequently monitor the vital signs, observing for wound hemorrhage caused by coagulation deficiency
7. Administer vitamin K parenterally as ordered
8. Encourage coughing, turning, and deep breathing
9. Monitor urinary output

10. Observe for chemotherapeutic and radiation side effects (e.g., skin irritation, anorexia, nausea, vomiting)
11. Maintain skin markings for radiation therapy
12. Support natural defense mechanisms of the client by encouraging frequent and supplemental feedings of high nutrient density foods as tolerated; stress the immune-stimulating nutrients, especially vitamins A, C, and E, and the mineral selenium
13. Control nausea and vomiting before feedings, if possible
14. Administer vitamin supplements, bile salts, and pancreatic enzymes, as ordered
15. Provide oral hygiene and maintain an esthetic environment, especially at mealtime

D. EVALUATION/OUTCOMES

1. States that pain is controlled
2. Maintains adequate nutritional status
3. States a reduction in pruritis
4. Discusses feelings and concerns
5. Adheres to medical regimen

▼ HEPATITIS

Data Base

A. Etiology and pathophysiology
1. Type A hepatitis (infectious hepatitis)
   a. Caused by type A hepatitis virus (HAV)
   b. Transmitted via fecal-oral route, contact with blood, or contaminated food (e.g., shellfish)
   c. Excreted in large quantities in feces 2 weeks before and 1 week after the onset of symptoms
   d. Incubation period is 30 to 40 days
   e. Confers immunity on individual
   f. Serum studies reveal anti–HAV-IgM (current infection) or anti–HAV-IgG (resolved infection)
2. Type B hepatitis (serum hepatitis)
   a. Caused by type B hepatitis virus (HBV)
   b. Transmitted by:
      (1) Contaminated blood products or articles (e.g., toothbrush, razor, needle)
      (2) Other body secretions (e.g., saliva, semen, urine)
      (3) Introduction of infectious material into eye, oral cavity, lacerations, or vagina
      (4) Contaminated needles
         (a) During administration of medication
         (b) Shared by drug users
   c. Incubation period is 40 to 180 days

d. Serum studies reveal HBs Ag (current or chronic infection), HBe Ag (increased infection), anti-HBc and anti-HBe (decreased infection), anti-HBs (antibody produced in response to HBV vaccine)

3. Type C (non-A, non-B) hepatitis
   a. Caused by a virus similar to HBV
   b. Transmitted through blood and blood products
   c. Symptoms occur after 40 to 100 days following exposure
   d. Serum studies reveal anti-HCV

4. Type D (delta agent) hepatitis
   a. Virus HDV must have HBV for cell replication
   b. Transmitted through blood and blood products and close personal contact
   c. Most common in Mediterranean countries
   d. Serum studies reveal anti–HDV-IgM (current infection) or anti–HDV-IgG (resolved infection)

5. Phases of disease
   a. Prodromal or preicteric
   b. Icteric
   c. Recovery (may take 4 months)

6. Progression to cirrhosis, hepatic coma, and death may occur, although this is rare

7. Other causes of hepatitis include chemical agents such as halothane (an anesthetic agent), carbon tetrachloride, gold compounds, and arsenic

B. Clinical findings
1. Prodromal (preicteric) phase
   a. Malaise
   b. Weight loss
   c. Anorexia, nausea, and vomiting
   d. Symptoms of upper respiratory tract infection
   e. Intolerance for smoking

2. Icteric phase
   a. Jaundice
   b. Bile-colored urine that foams when shaken
   c. Acholic (clay-colored) stools

3. Recovery phase: easy fatigability

C. Therapeutic interventions
1. Rest
2. Abstinence from alcohol
3. Diet therapy
   a. High protein: healing of liver tissue vital; daily intake should include 1.14 L milk; 2 eggs; 225 g lean meat, fish, or cheese; total should approximate 75 to 100 g protein
   b. High carbohydrate: energy needs, restore glycogen reserves; use daily 4 servings vegetables, including potato, 4 servings fruit with frequent juices, 6 to 8 servings bread or cereal; total carbohydrate should be 300 to 400 g

c. Moderate fat: 30 to 60 ml butter or fortified margarine, sufficient for making food palatable; a moderate amount of easily digestible foods such as whole milk, cream, butter, margarine, or vegetable oil is beneficial; total fat should be 100 to 150 g daily

d. High calorie: increased energy needs for disease process and tissue regeneration and to spare protein for healing; these food amounts should provide about 2500 to 3000 calories daily

e. Vitamins A and E should be given when steatorrhea is present; also mineral supplements of calcium and zinc

Nursing Care of Clients with Hepatitis

A. DATA COLLECTION
1. History of exposure to virus
2. History of employment over previous 6 months
3. Right upper quadrant for liver tenderness, firmness
4. Presence of jaundice in skin, sclera, and mucous membranes
5. Temperature to determine presence of fever (associated with type A) or low-grade fever (associated with types B and C)

B. ANALYSIS AND INTERPRETATION
Refer to General Nursing Diagnoses for Clients with Gastrointestinal System Disorders for the following diagnoses: A, B 1, J 2, M 1, N 1, O 1, R 1, and S 1

C. PLANNING/IMPLEMENTATION
1. Encourage quiet activities
2. Attempt to stimulate the appetite
   a. Provide oral hygiene
   b. Select foods based on the client's preferences
   c. Provide a pleasant, unhurried atmosphere for eating
   d. Provide small, frequent feedings that are usually tolerated better than large meals
3. Use precautions to prevent the spread of hepatitis to others
   a. Use standard (universal) precautions
   b. For a client with type A hepatitis, use contact precautions when exposed to the client's feces
4. Teach prevention
   a. Thorough hand washing
   b. Utilization of contact precautions when exposure to feces, blood, or body secretions is expected
   c. Careful handling of needles (dispose of needles without recapping to prevent self-injury and contamination, dispose of needles in hard-sided container)

d. Administration of immune serum globulin (ISG) after exposure to type A hepatitis

e. Vaccination of individuals at risk for type B hepatitis (Hep-B, Recombivax HB)

f. When client has hepatitis that can be transmitted sexually, encourage the use of condoms

D. EVALUATION/OUTCOMES

1. Maintains rest
2. Adheres to prescribed diet
3. Discusses feelings related to illness, restrictions, and prognosis
4. Verbalizes decrease in pain
5. Client and family follow appropriate precautions to prevent transmission

▼ HEPATIC CIRRHOSIS

Data Base

A. Etiology and pathophysiology

1. Irreversible fibrosis and degeneration of the liver
2. Several types of cirrhosis; Laënnec's (alcoholic cirrhosis, nutritional cirrhosis) most common
3. Incidence higher in alcoholics, who are often malnourished, and in those who have had hepatitis
4. Pressure rises in the portal system (which drains blood from the digestive organs), causing stasis and backup in digestive organs
5. As liver failure progresses, there is increased secretion of aldosterone, decreased absorption and utilization of the fat-soluble vitamins (A, D, E, K), and ineffective detoxification of protein wastes
6. Hepatic coma may result from high blood ammonia levels (hepatic encephalopathy) when the liver is unable to convert the ammonia to urea

B. Clinical findings

1. Subjective
   a. Nausea
   b. Weakness, fatigue
   c. Anorexia
   d. Abdominal discomfort
   e. Pruritis
2. Objective
   a. Weight loss
   b. Ascites
   c. Esophageal varices as a result of portal hypertension
   d. Hemorrhoids
   e. Edema of extremities
   f. Hematemesis
   g. Hemorrhage due to decreased formation of prothrombin

h. Jaundice; elevated serum bilirubin

i. Delirium caused by rising blood ammonia levels

j. Elevated liver enzymes (aspartate aminotransferase [AST], alanine aminotransferase [ALT], alkaline phosphatase [ALP], gamma-glutamyl transferase [GGT])

k. Decreased serum albumin

C. Therapeutic interventions

1. Rest
2. Restriction of alcohol intake
3. Vitamin therapy: especially A, D, E, and K
4. Diuretics to control ascites and edema
5. Neomycin and lactulose may be prescribed for elevated blood ammonia levels
6. If respiratory distress occurs as a result of ascites, a paracentesis is done; slow removal of fluid from the peritoneal cavity will relieve acute symptoms
7. Surgical intervention for portal hypertension: a portal-caval shunt, in which the circulation from the portal vein bypasses the liver and enters the vena cava, usually decreases portal hypertension
8. Blakemore-Sengstaken tube is utilized in the treatment of bleeding esophageal varices to apply direct pressure to the varices; vasopressin may be administered IV to control GI bleeding
9. Dietary modification
   a. Cirrhosis
      (1) Protein according to tolerance: with increasing liver damage, protein metabolism is hindered; hold to 80 to 100 g as long as tolerated; reduce as necessary
      (2) Continue high carbohydrate, moderate fat as in hepatitis to supply energy; vitamin supplements, especially B complex and vitamins A and E; mineral supplements of calcium and zinc
      (3) Low sodium: usually restricted to 500 to 1000 mg daily by eliminating salt and controlling foods processed with salt or sodium-based preservatives; sodium restriction helps to control the increasing ascites
      (4) Soft foods: if esophageal varices are present, to prevent danger of rupture and bleeding
      (5) Alcohol strictly forbidden to avoid continued irritation and malnutrition
   b. Hepatic coma
      (1) Low protein: reduced according to tolerance, 15 to 30 g
      (2) High calories and vitamins according to need: about 1500 to 2000 calories, sufficient to prevent tissue catabolism and the liberation of additional nitrogen

(3) Fluid carefully controlled according to output

Nursing Care of Clients with Hepatic Cirrhosis

A. DATA COLLECTION

1. History of anorexia, dyspepsia, and weight loss
2. Presence of abdominal pain and liver tenderness
3. Skin for presence of jaundice, dryness, petechiae, ecchymosis, spider angiomas, and palmar erythema
4. Presence of dullness when percussing over enlarged liver
5. Abdominal girth measurements for baseline data relative to ascites

B. ANALYSIS AND INTERPRETATION

Refer to General Nursing Diagnoses for Clients with Gastrointestinal System Disorders for the following diagnoses: A, B 1, B 2, D 1, I 1, J, L 1, M 1, N 1, O 1, O 6, R 1, S 1, U, and V

C. PLANNING/IMPLEMENTATION

1. Observe the client for objective signs of disease
2. Observe mental status, which may vary
3. Observe for bleeding
4. Provide special skin care and keep nails trimmed because pruritis is associated with jaundice
5. Maintain the client in a semi-Fowler's position to prevent ascites from causing dyspnea
6. Monitor intake and output, abdominal girth, and daily weight to assess fluid balance
7. Assist with paracentesis (see procedure)
8. Provide care when a Blakemore-Sengstaken tube is in place
   a. Maintain traction once the tube is passed and the gastric balloon is inflated to ensure proper placement
   b. Maintain the esophageal balloon at inflated level (30 to 35 mm Hg)
   c. If ordered, deflate the balloon for a few minutes at specific intervals to prevent necrosis
   d. Irrigate with saline if ordered
   e. Suction orally as necessary because the client is unable to swallow saliva
9. Teach dietary modifications since ability of client to understand and remember instructions is often impaired due to hepatic encephalopathy
   a. Focus teaching efforts on the family
   b. Limit high-protein foods
   c. Emphasize the use of carbohydrate foods such as pasta, rice, and potatoes to supply needed energy
   d. Limit salt intake
   e. Inform client that fats can be used to supply calories and improve food palatability unless steatorrhea occurs

   f. Repeat instructions to reinforce teaching

D. EVALUATION/OUTCOMES

1. Complies with dietary regimen
2. Abstains from alcohol
3. Maintains fluid balance
4. Reports reduction in pain
5. Remains free from injury

▼ CANCER OF THE LIVER

Data Base

A. Etiology and pathophysiology
   1. May be primary or metastatic carcinoma; primary carcinoma of the liver is rare
   2. Generally lethal within a few months
B. Clinical findings
   1. Subjective
      a. Anorexia
      b. Ache in epigastric area
   2. Objective
      a. Weight loss
      b. Anemia
      c. Jaundice; increased serum bilirubin
      d. Ascites
      e. Bleeding
      f. Increased alkaline phosphatase
C. Therapeutic interventions
   1. Generally palliative
   2. Hepatic lobectomy if the tumor is confined (the liver has extraordinary regenerative capacity)
   3. Percutaneous infusions with cytotoxic agents
   4. External radiation therapy

Nursing Care of Clients with Cancer of the Liver

A. DATA COLLECTION

1. Skin for jaundice, bleeding, and pallor
2. Presence of dullness when percussing over liver
3. Detailed history including exposure to any known causative agents

B. ANALYSIS AND INTERPRETATION

Refer to General Nursing Diagnoses for Clients with Gastrointestinal System Disorders for the following diagnoses: B 1, B 2, J , L 1, L 2, M 1, O 1, O 4, O 6, R 1, and S 1

C. PLANNING/IMPLEMENTATION

1. Provide comfort
2. Be available to both the client and family members to discuss their feelings
3. Provide care following hepatic surgery
   a. Maintain fluid and electrolyte balance with IV therapy
   b. Monitor intake and output

c. Observe for signs of bleeding, hypoglycemia, and other metabolic dysfunctions resulting from impaired liver function

d. Have the client cough, deep breathe, and change position frequently to prevent pulmonary and circulatory complications

e. Because the thoracic cavity may be entered during surgery, be aware of the care of a client with chest tubes (see procedure for chest tubes)

D. EVALUATION/OUTCOMES
1. Maintains adequate nutritional status
2. Complies with treatment protocol
3. States pain is reduced
4. Verbalizes feelings about prognosis

▼ MALABSORPTION SYNDROME

Data Base

A. Etiology and pathophysiology
1. Etiology unknown; possible hereditary factor
2. Nontropical sprue similar to celiac disease in children and is characterized by intolerance to gluten, abnormalities in the structure of the small intestine, and malabsorption
3. Tropical sprue is endemic in the Indian subcontinent and the Caribbean and is thought to be due to infection rather than diet
4. Intolerance to gluten results in blunting of the intestinal villi, which reduces absorptive surface of the intestinal mucosa

B. Clinical findings
1. Subjective
   a. Anorexia
   b. Fatigability; weakness
   c. Abdominal discomfort
2. Objective
   a. Weight loss
   b. Anemia (macrocytic)
   c. Diarrhea
   d. Steatorrhea
   e. Visualization of the small bowel demonstrates flat, blunt villi
   f. Tetany
   g. Demineralization of the skeletal system

C. Therapeutic interventions
1. Tropical sprue may respond to a high-protein, normal-fat diet with supplemental vitamin B_{12}, A, D, E, K, folic acid, and iron; in addition, antibiotics such as tetracycline for at least 6 months may be helpful
2. Nontropical sprue may respond to a high-protein, normal-fat, gluten-gliadin-free diet and vitamin supplements of A, D, K, B complex, and folic acid, as well as iron and calcium

3. Whenever the disease does not respond to diet, corticosteroids may be used
4. Fluid and electrolyte imbalances must be resolved

Nursing Care of Clients with Malabsorption Syndrome

A. DATA COLLECTION
1. History of symptoms and causative factors
2. History of bowel habits
3. Stool for diarrhea and steatorrhea
4. Presence and extent of bowel sounds

B. ANALYSIS AND INTERPRETATION
Refer to General Nursing Diagnoses for Clients with Gastrointestinal System Disorders for the following diagnoses: B 1, B 2, H 1, I 1, M 1, M 2, N 1, N 2, O 1, and O 3

C. PLANNING/IMPLEMENTATION
1. Teach the client and family how to modify the diet to comply with medical management
2. Instruct family that rice, corn, and soy flours should be used in place of wheat, rye, barley, and oats
3. Inform the client of the importance of reading labels, because gluten-containing grains are added to many products, and of the need to question the contents of foods in restaurants
4. Advise the client as to the importance of follow-up care for disease management
5. Provide an opportunity for the client and family to verbalize feelings about the illness
6. Observe the client for signs of electrolyte imbalance
7. Record weight on a regular basis

D. EVALUATION/OUTCOMES
1. Maintains or regains weight appropriate for height, age, and frame
2. Reports decreased number of bowel movements
3. Maintains fluid and electrolyte balance
4. Client and family verbalize feelings
5. Follows dietary recommendations

▼ APPENDICITIS

Data Base

A. Etiology and pathophysiology
1. Compromised circulation and inflammation of the vermiform appendix
2. Causes include obstruction by a fecalith, foreign body, or kinking
3. Inflammation may be followed by edema, necrosis, and rupture

B. Clinical findings
1. Subjective

a. Anorexia
b. Nausea
c. Right lower quadrant pain (McBurney's point)
d. Rebound tenderness
e. Abdominal distention and paralytic ileus if appendix is ruptured
  2. Objective
a. Vomiting
b. Fever
c. Leukocytosis
C. Therapeutic interventions
  1. Surgical removal of the appendix without delay to decrease the chance of rupture and the risk of peritonitis
  2. Prophylactic use of antibiotics postoperatively
  3. Fluid and electrolyte maintenance
  4. Analgesics for pain

Nursing Care of Clients with Appendicitis

A. DATA COLLECTION

1. History of characteristics of pain and presence of nausea and vomiting
2. Presence of anorexia or the urge to pass flatus
3. Presence of rebound tenderness when palpating abdomen
4. Presence of tenderness/rigidity when palpating McBurney's point
5. Temperature for baseline data
6. Presence and extent of bowel sounds

B. ANALYSIS AND INTERPRETATION

Refer to General Nursing Diagnoses for Clients with Gastrointestinal System Disorders for the following diagnoses: B 2, I 1, O 1, O 5, O 6, R 1, and R 3

C. PLANNING/IMPLEMENTATION

1. Provide emotional support because this condition is unanticipated and the individual needs to ventilate any fear of surgery
2. Monitor fluid and electrolyte balance
3. Assess the client for signs of infection; maintain a semi-Fowler's position to help localize infection if the appendix ruptures
4. Encourage early ambulation, if not contraindicated by the client's condition, to prevent complications
5. Assess the client's return of bowel function (bowel sounds, flatus, bowel movement)

D. EVALUATION/OUTCOMES

1. States pain is alleviated
2. Maintains adequate fluid balance
3. Verbalizes feelings

▼ REGIONAL ENTERITIS

Data Base

A. Etiology and pathophysiology
  1. Etiology unknown
  2. Usually occurs in young adults, but can occur at any age
  3. Inflammatory changes involving any part of the alimentary tract but usually demarcated segments of the small bowel
  4. Ulceration of the intestinal submucosa accompanied by congestion, thickening of the small bowel, and fissure formations
  5. Enlargement of regional lymph nodes
  6. Fibrosis and narrowing of the intestinal wall
  7. Abscesses and fistulas of the abdominal wall, bladder, and vagina
B. Clinical findings
  1. Subjective
a. Pain in the lower right quadrant, cramping, and spasms
b. Nausea
c. Exacerbations related to emotional upsets or dietary indiscretions with milk, milk products, and fried foods
  2. Objective
a. Borborygmus (rumbling, gurgling sound in the intestines), flatulence
b. Weight loss
c. Fever
d. Electrolyte disturbance
e. Diarrhea
f. Gastrointestinal x-ray series to detect and outline the congested, thickened, fibrosed, and narrowed appearance of the intestinal wall; also abscesses and fistulas, partial bowel obstruction, and ulceration of the mucosa
g. Proctosigmoidoscopy is performed to exclude other diseases, such as ulcerative colitis and diverticulitis
h. Stools are examined for the presence of blood, fat, protein, parasites, or ova
i. Fecal fat test is performed to determine fat content, an abnormal amount of which is significant in malabsorptive disorders or hypermotility
j. D-xylose tolerance test is performed to determine absorptive ability of upper intestinal tract
C. Therapeutic interventions
  1. Nothing by mouth in the presence of vomiting
  2. Clear fluid diet progressing to bland, low-residue, low-fat diet, but increased calories, proteins, vitamins (especially vitamin K), and carbohydrates

3. Total parenteral nutrition (TPN) may be ordered when oral intake is inadequate
4. Medications such as:
   a. Antiemetics
   b. Vitamins and minerals
   c. Anticholinergics
   d. Antidiarrheals
   e. Antiinflammatories
   f. Antiinfectives
5. Surgery (resection of diseased part) if the client does not respond to medical therapy or if complications such as obstruction, abscesses, or fistulas occur

Nursing Care of Clients with Regional Enteritis

A. DATA COLLECTION
1. Increased bowel motility on auscultation
2. Weight for baseline data
3. History of frequency, color, and consistency of stools
4. Presence and extent of bowel sounds

B. ANALYSIS AND INTERPRETATION
Refer to General Nursing Diagnoses for Clients with Gastrointestinal System Disorders for the following diagnoses: H 1, I 2, O 6, R 1, and S 2

C. PLANNING/IMPLEMENTATION
1. Monitor intake and output
2. Offer clear liquids hourly as ordered once the client ceases to experience nausea and vomiting
3. Encourage high-calorie, high-protein, high-carbohydrate diet supplemented with vitamins and potassium as ordered
4. Assist with total parenteral nutrition (TPN) if ordered (see procedure)
5. Offer small, frequent feedings considering client preference, types of food allowed, and esthetic factors
6. Record weight daily
7. Observe for signs of complications such as elevated temperature, increasing nausea and vomiting, abdominal rigidity
8. Communicate concern and awareness regarding the client's discomfort and emotional lability during exacerbations of this chronic illness
9. Teach the client:
   a. To avoid taking laxatives and salicylates that irritate the intestinal mucosa
   b. How to take antidiarrheals and mucilloid drugs effectively and the observations to make during their use
   c. Skin care if the perineal area is irritated
   d. The importance of seeking help early when exacerbations occur

D. EVALUATION/OUTCOMES
1. Reports a reduction in pain
2. Has a decrease in the number of bowel movements

3. Maintains adequate nutritional status
4. Maintains fluid and electrolyte balance
5. Maintains perianal skin integrity

▼ ULCERATIVE COLITIS

Data Base
A. Etiology and pathophysiology
   1. May be caused by emotional stress, an autoimmune response, or a genetic predisposition
   2. Edema of the mucous membrane of the colon leads to bleeding and shallow ulcerations
   3. Abscess formation occurs, and the bowel wall shortens and becomes thin and fragile
   4. Associated with increased risk of colon cancer
B. Clinical findings
   1. Subjective
      a. Weakness, debilitation
      b. Anorexia
      c. Nausea
   2. Objective
      a. Dehydration with tenting of skin (poor skin turgor)
      b. Passage of bloody, purulent, mucoid, watery stools
      c. Anemia
      d. Low-grade fever
C. Therapeutic interventions
   1. Dietary management
      a. Diet plays a major role in the management of colitis; emphasis has changed from a low-residue diet to a more liberal diet (restricted roughage may be useful during more acute attacks of severe cramps, diarrhea, and bleeding, but seems to have little effect on preventing relapses); supplementing diet with raw bran has been shown to be effective in controlling bouts of diarrhea and constipation
      b. If tolerated, unrestricted fluid intake; high-protein, high-calorie diet; avoidance of food allergens, especially milk
   2. Pharmacologic management
      a. Antiemetics
      b. Anticholinergics
      c. Corticosteroids
      d. Antibiotics
      e. Sedatives, analgesics, and tranquilizers
      f. Antidiarrheals
   3. Replacement of fluids and electrolytes that are lost because of diarrhea
   4. A temporary ileostomy, a partial colectomy, or a total colectomy with a permanent ileostomy may be performed when:
      a. No response to medical treatment is evident

b. Course of the disease is downhill
c. Massive hemorrhage or colonic obstruction occurs
d. Cancer is suspected

Nursing Care of Clients with Ulcerative Colitis
A. DATA COLLECTION
1. Localized areas of tenderness found over diseased bowel on palpation
2. History of patterns and characteristics of bowel elimination
3. Feces for color, consistency, and characteristics
4. Temperature and weight for baseline data
5. Presence and extent of bowel sounds

B. ANALYSIS AND INTERPRETATION
Refer to General Nursing Diagnoses for Clients with Gastrointestinal System Disorders for the following diagnoses: A, B 1, D 2, H 1, I 2, M 1, M 2, N 1, N 2, O 1, O 3, O 6, R 1, and S 2

C. PLANNING/IMPLEMENTATION
1. Instruct client to adhere to the following dietary program
   a. Eat small, frequent feedings of high-protein, high-calorie foods (low fat helps decrease steatorrhea, which is common with ileal involvement; if steatorrhea is present, vitamins A and E may be required as supplements)
   b. Avoid irritating spices such as red or black pepper
   c. Replace iron, calcium, and zinc losses with supplements; if there is ileal involvement, intramuscular injections of vitamin B_{12} may be prescribed monthly
   d. Avoid all food allergens, especially milk (milk has been implicated as a direct cause of colitis in infants and is often associated with diarrhea in adults); milk may be reintroduced when client is relatively asymptomatic; however, lactose intolerance is common in this condition and dairy restrictions may be permanent (some lactose-intolerant individuals can manage yogurt, buttermilk, and hard cheeses; lactase enzyme preparations are available that can be added to milk products to hydrolyze lactose)
2. Teach importance of diet in controlling and/or minimizing symptoms
3. Involve the client in dietary selection, recognizing preferences as much as possible
4. Initiate accurate administration and recording of fluid, electrolyte, or blood replacements as ordered by the physician
5. Plan nursing care to allow the client complete bed rest and the maximum number of rest periods

6. Provide gentle, thorough perineal care as required
7. Observe for complications such as rectal hemorrhage, fever, dehydration
8. Allow the client and family time to verbalize feelings and participate in care; encourage participation in the Crohn's and Colitis Foundation of America
9. If an ileostomy is performed, help the client accept the changes of body image and function involved (see Ileostomy Care)

D. EVALUATION/OUTCOMES
1. Maintains or regains weight
2. Reports decrease in pain
3. Adheres to medical regimen
4. Maintains skin integrity
5. Establishes an acceptable pattern of soft, formed bowel movements
6. Client or family member demonstrates ability to perform ostomy care

▼ CROHN'S DISEASE

Data Base
A. Etiology and pathophysiology
   1. Although the causative mechanisms are unknown, there are various theories involving genetic predisposition, autoimmune reaction, or environmental causes
   2. Cobblestone ulcerations form along the mucosal wall of the terminal ileum, cecum, and ascending colon, which form scar tissue and inhibit food and water absorption in the area
   3. Ulcerations may perforate through the intestinal wall and form fistulas with adjoining organs
B. Clinical findings
   1. Subjective
      a. Severe pain in the right lower quadrant
      b. Malaise
   2. Objective
      a. Moderate fever
      b. Elevated WBCs
      c. Mild diarrhea with mucus but no blood
      d. Anemia
C. Therapeutic interventions
   1. High-calorie, high-protein diet
   2. Vitamin supplements, including B_{12}, if a large portion of ileum is involved
   3. Pharmacologic management
      a. Anticholinergics
      b. Analgesics
      c. Intestinal antibiotics
      d. Immunosuppressives

4. Surgery when fistulas or intestinal obstruction occurs; the involved area of intestine is removed and the ends are anastomosed, if possible; an ostomy is indicated if large areas of intestine are involved

Nursing Care of Clients with Crohn's Disease

A. DATA COLLECTION

1. Weight and temperature for baseline data
2. Feces for color, consistency, and steatorrhea
3. Tenderness and guarding of the abdomen, especially in the right lower quadrant
4. Presence and extent of bowel sounds

B. ANALYSIS AND INTERPRETATION

Refer to General Nursing Diagnoses for Clients with Gastrointestinal System Disorders for the following diagnoses: A, B 1, B 2, D 2, H 1, I 2, M 1, M 2, N 1, N 2, O 3, R 1, and S 2

C. PLANNING/IMPLEMENTATION

1. Provide an emotionally therapeutic environment in which client can communicate concerns and stresses resulting from this illness; encourage client and family to participate in the Crohn's and Colitis Foundation of America
2. Instruct client regarding dietary restrictions and modifications (see Ulcerative Colitis)
3. Observe client for signs of fluid and electrolyte imbalances

D. EVALUATION/OUTCOMES

1. Reports decreased frequency of stool
2. Maintains or regains weight
3. Describes decrease in pain
4. Complies with treatment regimen
5. Reports reduced feelings of stress
6. Remains free from infection
7. Client or family member demonstrates ability to perform ostomy care

---

▼ INTESTINAL OBSTRUCTION

Data Base

A. Etiology and pathophysiology
   1. Interference with normal peristaltic movement of intestinal contents due to neurologic or mechanical impairments
   2. Causes
      a. Carcinoma of the bowel
      b. Hernias
      c. Adhesions (scar tissue that forms abnormal connections after surgery or inflammation)
      d. Intussusception (telescoping of the bowel on itself)
      e. Volvulus (twisting of the intestines)
      f. Paralytic ileus (interference with neural innervation of the intestines resulting in a decrease in or absence of peristalsis; may be caused by surgical manipulation, electrolyte imbalance, or infection)
B. Clinical findings
   1. Subjective
      a. Colicky abdominal pain
      b. Constipation
   2. Objective
      a. Abdominal distention
      b. Vomiting; may contain fecal matter
      c. Decreased or absent bowel sounds
      d. Signs of dehydration and electrolyte imbalance
      e. Flat plate of the abdomen shows the bowel distended with air
      f. Obstipation
C. Therapeutic interventions
   1. Restriction of oral intake; administration of parenteral fluid and electrolytes
   2. Surgical correction of cause (e.g., hernias, adhesions)
   3. Colostomy, cecostomy, or ileostomy as necessary
   4. Drugs such as pantothenyl alcohol (Ilopan) and neostigmine (Prostigmin) to stimulate the passage of flatus
   5. Gastric decompression by means of a nasogastric, Cantor, or Miller-Abbott tube

Nursing Care of Clients with Intestinal Obstruction

A. DATA COLLECTION

1. Detailed history to determine risk and causative factors
2. Abdomen for peristaltic waves
3. Presence and characteristics of bowel sounds
4. Abdomen for distention
5. Patterns and characteristics of bowel elimination

B. ANALYSIS AND INTERPRETATION

Refer to General Nursing Diagnoses for Clients with Gastrointestinal System Disorders for the following diagnoses: D 2, G 4, I 1, L 3, M 1, M 2, N 1, N 2, O 5, and R 1

C. PLANNING/IMPLEMENTATION

1. Assess the client for dehydration and electrolyte imbalance
2. Monitor intake and output
3. Auscultate for bowel sounds; note the passage of flatus
4. Administer mouth care frequently
5. Measure abdominal girth daily to assess distention

6. Provide special care for the client with a Miller-Abbott or Cantor tube
   a. Once the lubricated tube is inserted, position the client first on the right side, to facilitate passage of tube through the pylorus, and then in a semi-Fowler's position, to continue the gradual advance into the intestines
   b. Coil and loosely attach extra tubing to the client's gown to avoid tension against peristaltic action
   c. Irrigate as ordered to maintain patency
   d. Frequently assess placement of the tube; record the level of advancement
   e. When the tube is discontinued by the physician, remove the tube gradually because it is being pulled against peristalsis

D. **EVALUATION/OUTCOMES**
   1. Establishes a regular pattern of bowel elimination
   2. Maintains adequate nutritional/fluid intake
   3. States pain is reduced
   4. Remains free of complications

▼ DIVERTICULAR DISEASE

Data Base
A. Etiology and pathophysiology
   1. Diverticulosis: presence of multiple diverticula, which are pouchlike herniations of intestinal mucosa, as a result of weakness and increased intraabdominal pressure; client may be asymptomatic
   2. Diverticulitis: inflammation caused by food or feces trapped in a diverticulum; may lead to bleeding, perforation, peritonitis, and bowel obstruction
   3. Most commonly occurs in the sigmoid colon, but could occur anywhere along the GI tract
   4. Incidence increases with age; inadequate dietary fiber, history of constipation with straining at stool, and congenital predisposition are risk factors
B. Clinical findings
   1. Subjective
      a. Cramping, colicky pain in left lower quadrant
      b. Nausea
      c. Malaise
   2. Objective
      a. Altered bowel elimination: diarrhea or constipation
      b. Abdominal distention
      c. Fever

   d. Leukocytosis
   e. Presence of blood in stool
   f. Diagnostic tests: CT scan, barium enema, and sigmoidoscopy provide direct evidence of the disease
C. Therapeutic interventions
   1. High-fiber diet and bulk laxatives to prevent diverticulitis
   2. Nothing by mouth or clear liquids during acute diverticulitis
   3. Analgesics; morphine sulfate is avoided because it can increase intracolonic pressure
   4. Fluid and electrolyte replacement
   5. Antibiotic therapy
   6. Surgery
      a. Colon resection with an anastomosis
      b. Temporary loop colostomy

Nursing Care of Clients with Diverticular Disease
A. **DATA COLLECTION**
   1. History of constipation and/or diarrhea with progression of symptoms
   2. Vital signs
   3. Stool for consistency and presence of blood
   4. Abdomen for distention
   5. Presence and extent of bowel sounds
B. **ANALYSIS AND INTERPRETATION**
   Refer to General Nursing Diagnoses for Clients with Gastrointestinal System Disorders for the following diagnoses: B 1, B 2, D 2, F, G 1, G 4, H 1, I 2, K, M 1, M 2, N 1, N 2, O 1, O 5, R 1, and V
C. **PLANNING/IMPLEMENTATION**
   1. Teach importance of high-fiber and high-fluid intake to prevent diverticulitis
   2. Administer bulk laxatives and stool softeners as prescribed
   3. Restrict oral intake if inflammation is present
   4. Monitor for signs of peritonitis: pain, hypotension, abdominal rigidity, abdominal distention, and leukocytosis
   5. Administer fluid and electrolyte replacement
   6. Teach client the importance of completing antibiotic regimen
   7. Provide care related to bowel surgery (see Nursing Care of Clients with Cancer of the Small Intestine, Colon, and Rectum)
D. **EVALUATION/OUTCOMES**
   1. Exhibits normal pattern of soft, formed bowel movements
   2. Increases intake of high-fiber foods
   3. Reports relief from pain
   4. Maintains fluid and electrolyte balance
   5. Client or family member demonstrates ability to perform ostomy care

▼ CANCER OF THE SMALL INTESTINE, COLON, AND RECTUM

Data Base

A. Etiology and pathophysiology
1. Cancer of the colon and rectum: can cause a narrowing of the lumen of the bowel, ulcerations, necrosis, or perforation
2. Predisposing factors include familial polyps, chronic ulcerative colitis, and possibly bowel stasis or ingestion of food additives
3. A high-fat, low-fiber diet has been implicated as a causative factor in colon cancer; it is thought that fat and/or bile is chemically altered by intestinal bacteria producing carcinogens that are responsible for the development of cancer; absence of dietary fiber tends to slow the passage of stool through the colon, giving carcinogens more time in contact with the surface of the mucosa
4. Cancer of the colon: more common in males, and incidence increases after 50 years of age
5. Cancer of the small intestine is rare; adeno-carcinoma of the large intestine is relatively common

B. Clinical findings
1. Subjective
   a. Abdominal discomfort or pain
   b. Weakness and fatigue
2. Objective
   a. Alterations in usual bowel function (constipation or diarrhea or alternating constipation and diarrhea)
   b. Blood in stool
   c. Abdominal distention
   d. Changes in shape of stool (pencil- or ribbon-shaped)
   e. Weight loss
   f. Secondary anemia

C. Therapeutic interventions
1. Diagnostic measures
   a. Digital examination of the rectum to detect any palpable masses
   b. Proctosigmoidoscopy to visualize the bowel directly to determine the presence of abnormalities and to perform a biopsy
   c. Stool examination to test for occult blood
   d. Cytologic examination of tissue from GI tract to detect malignant cells
   e. Hemoglobin level to detect anemia
   f. Alkaline phosphatase and AST levels to detect metastasis to the liver
   g. Serum carcinoembryonic antigen (CEA): measure to screen for carcinoma of the colon

2. After diagnosis is established, the physician may prepare the client for surgery by:
   a. Prescribing antibiotics to reduce bacteria in the bowel
   b. Typing and cross-matching of blood for transfusions to correct the anemia
   c. Ordering vitamin supplements to improve the nutritional status
   d. Inserting a Cantor or Miller-Abbott tube with suction to decompress the colon
3. Surgical intervention to remove the mass and restore bowel function (e.g., hemicolectomy, resection of the transverse colon, abdominal perineal resection)
4. Radiation in nonsurgical situations may be used in an attempt to relieve symptoms; may be used preoperatively to reduce size of tumor or postoperatively to limit metastases
5. Chemotherapy orally or parenterally in an attempt to reduce the lesion and limit metastases
6. Postoperatively
   a. Antibiotic therapy to prevent infection
   b. Parenteral fluids and electrolytes to maintain balance
   c. Cholinergics to stimulate peristalsis
   d. Cantor or Miller-Abbott tube clamped for regular, increasing periods; removed when the client is able to tolerate clamping and when bowel sounds have returned
   e. Sips of water progressing to clear liquid diet and to low-residue diet as tolerated
7. If colostomy has been performed
   a. Colostomy irrigations and care as required (see procedure)
   b. Irrigations of perineal incision if present
   c. Skin care to prevent breakdown around stoma

Nursing Care of Clients with Cancer of the Small Intestine, Colon, and Rectum

A. DATA COLLECTION
1. Detailed history of symptoms and risk factors
2. Stool for frequency, color, consistency, and shape
3. Weight for baseline data
4. Areas of abdominal discomfort on palpation
5. Presence and extent of bowel sounds

B. ANALYSIS AND INTERPRETATION
Refer to General Nursing Diagnoses for Clients with Gastrointestinal System Disorders for the following diagnoses: B 1, B 2, D 1, D 2, G 4, L 2, L 3, M 1, M 2, N 1, N 2, O 3, O 4, O 5, R 1, R 3, and S 2

C. PLANNING/IMPLEMENTATION
1. Observe vital signs, increasing abdominal pain, nausea, and vomiting to detect early signs of complications

2. Monitor patency of the Cantor or Miller-Abbott tube to ensure that accumulated air and fluid are decreased and distention is minimized; instill or irrigate the tube with normal saline as ordered

3. Note the character of drainage from the decompression tube

4. Implement measures for mechanical cleansing and intestinal antisepsis preoperatively (e.g., enemas, colonic irrigations, antibacterial therapy such as neomycin or sulfonamides)

5. Administer chemotherapeutic drugs if ordered and observe for significant side effects such as stomatitis (ulceration of the mouth), dehydration, nausea and vomiting, diarrhea, leukopenia

6. Administer electrolyte and parenteral fluid replacement as ordered in situations of bleeding, vomiting, and/or obstruction

7. Carefully note the client's tolerance to the introduction of oral fluids and foods while the intestinal tube is clamped

8. Teach the client and family dietary modifications, including low-residue, non–gas-forming foods, avoidance of stimulants, adequate fluid intake; diet should be as close to the client's normal as possible; encourage a positive attitude

9. Teach client the importance of diet in supporting the body's natural defense mechanisms; diet should emphasize high nutrient density foods from the fruits, vegetables, cereal grains, and legumes groups with some lean meat, fish, and poultry; encourage client to eat as great a variety of foods as can be tolerated; vitamin and mineral supplements can be encouraged, especially the immune-stimulating factors

10. Provide colostomy care using medical aseptic technique (see procedure)

11. Recognize that the client with a colostomy may experience sadness, withdrawal, depression, and suicidal thoughts as a result of body-image changes

12. Assess the client's reaction to the colostomy, recognizing that a great deal will depend on how the client sees it is affecting life-style, physical and emotional status, social and cultural background, and place and role in the family

13. Encourage involvement in colostomy care as soon as physical and emotional status permits

14. Encourage visiting by family members, stressing the client's increased need for love and acceptance

15. Recognize that the client with a cecostomy or colostomy is especially sensitive to gestures, odors, facial expressions, and the amount of attention given

16. Teach the client and family care of the colostomy, measures to facilitate acceptance and adjustment, resumption of activities, and the need for regular medical supervision

17. Teach the client that colostomy drainage can be controlled by following a regular irrigation schedule and dietary modifications

18. Arrange for follow-up care with community agencies as required (e.g., Public Health, Home Care Programs, Cancer Society, ostomy resource person)

D. EVALUATION/OUTCOMES

1. Maintains adequate fluid and nutrient intake

2. Resumes a regular pattern of bowel elimination

3. Complies with treatment protocol

4. Avoids complications related to treatment/disease

5. Client or family member demonstrates ability to perform colostomy care

6. Discusses feelings concerning colostomy

▼ PERITONITIS

Data Base

A. Etiology and pathophysiology
  1. Inflammation of the peritoneum
  2. Generally caused by infection from perforation of GI tract or by chemical stress, as in pancreatitis

B. Clinical findings
  1. Subjective
    a. Abdominal pain, rebound tenderness
    b. Malaise
    c. Nausea
  2. Objective
    a. Abdominal muscle rigidity
    b. Elevated temperature and WBCs
    c. Vomiting

C. Therapeutic interventions
  1. Bed rest in a semi-Fowler's position to localize drainage to the dependent portion of the abdominal cavity
  2. Nasogastric tube attached to suction and left in place until the client passes flatus
  3. Fluids and electrolytes replaced parenterally
  4. Antibiotic therapy
  5. Surgery to correct the cause of peritonitis (e.g., appendectomy, incision and drainage of abscesses, closure of a perforation)

Nursing Care of Clients with Peritonitis

A. DATA COLLECTION

1. Temperature for baseline data

2. Guarded movements and/or self-splinting

3. Reduction or absence of bowel sounds
4. Presence and characteristics of abdominal pain

B. ANALYSIS AND INTERPRETATION

Refer to General Nursing Diagnoses for Clients with Gastrointestinal System Disorders for the following diagnoses: B 1, B 2, G 6, O 5, and R 1

C. PLANNING/IMPLEMENTATION

1. Maintain the semi-Fowler's position to help localize infection in the pelvic area
2. Assess the client's temperature, vital signs, and pain
3. Monitor IV therapy and gastrointestinal decompression
4. Monitor intake and output
5. Auscultate for bowel sounds; note the passage of flatus

D. EVALUATION/OUTCOMES

1. Reports absence of pain
2. Maintains fluid balance
3. Reestablishes regular pattern of bowel elimination
4. Maintains adequate nutritional intake

▼ HEMORRHOIDS

Data Base

A. Etiology and pathophysiology
   1. Varicosities of the rectum that can be internal or external
   2. Constipation, prolonged sitting or standing, straining at defecation, and pregnancy increase the risk of developing hemorrhoids
   3. Prevention can often be achieved by high-fiber diets; soluble fibers such as pectin and guar gums are particularly effective

B. Clinical findings
   1. Subjective
      a. Anal pain
      b. Pruritus
   2. Objective
      a. Protrusion of varicosities around the anus
      b. Rectal bleeding and mucus discharge

C. Therapeutic interventions
   1. High-fiber diet (especially pectin-containing fruits and vegetables) to prevent constipation
   2. Low-roughage diet (elimination of raw fruits and vegetables) during acute exacerbations
   3. Use of laxatives and stool softeners to regulate bowel habits
   4. Analgesic suppositories and ointments may be prescribed in addition to sitz baths or ice compresses to alleviate discomfort
   5. Internal hemorrhoids may be ligated with rubber bands; as necrosis occurs, the tissue sloughs off

6. Hemorrhoidectomy: surgical removal of hemorrhoids

Nursing Care of Clients with Hemorrhoids

A. DATA COLLECTION

1. History of causative factors
2. Presence and characteristics of pain
3. Presence of hemorrhoids in perianal area

B. ANALYSIS AND INTERPRETATION

Refer to General Nursing Diagnoses for Clients with Gastrointestinal System Disorders for the following diagnoses: B 2, G 5, K, and R 1

C. PLANNING/IMPLEMENTATION

1. Administer medication as ordered to relieve discomfort
2. Provide privacy and sufficient time for defecation
3. Educate client concerning appropriate dietary and bowel habits
   a. Encourage generous daily intake of high-fiber foods including fresh fruits and vegetables, whole-grain breads, and cereals and legumes
   b. Promote intake of at least 8 glasses of fluid per day
   c. Discourage routine use of laxatives, which results in dependency; bulking agents such as Metamucil may be prescribed
4. Assist the client with sitz baths or ice compresses as ordered
5. Provide care for the client having a hemorrhoidectomy
   a. Administer cleansing enemas and prepare the perineal area preoperatively
   b. Observe for rectal hemorrhage and urinary retention postoperatively
   c. Administer a retention enema on the second or third postoperative day if ordered to stimulate defecation and soften the stool
   d. Explain that postoperatively a small amount of bleeding with a bowel movement is normal

D. EVALUATION/OUTCOMES

1. Reports increased comfort, particularly on defecation
2. Complies with treatment regimen
3. Remains free from infection

▼ HERNIAS

Data Base

A. Etiology and pathophysiology
   1. Protrusion of an organ or structure through a weakening in the abdominal wall; may contain fat, intestine, or an organ, such as the bladder

2. Abdominal wall can become weakened due to a congenital or acquired defect
3. If the protruding structure can be manipulated back in place, the hernia is said to be reducible; if it cannot, it is considered incarcerated
4. Strangulation occurs when blood supply to the tissues within the hernia is disrupted; this is an emergency situation, since gangrene occurs
5. Hernias are named according to location
   a. Incisional: due to failure of fascia or muscles to heal postoperatively; intraabdominal pressure causes herniation through the scar tissue
   b. Umbilical: due to failure of the umbilicus to close at birth or to a congenital weakness of the musculature in the area; increased intraabdominal pressure due to obesity, pregnancy, or chronic cough causes herniation through the umbilicus
   c. Femoral: when a loop of intestine herniates through the femoral canal due to a weakness in the femoral ring; more common in women than men; strangulation is a common complication
   d. Inguinal: when a loop of intestine herniates through a weakened abdominal ring (frequently through the spermatic cord) into the inguinal canal; more common in men than women

B. Clinical findings
   1. Subjective
      a. History of the appearance of swelling after lifting, coughing, or vigorous exercise
      b. Pain (may be due to irritation or strangulation)
      c. Nausea can accompany strangulation
   2. Objective
      a. Swelling (lump) in the groin or umbilicus, or near an old surgical incision, that may subside when the client is in a recumbent position
      b. Vomiting and abdominal distention may develop when strangulation occurs

C. Therapeutic interventions
   1. Manual reduction by gently pushing the mass back into the abdominal cavity
   2. When the client is a poor surgical risk, use of a truss (pad worn next to skin held in place under pressure by a belt)
   3. Herniorrhaphy (surgical repair of the defect in the abdominal musculature or fascia)
   4. Hernioplasty to prevent recurrence (wire, mesh, or plastic may be inserted to strengthen the abdominal wall)

Nursing Care of Clients with Hernias

A. **DATA COLLECTION**
   1. History of potential causative factors
   2. Presence or absence of bowel sounds on auscultation
   3. Abdomen with client in standing and lying positions to determine if hernia reduces with positional change

B. **ANALYSIS AND INTERPRETATION**
   Refer to General Nursing Diagnoses for Clients with Gastrointestinal System Disorders for the following diagnoses: L 3, R 1, and R 3

C. **PLANNING/IMPLEMENTATION**
   1. Avoid abdominal palpation if hernia is strangulated
   2. Teach the client using a truss that it should be applied prior to getting out of bed
   3. Provide care following surgery
      a. Observe the client for signs of respiratory infection; administer cough suppressants as ordered to prevent stress on the incision
      b. Instruct client to avoid coughing if possible; use deep breathing and incentive spirometry to prevent respiratory complications
      c. Instruct the client to self-splint when coughing and turning to provide incisional support
      d. When spinal or local anesthesia is used, peristalsis is not interfered with and postoperative diet can be normal; when general anesthesia is used, nasogastric decompression may be employed until peristalsis returns
      e. Administer mild cathartics as ordered to prevent straining and increased intraabdominal pressure at defecation
      f. Apply an ice bag and scrotal support with a rolled towel or suspensory if the scrotum is edematous postoperatively to reduce the edema and pain
      g. Administer medication for pain as ordered when necessary
      h. Instruct the client to avoid lifting or strenuous exercise on discharge until permitted by the surgeon

D. **EVALUATION/OUTCOMES**
   1. Reports decreased pain
   2. Restates discharge instructions

EATING DISORDERS

See Eating Disorders in Psychiatric/Mental Health Nursing (Chapter 4)

FOOD POISONING

▼ STAPHYLOCOCCUS AUREUS

Data Base

A. Etiology and pathophysiology
1. Gram-positive *Staphylococcus* strain that clots plasma (coagulase positive) is the most virulent type and causes a variety of infections
2. Most food poisoning resulting in GI upset occurs as a result of this bacterium
3. Organism is found in unrefrigerated creams, mayonnaise, stuffing, meats, and fish
4. Bacteria usually are transmitted to food on the hands of food handlers
5. Incubation period is 1 to 6 hours after ingestion of contaminated food, with symptoms lasting 24 to 48 hours

B. Clinical findings
1. Subjective
   a. Nausea
   b. Malaise
   c. Abdominal cramps and pain
2. Objective
   a. Diarrhea 1 to 8 hours after ingestion
   b. Subnormal temperature
   c. Vomiting

C. Therapeutic interventions
1. Supply with adequate fluid and electrolytes orally or parenterally
2. Bed rest

Nursing Care of Clients with *Staphylococcus Aureus*

A. DATA COLLECTION
1. History of food ingested over the last 18 hours
2. Frequency and characteristics of stool
3. Temperature for baseline data
4. Presence of nausea and vomiting

B. ANALYSIS AND INTERPRETATION

Refer to General Nursing Diagnoses for Clients with Gastrointestinal System Disorders for the following diagnoses: H 4, I 2, and O 6

C. PLANNING/IMPLEMENTATION
1. Obtain stool specimen for culture
2. Offer fluids in small amounts as tolerated
3. Administer intravenous fluids to restore fluid and electrolyte balance
4. Teach the importance of eating foods that are properly prepared and stored

D. EVALUATION/OUTCOMES
1. Reports decreased bowel activity
2. Maintains fluid balance
3. Maintains nutritional status

▼ BOTULISM

Data Base

A. Etiology and pathophysiology
1. *Clostridium botulinum*: large, gram-positive bacillus; an obligate anaerobe; its exotoxin, the most powerful biologic toxic known, is responsible for botulism
2. Organism causes the most serious, often fatal, form of food poisoning
3. Toxins found in improperly processed foods (mostly canned foods) that have been infected with the anaerobic bacillus *Clostridium botulinum*
4. Toxins block neuromuscular transmission in cholinergic nerve fibers by possibly binding with acetylcholine
5. Incubation period usually 12 to 72 hours after ingestion of contaminated food, but may be as long as 4 to 8 days

B. Clinical findings
1. Subjective
   a. Lassitude and fatigue
   b. Diplopia
   c. Weakness of muscles in the extremities
   d. Dysphasia and dysphagia
2. Objective
   a. Diminished visual acuity
   b. Loss of pupillary light reflex
   c. Diminished gag reflex

C. Therapeutic interventions
1. Keep the client in a darkened room
2. IV feedings to prevent aspiration
3. Tracheostomy and other supportive measures as necessary
4. Cathartics and cleansing enemas to remove toxins from the body
5. Trivalent antitoxins as necessary
6. Gastric lavage

Nursing Care of Clients with Botulism

A. DATA COLLECTION
1. History of ingestion of contaminated foods
2. Extent of weakness
3. Neurologic status for baseline data
4. Presence or absence of gag reflex

B. ANALYSIS AND INTERPRETATION

Refer to General Nursing Diagnoses for Clients with Gastrointestinal System Disorders for the following diagnoses: A, C 1, I 1, L 4, and O 2

C. PLANNING/IMPLEMENTATION
1. Obtain stool specimen for culture
2. Prevent aspiration pneumonia by proper positioning; keep suction equipment available at the bedside
3. Carefully observe the client's neurologic status to determine progression of the disease

4. Prevent contractures and emboli by the use of range-of-motion exercises
5. Provide emotional support to the client and family in an attempt to reduce anxiety

D. EVALUATION/OUTCOMES
1. Maintains fluid balance
2. Maintains nutritional status
3. Demonstrates respiratory rate and characteristics within normal limits

SALMONELLOSIS

Data Base

A. Etiology and pathophysiology
1. Many species of *Salmonella* cause a local GI infection in which organisms do not enter blood (unlike *S. typhosa* and *S. paratyphi*); such infections are referred to as salmonellosis or salmonella food poisoning
2. Organisms found in inadequately cooked meats
3. Multiply in the intestines, causing GI upset and infection
4. Incubation period usually 10 to 24 hours after ingestion of contaminated food, and symptoms usually last 2 to 3 days

B. Clinical findings
1. Subjective
   a. Nausea
   b. Malaise
   c. Abdominal cramps and pain
2. Objective
   a. Chills and fever
   b. Vomiting

C. Therapeutic interventions
1. Bed rest
2. Fluid and electrolyte replacement

Nursing Care of Clients with Salmonellosis

A. DATA COLLECTION
1. History of causative factors
2. Temperature for baseline data
3. Presence of nausea, malaise, abdominal cramps, and pain

B. ANALYSIS AND INTERPRETATION
Refer to General Nursing Diagnoses for Clients with Gastrointestinal System Disorders for the following diagnoses: A, I 1, O 6, and R 1

C. PLANNING/IMPLEMENTATION
1. Obtain stool specimen for culture
2. Offer the client small amounts of fluids as tolerated
3. Teach the client the importance of eating foods that have been cooked properly

D. EVALUATION/OUTCOMES
1. Reports decreased pain
2. Maintains fluid balance
3. Maintains nutritional status

NEUROMUSCULOSKELETAL SYSTEMS

REVIEW OF ANATOMY AND PHYSIOLOGY OF THE NEUROMUSCULOSKELETAL SYSTEMS

Structures and Functions of the Nervous System

Overview of the Nervous System
A. Neurons (nerve cells) are basic structural and functional units; about 10 billion in the human brain
B. Central nervous system (CNS): spinal cord and brain
C. Peripheral nervous system (PNS): nerves and ganglia
D. Autonomic nervous system (ANS): sympathetic and parasympathetic
E. Sense organs
F. Definitions
1. White matter: bundles of myelinated nerve fibers
2. Gray matter: clusters of mainly neuronal cell bodies
3. Nerves: bundles of myelinated nerve fibers located outside the CNS
4. Tracts: bundles of myelinated nerve fibers located within the CNS
5. Ganglia (singular: ganglion): microscopic structures consisting of neuron cell bodies; mainly located outside the CNS

Neurons
A. General properties and functions
1. Irritability: response to stimulus
2. Conductivity: conduct electrical energy (nerve impulse); basis for body's rapid communication and integration network
3. Types
   a. Sensory (afferent) neurons: transmit impulses to spinal cord or brain
   b. Motoneurons (motor or efferent neurons): transmit impulses away from brain or spinal cord toward or to muscles or glands
   (1) Somatic motoneurons: transmit impulses from the cord or brain stem to skeletal muscle
   (2) Visceral or autonomic motoneurons: transmit impulses from the cord or brainstem to smooth muscle, cardiac muscle, or glands

c. Interneurons (internuncial or intercalated neurons): transmit impulses from sensory neurons to motoneurons

4. Neurons cannot be replaced if lost, but neuronal contents are constantly being replenished; a system of axonal flow distributes neural components to all regions from the cell body, where most synthesis occurs

B. Structure: well suited to transmitting impulses over distances
   1. Cell body contains a nucleus and other cytoplasmic organelles
   2. Axon and dendrites: cellular extensions; single axon or dendrite referred to as a nerve fiber
      a. Axon: one per neuron; carries impulse away from cell body; longer and thinner than dendrites; transmits only at end where it communicates with other neurons, muscles, or glands; may be over 1 m in length and may communicate with 1000 other neurons
      b. Dendrites: delicate cellular extensions carry impulses toward cell body; several per neuron; each repeatedly branches, forming complex, bushlike network around cell body; increases surface area for reception by neuron of incoming electric signals; dendrite of sensory neurons exceptional in being extremely long, extending to periphery from ganglia near brain and spinal cord
   3. Supportive coverings and sheaths
      a. Myelin: multiple, dense layers of membrane wrapped around an axon or dendrite; gaps in myelin every millimeter or so along the fiber are called nodes of Ranvier; myelinated nerve fibers transmit nerve impulses more rapidly than nonmyelinated fibers of same diameter
      b. Neurilemma: sheath of cells (Schwann cells) forming an envelope around axons and some dendrites
         (1) Responsible for effective regeneration of a nerve fiber after injury in the peripheral nervous system; the neurilemma forms a cellular tube down which the regenerating fiber travels
         (2) Forms the myelin sheath
   4. Neuronal cell membrane: similar in lipid content to cell membranes of all other body cells; however, specific proteins embedded in and attached to the surface of the lipid provide special characteristics; membrane proteins can be grouped into five classes:
      a. Pumps: actively transport ions (notably sodium and potassium) between intracellular and interstitial fluid; establish ionic conditions for resting potential and nerve impulse
      b. Channels: provide selective pathways for diffusion of specific ions, as in neuronal depolarization and repolarization; channels open and close (gating mechanisms) in response to voltage changes and chemicals
      c. Receptors: depolarization and repolarization; channels provide specific binding sites for various naturally occurring transmitters and drugs
      d. Enzymes: catalyze chemical reactions on the membrane surface
      e. Structural proteins: interconnect cells to form tissues and organs; hold cell parts together
   5. Synapse: point of contact between one neuron and another
      a. Typical neuron may have between 1000 and 10,000 synapses
      b. Most often occurs between axon of one cell and dendrite of another; also commonly between axon and the cell body of another
      c. Physical gap (synaptic cleft) separates the terminal axonal branches and dendrite or cell body of the next neuron
      d. At the synapse, the axon terminals enlarge to form a terminal button (bouton), which is the information-delivering part of the synapse; some synapses are excitatory and others inhibitory
   6. Neuroglia take up most of the space in the nervous system not occupied by neurons; they support, defend, and nourish neurons; chief source of CNS tumors; unlike neurons, neuroglia retain the ability to divide; astrocytes, a type of neuroglia cell, provide framework of cells and fibers that suspend neurons and help provide the blood-brain barrier

Brain

A. General considerations
   1. Most active of all body organs in energy consumption; has large blood supply and high oxygen consumption, which increases even further during dreaming stage of sleep
   2. Unlike other cells of body, neurons can only utilize glucose for energy metabolism; therefore hypoglycemia can seriously alter brain function and lead to coma
   3. Brain cells protected by the blood-brain barrier, a selective filtration system that isolates the brain from substances in the general circulation; barrier is based on the relative impermeability of blood vessels in the brain and the tight wrapping of neuroglial cells around the neurons and blood vessels of the brain; only

selected brain regions designed to monitor the chemical composition of blood are not protected by the blood-brain barrier

4. Ease of drug entry into the brain depends on size and fat solubility; the smaller the molecule and the greater the fat solubility, the more easily the drug enters brain tissue

5. Overall function of the brain and spinal cord is to channel sensory input to a variety of neural structures whose analysis culminates in the convergence of impulses on various motor neurons, which effect movements of all types of muscles and activity of glands

B. Regions of brain and their functions
1. Basic tissue types
   a. Gray matter: aggregations of neuron cell bodies
   b. White matter: composed primarily of tracts of fibers (axons) interconnecting neurons in different regions of the CNS
2. Basic cellular types in the CNS
   a. Association (intercalated) neurons: about 99.9% of all the neurons in the CNS
   b. Motor neurons: several million found in the CNS
3. Gross anatomic regions
   a. Hindbrain (brainstem): lowermost brain division; formed by enlargement of the spinal cord as it enters the cranial cavity
      (1) Medulla: lowest portion of the hindbrain
         (a) Consists mainly of white matter (sensory and motor tracts); also contains reticular formation (mixture of gray and white matter); some important reflex centers located in reticular formation: cardiac, vasomotor, respiratory, and swallowing centers
         (b) Functions: contains centers for vital heart, blood vessel diameter (blood pressure), and respiratory reflexes; also centers for vomiting, coughing, swallowing, etc.; conducts impulses between the cord and brain (both sensory and motor)
      (2) Pons
         (a) Part of the brain located just above the medulla; consists mainly of white matter (sensory and motor tracts) interspersed with gray matter (reflex centers)
         (b) Conducts impulses between the cord and various parts of the brain and contains reflex centers for cranial nerves V, VI, VII, and VIII (trigeminal, abducent, facial, and acoustic)

b. Cerebellum: dorsal appendage of the hindbrain
   (1) Structure: second largest part of the human brain; surface marked with sulci (grooves) and very slightly raised, slender convolutions; internal white matter forms pattern suggestive of veins of a leaf
   (2) Functions
      (a) Cerebellum exerts synergic control over the skeletal muscles; this means that impulses conducted by cerebellar neurons regulate and modulate output of the somatomotor region of the neocortex, which results in coordination of skeletal muscle contractions to produce smooth, steady, and precise movements
      (b) Because it coordinates skeletal muscle contractions, the cerebellum plays an essential part in producing normal postures and maintaining equilibrium
c. Midbrain: part of the brain located between the pons, which lies below it, and the diencephalon and cerebrum, which lie above it; consists mainly of white matter (cerebral peduncles) with scattered bits of gray matter
   (1) Superior and inferior colliculi (corpora quadrigemina): integrate and analyze sensory input from the ears, eyes, and various regions of the cerebral cortex; put out motor information to lower motor system
   (2) Reflex centers for cranial nerves III (oculomotor) and IV (trochlear): pupillary reflexes and eye movements
   (3) Pineal body: precise function unknown; may be part of endocrine system, helping to regulate secretion of gonadotropins from the hypophysis cerebri
d. Forebrain
   (1) Optic vesicles: develop into the retinas connected to base of the forebrain by their stalks, the optic nerves
   (2) Diencephalon: unpaired division of the forebrain; cerebral hemispheres diverge from this structure
      (a) Thalamus: mass of gray matter in each cerebral hemisphere:
         • Processes incoming sensory information prior to distribution to the somatosensory cortex; crudely translates sensory impulses into sensations but does not localize them on a body region

- Ventral nucleus of the thalamus processes motor information from the cerebral cortex and cerebellum and projects its analysis back to the motor cortex
- Contributes to the concentrating ability by filtering out distracting sensory input
- Contributes to emotional component of sensations (pleasant or unpleasant)

(b) Hypothalamus: gray matter that forms floor of third ventricle and lower part of its lateral walls:
- Contains many higher autonomic reflex centers; these centers integrate autonomic functions by sending impulses to each other and to the lower autonomic centers; they form a crucial part of the neural path by which emotions and other cerebral functions can alter vital, automatic functions such as the heartbeat, blood pressure, peristalsis, and secretion by glands producing psychophysiologic diseases; neural path for psychophysiologic disease: impulses from the cerebral cortex to autonomic centers in the hypothalamus, to lower autonomic centers in the brainstem and cord, to visceral effectors (e.g., heart, smooth muscle, glands)
- Helps control the anterior pituitary gland; certain neurons in the hypothalamus secrete neuropeptides into the pituitary portal veins, which transport them to the anterior pituitary gland where they influence secretion of various important hormones; for example, TRH and LH-RH regulate the pituitary secretions of TSH and gonadotropic hormones, respectively
- Neurons in the supraoptic nucleus of the hypothalamus synthesize ADH and oxytocin; from the cell bodies of these neurons, ADH and oxytocin are transmitted down their axons into the posterior pituitary gland, from which they are released into the blood; in short, hypothalamic neurons make ADH and oxytocin, but the posterior pituitary gland secretes them
- Certain hypothalamic neurons serve as an appetite center and others function as a satiety center; together these centers regulate appetite and food intake
- Certain hypothalamic neurons serve as heat-regulating centers by relaying impulses to lower autonomic centers for vasoconstriction, vasodilation, and sweating, and to somatic centers for shivering
- Maintains waking state; constitutes part of the arousal or alerting neural pathway

(c) Corpus callosum: mass of white matter (nerve tracts) that interconnects the two cerebral hemispheres

(d) Optic chiasm: the point of crossing over (decussation) of optic nerve fibers from the nasal half of each retina to the opposite side, where they join optic nerve fibers from the lateral half of the other eye's retina to form the optic tracts

(3) Paired cerebral hemispheres (telencephalon): longitudinal fissure divides the cerebrum into two hemispheres connected only by the corpus callosum; each cerebral hemisphere divided by fissures into four major lobes: frontal, parietal, temporal, occipital; also contains deeper regions of gray matter and fiber tracts

(a) Cerebral cortex is outer layer of gray matter forming folds (convolutions) composed of hills (gyri) and valleys (sulci)

(b) Frontal lobes:
- Influence abstract thinking, sense of humor, and uniqueness of personality
- Control contraction of skeletal muscles and synchronization of muscular movements
- Exert control over hypothalamus; influence basic biorhythms
- Control muscular movements necessary for speech; found only in one cerebral hemisphere

(c) Parietal lobes:
- Translate nerve impulses into sensations (e.g., touch, temperature)
- Interpret sensations; provide appreciation of size, shape, texture, and weight

- Interpret sense of taste
  (d) Temporal lobes:
  - Translate nerve impulses into sensations of sound and interpret sounds
  - Interpret sense of smell
  - Control behavior patterns
  (e) Occipital area
  - Translates nerve impulse into sights and interprets sights
  - Provides appreciation of size, shape, and color
  (f) Angular gyrus: analysis and integration of sights, sounds, and somatic sensations
  (g) Amygdala: controls patterns of emotional behavior
  (h) Corpus striatum: helps regulate muscle contraction and emotional reactions
  (i) Cerebral tracts: bundles of axons compose the white matter in the interior of the cerebrum; ascending projection tracts transmit impulses toward the cerebral cortex; descending projection tracts transmit impulses from cerebral cortex; commissural tracts transmit from one hemisphere to the other; association tracts transmit from one convolution to another in the same hemisphere

4. Brain and spinal cord coverings
   a. Bony: vertebrae around the cord; cranial bones around the brain
   b. Membranous: called meninges; consist of three layers
      (1) Dura mater: white fibrous tissue, outer layer
      (2) Arachnoid membrane: cobwebby middle layer
      (3) Pia mater: innermost layer; adheres to outer surface of the cord and brain; contains blood vessels

5. Cord and brain fluid spaces
   a. Subarachnoid space around the cord and extending beyond the cord into the fourth and fifth lumbar vertebrae
   b. Subarachnoid space around the brain
   c. Central canal inside the cord
   d. Ventricles and cerebral aqueduct inside the brain; four cavities
      (1) First and second (lateral) ventricles: large cavities, one in each cerebral hemisphere
      (2) Third ventricle: vertical slit in the cerebrum beneath the corpus callosum and longitudinal fissure

      (3) Fourth ventricle: diamond-shaped space between the cerebellum and medulla and pons; expansion of the central canal of the cord

6. Formation and circulation of the cerebrospinal fluid (CSF)
   a. Formed by plasma filtering from the network of capillaries (choroid plexus) in each ventricle; active transport of plasma also involved
   b. Circulates from the lateral ventricles to the third ventricle, cerebral aqueduct, fourth ventricle, central canal of the cord, and the subarachnoid space of the cord and brain; returns to blood via venous sinuses of the brain

Cranial Nerves: 12 Pairs

See Table 6-13

Spinal Cord

A. Location: in the spinal cavity, from the foramen magnum to the first lumbar vertebra
B. Structure
   1. Deep groove (anterior median fissure) and more shallow groove (posterior median sulcus) incompletely divide the cord into right and left symmetric halves
   2. Inner core of the cord consists of gray matter shaped like a three-dimensional H
   3. Long columns of white matter surround the cord's inner core of gray matter; namely, right and left anterior, lateral, and posterior columns; composed of numerous sensory and motor tracts (Fig. 6-14, *A* and *B*)
C. Functions
   1. Sensory tracts conduct impulses up cord to brain; motor tracts conduct impulses down cord from brain
   2. Gray matter of cord contains reflex centers for all spinal cord reflexes

Spinal Nerves: 31 Pairs

A. Each nerve attaches to the cord by two short roots, anterior and posterior; the posterior roots are marked by a swelling, the spinal ganglion
B. Branches of the spinal nerves form plexuses or intricate networks of fibers (e.g., brachial plexus), from which nerves emerge to supply various parts of the skin, mucosa, and skeletal muscles
C. All spinal nerves are mixed nerves composed of both sensory dendrites and motor axons; they function in both sensations and movements
D. Nerve consists of bundles of nerve fibers (axons and dendrites) supported by connective tissue

Autonomic Nervous System

A. Definition: division of the nervous system that conducts impulses from the brainstem or cord out to visceral effectors: cardiac muscle, smooth muscle, and glandular tissue

TABLE 6-13 Distribution and function of cranial nerve pairs

Name and number	Distribution	Function
Olfactory (I)	Nasal mucosa, high up along the septum especially	Sense of smell (sensory only)
Optic (II)	Retina of eyeball	Vision (sensory only)
Oculomotor (III)	Extrinsic muscles of eyeball, except superior oblique and external rectus; also intrinsic eye muscles (iris and ciliary)	Eye movements; constriction of pupil and bulging of lens, which together produce accommodation for near vision
Trochlear (IV), smallest cranial nerve	Superior oblique muscle of eye	Eye movements
Trigeminal (V) (or trifacial), largest cranial nerve	Sensory fibers to skin and mucosa of head and to teeth; muscles of mastication (sensory and motor fibers)	Sensation in head and face; chewing movements
Abducent (VI)	External rectus muscle of eye	Abduction of eye
Facial (VII)	Muscles of facial expression; taste buds of anterior two thirds of tongue; motor fibers to submaxillary and sublingual salivary glands	Facial expressions; taste; secretion of saliva
Acoustic (VIII) (vestibulocochlear)	Inner ear	Hearing and equilibrium (sensory only)
Glossopharyngeal (IX)	Posterior third of tongue; mucosa and muscles of pharynx; parotid gland; carotid sinus and body	Taste and other sensations of tongue; secretion of saliva; swallowing movements; function in reflex arcs for control of blood pressure and respiration
Vagus (X) (or pneumogastric)	Mucosa and muscles of pharynx, larynx, trachea, bronchi, esophagus; thoracic and abdominal viscera	Sensations and movements of organs supplied; for example, slows heart, increases peristalsis and gastric and pancreatic secretion; voice production
Spinal accessory (XI)	Certain neck and shoulder muscles (muscles of larynx, sternocleidomastoid, trapezius)	Shoulder movements; turns head; voice production; muscle sense
Hypoglossal (XII)	Tongue muscles	Tongue movements, as in talking; muscle sense

Note: The first letters of the words in the following sentence are the first letters of the cranial nerves, and many generations of anatomy students have used it as an aid to memorizing the names: "*On Old Olympus' Towering Tops, A Finn and German Viewed Some Hops.*" (There are several slightly different versions of the mnemonic.)

B. Divisions: consists of two divisions: the sympathetic (thoracolumbar) system and the parasympathetic (craniosacral) system
  1. Sympathetic system
    a. Sympathetic ganglia: two chains of 21 or 22 ganglia located immediately in front of the spinal column, one chain to the right, one to the left
    b. Collateral ganglia: located a short distance from the cord (e.g., celiac ganglia [solar plexus], superior and inferior mesenteric ganglia)
    c. Sympathetic nerves: (e.g., splanchnic nerves, cardiac nerves)
  2. Parasympathetic system
    a. Parasympathetic ganglia: located some distance from the spinal column, in or near the visceral effectors (e.g., ciliary ganglion in posterior part of the orbit, near the iris and ciliary muscle)

    b. Parasympathetic nerves: (e.g., vagus nerve, called the great parasympathetic nerve of the body)
C. Neurons
  1. Preganglionic sympathetic neurons: dendrites and cell bodies lie in the lateral gray columns of thoracic and lumbar segments of the cord; their axons conduct from the cord to the sympathetic ganglia or the collateral ganglia (see D 3, which follows)
  2. Postganglionic sympathetic neurons: dendrites and cell bodies lie in the sympathetic ganglia or the collateral ganglia; their axons conduct to visceral effectors
  3. Preganglionic parasympathetic neurons: dendrites and cell bodies of some of these neurons lie in gray matter of the brainstem; others exit at sacral segments of the cord; conduct impulses from the brainstem or cord to the parasympathetic ganglia (see D 3, which follows)

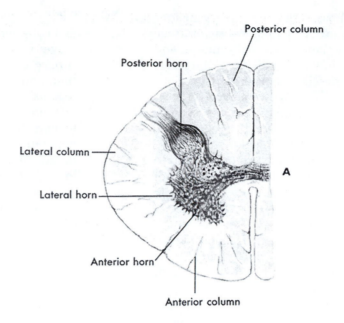

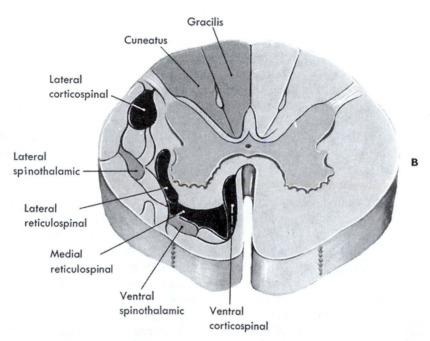

FIGURE 6-14 A, Distribution of gray matter (horns) and white matter (columns) in a section of the spinal cord at the thoracic level. **B**, Location in the spinal cord of some major projection tracts. Black areas are descending motor tracts. Shaded areas are ascending sensory tracts. (From Anthony CP and Thibodeau GA: *Textbook of anatomy and physiology*, ed 13, St. Louis, 1989, Mosby.)

4. Postganglionic parasympathetic neurons: dendrites and cell bodies lie in the parasympathetic ganglia; their axons conduct to visceral effectors (see D 3, which follows)

D. Principles about the autonomic nervous system
 1. Dual autonomic innervation: both sympathetic and parasympathetic fibers supply most visceral effectors

2. Single autonomic innervation: only sympathetic fibers supply sweat glands and probably the smooth muscles of hairs and of most blood vessels; preganglionic sympathetic fibers terminate in adrenal medulla (not postganglionic fibers as in other glands)

3. Autonomic chemical transmitters: all preganglionic axons are cholinergic fibers, as are most

(or perhaps all) parasympathetic postganglionic axons and a few sympathetic postganglionic axons (to sweat glands, external genitalia, and smooth muscle in walls of blood vessels located in skeletal muscles); sympathetic postganglionic axons are the only adrenergic (i.e., norepinephrine-releasing) fibers; but, as just mentioned, a few of them are cholinergic

4. Autonomic antagonism and summation: sympathetic and parasympathetic impulses tend to produce opposite effects; the algebraic sum of two opposing tendencies determines the response made by dually innervated visceral effectors (Table 6-14)

5. Principle of parasympathetic dominance of the digestive tract: normally, parasympathetic impulses to digestive tract glands and smooth muscle dominate over sympathetic impulses to these effectors; the dominance of parasympathetic impulses promotes digestive gland secretion, peristalsis, and defecation

6. Principle of sympathetic dominance in stress situations: under conditions of stress, sympathetic impulses to the visceral effectors usually increase greatly and dominate over parasympathetic impulses; however, in some individuals under stress, parasympathetic impulses via the vagus nerve to glands and smooth muscle of the stomach greatly increase, causing increased hydrochloric acid secretion and increased gastric motility; this can eventually cause peptic ulcer, a condition that may aptly be called the great parasympathetic stress disease

7. In general, when the sympathetic system dominates control of visceral effectors, it causes them to function in ways that enable the body to expend maximum energy as is necessary in strenuous exercise and other types of stress (see Table 6-14 for sympathetic action on specific visceral effectors)

8. Principle of nonautonomy: the autonomic nervous system is neither anatomically nor physiologically independent of the rest of the nervous system; all parts of the nervous system work together as a single, functional unit; that is, dendrites and cells of all preganglionic neurons in gray matter of the brainstem or cord (lower autonomic centers) are influenced by impulses conducted to them from higher autonomic centers, notably the hypothalamus

9. Importance of autonomic nervous system: plays a major role in maintaining physiologic balance; under usual conditions, autonomic impulses regulate activities of the visceral effectors so they maintain or quickly restore this balance; under highly stressful conditions, problems may occur

Nerve Impulses: Conduction

A. General considerations
1. Wave of electrical energy that flows over the surface of neurons and permits communication and integration between distant body regions
2. The larger the nerve fiber and the thicker the myelin sheath, the greater the velocity of the nerve impulse
3. Based on concentration differences between ions in the intracellular fluid of neuron and surrounding interstitial fluid
4. Ionic differences depend on ion pumps: most often studied is the sodium pump
   a. Requires ATP to work
   b. Pumps three sodium ions out of the cell in exchange for two potassium ions taken into the cell
   c. Due to action of the sodium pump, intracellular fluid is about 10 times richer in potassium ions than is interstitial fluid, and interstitial fluid is about 10 times richer in sodium ions than is intracellular fluid

B. Impulse generation
1. Resting potential: after the sodium pump establishes ionic gradients, some potassium diffuses out of the cell through permanently open potassium channels; such potassium flow results in an excess of positive charge on the membrane's outer surface and a deficit of positive charge on the membrane's inner surface; the result is a voltage difference of 70 millivolts (mV) with the cell interior being negative; this is the resting potential
2. Action potential: change in voltage across the neuronal membrane activates (opens) specific sodium ion channels in the membrane, allowing sodium ions to enter the cell and reverse the membrane's charge (inside becomes positive and outside becomes negative); as depolarization proceeds, the sodium channel closes and a voltage-gated potassium channel opens so that repolarization occurs with the voltage difference returning to the resting potential
3. Nerve impulse: action potential, composed of depolarization and repolarization, propagates itself down the axon or dendrite and is known as the nerve impulse

C. Basic route of impulse conduction: reflex arc
1. Description: impulse conduction
   a. Starts in receptors
   b. Continues over reflex arc(s)
   c. Terminates in effectors (muscles and glands)
   d. Results in a reflex: response by muscles or glands in which the impulse terminates; a reflex, therefore, is either contraction of muscle or secretion by gland

TABLE 6-14 Autonomic functions

Autonomic effector	Effect of sympathetic stimulation (neurotransmitter: norepinephrine unless otherwise stated)	Effect of parasympathetic stimulation (neurotransmitter: acetylcholine)
CARDIAC MUSCLE	Increased rate and strength of contraction (beta receptors)	Decreased rate and strength of contraction
SMOOTH MUSCLE OF BLOOD VESSELS		
Skin blood vessels	Constriction (alpha receptors)	No effect
Skeletal muscle blood vessels	Dilation (beta receptors)	No effect
Coronary blood vessels	Constriction (alpha receptors) Dilation (beta receptors)	Dilation
Abdominal blood vessels	Constriction (alpha receptors)	No effect
Blood vessels of external genitals	Constriction (alpha receptors)	Dilation of blood vessels causing erection
SMOOTH MUSCLE OF HOLLOW ORGANS AND SPHINCTERS		
Bronchioles	Dilation (beta receptors)	Constriction
Digestive tract, except sphincters	Decreased peristalsis (beta receptors)	Increased peristalsis
Sphincters of digestive tract	Constriction (alpha receptors)	Relaxation
Urinary bladder	Relaxation (beta receptors)	Contraction
Urinary sphincters	Constriction (alpha receptors)	Relaxation
Reproductive ducts	Contraction (alpha receptors)	Relaxation
Eye		
Iris	Contraction of radial muscle; dilated pupil	Contraction of circular muscle; constricted pupil
Ciliary	Relaxation; accommodates for far vision	Contraction; accommodates for near vision
Hairs (pilomotor muscles)	Contraction produces goose pimples, or piloerection (alpha receptors)	No effect
GLANDS		
Sweat	Increased sweat (neurotransmitter: acetylcholine)	No effect
Lacrimal	No effect	Increased secretion of tears
Digestive (salivary, gastric, etc.)	Decreased secretion of saliva; not known for others	Increased secretion of saliva
Pancreas, including islets	Decreased secretion	Increased secretion of pancreatic juice and insulin
Liver	Increased glycogenolysis (beta receptors); increased blood sugar level	No effect
*Adrenal medulla**	Increased epinephrine secretion	No effect

*Sympathetic preganglionic axons terminate in contact with secreting cells of the adrenal medulla. Thus the adrenal medulla functions, to quote someone's descriptive phrase, as a "giant sympathetic postganglionic neuron." (From Thibodeau GA and Patton K: *Anatomy and physiology*, ed 2, St. Louis, 1993, Mosby.)

e. Not all impulses result in reflexes; many are inhibited at some point along the reflex arc

2. Types of reflex arcs
   a. Two-neuron (monosynaptic) reflex arc: simplest arc possible; consists of at least one sensory neuron, one synapse, and one motoneuron (motor neuron); synapse is a region of contact between axon terminals of one neuron and dendrites or the cell body of another neuron

   b. Three-neuron arc (Fig. 6-15): consists of at least one sensory neuron, one synapse, one interneuron, one synapse, and one motoneuron
   c. Complex multisynaptic neural pathways also exist; many not yet mapped

D. Conduction across synapses
   1. Given synapse can transmit only one type of transmitter substance

2. There are 30 different types of neurotransmitters, including
   a. Monoamines (norepinephrine, dopamine, serotonin, acetylcholine); axons that release acetylcholine are called cholinergic; those that release norepinephrine are called adrenergic
   b. Amino acids (gamma-aminobutyric acid [GABA], glutamic acid, glycine, taurine); GABA is the most common inhibitory transmitter in the brain
   c. Neuropeptides (hormone-releasing hormones, enkephalins, and endorphins); some influence hormone levels and some influence perception and integration of pain and emotional experience
   d. Prostaglandins: high levels in brain tissue; some inhibit and some excite; may moderate the action of other transmitters by influencing the neuronal membrane

3. Overall response of the neuron: sum or average of excitatory and inhibitory inputs determines whether the cell will fire and the rate at which it will fire; the neuron is seen to be an evaluator of signals, not just a passive transmitter; the result of its evaluation is its individual rate of impulse transmission

Sensorineural Pathways (from Periphery to Cerebral Cortex)

A. Sensory pathways to the cerebral cortex from the periphery consist of relays of at least three neurons, which are identified by Roman numerals
   1. Sensory neuron I: conducts from the periphery to the cord or to the brainstem
   2. Sensory neuron II: conducts from the cord or brainstem to the thalamus

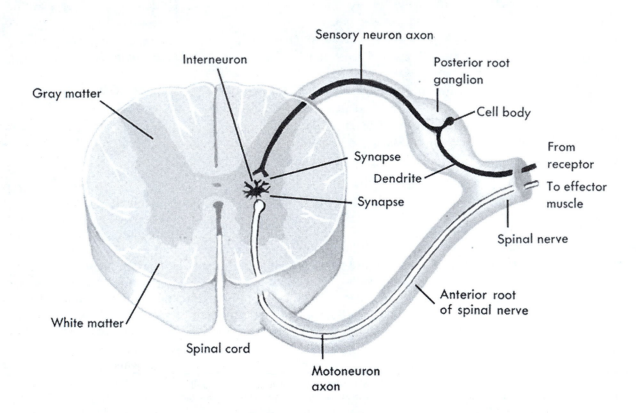

FIGURE 6-15 Three-neuron ipsilateral reflex arc, consisting of an afferent (sensory) neuron, an interneuron, and an efferent (motor) neuron (motoneuron). Note the presence of two synapses in this arc: (1) between sensory neuron axon terminals and interneuron dendrites and (2) between interneuron axon terminals and motoneuron dendrites and cell bodies (located in the anterior gray matter). Nerve impulses traversing such arcs produce many spinal reflexes (e.g., withdrawing the hand from a hot object). (From Anthony CP and Thibodeau GA: *Textbook of anatomy and physiology*, ed 13, St. Louis, 1989, Mosby.)

3. Sensory neuron III: conducts from the thalamus to the somatosensory area of the cerebral cortex

B. Crude awareness of sensations occurs when impulses reach the thalamus

C. Full consciousness of sensations with accurate localization and discrimination of fine details occurs when impulses reach the cerebral cortex

D. Most sensory neuron II axons decussate; so one side of the brain registers most of the sensations for the opposite side of the body

E. Principle of divergence applies to the sensorineural pathways; each sensory neuron synapses with many neurons, and therefore impulses may diverge from any sensory neuron and be conducted to many brain regions, including the cerebellum, reticular formation, and also, more directly, the motoneurons

F. Impulses that produce pain and an awareness of temperature are conducted up the cord to the thalamus by the lateral spinothalamic tracts

G. Impulses that produce touch and pressure sensations are conducted up the cord to the thalamus by the following two pathways:
   1. Impulses that result in discriminating touch and pressure sensations (e.g., stereognosis, precise localization, vibratory sense) are conducted by the tracts of the posterior white columns of the cord to the medulla and from there are transferred to the thalamus
   2. Impulses that result in crude touch and pressure sensations are conducted up the cord to the thalamus by fibers of the ventral spinothalamic tracts

H. Sensory impulses that result in conscious proprioception or kinesthesia (sense of position or movement of body parts) are conducted over the same pathway as are impulses that result in discriminating touch and pressure sensations

I. Sensory impulses, in addition, are also conducted to the cerebral cortex via complex multineuron pathways known as the reticular activating system; spinoreticular tracts relay sensory impulses up the cord to the brainstem reticular gray matter, and from there other neurons relay them to the hypothalamus, thalamus, and probably other parts of the brain, then finally to the cerebral cortex; conduction by the reticular activating system is essential for producing and maintaining consciousness; presumably, general anesthetics produce unconsciousness by inhibiting conduction by the reticular activating system; conversely, amphetamines and norepinephrine are thought to produce wakefulness by stimulating the reticular activating system

Motoneural Pathways (from Cerebral Cortex to Periphery)

A. Principle of the final common path: the final common path for impulse conduction to skeletal muscles consists of anterior horn neurons (i.e., motoneurons whose dendrites and cell bodies lie in the anterior gray columns of the cord and whose axons extend out through the anterior roots of spinal nerves and their branches to terminate in skeletal muscles); besides being referred to as the final common path and as anterior horn cells, these neurons are also called lower motoneurons, somatic motoneurons, and lower motor system

B. Principle of convergence: axons of many neurons converge on (i.e., synapse with) each anterior horn motoneuron

C. Motor pathways from the cerebral cortex to anterior horn cells are classified according to the route by which the fibers enter the cord
   1. Pyramidal tracts (corticospinal tracts): axons of neurons whose dendrites and cell bodies lie in the cerebral cortex; axons descend from cortex through internal capsule, pyramids of medulla, and spinal cord; a few of these axons synapse with anterior horn cells, but most of them synapse with internuncial neurons that synapse with anterior horn cells; conduction by pyramidal tracts is necessary for willed movements to occur; hence one cause of paralysis is interruption of pyramidal tract conduction
   2. Extrapyramidal tracts: all tracts that conduct between the motor cortex and the anterior horn cells, except the pyramidal tracts; upper extrapyramidal tracts relay impulses between the cortex, basal ganglia, thalamus, and brainstem; reticulospinal tracts (the main lower extrapyramidal tracts) relay impulses from the brainstem to the anterior horn cells in the cord; impulse conduction via extrapyramidal tracts is essential for producing large, automatic movements (e.g., walking, swimming) and for producing facial expressions and movements that characterize many emotions

D. Motor conduction pathway from the primary motor area of the cerebral cortex to skeletal muscles via pyramidal tracts consists of a two-neuron relay; an upper motoneuron conducts impulses from cerebrum to cord and a lower motoneuron (anterior horn cell) conducts from cord to skeletal muscle (Fig. 6-16)

E. Motor conduction pathway from the cerebral cortex via the extrapyramidal tracts consists of complex multineuron relays; several upper motoneurons relay impulses through the basal ganglia, thalamus, and brainstem down the cord to the lower motoneuron

F. Motor pathways from the cerebral cortex to anterior horn cells classified according to their influence on anterior horn cells as follows:

1. Facilitatory tracts: conduct impulses that have a facilitating or stimulating effect on anterior horn cells; main facilitatory tracts are the pyramidal tracts and the facilitatory reticulospinal tracts

2. Inhibitory tracts: conduct impulses that have an inhibiting effect on anterior horn cells; main inhibitory tracts are the inhibitory reticulospinal tracts; interruption of inhibitory reticulospinal tracts results in spasticity and rigidity

G. Ratio of facilitatory and inhibitory impulses impinging on anterior horn cells determines their activity (whether they are facilitated, stimulated, or inhibited)

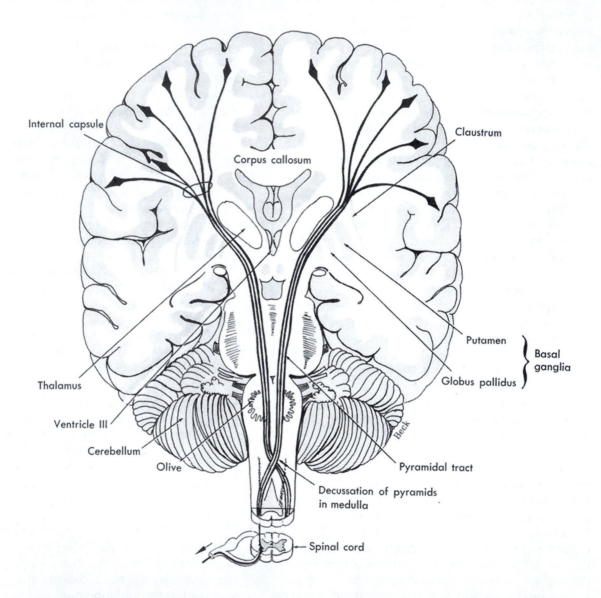

FIGURE 6-16 Cross pyramidal (lateral corticospinal) tracts, the main motor tracts of the body. Axons that compose the pyramidal tracts come from neuron cell bodies in the cerebral cortex. After they descend through the internal capsule of the cerebrum and the white matter of the brainstem, about three/fourths of the fibers decussate—cross over from one side to the other—in the medulla, as shown here. Then they continue downward in the lateral corticospinal tract on the opposite side of the cord. Each lateral corticospinal tract, therefore, conducts motor impulses from one side of the brain to skeletal muscles on the opposite side of the body. (From Anthony CP and Thibodeau GA: *Textbook of anatomy and physiology*, ed 13, St. Louis, 1989, Mosby.)

Sense Organs

Millions of receptors distributed widely throughout the skin and mucosa; muscles, tendons, joints, and viscera are sense organs of body (Table 6-15)
A. General considerations
1. Receptors monitor internal and external environment
2. Stimuli are interpreted and converted to nerve impulses, which are conducted through sensory neurons to the brain
3. Receptors' degrees of depolarization depend on the strength of the stimulus; the variable degree of depolarization is called the generator potential
4. Generator potential determines the frequency of nerve impulses sent to the CNS by afferent nerve fibers attached to receptors
5. Most receptors display sensory adaptation: steady and prolonged stimulus results in a steady decrease in strength of generator potential
B. Types of receptors
1. Exteroceptors of skin and mucosa: consist of receptors for spinal or cranial nerve branches; different types of receptors for different sensations such as heat, cold, pain, touch, and pressure
2. Proprioceptors of muscles, tendons, and joints: stretching of muscles or tendons during movements initiates stretch reflexes
3. Visceroceptors: pressoreceptors (baroreceptors) respond to stretch in walls of the aorta and carotid arteries, providing the brain with information on blood pressure; oxygen chemoreceptors in the aortic and carotid bodies monitor O$_2$ levels; carbon dioxide chemoreceptors in the respiratory center (in medulla) help control the rate and depth of respirations

4. Taste
   a. Taste buds consist of groups of receptor cells bundled together with sensory hairs protruding from a pore in the taste bud and connected to the facial and glossopharyngeal nerves (VII and IX)
   b. Respond to chemicals: sweet at tongue tip; sour and salt at tip and sides; bitter at back; receptors for bitter most sensitive
   c. Olfaction intimately involved in the sense of taste
5. Olfaction
   a. Receptors in epithelium of the nasal mucosa
   b. Odors sensed as chemicals interact with receptor sites on sensory hairs of olfactory cells
   c. Olfactory neural pathways utilize cranial nerve I
6. Sight
   a. Coats of the eyeball
      (1) Outer: sclera proper and cornea
      (2) Middle: choroid proper, ciliary body, suspensory ligament holding lens, and iris
      (3) Inner: retina
   b. Cavities and humors of the eyeball
      (1) Anterior cavity with an anterior and posterior chamber; both contain aqueous humor
      (2) Posterior cavity has no divisions; contains vitreous humor
   c. Muscles of the eye (Table 6-16)
   d. Refractory media of the eye
      (1) Cornea
      (2) Aqueous humor
      (3) Crystalline lens (has greatest refractive power)
      (4) Vitreous humor

TABLE 6-15 Receptors

Kinds	Locations	Stimulated by	Functions
Exteroceptors	Skin, mucosa, ear, eye	Changes in external environment (e.g., pressure, heat, cold, light waves, sound waves)	Initiate reflexes; Initiate sensations of many kinds (e.g., pressure, heat, cold, pain, vision, hearing)
Visceroceptors (interoceptors)	Viscera	Changes in internal environment (e.g., pressure, chemical)	Initiate reflexes; Initiate sensations of many kinds (e.g., hunger, sex, nausea, pressure)
Proprioceptors	Muscles, tendons, joints, semicircular canals of inner ear	Pressure changes	Initiate reflexes; Initiate muscle sense, or sense of position and movement of parts; also called kinesthesia

e. Accessory structures of the eye
   (1) Eyebrows and lashes
   (2) Eyelids or palpebrae: lined with mucous membrane (conjunctiva) that continues over surface of eyeball; corners of eyes, where upper and lower lids join, called inner and outer canthi
   (3) Lacrimal apparatus: lacrimal glands, ducts, sacs, and nasolacrimal ducts
f. Physiology of vision
   (1) Formation of an image on the retina, accomplished by:
       (a) Refraction: bending of light rays as they pass through the eye
       (b) Accommodation: bulging of the lens for viewing near objects
       (c) Constriction of pupils: occurs simultaneously with accommodation and in bright light
       (d) Convergence of the eyes for near objects so light rays from the object may fall on corresponding points of two retinas; necessary for single binocular vision
   (2) Stimulation of the retina: dim light causes breakdown of the chemical rhodopsin present in rods, thereby initiating impulse conduction by the rods; bright light causes breakdown of chemicals in the cones; rods considered receptors for night vision, cones receptors for daylight and color vision
   (3) Most cones concentrated in small region of the retina called fovea centralis; provides sharpest color vision
   (4) Conduction to visual area in occipital lobe of cerebral cortex by fibers of optic nerves and optic tract
7. Hearing
   a. External ear: consists of the auricle (or pinna), external acoustic meatus (ear opening), and external auditory canal
   b. Middle ear: separated from the external ear by the tympanic membrane; middle ear contains auditory ossicles (malleus, incus, stapes) and openings from the auditory (eustachian) tubes, mastoid cells, external ear, and internal ear; auditory tube is collapsible and lined with mucosa and extends from the nasopharynx to the middle ear; equalizes pressure on both sides of eardrum, as when tubes open during yawning, swallowing, or sucking
   c. Inner ear (or labyrinth): composed of a bony labyrinth that has a membranous labyrinth inside it; parts of the inner ear
       (1) Bony vestibule: contains the membranous utricle and saccule, each of which in turn contains a sense organ called the macula; vestibular nerve (branch of eighth cranial [acoustic or vestibulocochlear] nerve) supplies the maculae aousticae; these sense organs give information about equilibrium, position of the head, and acceleration and deceleration
       (2) Bony, semicircular canals: contain the membranous semicircular canals in which are located the crista ampullaris, the sense organ for sensations of equilibrium and head movements; vestibular nerve supplies the crista as well as the macula
       (3) Bony cochlea: contains the membranous cochlear duct in which is located the organ of Corti, the hearing sense organ; cochlear nerve (branch of eighth cranial nerve) supplies the organ of Corti
   d. Physiology of hearing
       (1) Sound waves moving through the air enter the ear canal and move down it to

TABLE 6-16 Eye muscles			
Location	Kind of muscle	Names	Functions
Extrinsic—attached to outside of eyeball and to bones of orbit	Skeletal (voluntary striated)	Superior rectus Inferior rectus Lateral rectus Medial rectus Superior oblique Inferior oblique	Move eyeball in various directions
Intrinsic—within eyeball	Visceral (involuntary, smooth)	Iris Ciliary muscle	Regulate size of pupil Control shape of lens, making possible accommodation for near and far objects

strike against the tympanic membrane, causing it to vibrate

(2) Vibrations of the tympanic membrane move the malleus, whose handle is attached to the membrane

(3) Movement of the malleus moves the incus, to which the head of the malleus attaches

(4) Incus attaches to the stapes; so, as the incus moves, it moves the stapes against the oval window, into which it fits; as the stapes presses inwardly on the perilymph around the cochlear duct, it starts a ripple in the perilymph

(5) Movement of the perilymph is transmitted to the endolymph inside the cochlear duct and stimulates the organ of Corti, which projects into the endolymph

(6) Cochlear nerve conducts impulses from the organ of Corti to the brain; hearing occurs when impulses reach the auditory area in the temporal lobe of the cerebral cortex

Structures and Functions of the Muscular System

Overview of the Muscular System

A. Purpose
1. Movement
2. Posture
3. Heat production: metabolism in muscle cells produces relatively large share of body heat

B. Types of muscles and neural control
1. Striated: controlled by voluntary nervous system via somatic motoneurons in spinal and some cranial nerves
2. Smooth: controlled by autonomic nervous system via autonomic motoneurons in autonomic, spinal, and some cranial nerves; not under voluntary control (with rare exceptions)
3. Cardiac: control is identical to that of smooth muscle

C. Origins, insertions, and functions of main skeletal muscles grouped according to functions (Table 6-17)

D. Bursae

E. Tendon sheaths

Skeletal Muscles

A. Characteristics
1. Typically spindle shaped; composed of long muscle cells referred to as muscle fibers; invested by coating of fibrous connective tissue (fascia), which binds muscle to surrounding tissues
2. Arranged in bundles or fasciculi; each muscle contains several fasciculi
3. Contains rich blood supply; numerous capillary beds provide nutrients to and remove wastes from muscle
4. Individual skeletal muscle fibers
   a. Generally long and spindle shaped
   b. Multinucleate; called a syncytium
   c. Cell membrane called sarcolemma; endoplasmic reticulum called sarcoplasmic reticulum; mitochondria may be referred to as sarcosomes
   d. Contain myofibrils specialized for contraction; composed of two types of protein myofilaments, actin and myosin

B. Metabolism of skeletal muscle
1. Hypertrophy is physical enlargement of the muscle due to the addition of more myofibrils to muscle fibers, making them swell; muscle fibers do not divide to produce new fibers
2. Atrophy is reduction in size of muscle due to decrease in number of myofibrils in muscle fiber
3. Treppe (staircase phenomenon): when a muscle has contracted a few times, subsequent contractions are more powerful; may be related to the release of increased quantities of calcium ions from sarcoplasmic reticulum after the first few contractions
4. Shivering: rapid, repeating, involuntary skeletal muscle contractions; caused by hypothalamic temperature regulating center; makes use of inefficiency of muscle contraction (i.e., most of the energy of ATP is converted to heat; a smaller part goes into the mechanical motion of contraction)
5. Rigor mortis: ATP must combine with myosin to effect release of actin from myosin, which permits relaxation; after death, ATP is depleted from muscle fibers, and actin and myosin strongly associate, producing rigor mortis; subsequent bacterial decomposition of muscle proteins brings about relaxation; body enters rigor state about 24 hours after death and comes out of rigor about 24 hours later

C. Basic principles of skeletal muscle action
1. Skeletal muscles contract only if stimulated; a skeletal muscle and its motor nerve function as a physiologic unit (motor unit); either is useless without the other's functioning; for this reason anything that prevents impulse conduction to a skeletal muscle paralyzes the muscle
2. Most skeletal muscles attach to at least two bones; as a muscle contracts and pulls on its bones, it mobilizes the bone that moves most easily; the bone that moves is called the muscle's insertion bone, and that which remains stationary is its origin bone
3. Bones serve as levers, and joints as fulcrums of these levers; a muscle's contraction exerts a

Part of body moved	Movement	Muscle	Origin	Insertion
Upper arm	Flexion	Pectoralis major	Clavicle (medial half) Sternum Costal cartilages of true ribs	Humerus (greater tubercle)
	Extension	Latissimus dorsi	Vertebrae (lower thoracic, lumbar, and sacral) Ilium (crest) Lumbodorsal fascia	Humerus (intertubercular groove)
	Abduction	Deltoid	Clavicle Scapula (spine and acromion)	Humerus (lateral side on deltoid tubercle)
	Adduction	Latissimus dorsi contracting with pectoralis major	See above (Latissimus dorsi) See above (Pectoralis major)	Humerus (greater tubercle) Humerus (intertubercular groove)
Shoulder	Shrugging, elevating	Trapezius	Occipital bone Vertebrae (cervical and thoracic)	Scapula (spine and acromion) Clavicle
	Lowering	Pectoralis minor Serratus anterior	Ribs (second to fifth) Ribs (upper 8 or 9)	Scapula (coracoid) Scapula (anterior surface)
Lower arm	Flexion With forearm supinated With forearm pronated With forearm semisupinated or semipronated	Biceps brachii Brachialis	Scapula (supraglenoid tuberosity) Scapula (coracoid) Humerus (distal half, anterior surface)	Radius (tubercle at proximal end) Ulna (front of coronoid process)
		Brachioradialis	Humerus (above lateral epicondyle)	Radius (styloid process)
	Extension	Triceps brachii	Scapula (infraglenoid tuberosity) Humerus (posterior surface–lateral head above radial groove; medial head, below)	Ulna (olecranon process)
Thigh	Flexion	Iliopsoas (iliacus and psoas major)	Ilium (iliac fossa) Vertebrae (bodies of twelfth thoracic to fifth lumbar)	Femur (small trochanter)
		Rectus femoris	Ilium and anterior inferior iliac spine	Tibia (by way of patellar tendon)
	Extension	Gluteus maximus	Ilium (crest and posterior surface) Sacrum and coccyx (posterior surface)	Femur (gluteal tuberosity) Iliotibial tract
		Hamstring group (see below)	Ischium (tuberosity) Femur (linea aspera)	Fibula (head of) Tibia (lateral condyle, medial condyle, and medial surface)
	Abduction	Gluteus medius and minimus	Ilium (lateral surface)	Femur (greater trochanter)
		Tensor fasciae latae	Ilium (anterior part of crest)	Iliotibial tract
	Adduction	Adductor group Brevis Longus Magnus	Pubic bone	Femur (linea aspera)
Lower leg	Flexion	Hamstring group Biceps femoris Semitendinosus Semimembranosus	Ischium (tuberosity) Femur (linea aspera)	Fibula (head of) Tibia (lateral condyle, medial condyle, and medial surface)
		Gastrocnemius	Femur (condyles)	Tarsal bone (calcaneus by way of tendo calcaneus)

Continued.

Part of body moved	Movement	Muscle	Origin	Insertion
Lower leg—cont'd	Extension	Quadriceps femoris group	Ilium (anterior inferior spine)	Tibia (by way of patellar tendon)
		Rectus femoris	Femur (linea aspera and anterior surface)	
		Vastus lateralis		
		Vastus medialis		
		Vastus intermedius		
Foot	Flexion (dorsiflexion)	Tibialis anterior	Tibia (lateral condyle)	First cuneiform tarsal Base of first metatarsal
	Extension (plantar flexion)	Gastrocnemius	Femur (condyles)	Calcaneus (by way of tendo calcaneus)
		Soleus	Tibia	Same as gastrocnemius, but underneath
Head	Flexion	Sternocleidomastoid	Sternum Clavicle	Temporal bone (mastoid process)
	Extension	Trapezius	Vertebrae (cervical) Scapula (spine and acromion) Clavicle	Occiput
Abdominal wall	Compresses abdominal cavity; therefore assists in straining, defecation, forced expiration, childbirth, posture, etc.	External oblique	Ribs (lower 8)	Innominate bone (iliac crest and pubis by way of inguinal ligament) Linea alba
		Internal oblique	Innominate bone (iliac crest, inguinal ligament) Lumbodorsal fascia	Ribs (lower 3) Pubic bone Linea alba
		Transversus	Ribs (lower 6) Innominate bone (iliac crest, inguinal ligament) Lumbodorsal fascia	Pubic bone Linea alba
		Rectus abdominis	Innominate bone (pubic bone and symphysis pubis)	Ribs (costal cartilage of fifth, sixth, seventh)
Chest wall	Elevates ribs, thereby enlarging anteroposterior and anterolateral dimensions of chest and causing inspiration	External intercostals	Ribs (lower border of all but twelfth)	Ribs (upper border of rib below origin)
	Depresses ribs	Internal intercostals	Ribs (inner surface, upper border of all except first)	Ribs (lower border of rib above origin)
	Pulls floor of thorax downward, thereby enlarging vertical dimension of chest and causing inspiration	Diaphragm	Lower circumference of rib cage	Central tendon of diaphragm
Trunk	Flexion	Iliopsoas	Femur (small trochanter)	Ilium Vertebrae (bodies of twelfth thoracic to fifth lumbar)

	Extension	Sacrospinalis
		  Iliocostalis (lateral)
		  Longissimus (medial)
			Vertebrae (posterior surface of sacrum, spinous processes of lumbar, and last 2 thoracic)
			
			Ilium (posterior part of crest)
				Ribs (lower 6)
				Vertebrae (transverse processes of thoracic)
				Ribs
				Vertebrae (spines of thoracic)

		Quadratus lumborum	Ilium (posterior part of crest) Vertebrae (lower 3 lumbar)	Ribs (twelfth) Vertebrae (transverse processes of first 4 lumbar)

pulling force on its insertion bone at the point where it inserts, pulling that point nearer the muscle's origin bone

4. Skeletal muscles almost always act in groups rather than singly; members of groups are classified as follows:
   a. Prime movers: muscle or muscles whose contraction actually produces the movement
   b. Synergists: muscles that contract at the same time as the prime mover, helping it produce the movement or stabilizing the part (i.e., holding it steady) so the prime mover can produce a more effective movement
   c. Antagonists: muscles that relax while the prime mover is contracting (exception: antagonist contracts at the same time as the prime mover when a part needs to be held rigid, as the knee joint does in standing); antagonists are usually located directly opposite the bones they move; for example, muscle that flexes the lower arm lies on anterior surface of the upper arm bone, whereas that which extends the lower arm lies on posterior surface of the upper arm

5. Body of a muscle usually does not lie over the part moved by the muscle; instead it lies above or below, or anterior or posterior to, the part; thus the body of a muscle that moves the lower arm will not be located in the lower arm but in the upper arm; e.g., biceps and triceps brachii muscles

6. Contraction of a skeletal muscle either shortens the muscle, producing movement, or increases the tension (tone) in the muscle; contractions are classified according to whether they produce movement or increase muscle tone as follows:
   a. Tonic contractions: produce muscle tone; do not shorten the muscle so do not produce movements; only a few fibers contract at one time, and this produces a moderate degree of muscle tone; in the healthy, awake body all muscles exhibit tone
   b. Isometric contractions: increase the degree of muscle tone; do not shorten the muscle so do not produce movements; daily repetition of isometric contractions gradually increases muscle strength
   c. Isotonic contractions: the muscle shortens, thereby producing movement; all movements are the result of isotonic contractions

D. Muscle fiber contraction
1. Electrical energy flows deep into muscle fiber along transverse intracellular tubules associated with sarcoplasmic reticulum
2. Calcium ions released by flow of electrical energy inactivate troponin, which normally

blocks the interaction between actin and myosin
3. Myosin releases and uses energy from ATP to cause actin to slide along myosin filaments (contraction); cessation of impulses leaves actin and myosin in a relaxed unassociated phase
4. Energy for contraction: immediate energy is ATP; creatine phosphate, a high-energy molecule stored in abundance in muscle, replenishes supply of ATP as needed; the ultimate source of energy is glucose and fatty acids oxidized aerobically to carbon dioxide and water, with the release of energy
5. Anaerobic breakdown of glucose during prolonged and vigorous muscle contraction results in lactic acid buildup associated with fatigue and an aching feeling; this oxygen debt is paid off during rest, when oxygen is plentiful

E. Neuromuscular junction
1. Axon terminal forms junction with the sarcolemma of muscle fiber; tiny synaptic cleft separates the presynaptic membrane (axon) from postsynaptic membrane (sarcolemma)
2. Axon terminals contain tiny sacs, synaptic vesicles; these contain the neurotransmitter acetylcholine
3. When a nerve impulse reaches the axon terminal, acetylcholine is released from synaptic vesicles into synaptic cleft; acetylcholine diffuses across synaptic cleft and attaches to receptor sites on sarcolemma; receptor sites are attached to channels in the membrane; when acetylcholine binds to the receptor site, a channel opens and sodium and potassium ions flow down their concentration gradients; the sarcolemma is depolarized, and electrical energy flows into the muscle fiber.
4. The enzyme cholinesterase, found in the synaptic cleft, inactivates acetylcholine; additional stimulation of muscle requires release of more acetylcholine

Bursae
A. Definition: small sacs lined with synovial membrane and containing synovial fluid
B. Locations: wherever pressure is exerted over moving parts
   1. Between skin and bone
   2. Between tendons and bone
   3. Between muscles or ligaments and bone
C. Names of bursae that frequently become inflamed (bursitis)
   1. Subacromial: between the acromion and the capsule of the shoulder joint
   2. Olecranon: between the olecranon process of the ulna and the skin; inflammation called student's elbow

3. Prepatellar: between the patella and the skin; inflammation called housemaid's knee
D. Function: act as cushions, relieving pressure between moving parts

Tendon Sheaths

A. Definition and location: tube-shaped structures that enclose certain tendons, notably those of wrist and ankle; made of connective tissue lined with synovial membrane
B. Function: facilitate gliding movements of tendons

Structures and Functions of the Skeletal System

Overview of the Skeletal System

A. Purpose
   1. Furnishes supporting framework
   2. Affords protection for the viscera, brain, and hemopoietic system
   3. Provides levers for the muscles to pull on to produce movements
   4. Hemopoiesis by red bone marrow: formation of all kinds of blood cells; note that some lymphocytes and monocytes are formed in lymphatic tissue
   5. Mineral storage: calcium, phosphorus (in the form of phosphates), and sodium are stored in bone
B. Structure of long bones (Fig.6-17)
C. Names and numbers of bones (Table 6-18)
D. Joints
E. Differences between male and female skeletons
   1. Male skeleton larger and heavier than female skeleton
   2. Male pelvis deep and funnel shaped with narrow pubic arch; female pelvis shallow, broad, and flaring with wider pubic arch
F. Age changes in skeleton
   1. From infancy to adulthood, not only do bones grow but their relative sizes change as well; the head becomes proportionately smaller, the pelvis relatively larger, the legs proportionately longer, etc.
   2. From young adulthood to old age, bone margins and projections change gradually; bone piles up along them (marginal lipping and spurs), thereby restricting movement; such continuing growth is due, in part, to stimulation of somatotrophic hormone
   3. Osteoporosis may occur in postmenopausal women; related to decreased estrogen production, lack of exercise that stresses skeleton, and inadequate intake of calcium, magnesium, and vitamins A, C, and D

Nature of Bone Substance

A. Organic matter: makes up about 33% of bone by weight
   1. Cells

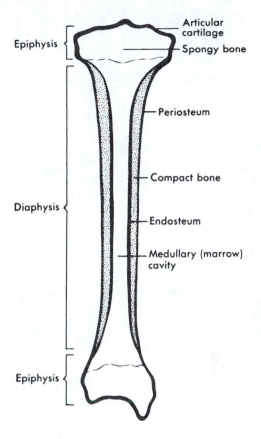

FIGURE 6-17 Diagram to show the structure of a long bone as seen in longitudinal section. (From Anthony CP and Thibodeau GA: *Textbook of anatomy and physiology*, ed 13, St. Louis, 1989, Mosby.)

   a. Osteoblasts: bone-producing cells
   b. Osteoclasts: bone-dissolving cells
   c. Osteocytes: former osteoblasts embedded in and maintaining bone substance
   2. Collagen: collagen fibers make up about 97% of organic matter of bone; give bone tough and somewhat flexible quality; responsible for high tensile strength of bone
   3. Polysaccharides: part of ground substance of bone consists of polysaccharides such as hyaluronic acid and sialic acid
   4. Protein: polysaccharide complexes such as chondroitin sulfate are part of ground substance of bone
B. Inorganic matter: makes up about 67% of bone by weight
   1. Apatite salts: apatite, a complex ion composed of calcium and phosphates, forms hydroxyapatite, carbonate apatite, and fluoride apatite; makes bone hard and is responsible for the high compressional strength of bone
   2. Magnesium and sodium ions are part of bone matrix

TABLE 6-18 Bones of the body

Parts of body	Name of bone	Number	Description
1. Axial skeleton			
a. Skull*			
(1) Cranium	1. Frontal	1	1. Forehead bone
	2. Parietal	2	2. Bulging bones that form top sides of cranium
	3. Temporal	2	3. Form lower sides of cranium and part of cranial floor
	4. Occipital	1	4 Forms posterior part of cranial floor and walls
	5. Sphenoid	1	5. Forms midportion of cranial floor
	6. Ethmoid	1	6. Composes part of anterior portion of cranial floor; lies anterior to sphenoid, posterior to nasal bones
(2) Face	1. Nasal	2	1. Form upper part of bridge of nose
	2. Maxillary	2	2. Upper jaw bones
	3. Zygomatic (malar)	2	3. Cheek bones
	4. Mandible	1	4. Lower jaw bone
	5. Lacrimal	2	5. Fingernail-shaped bones posterior and lateral to nasal bones, in medial wall of orbit
	6. Palatine	2	6. Form posterior part of hard palate
	7. Inferior conchae (turbinates)	2	7. Thin scroll of bone along inner surface of side wall of nasal cavity
	8. Vomer	1	8. Lower, posterior part of nasal septum
(3) Ear ossicles	1. Malleus (hammer)	2	Tiny bones in middle ear in temporal bone; resemble, respectively, miniature hammer, anvil, and stirrup
	2. Incus (anvil)	2	
	3. Stapes (stirrup)	2	
b. Hyoid bone		1	U-shaped bone in neck between mandible and upper part of larynx; only bone in body that forms no joints with any other bones
c. Vertebral column	1. Cervical vertebrae	7	1. Upper seven vertebrae
	2. Thoracic vertebrae	12	2. Next 12 vertebrae; ribs attached to these
	3. Lumbar vertebrae	5	3. Next five vertebrae, located in "small" of back
	4. Sacrum	1	4. In embryo, five separate vertebrae, but fused in adult into one wedge-shaped bone
	5. Coccyx	1	5. In embryo, four or five separate vertebrae, but fused in adult into one bone
d. Ribs and sternum	1. True ribs	7 pairs	1. Upper seven pairs fastened to sternum by costal cartilages
	2. False ribs	5 pairs	2. Do not attach to sternum directly; upper three pairs of false ribs attached by means of costal cartilage of seventh ribs; last two pairs not attached at all and therefore called "floating" ribs
	3. Sternum	1	3. Breast bone
2. Appendicular skeleton			
a. Upper extremities	1. Clavicle	2	1. Shoulder girdle fastened to axial skeleton by articulation of clavicle with sternum
	2. Scapula	2	2. Shoulder blade
	3. Humerus	2	3. Long bone of upper arm
	4. Radius	2	4. Thumb side of forearm
	5. Ulna	2	5. Little finger side of forearm
	6. Carpals	16	6. Wrist bones; arranged in two rows at proximal end of hand
	7. Metacarpals	10	7. Long bones; form framework of palm of hand
	8. Phalanges	28	8. Miniature long bones of fingers; three in each finger, two in each thumb
b. Lower extremities	1. Os coxae, or pelvic bone	2	1. Large hip bones; lower extremities attached to axial skeleton by articulation of pelvic bones with sacrum
	2. Femur	2	2. Thigh bone
	3. Patella	2	3. Kneecap
	4. Tibia	2	4. Shin bone
	5. Fibula	2	5. Long, slender bone of lateral side of lower leg
	6. Tarsals	14	6. "Ankle" bones; form heel and proximal end of foot
	7. Metatarsals	10	7. Long bones of feet
	8. Phalanges	28	8. Miniature long bones of toes
	Total	206†	

* Paranasal sinuses—holes in frontal, sphenoidal, maxillary, and ethmoid bones reduce weight of skull, serve as resonating chambers in speech, produce mucus, and often become inflamed due to allergic responses and viral or bacterial infection.

† Sesamoid bones (rounded bones found in various tendons) have not been counted except for patellae, which are largest sesamoid bones; number of these bones varies greatly among individuals. Wormian bones (small islets of bone in some cranial sutures) have not been counted because of variability of occurrence.

3. Certain radioactive isotopes accumulate in bone (e.g., strontium 90, calcium 45, phosphorus 32, plutonium 259); may increase likelihood of bone tumors and leukemia

Bone Formation

A. Intramembranous ossification: fibrous membranes composing certain parts of fetal skeleton, such as skull bones and lower jaw, are converted to bone

B. Endochondral ossification: conversion of cartilage bone models into actual bone in fetus; most of fetal skeletal system ossifies by endochondral ossification

C. Ossification: end result of either intramembranous or endochondral ossification is the same, cancellous (spongy) bone; the denser type of bone substance, compact bone, forms later in development through conversion of selected regions of cancellous bone into compact bone
   1. Distribution of cancellous and compact bone
      a. Outer surface of all bones, except at joints, composed of compact bone
      b. Interior of short, flat, and irregular bones (all bones except long bones) composed of cancellous bone; epiphyses of long bones composed of cancellous bone in their interior
      c. Diaphyses of long bones hollow; walls of diaphysis composed of compact bone
   2. Ossification process
      a. Formation of bone matrix (the intercellular substance of bone), made up of collagen fibers and a cementlike ground substance composed of polysaccharides and protein-polysaccharide complexes; the osteoblasts (bone-forming cells) synthesize collagen and cement substance from proteins provided by the diet; vitamin C promotes the formation of bone matrix; exercise and estrogens act to stimulate osteoblasts to form bone matrix
      b. Calcification of bone matrix: calcium salts deposited in the bone matrix; vitamin D promotes calcification by stimulating calcium uptake in small intestine
   3. Bone growth
      a. In length: by continual thickening of epiphyseal cartilage followed by ossification; as long as bone growth continues, epiphyseal cartilage grows faster than it can be replaced by bone; therefore line of cartilage persists between diaphysis and epiphyses and can be seen on x-ray film; during adolescence cartilage is completely transformed into bone, at which time bone growth is complete
      b. In diameter: osteoclasts destroy bone surrounding the medullary cavity, thereby enlarging the cavity; at the same time, osteoblasts add new bone around outer surface of the bone; bones may thicken throughout life, depending on the stresses placed on the bone; the more prolonged the stress (walking, running, weight lifting), the thicker the bones become (within physiologic limits)

D. Repair of skeleton
   1. When bone is fractured, connective tissue called a callus grows into and around the broken region
   2. Macrophages reabsorb dead and damaged cells
   3. Osteoclasts dissolve bone fragments
   4. Osteoblasts produce new bone substance and fuse bone together
   5. Final bone shape slowly remodeled; the complete process takes several months; much slower than epithelial tissue, which has a higher metabolic rate and richer blood supply

E. Nutrients required for growth, maintenance, and remodeling of bone
   1. Vitamin A: promotes chondrocyte function and synthesis of lysosomal enzymes for osteoclast activity
   2. Vitamin C: promotes synthesis of collagen
   3. Vitamin D: promotes calcium and phosphorus absorption
   4. Calcium: needed to form calcium phosphate and hydroxyapatite
   5. Magnesium: important enzyme activator in the mineralization process
   6. Phosphorus: needed to form calcium phosphate and hydroxyapatite

Joints

A. Synarthrotic: generally nonmovable joints; also called fibrous joints; no joint cavity or capsule; joining bones held together by fibrous tissue
   1. Sutures: bind skull bones together
   2. Syndesmoses: bind tibia and fibula; also the diaphyses of the radius and ulna

B. Amphiarthrotic: slightly movable joints; also called cartilaginous joints; no joint cavity or capsule; joining bones held together by cartilage and ligaments
   1. Symphyses: disc of cartilage between bones, as between vertebrae or at the pubic symphysis
   2. Synchondroses: costal cartilages bind ribs to the sternum

C. Diarthrotic: freely movable joints; the joint cavity or space between articular surfaces of two bones is lined by a thin layer of hyaline cartilage covering the articular surfaces of the joining bones; the bones are held together by a fibrous capsule lined with synovial membrane and ligaments
   1. May be ball and socket (as in hip), hinge (as in elbow), condyloid (as at wrist), pivot, gliding, or saddle

2. Kinds of movement possible at diarthrotic joints
   a. Flexion: bending one bone on another; (e.g., bending forearm on upper arm)
   b. Extension: stretching one bone away from another (e.g., straightening lower arm out from a flexed position)
   c. Abduction: moving bone away from body's midline (e.g., moving arms straight out from sides)
   d. Adduction: moving bone back toward the body's midline (e.g., bringing arms back to sides of body from an outstretched, or abducted, position)
   e. Rotation: pivoting bone on its axis (e.g., partial rotation such as turning the head from side to side)
   f. Circumduction: describing surface of a cone with the moving part (e.g., moving arm around so the hand describes a circle)
   g. Supination: forearm movement turning the palm forward
   h. Pronation: forearm movement turning the back of the hand forward
   i. Inversion: ankle movement turning the sole of the foot inward
   j. Eversion: ankle movement turning the sole outward
   k. Protraction: moving a part, such as the lower jaw, forward
   l. Retraction: pulling a part back; opposite of protraction
   m. Plantar flexion: pointing the toes (as a ballerina) away from the body
   n. Dorsiflexion: pointing toes toward the body

REVIEW OF PHYSICAL PRINCIPLES RELATED TO THE NEUROMUSCULOSKELETAL SYSTEMS

Principles of Mechanics

A. Applications of energy laws—machines: apart from friction, the work output of a machine is equal to the work input to the machine; the first law of thermodynamics indicates that energy cannot be created or destroyed; a machine can multiply force, that is, provide a mechanical advantage, but at the expense of distance
   1. Lever: rigid bar that moves about a fixed point known as the fulcrum; a small force is applied through a large distance and the other end of the lever exerts a large force over a small distance; the musculoskeletal system operates through lever systems
      a. First-class lever: fulcrum between resistance and effort (e.g., scissors, hemostat, bending head backward or forward)
      b. Second-class lever: resistance between fulcrum and effort (e.g., wheelbarrow, oxygen tank carrier)
      c. Third-class lever: effort between resistance and fulcrum (e.g., forceps, bending over and using your back muscles to lift an object with your hips acting as the fulcrum; swinging the arm when using a tennis racquet)
   2. Pulleys: can multiply force at the expense of distance; the use of a number of pulleys together, as in a block and tackle, provides a mechanical advantage equal to the number of ropes excluding the pull rope; thus a block and tackle with two ropes gives a mechanical advantage of two; a 100-lb weight can be lifted by application of a force of 50 lbs (e.g., traction, lifting heavy objects like engines; pulleys used to change direction of a force); used in traction to apply tension in back injuries

B. Center of gravity
   1. Position in a body where all the weight is considered to be located; sphere, such as a rubber ball, has its center of gravity in its center
   2. Object is stable (will not topple over) as long as a line dropped from its center of gravity to the ground is within the base of the object; in a human the center of gravity is in the pelvic cavity, and for upright balance the line drawn from this point to the ground must fall somewhere between the legs
      a. When lifting a client, the back should be kept straight to keep torque at a minimum; in addition, when bending over, the body's center of gravity shifts from a stable position between the legs to an unstable position outside the legs; the back muscles must then work even harder to prevent the body from toppling over
      b. When walking and carrying a load, the load should be carried as close to the body (center of gravity) as possible to maintain balance and to avoid strain

Principles of Physical Properties of Matter

A. Pascal's principle: when pressure is applied to a fluid in a closed, nonflexible container, it is transmitted undiminished throughout all parts of the fluid and acts in all directions
   EXAMPLES: Cerebrospinal fluid: abnormal increase of pressure on this fluid is transmitted to all parts of the central nervous system containing the fluid
   1. Brain tumor: mass of tissue displaces fluid and increases the pressure of the cerebrospinal fluid
   2. Hydrocephalus: blockage in the canal of Sylvius or overactivity of the choroid plexuses results in a tremendous collection of fluid and increased pressure

B. Electromagnetic fields
  1. Magnetic resonance imaging (MRI): the client lies within a strong magnetic field while areas of the body are stimulated by radio frequency (RF) waves that cause energy changes at the sites being assessed; these changes are measured by the MRI computer to generate images; no radiation is emitted
  EXAMPLE: MRI of the brain produces multiple cross-sectional images of the brain
  2. X-ray: high-energy electromagnetic radiation produced when electrons, traveling at high speeds, strike certain materials, particularly heavy metal; may be used for both diagnostic and treatment purposes; exposes client to radiation
  EXAMPLES:
    a. X-ray of skeletal system
    b. Radiation therapy for cancer of the bone
  3. Computerized tomography (CT) scan: x-ray beam with computer analysis; produces a computerized image from simultaneous scans in more than one plane
  EXAMPLE: CT of brain to identify size and location of tumors
  4. Radiation hazards: individuals working with x-rays should leave the room, stand behind a lead shield, or wear a lead apron when activating the x-ray machine, since there is some scattering of radiation in all directions even though the x-ray beam is aimed at a particular area; film badges (photographic film) should be worn when working near sources of radiation to provide a record of the individual's overall exposure to the radiation
C. Sound: mechanical vibration; cannot occur in a vacuum; propagated best through solids, and through liquids better than gases; travels in waves from vibrating source such as vocal cords, loudspeaker, or dropped object
  1. Properties of waves
    a. Transverse waves: particles of the medium vibrate at right angles to the direction of the wave (e.g., waves on the surface of liquids and all electromagnetic waves [light, infrared, and ultraviolet])
    b. Longitudinal waves: particles of the medium vibrate back and forth along the same direction as the wave (e.g., sound waves)
    c. Frequency: number of complete vibrations (or waves) generated or moving along per second; units of frequency are cycles per second or a hertz (Hz)
    d. Passage of a wave through a medium (gas, liquid, solid, or plasma) is actually the passage of a disturbance in the medium, not a flowing of the medium itself; the wave represents sequential vibration or swinging of the molecules of the medium from the vibrating source to the ears
    e. Refraction of sound waves: sound travels faster in warm air than in cool air; in warm air the average kinetic energy of the air molecules is higher than in cool air, and the wave can be propagated more quickly
    f. Reflection of sound waves: many solid objects reflect sound waves from their surfaces resulting in an echo; a reverberation is a series of echoes
    g. Energy of sound waves: all waves possess energy but to differing degrees; ultraviolet waves and gamma radiation possess high energy, whereas sound waves possess little energy; the structure of the ear reflects the need to amplify the relatively weak energy of sound waves into more energetic waves capable of stimulating the liquid-filled organ of hearing, the cochlea in the inner ear
    h. Velocity of sound: frequency of the wave multiplied by the length of the wave; the velocity of sound waves varies with the nature and temperature of the medium; since light travels much faster than sound, lightning is seen before thunder is heard
  2. Interpretation of sounds
    a. Loudness: neurologic or psychologic interpretation of intensity; although the exact relationship is complex, one could say that the greater the intensity of the sound waves stimulating the organ of Corti, the greater will be the size of nerve impulses reaching the auditory centers of the brain, and the louder the sound seems to be
      (1) Noise level is measured in decibels (dB); a normal conversation is about 65 dB, amplified rock music about 120 dB, and the sound of a nearby jet airplane about 140 dB; the decibel scale is logarithmic so that 120 dB is 1 million times more intense than 60 dB
      (2) Excessive noise can result in hearing loss at certain frequencies of sound; noise levels of about 85 dB and over can damage the organ of Corti; damage increases with the length and intensity of noise and is irreversible
      (3) Doppler effect: when a vibrating source and a receiver of sound move toward each other, the pitch or frequency of the sound produced by the source becomes higher; as the vibrating source

and the receiver move away from each other, the frequency of the sound becomes lower

(4) Speech audiometry: this technique detects the threshold of hearing of actual speech for individuals by presenting groups of two-syllable words at successively lower levels until the person fails to hear; these data are presented as a speech reception threshold (SRT) in decibels; phonetically balanced single-syllable words can also be presented; these words represent a frequency of sounds of speech that approximates a typical conversation; the percentage of words repeated correctly is the Davis Social Adequacy Index (SAI); a score of 94% to 100% is considered normal

b. Pitch: corresponds to frequency; the higher the frequency, the higher the pitch of the sound

(1) Humans can potentially hear sounds whose frequencies range from 16 to 20,000 Hz; with increasing age, the upper range decreases slightly, which presents no problem in hearing speech, since speech falls in the range of 85 to 1050 Hz

(2) Audiometers are capable of electronically producing sounds at a variety of frequencies as well as intensities and are used to measure hearing loss

c. Quality: people have different and distinct qualities or timbres to their voices; similarly, the sounds of different musical instruments are easily recognized; a musical sound or a voice rarely represents a pure tone but usually many frequencies occurring simultaneously

d. Ultrasonic sound: vibrational frequencies exceeding the upper level of human hearing (20,000 Hz)

(1) Can be used in cleaning metal parts; the high-frequency vibrations shake the solution and produce bubbles that help in the cleaning process

(2) Low-intensity ultrasonic waves have been used to treat arthritis and bursitis, to break kidney stones, and to help dissolve scars

(3) Ultrasonic dental drills can quickly drill into teeth without the pain associated with tooth vibrations, which stimulate the nerve of the tooth

(4) Sonograms are pictures of the body derived through differential reflection or transmission of sound waves

e. Deafness: condition wherein sound vibrations are not transmitted to the brain for interpretation

(1) Perforation or tear of the tympanic membrane

(2) Inflexibility of the three middle-ear bones or ossicles; vibrations are thus only poorly transmitted to the oval window

(3) Otosclerosis: abnormal bone formation over the oval window immobilizes the stapes

(a) Surgery can remove the abnormal bony tissue in the early stages of the disease

(b) In later stages the stapes may be removed and a prosthesis implanted

(c) If the oval window is ossified, a new opening in the cochlea is made to replace the oval window (fenestration)

(d) Bone-conduction hearing aids can essentially bypass the middle ear

(4) Deafness caused by auditory nerve damage; the nerve cannot be regenerated nor can hearing be helped by hearing aids

f. Hearing aids: electronic devices that amplify sounds and assist partially deaf persons to hear; a miniature microphone picks up the sound, sends it to an amplifier, and then to a miniature loudspeaker fitted in or behind the ear

(1) Air-conduction type sends an amplified sound wave into the ear, thus utilizing the person's own middle ear

(2) Bone-conduction type bypasses the middle ear and transmits amplified vibrations to the skull bones, which in turn produce vibrations in the inner ear

D. Light
1. Basic concepts
a. Visible light is a type of electromagnetic radiation; all electromagnetic radiation consists of oscillating electric and magnetic fields that come into existence because of the vibrations of electrically charged particles

b. All types of electromagnetic radiation have the same electric and magnetic nature and travel at the same constant velocity: 186,000 miles per second (speed of light)

c. Electromagnetic spectrum varies from extremely long AM and FM radio waves measured in miles to very short gamma and cosmic rays measured in tenths of picometer

d. Product of the frequency of vibration and the wavelength is constant (the velocity of light); the lower the frequency of vibration of the wave, the longer will be the wavelength, and the higher the frequency, the shorter the wavelength

e. The higher the frequency (or the shorter the wavelength) of electromagnetic radiation, the greater will be the energy content of the radiation

2. Wavelengths of electromagnetic radiation

a. Wavelengths can be measured in millimicrons or Angström units

   (1) A millimicron is one thousandth of a micron; a micron is one millionth of one meter

   (2) An Angström unit is one tenth of a millimicron

b. Wavelengths of visible light possess just the right amount of vibrational energy to excite the photoreceptor cells (rods and cones) of the retina

c. Different wavelengths of light are bent or refracted to slightly different degrees and appear to the eyes and brain as different colors; this principle of dispersion is responsible for a rainbow

d. Emission of light: atoms can be excited by absorbing energy that causes orbiting electrons to jump to higher energy levels within the atom; as the electrons fall back to their lower (more stable) energy levels (deexcitation), the energy of excitation is released and may appear as visible light (e.g., advertising signs, mercury vapor street lamps)

   (1) Characteristic pattern of wavelengths of light (a discontinuous spectrum) is emitted from every element in the vapor state; this pattern is best seen by means of a spectroscope

   (2) Fluorescence: property of absorbing radiation of one frequency and emitting radiation of a lower frequency and energy; a substance is said to be fluorescent if it emits visible light when energized or bombarded with ultraviolet (UV) light; high-intensity fluorescent light bulbs have been used to treat jaundice in newborn infants; the excess bilirubin in the blood, which is responsible for the jaundice, is oxidized by exposure to the bright light as blood passes through the vessels of the thin skin

   (3) Phosphorescence: atoms of a phosphorescent substance become deexcited a relatively long time after being excited; the phosphorescent atoms in the dial of a luminous clock are excited during the day by the visible light striking them; the dial then glows throughout the night as billions of excited atoms gradually become deexcited, releasing their energy as visible light

3. Laser

a. Acronym for light amplification by stimulated emission of radiation; a laser produces monochromatic coherent light, which means that the light waves are all of the same frequency, are all in phase with each other (peak with peak, trough with trough), and are all traveling in the same direction; in coherent light, millions of light waves become additive and form a single, concentrated beam of light that travels in a straight line without spreading out and that can be precisely focused on minute areas

b. As coherent light leaves the laser (one type of laser uses a ruby crystal), it can be utilized for a variety of purposes

   (1) Eye surgery: energy in the coherent light produced by a laser is used to fuse minute areas of the retina to the surrounding choroid coat; an ophthalmoscope is used to focus the coherent light precisely on specific, tiny areas of the retina; a detached retina can thus be reattached, and the fusion points are so tiny that there is no apparent loss of light-sensitive retinal tissue; the machine used in this type of surgery is called a photocoagulator and uses a ruby laser

   (2) Cancer therapy: laser has been used in the selective treatment of pigmented skin cancers, which apparently absorb the light more readily than do surrounding, less pigmented, normal tissues

4. Color

a. Perception of color is the result of the translation and interpretation of certain nerve impulses in the brain that come from the retina; the frequency of light determines the color that is seen; the lowest frequency stimulating the retina is red, the highest is violet, in between are all the colors of nature

b. Objects may appear to be colored because they emit electromagnetic radiation that falls within the visible range; may also appear colored not because they emit light, but because of selective reflection

c. Color mixing

(1) Red, green, and blue are the additive primaries; any color in the spectrum can be obtained with the proper blend of these three; equal amounts of the three produce white light

(2) Magenta, yellow, and cyan (turquoise) are the subtractive primaries; any color in the spectrum can be obtained using the proper blend of these three; they are sometimes loosely called red, yellow, and blue

(3) Complementary colors are any two colors that, when added together, produce white: red and cyan, magenta and green, and yellow and blue

d. Perception of color is believed to depend on the cones of the retina, which are located most densely at the part of the retina called the fovea centralis; one type of cone detects red, another detects green, and another blue; it is generally thought that the brain blends nerve impulses from these three types of cones to produce our perception of all the colors of nature

(1) Faulty color vision is thought to be caused by cones that are either missing or not functioning properly; red-green color blindness is the most common type and is a genetically inherited trait that causes individuals to see red and green objects as shades of gray; more men are affected than women, since the trait appears to be sex linked

(2) Color and emotion: even though red light has a lower frequency and therefore less energy than a quantum of blue light, the human mind generally associates red with warmth, excitement, and mental stimulation, and blue with coolness and calmness; for many individuals the color of an object or a room determines to a great extent whether they will keep and use the object or stay in the room; thus color has a physical basis in the electromagnetic radiation but involves complex interpretation by the human mind

5. Reflection and refraction

a. General principles

(1) Source of light: sun is the primary outdoor source; incandescent and fluorescent bulbs are indoor sources

(2) Most objects are visible because they reflect light emitted from various sources

(3) Pane of glass is transparent if it allows light to pass through it in straight lines

(4) Thin cloth window shade or a piece of paper is translucent if it allows light to pass through it in a diffused manner so objects cannot be seen; in hospitals, shades or blinds diffuse light and cut down on harsh glare

(5) Heavy pair of curtains is opaque if light cannot pass through them

(6) Light traveling in any single medium travels in straight lines; each straight line called a ray

b. Reflection

(1) When light strikes a surface off which it can reflect, the angle of incidence equals the angle of reflection as measured from the normal (a line perpendicular to the plane of the reflecting surface)

(a) When successive elevations of any surface are less than about one fourth the wavelength of the incident light, the light reflected from the surface travels mainly in one direction and the surface is polished

(b) Light reflected from rougher surfaces travels in many directions and is diffusely reflected; it is easier to read a page of text printed on paper that provides a more diffuse than polished reflection, since glare is eliminated

(c) The word ambulance is often printed backward on the front of these vehicles so that motorists seeing the lettering via reflected light through their rearview mirrors will be able to read the lettering correctly

(2) Virtual images: as light reflects off a mirror, the angles of incidence and reflection are equal; the reflected rays of light appear to come from a point behind the mirror; because the light rays do not actually come from this point, the image is referred to as a virtual image as opposed to a real image; the virtual image of a plane mirror is as far behind the mirror as the object is in front of the mirror

c. Refraction

(1) Refraction: bending of an oblique ray of light as it travels from one transparent

medium into another; refraction is caused by the change in velocity of light as it passes through the medium

(2) Index of refraction: average speed of light varies in different transparent media; the average speed of light in water is only 75% of its average speed in a vacuum; the average speed in a diamond is 41% of its average speed in a vacuum; the index of refraction is a measure of how much the average speed of light differs from its speed in a vacuum; index of refraction equals the speed of light in a vacuum divided by its speed in a medium; the higher the index of refraction, the slower the speed of light through the medium

EXAMPLES

(a) Thermometer or syringe half immersed in a beaker of water appears to be bent at the point of immersion

(b) Object in water appears to be nearer the surface than it actually is; thus it seems larger because it is magnified

(c) Mirage: average speed of light is slightly greater in hot air than in cool air; on a hot, paved road or a desert, the light reflected from an object is refracted upward, away from the hot surface, and may then produce an upside-down virtual image to an individual some distance away; the wet, shimmering look of a hot road is refracted light from the sky reaching a motorist's eye after passing through hot air layers

(d) Total internal reflection: at a certain critical angle, light between two media is not refracted (or bent) but is reflected back into the first medium provided the first medium has a higher index of refraction than the second medium:

- This phenomenon permits viewing of the interior walls of the stomach, intestines, and blood vessels
- Dentist's flashlight will "curve" the light (via total internal reflection) to the appropriate part of an individual's mouth
- Total internal reflection via the paired prisms in a pair of binoculars permits higher magnifications in a short optic tube

6. Diffraction
Bending of light or any type of electromagnetic wave around corners; the longer the wavelength of electromagnetic radiation, the larger the object that it can be bent around

EXAMPLES

a. AM radio waves, some of which are more than 5 km long, easily bend around objects, thereby allowing AM broadcasts to come in clearly even in cities having many tall buildings and mountainous regions

b. FM radio waves, which are from 2.7 to 3.6 m long, cannot easily bend around large objects; consequently, a specific location in a city or suburban area with large obstructing objects can determine the quality of the reception of FM broadcasts

c. Some spectrophotometers used in certain laboratory analyses of blood and urine rely on diffraction gratings to disperse white light into its component wavelengths and to utilize these specific wavelengths in the analytic procedure

d. X-ray diffraction: because of their very short wavelengths, x-rays diffract around the atoms in large molecules and produce diffraction patterns on photographic plates; analyses of these patterns can reveal the details of the arrangement of the atoms in a molecule; used in DNA analysis

7. Polarization
Certain naturally occurring crystals, like tourmaline, absorb light waves striking them in all planes but one; the light transmitted through and emerging from the crystal vibrates in only one plane; this is called plane-polarized light

EXAMPLES

a. Polaroid filters contain synthetic molecules, that will permit only light vibrating in a single plane to pass through; when used in sunglasses, they cut down on glare and eye strain; much of the light reflected from nonmetallic surfaces, such as water, glass, or roadways, is already polarized because these surfaces tend to transmit light waves perpendicular to their surfaces and to reflect light waves parallel to their surfaces; when this polarized light strikes the Polaroid filters in the sunglasses, many of the light waves are absorbed; thus fewer waves are transmitted and the harsh glare is reduced

b. Polarizing filters for cameras cut down on glare in photographs and also have the effect of deepening the blue color of the sky

c. Polarizing microscopes are used in research laboratories to analyze the molecular structure of many substances

8. Lenses
   a. Refraction of light through transparent glass (or quartz or fluorite) lenses is of great practical importance; magnification of objects is possible using simple lenses as well as groups of lenses arranged in telescopes and microscopes; the principal axis of a lens is the line joining the two points that represent the centers of curvature of the curved surfaces of a given lens
   b. Convex lenses (converging or positive lenses) converge light rays passing through them; concave lenses (diverging or negative lenses) diverge light rays passing through them
   c. When light rays parallel with the principal axis pass through a converging lens, they converge on the focal point; parallel light rays that are not parallel with the principal axis converge in a series of points above and below the focal point, making up the focal plane
      (1) Converging lens will magnify an object (acting as a simple magnifying glass) if it is held inside the focal point of the lens; the image is enlarged, right side up, and virtual; this means that the image only appears to exist but has no physical reality
      (2) When an object is placed outside the focal point of a converging lens, a real, inverted image is obtained that can be focused on a screen; whenever a real image is formed, the object and image are on opposite sides of the lens
         EXAMPLES
         (a) Motion pictures utilize converging lenses, and the movie screen is the plane where light rays are converged; slide projectors also operate under the same principle
         (b) In cameras the film is flattened out and placed in the focal plane of the camera's lens; in popular single-lens reflex (SLR) cameras, a mirror diverts the light to a prism, which erects the image, allowing the viewer to see exactly what will be focused on the film; when the shutter button is pushed and the mirror flips out of the way, light is focused on and exposes the photographic film
         (c) Diverging lenses used alone produce smaller, virtual images; they are used on some cameras (not SLR cameras) as "finders," since the virtual image seen approximates the proportions of the photograph; whenever a virtual image is formed, the object and the image are on the same side of the lens

9. Lens defects
   Distortions in an image produced by a given lens are called aberrations; combining a number of lenses as a system can usually minimize aberrations; this is the reason that microscopes and telescopes employ compound lenses in their construction
   a. Spheric aberration: unsharp (uncrisp) images are formed because light refracted from the outer edges of the lens is focused at a point slightly different from the point at which light refracted from more central areas of the lens is focused
      (1) In cameras and microscopes this is corrected by using more than one lens and also by using diaphragms to cover the outer regions of the lens
      (2) In the human eye, the iris is generally contracted to varying degrees and acts, in effect, like a diaphragm to block light from being refracted through the outer regions of the lens
   b. Chromatic aberration: each wavelength of visible light refracts through lenses at different angles; thus each wavelength (color) of white light is brought to focus at a slightly different point; the result of this is that objects take on colors that they do not possess; this is corrected in cameras, microscopes, and telescopes by using combinations of simple lenses made of different types of glass called achromatic lenses; in the human eye, vision is sharpest when the pupil is the smallest; cutting down on light moving through the periphery of the lens minimizes chromatic as well as spheric aberration
   c. Astigmatism: human eye astigmatism is a type of aberration caused by the surface of the cornea possessing irregular curves; since the cornea, in addition to the lens, is important in refracting (focusing) light on the retina, the result of astigmatism is blurred vision, which can be corrected by using lenses that have variable curvature to compensate for the irregular curvature of the cornea

10. Focusing: camera focuses on objects at varying distances by changing the distance between the lens and the film; the human eye focuses on objects at varying distances by changing the degree of curvature of the lens; this ability of

the human eye to change the focal length of the lens is called accommodation; whereas the cornea, aqueous humor, and vitreous humor all help to focus light on the retina, only the crystalline lens is able to accommodate; the muscle responsible for accommodation is the ciliary body; when the ciliary body contracts, the suspensory ligaments loosen and the lens rounds out and is in position for focusing on near objects; when the ciliary body relaxes, the suspensory ligaments pull the lens into a flattened position, which allows for focusing on distant objects; the limit for accommodation is represented by the near point; objects closer to the eye than the near point (about 15 cm from the surface of a normal eye) cannot be clearly focused on the retina

a. Emmetropia: normal refractive state of the eye

b. Ametropia: any abnormality in refractive ability of the eye

(1) Myopia: eye focuses light anterior to the retina (somewhere in the vitreous humor); from this abnormal focal point, light rays diverge and produce a blurred image on the retina; however, if objects are held about 2.5 cm from the eye, they will focus on the retina; for this reason, myopia is also called near-sightedness; glasses containing diverging lenses correct this condition

(2) Hyperopia: eye focuses light posterior to the retina; thus a circle of not-yet-converged light strikes the retina, producing a blurred image; hyperopia is also called far-sightedness and can be corrected using glasses containing converging lenses

c. Contact lenses: thin lenses that are molded to the shape of the outer surface of the cornea; this can correct near-sightedness, far-sightedness, and astigmatism; the lens is applied to the surface of the eye using a saline solution that helps adhere the lens to the eye's surface

11. Eye examination with the ophthalmoscope and the retinoscope

a. Ophthalmoscope: permits visualization of the interior of the eye; thus the examiner can study a client's vision with this instrument; light shone into an eye with normal refractive ability will be focused on the retina and reflected back to the examiner's eye; persons with myopia or hyperopia will not converge the light on the retina, and the examiner will not clearly see the eye's interior; then by using lenses of varying refractive abilities the examiner can compensate for the person's abnormal refraction, study the interior of the eye, and determine the state of vision

b. Retinoscope: permits diagnosis and evaluation of the refractive state of the eye; a beam of light shone into the eye is reflected from the retina as it leaves the pupil; by observing its distribution as it leaves the pupil, the examiner can determine the refractive error in the eye

12. Binocular vision: visual fields of the two human eyes overlap; although each eye sees some areas of the environment that the other eye cannot see, both eyes also see large areas in common; the human brain interprets these overlapping fields in terms of depth; the environment appears in three dimensions, as opposed to the visual effect of a movie projected on a flat screen; the blind spot of the right eye can be seen by the left eye and vice versa; therefore no gaps in the field of vision exist

REVIEW OF CHEMICAL PRINCIPLES RELATED TO THE NEUROMUSCULOSKELETAL SYSTEMS

Amines

A. Organic compounds containing an amino group (NH_2) that can be considered derivatives of ammonia

B. Reactions of the amines
1. Basic, in water solution
2. Like a base with acids, forming complex ions

C. Important amines
1. Monoamines such as norepinephrine, dopamine, serotonin, acetylcholine, and histamine serve as transmitter chemicals in the nervous system
2. Amino acids such as gamma-aminobutyric acid (GABA) and glycine act as inhibitors; glutamic acid has an excitatory influence on the nervous system

Lipids

Phospholipids, lecithin, cephalins, and sphingomyelins are important components of nerve membranes and sheaths

Proteins

Actin, myosin, and troponin are important in muscle contraction

Group I A Alkali Metals

A. Sodium: in the extracellular fluid these ions are responsible for action potentials of nervous and muscular tissue; after some stimulus, it is the diffusion of sodium from the interstitial fluid into the intracellular fluid of neurons and muscle fibers that brings about depolarization; thus sodium ions are basic to the functioning of the body's communication system, the nervous system, and all muscular movements

B. Potassium
  1. Resting polarization of neurons, all types of muscle fibers (e.g., smooth, cardiac, striated), and most cells of the body is caused by the continual diffusion of potassium from the intracellular fluid to the interstitial fluid; similarly, repolarization of neurons and muscle fibers is caused by the outward diffusion of potassium to the interstitial fluid from the intracellular fluid
  2. Several important cellular enzymes functioning in glucose and amino acid metabolism require K^+ as a cofactor

Group II A Alkali Earth Metals

A. Magnesium
  1. Activator for many enzymes
  2. Present in bones
B. Calcium
  1. Gives hardness to bones and teeth by forming phosphate, carbonate, and fluoride salts
  2. Important in muscle contraction; ATP must combine with calcium before its energy can be used to slide actin and myosin filaments together
  3. Extracellular calcium concentration must be precisely regulated (through the parathyroid glands) for normal body functioning; hypocalcemia can result in tetany; hypercalcemia can result in depression of the nervous system
C. Strontium
  1. May substitute for calcium in body
  2. Radioactive isotope (strontium 90) can be a health hazard, forming pockets of radiation in tissues

Group VI A Halogens

Fluorine: prevents tooth decay when added to water supply

Group I B Metals

A. Silver: filling for teeth, surgical mending of bone, photography
B. Gold: filling for teeth

REVIEW OF MICROORGANISMS RELATED TO THE NEUROMUSCULOSKELETAL SYSTEMS

A. Bacterial pathogens
  1. *Clostridium tetani*: large, gram-positive, motile bacillus forming large terminal spores; like all clostridia, it is an obligate anaerobe; causes tetanus (lockjaw)
  2. *Haemophilus aegyptius* (Koch-Weeks bacillus): indistinguishable morphologically from *Haemophilus influenzae*; causes a common conjunctivitis called pinkeye
  3. *Neisseria meningitidis*: gram-negative diplococcus; causes epidemic (meningococcic) meningitis
B. DNA viruses: herpes viruses; spheric and 150 to 200 nm in diameter; cause herpes simplex, varicella (chickenpox), herpes zoster (shingles), infectious mononucleosis, and cytomegalic inclusion disease
C. RNA viruses: togaviruses; spheric and 40 to 60 nm in diameter; mostly borne by mosquitoes and ticks; cause eastern equine encephalomyelitis, western equine encephalomyelitis, Venezuelan equine encephalomyelitis, and a number of other infections
D. Fungal pathogen: *Cryptococcus neoformans*—pathogenic yeast with a characteristic large capsule around the cell; causes cryptococcosis (torulosis, European blastomycosis), a serious infection involving the lungs and central nervous system
E. Protozoa: Trypanosoma—flagellated ribbonlike protozoa; *T. gambiense* and *T. rhodesiense* cause African sleeping sickness (transmitted by tsetse flies), and *T. cruzi* causes South American trypanosomiasis or Chagas' disease (transmitted by reduviid bugs)
F. Worm: *Trichinella spiralis*—one of smallest parasitic nematodes (about 1.5 mm in length), causes trichinosis (muscle infestation with trichina)

PHARMACOLOGY RELATED TO NEUROMUSCULOSKELETAL SYSTEMS DISORDERS

Anticonvulsants

A. Description
  1. Used to decrease the occurrence, frequency, and/or severity of convulsive episodes; end result of anticonvulsant therapy is the control of seizures
  2. Act by modifying bioelectric activity at subcortical and cortical sites by stabilizing the nerve cell membrane and/or raising the seizure threshold to incoming stimuli
  3. Available in oral and parenteral (IM, IV) preparations
B. Examples
  1. Control of tonic-clonic (grand mal) seizures
    a. Carbamazepine (Tegretol): also used for partial seizures
    b. Diazepam (Valium): used IV for status epilepticus
    c. Magnesium sulfate

d. Phenytoin (Dilantin): also used for partial seizures

e. Phenobarbital (Gardenal)

2. Control of absences (petit mal seizures)

a. Ethosuximide

b. Methsuximide

c. Paramethadione

d. Trimethadione

C. Major side effects

1. Dizziness, drowsiness (CNS depression)

2. Nausea, vomiting (irritation of gastric mucosa)

3. Skin rash (hypersensitivity)

4. Blood dyscrasias (decreased RBCs, WBCs, platelet synthesis)

5. Phenytoin

a. Ataxia (neurotoxicity)

b. Gingival hyperplasia (gum irritation leading to tissue overgrowth)

c. Hirsutism (virilism)

d. Hypotension (decreased atrial and ventricular conduction)

D. Nursing care

1. Administer with food to reduce GI irritation

2. Provide care for the client having a seizure

a. Maintain airway; place in side-lying position after seizure

b. Protect client from injury

c. Assess the type and duration of seizure

3. Instruct client to:

a. Avoid alcohol and other CNS depressants

b. Notify physician if fever, sore throat, or skin rash develops

c. Carry medical alert card

4. Teach client receiving barbiturates to:

a. Avoid engaging in hazardous activities

b. Assess for cardiac and respiratory depression

5. Care for the client receiving phenytoin (Dilantin)

a. Provide oral hygiene; inspect oral mucosa for infection

b. Avoid mixing with other IV infusions

c. Assess for potentiation of anticoagulant effect

d. Assess urine; drug may discolor urine pink to red-brown

e. Assess for therapeutic blood levels (40 to 80 μmol/L)

6. Encourage diet rich in nutrient-dense foods such as fruits, vegetables, whole grains, and legumes to improve and maintain nutritional status and prevent possible drug-induced nutrient deficiencies

7. Evaluate client's response to medication and understanding of teaching

Osmotic Diuretics

A. Description

1. Reduce cerebral edema and intraocular pressure by increasing the osmotic pressure within the vasculature, thus causing fluid to leave the tissues and be excreted in the urine

2. Used to treat increased intracranial pressure

3. Available in parenteral (IV) preparations

B. Examples

1. Mannitol (Osmitrol)

2. Urea (Ureaphil)

C. Major side effects

1. Headache (dehydration)

2. Nausea (fluid and electrolyte imbalance)

3. Chills (fluid and electrolyte imbalance)

4. Rebound edema when discontinued (fluid and electrolyte imbalance)

5. Fluid/electrolyte imbalances (hyponatremia, hypokalemia) (promotion of sodium and potassium excretion)

D. Nursing care

1. Monitor intake and output during therapy

2. Avoid administration in clients with congestive heart failure or impaired renal function

3. Elevate head of bed during therapy

4. Monitor daily weight and serum electrolytes during course of therapy

5. Assess client for signs of increased intracranial pressure (decreasing pulse rate, widening pulse pressure, increasing systolic pressure, unequal pupils, change in level of consciousness)

6. Evaluate client's response to medication and understanding of teaching

Calcium Enhancers

A. Description

1. Used to restore calcium ion balance

2. Serum calcium concentration is increased through:

a. Direct calcium ion replacement

b. Vitamin D replacement, which improves the absorption of calcium from the intestines

3. Available in oral and parenteral (IM, IV) preparations

B. Examples

1. Calcium ion replacement

a. Calcium carbonate (Os-Cal)

b. Calcium chloride: IV administration only

c. Calcium gluconate

2. Vitamin D replacement

a. Calcitriol

b. Cholecalciferol

c. Dihydrotachysterol

C. Major side effects

1. Nausea, vomiting (hypercalcemia)

2. Constipation (increased serum calcium delays passage of stool in GI tract)

3. Renal calculi (hypercalcemia)

4. Muscle flaccidity (hypercalcemia)

5. Calcium preparations: cardiac disturbances (stimulation of cardiac conduction)
6. Vitamin D: dry mouth; metallic taste (early vitamin D toxicity associated with hypercalcemia)

D. Nursing care
1. Assess client for signs of tetany and hypercalcemia
2. Encourage increased fluid intake and acid ash diet to reduce potential of renal calculi and constipation; stress vitamin D and calcium-rich foods such as eggs, cheese, whole-grain cereals, and cranberries; limit milk, fruits, and vegetables
3. Monitor serum electrolytes during course of therapy
4. Calcium preparations: assess for potentiation of digitalis effect
5. Evaluate client's response to medication and understanding of teaching

Antiparkinson Agents

A. Description
1. Anticholinergic drugs act at central sites to inhibit cerebral motor impulses and to block efferent impulses that cause rigidity of the musculature
2. Levodopa preparations and others supply or cause the release of dopamine required for norepinephrine synthesis and maintenance of the neurohormonal balance at subcortical, cortical, and reticular sites that control motor function
3. Used to control the symptoms of Parkinson's disease
4. Available in oral and parenteral (IM, IV) preparations

B. Examples
1. Anticholinergic drugs
   a. Benztropine mesylate (Cogentin)
   b. Ethopropazine HCl (Parsidol)
   c. Trihexyphenidyl HCl (Apo-Trihex)
2. Other drugs
   a. Amantadine HCl (Symmetrel)
   b. Carbidopa-levodopa (Sinemet)
   c. Levodopa
   d. Selegiline HCl

C. Major side effects
1. Anticholinergic drugs (decrease parasympathetic stimulation)
   a. Dry mouth (decreased salivation)
   b. Blurred vision (pupillary dilation)
   c. Constipation (decreased peristalsis)
   d. Urinary retention (decreased muscle tone)
2. Other drugs
   a. Orthostatic hypotension (loss of compensatory vasoconstriction with position change)
   b. Ataxia (neurotoxicity)
   c. CNS disturbances and emotional disturbances (CNS effect)
   d. Nausea, vomiting (irritation of gastric mucosa)

D. Nursing care
1. Instruct client to:
   a. Avoid discontinuing drug suddenly
   b. Understand that treatment controls symptoms but is not a cure
   c. Keep all scheduled appointments; medical supervision is necessary
2. Offer emotional support to client at this time; therapy is usually for life
3. Care for the client receiving anticholinergic drugs
   a. Offer sugar-free chewing gum and hard candy to increase salivation
   b. May interfere with ability to perform potentially hazardous activities
4. Care for the client receiving levodopa
   a. Eliminate vitamin B$_6$ from diet
   b. Inform client regarding dosage and "holiday" periods
5. Encourage diet rich in nutrient-dense foods such as fruits, vegetables, whole grains, and legumes to improve and maintain nutritional status and prevent possible drug-induced nutrient deficiencies; clients taking levodopa should limit intake of foods high in vitamin B$_6$ (e.g., pork, glandular meats, lamb, veal, legumes, potatoes, oatmeal, wheat germ, and bananas)
6. Care for the client receiving selegiline HCl
   a. Use safety precautions because drug can cause orthostatic hypotension
   b. Avoid foods containing tyramine such as wine, cheese, and chocolate because this drug is an MAO inhibitor; ingestion of these foods can cause a hypertensive crisis
7. Evaluate client's response to medication and understanding of teaching

Cholinesterase Inhibitors

A. Description
1. Used to diagnose and treat myasthenia gravis
2. Act by:
   a. Preventing enzymatic breakdown of acetylcholine at nerve endings, thus allowing accumulation of the neurotransmitter
   b. Improving the strength of contraction in all muscles, including those involved with the process of respiration
3. Available in oral and parenteral (IM, IV) preparations

B. Examples
  1. Ambenonium chloride
  2. Edrophonium chloride (Tensilon): for diagnostic purposes
  3. Neostigmine bromide (Prostigmin)
  4. Pyridostigmine bromide (Mestinon)
C. Major side effects
  1. Nausea, vomiting (irritation of gastric mucosa)
  2. Diarrhea (increased peristalsis)
  3. Hypersalivation (increased parasympathetic stimulation)
  4. Muscle cramps (increased skeletal muscle contraction)
  5. CNS disturbances (CNS effect)
  6. Acute toxicity: pulmonary edema and respiratory failure (bronchial constriction)
D. Nursing care
  1. Monitor client closely; dosage is adjusted according to needs
  2. Have atropine sulfate available for treatment of overdosage
  3. Administer medications exactly according to schedule
  4. Administer with food to reduce GI irritation
  5. Instruct client to:
    a. Carry a medical alert card
    b. Take medication before meals to improve chewing and swallowing
    c. Encourage diet rich in nutrient-dense foods such as fruits, vegetables, whole grains, and legumes to improve and maintain nutritional status and prevent possible drug-induced nutrient deficiencies
  6. Evaluate client's response to medication and understanding of teaching

Skeletal Muscle Relaxants

A. Description
  1. Used to relieve inappropriate and abnormal muscle contraction
  2. Central agents act by CNS depression to bring about relaxation of voluntary muscles
  3. Peripheral agents block nerve-impulse conduction at the myoneural junction
  4. Available in oral and parenteral (IM, IV) preparations
B. Examples
  1. Central agents
    a. Carisoprodol
    b. Chlorzoxazone
    c. Cyclobenzapine (Flexeril)
    d. Diazepam (Valium)
    e. Methocarbamol (Robaxin)
    f. Orphenadrine (Norflex)
  2. Peripheral agents
    a. Gallamine triethiodide
    b. Pancuronium bromide (Pavulon)

c. Succinylcholine chloride (Anectine)
    d. Tubocurarine chloride
C. Major side effects
  1. Central agents
    a. Dizziness, drowsiness (CNS depression)
    b. Nausea (irritation of gastric mucosa)
    c. Headache (central antimuscarinic effect)
    d. CNS disturbances (direct CNS effect)
    e. Tachycardia (brain stem stimulation)
  2. Peripheral agents
    a. Hypotension (increased vagal stimulation; increased release of histamine; ganglionic blockade)
    b. Respiratory depression (neuromuscular blockade)
    c. Dysrhythmias (increased vagal stimulation)
D. Nursing care
  1. Provide care for the client receiving central agents
    a. Utilize safety precautions (supervise ambulation; side rails up) during initial therapy
    b. Instruct client to:
      (1) Avoid concurrent use of alcohol and other CNS depressants
      (2) Avoid engaging in potentially hazardous activities
  2. Provide care for the client receiving peripheral agents
    a. Have O_2 and emergency resuscitative equipment available
    b. Assess vital signs before, during, and after administration
    c. Administer under direct medical supervision
  3. Encourage diet rich in nutrient-dense foods such as fruits, vegetables, whole grains, and legumes to improve and maintain nutritional status and prevent possible drug-induced nutrient deficiencies
  4. Evaluate client's response to medication and understanding of teaching

Nonsteroidal Antiinflammatory Drugs (NSAIDs)

A. Description
  1. Used to alleviate the inflammation and subsequent discomfort of rheumatoid conditions
  2. Act by interfering with prostaglandin synthesis in the body
  3. Available in oral and parenteral (IM) preparations
B. Examples
  1. Ibuprofen (Motrin)
  2. Indomethacin (Indocid)
  3. Ketorolac tromethamine (Torodol)
  4. Naproxen (Naprosyn)
  5. Oxaprozin

6. Piroxicam (Novo-Pirocam)
7. Salicylates (ASA)
8. Sulindac

C. Major side effects
1. GI irritation (local effect)
2. Skin rash (hypersensitivity)
3. Blood dyscrasias (decreased RBCs, WBCs, platelet synthesis)
4. CNS disturbances (neurotoxicity)
5. Indomethacin: drowsiness (CNS effect)

D. Nursing care
1. Administer with meals to reduce GI irritation
2. Monitor blood work during therapy
3. Assess vital signs during course of therapy
4. Instruct client to report the occurrence of any side effects to the physician
5. Inform client taking Indomethacin that it may interfere with ability to engage in hazardous activities
6. Encourage diet rich in nutrient-dense foods such as fruits, vegetables, whole grains, and legumes to improve and maintain nutritional status and prevent possible drug-induced nutrient deficiencies
7. Evaluate client's response to medication and understanding of teaching

Antigout Agents

A. Description
1. Used to prevent and arrest gout attacks that are caused by high levels of uric acid in the blood
2. Act by:
   a. Increasing the excretion of uric acid (uricosuric agent)
   b. Decreasing uric acid formation by the body
3. Available in oral and parenteral (IV) preparations

B. Examples
1. Allopurinol (Purinol): blocks formation of uric acid within the body
2. Colchicine: decreases uric acid crystal deposits by inhibiting lactic acid production by leukocytes; used for acute attacks
3. Probenecid (Benemid): prevents formation of tophi by inhibiting the reabsorption of uric acid by the kidneys

C. Major side effects
1. Nausea, vomiting (irritation of gastric mucosa)
2. Blood dyscrasias (decreased RBCs, WBCs, and platelet synthesis)
3. Liver damage (hepatotoxicity)
4. Skin rash (hypersensitivity)

D. Nursing care
1. Administer antiinflammatory drugs (Prednisone, Indocin) in addition to drugs that will lower serum uric acid during the acute phase
2. Increase fluids to discourage the formation of renal calculi
3. Encourage weight reduction
4. Monitor serum urate levels to determine effectiveness of treatment
5. Administer with meals to reduce GI irritation
6. Instruct client to avoid high-purine foods such as organ meats, anchovies, sardines, and shellfish; encourage diet rich in nutrient-dense foods such as fruits, vegetables, and whole grains, as well as milk, cheese, and eggs; teach Canada's Food Guide and importance of preventing drug-induced nutrient deficiencies with improved diet
7. Monitor blood work during therapy
8. Evaluate client's response to medication and understanding of teaching

Ophthalmic Agents

A. Description
1. Used to treat conditions affecting the eyes
2. Produce effects ranging from antibiotic to antiinflammatory; play significant roles in medical and surgical diagnosis and treatment
3. Available in a variety of topical preparations; drugs having a systemic action are available in oral and parenteral (IM, IV) preparations

B. Examples
1. Miotics: constrict the pupil, pulling the iris away from the filtration angle and improving outflow of aqueous humor
   a. Carbachol
   b. Physostigmine
   c. Pilocarpine HCl
   d. Timolol maleate (Timoptic)
2. Anticholinergics: dilate the pupil (mydriasis) by relaxing the ciliary muscle and the sphincter muscle of the iris; paralyze accommodation (cycloplegia); thus facilitating eye examination
   a. Atropine sulfate
   b. Homatropine HBr
   c. Scopolamine HBr
   d. Tropicamide (Mydriacyl)
3. Mydriatics: dilate pupil (mydriasis) by causing contraction of the dilator muscle of iris with minimal effect on ciliary muscle, which lessens the effect on accommodation
   Phenylephrine HCl (Neo-Synephrine)
4. Carbonic anhydrase inhibitors: decrease inflow

of aqueous humor in control of intraocular pressure

    a. Acetazolamide (Diamox)

    b. Methazolamide (Neptazane)

5. Osmotic agents: administered systemically to decrease blood osmolality, which mobilizes fluid from the eye to reduce volume of intraocular fluid

    a. Glycerin

    b. Mannitol (Osmitrol)

    c. Urea (Ureaphil)

C. Major side effects

1. Miotics

    a. Twitching of eyelids (increased cholinergic stimulation)

    b. Brow ache (increased cholinergic stimulation)

    c. Headache (vasodilation)

    d. Conjunctival pain (irritation of conjunctiva)

    e. Contact dermatitis (local irritation)

2. Anticholinergics (decreased parasympathetic stimulation)

    a. Dry mouth (decreased salivation)

    b. Flushing, fever (CNS effect)

    c. Blurred vision (pupillary dilation)

    d. Skin rash (hypersensitivity)

    e. Tachycardia (decreased vagal stimulation)

    f. Ataxia (CNS effect)

3. Mydriatics

    a. Brow ache (vasoconstrictor effect)

    b. Headache (vasoconstrictor effect)

    c. Blurred vision (pupillary dilation)

    d. Tachycardia (increased sympathetic stimulation)

    e. Hypertension (vasoconstrictor effect)

4. Carbonic anhydrase inhibitors

    a. Diuresis (increased excretion of sodium and water in renal tubule)

    b. Paresthesia (fluid-electrolyte imbalance)

    c. Nausea, vomiting (GI irritation)

    d. CNS disturbances (CNS effect)

5. Osmotic agents

    a. Headache (cerebral dehydration)

    b. Nausea, vomiting (fluid-electrolyte imbalance)

D. Nursing care

1. Instruct client regarding:

    a. Effects of drug prior to administration

    b. Proper method of application

    c. Need for medical supervision during therapy

2. Provide care for the client receiving mydriatics

    a. Caution client that vision will be blurred temporarily

    b. Advise client that sunglasses will relieve photophobia

    c. Have client avoid engaging in hazardous activities

3. Assess for occurrence of side effects and/or worsening of condition

4. Encourage diet rich in nutrient-dense foods such as fruits, vegetables, whole grains, and legumes to improve and maintain nutritional status and prevent possible drug-induced nutrient deficiencies

5. Evaluate client's response to medication and understanding of teaching

PROCEDURES RELATED TO THE NEUROMUSCULOSKELETAL SYSTEMS

Arthroscopic Examination

A. Definition: direct visualization of a joint with a fiber-optic scope inserted through a small skin incision

B. Purposes

1. Allow for evaluation of changes in joint structures

2. Permit removal of torn cartilage and repair of torn ligaments

3. Reduce period required for rehabilitation because adjacent muscles and ligaments are not disrupted

C. Nursing care

1. Explain procedure to client and obtain consent

2. Maintain sterile technique when changing postoperative dressing

3. Apply prescribed ace bandages to minimize swelling and stabilize joint

4. Maintain limb in position as ordered

5. Assist client with ambulation as ordered

6. Evaluate client's response to procedure

Bárány's Caloric Test

A. Definition

1. Used to assess vestibular labyrinthine function

2. Warm or cold water is instilled rapidly into the auditory canal, causing motion of the endolymph within the semicircular canals and normally resulting in vertigo, nystagmus, and nausea

3. Eyes deviate toward the stimulated ear if cold water is used and away if warm water is used

B. Nursing care

1. Explain procedure to the client

2. Assemble equipment for the procedure

3. Assist the physician and support the client during irrigation

4. Observe and record reaction of the client

5. Evaluate client's response to procedure

Computerized Tomography (CT)

A. Definition
  1. Cross-sectional visualization of the brain determined by computer analysis of relative tissue density as an x-ray beam passes through; also known as computerized axial tomography (CAT) scan
  2. Provides valuable information about location and extent of tumors, infarcted areas, atrophy, and vascular lesions
  3. May be done with or without intravenous injection of dye for contrast enhancement
B. Nursing care
  1. Explain procedure; inform the client that it will be necessary to lie still and that the equipment is complex but will cause no pain or discomfort
  2. If the facility is small, arrange transportation to a larger facility that has the required equipment
  3. Evaluate for possible allergy to iodine, a component of the contrast material
  4. Withhold food for approximately 4 hours prior to testing; dye may cause nausea in sensitive patients
  5. Remove wigs, clips, and pins prior to the test
  6. Evaluate client's response to procedure

Cerebral Angiography

A. Definition: visualization of the cerebral vasculature with a contrast dye and x-ray projection
B. Nursing care (see Angiography under Procedures Related to the Circulatory System)

Continuous Passive Motion Devices (CPM)

A. Definition: a machine that provides for passive range of motion
B. Purposes
  1. Move joint without weight bearing or straining muscles following orthopedic surgery
  2. Stimulate regeneration of articular tissues
  3. Enhance joint mobility
C. Nursing care
  1. Adjust device according to length of client's extremity (the thigh and lower leg are measured for the CPM of the hip and knee)
  2. Set foot cradle at the angle ordered by the physician
  3. Set flexion, extension, and speed dials as ordered by the physician; these are generally increased gradually as tolerated to maximize mobility
  4. Demonstrate use of control cord to client
  5. Align extremity in padded CPM device
  6. Evaluate client's response to procedure

Electroencephalography (EEG)

A. Definition
  1. Measurement and recording of electrical activity of the brain in the form of waves
  2. Provides information about seizure disorders, local tumors, infections of the central nervous system, and chemical toxicity
  3. May be done at the bedside with portable equipment but generally is done in a special room to decrease distractions and interference
  4. The client may be asked to hyperventilate, or flashing lights may be utilized to trigger any abnormal wave pattern
B. Nursing care
  1. Explain procedure; common misconceptions include fear of receiving electrical shock and fear that personal thoughts will be revealed
  2. Provide the client with a normal meal to avoid hypoglycemia; stimulants such as coffee or tea and depressants are withheld because of their effect on the EEG; withhold anticonvulsants if ordered
  3. Shampoo hair after the test to remove collodion, the conducting jelly
  4. Evaluate client's response to procedure

Electromyography (EMG)

A. Definition
  1. Measurement and recording of the electrical activity of specific muscles into which needle electrodes have been inserted
  2. In addition to providing information about primary muscle disease, it helps differentiate between motor symptoms that are secondary to neurologic disturbances; contraindicated in clients with dysrhythmias
B. Nursing care
  1. Explain procedure to the client
  2. Evaluate client's response to procedure

Instillation of Eye Medications

A. Purpose: to provide therapeutic effect of medication ordered
B. Nursing care
  1. Explain procedure to the client
  2. Position the client with the head slightly backward
  3. Pull lower eyelid down and place ointment or solution in the center of the cul-de-sac of the eye that is to be medicated (check order: OD—right eye, OU—both eyes, OS—left eye)
  4. Allow the client to close the eyes gently and instruct that they should not be rubbed
  5. Apply pressure to the nasolacrimal duct if necessary
  6. Record administration of medication
  7. Evaluate client's response to procedure

Irrigations of the Ear

A. Definition
  1. Introduction of fluid into the external auditory canal
  2. Usually done for cleansing purposes but can be used to apply antiseptic solutions

B. Nursing care
  1. Explain procedure to the client
  2. Assemble equipment: irrigating solution, sterile irrigating syringe, cotton balls, cotton-tipped applicators, towel
  3. Assist the client to sitting position with the head tilted to affected side to facilitate drainage
  4. Gently pull up and back on the external ear of an adult, down and forward on a child, to straighten the canal
  5. Direct solution into the canal without exerting excessive force; collect returns in a basin
  6. Dry the outer ear and have client lie on the affected side
  7. Record the procedure, type of drainage, etc.
  8. Evaluate client's response to procedure

Lumbar Puncture

A. Definition: involves the introduction of a needle into the subarachnoid space, usually between L_3 and L_4 or L_4 and L_5, to prevent injury to the spinal cord above this level

B. Purposes
  1. Withdrawal of spinal fluid for diagnostic purposes or to reduce spinal pressure (normal is 70 to 200 mm H_2O)
  2. Measurement of spinal pressure (Queckenstedt's test involves compression of the jugular veins; normally pressure will rise; but if blockage exists, pressure will not change)
  3. Injection of air or dye for diagnostic x-ray examination
  4. Injection of medication such as anesthetics

C. Nursing care
  1. Explain procedure to the client and obtain a signed consent
  2. Set up a sterile field
  3. Assist the client into a position that will enlarge the opening between the vertebrae
     a. Lying on side with feet drawn up and head lowered to chest; back near edge of mattress
     b. Sitting over side of bed, leaning on overbed table, feet supported on a stool
  4. Observe for signs of shock, such as tachycardia, diaphoresis, and pallor
  5. After procedure assist the client into a recumbent position; the client should remain recumbent up to 24 hours, depending on the physician's orders
  6. Label specimens and send to laboratory

7. Note color and amount of spinal fluid, as well as the client's condition, and record
8. Administer fluids unless contraindicated
9. Evaluate client's response to procedure

Mobility: Use of Braces or Splints

A. Purposes
  1. Support and protect weakened muscles
  2. Prevent and correct anatomic deformities
  3. Aid in controlling involuntary muscle movements
  4. Immobilize and protect a diseased or injured joint
  5. Provide for improvement of function

B. Nursing care
  1. Keep equipment in good repair (e.g., oil joints, replace straps when worn, wash with saddle soap)
  2. Provide adequate shoes (e.g., keep in good repair, heels low and wide, high top to hold the heel in the shoe)
  3. Examine the skin daily for evidence of breakdown at pressure points
  4. Check alignment of the braces (e.g., leg braces: joints should coincide with body joints; back brace: upright bars in center of back, brace should grip the pelvis and trochanter firmly, lacing should begin from the bottom)
  5. Evaluate client's response to procedure

Mobility: Use of a Cane

A. Purposes
  1. Improve stability of the client with a lower limb disability
  2. Maintain balance
  3. Prevent further injury
  4. Provide security while developing confidence in ambulating
  5. Relieve pressure on weight-bearing joints
  6. Assist in increasing speed of ambulation with less fatigue
  7. Provide for greater mobility and independence

B. Nursing care
  1. Ascertain that the client is able to bear weight on the affected extremity
  2. Ensure that the client is able to use the upper extremity opposite the affected lower extremity
  3. Measure to determine the length of cane required
     a. Highest point should be approximately level with the greater trochanter
     b. Handpiece should allow 30 degrees of flexion at the elbow with the wrist held in extension

4. Explain the proper techniques in using a cane
   a. Hold in the hand opposite the affected extremity
   b. Advance the cane and the affected extremity simultaneously, and then the unaffected leg
   c. Keep the cane close to the body
   d. When climbing, step up with the unaffected extremity and then place the cane and the affected lower extremity on the step; when descending, reverse the procedure
5. Observe for incorrect use of the cane
   a. Leaning the body over the cane
   b. Shortening the stride on the unaffected side
   c. Inability to develop a normal walking pattern
   d. Persistence of the abnormal gait pattern after the cane is no longer needed
6. Evaluate client's response to procedure

Mobility: Crutch Walking

A. Purposes
   1. Support body weight, assist weak muscles, and provide joint stability
   2. Relieve pain
   3. Prevent further injury and provide for improvement of function
   4. Allow for greater independence
B. Nursing care
   1. Ensure proper fit of crutches by measuring the distance from the anterior fold of the axilla to a point 15 cm out from the heel
      a. Axillary bars must be 5 cm below the axillae and should be padded
      b. Hand bars should allow almost complete extension of the arm with the elbow flexed about 30 degrees when the client places weight on the hands
      c. Rubber crutch tips should be in good condition, about 5.1 to 7.6 cm in height, with a circumference of 3.8 to 4.4 cm
   2. Assist in use of proper technique, depending on ability to bear weight and to take steps with either one or both of the lower extremities
      a. Four-point alternate crutch gait
         (1) Right crutch, left foot, left crutch, right foot
         (2) Equal but partial weight bearing on each limb
         (3) Slow but stable gait; there are always three points of support on the floor
         (4) The client must be able to manipulate both extremities and get one foot ahead of the other (e.g., persons with polio, arthritis, cerebral palsy)
      b. Two-point alternate crutch gait
         (1) Right crutch and left foot simultaneously
         (2) There are always two points of support on the floor
         (3) This is a more rapid version of the four-point gait and requires more balance and strength (e.g., a bilateral amputee)
      c. Three-point gait
         (1) Advance both crutches and the weaker lower extremity simultaneously, then the stronger lower extremity
         (2) Fairly rapid gait, but requires more balance and strength in the arms and the good lower extremity
         (3) Used when one leg can support the whole body weight and the other cannot take full weight bearing (e.g., a client with a fractured hip)
      d. Swing crutch gaits
         (1) Swing-to gait
            (a) Place both crutches forward, lift and swing the body up to the crutches, then place crutches in front of the body and continue
            (b) There are always two points of support on the floor
            (c) This technique is indicated for anyone with adequate power in the upper arms
         (2) Swing-through gait
            (a) Place both crutches forward, lift and swing the body through the crutches, then place crutches in front of the body and continue
            (b) Very difficult gait, because as the client swings through the crutches it necessitates rolling the pelvis forward and arching the back to get the center of gravity in front of the hips
            (c) Indicated for the client who has power in the trunk and upper extremities, excellent balance, self-confidence, and a dash of daring (e.g., a bilateral amputee, a paraplegic with braces)
      e. Tripod crutch gaits
         (1) Tripod alternate gait
            (a) Right crutch, left crutch, drag the body and legs forward
            (b) The client constantly maintains a tripod position: both crutches are held fairly widespread out front while both feet are held together in the back
            (c) Necessary for the individual who cannot place one extremity ahead of the other (e.g., a person with flaccid paralysis from poliomyelitis, one with spinal cord injuries)

(2) Tripod simultaneous gait
  (a) Place both crutches forward, drag the body and legs forward
  (b) Because the tripod must have a large base, the client's body must be inclined forward sufficiently to keep the center of gravity in front of the hips
3. Observe for incorrect use of crutches
  a. Using the body in poor mechanical fashion
  b. Hiking hips with abduction gait (common in amputees)
  c. Lifting crutches while still bearing down on them
  d. Walking on ball of foot with foot turned outward and flexion at hip or knee level
  e. Hunching shoulders (crutches usually too long) or stooping with shoulders (crutches usually too short)
  f. Looking downward while ambulating
  g. Bearing weight under arms; should be avoided to prevent injury to the nerves in the brachial plexus; damage to these nerves can cause paralysis and is known as crutch palsy
4. Evaluate client's response to procedure

Mobility: Transfer of Client

A. Purpose
  1. Move a client from one surface to another (e.g., bed to wheelchair, wheelchair to commode)
    a. Weight-bearing transfers: by clients who have at least one stable lower extremity (e.g., hemiplegics, clients who have undergone a unilateral lower extremity amputation, clients with a fractured hip)
    b. Non–weight-bearing transfers: by clients who do not have a stable lower extremity (e.g., paraplegics not wearing braces, clients with double lower extremity amputations)
  2. Move client who cannot move self
B. Nursing care
  1. Assess the client's abilities (e.g., sitting tolerance, balance, weight-bearing potential, strength, motivation, understanding of principles of transfer)
  2. Identify need for and selection of assistive devices (e.g., slide board, trapeze, transfer belt, wheelchair with a removable arm, hydraulic lift)
  3. Select most appropriate transfer method and teach and assist the client with this new technique
  4. Provide for client safety (e.g., encourage use of low-heeled shoes, lock wheelchair brakes during transfer, remove hazards [scatter rugs, slippery floors, stepstools], ensure adequate assistance)
  5. Communicate individualized transfer techniques by instructing the client and family and informing the entire health team
  6. Consider the client's abilities and disabilities when deciding appropriate transfer technique and need for assistive devices (e.g., hemiplegia: place the wheelchair on the side opposite the affected extremities; paraplegia: may use trapeze, slide board, or wheelchair with removable arm)
  7. Maintain correct proximity and visual relationship of wheelchair to the bed (e.g., paraplegia: place the wheelchair lateral or perpendicular to the bed; hemiplegia: place the wheelchair at a 30-degree angle to the bed on the unaffected side)
  8. Evaluate client's response to procedure

Mobility: Use of a Walker

A. Purposes
  1. Maintain balance
  2. Provide additional support because of wide area of contact with floor
  3. Allow for some ambulatory independence
B. Nursing care
  1. Assist in selecting a walker
    a. Device should not be used unless the client will never be able to ambulate with a cane or crutches
    b. Measurements for a walker are the same as for a cane
    c. The client must have strong elbow extensors and shoulder depressors and partial strength in the hands and the wrist muscles
    d. The client needs maximum support to ensure security and enhance confidence
    e. Device is ordinarily limited to the home because it cannot be used on steps
  2. Assist in ambulating with the walker
    a. Lift the device off the floor and place forward a short distance, then advance between the walker
    b. Two-wheeled walkers: raise back legs of the device off the floor, roll walker forward, then advance to it
    c. Four-wheeled walkers: push device forward on floor and then walk to it
  3. Observe for incorrect use of the walker
    a. Keeping arms rigid and swinging through to counterbalance the position of the lower extremity
    b. Tending to lean forward with abnormal flexion at the hips
    c. Tending to step forward with the unaffected leg and shuffle the affected leg up to the bar
  4. Evaluate client's response to procedure

Mobility: Use of a Wheelchair

A. Purpose
  1. Move a client on a special chair that has wheels or casters; the client is propelled or propels himself or herself
  2. Support the body
  3. Decrease cardiac workload
  4. Promote independence and stimulate activities
  5. Provide mobility for those who cannot ambulate or those who can ambulate but whose ambulation is unsteady, unsafe, or too strenuous

B. Nursing care
  1. Instruct the client that prolonged sitting in one position can cause flexion contractures of the hips and knees and ischial decubiti (encourage the client to change body positions and to use padded cushions and exercises such as push-ups every hour to relieve pressure)
  2. Ensure that specific devices necessary for client safety (e.g., wheel brakes, arm locks, seat belts, swing foot rests) are in operating condition
  3. Alert the wheelchair-bound client to the accessories that meet the client's specific needs (e.g., removable arms, lap boards, knobs on the handrims, extra-long leg panels, battery or motor propulsion)
  4. Evaluate client's response to procedure

Myelography

A. Definition: visualization of the spinal canal after it has been injected with radiopaque dye

B. Nursing care
  1. Explain procedure to the client and obtain a signed consent
  2. Maintain the NPO status prior to the test
  3. Remove dentures and metal objects
  4. Administer a sedative as ordered prior to the procedure
  5. Care for the client following the procedure
    a. Observe for neurologic signs
    b. Keep the client in a recumbent position for 24 hours
    c. Encourage fluid intake
  6. Evaluate client's response to procedure

Neurologic Assessment

A. Definition: systematic evaluation of the cranial nerves, motor and sensory functioning, and mental status to detect neurologic abnormalities
  1. Critical aspects of a complete neurologic assessment are generally extracted and compose a "neuro checklist," which is used when the nature of the situation does not warrant complete evaluation

2. See Review of Anatomy and Physiology of the Neuromusculoskeletal Systems

B. Nursing care
  1. Perform assessment as dictated by the client's needs
    a. Cranial nerves
      (1) Olfactory (I): ability to identify familiar odors such as mint or alcohol with eyes closed and one nostril occluded at a time
      (2) Optic (II): visual acuity measured by use of Snellen chart or by gross estimation with reading material; gross comparison of visual fields with those of examiner; color perception
      (3) Oculomotor (III), trochlear (IV), and abducent (VI): ability of the pupils to react equally to light and to accommodate to varying distances; normal range of extraocular movement (EOM) evaluated by asking the client to follow a finger or object with the eyes; should also include assessment for nystagmus (jerking motion of eyes), particularly when eyes are directed laterally
      (4) Trigeminal (V): sensations of the face evaluated by lightly stroking cotton across forehead, chin, and cheeks while the client's eyes are closed; ability to clench the teeth (jaw closure)
      (5) Facial (VII): symmetry of the facial muscles as the client speaks or is asked to make faces
      (6) Acoustic or vestibulocochlear (VIII): hearing acuity determined by a watch tick or whispered numbers; Weber's test may be performed by holding the stem of a vibrating tuning fork at midline of the skull (should be heard equally in both ears)
      (7) Glossopharyngeal (IX) and vagus (X): uvula should hang in midline; swallow and gag reflexes should be intact
      (8) Spinal accessory (XI): symmetric ability to turn the head or shrug the shoulders against counterforce of the examiner's hands
      (9) Hypoglossal (XII): ability to protrude the tongue without deviation to left or right, and without tremors
    b. Motor function (including cerebellar function)
      (1) Balance
        (a) Observation of gait
        (b) Romberg test: positive if the client fails to maintain an upright position

with feet together when the eyes are closed

    (2) Coordination: ability to touch the finger to the nose when arms are extended or to perform similar tasks smoothly

    (3) Muscle strength: evaluated by having the client move major muscle groups against opposition supplied by the examiner

  c. Sensory function: bilateral testing of the response to light touch with cotton, superficial pinprick, vibration of a tuning fork

  d. Mental status of cerebral functioning

    (1) Level of consciousness: determined by the response to stimuli (e.g., verbal or physical); a client may be in any state, ranging from alert to comatose; Glasgow Coma Scale may be used

    (2) Orientation to person, place, and time: determined by general conversation and direct questioning

    (3) Judgment, memory, and ability to perform simple calculations

    (4) Appropriateness of behavior and mood

  e. Reflexes

    (1) Deep tendon (biceps, triceps, patellar, Achilles reflexes) with a reflex hammer; classification from 0 (absent) to 4+ (signifying hyperactive)

    (2) Plantar: plantar flexion of the foot when the sole is stroked firmly with a hard object such as a tongue blade; abnormal adult response (dorsiflexion of the foot and fanning of the toes) is described as a positive Babinski and is indicative of corticospinal tract disease

2. Accurately record findings
3. Report any deviations that warrant immediate treatment
4. Explain and reassure the client when the examination must be repeated frequently (e.g., after head trauma)
5. Evaluate client's response to procedure

Coma Assessment with the Glasgow Coma Scale

A. Definition

1. Technique of objectifying a client's level of responses
2. Areas of assessment
  a. Eye-opening ability
  b. Motor response
  c. Verbal response
3. Client's best response in each area is given a numerical value, and the three values are totaled; a numerical value of 3 would be least

responsive and a value of 15 would be most responsive

B. Nursing care

1. Perform the assessment at appropriate intervals to determine current level of changes in client's level of consciousness; usually every 2 to 4 hours
2. A score of 7 or less indicates "coma"
3. Assess other indicators such as vital signs, pupillary reaction, movement of extremities, strength, etc.
4. Document findings

Magnetic Resonance Imaging (MRI)

A. Definition

1. This procedure utilizes magnetism and radio waves to produce images of cross-sections of the body
2. The MRI machine registers the existence of odd-numbered atoms in the cross sections of the body, yielding data about the chemical makeup of the tissues
3. MRI can produce accurate images of blood vessels, bone marrow, gray and white brain matter, the spinal cord, the globe of the eye, the heart, abdominal structures, and breast tissue, and can monitor blood velocity

B. Nursing care

1. Assess ability to withstand confining surroundings because client must remain in the tunnel-like machine for up to 90 minutes; open MRI may be an option for clients who cannot tolerate closed spaces
2. Instruct client to toilet prior to test, since this will be impossible during the procedure
3. Advise client to remove jewelry, clothing with metal fasteners, dentures, hearing aids, and glasses prior to entering scanner
4. Since this procedure is contraindicated for certain clients, before the test assess for:
  a. Metal prostheses, such as orthopedic screws, since the magnetic force can dislodge the devices
  b. Pacemakers, since the scanner deactivates pacemaker
  c. Dysrhythmias, because the magnetic field can affect the conduction system of the heart
  d. Unstable medical conditions, since monitoring of the client is limited during the test
5. Evaluate client's response to procedure

Positron Emission Tomography (PET SCAN)

A. Definition

1. This test registers glucose metabolism in a cross-section of the brain; glucose metabolism increases in areas of the brain that are active

2. Utilized to diagnose Alzheimer's disease, depression, dementia, and brain tumors

B. Nursing care
1. Instruct client to abstain from alcohol, tobacco, and caffeine 24 hours prior to test
2. Allow client to eat a meal 3 hours prior to test; diabetic clients should have a dose of long-acting insulin prior to this meal
3. Provide tranquil environment since anxiety can affect test results
4. Instruct client about what to expect during test
   a. Two IVs will be utilized: one for drawing blood samples and one for infusing the radioactive material
   b. A blindfold may be applied and cotton plugs may be placed in the ears during the test
   c. Certain mental activities may have to be performed during the test
   d. The scan will take 60 to 90 minutes and client must remain still
5. Following test, encourage client to void to clear radioactive isotope from the body
6. Evaluate client's response to procedure

Special Beds for Positioning Clients

A. Beds and their purposes
1. Beds to promote turning
   a. Purpose
      (1) Immobilizes the vertebral column
      (2) Facilitates turning
      (3) Promotes body functions (circulation, respiration, elimination)
   b. Examples
      (1) Turning frames
         (a) Stryker or Foster frames: allow for horizontal turning of the client
         (b) CircOlectric bed: allows for vertical turning; the client can be placed in a variety of positions (Trendelenburg, prone, standing, supine); one nurse can turn the client, with the electric motor providing the power; attachments permit application of traction and other accessories
      (2) Oscillating beds (e.g., Rotokinetic treatment table): uses a continual side-to-side rotation with the client in constant motion
2. Beds to promote skin integrity
   a. Purpose
      (1) Relieves pressure by distributing body weight
      (2) Limits friction
      (3) Promotes circulation of air under client
   b. Examples
      (1) Air-fluidized beds (e.g., Clinitron bed):

uses flow of temperature-controlled air through small ceramic spheres to evenly distribute client's weight
      (2) Air mattresses (e.g., Flexicare bed): uses an automatic airbag system that adjusts to individual's weight and activity to evenly distribute client's weight

B. Nursing care
1. Care for a client on a turning frame
   a. Turn the client all in one piece (log roll)
   b. Because frames are narrow, for safety purposes do not permit the client to sit up, roll over, or reach out to the side; do not place extremely obese or disoriented clients on a frame
   c. Since only the prone and supine positions can be used, strict attention must be paid to prevention of decubiti
   d. Before releasing pivot pins, secure all bolts and straps to ensure client safety
   e. When turning the CircOlectric bed, do so slowly so that the client's cerebral circulation can adjust to the new position; observe for signs of hypotension
2. Care for a client on a bed that promotes skin integrity
   a. Use only the incontinence pads recommended by the manufacturer
   b. With air-fluidized beds:
      (1) Assess the client for signs of dehydration because air flow promotes evaporation
      (2) Use foam wedges when positioning the client
   c. With oscillating beds assess the client for agitation and motion sickness
3. Call company representative for regular servicing of bed
4. Evaluate client's response to procedure

GENERAL NURSING DIAGNOSES FOR CLIENTS WITH NEUROMUSCULOSKELETAL SYSTEMS DISORDERS

A. Decreased adaptive capacity: intracranial related to:
1. Sustained increase in intracranial pressure
2. Decreased cerebral perfusion
B. Risk for aspiration related to decreased or absent gag reflex
C. Body image disturbance related to actual change in function
D. Bowel incontinence related to:
1. Impaired neuromuscular control
2. Impaired thought process
E. Ineffective breathing pattern related to muscle weakness

F. Chronic confusion related to cognitive impairment
G. Constipation related to:
   1. Immobility
   2. Loss of innervation
H. Risk for disuse syndrome related to:
   1. Immobilization
   2. Pain
I. Diversional activity deficit related to:
   1. Long-term hospitalization
   2. Immobility
   3. Bed rest
   4. Impaired sensory function
J. Dysreflexia related to spinal cord injury T 7 or above
K. Altered family processes related to role changes
L. Fear related to anticipation of pain
M. Risk for injury related to:
   1. Cognitive impairment
   2. Sensory impairment
   3. Neuromusculoskeletal impairment
   4. Seizure activity
N. Ineffective management of therapeutic regimen (families) related to:
   1. Complexity of regimen
   2. Excessive demands on family members
O. Ineffective management of therapeutic regimen (individual) related to:
   1. Complexity of the regimen
   2. Cognitive impairments
   3. Excessive demands on the individual
P. Altered nutrition: less than body requirements related to inability to ingest
Q. Pain related to:
   1. Inflammatory process
   2. Pressure
R. Impaired physical mobility related to:
   1. Inability to move purposefully
   2. Impaired coordination
   3. Limited range of motion
   4. Imposed restrictions
S. Reflex incontinence related to impaired neuromuscular control
T. Altered role performance related to interruption of neuromusculoskeletal functioning
U. Self-care deficit (bathing/hygiene, dressing/grooming, feeding, toileting) related to:
   1. Neuromuscular impairment
   2. Cognitive impairment
   3. Musculoskeletal impairment
V. Sensory/perceptual alteration related to:
   1. Visual impairment
   2. Diminished sense of touch
   3. Hearing loss
W. Sexual dysfunction related to actual or perceived limitation imposed by disease and/or therapy
X. Situational low self-esteem related to actual change in function

Y. Risk for impaired skin integrity related to immobility
Z. Impaired social interaction related to decreased sensory function
AA. Impaired swallowing related to weakness or paralysis
BB. Ineffective thermoregulation related to head trauma
CC. Altered thought processes related to impaired cerebral function
DD. Impaired verbal communication related to:
   1. Impaired articulation
   2. Disorientation/confusion

MAJOR DISORDERS OF THE NEUROMUSCULOSKELETAL SYSTEMS

▼ MIGRAINE HEADACHES

Data Base
A. Etiology and pathophysiology
   1. Caused by constriction and then dilation of the cerebral arteries
   2. Individuals who have migraines are frequently described as perfectionists, inflexible, and ambitious
   3. Incidence higher in females; familial tendency
B. Clinical findings
   1. Subjective
      a. Severe, throbbing pain, often in temporal or supraorbital area, that lasts several hours to several days
      b. Fatigue and irritability may precede headache
      c. Nausea
      d. Visual disturbances
      e. Aura consisting of a neurologic symptom
   2. Objective
      a. Pallor
      b. Vomiting
C. Therapeutic interventions
   1. Methysergide maleate (Sansert) to prevent attacks; should not be continued for more than 6 to 12 months consecutively; then, should be omitted for a few months before it is resumed
   2. Beta blockers such as propranolol hydrochloride (Inderal) to prevent attacks
   3. Ergotamine tartrate (Gynergen) or ergotamine with caffeine (Cafergot) to relieve migraines
   4. Sumatriptan (Imitrex) for treatment of acute migrain; SC injection and oral tablets
   5. Elimination of factors (physical, psychologic, environmental) that precipitate illness
   6. Dietary exclusion of headache-precipitating foods, such as those containing tyramines (red wine), monosodium glutamate, nitrates, or milk products

Nursing Care of Clients with Migraine Headaches

A. DATA COLLECTION

1. History to identify situations that may precipitate attacks
2. Detailed description of aura and pain

B. ANALYSIS AND INTERPRETATION

Refer to General Nursing Diagnoses for Clients with Neuromusculoskeletal Systems Disorders for the following diagnoses: L, P, Q 2, and X

C. PLANNING/IMPLEMENTATION

1. Assist the client in identifying situations that seem to precipitate attacks
2. Support the client in modification of life-style and development of insight
3. Provide a dark, quiet environment when migraine begins
4. Provide care for the nauseated client
   a. Administer an antiemetic if ordered
   b. Offer small, frequent sips of fluid as tolerated
   c. Assist with mouth care
5. Explain medications and their side effects

D. EVALUATION/OUTCOMES

1. Reduces frequency of attacks, which are less painful and of shorter duration
2. Establishes regular routine of rest and exercise
3. Avoids stressful situations
4. Reduces or eliminates intake of potential headache-causing foods

▼ HEAD INJURIES

Data Base

A. Etiology and pathophysiology
   1. Result from trauma, frequently seen after motor vehicle accidents
   2. Fractures
      a. Linear: simple break in the bone
      b. Depressed: break that results in fragments of bone penetrating the brain tissue
   3. Hemorrhages
      a. Epidural: hematoma forms between the dura and the skull; may result from a laceration of the middle meningeal artery
      b. Subdural: hematoma forms between the dura and arachnoid layers; generally follows venous damage
   4. Concussion: temporary disruption of synaptic activity
   5. Contusions: bruising of brain tissue, with slight bleeding of small cerebral vessels into surrounding tissues at site of impact (coup) or opposite to site (contracoup) as a result of rebound reaction

B. Clinical findings
   1. Subjective
      a. Lethargy
      b. Indifference to surroundings
      c. Altered sensory function
   2. Objective
      a. Signs of increased intracranial pressure (ICP) (see Provide care for the client requiring brain surgery under Brain Tumor)
      b. Lack of orientation to time and place
      c. Restlessness
      d. Labored respirations
      e. Positive Babinski sign (stroking bottom of the foot causes dorsiflexion of the toes)
      f. Decreased level of consciousness
      g. Dilation and fixation of pupils
      h. Seepage of cerebral spinal fluid from the nose or ears; usually is indicative of basal cell fracture

C. Therapeutic interventions
   1. Control seizures with anticonvulsants
   2. Mechanical ventilation; hyperventilation will constrict cerebral vessels lowering ICP
   3. Reduce cerebral edema with glucocorticoids and loop diuretics; there is disagreement regarding their efficacy
   4. Maintain adequate fluid and electrolyte balance
   5. Surgical intervention in cases of depressed skull fractures or hematomas

Nursing Care of Clients with Head Injuries

A. DATA COLLECTION

1. Airway and breathing pattern
2. Neurologic status (see Neurologic Assessment and Coma Assessment with the Glasgow Coma Scale under Procedures Related to the Neuromusculoskeletal System)
3. Signs of increased intracranial pressure
4. Circumstances of injury
5. Presence of glucose in clear drainage from nose or ear, which indicates cerebrospinal fluid

B. ANALYSIS AND INTERPRETATION

Refer to General Nursing Diagnoses for Clients with Neuromusculoskeletal Systems Disorders for the following diagnoses: A, B, C, D 1, D 2, F, G 1, I 1, I 2, I 3, I 4, K, M 1, M 2, M 3, N 1, N 2, O 1, O 2, O 3, P, R 1, T, U 1, U 2, AA, BB, CC, DD 1, and DD 2

C. PLANNING/IMPLEMENTATION

1. Observe for signs of increased intracranial pressure; institute neurologic assessments every 15 minutes for several hours, progressing to every hour and then every 4 hours
2. Maintain airway by suctioning as necessary (coughing increases intracranial pressure); use an airway or endotracheal tube

3. Keep the client's head slightly elevated to reduce venous pressure within the cranial cavity
4. Administer glucocorticoids and/or diuretics if ordered
5. Institute seizure precautions; administer anticonvulsants if ordered
6. Monitor for fluid or electrolyte imbalances; diabetes insipidus or syndrome of inappropriate antidiuretic hormone may occur
7. If the client's eyes remain open, protect the corneas with moistened pads, mineral oil, or ointment as ordered
8. Support client's nutritional needs; administer tube feedings or assist with small frequent meals
9. Position the client to prevent pressure areas from forming decubiti
10. Provide range-of-motion exercises and splints to prevent contractures
11. Provide auditory and tactile stimulation
12. Assist client to avoid activities that increase ICP such as Valsalva's maneuver, lifting, sneezing, and flexion of head
13. Utilize hypothermia as ordered to reduce temperature and metabolic demands
14. Encourage client and family to participate in planning and care
15. Provide opportunity for expression of grief

D. EVALUATION/OUTCOMES
1. Maintains a patent airway
2. Improves level of consciousness
3. Remains free from injury
4. Participates in decisions about administration of care
5. Maintains ideal body weight for age and frame
6. Identifies new coping skills to deal with changes in life-style

▼ BRAIN TUMORS

Data Base

A. Etiology and pathophysiology
1. Either benign or malignant; they require intervention, since the skull cannot accommodate the increasing size of the tumor, and intracranial pressure rises
2. Classified according to tissue of origin
   a. Meningioma: occurs outside the brain from the covering meninges; usually benign
   b. Acoustic neuroma and optic nerve spongioblastoma: occur from the cranial nerves
   c. Gliomas: originate in neural tissue; usually malignant
      (1) Astrocytoma
      (2) Glioblastoma
      (3) Oligodendroglioma
   d. Hemangioblastomas and angiomas: occur from within blood vessels
   e. Metastatic tumors: originate elsewhere in the body, most commonly the lung and breast
B. Clinical findings
1. Subjective
   a. Headache that increases with stooping
   b. Lethargy
2. Objective
   a. Vomiting
   b. Papilledema (noted on ophthalmoscopy)
   c. Abnormal brain waves on the EEG
3. Symptoms may vary depending on location of tumor
   a. Frontal lobe: personality changes, focal seizures, blurred vision, hemiparesis, aphasia
   b. Temporal lobe: seizures, headache, papilledema, aphasia
   c. Parietal lobe: jacksonian convulsions, visual loss
   d. Occipital region: focal seizures, visual hallucinations
   e. Cerebellar region: loss of coordination, papilledema
   f. Signs of increased intracranial pressure
   g. Motor and sensory deficits
C. Therapeutic interventions
1. Radiation therapy and/or chemotherapy
2. Surgery for partial or complete removal of the lesion
   a. Craniotomy with removal of lesion and invaded tissue
   b. Stereotaxic laser surgery; employs computer-directed laser to eradicate tissue
3. Steroids, anticonvulsives, and osmotic diuretics to control symptoms may be ordered

Nursing Care of Clients with Brain Tumors

A. DATA COLLECTION
1. History from client and family to identify behavioral changes, coping skills, and neurologic deficits
2. Neurologic status (see Neurologic Assessment and Coma Assessment with the Glasgow Coma Scale under Procedures Related to the Neuromusculoskeletal Systems)
3. Signs of increased intracranial pressure

B. ANALYSIS AND INTERPRETATION
Refer to General Nursing Diagnoses for Clients with Neuromusculoskeletal Systems Disorders for the following diagnoses: A, B, C, D 1, D 2, F, G 1,

H 1, H 2, I 1, I 2, I 3, I 4, K, M 1, M 2, N 1, N 2, O 1, O 2, O 3, P, R 1, R 2, T, U 1, U 2, W, X, Y, Z, AA, BB, and CC

C. PLANNING/IMPLEMENTATION

1. Provide emotional support for the client and family; refer to additional resources such as clergy and support groups
2. Maintain the client as comfortably as possible with analgesics and antiemetics as ordered
3. Support client's nutrition with small, frequent feedings, supplements, and oral hygiene
4. Provide care for the client requiring brain surgery
   a. Obtain consent for surgery and removal of hair (save the hair)
   b. After surgery keep the client's head elevated 30 degrees to aid drainage
   c. Support respiratory function by encouraging deep breathing, appropriate positioning, and suctioning to maintain the airway
   d. Assess the client's level of consciousness and neurologic status for changes
   e. Observe for signs of increased intracranial pressure (ICP)
      (1) Decreased level of consciousness
      (2) Restlessness
      (3) Weakness or paralysis
      (4) Visual and other sensory disturbances
      (5) Increased systolic pressure; widening pulse pressure
      (6) Decreased pulse rate
      (7) Changes in respiratory pattern
      (8) Unilateral nonreactive and/or dilated pupil progressing to bilateral
      (9) Headache
      (10) Rapid rise in body temperature
      (11) Vomiting
      (12) Seizures
      (13) Papilledema
   f. Use strict aseptic technique with ICP monitoring
   g. Observe dressings for cerebrospinal spinal (CSF) leakage or hemorrhage
   h. Maintain accurate intake and output records
   i. Utilize hypothermia as ordered if the client is febrile; fever increases metabolic needs of the brain
5. Assist client to focus on abilities rather than disabilities
6. Emphasize need for continued medical follow-up

D. EVALUATION/OUTCOMES

1. Maintains adequate respiratory function
2. Maintains stable vital signs
3. Demonstrates awareness of surroundings
4. Maintains skin integrity
5. Develops interests consistent with ability
6. Establishes effective communication with family
7. Complies with medical regimen
8. Participates in care

▼ BRAIN ABSCESS

Data Base

A. Etiology and pathophysiology
   1. Occurs when there is an infection in another region of the body that spreads to the brain or after a penetrating head wound
   2. Results from invasion of the brain causing formation and collection of exudate within the brain tissue
B. Clinical findings
   1. Subjective
      a. Headache
      b. Malaise
      c. Anorexia
   2. Objective
      a. Fever
      b. Vomiting
      c. Weight loss
      d. Focal deficits based on site: vision loss, paresis, seizures, personality change
C. Therapeutic interventions
   1. Large doses of antibiotics
   2. In severe cases, a craniotomy may be performed to allow removal of the abscess
   3. Anticonvulsants to control seizures

Nursing Care of Clients with Brain Abscesses

A. DATA COLLECTION

1. Neurologic status for baseline data
2. History of potential etiologic factors
3. Weight for baseline data

B. ANALYSIS AND INTERPRETATION

Refer to General Nursing Diagnoses for Clients with Neuromusculoskeletal Systems Disorders for the following diagnoses: M 1, M 2, P, Q 1, Q 2, and T

C. PLANNING/IMPLEMENTATION

1. Continue neurologic assessment
2. Encourage nutrient-dense diet to compensate for antibiotic impact on nutritional status (see Pharmacology Related to Infection)
3. Provide care for the client requiring brain surgery (see Nursing Care of Clients with Brain Tumors)
4. Explain the need to complete prescribed therapy of antibiotics and continue anticonvulsant therapy

5. Instruct client to seek prompt treatment for otitis media, sinusitis, and dental and other infections

D EVALUATION/OUTCOMES
1. Exhibits normal neurologic function
2. Reports relief of headache
3. Complies with medical regimen

▼ CEREBRAL ANEURYSM

Data Base

A. Etiology and pathophysiology
1. Sac formed by dilation of the walls of an artery within the cranial cavity
2. May be the result of a congenital weakness in the vessel, trauma, or arteriosclerosis
3. Symptoms occur when the aneurysm compresses nearby nerves or when it ruptures

B. Clinical findings
1. Subjective
   a. Unilateral headache
   b. Pain in the eye
   c. Diplopia
   d. Tinnitus
2. Objective
   a. Rigidity of the back of the neck and spine
   b. Ptosis of the eyelid
   c. Hemiparesis
   d. Decreased level of consciousness
   e. Deviations from normal results in CT scan and lumbar puncture
   f. Signs of increased ICP if rupture occurs

C. Therapeutic interventions
1. Attempt to keep the client hypotensive
2. If there is a stalk connecting the aneurysm, clips may be inserted surgically to cut off blood supply to the aneurysm permanently

Nursing Care of Clients with Cerebral Aneurysms

A. DATA COLLECTION
1. Neurologic status (see Neurologic Assessment under Procedures Related to the Neuromusculoskeletal Systems)
2. Presence of signs of increased ICP

B. ANALYSIS AND INTERPRETATION
Refer to General Nursing Diagnoses for Clients with Neuromusculoskeletal Systems Disorders for the following diagnoses: K, M 3, Q 2, R 4, T, and CC

C. PLANNING/IMPLEMENTATION
1. Continue neurologic assessment
2. Assist with lumbar puncture (see Lumbar Puncture under Procedures Related to the Neuromusculoskeletal Systems)

3. Provide care for the client requiring brain surgery (see Nursing Care of Clients with Brain Tumors)
4. Provide care based on neurologic deficits (see Nursing Care of Clients with Cerebral Vascular Accidents)
5. Teach client the need to continue antihypertensive medications
6. Teach client to avoid straining, lifting, exerting, and acutely flexing the neck
7. Provide opportunities for client and family to discuss fears
8. Encourage the need for continued medical supervision

D. EVALUATION/OUTCOMES
1. Exhibits normal neurologic function
2. Complies with medical regimen
3. Expresses realistic fears

▼ CEREBRAL VASCULAR ACCIDENT (CVA OR STROKE)

Data Base

A. Etiology and pathophysiology
1. Term applied to destruction (infarction) of brain cells caused by a reduction in the oxygen supply
2. Caused by a sudden or gradual interruption in the blood supply following an intracerebral hemorrhage, blockage of vessels by thrombi or emboli, or vascular insufficiency
3. Symptoms depend on the area of the brain involved and extent of damage
4. Conditions that predispose to a CVA include cerebral arteriosclerosis, syphilis, dehydration, trauma, and hypertension
5. Transient ischemic attacks (TIA) may also occur without causing permanent damage; these usually last only a few minutes
6. Incidence increases with age

B. Clinical findings
1. Subjective
   a. Syncope
   b. Changes in level of consciousness
   c. Transient paresthesias (with TIAs)
   d. Headache
   e. Mood swings
2. Objective
   a. Convulsions
   b. Nuchal rigidity (if caused by subarachnoid or intracerebral hemorrhage)
   c. Hemiplegia on side opposite the lesion (initially flaccid)
   d. Aphasia: brain unable to fulfill its communicative functions because of damage to its

input, integrative, or output centers; a disturbance of language function that may involve impairment of the ability to read, write, speak, or interpret messages

   (1) Expressive aphasia: difficulty making thoughts known to others; speaking and writing is most affected

   (2) Receptive aphasia: difficulty understanding what others are trying to communicate; interpretation of speech and reading is most affected

   (3) Expressive-receptive aphasia: equal difficulty with speaking, writing, interpreting speech, and reading

   e. Hemianopia (loss of half of visual field)
   f. Sensory changes
   g. Alterations in reflexes
   h. Functional disorders of the bladder and bowel
   i. CSF is bloody if cerebral or subarachnoid hemorrhage is present
   j. Abnormal EEG
   k. Cerebral angiography may reveal vascular abnormalities such as aneurysms, narrowing, or occlusions
   l. If increased intracranial pressure exists, as with hemorrhage, there may be elevated blood pressure and bounding pulse

C. Therapeutic interventions
   1. Complete bed rest with sedation as needed
   2. Maintenance of oxygenation by oxygen therapy or mechanical ventilation
   3. Maintenance of nutrition, by the parenteral route or nasogastric feedings, if the client is unable to swallow
   4. Anticoagulant therapy if thrombus or embolus is present
   5. Antihypertensive agents if indicated
   6. Surgical intervention
      a. To relieve pressure and control bleeding if hemorrhage is present
      b. Carotid endarterectomy, to improve cerebral blood flow when carotid arteries are narrowed by arteriosclerotic patches, may be done on a client in stable condition

Nursing Care of Clients with Cerebral Vascular Accidents

A. DATA COLLECTION
   1. Adequacy of airway and respiratory function
   2. Neurologic status (see Neurologic Assessment and Coma Assessment with Glasgow Coma Scale under Procedures Related to the Neuromusculoskeletal Systems)
   3. Presence of signs of increased ICP (see Planning/Implementation under Nursing Care of Clients with Brain Tumors)

B. ANALYSIS AND INTERPRETATION
Refer to General Nursing Diagnoses for Clients with Neuromusculoskeletal Systems Disorders for the following diagnoses: A, B, C, D 1, D 2, F, G 1, G 2, H 1, I 2, I 4, K, M 1, M 2, M 3, N 1, N 2, O 1, O 2, O 3, P, R 1, R 2, T, U 1, U 2, V 1, V 2, W, X, Y, AA, CC, DD 1, and DD 2

C. PLANNING/IMPLEMENTATION
   1. Assist with lumbar puncture if performed; may be performed if hemorrhage is suspected (see Lumbar Puncture under Procedures Related to the Neuromusculoskeletal Systems)
   2. Monitor respiratory functioning (vital signs, type and rate of respirations, color, blood gases, etc.)
   3. Evaluate swallowing and gag reflexes
   4. Maintain patency of the airway by positioning, suctioning, and inserting an artificial airway
   5. Provide for drainage and expansion of lungs by placing client in a low semi-Fowler's position with the head turned to the side
   6. Provide oxygen as necessary
   7. Provide frequent oral hygiene
   8. Encourage the client to breathe deeply and cough; utilize mechanical ventilation if ordered
   9. Continue neurologic assessments, noting signs of increased ICP
   10. Keep the side rails in place or use safety straps
   11. Provide for frequent nursing observations, since the client may be unable to signal for assistance
   12. Institute seizure precautions
   13. Utilize artificial tears if blink reflex is absent
   14. Provide elastic stockings for both legs
   15. Prevent decubiti
      a. Provide special care to the back and bony prominences; keep the client clean and dry
      b. Relieve pressure by use of mechanical and supportive devices and beds
      c. Turn the client every 2 hours
      d. Provide adequate hydration to maintain skin turgor
   16. Prevent muscle atrophy and contractures
      a. Provide for active and passive range-of-motion and other exercises
      b. Use devices to prevent footdrop, flexion of fingers, external rotation of hips, adduction of shoulders and arms
   17. Provide the client with tube feedings if swallowing and gag reflexes are depressed or absent
   18. Provide food in a form that is easily swallowed; encourage intake of nutrient-dense foods; when client is capable of chewing, introduce dietary fiber to promote normal bowel function

19. Assist with feeding (e.g., use a padded spoon handle; feed on the unaffected side of mouth; feed in as close to a sitting position as possible)
20. Encourage the aphasic client to communicate
    a. Be aware of own reactions to the speech difficulty
    b. Evaluate extent of the client's ability to understand and express self at a simple level
    c. Include the health team, especially the speech therapist, in planning care
    d. Involve the family as much as possible
    e. Convey that there is a problem with communication, not with intelligence
    f. Try to eliminate anxiety and tension related to communication attempts (e.g., be consistent; give the client time to respond; employ a calm, accepting, and deliberate manner)
    g. Help the client set attainable goals
    h. Stimulate communication without pushing to point of frustration
    i. Keep distractions at a minimum, since they interfere with the reception and integration of messages (e.g., one-to-one conversations rather than group conversations; shut off the radio when speaking)
    j. Speak slowly, clearly, and in short sentences, and do not raise voice
    k. Use alternate means of communication (e.g., gestures, writing, picture board)
    l. Involve the client in social interactions (e.g., encourage socialization, do not anticipate all needs, ask questions and expect answers, do not ignore the client in group conversations)
    m. Make a definite transition between tasks to prevent or reduce confusion
    n. Be alert for clues and gestures when speech is garbled (e.g., continue to listen, nod, and make occasional neutral statements, let the client know when you cannot understand)
    o. Provide for periodic reevaluation to demonstrate the effect and nature of progress to the client and health team
21. Attempt to prevent fecal impaction and/or urinary tract problems
    a. Provide adequate fluid intake
    b. Provide a diet with enough roughage for sufficient quantity of bowel content and proper consistency for evacuation
    c. Avoid preoccupation with elimination
    d. Avoid the overt encouragement of incontinence (e.g., through the routine use of incontinence pads and other depersonalizing devices)
    e. Stimulate normal elimination by exercise and activity
    f. Help the client develop regular bowel and bladder patterns
    g. Respect the individual (e.g., provide for privacy, individuality of routine, avoidance of delay); encourage the client to make decisions
    h. Utilize physical and psychologic techniques to stimulate elimination (e.g., run water, place the client's hands in warm water, place the client in as normal a position as possible for elimination)
    i. Create an environment that keeps sensory monotony to a minimum (e.g., orient to time and place, use a radio and television selectively, increase the client's social contacts, provide visual stimuli, extend environment beyond the client's room)
    j. Provide for self-esteem (e.g., encourage the client to wear own clothes, do self-care activities, make decisions)
    k. Accept and explore the client's feelings of fear, anger, and depression; a disabled person has few avenues by which to express anger; incontinence is often used in this manner
22. Provide realistic encouragement and praise
23. Accept mood swings and emotional outbursts
24. Assist the client and family to set realistic goals
25. Help the client to adjust to change in body image and altered self-concept

D. EVALUATION/OUTCOMES
1. Maintains respiratory function
2. Communicates needs effectively
3. Remains free of complications of immobility
4. Performs own activities of daily living within ability
5. Expresses acceptance of limitations
6. Family and client participate in decisions and care

▼ EPILEPSY (SEIZURE DISORDERS)

Data Base
A. Etiology and pathophysiology
1. Abnormal discharge of electric impulses by the nerve cells in the brain from idiopathic or secondary causes resulting in the typical manifestation of seizures
2. Onset of idiopathic epilepsy generally before age 30
3. Other conditions associated with seizures include brain tumor, CVA, hypoglycemia, and head trauma
4. Types of seizures
   a. Partial seizures (seizures beginning locally)

(1) Simple: focal motor or sensory effect; no loss of consciousness

(2) Complex: cognitive, psychosensory, psychomotor, or affective effect; brief loss of consciousness

b. Generalized seizures (bilaterally symmetric and without local onset)

(1) Absence (petit mal): brief transient loss of consciousness with or without minor motor movements of eyes, head, or extremities

(2) Myoclonic: brief, transient rigidity or jerking of extremities, singly or in groups

(3) Tonic-clonic (grand mal): aura, loss of consciousness, rigidity followed by tonic and clonic movements, interruption of respirations, loss of bladder and bowel control

c. Status epilepticus: prolonged partial or generalized seizures without recovery between attacks; may completely exhaust the client and lead to death

B. Clinical findings (tonic-clonic seizures)

1. Subjective

a. Aura or warning sensation such as seeing spots or feeling dizzy often precedes a tonic-clonic seizure

b. Loss of consciousness during seizure

c. Lethargy often follows return to consciousness (postictal phase)

d. Dyspnea

2. Objective

a. Pupils become fixed and dilated

b. Often the client cries out as seizure begins or as air is exhaled forcefully

c. Tonic and clonic movement of the muscles

d. Incontinence

e. Abnormal EEG

C. Therapeutic interventions

1. Anticonvulsant therapy continued throughout life

a. Phenytoin sodium (Dilantin), carbamazepine (Tegretol), valproic acid (Depakene), mephenytoin (Mesantoin) and primidone (Mysoline) often used to control tonic-clonic seizures

b. Trimethadione, phensuximide, and ethosuximide to control absence seizures

c. Diazepam (Valium) given IV to treat status epilepticus

2. Sedatives (e.g., phenobarbital) used to reduce emotional stress

3. Neurosurgery is sometimes indicated if seizures are caused by tumors, abscesses, or vascular problems

Nursing Care of Clients with Epilepsy

A. DATA COLLECTION

1. History of type, frequency, and duration of seizures
2. History to identify precipitating factors
3. Sensations associated with the seizure that may constitute an aura
4. Detailed list of client's medications

B. ANALYSIS AND INTERPRETATION

Refer to General Nursing Diagnoses for Clients with Neuromusculoskeletal Systems Disorders for the following diagnoses: B, M 4, X, and CC

C. PLANNING/IMPLEMENTATION

1. Provide protection for the client during and after the seizure by maintaining and protecting from injury; nothing should be forced into a client's mouth since this may cause the tongue to occlude the airway or may loosen teeth
2. Help the client who can identify an aura to prepare and provide some protection before the seizure develops
3. Encourage the client to carry and wear a medical alert tag
4. Help the client plan a schedule that provides for adequate rest and a reduction of stress
5. Instruct the client to refrain from excessive use of alcohol, since it is contraindicated with the medications
6. Teach the client and family to observe the aura, initial point of seizure, type of seizure, level of consciousness, loss of bladder and bowel control, progression of seizure, and postictal condition
7. Encourage the client to express feelings about illness and the necessary changes in life-style and self-image
8. Assist the client and family to accept the diagnosis and develop some understanding of the disease process
9. Help the client understand that medication must be taken continuously for the remainder of life under continued medical supervision
10. Refer the client for job counseling as needed
11. Encourage the client and family to attend meetings of the local epilepsy association
12. Refer client to individual state laws regarding driving
13. Teach client about anticonvulsant therapy (see Nursing Care under Anticonvulsants in Pharmacology Related to Neuromusculoskeletal Systems Disorders)

D. EVALUATION/OUTCOMES

1. Remains free from injury
2. Experiences a reduction in frequency of seizures

3. Verbalizes willingness to follow lifelong medication regimen
4. Lists activities sponsored by the local epilepsy association

▼ MONONEURITIS, POLYNEURITIS, AND CARPAL TUNNEL SYNDROME

Data Base

A. Etiology and pathophysiology
   1. May involve only one nerve (mononeuritis) or several peripheral nerves (polyneuritis)
   2. Mononeuritis occurs when there is trauma to the trunk of a nerve, such as from pressure of a tumor, dislocation of a joint, or infection; the nerve involved near the area of injury becomes part of the scar tissue or callus of bone
   3. Polyneuritis occurs when there is a deficiency of B vitamins (e.g., alcoholism) and subsequent disturbances in metabolism of nerve tissue
   4. Carpal tunnel syndrome occurs when the median nerve becomes compressed as a result of inflammation and swelling of the synovial lining of tendon sheaths surrounding the nerve
B. Clinical findings
   1. Subjective
      a. Pain that increases after any body movement that stretches nerve involved
      b. Burning pain along the injured nerve in mononeuritis
      c. Diminished sensation, paresthesias
      d. With carpal tunnel syndrome, there may be difficulty grasping or holding small or heavy objects
   2. Objective
      a. Swelling over the affected nerve in mononeuritis
      b. Paresis or paralysis of the affected limb in polyneuritis
      c. With carpal tunnel syndrome, symptoms can be elicited by tapping the median nerve at the wrist (Tinel's sign)
      d. With carpal tunnel syndrome, there may be atrophy of the padded area below the thumb (thenal eminence)
C. Therapeutic interventions
   1. Mononeuritis
      a. Sympathetic nerve block
      b. Physical therapy
      c. Analgesics
      d. Steroid therapy
   2. Polyneuritis
      a. Thiamine replacement
      b. Bed rest
      c. Analgesics

3. Carpal tunnel syndrome
      a. Splinting and resting the wrist
      b. Steroid injections into the area
      c. Surgery to release the transverse carpal ligament to reduce compression of the median nerve

Nursing Care of Clients with Mononeuritis, Polyneuritis, and Carpal Tunnel Syndrome

A. DATA COLLECTION
   1. History of factors associated with neuritis such as trauma, alcoholism, diabetes mellitus, renal failure, peripheral vascular disease, AIDS, and certain medications or chemicals; history of factors associated with carpal tunnel syndrome such as prolonged flexion of the wrist, repetitive tasks using the hand and wrist, and arthritis
   2. Dietary history
   3. Status of extremities including color, peripheral pulses, motor strength, sensation, pain, and atrophy

B. ANALYSIS AND INTERPRETATION
Refer to General Nursing Diagnoses for Clients with Neuromusculoskeletal Systems Disorders for the following diagnoses: H 1, H 2, M 2, Q 1, Q 2, and R 3

C. PLANNING/IMPLEMENTATION
   1. Administer pain medications as ordered
   2. Teach client alternative methods of pain control including distraction, relaxation techniques, and imagery
   3. Provide emotional support for the client during the course of hospitalization
   4. Encourage diet rich in nutrient-dense foods such as fruits, vegetables, whole grains, and legumes to improve and maintain nutritional status and prevent possible drug-induced nutrient deficiencies
   5. Teach importance of avoiding injury to extremities because of altered sensation
   6. Instruct client regarding resting and splinting the wrist

D. EVALUATION/OUTCOMES
   1. Reports decreased severity of pain
   2. Consumes nutritionally balanced diet
   3. Avoids exposing extremities with diminished sensation to heat or other environmental hazards
   4. Demonstrates correct use of splints

▼ BELL'S PALSY (FACIAL PARALYSIS)

Data Base

A. Etiology and pathophysiology
   1. Paralysis that occurs on one side of the face as

a result of an inflamed seventh cranial (facial) nerve; generally lasts only 2 to 8 weeks but may last longer in older clients
2. Cause is unknown; may be linked to viral disease
3. Most common between ages 20 to 50 years

B. Clinical findings
1. Subjective
   a. Facial pain
   b. Difficulty eating
   c. Altered taste
2. Objective
   a. Distortion of face
   b. Difficulty with articulation
   c. Diminished blink reflex
   d. Increased lacrimation

C. Therapeutic interventions
1. Prednisone therapy
2. Heat, massage, and electric stimulation are used to maintain circulation and muscle tone
3. Prevention of corneal irritation with eyedrops and the use of a protective eye shield

Nursing Care of Clients with Bell's Palsy

A. DATA COLLECTION
1. Presence or absence of blink reflex and ability to close the eye
2. Facial pain
3. Nutritional intake and the ability to chew and swallow
4. Extent of facial paralysis

B. ANALYSIS AND INTERPRETATION
Refer to General Nursing Diagnoses for Clients with Neuromusculoskeletal Systems Disorders for the following diagnoses: C, M 3, P, Q 1, and DD 1

C. PLANNING/IMPLEMENTATION
1. Explain to the client that in most cases recovery occurs within 2 to 8 weeks
2. Teach client to prevent corneal irritation by using artificial tears, manually closing the eye, and applying an eye shield
3. Teach client to keep the face warm
4. Teach the client to massage the face gently and perform simple exercises such as blowing
5. Encourage ventilation of feelings because self-image may be affected
6. Support client's nutritional status by providing privacy and small, frequent feedings and encouraging the client to favor the unaffected side while eating

D. EVALUATION/OUTCOMES
1. Maintains corneal integrity
2. Improves facial muscle tone
3. Expresses a positive body image
4. Consumes a nutritionally adequate diet

▼ TRIGEMINAL NEURALGIA (TIC DOULOUREUX)

Data Base
A. Etiology and pathophysiology
1. Disorder of the fifth cranial (trigeminal) nerve characterized by excruciating knifelike pain along the branches of the nerve
2. Etiology unknown
3. Incidence higher in women of middle and older age

B. Clinical findings
1. Subjective
   a. Burning or knifelike pain lasting 1 to 15 minutes, usually over the lip or chin and in teeth
   b. Pain precipitated by stimulation of trigger zones during activities such as brushing hair and eating or when sitting in a cold draft
2. Objective
   a. Sudden closure of an eye
   b. Twitching of the mouth

C. Therapeutic interventions
1. Carbamazepine (Tegretol) to relieve and prevent pain
2. Antiepileptic drugs
3. Injection of alcohol into the ganglion to relieve pain for several months or years until nerve regenerates
4. Surgical intervention requiring intracranial approach
   a. Severing of the sensory root of the nerve, which will cause loss of all sensation in the area supplied by the nerve
   b. Microscopic relocation of arterial loop that may cause vascular compression of the trigeminal nerve
5. Percutaneous radio frequency trigeminal gangliolysis: thermal lesion created by current destroys nerve, providing permanent relief for most clients

Nursing Care of Clients with Trigeminal Neuralgia

A. DATA COLLECTION
1. Descriptions of pain
2. Specific factors that trigger attacks
3. How condition affects behavior such as avoiding eating, shaving, washing the face, or brushing the teeth because of fear of precipitating an attack

B. ANALYSIS AND INTERPRETATION
Refer to General Nursing Diagnoses for Clients with Neuromusculoskeletal Systems Disorders for the following diagnoses: L, M 2, P, and Q 1

C. PLANNING/IMPLEMENTATION

1. Instruct client to avoid factors that can trigger an attack
   a. Avoid foods that are too cold or too hot
   b. Chew foods on the unaffected side
   c. Use cotton pads to gently wash face
   d. Keep the room free of drafts
   e. Avoid jarring
2. Provide teaching to clients who have sensory loss as a result of treatment
   a. Inspection of the eye for foreign bodies, which the client will not be able to feel, should be done several times a day
   b. Warm normal saline irrigation of the affected eye two or three times a day is helpful in preventing a corneal infection
   c. Dental checkups every 6 months, since dental caries will not produce pain; avoid rubbing
3. Explain drugs, their side effects, and the need for continued medical supervision (see Anticonvulsants in Pharmacology Related to Neuromusculoskeletal Systems Disorders)

D. EVALUATION/OUTCOMES

1. Reports decreased severity of attacks
2. Consumes nutritionally balanced diet
3. Develops coping mechanisms to realistically deal with fear

▼ PARKINSON'S DISEASE (PARALYSIS AGITANS)

Data Base

A. Etiology and pathophysiology
1. Progressive disorder in which there is a destruction of nerve cells in the basal ganglia and substantia nigra of the brain, which results in a generalized degeneration of muscular function
2. Suspected causes include neuromuscular imbalance (dopamine and acetylcholine), unknown virus, cerebral vascular disease, and chemical or physical trauma

B. Clinical findings
1. Subjective
   a. Mild, diffuse, muscular pain
   b. Feelings of stiffness and rigidity, particularly of large joints
   c. Defects in judgment and emotional lability may be present, but intelligence is usually not impaired
   d. Depression
   e. Cognitive and memory deficits
2. Objective
   a. Increased difficulty in performing usual activities such as writing, dressing, and eating
   b. Generalized tremor commonly accompanied by "pill-rolling" movements of the thumb against the fingers; non-intention tremors usually reduced by purposeful movements
   c. Various disorders of locomotion (e.g., bent posture, difficulty in rising from a sitting position, shuffling propulsive gait, loss of rhythmic arm swing when walking, bradykinesia)
   d. Masklike facial expression with unblinking eyes
   e. Low-pitched, slow, poorly modulated, poorly articulated speech
   f. Drooling because of difficulty in swallowing saliva
   g. Various autonomic symptoms (e.g., lacrimation, constipation, incontinence, decreased sexual capacity, excessive perspiration)
   h. In the elderly, dementia, confusion, and psychosis

C. Therapeutic interventions
1. Medical regimen is palliative rather than curative
2. Levodopa may be utilized to alleviate dopamine deficiency and decrease dyskinesia and rigidity
3. Anticholinergic agents that counteract the action of acetylcholine in the central nervous system
4. Medications to relieve related symptoms (e.g., antispasmodics, antihistamines, analgesics, sedatives)
5. Amantadine HCl to reduce rigidity and tremor
6. MAO inhibitors such as Elepryl to inhibit dopamine breakdown
7. Physiotherapy to reduce rigidity of muscles and prevent contractures
8. Surgical intervention using alcohol, freezing (cryosurgery), electric cautery, ultrasound, etc. to destroy the globus pallidus (to relieve rigidity), and/or the thalamus (to relieve tremor) portions of the brain; less common

Nursing Care of Clients with Parkinson's Disease

A. DATA COLLECTION

1. History of onset and progression of symptoms
2. Observations of tremors, gait, facial expression, and bradykinesia
3. Nutritional status
4. Elimination status
5. Blood pressure in horizontal and vertical positions to identify postural hypotension

B. ANALYSIS AND INTERPRETATION

Refer to General Nursing Diagnoses for Clients with Neuromusculoskeletal Systems Disorders for the following diagnoses: B, C, D 1, D 2, F, G 1, K, M 3, N 1, N 2, O 1, O 2, O 3, P, R 2, R 3, T, U 1, X, AA, and DD 1

C. PLANNING/IMPLEMENTATION

1. Provide a safe environment
2. Teach the client or family to cut food into small bite-sized pieces or alter the consistency to prevent choking
3. Provide small, frequent meals, prepared so they can be easily masticated
4. Encourage an adequate intake of roughage and fluids to avoid constipation
5. Teach the client activities to limit postural deformities (e.g., use firm mattress without a pillow, periodically lie prone, keep head and neck as erect as possible, consciously think about posture when walking)
6. Teach the client activities to maintain gait as normal as possible; utilize cane or walker if necessary
7. Teach and encourage daily physical therapy to limit rigidity and prevent contractures (e.g., warms baths, passive and active exercises)
8. Attempt to administer care when the client is able to accept it emotionally, and avoid rushing the client since he or she is unable to function under pressure
9. Encourage the client to continue taking medications even though results may be minimal
10. Advise client to report side effects to physician (see Antiparkinson Agents in Pharmacology Related to Neuromusculoskeletal Systems Disorders)
11. Encourage diet rich in nutrient-dense foods such as fruits, vegetables, whole grains, and legumes to improve and maintain nutritional status and prevent possible drug-induced nutrient deficiencies
12. Teach clients taking levodopa to limit intake of foods high in vitamin B_6, such as pork, glandular meats, lamb, veal, legumes, potatoes, oatmeal, wheat germ, and bananas
13. Assist client in setting achievable goals to improve self-esteem
14. Suction when necessary to maintain an adequate airway (usually advanced stages)

D. EVALUATION/OUTCOMES

1. Participates in daily exercise program
2. Complies with prescribed medical therapy
3. Establishes regular pattern of bowel elimination
4. Maintains ideal body weight
5. Ambulates without falling
6. Expresses a positive self-image
7. Remains oriented to person, place, and time

▼ MULTIPLE SCLEROSIS (DISSEMINATED SCLEROSIS)

Data Base

A. Etiology and pathophysiology
  1. Chronic, debilitating, progressive disease with periods of remission and exacerbation characterized by randomly scattered patches of demyelination in the brainstem, cerebrum, cerebellum, and spinal cord
  2. Cause unknown; viral and immunologic causes have been implicated
  3. Onset in early adult life (20 to 40 years)
  4. Fatigue, stress, and heat tend to increase symptoms
B. Clinical findings
  1. Subjective
     a. Paresthesia
     b. Altered position sense
     c. Dysphagia
     d. Ataxia
     e. Weakness
     f. Diplopia
     g. Blurred vision
     h. Inappropriate emotional affect (euphoria occurs in later stages)
  2. Objective
     a. Nystagmus
     b. Blindness
     c. Intention tremors
     d. Slurred or scanning speech
     e. Spastic paralysis and gait
     f. Impaired bowel function
     g. Impaired bladder function
     h. Impotence
     i. Cognitive loss (a late sign)
     j. Increased deep tendon reflexes
     k. Pallor of optic discs evident on examination with ophthalmoscope
     l. Increased gamma globulin levels in the CSF
C. Therapeutic interventions
  1. Generally palliative
  2. Corticosteroids or ACTH
  3. Baclofen is used to control spasticity
  4. Interferon beta-1b, recombinant (Betaseron)
  5. Physiotherapy, rehabilitation, and psychotherapy
  6. Nerve blocks may be used for severe spasticity
  7. Immunosuppressive drugs are being investigated as treatment

Nursing Care of Clients with Multiple Sclerosis

A. DATA COLLECTION

1. History of onset and progression of motor and sensory loss
2. Factors that intensify symptoms

3. Neurologic status (see Neurologic Assessment in Procedures Related to Neuromusculoskeletal Systems Disorders)

B. ANALYSIS AND INTERPRETATION

Refer to General Nursing Diagnoses for Clients with Neuromusculoskeletal Systems Disorders for the following diagnoses: B, C, D 1, G 1, G 2, H 1, I 1, I 2, I 3, I 4, K, M 2, M 3, N 1, N 2, O 1, O 3, R 1, R 2, R 3, T, U 1, V 1, V 2, W, X, Y, AA, CC, and DD 1

C. PLANNING/IMPLEMENTATION

1. Incorporate frequent rest periods
2. Avoid hot baths, which can increase symptoms
3. Teach the client to use assistive devices when carrying out activities of daily living
4. Assist the family to understand why the client should be permitted and encouraged to be active
5. Assist the client and family to plan and implement a bowel and bladder regimen
6. Explain the disease process to both the client and the family in understandable terms
7. Do not encourage false hopes during periods of remission
8. Spend time listening to both the client and the family, and encourage them to ventilate feelings
9. Attempt to refer the client and family to the National Multiple Sclerosis Society
10. Encourage the client to seek counseling and rehabilitation
11. Explain to the client and family that mood swings and emotional alterations are part of the disease process
12. Help the client reestablish a realistic self-image
13. Teach the client to compensate for problems with gait (walk with feet farther apart to broaden base of support, use low-heeled shoes), and provide assistive devices when necessary (tripod cane, walker, wheelchair)
14. Teach the client to compensate for loss of sensation by using a thermometer to test water temperature, avoiding constricting stockings, using protective clothing in cold weather, changing position frequently
15. Teach the client to compensate for difficulty in swallowing by taking small bites, chewing well, using a straw with liquids, using foods of more solid consistency
16. Provide a diet rich in nutrient-dense foods such as fruits, vegetables, whole grains, and legumes to improve and maintain nutritional status and compensate for nutrient interactions of corticosteroid medications
17. Provide care to prevent decubiti and contractures

a. Provide special skin care to prevent the formation of decubiti; turn frequently
b. Provide special attention to joints and attempt to prevent dysfunctional contractures; provide range-of-motion exercises; splints

D. EVALUATION/OUTCOMES

1. Establishes exercise/activity and rest/sleep routine that avoids fatigue
2. Remains free from injury
3. Maintains bowel control
4. Maintains bladder control
5. Establishes satisfying sexual relationship
6. Exerts control over decisions about care
7. Maintains effective communication with others

▼ MYASTHENIA GRAVIS

Data Base

A. Etiology and pathophysiology
1. Neuromuscular disorder in which there is a disturbance in the transmission of impulses at the myoneural junction resulting in profound weakness
2. Dysfunction thought to be caused by a reduced number of acetylcholine receptors (AChR) and the normal folded pattern of the postsynaptic membrane of the muscle end-plate is altered
3. Findings support the theory that it is caused by an autoimmune process; it is believed that complement and antibodies to AChR cause accelerated destruction and blockade of the AChR
4. Highest incidence in young adult females
5. Myasthenic crisis refers to the sudden inability to swallow or maintain respirations due to weakness of the muscles of respiration

B. Clinical findings
1. Subjective
   a. Extreme muscle weakness, which becomes progressively worse as the muscle is used, but disappears with rest
   b. Dysphagia (difficulty chewing and swallowing)
   c. Diplopia
   d. Dysarthria (difficulty speaking)
   e. Dyspnea
2. Objective
   a. Ptosis of the eyelid
   b. Weak voice (dysphonia)
   c. Myasthenic smile (snarling, nasal smile)
   d. Strabismus
   e. Diagnostic measures include administration of neostigmine (Prostigmin) subcutaneous or IV administration of edrophonium (Ten-

silon) to provide spontaneous relief of symptoms; edrophonium is also used to distinguish myasthenic crisis from cholinergic crisis (toxic effects of excessive neostigmine)

C. Therapeutic interventions
1. Specific medications that block the action of cholinesterase at the myoneural junction (see Cholinesterase Inhibitors in Pharmacology Related to Neuromusculoskeletal Systems Disorders)
   a. Neostigmine (Prostigmin)
   b. Pyridostigmine bromide (Mestinon)
   c. Ambenonium chloride (Mytelase)
2. X-ray therapy or surgical removal of the thymus may cause partial remission
3. Corticosteroids or ACTH
4. Tracheostomy with mechanical ventilation is often necessary in myasthenic crisis
5. Plasma exchange to temporarily reduce the titer of circulating antibodies

Nursing Care of Clients with Myasthenia Gravis

A. DATA COLLECTION
1. History of onset and progression of motor and sensory loss
2. Factors that intensify symptoms
3. Neurologic status (see Neurologic Assessment in Procedures Related to Neuromusculoskeletal Systems Disorders)

B. ANALYSIS AND INTERPRETATION
Refer to General Nursing Diagnoses for Clients with Neuromusculoskeletal Systems Disorders for the following diagnoses: B, E, K, M 3, N 1, N 2, O 3, P, R 1, T, U 1, V 1, W, X, Y, AA, and DD 1

C. PLANNING/IMPLEMENTATION
1. Administer medications on strict time schedule to prevent onset of symptoms; instruct the client and family to do the same
2. Observe for signs of dyspnea, dysphagia, and dysarthria, which may indicate myasthenic crisis
3. Have an emergency tracheostomy set at bedside
4. Plan activity to avoid fatigue based on the individual's tolerance
5. Instruct the client to avoid people with upper respiratory tract infections, since pneumonia may develop as a result of fatigued respiratory muscles
6. Encourage the client to carry a medical alert card or identification stating condition
7. Do not administer morphine to clients receiving anticholinesterases, since these drugs potentiate the effects of morphine and may cause respiratory depression
8. Provide emotional support and close contact with the client to allay anxiety
9. Administer tube feedings when necessary if the client has difficulty swallowing so that aspiration will not occur
10. Administer artificial tears to keep cornea moist if client has difficulty closing eyes
11. Encourage client and family to participate in planning care
12. Ensure that client understands the signs and symptoms of myasthenic and cholinergic crises
13. Refer client and family to the Myasthenia Gravis Foundation and local self-help groups
14. In severe instances anticipate all needs, since the client is too weak to turn, drink, or even request assistance
15. Maintain a patent airway; suction as necessary; provide tracheostomy care; maintain mechanical ventilation as ordered

D. EVALUATION/OUTCOMES
1. Completes activities of daily living without fatigue
2. Maintains effective respiratory function
3. Adheres to strict schedule of medications
4. Identifies signs and symptoms of crises
5. Maintains ideal body weight
6. Learns of community resources

▼ GUILLAIN-BARRÉ SYNDROME (POLYRADICULONEURITIS)

Data Base
A. Etiology and pathophysiology
1. Cause unknown; thought to be linked to immunologic status; often follows respiratory or gastrointestinal infection
2. Changes in the motor cells of the spinal cord and medulla with areas of demyelination
3. After initial and plateau periods, recovery may take up to a year; while most recover, some experience residual deficits or die of complications
B. Clinical findings
1. Subjective
   a. Generalized weakness
   b. Paresthesia
   c. Diplopia
2. Objective
   a. Paralysis begins in lower extremities; ascends within the body, usually 24 to 72 hours
   b. Respiratory paralysis
   c. Hypertension, tachycardia, and low-grade fever
   d. Incontinence
C. Therapeutic interventions
1. Steroids

2. Plasmapheresis
3. Support of vital functions

Nursing Care of Clients with Guillain-Barré Syndrome

A. DATA COLLECTION

1. Respiratory function including airway, respiratory rate, vital capacity, breath sounds, and arterial blood gases
2. Neurologic status (see Neurologic Assessment in Procedures Related to Neuromusculoskeletal Systems Disorders)
3. History of any recent illness (particularly viral infections)
4. Onset and progression of symptoms

B. ANALYSIS AND INTERPRETATION

Refer to General Nursing Diagnoses for Clients with Neuromusculoskeletal Systems Disorders for the following diagnoses: B, E, K, M 3, O 3, P, R 1, T, U 1, V 1, W, X, Y, and DD 1

C. PLANNING/IMPLEMENTATION

1. Monitor vital signs, vital capacity, breath sounds, and arterial blood gases
2. Keep airway and tracheostomy set at the bedside
3. Suction, provide fluid replacement therapy, and monitor functioning of the respirator as required
4. Provide emotional support to the client and family because of the severity and lengthy convalescent period
5. Prevent complications of immobility
   a. Skin care
   b. Range-of-motion exercises
   c. Position changes
   d. Coughing and deep breathing
   e. Antiembolism stockings
6. Provide explanations of disease process and care
7. Refer client and family to the Guillain-Barré Foundation for additional information and community resources

D. EVALUATION/OUTCOMES

1. Maintains effective respiratory function
2. Participates in prescribed therapy (physical therapy, occupational therapy, speech therapy)
3. Performs procedures to prevent complications
4. Performs activities of daily living
5. Focuses on abilities rather than disabilities
6. Discusses feelings with family members or other health-team members

▼ AMYOTROPHIC LATERAL SCLEROSIS (ALS)

Data Base

A. Etiology and pathophysiology
   1. Cause unknown
   2. Progressive degenerative process involving the spinal, corticobulbar, and lower motor neurons, with subsequent atrophic and spastic changes in the cranial as well as the spinal nerves
   3. Occurs more frequently in men than in women in the fourth and fifth decades of life
B. Clinical findings
   1. Subjective
      a. Muscular weakness
      b. Malaise and fatigue
   2. Objective
      a. Irregular spasmodic twitching in small muscle groups (fasciculations)
      b. Atrophy
      c. Spasticity
      d. Difficulty in chewing, swallowing, speaking
      e. Outbursts of laughter or crying
C. Therapeutic interventions
   1. Physiotherapy may be helpful in relieving spasticity
   2. Support respiratory functions

Nursing Care of Clients with Amyotrophic Lateral Sclerosis

A. DATA COLLECTION

1. History of onset and progression of symptoms
2. Neurologic status (see Neurologic Assessment in Procedures Related to Neuromusculoskeletal Systems Disorders)
3. Respiratory status including rate, depth, and effort

B. ANALYSIS AND INTERPRETATION

Refer to General Nursing Diagnoses for Clients with Neuromusculoskeletal Systems Disorders for the following diagnoses: B, C, E, G 1, G 2, H 1, I 1, I 2, I 3, K, M 3, N 1, N 2, O 1, O 3, R 1, T, U 1, W, X, Y, AA, and DD 1

C. PLANNING/IMPLEMENTATION

1. Encourage client to remain active as long as possible, employing supportive devices as needed
2. Encourage range-of-motion exercises
3. Monitor swallowing ability; positioning and altered consistency of diet help prevent aspiration
4. Provide alternate means of communication as speech declines
5. Allow client to discuss feelings about artificial

life support while still able to speak

6. Monitor respiratory function; increased fluids, positioning, chest physiotherapy, coughing and deep breathing exercises, and suctioning help prevent complications
7. Support natural defense mechanisms; encourage a diet consisting of high nutrient-dense foods, especially those rich in the immune-stimulating nutrients selenium and vitamins A, C, and E
8. Teach the avoidance of situations that may contribute to infection
9. Provide emotional support for the client and family
10. Refer client and family to ALS Association

D. EVALUATION/OUTCOMES
1. Utilizes supportive equipment to maintain mobility
2. Develops interests consistent with abilities
3. Discusses decisions about health care options with family and other health team members
4. Maintains communication as ability to speak declines
5. Performs breathing exercises as prescribed
6. Maintains effective respiratory function

▼ HUNTINGTON'S CHOREA

Data Base

A. Etiology and pathophysiology
1. Inherited disorder, considered autosomal dominant
2. Progressive atrophy of the basal ganglia and some portions of the cerebral cortex
3. Appears during the middle adult years

B. Clinical findings
1. Subjective
   a. Memory loss
   b. Disorientation
   c. Eventual dementia
2. Objective
   a. Uncontrolled jerky movements of the extremities, trunk, face, or tongue
   b. Disorganized gait
   c. Uncontrolled periods of anger
   d. Hesitant or explosive patterns of speech
   e. Grimacing facial movements
   f. Impaired chewing and swallowing
   g. Incontinence

C. Therapeutic interventions
1. Control of jerky movements with phenothiazines, butyrophenones, and thioxanthenes
2. Reserpine may be used to decrease presynaptic dopamine and tetrabenzine to reduce dopaminergic transmission
3. Symptoms are treated as they occur

Nursing Care of Clients with Huntington's Chorea

A. DATA COLLECTION
1. Neurologic status (see Neurologic Assessment in Procedures Related to Neuromusculoskeletal Systems Disorders), noting uncontrolled movements and cognitive ability
2. Family history of Huntington's chorea

B. ANALYSIS AND INTERPRETATION
Refer to General Nursing Diagnoses for Clients with Neuromusculoskeletal Systems Disorders for the following diagnoses: B, C, D 1, D 2, F, K, M 1, M 3, N 1, N 2, O 2, O 3, P, R 1, T, U 1, U 2, W, X, Y, AA, CC, and DD 1

C. PLANNING/IMPLEMENTATION
1. Provide emotional support for client and family
2. Allow client and family to express feelings about progressive deterioration and ultimate death
3. Encourage family members to seek genetic counseling
4. Modify environment to increase safety
5. Assess ability to swallow; provide nutritional support as needed
6. Encourage client to remain as active as possible
7. Provide respiratory support based on changing needs of client (airway, suctioning, oxygenation)
8. Utilize community agencies to provide situational support

D. EVALUATION/OUTCOMES
1. Remains free from complications of immobility
2. Modifies activities to prevent injury
3. Verbalizes feelings with family members and other members of the health team
4. Encourages family members to seek genetic counseling

▼ RHEUMATOID ARTHRITIS

Data Base

A. Etiology and pathophysiology
1. Chronic disease characterized by inflammatory changes in the body's connective tissue, particularly areas that have a cavity and easily moving surfaces
2. Cause unknown, although theories include autoimmunity, heredity, and psychophysiologic factors
3. Exacerbations are linked to physical and emotional stress

B. Clinical findings
1. Subjective
   a. Fatigue
   b. Malaise
   c. Joint pain

d. Stiffness after periods of inactivity, particularly in the morning

e. Paresthesia

f. Anorexia

2. Objective

a. Anemia

b. Weight loss

c. Joint inflammation and deformity

d. Subcutaneous nodules

e. Elevated sedimentation rate

f. Low-grade fever

g. Presence of rheumatoid factors in serum identified by latex fixation test

h. Positive C-reactive protein and antinuclear antibody (ANA) tests

C. Therapeutic interventions

1. Corticosteroids, antiinflammatories, analgesics, immunosuppressive drugs; aspirin is drug of choice followed by the addition of nonsteroidal antiinflammatory drugs and then gold or penicillamine, an oral chelating agent; corticosteroids are reserved for acute inflammation, if possible

2. Physiotherapy to minimize deformities

3. Surgical intervention to remove severely damaged joints (e.g., hip replacement)

4. Application of heat or cold; paraffin dips of affected extremity for relief of joint pain by providing uniform heat

5. Plasmapheresis may be used when the disease is advanced

Nursing Care of Clients with Rheumatoid Arthritis

A. DATA COLLECTION

1. History of onset and progression of symptoms, noting degree to which pain interferes with normal activities

2. Family history of rheumatoid arthritis

3. General physical health

4. Coping skills

B. ANALYSIS AND INTERPRETATION

Refer to General Nursing Diagnoses for Clients with Neuromusculoskeletal Systems Disorders for the following diagnoses: C, H 2, K, L, M 3, Q 1, R 3, U 3, W, X, and Y

C. PLANNING/IMPLEMENTATION

1. Administer analgesics and other medications as ordered

2. Teach the client to take medications as ordered and observe for aspirin toxicity (tinnitus, bleeding) and other adverse effects of medications

3. Apply heat and cold as ordered; heat paraffin to 52° to 54° C

4. Promote rest and position to ease joint pains

5. Provide for range-of-motion exercises up to the point of pain, recognizing that some discomfort is always present

6. Emphasize the need to remain active, but incorporate rest periods to avoid fatigue

7. Encourage the client to verbalize feelings

8. Help set realistic goals, focusing on strengths

9. Encourage use of supportive devices to help client conserve energy and maintain independence

10. Provide care for the client following joint replacement (see Nursing Care of Clients with Fractured Hips)

11. Encourage diet rich in nutrient-dense foods such as fruits, vegetables, whole grains, and legumes to improve and maintain nutritional status and compensate for nutrient interactions of corticosteroid and other treatment medications

D. EVALUATION/OUTCOMES

1. Experiences a reduction in pain

2. Completes activities of daily living using supportive devices as needed

3. Accepts life-style consistent with abilities

4. Maintains or improves range of motion of involved joints

▼ OSTEOARTHRITIS (DEGENERATIVE JOINT DISEASE)

Data Base

A. Etiology and pathophysiology

1. Etiology relates to wear and tear of joints; predisposing factors include obesity, aging, and joint trauma

2. A degeneration and atrophy of the cartilages and calcification of the ligaments

3. Primarily affects weight-bearing joints, spine, and hands

B. Clinical findings

1. Subjective

a. Pain after exercise

b. Stiffness of joints

2. Objective

a. Heberden's and Bouchard's nodes symmetrically occurring on fingers (bony hypertrophy)

b. Decreased range of motion

c. Crepitus when joint is moved

C. Therapeutic interventions

1. Weight reduction in instances of obesity

2. Local heat to affected joints

3. Medications to reduce symptoms, such as analgesics, antiinflammatory agents, and steroids

4. Exercise of affected extremities

5. Surgical intervention
   a. Synovectomy: removal of the enlarged synovial membrane before bone and cartilage destruction occurs
   b. Arthrodesis: fusion of a joint performed when the joint surfaces are severely damaged; this leaves the client with no range of motion of the affected joint
   c. Reconstructive surgery: replacement of a badly damaged joint with a prosthetic device (see Fractures of the Hips)

Nursing Care of Clients with Osteoarthritis
A. DATA COLLECTION
1. History for risk factors such as obesity, trauma, athletic involvement, and occupation
2. Joints, noting evidence of deformities, inflammation, and muscle atrophy
3. Extent of range of motion of involved joints

B. ANALYSIS AND INTERPRETATION
Refer to General Nursing Diagnoses for Clients with Neuromusculoskeletal Systems Disorders for the following diagnoses: C, H 2, K, L, M 3, Q 1, R 3, U 3, W, X, and Y

C. PLANNING/IMPLEMENTATION
1. Assist client in activities that require using affected joints; allow for rest periods
2. Maintain functional alignment of joints
3. Attempt to relieve the client's discomfort by the use of medications or the application of heat as ordered
4. Allow client ample time to verbalize feelings regarding limited motion and changes in lifestyle
5. Support client through weight loss program if indicated
6. Encourage client to follow physical therapist's instruction regarding regular exercise program and use of supportive devices
7. Provide care for the client requiring joint replacement (see Nursing Care of Clients with Fractures of the Hips)
8. Refer client and family to the Arthritis Foundation

D. EVALUATION/OUTCOMES
1. Reports a reduction in pain
2. Completes activities of daily living using supportive devices as needed
3. Develops life-style consistent with limitations
4. Follows daily program of prescribed exercise
5. Complies with weight-loss program

▼ GOUTY ARTHRITIS (GOUT)

Data Base
A. Etiology and pathophysiology

1. Disorder in purine metabolism that leads to high levels of uric acid in the blood and the deposition of uric acid crystals (tophi) in tissues, especially joints; followed by an inflammatory response
2. Incidence highest in males; a familial tendency has been demonstrated
3. Renal urate lithiasis (kidney stones) may result from precipitation of uric acid in the presence of a low urinary pH

B. Clinical findings
1. Subjective
   a. Sudden onset of asymmetric joint pain usually in the metatarsophalangeal joint of the great toe
   b. Local pruritus
   c. Malaise
   d. Headache
   e. Anorexia
2. Objective
   a. Elevated serum uric acid (greater than 7 mg/dl)
   b. Signs of inflammation of joint including swelling, heat, and redness
   c. Tophi in outer ear, hands, and feet

C. Therapeutic interventions
1. Administration of antiinflammatory and uricosuric (antigout) agents (see Pharmacology Related to the Neuromusculoskeletal Systems Disorders)
2. Alkaline-ash diet to increase the pH of urine to discourage precipitation of uric acid and enhance the action of drugs such as probenicid
3. Elimination of foods high in purines such as organ meats and shellfish
4. Weight loss is encouraged if indicated

Nursing Care of Clients with Gouty Arthritis
A. DATA COLLECTION
1. History of onset and progression of symptoms
2. Factors from history that contribute to hyperuricemia including diet, use of thiazide diuretics, conditions such as multiple myeloma
3. Involved joints for presence of tophi and signs of inflammation
4. Renal function to determine if affected by hyperuricemia

B. ANALYSIS AND INTERPRETATION
Refer to General Nursing Diagnoses for Clients with Neuromusculoskeletal Systems Disorders for the following diagnoses: L, M 3, Q 1, R 3, T, U 3, X, and Y

C. PLANNING/IMPLEMENTATION
1. Instruct the client to rest the joint during attacks

2. Use a bed cradle during the acute phase to keep pressure of sheets off joints
3. Administer nonsteroidal antiinflammatory drugs such as ibuprofen (Motrin), or indomethacin (Indocid) with antacids or milk to help prevent peptic ulcers; observe therapeutic response (see Nonsteroidal Antiinflammatory Drugs [NSAIDs] in Pharmacology Related to Neuromusculoskeletal Systems Disorders)
4. Administer prescribed antigout agents; monitor uric acid level and CBC (see Antigout Agents in Pharmacology Related to Neuromusculoskeletal Systems Disorders)
5. Carefully align joints so they are slightly flexed during acute stage; encourage regular exercise, which is important for long-term management
6. Increase fluid intake to 2000 to 3000 ml daily to prevent formation of calculi
7. Instruct client to avoid high-purine foods such as organ meats, anchovies, sardines, and shellfish; encourage diet rich in nutrient-dense foods of the fruit, vegetable, and whole-grain groups, as well as milk, cheese, and eggs; teach Food Guide Pyramid and importance of preventing drug-induced nutrient deficiencies with improved diet
8. Provide education regarding drug therapy and avoidance of excess alcohol intake

D. **EVALUATION/OUTCOMES**
1. Reports a reduction in pain
2. Engages in a regular program of exercise
3. Identifies side effects of medications
4. Prevents the development of urolithiasis

▼ OSTEOMYELITIS

Data Base

A. Etiology and pathophysiology
1. Occurs as the result of bacterial invasion of the bone most commonly by *Staphylococcus aureus*; other organisms include *Pseudomonas aeruginosa* and *Escherichia coli*
2. Infection of the bone results from trauma or systemic infection and involves the entire bone and surrounding soft tissue

B. Clinical findings
1. Subjective
   a. Pain and tenderness of the bone
   b. Malaise
   c. Difficulty in weight bearing
2. Objective
   a. Fever

b. Swelling and erythema over the affected bone
c. Signs of sepsis
d. Positive culture from bone biopsy
e. Nuclear bone scan demonstrates increased uptake of the isotope

C. Therapeutic interventions
1. Antibiotic therapy
2. Incision and drainage of a bone abscess
3. Sequestrectomy: surgical removal of the dead, infected bone and cartilage

Nursing Care of Clients with Osteomyelitis

A. **DATA COLLECTION**
1. History of trauma or infections
2. Involved tissue for signs of inflammation
3. Onset and characteristics of pain
4. Vital signs for baseline data

B. **ANALYSIS AND INTERPRETATION**
Refer to General Nursing Diagnoses for Clients with Neuromusculoskeletal Systems Disorders for the following diagnoses: C, L, M 3, Q 1, and R 4

C. **PLANNING/IMPLEMENTATION**
1. Review results of culture and white blood cell count reports
2. Monitor neurovascular status of involved extremity
3. Administer pain medications and antibiotics as ordered
4. Use surgical aseptic technique when changing dressings
5. Maintain functional body alignment and promote comfort
6. Use room deodorizer if a foul odor is apparent
7. Allow the client ample time to express feelings about long-term confinement
8. Encourage nutrient-dense diet to compensate for antibiotic impact on nutritional status (see Pharmacology Related to Infection)

D. **EVALUATION/OUTCOMES**
1. Reports a reduction in pain
2. Participates in self-care
3. Utilizes surgical asepsis when changing own dressing
4. Remains free from additional infections
5. Remains free from injury

▼ OSTEOGENIC SARCOMA

Data Base

A. Etiology and pathophysiology
1. Malignant bone tumor that usually begins in the long bones, especially around the knee
2. Metastasis to the lungs common and occurs early; prognosis is poor

3. Highest incidence between 20 and 30 years of age

B. Clinical findings
   1. Subjective
      a. Pain
      b. Limited motion
      c. Malaise
   2. Objective
      a. Local swelling
      b. Weight loss
      c. Anemia
      d. Elevated serum alkaline phosphatase
      e. Fever
      f. Microscopic evaluation of biopsy reveals neoplastic cells
C. Therapeutic interventions
   1. Amputation of limb or resection of tumor with reconstruction
   2. Chemotherapy
   3. Radiation

Nursing Care of Clients with Osteogenic Sarcoma

A. DATA COLLECTION

1. Description of onset and progression of symptoms
2. Characteristics of pain
3. Presence of bony mass, noting swelling, redness, and tenderness
4. Strength and weaknesses of support system and home environment

B. ANALYSIS AND INTERPRETATION

Refer to General Nursing Diagnoses for Clients with Neuromusculoskeletal Systems Disorders for the following diagnoses: C, G 1, K, L, M 3, Q 1, Q 2, R 3, U 3, X, and Y

C. PLANNING/IMPLEMENTATION

1. Maintain safe environment to decrease risk of pathologic fractures
2. Help client control pain by relaxation, imagery, distraction, and use of medication
3. Be available for the client and family to discuss fears, concerns, and treatment
4. Support natural defense mechanisms; encourage a diet of nutrient-dense foods, especially those rich in the immune-stimulating nutrients selenium and vitamins A, C, and E, as well as protein
5. Administer special nursing care following surgery (see Amputation)
6. Provide care for the client receiving radiation or chemotherapy (see Nursing Care of Clients with Neoplastic Disorders Receiving Either Chemotherapy or Radiation Therapy)
7. Refer client and family to cancer support groups

D. EVALUATION/OUTCOMES

1. Reports reduction in pain
2. Remains free from injury
3. Participates in self-care activities
4. Verbalizes fears with family members and health care providers

▼ MULTIPLE MYELOMA

Data Base

A. Etiology and pathophysiology
   1. Cause unknown, although genetic and viral factors are being closely considered
   2. Malignant overgrowth of plasma cells and malignant tumor growth in bone and bone marrow
   3. Occurs primarily in middle-aged men
B. Clinical findings
   1. Subjective
      a. Bone pain
      b. Progressive weakness
      c. Low back pain
   2. Objective
      a. Anemia
      b. Cachexia
      c. Idiopathic bone fractures
      d. Macroglobulinemia
      e. Platelet deficiency with resultant bleeding tendency
      f. Punched-out appearance of the bones at x-ray examination
      g. Presence of Bence-Jones protein in urine
      h. Hypercalcemia
      i. Hyperuricemia
C. Therapeutic interventions
   1. Chemotherapeutic agents, especially melphalan
   2. Radiation therapy
   3. Analgesics and narcotics for pain
   4. Supportive therapy such as transfusions as indicated

Nursing Care of Clients with Multiple Myeloma

A. DATA COLLECTION

1. Description of onset and progression of symptoms
2. Characteristics of pain
3. Neurovascular status of extremities if spine is involved
4. Renal function; precipitation of protein, calcium, and uric acid may cause renal damage

B. ANALYSIS AND INTERPRETATION

Refer to General Nursing Diagnoses for Clients with Neuromusculoskeletal Systems Disorders for the following diagnoses: C, G 1, H 2, I 1, K, L, M 3, N 2, O 3, Q 1, Q 2, R 1, T, U 3, W, X, and Y

C. PLANNING/IMPLEMENTATION

1. Allow the client ample time to express feelings about the disease and related therapies
2. Allow the client to participate in planning nursing care to aid in self-esteem and promote a feeling of self-control
3. Help the client control pain by relaxation, imagery, distraction, and use of analgesics
4. Carefully ambulate the client to prevent pneumonia and reduce pathologic fractures
5. Increase fluid intake to reduce renal damage
6. Provide care for the client receiving radiation or chemotherapy (see Nursing Care of Clients with Neoplastic Disorders Receiving Either Chemotherapy or Radiation Therapy)
7. Support natural defense mechanisms; encourage diet high in nutrient-dense foods, especially those rich in the immune-stimulating nutrients selenium and vitamins A, C, and E, as well as protein

D. EVALUATION/OUTCOMES

1. Reports decrease in pain
2. Maintains integrity of the skeletal system
3. Participates in self-care activities
4. Adheres to treatment regimen
5. Identifies side-effects of therapy
6. Remains free from renal damage

▼ INTRACTABLE PAIN

Data Base

A. Etiology and pathophysiology
   1. Pain not relieved by conventional treatment
   2. Causes include cancer, neuralgia, tic douloureux, and ischemia
B. Clinical findings
   1. Subjective
      a. Pain
      b. Fatigue
      c. Irritability or withdrawal
   2. Objective
      a. Evidence of a related disease process
      b. Pallor
C. Therapeutic interventions
   1. Surgical intervention
      a. Rhizotomy: posterior spinal nerve root is resected between the ganglion and the cord, resulting in permanent loss of sensation; the anterior root may be cut to alleviate painful muscle spasm
      b. Cordotomy: to alleviate intractable pain in the trunk or lower extremities; the transmission of pain and temperature sensation is interrupted by creation of a lesion in the ascending tracts, percutaneously using an electrode or surgically via laminectomy

   c. Sympathectomy: to control pain of vascular disturbances and phantom limb pain
   2. Acupuncture therapy
   3. Biofeedback to help the client develop control over anxiety and physiologic function
   4. Electronic stimulation may alter the electric potential of the nerve to prevent complete depolarization or block the transmission of pain sensations to the brain
      a. Transcutaneous Electric Nerve Stimulation (TENS): electrodes applied over the painful area or along the nerve pathway
      b. Dorsal column stimulator and peripheral nerve implant: involve direct attachment of an electrode to the sensory nerve; a transmitter attached to the electrode is carried by the client so electric stimulation can be administered as needed
   5. Patient-controlled analgesia (PCA): infusion pump is programmed for dose and time interval, allowing client to control administration without overdose; may be intravenous, subcutaneous, or epidural

Nursing Care of Clients with Intractable Pain

A. DATA COLLECTION

1. Characteristics of pain: location, type, intensity, and influencing factors
2. Baseline vital signs; acute pain is more likely to increase vital signs than is chronic pain
3. Methods of pain control the client has tried and extent of effectiveness

B. ANALYSIS AND INTERPRETATION

Refer to General Nursing Diagnoses for Clients with Neuromusculoskeletal Systems Disorders for the following diagnoses: C, K, L, Q 1, Q 2, R 4, T, and U 1

C. PLANNING/IMPLEMENTATION

1. Eliminate factors from the environment that seem to intensify pain
2. Support the client and family, since the client frequently will withdraw
3. Educate the client and family about treatments available and the potential side effects
4. Teach the client to utilize relaxation, imagery, or self-hypnosis in conjunction with other treatment
5. Instruct the client utilizing TENS to:
   a. Cleanse skin to decrease irritation and improve conduction
   b. Place electrodes over site using conducting gel
   c. Rotate electrode placement to avoid skin irritation
   d. Increase amplitude until sensation is experienced in underlying tissue
   e. Maintain log of use and effectiveness

6. Utilize other methods of cutaneous stimulation as ordered, such as pressure, massage, heat, and cold
7. Provide postoperative care
   a. Nursing care for a client undergoing a cordotomy or rhizotomy or implantation of a dorsal column stimulator (see Intervertebral Disc Disease [Herniated Nucleus Pulposus])
   b. Neurologically assess the extremities for movement, sensation, and skin temperature
   c. Carefully inspect skin, since the client will not feel pain of ulceration
   d. Instruct the client to avoid extreme environmental conditions and the use of heating pads, and to check the temperature of bath water, since temperature sensitivity is absent

D. EVALUATION/OUTCOMES
1. Reports a reduction in pain
2. Participates in self-care activities
3. Utilizes pain reduction techniques
4. Identifies side effects of analgesics or other prescribed treatments

▼ INTERVERTEBRAL DISC DISEASE (HERNIATED NUCLEUS PULPOSUS)

Data Base
A. Etiology and pathophysiology
   1. Involves protrusion of the nucleus pulposus into the spinal canal with subsequent compression of the cord or nerve roots; usually occurs as a result of trauma
   2. Most common site is lumbosacral area (between L4 and L5), but herniation can also occur in the cervical region (between C5 and C6 or C6 and C7)
B. Clinical findings
   1. Subjective
      a. Lumbosacral disc
         (1) Acute pain in lower back, radiating across the buttock and down the leg (sciatic pain)
         (2) Pain when raising the unflexed leg on the affected side (Lasègue's sign)
         (3) Weakness of the foot
      b. Cervical disc
         (1) Neck pain that may radiate down arm to the hand
         (2) Weakness of the affected upper extremity
   2. Objective
      a. Straightening of the normal lumbar curve with scoliosis away from the affected side (lumbosacral disc)
      b. Atrophy of the biceps and triceps may be present (cervical disc)

c. Elevated CSF protein
d. Myelogram and CT scans show impingement on the spinal cord
e. Electromyography (EMG) can help localize the site of a herniated disc

C. THERAPEUTIC INTERVENTIONS
1. Bed rest with traction to the lower extremities (lumbosacral disc) or cervical traction (cervical disc)
2. Back brace or support; cervical collar
3. Local application of heat
4. Muscle relaxants, analgesics, antiinflammatory agents
5. Surgical intervention
   a. Laminectomy: excision of the ruptured portion of the nucleus pulposus through an opening created by removal of part of the vertebra
   b. Discectomy: entire disc and cartilaginous plate are removed
   c. Microdiscectomy: utilizes a magnifying lens to facilitate removal of pieces of disc that press on nerve; incision is generally 1 inch
   d. Laminotomy: incision into the lamina
   e. Spinal fusion: if three or more discs are involved, the affected vertebrae are permanently fused to stabilize the spine
   f. Chemonucleolysis: injection of chymopapain, an enzyme from papaya, to dissolve disc

Nursing Care of Clients with Intervertebral Disc Disease
A. DATA COLLECTION
1. Characteristics of pain
2. Contributing factors such as trauma, obesity, degenerative joint disease, scoliosis
3. Posture and gait alterations
4. Extent of muscle strength and sensory function of involved extremities

B. ANALYSIS AND INTERPRETATION
Refer to General Nursing Diagnoses for Clients with Neuromusculoskeletal Systems Disorders for the following diagnoses: G 1, L, M 3, Q 1, Q 2, R 4, T, U 1, X, and Y

C. PLANNING/IMPLEMENTATION
1. Administer analgesics and other medications as ordered
2. Use a firm mattress and bed board under the client
3. Make certain that traction and/or braces are correctly applied and maintained and that weights hang freely
4. Use the fracture bedpan to avoid lifting of hips
5. Give frequent and extensive back care to relax muscles and promote circulation
6. Support body alignment at all times

7. Use log-rolling method to turn the client (instruct the client to fold arms across the chest, bend the knee on the side opposite the direction of the turn, and then roll over)
8. Teach the importance of weight loss, wearing low-heeled shoes, and appropriate body mechanics
9. Increase fluid intake and encourage diet rich in nutrient-dense foods such as fruits, vegetables, whole grains, and legumes to improve and maintain nutritional status as well as prevent constipation; if necessary use stool softeners to prevent straining
10. Provide special care for the client undergoing a laminectomy
    a. Explain that pain may persist postoperatively for some time because of edema
    b. Place the bedside table, phone, and call bell within reach to prevent twisting
    c. Observe the dressing for hemorrhage and leakage of spinal fluid; notify the physician immediately if either occurs
    d. Observe for inadequate ventilation, especially in clients who have undergone a cervical laminectomy
    e. Assess the client for changes in neurologic functioning
11. Allow the client to be dependent, but foster independence
12. Encourage client to perform exercises as prescribed to strengthen abdominal muscles for back support
13. Encourage the client to express feelings about altered functioning and self-image
14. Encourage the client to verbalize fears about the present condition and future disability

D. EVALUATION/OUTCOMES
1. Reports a reduction in pain
2. Demonstrates increased mobility
3. Participates in self-care activities
4. Avoids complications of immobility
5. Utilizes body mechanics
6. Participates in an exercise program

▼ FRACTURES OF THE EXTREMITIES

Data Base
A. Etiology and pathophysiology
1. Breaks in the continuity of bone, usually accompanied by localized tissue response and muscle spasm
2. Cause usually trauma, but pathologic fractures may occur as a result of osteoporosis, multiple myeloma, or bone tumors, which weaken bone structure

3. Types
   a. Complete fracture: bone completely separated into two parts; may be transverse or spiral
   b. Incomplete fracture: only part of the bone broken
   c. Comminuted fracture: bone broken into several fragments
   d. Greenstick fracture: splintering on one side of the bone, with bending of the other side; occurs only in pliable bones, usually in children
   e. Simple (closed) fracture: bone broken but no break in the skin
   f. Compound (open) fracture: break in the skin at the time of fracture with or without protrusion of the bone
4. Stages of healing include formation of a hematoma followed by cellular proliferation and callus formation by the osteoblasts; finally ossification and remodeling of the callus

B. Clinical findings
1. Subjective
   a. Pain aggravated by motion
   b. Tenderness
2. Objective
   a. Loss of motion
   b. Edema
   c. Crepitus (grating sound heard when fractured limb is moved)
   d. Ecchymosis
   e. X-ray examination reveals break in continuity of bone
   f. Deformity caused by change in bone alignment; often results in shortening of extremity

C. Therapeutic interventions
1. Traction may be used to reduce the fracture or to maintain alignment of bone fragments until healing occurs
   a. Skin traction: weights attached to adhesive, which is applied to the skin
      (1) Buck's extension: exerts a straight pull on a limb; often used temporarily to immobilize the leg when a client fractures a hip
      (2) Bryant's traction: both lower limbs extended vertically; used to align fractured femurs in young children
      (3) Russell traction: balanced traction in which the lower leg is supported in a hammock, which is attached to rope and pulleys on a Balkan frame; used to treat fractures of the femur (the foot of the bed is usually elevated for countertraction)

b. Skeletal traction applied to the bone
   (1) Steinmann pin or Kirschner's wire may be inserted through the bone and skin
   (2) Weights are then attached to a spreader, which is attached to both ends of the pin or wire (this may be used in conjunction with a cast)
2. Surgical intervention to align the bone (open reduction), often with plates and screws to hold fracture in alignment
3. Manipulation to reduce fracture (closed reduction)
4. Application of cast to maintain alignment and immobilize limb
   a. Plaster
   b. Fiberglass
5. Application of an external fixation device when fractures accompany soft tissue injury

Nursing Care of Clients with Fractures of the Extremities

A. DATA COLLECTION
1. Ability of client to move extremity
2. Altered appearance of involved body part
3. Neurovascular assessment; soft tissue injury or edema may compromise circulatory or neurologic functioning
4. Factors precipitating injury
5. Nutritional status

B. ANALYSIS AND INTERPRETATION
Refer to General Nursing Diagnoses for Clients with Neuromusculoskeletal Systems Disorders for the following diagnoses: C, G 1, L, M 3, Q 1, R 3, R 4, T, U 3, and Y

C. PLANNING/IMPLEMENTATION
1. Provide emergency care
   a. Evaluate the client's general physical condition
   b. Treat for shock
   c. Splint extremity in position found before moving the client; consider all suspected fractures to be fractures until x-ray films are available
   d. Cover open wound with sterile dressing if available
2. Observe for signs of emboli (fat or blood clot): severe chest pain, dyspnea, pallor, diaphoresis
3. Provide special care for a client with a cast
   a. Observe for signs of circulatory impairment: change in skin temperature or color, numbness or tingling, unrelieved pain, decrease in pedal pulse, prolonged blanching of toes after compression; compartment syndrome is a serious problem caused by compromised circulation to the muscle; ischemia leads to edema, which further compromises circulation

   b. Protect the cast from damage until dry by elevating it on a pillow; handle with palms of hands only
   c. Promote drying of the cast by leaving it uncovered; a light may be used with care to promote drying
   d. Maintain bed rest until the cast is dry and ambulation is permitted
   e. Observe for signs of hemorrhage and measure extent of drainage on cast when present
   f. Observe for irritation caused by rough cast edges, and pad as necessary for comfort and to prevent soiling
   g. Observe for swelling and notify the physician if necessary
   h. Administer analgesics judiciously and report unrelieved pain
   i. Observe for signs of infection (e.g., elevated temperature, odor from cast, swelling)
4. Provide special care for a client in traction
   a. Check that weights are hanging freely and that the affected limb is not resting against anything that will impede the pull of the traction
   b. Maintain in proper alignment
   c. Observe for foot-drop in clients with Russell traction or Buck's extension, since this may be indicative of nerve damage
   d. Observe for signs of thrombophlebitis; this is a more common complication of Russell traction because there is pressure on the popliteal space in addition to the stress of immobility
   e. Provide skin care
   f. Observe skin for irritation and observe site of insertion of skeletal traction for signs of infection
   g. Use aseptic technique when cleansing the site of insertion of skeletal traction (frequently an antiseptic ointment is also ordered)
5. Encourage high-protein, high-vitamin diet to promote healing; high-calcium diet is not recommended for the client confined to prolonged bed rest, since decalcification of the bone will continue until activity is restored, and a high calcium intake could lead to formation of renal calculi
6. Encourage fluids to help prevent complications of constipation, renal calculi, and urinary tract infection
7. Teach isometric exercises to promote muscle tone
8. Teach appropriate crutch-walking technique; non–weight bearing (three-point swing-

through); weight bearing (four point) progressing to use of cane (see procedures)

D. EVALUATION/OUTCOMES
1. Reports a reduction in pain
2. Maintains neurovascular functioning of extremities
3. Maintains skin integrity
4. Remains active participant in care without compromising treatment
5. Avoids complications of immobility
6. Regains complete mobility and function after healing

▼ FRACTURES OF THE HIPS

Data Base
A. Etiology and pathophysiology
1. Fractures of the head or neck of the femur (intracapsular fracture) or trochanteric area (extracapsular fracture)
2. Incidence highest in elderly females because of osteoporosis and degenerative joint disease
B. Clinical findings
1. Subjective
   a. Pain
   b. Changes in sensation
2. Objective
   a. Affected leg appears shorter
   b. External rotation of the affected limb
   c. X-ray examination reveals lack of continuity of the bone
C. Therapeutic interventions
1. Buck's extension or Russell traction as a temporary measure to relieve the pain of muscle spasm or if surgery is contraindicated
2. Closed reduction with a hip spica cast in fractures of the intertrochanteric region
3. Open reduction and internal fixation
   a. Austin Moore prosthesis
   b. Thompson prosthesis
   c. Smith-Petersen nail
   d. Jewett nail
   e. Zickel nail
4. Total hip replacement when joint degeneration will not permit an internal fixation

Nursing Care of Clients with Fractures of the Hips

A. DATA COLLECTION
1. Shortening and external rotation of leg
2. Degree and nature of pain
3. Baseline vital signs
4. Neurovascular status of involved extremity
5. Other health problems that may affect recovery

B. ANALYSIS AND INTERPRETATION
Refer to General Nursing Diagnoses for Clients with Neuromusculoskeletal Systems Disorders for the following diagnoses: G 1, L, M 3, Q 1, R 3, R 4, T, U 3, X, and Y

C. PLANNING/IMPLEMENTATION
1. See Nursing Care of Clients with Fractures of the Extremities
2. Encourage the use of a trapeze to facilitate movement
3. Use the fracture pan for elimination
4. Provide postoperative care
   a. Inspect dressing and linen for bleeding
   b. Use a trochanter roll to prevent external rotation of legs
   c. Do not turn client on the affected side unless specifically ordered; place pillow between legs when turning on the unaffected side
   d. Use pillows or abductor pillow to maintain the legs in slight abduction; after hip replacement it prevents dislodging of the prosthesis
   e. Encourage quadriceps setting exercises
   f. Assist the client to ambulate—first using a walker and eventually progressing to a cane; follow orders for extent of weight bearing permitted on affected extremity because this will depend on the type of surgery performed and the type of device inserted
   g. Avoid flexing the hips of a client with a total hip replacement; assist to a lounge chair position when permitted to sit
   h. Prevent complication of thromboembolism
      (1) Administer prescribed anticoagulants; observe for bleeding
      (2) Apply antiembolism stockings
      (3) Encourage dorsiflexion of feet
   i. Prevent pulmonary complication
      (1) Encourage coughing and deep breathing
      (2) Explain use of incentive spirometry
      (3) Assist with frequent position changes

D. EVALUATION/OUTCOMES
1. Reports reduction in pain
2. Maintains alignment of affected leg
3. Demonstrates improved mobility
4. Avoids complications of immobility

▼ SPINAL CORD INJURY

Data Base
A. Etiology and pathophysiology
1. Sudden impingements on the spinal cord as a result of trauma
2. Fractures of the vertebrae can cut, compress,

or completely sever the spinal cord if the client is not positioned and moved correctly at the scene of an accident; the symptoms depend on the location (lumbar, thoracic, cervical) and extent of the damage (complete transection, partial transection, compression) and may be temporary or permanent; the sensation and mobility of areas that are supplied by nerves below the level of the lesion are lost

B. Clinical findings
  1. Subjective
    a. Loss of sensation below the level of the injury
    b. Inability to move
  2. Objective
    a. Early symptoms of spinal shock
      (1) Absence of reflexes below the level of the lesion
      (2) Flaccid paralysis (immobility accompanied by weak, soft, flabby muscles) below the level of injury
      (3) Hypotonia (caused by disruption of neural impulses) results in bowel and bladder distention
      (4) Inability to perspire in affected parts
      (5) Hypotension
    b. Later symptoms of spinal cord injury
      (1) Reflex hyperexcitability (spastic paralysis): muscles below the site of injury become spastic and hyperreflexic
      (2) State of diminished reflex excitability (flaccid paralysis) below the site of injury follows the state of reflex hyperexcitability in all instances of total cord damage and may occur in some instances of partial cord damage
      (3) In total cord damage, since both upper and lower motoneurons are destroyed, the symptoms depend totally on the location of the injury; loss of motor and sensory function present at this time is usually permanent
        (a) Sacral region: paralysis (usually flaccid type) of the lower extremities (paraplegia) accompanied by atonic (autonomous) bladder and bowel with impairment of sphincter control
        (b) Lumbar region: paralysis of the lower extremities that may extend to the pelvic region (usually flaccid type) accompanied by a spastic (automatic) bladder and loss of bladder and anal sphincter control
        (c) Thoracic region: same symptoms as in the lumbar region except extends to the trunk below level of the

diaphragm
        (d) Cervical region: same symptoms as in the thoracic region except extends from the neck down and includes paralysis of all extremities (quadriplegia); if injury is above C4, respirations are depressed
      (4) In partial cord damage either the upper or the lower motoneurons, or both, may be destroyed; therefore the symptoms depend not only on the location but also on the type of neurons involved; destruction of lower motoneurons will result in atrophy and flaccid paralysis of the involved muscles, whereas destruction of upper motoneurons causes spasticity
      (5) Autonomic dysreflexia: exaggerated autonomic response to stimuli such as distended bowel or bladder; leads to severe hypertension, headache, flushed skin, diaphoresis, and nasal congestion

C. THERAPEUTIC INTERVENTIONS
  1. Neurologic assessment
  2. Maintenance of vertebral alignment by use of the following:
    a. Bed rest with supportive devices (bed board, sand bags, etc.)
    b. Bed rest with total immobilization (see Special Beds for Positioning Clients in Procedures Related to the Neuromusculoskeletal Systems)
    c. Traction (skeletal or skin traction); for example, Crutchfield tongs, Buck's extension, halo device
    d. Corsets, braces, and other devices when mobility is permitted
  3. Surgery to reduce pain or pressure and/or stabilize the spine (e.g., laminectomy, spinal fusion)
  4. Mechanical ventilation as needed
  5. Temperature control via hypothermia or tepid baths
  6. High doses of steroids to reduce the inflammatory process at the site of the injury
  7. Extensive rehabilitation therapy

Nursing Care of Clients with Spinal Cord Injuries

A. DATA COLLECTION
  1. Respiratory status
  2. Baseline vital signs
  3. Neurologic status
  4. Abdomen for bladder or bowel distention
  5. Circumstances of injury
  6. Health problems that can have an impact on recovery
  7. Client's coping skills and support systems

B. ANALYSIS AND INTERPRETATION

Refer to General Nursing Diagnoses for Clients with Neuromusculoskeletal Systems Disorders for the following diagnoses: C, D 1, E, G 1, G 2, H 1, I 1, I 2, J, K, M 2, M 3, N 1, N 2, O 1, O 3, R 1, S, T, U 1, V 2, W, X, Y and AA

C. PLANNING/IMPLEMENTATION

1. Maintain frequent observation of respiratory and neurologic functioning
2. Maintain spinal alignment at all times; when turning, use the log-rolling method, and make certain enough help is available to move the client as a single unit
3. Check safety locks on Stryker frames and CircOlectric beds before turning
4. Maintain surgical asepsis for the client with skeletal traction or spinal surgery
5. Provide skin care to back and bony prominences
6. Maintain body parts in a functional position; prevent dysfunctional contractures
7. Institute active and passive range-of-motion exercises as soon as approved by physician
8. Provide the client with simple explanations
9. Encourage the client to verbalize and accept feelings
10. Stay with the client when possible to provide assurance
11. Allow the client to be independent when possible
12. Include the client in decision-making process
13. Help the client to adjust to changes in body image and altered self-concept
14. Allow the client time to reorganize life-style
15. Set realistic short-term goals so the client can achieve some success
16. Test the temperature of bath water to avoid burns; teach the client to test water temperature in any water-related activity
17. Avoid bumps and bruises when involved in activities; utilize techniques to prevent pressure and examine skin for signs of pressure from positioning, braces, or splints
18. Provide an opportunity for the client to touch, grasp, and manipulate objects of different sizes, weights, and textures to stimulate tactile sensation
19. Encourage the client to be aware of all body segments: look at both extremities, comb both sides of the hair, shave both sides of the chin, put makeup on both sides of the face
20. Protect the affected limbs by proper positioning during transfer; use a sling when indicated
21. Teach the client to use the unaffected extremities to manipulate, move, and stabilize the affected ones

22. Attempt to reestablish a scheduled pattern of bowel function
    a. Understand what the individual's bowel functioning means to the client and family
    b. Involve the client, family, and entire health team in the development of a plan of care
    c. Review the client's bowel habits prior to illness as well as the current pattern of elimination
    d. Provide a diet with bowel-stimulating properties; emphasis should be placed on fruits, vegetables, cereal grains, and legumes, because these are rich sources of dietary fiber
    e. Encourage sufficient fluid intake: 2000 to 3000 ml per day
    f. Encourage the client to be as active as possible to develop the tone and strength of the muscles that can be used
    g. Establish a specific and definite time for the bowel movement; regularity is the most important aspect of bowel reeducation
       (1) Depends on the client's schedule
       (2) Depends on the client's past pattern
       (3) Consider scheduling evacuation after a meal to utilize the gastrocolic reflex (peristaltic wave in the colon induced by entrance of food into a fasting stomach)
    h. Determine if the client is aware of the need to defecate (e.g., feeling of fullness or pressure in the rectum, flatus, borborygmus)
    i. Provide privacy during toileting activities
    j. Encourage the client to assume a position most near the physiologic position for defecation (sitting the client up frequently assists in preparing for this)
    k. Utilize assistive measures to induce defecation by:
       (1) Teaching the client to bear down and contract abdominal muscles (Valsalva's maneuver should be avoided by people with cardiac problems)
       (2) Teaching the client to lean forward to increase intraabdominal pressure by compressing the abdomen against the thighs
       (3) Digital stimulation
       (4) Using suppository if necessary
       (5) Using enemas only as a last resort
    l. Provide for adaptation of equipment as necessary (e.g., elevated toilet seat, grab bars, padded backrest)
    m. Teach the family the bowel training program
23. Attempt to reestablish bladder function
    a. Determine the type of bladder problem
       (1) Neurogenic bladder: any disturbance in bladder functioning caused by a lesion of the nervous system

(2) Spastic bladder (reflex or autonomous): disorder caused by a lesion of the spinal cord above the bladder reflex center, in the conus medullaris; there is a loss of conscious sensation and cerebral motor control; the bladder empties automatically when the detrusor muscle is sufficiently stretched (about 500 ml)

(3) Flaccid bladder (atonic, nonreflex, or autonomous): disorder caused by a lesion of the spinal cord at the level of the sacral conus or below; the bladder continues to fill, becomes distended, and periodically overflows; the bladder muscle does not contract forcefully and therefore does not empty except with a conscious effort

b. Understand what the individual's bladder functioning means to the client and family

c. Involve the client, family, and entire health team in the development of a plan of care

d. Review the client's bladder habits prior to illness as well as the current pattern of elimination

e. Encourage activity

f. Encourage sufficient fluid intake
   (1) 3000 to 4000 ml per 24-hour period
   (2) Glass of water with each attempt to void
   (3) Reduce the amount of fluid as the day progresses and restrict fluid after 6 PM to limit the amount of urine in the bladder during the night

g. Provide for privacy during toileting activities

h. Encourage the client to assume as normal a position as possible for voiding

i. Establish a voiding schedule
   (1) Begin trial voiding at the time the client is most often incontinent
   (2) Attempt voiding every 2 hours all day and two to three times during the night
   (3) Time intervals between voiding should be shorter in the morning than later in the day
   (4) As the client's ability to maintain control improves, lengthen the time between attempts at voiding
   (5) Time of intervals is not as important as regularity

j. Determine whether the client is aware of need or act of urination (e.g., fullness or pressure, flushing, chilling, goose pimples, cold sweats)

k. Utilize assistive measures to induce urination by teaching the client to:
   (1) Use Credé maneuver: manual expression of the urine from the bladder with moderate external pressure, downward and backward, from the umbilicus to over the suprapubic area
   (2) Bend forward to increase intraabdominal pressure
   (3) Stimulate "trigger points": areas that, for the individual, will instigate urination (e.g., stroke the thigh, pull pubic hair, touch meatus)

l. Record intake, output, voiding times, and times of incontinence

m. Provide for adaptive equipment as necessary (e.g., elevated toilet seats, commode, urinals, drainage systems)

n. Teach the family the bladder-training program

24. Discuss need for sexual expression and options available; include discussion of penile implants

25. Care for the client experiencing autonomic dysreflexia
   (1) Place in a high-Fowler's position
   (2) Ensure patency of urinary drainage system
   (3) Assess for fecal impaction
   (4) Eliminate other potential stimuli such as drafts
   (5) Notify physician; administer prescribed antihypertensives

26. Refer client to national spinal cord injury association for information and support

D. EVALUATION/OUTCOMES
1. Maintains respiratory functioning
2. Avoids complications of immobility
3. Establishes program to maintain bowel function
4. Establishes program to maintain bladder function
5. Utilizes strengths to manage disabilities
6. Adjusts to changes in life-style
7. Functions satisfactorily sexually
8. Shares concerns with family members and health professionals

▼ AMPUTATION

Data Base
A. ETIOLOGY AND PATHOPHYSIOLOGY
1. Refers to the removal of a body part as a result of trauma or surgical intervention
2. Necessitated by:
   a. Malignant tumor
   b. Trauma
   c. Acute arterial insufficiency

B. CLINICAL FINDINGS
See Osteogenic Sarcoma and Peripheral Vascular Disease

C. THERAPEUTIC INTERVENTIONS
1. Below-the-knee amputation (BKA) common in peripheral vascular disease; facilitates successful adaptation to prosthesis because of retained knee function
2. Above-the-knee amputation (AKA) necessitated by trauma or extensive disease
3. Upper extremity amputation usually necessitated by severe trauma, malignant tumors, or congenital malformation

Nursing Care of Clients with Amputations
A. DATA COLLECTION
1. Neurovascular status of involved extremity
2. History to determine
   a. Causative factors
   b. Health problems that can compromise recovery
3. Client's understanding of the extent of the surgery
4. Client's coping skills
5. Client's support system

B. ANALYSIS AND INTERPRETATION
Refer to General Nursing Diagnoses for Clients with Neuromusculoskeletal Systems Disorders for the following diagnoses: C, G 1, I 2, K, L, M 3, R 2, T, U 3, X, and Y

C. PLANNING/IMPLEMENTATION
1. Provide care preoperatively
   a. Initiation of exercises to strengthen muscles of extremities in preparation for crutch walking
   b. Coughing and deep-breathing exercises
   c. Emotional support for anticipated alteration in body image
2. Monitor vital signs and stump dressing for signs of hemorrhage
3. Elevate stump for 12 to 24 hours to decrease edema; remove pillow after this time to prevent contractures
4. Provide stump care
   a. Maintain elastic bandage to shrink and shape stump in preparation for prosthesis
   b. When wound is healed, wash stump daily, avoiding the use of oils, which may cause maceration
   c. Apply pressure to end of stump with progressively firmer surfaces to toughen stump
   d. Encourage client to move the stump
   e. Place the client with a lower extremity amputation in a prone position twice daily to stretch the flexor muscles and prevent hip flexion contractures
5. Teach client about phantom limb sensation
   a. Phantom limb: physiologic reaction of the nerves in the stump causing an unpleasant feeling that the limb is still there; this response may or may not be precipitated by a psychologic overlay
   b. Phantom limb pain: when the unpleasant feelings become painful or disagreeable
   c. Characteristics of phantom limb: sensations may be constant or intermittent, and of varying severity
   d. Institute care that may help relieve phantom limb phenomenon: have the client look at the stump or close eyes and put the stump through range of motion as if the full limb were still there; if the client continues to have severe pain of long duration, the medical therapy may include:
      (1) Injecting the nerve endings in the stump with alcohol to give temporary relief
      (2) Surgical revision of the stump
6. Consider the special needs related to an upper extremity amputation
   a. Mastery of an upper extremity prosthesis is more complex than that of a lower extremity prosthesis
   b. The client must do bilateral shoulder exercises to prepare for fitting the prosthesis
   c. The artificial arm cannot be used above the head or behind the back because of the harnessing
   d. No artificial hand can duplicate all the fine movements of the fingers and thumb of the normal hand, although the development of electronic limbs does not negate this possibility for the future
   e. There is a loss of sensory feedback; therefore the client must use visual control at all times (a blind person could not adequately use a functional prosthesis)
7. Support client through fitting, application, and utilization of prosthesis
8. Encourage family to participate in care
9. Allow client to express emotional reactions

D. EVALUATION/OUTCOMES
1. Performs self-care activities
2. Verbalizes acceptance of altered body image
3. Demonstrates care of stump and prosthesis
4. Participates in rehabilitation program
5. Maximizes independence

▼ ANTERIOR SEGMENT DISORDERS OF THE EYE

Data Base
A. Etiology and pathophysiology
   1. Conjunctivitis: inflammation of the conjuncti-

va; can result from invasion by organisms, allergens, or irritants

2. Blepharitis: inflammation of the lid margins; classified as staphylococcal or seborrheic
3. Keratitis: inflammation of the cornea due to invasion of an organism
4. Uveitis: an inflammation of the iris, ciliary body, and/or the choroid
5. Pterygium: segment of thickened conjunctiva that can extend over the cornea
6. Trachoma: viral infection of the lids and conjunctiva that can result in corneal ulceration and blindness
7. Chalazion: sterile cyst of the meibomian gland that causes inflammation of the lid; cyst remains when the inflammation subsides
8. Hordeolum: infection of a follicle of the eyelash commonly caused by staphylococcal organisms
9. Dacryocystitis: infection of the lacrimal duct due to nasolacrimal duct obstruction

B. Clinical findings
1. Subjective
   a. Photophobia (keratitis, uveitis)
   b. Blurred vision (keratitis, uveitis, trachoma)
   c. Pain (keratitis, uveitis)
   d. Burning and itching of eyes (conjunctivitis, blepharitis, hordeolum)
2. Objective
   a. Scaling and crust formation of lids (conjunctivitis, blepharitis, keratitis, uveitus)
   b. Swelling and redness (conjunctivitis, blepharitis, keratitis, uveitis, hordeolum)
   c. Tearing (keratitis)
   d. Ciliary injection (uveitis)
   e. Purulent drainage (conjunctivitis)

C. Therapeutic interventions
1. Conjunctivitis, blepharitis, hordeolum, dacryocystitis
   a. Antibiotic ointments
   b. Warm compresses
2. Keratitis
   a. Culture analysis to determine causative organism
   b. Topical steroids and antibiotics
   c. If the cornea is badly damaged, corneal transplant
3. Uveitis
   a. Mydriatics to keep the iris at rest
   b. Topical steroids and antibiotics
   c. Dark glasses
4. Pterygium: surgical removal
5. Trachoma: oral antibiotics, usually tetracycline, for 3 to 5 weeks
6. Chalazion: usually surgical excision of cyst

Nursing Care of Clients with Anterior Segment Disorders of the Eye

A. DATA COLLECTION
1. Appearance of eye, noting the presence of any drainage
2. Visual acuity
3. Presence and characteristics of pain
4. Presence of light sensitivity

B. ANALYSIS AND INTERPRETATION
Refer to General Nursing Diagnoses for Clients with Neuromusculoskeletal Systems Disorders for the following diagnoses: C, I 4, M 2, and V 1

C. PLANNING/IMPLEMENTATION
1. Instruct the client on proper care of the eyes (hand washing, avoidance of rubbing, use of protective eye wear)
2. Administer antibiotic ointment and instruct client in its use
3. Apply soaks as ordered
4. Prepare the client for surgery, if indicated
5. Provide care for the client who has undergone a corneal transplant (keratoplasty)
   a. Maintain pressure patch on eye
   b. Explain the importance of avoiding Valsalva's maneuver and bending over during healing
   c. Explain that healing may take up to 6 months because the circulatory supply of the cornea is decreased
   d. Help client to organize environment to maintain safety

D. EVALUATION/OUTCOMES
1. Reports a reduction in pain
2. Maintains visual acuity
3. Demonstrates appropriate eye care
4. Remains free from injury
5. Performs self-care activities

▼ TUMORS OF THE EYE

Data Base

A. Etiology and pathophysiology
1. May be benign or malignant; can form in or metastasize to the eye
2. Retinoblastoma, a congenital malignant neoplasm found in children; spreads easily by extension to the brain
3. Melanoma common in the iris and choroid; grows slowly but metastasizes to the liver and lungs

B. Clinical findings
1. Subjective
   a. Headache
   b. Visual complaints
2. Objective

a. Redness and swelling of the conjunctiva

b. Decreased vision

c. In retinoblastoma, white pupillary reflex, strabismus, retinal detachment

d. Increased intraocular pressure

C. Therapeutic interventions

1. Chemotherapy

2. Radiation therapy

3. Enucleation (surgical removal of the eye)

Nursing Care of Clients with Eye Tumors

A. DATA COLLECTION

1. Description of onset and progression of symptoms

2. Visual acuity

3. Client's coping mechanisms

4. Client's support system

B. ANALYSIS AND INTERPRETATION

Refer to General Nursing Diagnoses for Clients with Neuromusculoskeletal Systems Disorders for the following diagnoses: C, I 4, M 2, V 1, and X

C. PLANNING/IMPLEMENTATION

1. Support the client and family as they attempt to cope with the diagnosis

2. Observe for side effects of medical therapy and attempt to limit their effects

3. Provide care for the client who has undergone an enucleation

   a. Maintain pressure dressings on the eye for 1 or 2 days to minimize hemorrhage

   b. Watch for signs of meningitis, which occurs as a complication, including headache or pain on the operative side

   c. Explain that monocularity results in the loss of depth perception, and activities that require this should be performed cautiously; turning head from side to side

   d. Explain that the artificial eye may be inserted when healing is complete, usually 1 to 2 months; support adaptation to changes in body image

   e. Instruct client about the care of the eye socket and prosthesis; cleanse eye prosthesis with warm water or saline

4. Support natural defense mechanisms; encourage intake of nutrient-dense foods, especially those rich in the immune-stimulating mineral selenium and vitamins A, C, and E, as well as protein

D. EVALUATION/OUTCOMES

1. Adapts to loss of eye without loss of positive body image

2. Remains active in satisfying activities

3. Remains free from injury

4. Cares for eye socket and prosthesis appropriately

▼ CATARACT

Data Base

A. Etiology and pathophysiology

1. Opacity of the crystalline lens or its capsule

2. Results from injury, exposure to heat, heredity, aging, or congenital factors that cause a diminution of sight

B. Clinical findings

1. Subjective

   a. Distortion of vision (e.g., haziness, cloudiness, diplopia)

   b. Photophobia

2. Objective

   a. Progressive loss of vision

   b. Usual black pupil appears clouded, progressing to milky white appearance

C. Therapeutic interventions

1. Mydriatics and ophthalmic antibiotics

2. Corrective lenses until surgery is needed as determined by the cataract

   a. Causing decreased vision that interferes with normal activities

   b. Obstructing view of the retina to diagnose other ocular disorders such as retinopathy

   c. Causing glaucoma

3. Surgical intervention to remove the opaque lens

   a. Surgical procedure is most frequently performed in an ambulatory surgery setting, but hospitalization may be required for some clients

   b. Extracapsular extraction involves removing the anterior capsule and lens through a small incision after the lens has been fragmented through a phacoemulsification technique; most common procedure

   c. Intracapsular extraction involves removal of the entire lens as a unit with a cryoprobe

   d. Intraocular lens implantation is generally performed at the time of cataract extraction

   e. Corrective lenses following cataract surgery when lens implants are not performed

      (1) Contact lenses

      (2) Aphakic spectacles

   f. Antiemetics, analgesics, and stool softeners postoperatively

Nursing Care of Clients with Cataracts

A. DATA COLLECTION

1. Description of onset and progression of symptoms

2. Visual acuity

3. Characteristics of pupil

4. Red reflex via ophthalmoscopic examination

B. ANALYSIS AND INTERPRETATION

Refer to General Nursing Diagnoses for Clients with Neuromusculoskeletal Systems Disorders for the following diagnoses: C, I 4, M 2, V 1, and X

C. PLANNING/IMPLEMENTATION

1. Provide thorough orientation to environment
2. Place call bell, phone, and other items on unaffected side
3. Avoid glaring lights
4. Provide auditory stimulation such as television, radio, and talking books
5. Remove environmental hazards
6. Provide care after cataract removal
   a. Instruct the client to prevent pressure on eyes by:
      (1) Not touching or rubbing the eyes
      (2) Not closing the eyes tightly
      (3) Avoiding coughing, sneezing, or bending from the waist (teach the client to open the mouth when coughing)
      (4) Lying on the back or the nonoperated side
      (5) Avoiding rapid head movements
      (6) Avoiding straining at stool or lifting
   b. Instruct the client to request prescribed analgesics and antiemetics as required
   c. Administer stool softeners
   d. Provide side rails to help in turning and preventing falls
   e. Assist the client with ambulation because of distortions in depth perception and extremely blurred vision
   f. Provide an easily accessible call bell
   g. Reduce the amount of light and encourage the use of sunglasses when the eye patch is removed
   h. Provide a quiet environment to promote rest
   i. Avoid substances that might precipitate coughing or sneezing (e.g., pepper, talcum powder)
   j. Observe for signs of increased intraocular pressure (e.g., pain, restlessness, increased pulse rate)
   k. Observe for signs of infection (e.g., pain, changes in vital signs)
   l. Encourage deep breathing
   m. Explain that depth perception will be altered but assure client that the corrective lenses will help to compensate for this distortion

D. EVALUATION/OUTCOMES

1. Remains free from injury
2. Demonstrates increased visual acuity with corrective lenses
3. Develops interests consistent with limitations
4. Continues medical follow-up

▼ GLAUCOMA

Data Base

A. Etiology and pathophysiology
   1. Condition in which the pressure within the eyeball is higher than normal
   2. Primary open-angle glaucoma
      a. Occurs when aqueous fluid does not drain properly from the eye related to pathologic changes in the trabecular meshwork of Schlemm's canal
      b. The intraocular pressure increases and destroys retinal nerve fibers, causing progressive vision loss in affected areas
      c. Most common type of glaucoma
   3. Closed-angle glaucoma or narrow-angle glaucoma
      a. Occurs when the iris lies close to drainage channels, creating a mechanical blockage of the trabecular meshwork that interferes with the exit of aqueous humor from the anterior chamber
      b. Trapped aqueous humor causes the intraocular pressure to rise suddenly
      c. Occurs more commonly in African Americans and people older than 60 years of age
B. Clinical findings
   1. Open-angle
      a. Subjective: haloes around lights
      b. Objective
         (1) Gradual loss of peripheral vision
         (2) Increased intraocular pressure (24 to 32mm Hg) as measured by a tonometer
   2. Closed-angle
      a. Subjective
         (1) Nausea
         (2) Halos around lights
         (3) Severe frontal headache
      b. Objective
         (1) Loss of peripheral vision
         (2) Steamy cornea
         (3) Conjunctival injection
         (4) Increased intraocular pressure (50 to 70 mm Hg) as measured with a tonometer
C. Therapeutic interventions
   1. Lowering the intraocular pressure with miotics or carbonic anhydrase inhibitors
   2. Surgical intervention to facilitate drainage of the aqueous humor is called a peripheral iridectomy; a surgical incision is made through the cornea to remove a portion of the iris to facilitate aqueous drainage
   3. Laser iridotomy

Nursing Care of Clients with Glaucoma

A. DATA COLLECTION

1. Description of onset and progression of symptoms
2. Visual acuity
3. Peripheral vision
4. Characteristics of sclera, pupil, and anterior chamber

B. ANALYSIS AND INTERPRETATION

Refer to General Nursing Diagnoses for Clients with Neuromusculoskeletal Systems Disorders for the following diagnoses: C, M 2, Q 2, T, and V 1

C. PLANNING/IMPLEMENTATION

1. Explain the importance of continued use of eye medications as ordered to prevent further visual loss
2. Explain the need for continued medical supervision for observation of intraocular pressure to ensure control of the disorder
3. Teach the client to avoid exertion, stooping, straining for a bowel movement, coughing, heavy lifting, or wearing constricting clothing, since these increase intraocular pressure
4. Instruct the client to report severe eye or brow pain and nausea to the physician

D. EVALUATION/OUTCOMES

1. Maintains present level of visual acuity
2. Complies with medical regimen
3. Identifies signs of increased intraocular pressure that must be reported
4. Remains free from injury
5. Participates actively in decision making and care

▼ DIABETIC RETINOPATHY

Data Base

A. Etiology and pathophysiology
   1. Involves pathologic changes in the retinal blood supply
   2. Stages
      a. Background retinopathy: microaneurysms form on retinal capillary walls and leak blood into retina or macula; this causes edema, decreased visual acuity, and color discrimination; as fluid is absorbed, yellow deposits form on the retina
      b. Preproliferative retinopathy: veins become engorged, "cotton wool" patches are noted on retina, and microvascular formations bypass vessels
      c. Proliferative retinopathy: neovascularization due to hypoxia; vessels are fragile and leak blood and protein into the vitreous and retina; if vessels grow into vitreous, traction may cause the vitreous to be pulled away and retinal detachment can occur
   3. Risk factors include insulin–dependent diabetes mellitus and non–insulin dependent diabetes mellitus of longer than 15 years' duration
   4. Diabetic retinopathy is a leading cause of blindness

B. Clinical findings
   1. Subjective
      a. Decreased color vision
      b. Decreased central vision
   2. Objective
      a. Cotton wool patches on retina
      b. Retinal hemorrhages
      c. Neovascularization

C. Therapeutic interventions
   1. Control of diabetes mellitus
   2. Laser photocoagulation: this causes small burns that seal off leaking retinal aneurysms and is performed in an outpatient setting
   3. Vitrectomy: surgical removal of the vitreous, which is replaced with saline or silicon oil; this supports the retina to allow scarring to occur
   4. See Detached Retina for additional therapeutic interventions

Nursing Care of Clients with Diabetic Retinopathy

A. DATA COLLECTION

1. History related to diabetic status, including type and duration
2. Description of onset of symptoms, including decreased color perception and diminished visual acuity
3. Visual acuity
4. Assessment of retina for cotton-wool patches, engorged vessels, yellow exudates, and edema

B. ANALYSIS AND INTERPRETATION

Refer to General Nursing Diagnoses for Clients with Neuromusculoskeletal Systems Disorders for the following diagnoses: I 4, M 2, T, V 1, and Z

C. PLANNING/IMPLEMENTATION

1. Teach the client the importance of regular eye examinations every 6 to 12 months through dilated pupils
2. Reinforce teaching related to management of diabetic condition
3. Teach client that dark glasses are important to decrease light sensitivity when pupils are dilated (after examination or following laser photocoagulation)
4. When the client has a vitrectomy with saline instillation, instruct as to the importance of maintaining a face-down position so that air instilled during the procedure floats against the retina until it is absorbed (4 to 5 days)

D. EVALUATION/OUTCOMES
1. Reports improved vision
2. Remains free from injury

▼ DETACHED RETINA

Data Base

A. Etiology and pathophysiology
1. May result from trauma, the aging process, or cataract surgery; also seen in clients with myopia or diabetes mellitus
2. Retina separates from the choroid, and vitreous humor seeps behind the retina
B. Clinical findings
1. Subjective
   a. Flashes of light
   b. Floaters
   c. Sensation of a veil in the line of sight
2. Objective
   a. Retinal separation noted on ophthalmoscopy
   b. Assessment of visual loss
C. Therapeutic interventions
1. Bed rest, with the area of detachment in a dependent position to promote healing
2. Tranquilizers to promote rest and reduce anxiety
3. Surgical intervention
   a. Cryosurgery: supercooled probe causes retinal scarring and healing of area
   b. Photocoagulation: laser beam through the pupil produces a retinal burn, which causes scarring of the involved area
   c. Scleral buckling: shortening of the sclera to force the choroid closer to the retina

Nursing Care of Clients with Detached Retinas

A. DATA COLLECTION
1. Description of onset and progression of symptoms
2. Visual acuity
3. Status of retina via ophthalmoscopic examination
4. History to identify contributing factors such as trauma or recent surgery of the eye

B. ANALYSIS AND INTERPRETATION
   Refer to General Nursing Diagnoses for Clients with Neuromusculoskeletal Systems Disorders for the following diagnoses: C, I 4, M 2, Q 1, Q 2, T, and V 1

C. PLANNING/IMPLEMENTATION
1. Provide accurate information in a calm voice; client's anxiety is high as a result of the sudden, unexpected vision loss
2. Keep the client on bed rest in position as ordered

3. Provide the client with a call bell and answer promptly
4. Maintain protective eye patch
5. Instruct client to avoid activities that increase intraocular pressure such as coughing, straining, and stooping
6. Observe for signs of hemorrhage postoperatively (severe pain, restlessness)
7. Diminish lights in the room
8. Explain that return to a sedentary occupation may occur in approximately 3 weeks and to a more active job in 6 to 8 weeks

D. EVALUATION/OUTCOMES
1. Reports absence of discomfort
2. Reports improved vision
3. Remains free from injury
4. Participates in planning and care
5. Expresses increased confidence in ability to provide self-care

▼ MACULAR DEGENERATION

Data Base

A. Etiology and pathophysiology
1. Growth of new blood vessels into the area of central retinal vision (macula) that obscures central vision
2. Etiology is unknown but it is believed to be a vascular response, since the macula is normally devoid of vessels
3. It is the leading cause of newly diagnosed legal blindness in persons older than 65 years of age in Canada
B. Clinical findings
1. Subjective
   a. Distortion of straight lines
   b. Scotoma or intermittent blurring of central vision that worsens over time
2. Objective
   a. Ophthalmoscopic examination reveals vessels on the macula
   b. Visual acuity is decreased
C. Therapeutic interventions
1. Laser photocoagulation in 10% of clients in early stage
2. Steroid therapy
3. Vitamin therapy, including zinc, has had questionable results

Nursing Care of Clients with Macular Degeneration

A. DATA COLLECTION
1. Description of onset and progression of symptoms
2. Visual acuity, particularly central vision

3. Status of retina via ophthalmoscopic examination

B. ANALYSIS AND INTERPRETATION

Refer to General Nursing Diagnoses for Clients with Neuromusculoskeletal Systems Disorders for the following diagnoses: C, I 4, M 2, T, and V 1

C. PLANNING/IMPLEMENTATION

1. Provide emotional support for client and family
2. Institute safety measures to prevent injury
3. Provide information related to medical management
4. Suggest alternatives for dealing with central vision loss that may interfere with reading and driving
5. Refer client and family to community agencies that provide information and support for the visually impaired

D. EVALUATION/OUTCOMES

1. Remains free from injury
2. Participates in satisfying activities that do not require central vision acuity
3. Maintains current visual function

▼ OTITIS MEDIA

Data Base

A. Etiology and pathophysiology
1. Inflammatory disease of the middle ear caused by bacterial invasion; usually begins in childhood
2. May be acute or chronic as a result of repeated attacks
3. Signs and symptoms caused by pressure of fluid
4. May permanently damage middle ear

B. Clinical findings
1. Subjective
   a. Hearing loss
   b. Feeling of fullness within the ear
   c. Pain (subsides in 6 to 9 hours)
2. Objective
   a. Drainage from the ear that may be foul smelling
   b. Bulging or perforation of the eardrum apparent during examination with an otoscope
   c. Conductive hearing loss

C. Therapeutic interventions
1. Systemic antibiotics
2. Antibiotic eardrops
3. Symptomatic relief with analgesics, antihistamines, and decongestants
4. Gentle irrigations to cleanse the ear
5. Myringotomy

Nursing Care of Clients with Otitis Media

A. DATA COLLECTION

1. History to identify prior episodes of otitis media and recent upper respiratory infections
2. Hearing acuity
3. Presence of inflammation of external ear structures
4. Presence of exudate from ear
5. Status of tympanic membrane via otoscopic examination
6. Baseline vital signs

B. ANALYSIS AND INTERPRETATION

Refer to General Nursing Diagnoses for Clients with Neuromusculoskeletal Systems Disorders for the following diagnoses: I 4, M 2, Q 1, Q 2, V 3, and Z

C. PLANNING/IMPLEMENTATION

1. Obtain a specimen of exudate for culture and sensitivity
2. Administer antibiotics and other drugs as prescribed
3. Instruct client to administer eardrops
4. Monitor temperature, drainage, pain, and hearing acuity to evaluate effectiveness of therapy
5. Teach client to avoid others with respiratory infections and delay air travel when and if such an infection is present
6. Face client, minimize distractions, enunciate clearly and/or provide written communication if hearing is diminished
7. Instruct the client to report headache or stiff neck immediately, since this may indicate complications of meningitis

D. EVALUATION/OUTCOMES

1. Reports a reduction in pain
2. Reports improved hearing acuity
3. Maintains effective communication

▼ MASTOIDITIS

Data Base

A. Etiology and pathophysiology
1. Disease of the mastoid process; may be acute or chronic
2. Generally occurs secondary to otitis media
3. Disruption of the intercellular construction of the bone; suppurative mastoiditis
4. May lead to meningitis or damage to select cranial nerves

B. Clinical findings
1. Subjective
   a. Tenderness over the mastoid process
   b. Headache and ear pain
   c. Anorexia
   d. Vertigo

2. Objective
   a. Drainage from the ear if perforated
   b. Elevated temperature
   c. Swelling over mastoid process
   d. Reddened, thick tympanic membrane with possible perforation
C. Therapeutic interventions
   1. Antibiotics: eardrops or systemic
   2. Cleansing of the ear
   3. Surgical intervention
      a. Mastoidectomy (radical or modified)
      b. Tympanoplasty

Nursing Care of Clients with Mastoiditis

A. DATA COLLECTION

1. Description of onset and progression of symptoms
2. History to determine previous episodes of otitis media
3. Status of tympanic membrane via otoscopic examination
4. Baseline vital signs

B. ANALYSIS AND INTERPRETATION

Refer to General Nursing Diagnoses for Clients with Neuromusculoskeletal Systems Disorders for the following diagnoses: M 2, Q 1, Q 2, and V 3

C. PLANNING/IMPLEMENTATION

1. Obtain specimen of exudate if present for culture and sensitivity
2. Instruct the client to seek treatment for any ear infections
3. Administer antibiotics as prescribed
4. Instruct client to administer eardrops
5. Observe for facial paralysis and report, since this may indicate damage to facial nerve
6. Instruct the client to report headache or stiff neck immediately because this may indicate meningitis
7. Utilize safety precautions such as side rails to prevent injury to the client who is experiencing vertigo
8. Position client on unaffected side postoperatively

D. EVALUATION/OUTCOMES

1. Reports a reduction in pain
2. Remains free from injury
3. Identifies signs and symptoms of complications such as meningitis or cranial nerve damage

▼ OTOSCLEROSIS

Data Base

A. Etiology and pathophysiology
   1. Fixation of the stapes caused by the growth of bone preventing transmission of vibrations

2. Cause unknown, but incidence higher in females; heredity a factor
B. Clinical findings
   1. Subjective
      a. Loss of hearing
      b. Ringing or buzzing in the ears
   2. Objective
      a. Use of a tuning fork shows bone conduction better than air conduction (Rinne test)
      b. Presence of spongy bone in the labyrinth
C. Therapeutic interventions
   1. Hearing aids to amplify sound
   2. Stapedectomy: removal of the diseased portion of the stapes, and replacement with a prosthetic implant to conduct vibrations from the middle to inner ear

Nursing Care of Clients with Otosclerosis

A. DATA COLLECTION

1. History of onset and progression of symptoms
2. Extent of hearing loss via audiometry
3. Rinne test to evaluate loss of air conduction

B. ANALYSIS AND INTERPRETATION

Refer to General Nursing Diagnoses for Clients with Neuromusculoskeletal Systems Disorders for the following diagnoses: C, I 4, M 2, V 3, and Z

C. PLANNING/IMPLEMENTATION

1. Position postoperatively according to the physician's preference
   a. Lying on the operated side facilitates drainage
   b. Lying on the nonoperated side helps prevent displacement of the graft
2. Instruct the client to alter position gradually to prevent vertigo
3. Question the client about pain, headache, vertigo, or unusual sensations in ear, and report these
4. Instruct the client to avoid sneezing and blowing nose, swimming, showering, and flying until permitted by the physician; if the client must sneeze, instruct to keep the mouth open to equalize pressure in the ear
5. Explain that because of edema from surgery and the presence of packing, hearing will be diminished but will improve

D. EVALUATION/OUTCOMES

1. Reports improved hearing ability
2. Remains free from injury
3. Establishes communication with family members and health care providers
4. Accepts and uses prescribed hearing aid

▼ MÉNIÈRE'S DISEASE (ENDOLYMPHATIC HYDROPS)

Data Base
A. Etiology and pathophysiology
1. Chronic disease of the inner ear causing severe vertigo
2. Cause unknown, but follows infections of the middle ear or trauma
3. Incidence highest in males between the ages of 40 and 60 years
B. Clinical findings
1. Subjective
a. Vertigo
b. Nausea
c. Headache
d. Sensitivity to loud sounds
e. Sensory hearing loss, usually unilateral
f. Tinnitus
2. Objective
a. Vomiting
b. Diaphoresis
c. Nystagmus during attacks
d. Weber test and auditory testing document unilateral hearing loss
C. Therapeutic interventions
1. Diuretics
2. Antihistamines
3. Diazepam (Valium)
4. Surgical destruction of the labyrinth or vestibular nerve, which will cause deafness in that ear
5. Surgical insertion of endolymphatic drainage shunt may relieve symptoms without loss of hearing
6. Salt-free diet

Nursing Care of Clients with Ménière's Disease
A. DATA COLLECTION
1. Description of onset and progression of symptoms
2. History of allergies or infections that may have contributed to the disorder
3. Extent of hearing loss via audiometry
4. Weber test to determine lateralization of hearing
5. Situations that seem to precipitate an attack

B. ANALYSIS AND INTERPRETATION
Refer to General Nursing Diagnoses for Clients with Neuromusculoskeletal Systems Disorders for the following diagnoses: C, I 4, M 2, R 2, T, V 3, X, and Z

C. PLANNING/IMPLEMENTATION
1. Support emotionally
2. To prevent the onset of symptoms, encourage the client not to move rapidly
3. Protect from injury during attack; use side rails; encourage the client to lie down during an attack
4. Instruct the client to pull off the road if driving when an attack occurs
5. Care for the client following a total labyrinthectomy
a. Maintain bed rest in the presence of severe vertigo
b. Instruct the client to avoid sudden movements
c. Explain that Bell's palsy may occur postoperatively but will subside within a few months
6. Teach client that foods high in salt, such as salted meats and fish, cheese, condensed milk, carrots, and spinach, should be avoided

D. EVALUATION/OUTCOMES
1. Reports a reduction in frequency and intensity of vertigo
2. Remains free from injury
3. Demonstrates increased interest in hygiene and other self-care activities
4. Establishes effective communication with family members and health care providers

MEDICAL-SURGICAL
REVIEW QUESTIONS

Growth and Development

1. When planning discharge teaching for a 22-year-old, the nurse should include the potential health problems common in this age group. The nurse can accomplish this by making the client aware of:
   1. Kidney dysfunction
   2. Cardiovascular diseases
   3. Accidents and their prevention
   4. Eye problems, such as glaucoma

2. Elderly people have a high incidence of hip fractures because of:
   1. Carelessness
   2. Fragility of bone
   3. Sedentary existence
   4. Rheumatoid diseases

3. The occurrence of chronic illness is greatest in:
   1. Older adults
   2. Adolescents
   3. Young children
   4. Middle-aged adults

4. The nurse would expect an elderly client with a hearing loss caused by aging to have:
   1. Copious, moist cerumen
   2. Tears in the tympanic membrane
   3. Difficulty hearing women's voices
   4. Overgrowth of the epithelial auditory lining

5. A test that should be included in the yearly physical examination of men during the late middle and older adult years is:
   1. PSA
   2. ELISA
   3. Western blot
   4. Serum triglycerides

Emotional Needs Related to Health Problems

6. A nursing diagnosis represents the:
   1. Proposed plan of care
   2. Client's health problems
   3. Assessment of client data
   4. Actual nursing intervention

7. The nurse who collaborates directly with the client to establish and implement a plan of care is the:
   1. Primary nurse
   2. Nurse clinician
   3. Clinical specialist
   4. Nurse coordinator

8. The determining factor in the revision of a nursing care plan is the:
   1. Time available for care
   2. Validity of the diagnoses
   3. Method for providing care
   4. Effectiveness of the interventions

9. Nursing process can be defined as the:
   1. Implementation of nursing care by the nurse
   2. Steps the nurse employs to provide nursing care
   3. Process the nurse uses to determine nursing goals
   4. Activities a nurse employs to identify a nursing problem

10. To utilize the nursing process, the nurse must first:
    1. Identify goals for nursing care
    2. State the client's nursing needs
    3. Obtain information about the client
    4. Evaluate the effectiveness of nursing actions

11. The effectiveness of nurse-client communication is best validated by:
    1. Client feedback
    2. Medical assessments
    3. Health team conferences
    4. Client's physiologic adaptations

12. While taking a nursing history from a client the nurse promotes communication by:
    1. Asking "why" and "how" questions
    2. Using broad, open-ended statements
    3. Reassuring the client that there is no cause for alarm
    4. Asking questions that can be answered by a "yes" or "no"

13. The best definition of a tort is:
    1. The application of force to the person of another by a reasonable individual
    2. An illegality committed by one person against the property or person of another
    3. Doing something that a reasonable person under ordinary circumstances would not do
    4. An illegality committed against the public and punishable by the law through the courts

14. Examples of intentional torts include:
    1. Malpractice and assault
    2. Malpractice and negligence
    3. False imprisonment and battery
    4. Negligence and invasion of privacy

15. Nurses are protected from all legal action when they:
    1. Offer health teaching regarding family planning
    2. Offer first aid at the scene of an automobile-bus accident
    3. Administer CPR measures on an unconscious child pulled from a swimming pool
    4. Report incidents of suspected child abuse to the appropriate authorities identified in legislation and policies

16. The primary purpose for the regulation of nursing practice is to protect:
    1. The public
    2. Practicing nurses
    3. The employing agency
    4. Professional standards

17. When obtaining consent for surgery, initially the nurse should:
    1. Explain the risks involved in the surgery
    2. Explain that obtaining the signature is routine for any surgery
    3. Evaluate if the client's knowledge level is sufficient to give consent
    4. Witness the signature because this is what the nurse's signature documents

18. A client is voluntarily admitted to the psychiatric unit. Later the client develops severe pain in the right lower quadrant and is diagnosed as having acute appendicitis. When preparing the client for an appendectomy the nurse should:
    1. Have two nurses witness the operative consent as the client signs it
    2. Have the surgeon and the psychiatrist sign for the surgery, since it is an emergency procedure

3. Phone the client's next of kin to come in to sign the consent form because the client is on the psychiatric unit
4. Ask the client to sign the preoperative consent form after being informed of the procedure and required care

19. A client is placed on a stretcher and restrained with Velcro straps while being transported to the x-ray department. A Velcro strap breaks, and the client falls to the floor, sustaining a fractured arm. Later the client states, "The Velcro strap was worn just at the very spot where the strap snapped." The nurse is:
    1. Exempt from any lawsuit because of the doctrine of *respondeat superior*
    2. Totally and singly responsible for the obvious negligence because of failure to report defective equipment
    3. Liable, along with the employer, for misapplication of equipment or use of defective equipment that harms the client
    4. Completely exonerated, since only the hospital, as principal employer, is primarily responsible for the quality and maintenance of equipment

20. The nurse insists that a medication for sleep be taken at 2100 h even though the client states, "I never went to sleep this early and I would like the medication later." Later the client awakens and is confused. The client tries to get out of bed and in so doing falls, fracturing a hip. Legally:
    1. The time the medication was given has nothing to do with the confusion
    2. Client's rights have precedence over hospital policy or physician's orders
    3. Hospital policy requires that sleep medications be given at 2100 h and *respondeat superior* applies
    4. When the physician orders a medication, it must be given at the scheduled time unless the nursing supervisor authorizes differently

21. The nurse will understand the emotional aspects of ulcerative colitis more readily by recognizing the stress-related functions of the:
    1. Cerebral cortex and thyroid gland
    2. Central nervous system and hypothalamus
    3. Sympathetic nervous system and pancreas
    4. Autonomic nervous system and adrenal glands

22. To give nursing care to a client, the nurse must first:
    1. Understand the client's emotional conflict

2. Develop rapport with the client's physician
3. Talk with the client's family or significant other
4. Recognize personal feelings toward this client

23. When a physically ill client is being overtly verbally hostile, the most appropriate nursing response would be a:
    1. Verbal defense of the staff's actions
    2. Reasonable exploration of the situation
    3. Silent acceptance of the client's behavior
    4. Complete withdrawal from the client

24. A client becomes openly hostile when learning that amputation of a gangrenous toe is being considered. The best indication that the nurse's interaction has been therapeutic would be:
    1. An increase in physical activity
    2. A relaxation of tensed muscles
    3. An absence of further outbursts
    4. A denial that further discussion is necessary

25. After being medicated for anxiety a client who has congestive heart failure says to the nurse, "I guess you are too busy to stay with me." The best response in this circumstance is:
    1 "I have to see other clients."
    2 "The medication will help you rest soon."
    3. "You will feel better; I will adjust your oxygen mask."
    4. "I have to go now, but I will come back in 10 minutes."

26. A 35-year-old executive secretary is hospitalized for treatment of severe hypertension. The physician orders Capoten and Xanax. The client quickly finds fault with the therapeutic regimen and nursing care. The nurse recognizes this behavior is probably a manifestation of the client's:
    1. Denial of illness
    2. Fear of the health problem
    3. Response to cerebral anoxia
    4. Reaction to hypertensive medications

27. A client with a history of hypertension is hospitalized with a transient ischemic attack (TIA). The client has been told to stop smoking. The nurse discovers a pack of cigarettes in the client's bathrobe. The best course of action to take at this time is to:
    1. Let the client know they were found
    2. Report the situation to the head nurse
    3. Call the physician and request directions
    4. Discard them without making a comment

28. The nurse is aware that characteristic behavior in the initial stage of coping with dying includes:
    1. Crying uncontrollably
    2. Criticizing medical care
    3. Refusing to receive visitors
    4. Asking for additional medical consultations

29. A client with cancer of the lung says to the nurse, "If I could just be free of pain for a few days, I might be able to eat more and regain strength." In reference to the stages of dying, the client indicates:
    1. Frustration
    2. Bargaining
    3. Depression
    4. Rationalization

30. When reaching the point of acceptance in the stages of dying, a client's behavior may reflect:
    1. Apathy
    2. Euphoria
    3. Detachment
    4. Emotionalism

31. A client who has reached the point of acceptance in the stages of dying appears happy but demonstrates a lack of involvement with the environment. The nurse can best deal with this client by:
    1. Ignoring the client's behavior when possible
    2. Pointing out the reality of the situation to the client
    3. Joining the client in denial because this is a defense
    4. Recognizing and accepting the client's behavior at this point

32. The family of a client who is terminally ill is likely to require more emotional nursing care than the client when the client reaches the stage of:
    1. Anger
    2. Denial
    3. Depression
    4. Acceptance

33. A client with a terminal illness reaches the stage of acceptance. The nurse can best help during this stage by:
    1. Allowing the client to cry
    2. Allowing unrestricted visiting
    3. Explaining all that is being done
    4. Being around though not necessarily speaking

34. A client asks the nurse, "Should I tell my husband I have AIDS?" The nurse's most appropriate response would be:
    1. "This is a decision you alone can make."
    2. "Do not tell him anything unless he asks."
    3. "You are having difficulty deciding what to say."
    4. "Tell him you feel you contracted AIDS from him."

35. A client who is scheduled for a hysterectomy for cervical cancer is upset about being unable to have more children. The nurse should:
    1. Evaluate her willingness to pursue adoption
    2. Encourage her to focus on her own recovery
    3. Emphasize that she does have two children already
    4. Ensure that all treatment options have been explored

36. A client who is scheduled to have a hysterectomy starts to sob and says, "I told my husband today that after this operation I will only be half a woman. He reassured me, but I know that was just a front." The most appropriate response would be:
    1. "It must be frightening to know that your husband rejects you as a woman."
    2. "You feel this operation will have an effect on how your husband feels about you as his wife?"
    3. "You know of course that this is silly. I wish you would not worry about such irrelevant things. The main thing is that you have to get well quickly."
    4. "I think I'll call your physician who may want to postpone the operation until you and your husband have adjusted better to the outcomes of a hysterectomy."

37. A male physician, who is found in a diabetic coma, has omitted information about a history of diabetes mellitus from his health record. This pertinent information has most likely been omitted because:
    1. Individuals with diabetes mellitus often have lapses of memory
    2. Physicians with diabetes are not accepted for residency in many hospitals
    3. He needs assistance in developing a more favorable adaptation to this stress
    4. He is unable to handle the psychologic stress related to alterations in body functioning

38. Despite initiation of therapy for peptic ulcer disease, a client continues to be apprehensive and restless. Nursing action should include:

1. Teaching the importance of rest
2. Administering antibiotics as ordered
3. Encouraging the expression of concerns
4. Explaining that everything will be all right

39. After having a transverse colostomy, the client asks what effect the surgery will have on future sexual relationships. The nurse should explain that:
    1. Sexual relationships must be curtailed for several weeks
    2. The client will be able to resume normal sexual relationships
    3. The surgery will temporarily decrease the client's sexual impulses
    4. The partner should be told about the surgery prior to any sexual activity

40. The nurse recognizes that the prognosis for a 25-year-old client with an acute attack of ulcerative colitis will remain guarded until:
    1. A high residue diet is followed
    2. The client's emotional conflicts are solved
    3. The client's endocrine activity decreases with age
    4. A surgical procedure is performed to remove the physiologic cause

41. When creating a therapeutic environment for a client who has just had a myocardial infarction, the nurse should provide for:
    1. Short family visits
    2. Telephone communication
    3. Television for short periods
    4. Daily papers in the morning

42. After being scheduled for a colostomy, a client's anxiety is overt and realistic. The most effective way for the nurse to help the client at this point would be to:
    1. Administer a prescribed prn sedative
    2. Encourage the client to express feelings
    3. Explain the procedure and postoperative course
    4. Reassure the client that many people cope with this problem

43. A client complains that low-salt food is very tasteless. The nurse's best response would be:
    1. "I know how difficult it is for you"
    2. "You miss your ham and cabbage?"
    3. "Salt can be very harmful to your health."
    4. "Ask the doctor if you can splurge occasionally."

44. While receiving a preoperative enema a client starts to cry and says, "I'm sorry you have to do

this messy thing for me." The best response by the nurse at this time would be:
1. "I don't mind it."
2. "You are upset."
3. "This is part of my job."
4. "Nurses get used to this."

45. The best approach for the nurse to use when helping a client express anxiety over a scheduled D&C and conization would be to:
1. Ask, "What are you really upset about?"
2. Explain that a conization and a D&C are considered minor surgery
3. Say, "I can tell that something is troubling you. It might help to talk about it."
4. Tell the client that it is normal to be anxious; everybody is fearful, even though there is no reason to worry

46. The emotional responses of a client with a left cerebral vascular accident (CVA) would be most influenced by the:
1. Care the client is receiving
2. Location of the client's lesion
3. Client's premorbid personality
4. Ability of the client to understand the illness

47. When helping a client with a CVA to develop independence, the nurse should:
1. Establish long-range goals for the client
2. Reinforce success in tasks accomplished
3. Point out errors in performance on which to focus
4. Demonstrate ways the client can regain independence in activities

48. When helping a client immobilized by the pain of rheumatoid arthritis toward self-reliance and independence, the nurse should approach the problem with:
1. A series of limited objectives
2. A positive attitude toward the eventual outcome
3. The understanding that little can be accomplished
4. The recognition that a nursing home type facility is needed

49. The spouse of a client with a CVA insists on doing everything for the client during visits. After these visits the client seems to be quite depressed. The nurse should assume that the client is probably:
1. Losing faith in the future
2. Feeling the loss of independence
3. Feeling guilty about being a burden
4. Experiencing the problem that is a natural part of this illness

50. The spouse of a client who has had a CVA seems unable to accept the idea that the client must be encouraged to participate in self-care. The nurse may be able to work around these feelings by:
1. Telling the spouse to let the client do things independently
2. Allowing the spouse to assume total responsibility for the client's care
3. Explaining that the nursing staff has full responsibility for client's activities
4. Asking the spouse for assistance in planning activities most helpful to the client

51. A client with hemiplegia is staring blankly at the wall and complains of feeling like half a person. Initially nursing care for this client should be directed at:
1. Distracting the client from self-pity
2. Including the client in all decisions
3. Helping the client explore personal feelings
4. Preventing the client from developing contractures

52. Immediately after a storm has passed, the rescue team with which the nurse is working is searching for injured people. A victim lying next to a broken natural gas main is not breathing and is bleeding heavily from a wound on the foot. The nurse's first step would be to:
1. Treat the victim for shock
2. Start rescue breathing immediately
3. Apply surface pressure to the foot wound
4. Remove the victim from the immediate vicinity

53. When a disaster occurs, the nurse may have to treat mass hysteria first. The person or persons to be cared for immediately would be those in:
1. Panic
2. Coma
3. Euphoria
4. Depression

Fluid and Electrolytes

54. A nurse administers an intravenous solution of 0.45% sodium chloride. With respect to human blood cells, this solution is:
1. Isotonic
2. Isomeric
3. Hypotonic
4. Hypertonic

55. Two body systems that interact with the bicarbonate buffer system to preserve the normal body fluid pH of 7.4 are the:
    1. Skeletal and nervous systems
    2. Circulatory and urinary systems
    3. Respiratory and urinary systems
    4. Muscular and endocrine systems

56. The statement that correctly compares blood plasma and interstitial fluid is:
    1. Both contain the same kinds of ions
    2. Plasma exerts lower osmotic pressure than does interstitial fluid
    3. Plasma contains slightly more of each kind of ion than does interstitial fluid
    4. The main cation in plasma is sodium, whereas the main cation in interstitial fluid is potassium

57. Ammonia is excreted by the kidney to help maintain:
    1. Osmotic pressure of the blood
    2. Acid-base balance of the body
    3. Low bacterial levels in the urine
    4. Normal red blood cell production

58. The nurse understands that a client with albuminuria has edema caused by a:
    1. Fall in tissue hydrostatic pressure
    2. Rise in plasma hydrostatic pressure
    3. Fall in plasma colloid oncotic pressure
    4. Rise in tissue colloid osmotic pressure

59. The percentage of water in the average adult human body is:
    1. 80%
    2. 60%
    3. 40%
    4. 20%

60. The receptors for the regulation of body water through detection of osmotic pressure are located in the:
    1. Blood
    2. Hypothalamus
    3. Kidney tubules
    4. Neurohypophysis

61. The major role in maintaining fluid balance in the body is performed by the:
    1. Liver
    2. Heart
    3. Lungs
    4. Kidneys

62. The weight of extracellular body fluid is approximately 20% of the total body weight of an average individual. The component of the extracellular fluid that contributes the greatest portion to this amount is the:
    1. Plasma fluid
    2. Interstitial fluid
    3. Fluid in dense tissue
    4. Fluid in body secretions

63. The most important electrolyte of intracellular fluid is:
    1. Sodium
    2. Calcium
    3. Chloride
    4. Potassium

64. The body fluids that make up 40% to 50% of the total body weight are:
    1. Interstitial
    2. Intracellular
    3. Extracellular
    4. Intravascular

65. When intravenous fluid is allowed to flow into a person by gravity:
    1. Potential energy is converted to kinetic energy
    2. Kinetic energy is converted to potential energy
    3. Chemical energy is converted to kinetic energy
    4. Potential energy is converted to chemical energy

66. A solution containing 1 gram-equivalent weight of solute in 1 L of solution is called:
    1. A molar solution
    2. A normal solution
    3. An isotonic solution
    4. A saturated solution

67. The coronary care unit nurse draws an arterial blood sample to assess a client for acidosis. A normal pH for arterial blood is:
    1. 7.0
    2. 7.30
    3. 7.42
    4. 7.50

68. The nurse must be alert for signs of respiratory acidosis in the client with emphysema because this individual has a long-term problem with oxygen maintenance and:
    1. The carbon dioxide is not excreted
    2. Hyperventilation occurs, even if the cause is not physiologic
    3. There is a loss of carbon dioxide from the body's buffer pool

4. Localized tissue necrosis occurs as a result of poor oxygen supply to the area

69. A client is in a state of uncompensated acidosis. The nurse would expect the arterial blood pH to be approximately:
   1. 6.9
   2. 7.2
   3. 7.45
   4. 7.48

70. Potassium chloride, 20 mEq, is to be added to 1 liter of IV solution of a client with diabetic ketoacidosis. The primary purpose for administering this drug is:
   1. Treatment of hyperpnea
   2. Prevention of flaccid paralysis
   3. Replacement of potassium deficit
   4. Treatment of cardiac dysrhythmias

71. Larger than normal amounts of acetoacetic acid have been entering the blood as one of the indirect results of a client's insulin deficiency. Like lactic acid and other nonvolatile acids, acetoacetic acid is buffered in the blood chiefly by:
   1. Potassium
   2. Bicarbonate
   3. Carbon dioxide
   4. Sodium chloride

72. The nurse must assess the client with gastric lavage or prolonged vomiting for:
   1. Acidosis
   2. Alkalosis
   3. Loss of oxygen from the blood
   4. Loss of osmotic pressure of the blood

73. The nurse explains to a client that it is not advisable to take bicarbonate of soda regularly. This statement is based on knowledge that bicarbonate of soda can cause:
   1. Gastric distention
   2. Metabolic alkalosis
   3. Chronic constipation
   4. Cardiac dysrhythmias

74. Following extensive, prolonged surgery it is most important that the nurse observe the client for the depletion of the electrolyte:
   1. Sodium
   2. Calcium
   3. Chloride
   4. Potassium

75. A client is admitted with diarrhea, anorexia, weight loss, and abdominal cramps, and a diagnosis of colitis is made. The symptoms of fluid and electrolyte imbalance caused by this condition that the nurse should report immediately are:
   1. Skin rash, diarrhea, and diplopia
   2. Extreme muscle weakness and tachycardia
   3. Development of tetany with muscle spasms
   4. Nausea, vomiting, and leg and stomach cramps

76. When an intestinal obstruction is suspected a client has a nasogastric tube inserted and attached to suction. Critical assessment of this client includes observation for:
   1. Edema
   2. Belching
   3. Dehydration
   4. Excessive salivation

77. When preparing an IV piggyback medication for a client the nurse is aware that it is essential to:
   1. Use strict sterile technique
   2. Rotate the bag after adding the medication
   3. Use exactly 100 ml of fluid to mix the medication
   4. Change the needle prior to adding the medication

78. An IV of 1000 ml 5% dextrose in water to be infused at 125 ml/hr is started on admission to correct fluid imbalance. The infusion set delivers 10 drops per milliliter. To regulate the rate of flow so that the solution would be infused over an 8-hour period, the nurse should set the rate of flow at:
   1. 20 drops per minute
   2. 40 drops per minute
   3. 60 drops per minute
   4. 160 drops per minute

79. The intake and output for a client over an 8-hour period is:
   0800: IV with D5W infusing and 900 ml left in bag
   0830: 150 ml urine voided
   0900-1500: 200 ml gastric tube formula and 50 ml water at q3h intervals; no aspirate obtained until final feeding; 25 ml at this time
   0800-1600: vitamin solution, 10 ml q4h
   1300: 220 ml voided
   1515: 235 ml voided
   1600: IV with 550 ml left in bag

   The nurse calculates the intake and output as:
   1. Intake, 930 ml; output, 650 ml
   2. Intake, 1050 ml; output, 680 ml
   3. Intake, 1080 ml; output, 595 ml
   4. Intake, 1130 ml; output, 630 ml

80. A serious complication of acute malaria is:
    1. Congested lungs
    2. Impaired peristalsis
    3. Anemia and cachexia
    4. Fluid and electrolyte imbalance

81. The nurse must assess a client experiencing excessive production of antidiuretic hormone for:
    1. Polyuria
    2. Dehydration
    3. Hyponatremia
    4. Hyperglycemia

82. In the emergent phase immediately after a severe burn injury, care is centered on replacement therapy by IV fluids. The nurse should question the physician's order if it is designed to provide:
    1. Water
    2. Potassium
    3. Lactated Ringer's
    4. Plasma expanders

83. The client is receiving 5% dextrose in water at a slow rate. The nurse should be aware that the longest period of time that one bag can be infused without producing untoward effects would be:
    1. 6 hours
    2. 12 hours
    3. 18 hours
    4. 24 hours

84. A client is to receive 2000 ml of IV fluid in 12 hours. The drop factor is 10 gtt/ml. The nurse should regulate the flow so the number of drops per minute is approximately:
    1. 27 to 29
    2. 30 to 32
    3. 40 to 42
    4. 48 to 50

85. The nurse is aware that ascites can be related to:
    1. Portal hypotension
    2. Kidney malfunction
    3. Diminished plasma protein
    4. Decreased production of potassium

86. The nurse is aware that negative nitrogen balance most directly occurs in a client receiving IV administration of 5% dextrose in water due to:
    1. Insufficient carbohydrate intake
    2. Lack of protein supplementation
    3. Insufficient intake of water-soluble vitamins
    4. Increased concentration of electrolytes in cells

87. A client has an IV infusion. If the IV infusion infiltrates, the nurse should first:
    1. Elevate the IV site
    2. Discontinue the infusion
    3. Attempt to flush the tube
    4. Apply warm, moist soaks

88. While a client is receiving albumin, the planned therapeutic effect will be greater if the infusion is regulated to run:
    1. Rapidly, and fluids are encouraged
    2. Slowly, and fluid intake is restricted
    3. Rapidly, and fluid intake is withheld
    4. Slowly, and fluids are encouraged liberally

89. The nurse administers serum albumin to a client to assist in:
    1. Clotting of blood
    2. Formation of red blood cells
    3. Activation of white blood cells
    4. Development of oncotic pressure

90. A client who is receiving furosemide (Lasix) and digoxin (Lanoxin) should be observed for symptoms of electrolyte depletion caused by:
    1. Diuretic therapy
    2. Sodium restriction
    3. Continuous dyspnea
    4. Inadequate oral intake

91. The nurse, recognizing that digitalis preparations promote diuresis, should evaluate clients for a depletion of:
    1. Sodium
    2. Calcium
    3. Potassium
    4. Phosphate

92. A client with hypokalemia is placed on a cardiac monitor to evaluate cardiac activity during IV potassium replacement. Before starting the IV, the nurse observes the monitor, which shows:
    1. Lowering of the T wave
    2. Elevation of the ST segment
    3. Shortening of the QRS complex
    4. Increased deflection of the Q wave

93. An IV solution containing potassium inadvertently infuses too rapidly. The physician prescribes insulin added to a 10% dextrose in water solution. The rationale for the order is:
    1. Potassium moves into body cells with glucose and insulin
    2. Increased insulin accelerates excretion of glucose and potassium
    3. Glucose and insulin increase metabolism and accelerate potassium excretion

4. Increased potassium causes a temporary slowing of pancreatic production of insulin

94. The nurse suspects hypokalemia is present when a client has:
1. Edema, bounding pulse, confusion
2. Spasms, diarrhea, irregular pulse rate
3. Apathy, weakness, abdominal distention
4. Sunken eyeballs, Kussmaul breathing, thirst

95. Intravenous orders state that the client is to receive 1000 ml of fluid every 8 hours. If the equipment delivers 15 drops/minute, the nurse should regulate the flow at approximately:
1. 15 drops/min
2. 23 drops/min
3. 31 drops/min
4. 60 drops/min

96. When taking the blood pressure of a client who has had a thyroidectomy, the nurse notices the client is pale and has spasms of the hand and notifies the physician. While awaiting the physician's orders, the nurse should prepare for the replacement of:
1. Calcium
2. Magnesium
3. Bicarbonate
4. Potassium chloride

97. An intravenous piggyback (IVPB) of cefazolin sodium (Ancef) 500 mg in 50 ml of 5% dextrose in water is to be administered over a 20-minute period. The tubing has a drop factor of 15 drops per milliliter. The nurse should regulate the infusion to run at:
1. 28 drops/min
2. 38 drops/min
3. 58 drops/min
4. 76 drops/min

Cardiovascular

98. The nurse identifies a commonality between the strain on a client's heart with prolonged anemia or polycythemia to be:
1. Pressure
2. Temperature
3. Cardiac output
4. Surface tension

99. A client with pyrexia will most likely demonstrate:
1. Dyspnea
2. Precordial pain
3. Increased pulse rate
4. Elevated blood pressure

100. Nursing care of a client with a fractured hip should include the assessment of pedal pulses. The important characteristics of pedal pulses are:
1. Contractility and rate
2. Color of skin and rhythm
3. Amplitude and symmetry
4. Local temperature and visible pulsations

101. The nurse assesses that a client's pulse pressure is decreasing. This would be evaluated by calculating the:
1. Force exerted against an arterial wall
2. Difference between the apical and radial rates
3. Difference between systolic and diastolic readings
4. Degree of ventricular contraction in relation to output

102. Infection with Group A beta-hemolytic streptococci is associated with:
1. Rheumatic fever
2. Hepatitis Type A
3. Spinal meningitis
4. Rheumatoid arthritis

103. In the post-anesthesia unit, while caring for a client who has received a general anesthetic, the nurse should notify the physician if the:
1. Client pushes out the airway
2. Client has snoring respirations
3. Respirations are regular but shallow
4. Systolic blood pressure drops from 130 to 100 mm Hg

104. Postural changes immediately after spinal anesthesia may result in hypotension because there is:
1. Dilation of capacitance vessels
2. Decreased response of baroreceptors
3. Decreased strength of cardiac contractions
4. Interruption of cardiac accelerator pathways

105. After abdominal surgery a client suddenly complains of numbness in the right leg and a "funny feeling" in the toes. The nurse should first:
1. Elevate the legs and tell the client to stay in bed
2. Tell the client to remain in bed and notify the physician
3. Rub the client's legs to start circulation and cover the client with a warm blanket
4. Tell the client about the dangers of staying in bed too much and encourage ambulation

106. Following a bilateral lumbar sympathectomy a client has a sudden drop in blood pressure but no evidence of bleeding. The nurse recognizes that this is most likely caused by:
    1. An inadequate fluid intake
    2. The after effects of anesthesia
    3. A reallocation of the blood supply
    4. An increased level of epinephrine

107. Prolonged bed rest after surgery appears to promote hemostasis, particularly in the deep veins of the calves. The most likely pathologic result of such hemostasis may be thrombus formation and:
    1. Cerebral embolism
    2. Coronary occlusion
    3. Pulmonary embolism
    4. Dry gangrene of a limb

108. The nurse understands that a pulmonary embolism is a most unlikely complication in the postoperative period following:
    1. Hysterectomy
    2. Prostatectomy
    3. Appendectomy
    4. Saphenous vein ligation

109. While convalescing from abdominal surgery a client develops thrombophlebitis. The sign that would indicate this complication to the nurse would be:
    1. Intermittent claudication
    2. Pitting edema of the lower extremities
    3. Severe pain on extension of an extremity
    4. Localized warmth and tenderness of the leg

110. To prevent a pulmonary embolus in a client on bed rest, the nurse should:
    1. Limit the client's fluid intake
    2. Encourage deep breathing and coughing
    3. Use the knee gatch when the client is in bed
    4. Teach the client to move the legs when in bed

111. A client is being instructed on the use of elastic stockings. The nurse should teach the client that the stockings should be:
    1. Alternately kept on 2 hours and off 2 hours
    2. Worn only at night when activity is lessened
    3. Put on before getting out of bed in the morning
    4. Left in place until the physician advises otherwise

112. The nurse should be aware that arteriosclerosis of blood vessels leading to the brain may not become evident until there is an extremely severe blockage or until a stroke occurs because of collateral blood circulation supplied through the:

    1. Circle of Willis
    2. Jugular vessels
    3. The bicarotid trunk
    4. Hypothalamic-hypophyseal portal system

113. After a client has an endarterectomy the nurse should plan to observe for a change in:
    1. Appetite
    2. Skin color
    3. Bowel habits
    4. Tissue turgor

114. The nurse should teach clients with peripheral vascular disease to stop smoking because nicotine:
    1. Constricts the superficial vessels, dilating the deep vessels
    2. Constricts the peripheral vessels and increases the force of flow
    3. Dilates the superficial vessels but constricts the collateral circulation
    4. Dilates the peripheral vessels, causing a reflex constriction of visceral vessels

115. With chronic occlusive arterial disease the precipitating cause for ulceration and gangrenous lesions often is:
    1. Emotional stress, which is short lived
    2. Poor hygiene and limited protein intake
    3. Stimulants such as coffee, tea, or cola drinks
    4. Trauma from mechanical, chemical, or thermal sources

116. When obtaining data from a client with thromboangiitis obliterans (Buerger's disease), the nurse would expect the client to demonstrate or report:
    1. Easy fatigue of extremities, continuous claudication
    2. General blanching of skin, intermittent claudication
    3. Intermittent claudication, burning pain after exposure to cold
    4. Burning pain precipitated by cold exposure, fatigue, blanching of skin

117. A simple test for varicose veins is the:
    1. Arteriography
    2. Babinski reflex
    3. Romberg's sign
    4. Trendelenburg test

118. Following a vein ligation and stripping, the client should be positioned:
    1. Flat with the knee gatch engaged
    2. Supine with the legs elevated at 30-degrees

3. In a semi-Fowler's position with the knees flexed
4. With the head elevated and the feet against a footboard

119. When considering the factors affecting the development of essential hypertension, the nurse understands its primary cause is thought to be:
   1. Kidney failure
   2. Unresolved grief
   3. Unexpressed rage
   4. Generalized arteriosclerosis

120. The nurse explains to a client that the mechanism mediating long-term blood pressure regulation is the:
   1. Capillary fluid shifts
   2. Fight or flight response
   3. Adjustment of urinary output
   4. Nervous system baroreceptors

121. To assess the effectiveness of a vasodilator administered to lower hypertension, the nurse should take the client's pulse and blood pressure:
   1. Prior to administering the drug
   2. Thirty minutes after giving the drug
   3. Immediately after the client gets out of bed
   4. After the client has been supine for 5 minutes

122. When teaching a client about orthostatic hypotension, the nurse should explain that it can be modified by:
   1. Wearing support hose continuously
   2. Lying down for 30 minutes after taking the drug
   3. Avoiding tasks that require high energy expenditures
   4. Sitting on the edge of the bed a short time before arising

123. To avoid an error of parallax when taking a client's blood pressure, the nurse should:
   1. Use a narrow cuff
   2. Read it at eye level
   3. Stand close to the manometer
   4. Elevate the client's arm on a pillow

124. A 2 g sodium diet is prescribed for a client with severe hypertension. The client does not like the diet, and the nurse hears the client tell a friend to bring in some "good home-cooked food." It would be most effective for the nurse to plan to:
   1. Call in the dietitian for client teaching
   2. Wait for the client's family and discuss the diet with the client and family

3. Tell the client that the use of salt is forbidden, because it will raise the blood pressure
4. Catch the family members before they go into the client's room and tell them about the diet

Client Case Scenario 1: Lily Johnson, a 64-year-old housewife, is admitted to the hospital with a diagnosis of anginal pain. **Items 125 to 131 refer to this client case scenario.**

125. Mrs. Johnson states that her anginal pain increases after activity. The nurse should realize that angina pectoris is a sign of:
   1. Mitral insufficiency
   2. Myocardial ischemia
   3. Myocardial infarction
   4. Coronary thrombosis

126. Mrs. Johnson asks what the coronary arteries have to do with angina. When determining the answer, the nurse should take into consideration that the coronary arteries:
   1. Supply blood to the endocardium
   2. Carry blood from the aorta to the myocardium
   3. Carry reduced-oxygen-content blood to the lungs
   4. Carry high-oxygen-content blood from the lungs toward the heart

127. The nurse realizes that the pain associated with a coronary occlusion is caused primarily by:
   1. Arterial spasm
   2. Ischemia of the heart muscle
   3. Blocking of the coronary veins
   4. Irritation of nerve endings in the cardiac plexus

128. Nitroglycerin SL is prescribed for Mrs. Johnson's anginal pain. When teaching how to use nitroglycerin, the nurse tells her to place 1 tablet under the tongue when pain occurs and to repeat the dose in 5 minutes if pain persists. The nurse should also tell Mrs. Johnson to:
   1. Place 2 tablets under the tongue when intense pain occurs
   2. Swallow 1 tablet and place 1 tablet under the tongue when pain is intense
   3. Place 1 tablet under the tongue 3 minutes before activity and repeat the dose in 5 minutes if pain occurs
   4. Place 1 tablet under the tongue when pain occurs and use an additional tablet after the attack to prevent recurrence

129. Cholesterol, frequently discussed in relation to atherosclerosis, is a substance that:
    1. May be controlled by eliminating food sources
    2. Is found in many foods, both plant and animal sources
    3. All persons would be better off without because it causes the disease process
    4. Circulates in the blood, the level of which responds usually to dietary substitutions of unsaturated fats for saturated fats

130. When cardiovascular disease is a concern, reduction of the saturated fat in the diet may be desired and substitutes made of polyunsaturated fat. When teaching about this diet the nurse should instruct Mrs. Johnson to avoid:
    1. Fish
    2. Corn oil
    3. Whole milk
    4. Soft margarine

131. When teaching Mrs. Johnson, who has been placed on a high-unsaturated fatty acid diet, the nurse should stress the importance of increasing the intake of:
    1. Enriched whole milk
    2. Red meats, such as beef
    3. Vegetables and whole grains
    4. Liver and other glandular organ meats

Client Case Scenario 2: William Topper, age 72, is admitted through emergency to the coronary care unit (CCU). He is suspected of having a myocardial infarction and scheduled for a heart catheterization. **Items 132 to 138 refer to this client case scenario.**

132. During a cardiac catheterization blood samples from the right atrium, right ventricle, and pulmonary artery are analyzed for their oxygen content. Normally:
    1. All contain less CO_2 than does pulmonary vein blood
    2. All contain more oxygen than does pulmonary vein blood
    3. The samples all contain about the same amount of oxygen
    4. Pulmonary artery blood contains more oxygen than the other samples

133. When caring for Mr. Topper after his cardiac catheterization, it is most important that the nurse:
    1. Provide for rest
    2. Administer oxygen
    3. Check the ECG every 30 minutes
    4. Check pulse distal to the insertion site

134. The nurse in the coronary care unit (CCU) should observe Mr. Topper for one of the more common complications of myocardial infarction, which is:
    1. Hypokalemia
    2. Anaphylactic shock
    3. Cardiac dysrhythmia
    4. Cardiac enlargement

135. When taking Mr. Topper's apical pulse the nurse should place the stethoscope:
    1. Just to the left of the median point of the sternum
    2. In the fifth intercostal space along the left midclavicular line
    3. Between the sixth and seventh ribs at the left midaxillary line
    4. Between the third and fourth ribs and to the left of the sternum

136. Which laboratory tests should the nurse expect the physician to order to confirm Mr. Topper's diagnosis of myocardial infarction?
    1. LD, CK, AST (GOT)
    2. Serum calcium, APPT
    3. Sedimentation rate, ALT
    4. Paul-Bunnell, serum potassium

137. During the acute phase following a myocardial infarction, the nurse should make Mr. Topper's bed by:
    1. Changing the top linen and only the necessary bottom linen
    2. Lifting rather than rolling the client from side to side while changing the linen
    3. Changing the linen from top to bottom without lowering the head of the bed
    4. Sliding the client onto a stretcher, remaking the bed, then sliding the client back to the bed

138. Mr. Topper is receiving digoxin (Lanoxin) and will continue taking the drug after discharge. The nurse should be primarily concerned with:
    1. Monitoring vital signs and encouraging gradual increase in activities of daily living
    2. Taking the apical pulse before drug administration and teaching Mr. Topper how to count the pulse rate
    3. Assessing Mr. Topper for changes in cardiac rhythm and planning activity at home based on tolerance
    4. Observing Mr. Topper for return of normal cardiac conduction patterns and for adverse effects of the drug

Client Case Scenario 3: Larry Green, a 76-year-old retired politician, is admitted with cerebral arteriosclerosis, complicated by polycythemia vera. **Items 139 to 141 refer to this client case scenario.**

139. Mr. Green is prescribed Heparin subcutaneously, q6h. If the anticoagulant therapy is effective, the nurse would expect:
    1. A PTT twice the normal value
    2. An absence of ecchymotic areas
    3. A decreased viscosity of the blood
    4. A reduction of confusion and weakness

140. When Mr. Green is receiving anticoagulants, the nursing care should include observations for:
    1. Nausea
    2. Epistaxis
    3. Headache
    4. Chest pain

141. Mr. Green is also receiving Dicumarol, a coumarin derivative. Which test would be most specific for calculating the daily dosage of this anticoagulant?
    1. Clotting time
    2. Bleeding time
    3. Prothrombin time
    4. Sedimentation rate

142. Following open heart surgery a client develops a temperature of 38.8° C. The nurse notifies the physician because elevated temperatures:
    1. Increase the cardiac output
    2. May indicate cerebral edema
    3. May be a forerunner of hemorrhage
    4. Cause diaphoresis and possible chilling

143. When preparing a client for discharge following surgery for a coronary artery bypass graft, the nurse should teach that there will be:
    1. No further drainage from the incisions after hospitalization
    2. A mild fever and extreme fatigue for several weeks following surgery
    3. Little incisional pain and tenderness after 3 to 4 weeks following surgery
    4. Some increase in edema in the leg used for the donor graft with increased activity

144. The nurse suspects a client is in cardiogenic shock. The nurse understands that this type of shock is:
    1. An irreversible phenomenon
    2. A failure of peripheral circulation
    3. Usually a fleeting reaction to tissue injury
    4. Generally caused by decreased blood volume

145. The nurse assists the physician in treating a client in shock. One modality of treatment that employs the physical law explaining the increased venous return accompanying mild vasoconstriction underlies the use of:
    1. Adrenalin in treating shock
    2. Digoxin to increase cardiac output
    3. Sympathectomy in treating hypertension
    4. Rotating tourniquets in pulmonary edema

146. The nurse finds an injured person, sitting in a chair obviously in shock. The nurse should:
    1. Keep the head elevated; give a stimulant in small sips
    2. Apply tourniquets to three extremities, rotating one every 15 minutes
    3. Surround the body with a warm blanket or chemical heating pads if available
    4. Place the person in the supine position, prevent chilling, and give fluids if possible

147. The nurse is to take central venous pressure (CVP) readings every 2 hours. The nurse is aware that:
    1. A normal reading is 60 to 120 mm of water
    2. A high reading may be indicative of dehydration
    3. The zero point of the manometer is level with the midaxilla
    4. The client must be kept flat in bed while the catheter is in place

148. When obtaining a central venous pressure reading the nurse should place the client:
    1. In a low-Fowler's position
    2. Supine in the contour position
    3. In the dorsal recumbent position
    4. On the side opposite to the manometer

149. The nurse prepares a client for insertion of a pulmonary artery catheter (e.g., Swan-Ganz catheter). The nurse teaches the client that the catheter will be inserted to provide information about:
    1. Stroke volume
    2. Cardiac output
    3. Venous pressure
    4. Left ventricular heart failure

Client Care Scenario 4: Patrick Evere, a 69-year-old retired musician, is admitted to the intensive care unit with a diagnosis of Adams-Stokes syndrome. **Items 150 to 156 refer to this client case scenario.**

150. Mr. Evere has a sudden episode of cyanosis and a change in respirations. The nurse starts oxygen administration immediately. In this situation:
    1. Oxygen had not been ordered and therefore should not be administered
    2. The nurse's observations were sufficient to begin administration of oxygen
    3. The symptoms were too vague for the nurse to diagnose a need for oxygen
    4. The physician should have been called for an order before oxygen was begun

151. The nurse institutes safety precautions for Mr. Evere while he is receiving oxygen because oxygen:
    1. Is flammable
    2. Supports combustion
    3. Has unstable properties
    4. Increases apprehension

152. When instituting oxygen therapy, the nurse recognizes that the method of oxygen administration least likely to increase Mr. Evere's apprehension is:
    1. Tent
    2. Mask
    3. Cannula
    4. Catheter

153. The adaptations of Mr. Evere, who has Adams-Stokes syndrome, would most likely include:
    1. Nausea and vertigo
    2. Flushing and slurred speech
    3. Cephalgia and blurred vision
    4. Syncope and low ventricular rate

154. The nurse is aware that the term bradycardia means:
    1. A grossly irregular heartbeat
    2. A heart rate of over 90 per minute
    3. A heart rate of under 60 per minute
    4. A heartbeat that has regular "skipped" beats

155. A permanent pacemaker is implanted in Mr. Evere. The nurse observes the cardiac monitor for the presence of a lethal dysrhythmia requiring immediate intervention. This lethal dysrhythmia is known as:
    1. Atrial fibrillation
    2. Sinus tachycardia
    3. Ventricular fibrillation
    4. Second-degree heart block

156. While a pacemaker catheter is being inserted, Mr. Evere's heart rate drops to 38. The drug the nurse should expect the physician to order is:
    1. Atropine sulfate
    2. Digoxin (Lanoxin)
    3. Lidocaine (Xylocaine)
    4. Procainamide (Pronestyl)

157. A client with a bundle branch block is on a cardiac monitor. The nurse would expect to observe:
    1. Sagging ST segments
    2. Absence of P wave configurations
    3. Inverted T waves following each QRS complex
    4. Widening of QRS complexes to 0.12 second or greater

158. The nurse would prioritize care and provide treatment first for a client with:
    1. Head injuries
    2. A fractured femur
    3. Ventricular fibrillation
    4. A penetrating abdominal wound

159. Cardioversion is a procedure used to convert certain dysrhythmias to normal rhythm. In addition to atrial fibrillation, cardioversion is most effective when the client demonstrates:
    1. Ventricular standstill
    2. Ventricular fibrillation
    3. Ventricular tachycardia
    4. Premature ventricular beats

160. When ventricular fibrillation occurs in a coronary care unit, the first person reaching the client should:
    1. Administer oxygen
    2. Defibrillate the client
    3. Initiate cardiopulmonary resuscitation
    4. Administer sodium bicarbonate intravenously

161. The nurse in the coronary care unit (CCU) understands that the portion of the cardiac monitor that is related to the alarm system for extremes in the heart rate is called the:
    1. Voltmeter
    2. Pacemaker
    3. Oscilloscope
    4. Synchronizer

162. A client who has a myocardial infarction is in the CCU on a cardiac monitor. The nurse observes ventricular irritability on the screen. The nurse should prepare to administer:
    1. Digoxin (Lanoxin)

2. Furosemide (Lasix)
3. Lidocaine (Xylocaine)
4. Norepinephrine bitartrate (Levophed)

163. A client is admitted to the CCU with atrial fibrillation and a rapid ventricular response. The nurse prepares for cardioversion. To overcome the potential danger of inducing ventricular fibrillation during cardioversion, the nurse should ensure that:
    1. The energy level is set at its maximum level
    2. The synchronizer switch is in the "on" position
    3. The skin electrodes are applied after the T wave
    4. The alarm system of the cardiac monitor is functioning simultaneously

Client Care Scenario 5: Stanley Everett has been admitted to the CCU with a tentative diagnosis of bundle branch block. **Items 164 to 167 refer to this client case scenario.**

164. Mr. Everett is to have a pacemaker inserted. The nurse explains that the catheter will be inserted into the subclavian vein and advanced to allow the electrode to be positioned in the:
    1. SA node
    2. Left atrium
    3. Right ventricle
    4. Superior vena cava

165. The nurse realizes that a pacemaker is used in some clients to serve the function normally performed by the:
    1. AV node
    2. SA node
    3. Bundle of His
    4. Accelerator nerves to the heart

166. The physician has inserted a permanent demand pacemaker in Mr. Everett. When teaching, the nurse should:
    1. Instruct Mr. Everett to sleep on two pillows
    2. Encourage him to reduce his former level of activity
    3. Instruct Mr. Everett to take his pulse daily and keep accurate records
    4. Inform him that the pacemaker will function continuously at a set rate

167. To evaluate the effectiveness of Mr. Everett's pacemaker, the nurse ensures that the pulse remains at least:
    1. In a regular rhythm
    2. Above the demand rate

3. Equal to the pacemaker
4. Palpable at distant sites

Client Case Scenario 6: Arturo Rush is admitted to the CCU with atrial fibrillation and a rapid ventricular response. **Items 168 to 172 refer to this client case scenario.**

168. The nurse observes Mr. Rush's cardiac monitor and identifies asystole. This dysrhythmia requires nursing attention because the heart is:
    1. Not beating
    2. Beating slowly
    3. Beating irregularly
    4. Beating very rapidly

169. Mr. Rush goes into cardiac arrest. During the cardiac arrest, the nurse and the arrest team must keep in mind the:
    1. Age of the client
    2. Time the client is anoxic
    3. Emergency medications available
    4. Heart rate of the client before the arrest

170. Mr. Rush has no carotid pulse or respirations. The nurse should:
    1. Initiate a code
    2. Check for a radial pulse
    3. Give four full lung inflations
    4. Compress the lower sternum 15 times

171. When performing cardiac compression on Mr. Rush, the nurse is aware that it is essential to exert vertical downward pressure, which depresses the lower sternum at least:
    1. 1.3 to 2 cm
    2. 2 to 2.5 cm
    3. 2.5 to 4 cm
    4. 4 to 5 cm

172. When performing external cardiac compression on Mr. Rush, the nurse should exert downward vertical pressure on the lower sternum by placing:
    1. The fleshy part of a clenched fist on the lower sternum
    2. The heels of each hand side by side, extending the fingers over the chest
    3. The fingers of one hand on the sternum and the fingers of the other hand on top of them
    4. The heel of one hand on the sternum and the heel of the other on top of it, interlocking the fingers

Client Case Scenario 7: Jane Harvey has an acute episode of right-sided heart failure and is receiving furosemide (Lasix). **Items 173 to 178 refer to this client case scenario.**

173. When taking Mrs. Harvey's admission history, the nurse would expect her to complain of:
   1. Dyspnea, edema, fatigue
   2. Fatigue, vertigo, headache
   3. Weakness, palpitations, nausea
   4. A feeling of distress when breathing

174. The nurse can best assess the degree of edema in an extremity by:
   1. Checking for pitting
   2. Weighing Mrs. Harvey
   3. Measuring the affected area
   4. Observing intake and output

175. When assessing Mrs. Harvey's lower extremities, the nurse expects pitting edema because of the:
   1. Increase in tissue colloid osmotic pressure
   2. Decrease in the plasma colloid osmotic pressure
   3. Increase in the tissue hydrostatic pressure at the arterial end of the capillary bed
   4. Elevation in the plasma hydrostatic pressure at the venous end of the capillary bed

176. The nurse should realize that Mrs. Harvey may develop ascites because of:
   1. Loss of cellular constituents in blood
   2. Rapid osmosis from tissue spaces to cells
   3. Increased pressure within the circulatory system
   4. Rapid diffusion of solutes and solvents into plasma

177. Mrs. Harvey has edematous ankles. To limit edema of the feet the nurse should prepare to:
   1. Restrict fluids
   2. Elevate the legs
   3. Apply elastic bandages
   4. Do range-of-motion exercises

178. The nurse suggests to Mrs. Harvey that air conditioning be used in the summer. This suggestion is made because:
   1. The internal body temperature drops below 37° C
   2. The increased circulation in the skin gives the heart the exercise it needs
   3. The increased circulation in the skin causes excess body heat to radiate away
   4. The heart is relieved of the strain of pumping blood through many miles of blood vessels in the skin

Client Case Scenario 8: Harold McNabb, a 65-year-old self-employed grocer, is admitted to hospital with congestive heart failure and pulmonary edema. **Items 179 to 185 refer to this client case scenario.**

179. When assessing Mr. McNabb with the following medical problems, the nurse would expect pulmonary edema to be associated with:
   1. Mitral stenosis
   2. Pulmonary valve stenosis
   3. Severe arteriosclerosis of the coronary arteries
   4. Calcification and incomplete closure of the tricuspid valve

180. When Mr. McNabb is admitted to the coronary care unit the nurse should be prepared for:
   1. Wet phlebotomy
   2. Postural drainage
   3. Respiratory therapy
   4. Rotating tourniquets

181. Oxygen is ordered for Mr. McNabb. The nurse would expect oxygen via nasal cannula to be set at:
   1. 2 L
   2. 6 L
   3. 8 L
   4. 10 L

182. The nurse attempts to allay Mr. McNabb's anxiety because restlessness:
   1. Increases the cardiac workload
   2. Interferes with normal respiration
   3. Produces an elevation in temperature
   4. Decreases the amount of oxygen available

183. To help alleviate Mr. McNabb's distress due to congestive heart failure and pulmonary edema, the nurse should:
   1. Elevate his lower extremities
   2. Encourage frequent coughing
   3. Place him in an orthopneic position
   4. Prepare him for modified postural drainage

184. Rotating tourniquets are used for Mr. McNabb. The nurse should remember that the:
   1. Tourniquets are rotated every 15 minutes
   2. Two tourniquets are moved at each interval
   3. Automatic tourniquets occlude arterial blood flow
   4. Tourniquets are simultaneously applied to four limbs

185. The nurse is aware that rotating tourniquets are effective for:
   1. Decreasing arterial flow of blood to the body
   2. Decreasing venous flow of blood to the heart

3. Increasing the flow of blood through the capillaries
4. Restricting visceral flow in the internal body cavities

186. A client has edema during the day, and it disappears at night. The client states it is not painful and is located in the lower extremities. The nurse should suspect:
    1. Lung disease
    2. Pulmonary edema
    3. Myocardial infarction
    4. Right ventricular heart failure

Blood and Immunity

187. An example of primary health care by the nurse would be:
    1. Prevention of disabilities
    2. Correction of dietary deficiencies
    3. Establishing goals for rehabilitation
    4. Assisting in immunization programs

188. In general, the higher the red blood cell count:
    1. The higher the blood pH
    2. The lower the hematocrit
    3. The greater the blood viscosity
    4. The less it contributes to immunity

189. The nurse understands that the only molecules that cannot pass through the capillary endothelium are:
    1. Blood gases
    2. Plasma proteins
    3. Glucose and ions
    4. Amino acids and water

190. When caring for a client with an impaired immune system, the nurse recognizes that the blood protein involved is:
    1. Albumin
    2. Globulin
    3. Thrombin
    4. Hemoglobin

191. Antibodies are produced by:
    1. Eosinophils
    2. Plasma cells
    3. Erythrocytes
    4. Lymphocytes

192. A client has a bone marrow aspiration performed. Immediately after the procedure, the nurse should:
    1. Position the client on the affected side
    2. Begin frequent monitoring of vital signs

3. Cleanse the site with an antiseptic solution
4. Briefly apply pressure over the aspiration site

193. When caring for a client who is HIV positive, a primary responsibility of the nurse is to explain how the client can prevent:
    1. AIDS
    2. Social isolation
    3. Other infections
    4. Kaposi's sarcoma

194. When a trauma victim expresses fear that AIDS may develop as a result of a blood transfusion, the nurse should explain that:
    1. Blood is treated with radiation to kill the virus
    2. Screening for the HIV antibodies has minimized this risk
    3. The ability to directly identify HIV has eliminated this concern
    4. Consideration should be given to donating own blood for transfusion

Client Case Scenario 9: Freda Martin, age 36 years, is diagnosed with AIDS and admitted to hospital. She has a 4-month-old daughter whom she has been caring for, even though she has not been feeling well. **Items 195 to 197 refer to this client case scenario.**

195. The nurse should ask Freda:
    1. If she is breastfeeding the baby
    2. If she has hugged or kissed the baby
    3. When the baby last received antibiotics
    4. How long she has been caring for the baby

196. During an AIDS education class, Freda Martin states, "Vaseline works great when I use condoms." The nurse recognizes that this statement indicates:
    1. An understanding of safer sex
    2. The ability to assume self-responsibility
    3. Ignorance concerning the transmission of HIV
    4. A lack of information concerning correct condom use

197. When providing discharge teaching to Freda Martin, the nurse should teach her:
    1. "You need to boil the dishes for 30 minutes after use."
    2. "You need to eat from paper plates and discard them."
    3. "Wash the dishes in hot soapy water as you usually do."
    4. "Let the dishes soak in hot water overnight before washing."

Client Case Scenario 10: Brad Johns is admitted to hospital for whole body radiation for Hodgkin's disease. **Items 198 to 200 refer to this client case scenario.**

198. With Hodgkin's disease the lymph nodes usually affected first are the:
    1. Axillary
    2. Inguinal
    3. Cervical
    4. Mediastinal

199. The highest incidence of Hodgkin's disease is in:
    1. Children
    2. Young adults
    3. Elderly persons
    4. Middle-aged persons

200. Mr. Johns is to have whole-body radiation. The nurse's teaching plan should center around the likely occurrence of increased:
    1. Blood viscosity
    2. Susceptibility to infection
    3. Red blood cell production
    4. Tendency for pathologic fractures

201. Mr. Johns may have destruction of bone marrow, making it unable to function normally. As a result of this, the nurse would expect him to develop:
    1. Increased blood viscosity
    2. Increased tendency for fractures
    3. Decreased number of erythrocytes
    4. Decreased susceptibility to infections

202. The increased tendency toward coronary and cerebral thromboses seen in individuals with polycythemia vera is attributable to the:
    1. Increased viscosity
    2. Fragility of the cells
    3. Elevated blood pressure
    4. Immaturity of red blood cells

203. A serum bilirubin is performed on a client who is weak, dyspneic, and jaundiced. A total plasma bilirubin level above 30 μmol/L could be indicative of:
    1. Hemolytic anemia
    2. Pernicious anemia
    3. Decreased rate of red cell destruction
    4. Low oxygen-carrying capacity of erythrocytes

204. A client with upper gastrointestinal bleeding develops a mild anemia. The nurse should expect the client to be treated with:
    1. Dextran
    2. Epogen
    3. Iron salts
    4. Vitamin B_{12}

Client Case Scenario 11: Myrna Partridge, age 19 years, is admitted to hospital as a result of a serious motor vehicle accident. She has multiple traumas including a ruptured spleen. **Items 205 to 207 refer to this client case scenario.**

205. A splenectomy is performed on Myrna Partridge because:
    1. The spleen is a highly vascular organ
    2. It is anatomically adjacent to the diaphragm
    3. The spleen is the largest lymphoid organ in the body
    4. Rupture of the spleen can cause diseases of the liver

206. In the immediate postoperative period following a splenectomy, the nurse specifically should observe Myrna Partridge for:
    1. Shock and infection
    2. Intestinal obstruction and bleeding
    3. Hemorrhage and abdominal distention
    4. Peritonitis and pulmonary complications

207. The nursing consideration that is of primary importance after Myrna Partridge's splenectomy is:
    1. Early ambulation
    2. Pulmonary embolism
    3. Adequate lung aeration
    4. Postoperative hemorrhage

208. A client is concerned about contracting malaria while visiting relatives in Southeast Asia. The nurse explains that the best way to prevent malaria is to avoid:
    1. Mosquito bites
    2. Untreated water
    3. Undercooked food
    4. Over-populated areas

209. The nurse is reviewing the physical examination and laboratory tests of a client with malaria. The nurse understands that an important finding in malaria is:
    1. Leukocytosis
    2. Erythrocytosis
    3. Splenomegaly
    4. Elevated sedimentation rate

210. When caring for a client with malaria, the nurse should know that:
    1. Seizure precautions must be followed
    2. Peritoneal dialysis is usually indicated
    3. Isolation is necessary to prevent cross infection

4. Nutrition should be provided between paroxysms

211. When teaching a client about drug therapy against *Plasmodium falciparum*, the nurse should include the fact that:
    1. The infections are controlled
    2. Immunity will prevent reinfestation
    3. The infections can generally be eliminated
    4. Transmission by the *Anopheles* mosquito can occur

212. Blackwater fever occurs in some clients with malaria; therefore, the nurse should observe a client with malaria for:
    1. Diarrhea
    2. Dark red urine
    3. Low-grade fever
    4. Coffee ground emesis

Client Case Scenario 12: Mary Fuller, age 46, was admitted to hospital with a compound fracture to her left radius. Items 213 to 217 refer to this client case scenario.

213. Fragments of cells in the bloodstream that break down on exposure to injured tissue and begin the chain reaction leading to a blood clot are known as:
    1. Platelets
    2. Leukocytes
    3. Erythrocytes
    4. Red blood cells

214. The nurse understands that thromboplastin, which initiates the clotting process, is found in:
    1. Bile
    2. Plasma
    3. Platelets
    4. Erythrocytes

215. When assessing Mrs. Fuller's wound 3 days following the accident, it exhibits signs of blood coagulation and healing. The nurse understands that the soluble substance that becomes an insoluble gel is:
    1. Fibrin
    2. Thrombin
    3. Fibrinogen
    4. Prothrombin

216. The nurse understands that blood clotting requires the presence of the catalyst:
    1. F^-
    2. Cl^-
    3. Ca^{++}
    4. Fe^{+++}

217. Vitamin K is essential for Mrs. Fuller to have normal blood clotting because it promotes:
    1. Platelet aggregation
    2. Ionization of blood calcium
    3. Fibrinogen formation by the liver
    4. Prothrombin formation by the liver

Client Care Scenario 13: Karl Bandway, age 21, experiences an anaphylactic reaction within the first 30 minutes after an IV infusion is established that contains penicillin. **Items 218 and 219 refer to this client case scenario.**

218. The nurse understands that Mr. Bandway's symptoms are the result of:
    1. Respiratory depression and cardiac standstill
    2. Constriction of capillaries and decreased cardiac output
    3. Bronchial constriction and decreased peripheral resistance
    4. Decreased cardiac output and dilation of major blood vessels

219. Occurrence of an anaphylactic reaction after receiving penicillin indicates that Mr. Bandway has:
    1. An acquired atopic sensitization
    2. Passive immunity to the penicillin allergen
    3. Antibodies to penicillin acquired after prior use of the drug
    4. Developed potent bivalent antibodies when the IV administration was started

220. When it is impossible to determine whether a client has been immunized against tetanus, the preparation of choice used to produce passive immunity for several weeks with minimal danger of allergic reactions is:
    1. DTP vaccine
    2. Tetanus toxoid
    3. Tetanus antitoxin
    4. Tetanus immune globulin

221. A client who is suspected of having tetanus asks the nurse about immunizations against tetanus. The nurse explains that the major benefit in using tetanus antitoxin is that it:
    1. Stimulates plasma cells directly
    2. Provides a high titer of antibodies
    3. Provides immediate active immunity
    4. Stimulates long-lasting passive immunity

222. A client who was exposed to hepatitis A is given gamma globulin to provide passive immunity, which:
1. Increases production of short-lived antibodies
2. Provides antibodies that neutralize the antigen
3. Accelerates antigen-antibody union at hepatic sites
4. Stimulates the lymphatic system to produce large numbers of antibodies

223. The spouse of a comatose client who has severe internal bleeding refuses to allow transfusions of whole blood because they are Jehovah's Witnesses. The nurse involved in this situation should:
1. Phone the physician for a special administrative order to give the blood under these circumstances
2. Have the spouse sign a treatment refusal form and notify the physician so a court order can be obtained
3. Gently explain to the husband why the transfusion is necessary, emphasizing the implications of not having the transfusion
4. Institute the blood transfusion anyway, since the physician ordered it and the client's survival depends on volume replacement

224. A client with hypothermia is brought to the emergency room. The family should be taught that treatment will include:
1. Core rewarming with warm fluids
2. Ambulation to increase metabolism
3. Frequent oral temperature assessment
4. Gastric tube feedings to increase fluids

Respiratory

225. A client is admitted and the physician suspects atelectasis. When assessing this individual, the nurse would expect:
1. Slow, deep respirations
2. A dry, unproductive cough
3. A normal oral temperature
4. Diminished breath sounds

226. The efficacy of the abdominal-thoracic thrust (Heimlich maneuver) to expel a foreign object in the larynx demonstrates the gas volume related to the individual's:
1. Tidal volume
2. Vital capacity
3. Residual volume
4. Inspiratory reserve volume

227. A client who undergoes a submucosal resection should be observed carefully for:
1. Periorbital crepitus
2. Occipital headache
3. Spitting up or vomiting of blood
4. White areas of healing sublingually

228. The nurse understands that in the absence of pathology, a client's respiratory center is stimulated by:
1. Oxygen
2. Lactic acid
3. Calcium ions
4. Carbon dioxide

229. Oxygen dissociation from hemoglobin and therefore oxygen delivery to the tissues are accelerated by:
1. A decreasing oxygen pressure in the blood
2. An increasing carbon dioxide pressure in the blood
3. A decreasing oxygen pressure and/or an increasing carbon dioxide pressure in the blood
4. An increasing oxygen pressure and/or a decreasing carbon dioxide pressure in the blood

230. A client is admitted with carbon monoxide poisoning. The nurse understands that the poisonous nature of carbon monoxide results from:
1. Its tendency to block CO_2 transport
2. The inhibitory effect it has on vasodilation
3. Its preferential combination with hemoglobin
4. The bubbles it tends to form in blood plasma

231. With an oxygen debt, muscle shows:
1. Low levels of ATP
2. High levels of calcium
3. High levels of glycogen
4. Low levels of lactic acid

232. Clients who are emotionally disturbed and upset may threaten to hold their breaths unless the staff meets their demands. The nurse understands that if the threats are carried out:
1. The individuals will soon die of suffocation
2. Increased N_2 concentration will have a toxic effect
3. Accumulated CO_2 will force resumption of breathing
4. Rising O_2 concentrations will stimulate the breathing center

233. A nurse initially will use an AmbuBag in the intensive care unit when:

1. A respiratory arrest occurs
2. The client is in ventricular fibrillation
3. The respiratory output must be monitored
4. A surgical incision with copious drainage is present

234. Cutting the left phrenic nerve results in:
1. Collapse of the right lung
2. Relief of pain in the left side of the chest
3. Paralysis of the left side of the diaphragm
4. Paralysis of the diaphragm on the opposite side

235. The nurse obtains a laboratory report that shows acid-fast rods in a client's sputum. These are presumed to be:
1. Influenza virus
2. Diphtheria bacillus
3. *Bordetella pertussis*
4. *Mycobacterium tuberculosis*

236. A client states that the physician said the tidal volume is slightly diminished and asks the nurse what this means. The nurse explains that tidal volume is the amount of air:
1. Exhaled forcibly after a normal expiration
2. Exhaled normally after a normal inspiration
3. Trapped in the alveoli that cannot be exhaled
4. Forcibly inspired over and above a normal inspiration

Client Case Scenario 14: Keith Singer, age 68, is admitted with severe dyspnea and hemoptysis. **Items 237 to 241 refer to this client case scenario.**

237. Mr. Singer is scheduled for a pulmonary function test. The nurse explains that during the test the respiratory therapist will ask him to breathe normally to measure the:
1. Tidal volume
2. Vital capacity
3. Expiratory reserve
4. Inspiratory reserve

238. Air rushes into the alveoli as a result of the:
1. Relaxation of the diaphragm
2. Rising pressure in the alveoli
3. Rising pressure in the pleura
4. Lowered pressure in the chest cavity

239. To facilitate maximum air exchange, Mr. Singer should be placed in the:
1. Supine position
2. Orthopneic position
3. High-Fowler's position
4. Semi-Fowler's position

240. The position in which Mr. Singer should be placed is:
1. Sims'
2. Supine
3. Orthopneic
4. Trendelenburg

241. Mr. Singer begins to expectorate blood. The nurse describes this episode as:
1. Hematuria
2. Hematoma
3. Hemoptysis
4. Hematemesis

242. The nurse must establish and maintain an airway in a client who has experienced a near drowning. The nurse should recognize that one danger of near drowning that must be assessed for is:
1. Alkalosis
2. Renal failure
3. Hypervolemia
4. Pulmonary edema

243. The common factor of puerperal sepsis, scarlet fever, otitis media, bacterial endocarditis, rheumatic fever, and glomerulonephritis is that all:
1. Are noncontagious, self-limiting infections by spirilla
2. Can be easily controlled through childhood vaccination
3. Are caused by parasitic bacteria that normally live outside the body
4. Result from streptococcal infections that enter via the upper respiratory tract

244. An example of a rapidly acting diuretic that can be administered intravenously to clients with acute pulmonary edema is:
1. Furosemide
2. Chlorothiazide
3. Chlorthalidone
4. Spironolactone

Client Case Scenario 15: Bill Rogers, with a long history of emphysema is now terminally ill with cancer of the esophagus. His plan of care includes a soft diet, modified postural drainage, and nebulizer treatments b.i.d. He is weak, dyspneic, emaciated, and apathetic. **Items 245 to 255 refer to this client case scenario.**

245. The nurse is aware that when emphysema is present there is a decreased oxygen supply because of:
    1. Pleural effusion
    2. Infectious obstructions
    3. Loss of aerating surface
    4. Respiratory muscle paralysis

246. The nursing care plan for Mr. Rogers should give priority to:
    1. Intake and output
    2. Diet and nutrition
    3. Hygiene and comfort
    4. Body mechanics and posture

247. When determining the method of oxygen administration for Mr. Rogers, the major concern is:
    1. Level of activity
    2. Facial anatomy
    3. Pathologic condition
    4. Age and mental capacity

248. The nurse administers oxygen at 2 L/minute via nasal cannula to Mr. Rogers. The nurse should observe him closely for:
    1. Cyanosis and lethargy
    2. Anxiety and tachycardia
    3. Hyperemia and increased respirations
    4. Drowsiness and decreased respirations

249. Because the alveoli lose their normal elasticity as a result of emphysema, the nurse teaches Mr. Rogers exercises that lead to effective use of the diaphragm because:
    1. Inspiration has been markedly prolonged and difficult
    2. The residual capacity of the lungs has been increased
    3. Mr. Rogers has an increase in the vital capacity of the lungs
    4. Abdominal breathing is an effective compensatory mechanism that is spontaneously initiated

250. To assist Mr. Rogers in obtaining maximum benefits after postural drainage, the nurse should:
    1. Administer the prn oxygen
    2. Place him in a sitting position
    3. Encourage him to cough deeply
    4. Encourage him to rest for 30 minutes

251. Mr. Rogers is visited frequently by his spouse, a 16-year-old daughter, and a 20-year-old son. In view of his extreme weakness and dyspnea, nursing care plans should include:
    1. Allowing self-activity whenever possible
    2. Encouraging family members to feed and assist him
    3. Limiting family visiting hours to the evening before he sleeps
    4. Planning all necessary care at one time with long rest periods in between

252. Mr. Rogers experiences a sudden episode of shortness of breath. The physician diagnoses a spontaneous pneumothorax. The nurse is aware that the probable cause of the spontaneous pneumothorax is a:
    1. Pleural friction rub
    2. Tracheoesophageal fistula
    3. Rupture of a subpleural bleb
    4. Puncture wound of the chest wall

253. When teaching Mr. Rogers about a spontaneous pneumothorax, the nurse bases the explanation on the understanding that:
    1. The heart and great vessels shift to the affected side
    2. The other lung will collapse if not treated immediately
    3. Inspired air will move from the lung into the pleural space
    4. There is a greater negative pressure within the chest cavity

254. Following a spontaneous pneumothorax, Mr. Rogers becomes extremely drowsy and his pulse and respirations increase. The nurse should suspect:
    1. Hypercapnia
    2. Hypokalemia
    3. An elevated PO_2
    4. Respiratory alkalosis

255. When assessing Mr. Rogers, the nurse should expect dyspnea and:
    1. Hematemesis
    2. Unilateral chest pain
    3. Increased chest motion
    4. Mediastinal shift toward the involved side

256. As a result of fractured ribs, the client may develop:
    1. Scoliosis

2. Pneumothorax
3. Obstructive lung disease
4. Herniation of the diaphragm

257. When a client suffers a complete pneumothorax, there is danger of a mediastinal shift. If such a shift occurs, it may lead to:
   1. Infection of the subpleural lining
   2. Decreased filling of the right heart
   3. Rupture of the pericardium or aorta
   4. Increased volume of the unaffected lung

258. The physician inserts a chest tube in a client who has been stabbed in the chest and attaches it to a two-chamber closed-drainage system. When caring for the client, the nurse should:
   1. Apply a thoracic binder to prevent tension on the tube
   2. Observe for fluid fluctuations in the waterseal chamber
   3. Clamp the tubing to prevent a rapid decline in pressure
   4. Administer morphine sulfate, because the client will be agitated

259. Complete lung expansion before the removal of chest tubes is evaluated by:
   1. Return of normal tidal volume
   2. Absence of additional drainage
   3. Decreased adventitious sounds
   4. Comparison of chest radiographs

Client Care Scenario 16: Kurt Psanka has a long history of asthma. He is admitted to hospital for an inguinal hernia repair. **Items 260 to 264 refer to this client case scenario.**

260. While receiving orciprenaline sulfate (Alupent) Mr. Psanka complains of palpitation, chest pain, and a throbbing headache. In view of these symptoms, the most appropriate nursing action would be to:
   1. Withhold the drug until additional orders are obtained from physician
   2. Tell him not to worry; these are expected side effects from the medicine
   3. Ask him to relax; then give instructions to breathe slowly and deeply for several minutes
   4. Reassure him that these effects are temporary and will subside as the body becomes accustomed to the drug

261. Mr. Psanka's pulmonary function studies are abnormal. The nurse should realize that one of the most common complications of chronic asthma is:
   1. Atelectasis

2. Emphysema
3. Pneumothorax
4. Pulmonary fibrosis

262. Mr. Psanka is scheduled for surgery. Preoperative teaching should include the fact that he:
   1. Will be quite prone to respiratory tract infections
   2. Can control and limit asthmatic attacks if desired
   3. Should try to limit coughing, because this causes distention of the chest
   4. Can control anxiety and decrease the severity of postoperative asthma attacks

263. The nurse should position Mr. Psanka recovering from general anesthesia in a:
   1. Supine position
   2. Side-lying position
   3. High-Fowler's position
   4. Trendelenburg position

264. During the immediate postoperative period the nurse should give the highest priority to:
   1. Observing for hemorrhage
   2. Maintaining a patent airway
   3. Recording the intake and output
   4. Checking the vital signs every 15 minutes

265. A client has seeds containing radium implanted in the pharyngeal area. When caring for this client, the nurse should:
   1. Have the client void q2h
   2. Maintain the client in isolation
   3. Spend as much time with the client as possible
   4. Use rubber gloves when giving the client a bath

266. The nurse can expect a client who has had a splenectomy to complain of:
   1. Pain on expiration
   2. Pain on inspiration
   3. Shortness of breath
   4. Excessively moist respirations

267. A client has a bronchoscopy in ambulatory surgery. To prevent laryngeal edema, the nurse should:
   1. Place ice chips in the client's mouth
   2. Offer the client liberal amounts of fluid
   3. Keep the client in the semi-Fowler's position
   4. Tell the client to suck on medicated lozenges

268. After a bronchoscopy because of suspected cancer of the lung, a client develops pleural effusion. This is most likely the result of:
    1. Excessive fluid intake
    2. Inadequate chest expansion
    3. Extension of cancerous lesions
    4. Irritation from the bronchoscopy

269. A client has a right pneumonectomy. During surgery the phrenic nerve is severed to:
    1. Produce an atonic diaphragm
    2. Limit the postoperative pain considerably
    3. Allow the diaphragm to partially fill the space
    4. Permit greater excursion of the thoracic cavity

270. The factor that would have little influence in predisposing an individual to cancer of the larynx would be:
    1. Air pollution
    2. Poor dental hygiene
    3. Heavy alcohol ingestion
    4. Chronic respiratory infections

271. When cleaning a tracheostomy tube that has an inner cannula, the nurse should plan to remove the inner cannula:
    1. And replace it with a sterile obturator
    2. In order to cleanse it with hydrogen peroxide
    3. After the high volume, low pressure cuff is deflated
    4. And use sterile applicators to cleanse the outer cannula

272. When suctioning a client with a tracheostomy the nurse must remember to:
    1. Use a new sterile catheter with each insertion
    2. Initiate suction as the catheter is being withdrawn
    3. Insert the catheter until the cough reflex is stimulated
    4. Remove the inner cannula before inserting the suction catheter

273. A client complains of severe pain 2 days following surgery. The nurse's initial action should be to:
    1. Have the client rest
    2. Take the client's vital signs
    3. Administer the prn analgesic
    4. Determine when the last analgesic was given

274. The nurse expects that the initial treatment for a client who has a leak of the thoracic duct following radical neck surgery would include inserting a:

1. Gastrostomy tube to drain the fluid, a high-fat diet, and bed rest
2. Chest tube to drain the fluid, total parenteral nutrition, and bed rest
3. Rectal tube to prevent distention, a low-fat diet, and increased activity
4. Nasogastric tube to drain the fluid, a moderate-fat diet, and increased activity

275. As a result of pulmonary tuberculosis, a client has a decreased surface area for gaseous exchange in the lungs. Oxygen and carbon dioxide are exchanged in the lungs by:
    1. Osmosis
    2. Diffusion
    3. Filtration
    4. Active transport

276. Before discontinuing airborne precautions (respiratory isolation) for a client with pulmonary tuberculosis, the nurse must determine that:
    1. The tuberculin skin test is negative
    2. The client no longer has the disease
    3. No acid-fast bacteria are in the sputum
    4. The client's temperature has returned to normal

277. A thoracentesis is performed. Following the procedure it is most important for the nurse to observe the client for:
    1. Periods of confusion
    2. Expectoration of blood
    3. Increased breath sounds
    4. Decreased respiratory rate

278. A client with a pulmonary embolus is intubated and placed on mechanical ventilation. When suctioning the endotracheal tube, the nurse should:
    1. Apply suction while inserting the catheter
    2. Hyperoxygenate with 100% oxygen before and after suctioning
    3. Use short, jabbing movements of the catheter to loosen secretions
    4. Suction two to three times in quick succession to remove all secretions

Endocrine

279. Glucose is an important molecule in a cell because this molecule is primarily used for:
    1. Extraction of energy
    2. Synthesis of proteins
    3. Building the genetic material
    4. Formation of cell membranes

280. The source of glucose for maintaining normal levels when the blood glucose begins to fall is:
1. Ingested food
2. Liver glycogen
3. Gluconeogenesis
4. Intestinal hydrolysis

281. The fuel glucose is delivered to the cells by the blood for production of energy. The hormone controlling use of glucose by the cell is:
1. Insulin
2. Thyroxine
3. Adrenal steroids
4. Growth hormone

282. When a client is first admitted with hyperglycemic hyperosmolar nonketotic coma (HHNC), the nurse's priority is to provide:
1. Oxygen
2. Carbohydrates
3. Fluid replacement
4. Dietary instruction

283. Ketone bodies appear in the blood and urine when fats are being oxidized in great amounts. This condition is associated with:
1. Starvation
2. Alcoholism
3. Bone healing
4. Positive nitrogen balance

284. Oral hypoglycemic agents may be used for clients with:
1. Ketosis
2. Obesity
3. Type I diabetes
4. Some insulin production

Client Case Scenario 17: Dr. Patrick Kinsey was found in a coma in his room at the large hospital where he has begun his residency. There is a strong odor of acetone on his breath. He is married, 28 years of age, and health records submitted did not reveal that Dr. Kinsey had diabetes mellitus. Emergency measures are instituted immediately. **Items 285 to 289 refer to this client case scenario.**

285. Diabetic coma results from an excess accumulation in the blood of:
1. Sodium bicarbonate, causing alkalosis
2. Ketones from rapid fat breakdown, causing acidosis
3. Nitrogen from protein catabolism, causing ammonia intoxication
4. Glucose from rapid carbohydrate metabolism, causing drowsiness

286. The most common cause of diabetic ketoacidosis is:
1. Emotional stress
2. Presence of infection
3. Increased insulin dose
4. Inadequate food intake

287. The primary treatment for Dr. Kinsey will include administration of:
1. IV fluids
2. Potassium
3. NPH insulin
4. Sodium polystyrene sulfonate (Kayexalate)

288. The insulin that would be administered to Dr. Kinsey is:
1. NPH
2. Regular
3. Globulin
4. Protamine zinc

289. A difference between diabetic coma and hyperglycemic hyperosmolar nonketotic coma (HHNC) is that Dr. Kinsey experiences:
1. Fluid loss
2. Glycosuria
3. Kussmaul respirations
4. Increased blood glucose

---

290. When glucagon is administered for reversal of the hypoglycemic state, it acts by:
1. Liberating glucose from hepatic stores of glycogen
2. Supplying glycogen to the brain and other vital organs
3. Competing for insulin and blocking its action at tissue sites
4. Providing a glucose substitute for rapid replacement of deficits

Client Case Scenario 18: Tony Ambro, age 34, is brought into hospital in a coma. It is discovered that he is diabetic. He is given an IV containing insulin, glucose, and potassium. A retention catheter is inserted. **Items 291 to 296 refer to this client case scenario.**

291. Mr. Ambro's acidosis is directly caused by an increased concentration in the serum of:
1. Ketones
2. Glucose
3. Lactic acid
4. Glutamic acid

292. Diabetic acidosis is precipitated by:
    1. Breakdown of fat stores for energy
    2. Ingestion of too many highly acidic foods
    3. Excessive secretion of endogenous insulin
    4. Increased concentrations of cholesterol in the extracellular compartment

293. A urine specimen for ketones should be removed from Mr. Ambro's retention catheter by:
    1. Disconnecting and draining it into a clean container
    2. Cleansing the drainage valve and removing it from the collection bag
    3. Wiping the catheter with alcohol and draining it into a sterile test tube
    4. Using a sterile syringe to remove it from a clamped, cleansed catheter

294. The nurse should expect laboratory tests performed on Mr. Ambro to reveal:
    1. Low serum glucose, increased acidity, high carbon dioxide
    2. Low serum glucose, decreased acidity, low carbon dioxide
    3. Elevated serum glucose, normal acidity, high carbon dioxide
    4. Elevated serum glucose, increased acidity, low carbon dioxide

295. Mr. Ambro's blood gases will reflect:
    1. Increased pH
    2. Decreased PO_2
    3. Increased PCO_2
    4. Decreased HCO_3

296. The type of insulin that is used for Mr. Ambro is:
    1. Regular insulin
    2. Insulin zinc suspension
    3. Isophane insulin suspension
    4. Insulin zinc suspension extended

Client Case Scenario 19: On the basis of diagnostic tests, Beatrice Hollens is said to have diabetes mellitus. **Items 297 to 304 refer to this client case scenario.**

297. Mrs. Hollens has a hypoglycemic reaction to insulin. The assessments that are indicative of this response include:
    1. Pallor, perspiration, tremors
    2. Excessive thirst, dry hot skin
    3. Fruity odor of breath, acetonuria
    4. Anorexia, glycosuria, tachycardia

298. The nurse knows that glucagon may be given in the treatment of hypoglycemia because it:
    1. Inhibits glycogenesis
    2. Stimulates release of insulin
    3. Increases blood sugar levels
    4. Provides more storage of glucose

299. The nursing intervention that should be instituted immediately to relieve Mrs. Hollens' symptoms include:
    1. Giving 250 ml of fruit juice
    2. Administering 5% dextrose solution IV
    3. Withholding a subsequent dose of insulin
    4. Providing a snack of cheese and dry crackers

300. The nursing plan includes that before discharge Mrs. Hollens will know how to self-administer insulin, adjust the insulin dosage, understand the exchange diet, and test the serum for glucose. Mrs. Hollens progresses well and is discharged 5 days following admission. Legally:
    1. The nurse was properly functioning as a health teacher
    2. The visiting nurse should do health teaching in the client's home
    3. A family member also should have been taught to administer the insulin
    4. The physician was responsible and the nurse should have cleared the care with the physician

301. When teaching about diabetes mellitus and diet, it is important that Mrs. Hollens and her family understand that the diet:
    1. Should be rigidly controlled to avoid emergencies
    2. Can be planned around a wide variety of commonly used foods
    3. Is based on nutritional requirements that are the same for all clients
    4. Must not include combination dishes and processed foods, since they have too many variable seasonings

302. The nurse should recognize that Mrs. Hollens needs further teaching when, after reviewing the dietary exchange system, she states that:
    1. 1 egg = 30 g meat
    2. 30 g cheese = 250 ml milk
    3. 1 slice bacon = 30 ml cream
    4. 1 scoop ice milk = 1 slice bread

303. Mrs. Hollens states, "I cannot eat big meals and I prefer to snack throughout the day." The nurse should carefully explain that:
    1. Regulated food intake is basic to control
    2. Salt and sugar restriction is the main concern
    3. Small, frequent meals are better for digestion
    4. Large meals can contribute to a weight problem

304. The best indication that Mrs. Hollens is successfully managing the disease after discharge is a:
1. Reduction in excess body weight
2. Stabilization of the serum glucose
3. Demonstrated knowledge of the disease
4. Statement by Mrs. Hollens that insulin orders are being followed

305. The primary use of glucagon is to treat:
1. Diabetic acidosis
2. Hyperinsulin secretion
3. Insulin-induced hypoglycemia
4. Idiosyncratic reactions to insulin

306. In addition to administering regular insulin to a client in diabetic ketoacidosis, the IV solution prescribed should contain potassium to replenish potassium ions in the extracellular fluid that are being:
1. Rapidly lost from the body by copious diaphoresis present during coma
2. Carried with glucose to the kidneys and excreted in the urine in increased amounts
3. Quickly used up during the rapid series of catabolic reactions stimulated by insulin and glucose
4. Moved into the intracellular fluid compartment because of the generalized anabolism induced by insulin and glucose

307. An independent nursing action that should be included in the plan of care for a client after an episode of ketoacidosis is:
1. Observing for signs of hypoglycemia as a result of treatment
2. Withholding glucose in any form until the ketoacidosis is corrected
3. Regulating insulin dosage according to the amount of ketones found in the urine
4. Giving fruit juices, broth, and milk as soon as the client is able to take fluids orally

308. A client with diabetes mellitus has an above-the-knee amputation because of severe peripheral vascular disease. Two days following surgery, when preparing the client for dinner, it is the nurse's primary responsibility to:
1. Assist the client out of bed into a chair
2. Check the client's serum glucose level
3. Ensure that the client's stump is elevated
4. Place the client in the high-Fowler's position

Client Case Scenario 20: Paula Sohl, age 52, develops symptoms of diabetes insipidus following head trauma. **Items 309 to 312 refer to this client case scenario.**

309. The assessment of Mrs. Sohl that would be most indicative of diabetes insipidus is:
1. Increased blood glucose
2. Low urinary specific gravity
3. Elevation of blood pressure
4. Decreased serum osmolarity

310. To understand diabetes insipidus, the nurse must be aware that an antidiuretic substance important for maintaining fluid balance is released by the:
1. Adrenal cortex
2. Adrenal medulla
3. Anterior pituitary
4. Posterior pituitary

311. Normally the antidiuretic hormone (ADH) influences kidney function by stimulating the:
1. Nephron tubules to reabsorb water
2. Nephron tubules to reabsorb glucose
3. Glomerulus to withhold the proteins from the urine
4. Glomerulus to control the quantity of fluid passing through it

312. The nurse knows that most of the hormones present in Mrs. Sohl's body at any given time were secreted from the endocrine glands:
1. 24 hours ago
2. 4 to 6 hours ago
3. 8 to 12 hours ago
4. More than 72 hours ago

Client Case Scenario 21: Arnold Pierce, a client who has acromegaly and diabetes mellitus, has had a hypophysectomy. **Items 313 to 315 refer to this client case scenario.**

313. Acromegaly is produced by an oversecretion of:
1. Testosterone
2. Growth hormone
3. Thyroid hormone
4. Thyroid-stimulating hormone

314. The nurse recognizes that further teaching about the hypophysectomy is necessary when Mr. Pierce states, "I know I will:
1. Be sterile for the rest of my life."
2. Require larger doses of insulin than I did preoperatively."
3. Have to take thyroxine (or a similar preparation) for the rest of my life."
4. Have to take cortisone (or a similar preparation) for the rest of my life."

315. Following a hypophysectomy the nurse specifically should observe Mr. Pierce for signs of:
    1. Urinary retention
    2. Respiratory distress
    3. Bleeding at the suture line
    4. Increased intracranial pressure

Client Case Scenario 22: Susan Louis is admitted to hospital with the diagnosis of Cushing's syndrome. **Items 316 to 323 refer to this client case scenario.**

316. The nurse understands that the cause of Cushing's syndrome is most commonly:
    1. Pituitary hypoplasia
    2. Insufficient ACTH production
    3. Hyperplasia of the adrenal cortex
    4. Deprivation of adrenocortical hormones

317. The nurse should be aware that glucocorticoids and mineralocorticoids are secreted by the:
    1. Gonads
    2. Pancreas
    3. Adrenal glands
    4. Anterior pituitary

318. Mrs. Louis may manifest signs of diabetes mellitus because:
    1. The cortical hormones created a too rapid weight loss
    2. Excessive ACTH secretion will damage pancreatic tissue
    3. A negative nitrogen balance resulted from the tissue catabolism
    4. The excessive glucocorticoids secreted by the adrenal gland caused excessive tissue catabolism and gluconeogenesis

319. When assessing Mrs. Louis, the nurse would expect:
    1. Dehydration and menorrhagia
    2. Buffalo hump and hypertension
    3. Pitting edema and frequent colds
    4. Migraine headaches and dysmenorrhea

320. In Cushing's syndrome excessive amounts of glucocorticoids and mineralocorticoids will increase Mrs. Louis':
    1. Urine output
    2. Glucose level
    3. Serum potassium
    4. Immune response

321. Mrs. Louis is to have a bilateral adrenalectomy. Prior to surgery, steroids are administered. The nurse understands the reason for this is to:

    1. Foster accumulation of glycogen in the liver
    2. Increase the inflammatory action to promote scar formation
    3. Facilitate urinary excretion of salt and water following surgery
    4. Compensate for sudden lack of these hormones following surgery

322. The medication the nurse would expect to administer to Mrs. Louis on the day of her surgery and in the immediate postoperative period is:
    1. ACTH
    2. Regular insulin
    3. Pituitary extract
    4. Hydrocortisone succinate (Solu-Cortef)

323. Until Mrs. Louis is regulated by steroid therapy, she may show symptoms of:
    1. Hypotension
    2. Hyperglycemia
    3. Sodium retention
    4. Potassium excretion

324. The administration of corticosteroids to control the symptoms of one disease can cause infections. A rationale that does not support this concept is that corticosteroids:
    1. Prevent the production of leukocytes
    2. Stop antibody production in lymphatic tissue
    3. Promote the growth and spread of enteric viruses
    4. Interfere with the inflammatory response of the body

325. Increased blood concentration of cortisol:
    1. Tends to accelerate wound healing
    2. Impairs gluconeogenesis in the liver
    3. Decreases the anterior pituitary secretion of ACTH
    4. Makes the body less able to resist stress successfully

326. In an emergency the rapid adjustments made by the body are associated with the increased activity of the:
    1. Thyroid gland
    2. Adrenal gland
    3. Pituitary gland
    4. Pancreas gland

Client Case Scenario 23: Lucy Thompson, age 39, was admitted to the hospital with Addison's disease. She exhibited the following signs and symptoms: muscular weakness, anorexia, emaciation, GI distress, generalized dark pigmentation, hypotension, hypoglycemia, low sodium and high potassium levels, and a loss of libido. **Items 327 to 332 refer to this client case scenario.**

327. Hypotension associated with Addison's disease involves a disturbance in the production of:
    1. Estrogens
    2. Androgens
    3. Glucocorticoids
    4. Mineralocorticoids

328. The nurse should observe Mrs. Thompson closely for signs of infectious complications because there is a disturbance in:
    1. Metabolic process
    2. Respiratory function
    3. Electrolytic balances
    4. Inflammatory effects

329. Mrs. Thompson's emaciation, muscular weakness, and fatigue are due to a disturbance in:
    1. Fluid balance
    2. Electrolyte levels
    3. Protein anabolism
    4. Masculinizing effects

330. An important nursing intervention specific for Mrs. Thompson is:
    1. Encouraging exercise
    2. Protecting from exertion
    3. Providing a variety of diversional activities
    4. Permitting as much activity as Mrs. Thompson desires

331. Therapy for Mrs. Thompson is aimed chiefly at:
    1. Decreasing eosinophils
    2. Increasing lymphoid tissue
    3. Restoring electrolyte balance
    4. Improving carbohydrate metabolism

332. Mrs. Thompson's treatment includes a high-protein, high-calorie diet with extra salt. As a means of encouraging her to eat, the nurse explains that:
    1. Increased amounts of potassium are needed to replace renal losses
    2. Increased protein is needed to heal the adrenal tissue and thus cure the disease
    3. Increased vitamins are needed to supply energy to assist in regaining lost weight
    4. Extra salt is needed to replace the amount being lost due to lack of sufficient aldosterone to conserve sodium

333. A client on fludrocortisone therapy for adrenal insufficiency should be taught to consult the physician in the event of:
    1. Unpredictable changes in mood
    2. Increased frequency of urination
    3. Fatigue, particularly in the afternoon
    4. Rapid weight gain and dependent edema

334. The gland that regulates the rate of oxygenation in all the body cells is the:
    1. Thyroid gland
    2. Adrenal gland
    3. Pituitary gland
    4. Pancreas gland

335. Underproduction of thyroxine produces:
    1. Myxedema
    2. Acromegaly
    3. Graves' disease
    4. Cushing's disease

336. As a result of low levels of T_3 and T_4 the nurse should expect a client to exhibit:
    1. Irritability
    2. Tachycardia
    3. Cold intolerance
    4. Profuse diaphoresis

Client Case Scenario 24: Julia McNeer has been diagnosed as having Graves' disease. Radioactive iodine is prescribed to decrease the activity of the thyroid, but this therapy is unsuccessful. She is scheduled for a thyroidectomy. **Items 337 to 343 refer to this client case scenario.**

337. The nurse knows that after radioactive iodine is administered to Mrs. McNeer, she is:
    1. Not radioactive and can be handled as any other individual
    2. Highly radioactive and should be isolated as much as possible
    3. Mildly radioactive and should be treated with routine safety precautions
    4. Not radioactive but may still transmit some dangerous radiations and must be treated with precautions

338. The most appropriate diet for Mrs. McNeer would be:
    1. Soft
    2. High-calorie
    3. Low sodium
    4. High-roughage

339. The nurse, recognizing the need to decrease the size and vascularity of the thyroid gland prior to a thyroidectomy, would expect the physician to order:
1. Propylthiouracil
2. Lugol's iodine solution
3. Potassium permanganate
4. Liothyronine sodium (Cytomel)

340. When preparing for Mrs. McNeer's return after surgery, the nurse should give priority to having available:
1. Sandbags
2. Hemostats
3. Tracheotomy tray
4. Nasogastric suction

341. When Mrs. McNeer returns from the recovery room following a subtotal thyroidectomy, the nurse should immediately:
1. Inspect the incision
2. Instruct Mrs. McNeer not to speak
3. Keep Mrs. McNeer supine for 24 hours
4. Place a tracheostomy set at the bedside

342. To evaluate possible laryngeal nerve injury following a thyroidectomy, the nurse on an hourly basis should:
1. Ask Mrs. McNeer to speak
2. Ask Mrs. McNeer to swallow
3. Have Mrs. McNeer hum a familiar tune
4. Swab Mrs. McNeer's throat to test her gag reflex

343. The nurse suspects an accidental removal of the parathyroid glands during Mrs. McNeer's thyroidectomy, which would cause:
1. Myxedema
2. Tetany and death
3. Hypovolemic shock
4. Adrenocortical stimulation

344. Thyroid storm is caused by:
1. Increased iodine in the blood
2. Removal of the parathyroid gland
3. Increased amount of thyroid hormone in the blood
4. A rebound increase in metabolism following anesthesia

345. When teaching a client with hyperthyroidism about the diagnostic tests to be done, the nurse should include:
1. T_4 and x-ray films
2. TSH assay and T_3
3. Thyroglobulin level and PO_2
4. Protein-bound iodine and SMA

Client Case Scenario 25: Paul Jackson, 47 years old, is admitted with a diagnosis of primary hyperparathyroidism as a result of a malignant neoplasm. **Items 346 to 349 refer to this client case scenario.**

346. The two interbalanced regulatory agents that control overall calcium balance in the body are:
1. Phosphorus and ACTH
2. Vitamin A and thyroid hormone
3. Ascorbic acid and growth hormone
4. Vitamin D and parathyroid hormone

347. The hormone that tends to decrease calcium concentration in the blood is:
1. Calcitonin
2. Aldosterone
3. Thyroid hormone
4. Parathyroid hormone

348. When assessing Mr. Jackson for complications of hyperparathyroidism, the nurse should monitor him for:
1. Tetany
2. Seizures
3. Graves' disease
4. Bone destruction

349. The nursing action that should be included in Mr. Jackson's plan of care is the:
1. Provision of a high-calcium diet
2. Assurance of a large fluid intake
3. Institution of seizure precautions
4. Maintenance of absolute bed rest

350. Following the removal of the parathyroid glands, calcium is required because parathormone is the hormone that tends to:
1. Decrease blood calcium concentration and relieve tetany
2. Accelerate bone breakdown with release of calcium into the blood
3. Increase blood phosphate concentration and decrease calcium levels
4. Increase calcium absorption into bone and remove calcium from the blood

Integumentary

351. The nurse realizes that sink faucets in a client's room are considered contaminated because:
1. They are not in sterile areas
2. They are opened with dirty hands
3. Large numbers of people use them
4. Water encourages bacterial growth

352. The most important aspect of hand washing is:
    1. Time
    2. Soap
    3. Water
    4. Friction

353. A moist sterile dressing placed on a cloth sterile field will be contaminated because of the principle of:
    1. Dialysis
    2. Diffusion
    3. Osmosis
    4. Capillarity

354. When changing a client's postoperative dressing, the nurse is careful not to introduce microorganisms into the surgical incision. This is an example of;
    1. Wound asepsis
    2. Medical asepsis
    3. Surgical asepsis
    4. Concurrent asepsis

355. To promote healing of a large surgical incision, a client's physician would most likely order daily doses of
    1. Vitamin A
    2. Vitamin K
    3. Ascorbic acid
    4. Vitamin B_{12} complex

356. The primary reason for the ease of penetration of the needle through the tissue when administering an IM injection is the:
    1. Long and slender shape of the needle
    2. Force used by the nurse when inserting the needle
    3. Softness of the tissue compared with the hardness of the needle
    4. High pressure developed at the tip of the needle due to its very small area

357. The temperature of water for a tepid bath should be:
    1. 12.8° C to 18.3° C
    2. 15.5° C to 20° C
    3. 21° C to 25.5° C
    4. 26.6° C to 33.8° C

358. Local hot and cold applications transfer temperature to and from the body by:
    1. Radiation
    2. Insulation
    3. Convection
    4. Conduction

359. Cholesterol is important in the human body for:
    1. Blood clotting
    2. Bone formation
    3. Muscle contraction
    4. Cellular membrane structure

360. The client with unresolved edema will most likely develop:
    1. Proteinemia
    2. Contractures
    3. Tissue ischemia
    4. Thrombus formation

361. The darkening of tissue seen in the various forms of gangrene is due to the breakdown of hemoglobin with subsequent formation of:
    1. Heme
    2. Ferric chloride
    3. Ferrous sulfide
    4. Insoluble proteins

362. A disease produced when a *Clostridium* organism enters wounds and produces a toxin causing crepitus is:
    1. Anthrax
    2. Tetanus
    3. Botulism
    4. Gangrene

Client Care Scenario 26: Alice Green is diagnosed with psoriasis and attends her local health clinic. **Items 363 and 364 refer to this client care scenario.**

363. The nurse should assess Mrs. Green for:
    1. Pruritic lesions
    2. Multiple petechiae
    3. Shiny, scaly lesions
    4. Erythematous macules

364. The nurse should explain to Mrs. Green that treatment usually involves:
    1. Avoiding exposure to the sun
    2. Topical application of steroids
    3. Potassium permanganate baths
    4. Debridement of necrotic placques

365. When caring for a client with scabies, the nurse should be aware that scabies is:
    1. Highly contagious
    2. A chronic problem
    3. Caused by a fungus
    4. Associated with other allergies

366. The nurse must help the client with pemphigus vulgaris deal with the resulting:
    1. Infertility
    2. Paralysis
    3. Skin lesions
    4. Impaired digestion

367. The assessment that is most indicative of systemic lupus erythematosus (SLE) is:
    1. A butterfly rash
    2. Firm skin fixed to tissue
    3. Muscle mass degeneration
    4. An inflammation of small arteries

368. Although no cause has been determined for scleroderma, it is thought to be caused by:
    1. Autoimmunity
    2. Ocular motility
    3. Increased amino acid metabolism
    4. Defective sebaceous gland formation

Client Care Scenario 27: Patrice Renee, a 32-year-old, is admitted to the emergency room with second-degree burns over 42% of her body and face, which she received when her nightgown caught fire. A urinary catheter is inserted. **Items 369 to 374 refer to this client care scenario.**

369. Miss Renee's condition would be considered:
    1. Fair
    2. Poor
    3. Good
    4. Critical

370. During the first few hours after Miss Renee is admitted to the burn unit, the nurse is least concerned with the client developing:
    1. Pain
    2. Leukopenia
    3. Hypovolemia
    4. Laryngeal edema

371. Miss Renee is placed on a circulating air bed primarily to:
    1. Increase mobility
    2. Prevent contractures
    3. Limit orthostatic hypotension
    4. Prevent pressure on peripheral blood vessels

372. To best evaluate Miss Renee's fluid loss, the nurse should monitor the:
    1. BUN
    2. Blood pH
    3. Hematocrit
    4. Sedimentation rate

373. When evaluating fluid loss in Miss Renee, the nurse should recognize that the relationship between body surface area and fluid loss is:
    1. Equal
    2. Unrelated
    3. Inversely related
    4. Directly proportional

374. Miss Renee requires intubation and is placed on a mechanical ventilator. Central venous pressure must be monitored. When caring for Miss Renee, the nurse understands that:
    1. The fluid level in the manometer fluctuates with each respiration
    2. The zero mark on the manometer should be at the level of the diaphragm
    3. Blood should not be easily aspirated from the central venous pressure line
    4. The client should not be taken off the ventilator for the central venous pressure readings

Client Care Scenario 28: Howard Anthony has second- and third-degree burns and receives a skin graft from his thigh over the third-degree burns of his arm. He may require further grafts after observation. **Items 375 to 377 refer to this client case scenario.**

375. A skin graft that is taken from Mr. Anthony's thigh is known as:
    1. An allograft
    2. An autograft
    3. A homograft
    4. A heterograft

376. A pigskin graft may be applied to Mr. Anthony's other burned areas. This graft is known as:
    1. An isograft
    2. An allograft
    3. A homograft
    4. A heterograft

377. The medication that the nurse should anticipate administering to Mr. Anthony as soon after admission as possible is:
    1. Tetanus toxoid
    2. Gamma globulin
    3. Isoproterenol (Isuprel)
    4. Vitamin K (Mephyton)

378. When teaching first aid, the nurse should explain that the best first-aid treatment for acid burns on the skin is to flush them with water and then apply a solution of sodium:
    1. Sulfate
    2. Chloride
    3. Hydroxide
    4. Bicarbonate

379. An effective first-aid treatment for an alkali burn is to flush it with water and then with:
    1. A weak acid
    2. A dilute base
    3. A salt solution
    4. An antibiotic solution

380. An elderly client is admitted to the surgical unit from a nursing home for treatment of a pressure ulcer. During the initial physical assessment, the nurse notes that the client is dehydrated and the skin is dry and scaly. The nurse immediately applies emollients to the client's skin and changes the dressing on the pressure ulcer. Legally:
    1. The nurse should have instituted a plan to increase activity
    2. The nurse provided supportive nursing care for the well-being of the client
    3. No treatment should have been instituted for the client until a physician ordered it
    4. Debridement of the pressure ulcer should have been done by the nurse before the dressing was applied

Client Case Scenario 29: Harriet Breen, an 84-year-old widow, is admitted with metastatic melanoma. **Items 381 and 382 refer to this client case scenario.**

381. The nurse should assess Mrs. Breen for the presence of:
    1. Oily skin
    2. Nikolsky's sign
    3. Lymphadenopathy
    4. Erythema of the palms

382. The physician suspects that Mrs. Breen also has primary cancerous lesions in the connective tissue. The nurse understands that these lesions are classified as:
    1. Sarcomas
    2. Carcinomas
    3. Collagenomas
    4. Osteoblastomas

383. The nurse should question clients with basal cell carcinoma about:
    1. Familial tendencies
    2. Their dietary patterns
    3. Their smoking history
    4. Ultraviolet radiation exposure

384. A client expresses concern about being exposed to radiation because it can cause cancer. When assisting the client to understand the treatment, the nurse should emphasize the:

    1. Dosage of radiation utilized
    2. Extent of the body irradiated
    3. Physical condition of the client
    4. Nutritional environment of the cells

385. The most effective first-aid treatment for a client who has been bitten by a raccoon involves:
    1. Administering an antivenin
    2. Maintaining a pressure dressing
    3. Cleansing the wound with soap and water
    4. Applying a tourniquet proximal to the wound

386. The physician performs a colostomy. During the early postoperative period nursing care should include:
    1. Withholding all fluids for 72 hours
    2. Limiting fluid intake for several days
    3. Having the client change the dressing
    4. Keeping the skin around the stoma clean and dry

Reproductive and Genitourinary
(For additional questions see Women's Health in Chapter 3, Childbearing and Women's Health)

Reproductive

387. During the ovulation phase of the menstrual cycle, ovulation is caused by secretion of:
    1. Estrogen
    2. Progesterone
    3. Luteinizing hormone
    4. Follicle-stimulating hormone

388. The large amount of progesterone secreted during the secretory phase of the menstrual cycle is responsible for:
    1. The onset of ovulation
    2. The regulation of menstruation
    3. The incidence of capillary fragility
    4. Sustaining the thick endometrium of the uterus

389. The hormones responsible for the proliferation phase of menstruation are:
    1. Luteinizing hormone and estrogen
    2. Luteinizing hormone and progesterone
    3. Lactogenic hormone and progesterone
    4. Follicle-stimulating hormone and estrogen

390. The main blood supply to the uterus is directly from the:
    1. Uterine and ovarian arteries
    2. Ovarian arteries and the aorta
    3. Uterine and hypogastric arteries
    4. Aorta and the hypogastric arteries

391. The hormones responsible for the menstrual cycle are:
    1. Gonadotropins
    2. Estrogen and progesterone
    3. Gonadotropins and estrogen
    4. Gonadotropins, estrogen, and progesterone

392. A woman menstruates regularly every 30 days. Her last menses started on January 1. She will most probably ovulate again on:
    1. January 5
    2. January 15
    3. January 17
    4. January 28

393. The term metrorrhagia refers to:
    1. Spotting or staining at time of ovulation
    2. Presence of occult blood in vaginal discharge
    3. Severe bleeding during each menstrual period
    4. Periods of bleeding in between menstrual periods

394. Spermatogenesis occurs:
    1. At the time of puberty
    2. At any time following birth
    3. Immediately following birth
    4. During embryonic development

395. The testes are suspended in the scrotum to:
    1. Protect the sperm from the acidity of urine
    2. Facilitate the passage of sperm through the urethra
    3. Protect the sperm from high abdominal temperatures
    4. Facilitate their maturation during embryonic development

396. A disease that can arise from normal microbial flora, especially after prolonged antibiotic therapy, is:
    1. Q fever
    2. Candidiasis
    3. Scarlet fever
    4. Herpes zoster

397. Gram-negative diplococci found in a vaginal smear are presumed to be:
    1. Gonococci
    2. Meningococci
    3. Pneumococci
    4. *Treponema pallidum*

398. The term *condylomata acuminata* refers to:
    1. Scabies
    2. Herpes zoster

3. Venereal warts
4. Cancer of the epididymis

399. Clients who develop general paresis as a complication of syphilis are usually treated with:
    1. Penicillin
    2. Major tranquilizers
    3. Behavior modification
    4. Electroconvulsive therapy

Client Case Scenario 30: Otto Strank is a 19-year-old university student who is diagnosed with gonorrhea in a sexually transmitted disease clinic. **Items 400 to 402 refer to this client case scenario.**

400. The nurse understands that the causative organism of gonorrhea is:
    1. Döderlein's bacillus
    2. *Treponema pallidum*
    3. *Neisseria gonorrhoeae*
    4. *Staphylococcus* organism

401. The nurse teaches Mr. Strank that gonorrhea is highly infectious and:
    1. Is easily cured
    2. Occurs very rarely
    3. Can produce sterility
    4. Is limited to the external genitalia

402. When Mr. Strank is diagnosed as having gonorrhea the nurse should expect the physician to order:
    1. Colistin
    2. Penicillin
    3. Actinomycin
    4. Chloramphenicol

Client Case Scenario 31: Cheryl Robbins, age 26, is diagnosed with a trichomonal infection on a routine physical examination at her doctor's office. **Items 403 to 407 refer to this client case scenario.**

403. The nurse understands that the organism that causes Miss Robbins' trichomonal infection is a:
    1. Yeast
    2. Fungus
    3. Protozoan
    4. Spirochete

404. For Miss Robbins, the nurse would expect the physician to order douches with:
    1. Vinegar to decrease the pH of the vagina
    2. Tap water to increase the pH of the vagina
    3. Physiologic saline to decrease the pH of the vagina
    4. Sodium bicarbonate to increase the pH of the vagina

405. The oral drug that is most likely to be prescribed to Miss Robbins is:
1. Penicillin
2. Gentian violet
3. Nystatin (Mycostatin)
4. Metronidazole (Flagyl)

406. The nurse administers a douche. The best position for Miss Robbins to assume would be the:
1. Sims'
2. Fowler's
3. Knee-chest
4. Dorsal recumbent

407. When teaching Miss Robbins how to self-administer a douche, the nurse should instruct her to direct the douche nozzle toward the:
1. Left
2. Right
3. Sacrum
4. Umbilicus

---

408. When counseling a client after a vasectomy, the nurse should advise him that:
1. Recanalization of the vas deferens is impossible
2. Some impotency is to be expected for several weeks
3. Unprotected coitus is possible within a week to 10 days
4. It requires at least 10 ejaculations to clear the tract of sperm

409. Torsion of the testes requires immediate surgical correction because:
1. There is no other way to control the pain
2. Irreversible damage occurs after a few hours
3. Swelling is excessive and the testicle may rupture
4. The reduction in testicular blood flow leads to rapid death of sperm

410. A 15-year-old client complains of persistent dysmenorrhea. The nurse should encourage her to:
1. Maintain daily activities
2. Have a gynecologic exam
3. Eat a nutritious diet containing iron
4. Practice relaxation of abdominal muscles

411. Acute salpingitis is most commonly the result of:
1. Syphilis
2. Abortion
3. Gonorrhea
4. Hydatidiform mole

412. The most therapeutic position for a client with pelvic inflammatory disease would be the:
1. Sims' position
2. Fowler's position
3. Lithotomy position
4. Supine position with knees flexed

Client Case Scenario 32: Mrs. Lort, age 41, is admitted to hospital with suspected procidentia (prolapse of the uterus). She is tentatively scheduled for a vaginoplasty. She has been experiencing severe abdominal cramps each month at the time of menstruation for almost 1 year. **Items 413 to 416 refer to this client case scenario.**

413. Because Mrs. Lort complains of exceptionally severe abdominal cramps for 1 or 2 days each month at the time of menstruation, the nurse should suspect:
1. Hypokalemia
2. Hypocalcemia
3. Hyperglycemia
4. Hypernatremia

414. The test that the physician might perform to determine the underlying cause of Mrs. Lort's uterine pain is:
1. Laparoscopy
2. Estradiol level
3. Tubal insufflation
4. Endometrial smear

415. Prior to surgery, the nurse plans to assess Mrs. Lort for:
1. Exudate
2. Swelling
3. Ulcerations
4. Vaginal discharge

416. Mrs. Lort is scheduled for a vaginoplasty. Preoperatively the nurse may expect to:
1. Encourage ambulation
2. Apply moist compresses
3. Elevate the foot of the bed
4. Manipulate the procidentia

Client Case Scenario 33: Mrs. Coral, age 56, is admitted to the women's center with erosion to her cervix. She undergoes cauterization. **Items 417 to 419 refer to this client case scenario.**

417. Erosions of the cervix are common when:
1. There has been a long labor
2. The normal acidity of the vagina is altered
3. The cervix is not dilated completely when delivery occurs
4. The cervix stretches during delivery and there is an unhealed laceration

418. The physician advises Mrs. Coral to douche with a solution of 2 L of water and 45 ml of vinegar following cauterization. This douche is ordered primarily to:
    1. Increase her comfort
    2. Alter the pH of the vagina
    3. Eliminate sloughed tissue
    4. Keep the vaginal canal free of bacteria

419. Early treatment of cervical erosion is performed for Mrs. Coral specifically to prevent:
    1. Metrorrhagia
    2. Cancer of the cervix
    3. Further erosions from occurring
    4. Infections of the reproductive system

420. The nurse knows that cervical polyps:
    1. Do not cause bleeding until they are malignant
    2. Are frequently the precursors of uterine cancer
    3. Are usually malignant, and curettage is always done
    4. Are usually benign, but curettage of the uterus is always done

421. A condyloma has been identified during a yearly gynecological examination. While awaiting the biopsy report prior to its removal, the client indicates to the nurse that she is fearful of cervical cancer. The best response by the nurse would be:
    1. "Worrying today is not going to help the situation."
    2. "It is very upsetting to have to wait for a biopsy report."
    3. "Of course you don't have cancer; a condyloma is always benign."
    4. "No operation is done without specimens being sent to the laboratory first."

Client Case Scenario 34: Kelly Garvin is admitted for treatment of cancer of the cervix. **Items 422 to 430 refer to this client case scenario.**

422. A manifestation of cancer of the cervix that may have brought Mrs. Garvin to the gynecologist is:
    1. Abdominal heaviness
    2. Foul-smelling discharge
    3. Pressure on the bladder
    4. Bloody spotting after intercourse

423. The most common site for cancer cell growth in the cervix is at the:
    1. External os and the regional nodes
    2. Internal os and the endocervical glands

    3. Junction of the cervix and lower uterine segment
    4. Columnosquamous junction of the internal and external ossa

424. Following a biopsy for suspected cervical cancer, the laboratory reports reveal a stage 0 lesion. According to the International Federation of Gynecology and Obstetrics, stage 0 is indicative of:
    1. Carcinoma in situ
    2. Early stromal invasion
    3. Parametrial involvement
    4. Carcinoma strictly confined to the cervix

425. Mrs. Garvin has a radium implant. Symptoms observed in Mrs. Garvin following radium insertion that are indicative of a radium reaction are:
    1. Nausea and vomiting
    2. Restlessness and irritability
    3. Vaginal discharge and excoriation
    4. Pain and elevation of temperature

426. When caring for Mrs. Garvin the nurse should:
    1. Spend time with Mrs. Garvin to alleviate her anxiety
    2. Wear a lead-lined apron while administering any care
    3. Limit Mrs. Garvin's activity so as not to dislodge the radium insert
    4. Use disposable sheets and towels to prevent exposure of laundry personnel

427. In regards to Mrs. Garvin's care, the nurse should also:
    1. Restrict visitors to a 10-minute stay
    2. Store urine in a lead lined container
    3. Wear a lead apron when giving care
    4. Avoid giving IM injections into the gluteal muscle

428. The nurse checking Mrs. Garvin's perineum finds the packing protruding from the vagina. The immediate action to take is to report this situation to the physician at once because the packing:
    1. Must be removed
    2. Has become radioactive
    3. Prevents excessive loss of blood
    4. Decreases rectal and bladder trauma

429. The doctor removes Mrs. Garvin's radium implant. Safety precautions include:
    1. Cleaning radium carefully in ether or alcohol
    2. Ensuring that long forceps are available for use
    3. Handling the radium carefully wearing foil-lined rubber gloves
    4. Charting the date and hour of removal and the total time of treatment

430. Before discharge the nurse should explain to Mrs. Garvin the importance of:
    1. Limiting daily fluid intake
    2. Continuing a low residue diet
    3. Returning for medical follow-up care
    4. Taking daily multivitamin supplements

431. A client's pathology report shows metastatic adenocarcinoma of the breast. The client is to receive doxorubicin (Adriamycin), which modifies the growth of cancer cells by:
    1. Preventing folic acid synthesis
    2. Changing the osmotic gradient in the cell
    3. Inhibiting RNA synthesis by binding DNA
    4. Increasing the permeability of the cell wall

432. A client expresses concern about having a hysterectomy at age 45 because she has heard from friends that she will undergo severe symptoms of menopause after surgery. The most appropriate response for the nurse would be:
    1. "This is something that does occur in older women on occasion, but you don't have to worry about it."
    2. "It's too bad you did not discuss this with your doctor. I really can't give you any kind of information about this."
    3. "You were misinformed. This never happens following this type of surgery. Your friend probably had a different diagnosis."
    4. "Some women occasionally experience exaggerated symptoms of menopause if in addition to their uterus, their ovaries are removed."

433. After a hysterectomy a client wants to know if it would be wise for her to take hormones right away to prevent symptoms of menopause. The most appropriate response would be:
    1. "It is best to wait; you may not have any symptoms at all."
    2. "You have to wait until symptoms are severe; otherwise, hormones will have no effect."
    3. "Isn't it comforting to know that hormones are available if you should need them?"
    4. "This is something you should discuss with your physician, since it is important for the physician to know how you feel and what your concerns are."

434. A client who had a mastectomy asks about the term ERP-positive. The nurse explains that tumor cells are evaluated for estrogen receptor protein to determine:
    1. If breast reconstruction is feasible
    2. The need for supplemental estrogen
    3. Potential response to hormone therapy
    4. The degree of metastasis that has occurred

435. The definitive diagnosis of benign prostatic hypertrophy is arrived at by:
    1. Rectal examination
    2. Biopsy of prostatic tissue
    3. Pap smear of prostatic fluid
    4. Serum phosphatase studies

436. With cancer of the prostate it is possible to follow the course of the disease by monitoring the serum level of:
    1. Creatinine
    2. Acid phosphatase
    3. Blood urea nitrogen
    4. Nonprotein nitrogen

437. The tests that would help indicate the effect of benign prostatic hypertrophy on the kidneys are:
    1. Microscopic porphyrins, urinalysis
    2. PSP, urea clearance, urine concentration
    3. Sulkowitch, catecholamines, urine dilution
    4. Bence Jones protein, urine concentration, albumin

438. A nurse should be aware that benign prostatic hypertrophy (BPH):
    1. Is a congenital abnormality
    2. Usually becomes malignant
    3. Predisposes to hydronephrosis
    4. Causes an elevated acid phosphatase

439. A client is diagnosed with herpes genitalis. To prevent cross-contamination the nurse should:
    1. Institute droplet precautions
    2. Arrange transfer to a private room
    3. Wear a gown and gloves when giving direct care
    4. Close the door and wear a mask when in the room

Client Case Scenario 35: Rhoda Fleming, 34 years old, is diagnosed with syphilis. **Items 440 to 442 refer to this client case scenario.**

440. Miss Fleming cannot understand how syphilis was contracted because there has been no sexual activity for several days. As part of teaching, the nurse explains that the incubation period for syphilis is about:
    1. 1 week
    2. 72 hours
    3. 2 months
    4. 2 to 6 weeks

441. Syphilis is not considered contagious in the:
    1. Tertiary stage
    2. Primary stage
    3. Incubation stage
    4. Secondary stage

442. Before Miss Fleming can be treated, the nurse must determine the:
    1. Portal of entry
    2. Size of the chancre
    3. Existence of allergies
    4. Names of sexual contacts

443. In relation to the public health implications of gonorrhea diagnosed in a 16-year-old, the nurse should be most interested in:
    1. Finding the client's contacts
    2. Interviewing the client's parents
    3. The reasons for the client's promiscuity
    4. Instructing the client about birth control measures

444. When teaching a client about the drug therapy for gonorrhea, the nurse should state that it:
    1. Cures the infection
    2. Prevents complications
    3. Controls its transmission
    4. Reverses pathologic changes

Genitourinary

445. An example of a purely objective piece of data is:
    1. "A history of alcohol abuse."
    2. "The large sacral pressure ulcer."
    3. "A urine specific gravity of 1.030."
    4. "The client's high level of anxiety."

446. When encouraging hospitalized clients to void, the most basic method for the nurse to employ is:
    1. Providing privacy
    2. Warming a bedpan
    3. Having the client listen to running water
    4. Placing the client's hands in warm water

447. When collecting a 24-hour urine specimen, the nurse should:
    1. Check if any preservatives need to be added
    2. Weigh the client before starting the collection
    3. Discard the last voided specimen of the 24-hour period
    4. Check the intake and output for the previous 24-hour period

448. The most important means of maintaining the fluid and electrolyte balance of the body is:
    1. Aldosterone
    2. The urinary system
    3. The respiratory system
    4. Antidiuretic hormone (ADH)

449. To better understand fluid balance the nurse needs to recognize that:
    1. Glomerular filtration occurs in the glomeruli, which are small arteries in the kidneys
    2. A decrease in blood protein concentration tends to increase the glomerular filtration rate
    3. The volume of urine secreted is regulated mainly by mechanisms that control the glomerular filtration rate
    4. An increase in the hydrostatic pressure in Bowman's capsule tends to increase the glomerular filtration rate

450. The reabsorption of water from glomerular filtrate (in the kidney tubules), the flow of water between the intracellular and interstitial compartments, and the exchange of fluid between plasma and interstitial fluid spaces are caused by:
    1. Dialysis
    2. Osmosis
    3. Diffusion
    4. Active transport

Client Case Scenario 36: John Higgs is admitted to hospital to have his urethra dilated by the physician. A urinary retention catheter is inserted following the procedure. **Items 451 to 456 refer to this client case scenario.**

451. A routine urinalysis is ordered for Mr. Higgs. If the specimen cannot be sent immediately to the laboratory, the nurse should:
    1. Take no special action
    2. Refrigerate the specimen
    3. Store on "dirty" side of utility room
    4. Discard and collect a new specimen later

452. The nurse understands that the structure that encircles the male urethra is the:
    1. Epididymis
    2. Prostate gland
    3. Seminal vesicle
    4. Bulbourethral gland

453. Mr. Higgs' Foley catheter operates by the principle of:
    1. Inertia
    2. Gravity
    3. Osmosis
    4. Diffusion

454. The nurse can best prevent the contamination from Mr. Higgs' retention catheter by:
1. Perineal cleansing
2. Encouraging fluids
3. Irrigating the catheter
4. Cleansing around the meatus periodically

455. When Mr. Higgs, who has a urinary retention catheter in place, complains of discomfort in the bladder and urethra, the nurse should first:
1. Notify the physician
2. Milk the tubing gently
3. Check the patency of the catheter
4. Irrigate the catheter with prescribed solutions

456. Mr. Higgs experiences difficulty in voiding after his indwelling urinary catheter is removed. This is probably related to:
1. Fluid imbalances
2. Mr. Higg's recent sedentary lifestyle
3. An interruption in normal voiding habits
4. Nervous tension following the procedure

Client Case Scenario 37: Helen Stewart is admitted to hospital with complaints of hematuria, frequency, urgency, and dysuria. **Items 457 to 460 refer to this client case scenario.**

457. Mrs. Stewart's signs and symptoms would most likely be associated with:
1. Pyelitis
2. Cystitis
3. Nephrosis
4. Pyelonephritis

458. Mrs. Stewart is receiving methenamine mandelate (Mandelamine) and ammonium chloride. The primary reason for administering the two drugs concurrently is that ammonium chloride:
1. Promotes healing of irritated bladder mucosa
2. Decreases bladder irritation by acidifying the urine
3. Improves methanamine mandelate's effect on bacteria by acidifying the urine
4. Interacts with methenamine mandelate to decrease crystal and stone formation

459. Mrs. Stewart has a higher risk of developing cystitis than does a male. This is due to:
1. Altered urinary pH
2. Hormonal secretions
3. Juxtaposition of the bladder
4. Proximity of urethra and anus

460. When assessing Mrs. Stewart's urine, each specimen of urine should be assessed for:

1. Clarity
2. Viscosity
3. Specific gravity
4. Sugar and acetone

461. A client with cancer of the prostate requests the urinal at frequent intervals but either does not void or voids in very small amounts. This is most likely caused by:
1. Edema
2. Dysuria
3. Retention
4. Suppression

462. When a urinary catheter is removed, the client is unable to empty the bladder. A drug used to relieve urinary retention is:
1. Carbachol injection
2. Neosporin GU irrigant
3. Bethanechol (Urecholine)
4. Pilocarpine hydrochloride (Pilocar)

463. The family of an elderly, aphasic client complain that the nurse failed to obtain a signed consent before inserting an indwelling catheter to measure hourly output. This is an example of:
1. A catheter inserted for the client's benefit
2. A treatment that does not need a separate consent form
3. Treatment without consent of the client, which is an invasion of rights
4. Inability to obtain consent for treatment because the client was aphasic

464. When caring for a client with a continuous bladder irrigation, the nurse should:
1. Monitor urinary specific gravity
2. Record urinary output every hour
3. Subtract irrigant from output to determine urine volume
4. Include irrigating solution in any 24-hour urine tests ordered

465. A client who is receiving hemodialysis for chronic renal failure is especially prone to develop:
1. Peritonitis
2. Renal calculi
3. Hepatitis Type B
4. Bladder infection

466. When teaching a female client with recurrent urinary tract infections, the nurse states that women are most susceptible because of:
1. Inadequate fluid intake
2. Poor hygienic practices
3. The length of the urethra
4. Continuity of the mucous membrane

467. A client in a nursing home is diagnosed with urethritis. Before initiating treatment orders, the nurse should plan to:
    1. Start a 24-hour urine collection
    2. Administer an oil-retention enema
    3. Prepare for urinary catheterization
    4. Obtain a urine specimen for culture and sensitivity

468. When a client has hematuria, the nurse should observe for:
    1. Diarrhea
    2. Acetone in urine
    3. Symptoms of peritonitis
    4. Gross blood in the urine

Client Case Scenario 38: Mrs. Hart, 81 years old, is admitted to hospital for a cystocele repair. **Items 469 to 472 refer to this client case scenario.**

469. A rectocele and cystocele are usually due to:
    1. Injury during childbirth
    2. Infection of the bladder
    3. Relaxation of musculature of the pelvic floor
    4. Trauma in repair of an episiotomy or laceration

470. When taking Mrs. Hart's health history, the nurse would expect her to report the occurrence of:
    1. Heavy leukorrhea, pruritus
    2. Sporadic bleeding accompanied by abdominal pain
    3. Stress incontinence, feeling of low abdominal pressure
    4. Change in acidity level of the vagina, leukorrhea, spotting

471. Mrs. Hart has surgery and returns from the post-anesthesia unit with an indwelling catheter in place. The primary reason for the catheter is to prevent:
    1. Retention
    2. Discomfort
    3. Loss of bladder tone
    4. Pressure on the suture line

472. Mrs. Hart complains of bladder irritability following the removal of her catheter. A sign of this complication would probably be:
    1. Dysuria
    2. Polyuria
    3. Dribbling
    4. Hematuria

Client Case Scenario 39: Andrew Carpenter, a 60-year-old laborer, is admitted to hospital with a bladder tumor and complaints of dysuria. **Items 473 to 475 refer to this client case scenario.**

473. The activity most often associated with bladder tumors is:
    1. Jogging 3 miles a day
    2. Drinking three cans of cola a day
    3. Smoking two packs of cigarettes a day
    4. Working with a jackhammer every day

474. A cystectomy and ileal conduit are scheduled for Mr. Carpenter. Preoperatively, the nurse plans to:
    1. Limit fluid intake for 24 hours
    2. Teach muscle-tightening exercises
    3. Teach the procedure for irrigation of the stoma
    4. Provide cleansing enemas and laxatives as ordered

475. The nurse recognizes that the major disadvantage of an ileal conduit is that:
    1. Peristalsis is greatly decreased
    2. Stool continuously oozes from it
    3. Urine continuously drains from it
    4. Absorption of nutrients is diminished

Client Case Scenario 40: Mrs. Cyr is hospitalized and undergoes a left nephrectomy. **Items 476 and 477 refer to this client case scenario.**

476. After a nephrectomy Mrs. Cyr arrives in the post-anesthesia unit with a plastic airway in place. When observing Mrs. Cyr for signs of hemorrhage, the nurse must be certain to:
    1. Turn Mrs. Cyr to observe the dressings
    2. Keep Mrs. Cyr's nail beds in view at all times
    3. Observe Mrs. Cyr for hemoptysis when suctioning
    4. Report any increase in Mrs. Cyr's blood pressure immediately

477. The most inaccurate method to estimate Mrs. Cyr's postoperative drainage after a nephrectomy would be by:
    1. Weighing saturated dressings
    2. Counting saturated 10 cm × 10 cm gauze pads
    3. Measuring drainage that has seeped through the dressing
    4. Wringing saturated 10 cm × 10 cm pads into a graduated container

Client Case Scenario 41: Mr. Sati has undergone a suprapubic prostatectomy. He has a Foley catheter. **Items 478 to 481 refer to this client case scenario.**

478. In addition to a Foley catheter, the nurse should expect Mr. Sati to have a:
1. Ureterostomy with gravity drainage
2. Nephrostomy tube with tidal drainage
3. Rectal incision and a ureteral catheter
4. Cystostomy tube and an abdominal incision

479. The most significant complication immediately after a suprapubic prostatectomy is:
1. Spasms
2. Impotence
3. Hemorrhage
4. Urinary incontinence

480. When irrigating Mr. Sati's indwelling urinary catheter the nurse should:
1. Obtain and use sterile equipment
2. Instill the fluid under high pressure
3. Warm the solution to body temperature
4. Aspirate immediately to ensure return flow

481. When Mr. Sati returns from the post-anesthesia care unit, he accidentally pulls out the urethral catheter. The nurse should:
1. Reinsert a new catheter
2. Notify the physician immediately
3. Check for bleeding by irrigating the suprapubic tube
4. Take no immediate action if the suprapubic tube is draining

482. After an anterior-posterior colporrhaphy in a client past menopause the nurse should teach the client how to prevent:
1. Pregnancy
2. Constipation
3. Incontinence
4. Rectovaginal fistulas

483. A palliative method of urinary divergence sometimes used for clients with advanced kidney disease is:
1. Ileostomy
2. Cecostomy
3. Nephrostomy
4. Ureterostomy

484. A client has a transurethral resection of the prostate. After the continuous bladder irrigation is discontinued, the indwelling catheter becomes obstructed. When preparing for the physician to irrigate the catheter, the nurse should obtain:
1. Sterile water
2. Isotonic saline
3. Hypotonic saline
4. Genitourinary irrigating solution

Client Case Scenario 42: Andy Lam, a 54-year-old engineer, is admitted to hospital with the diagnosis of renal calculi. **Items 485 to 488 refer to this client case scenario.**

485. The nurse would expect Mr. Lam to complain of:
1. Irritability and twitching
2. Dry, itchy skin and pyuria
3. Frequency and urgency on urination
4. Pain radiating from kidney to shoulder

486 When caring for Mr. Lam, the most important nursing action is to:
1. Strain all urine
2. Limit fluids at night
3. Record blood pressure
4. Administer analgesics every 3 hours

487. Diet therapy for Mr. Lam whose renal calculi are thought to be of calcium phosphate composition would probably be:
1. Low calcium and phosphorus, acid ash
2. High calcium and phosphorus, acid ash
3. Low purine and phosphorus, alkaline ash
4. High calcium and phosphorus, alkaline ash

488. Mr. Lam has surgery to remove his renal calculi. To obtain an accurate urine output for Mr. Lam, who has a continuous bladder irrigation (CBI), the nurse should:
1. Measure the contents of the bedside drainage bag
2. Stop the irrigation until the urine output is determined
3. Subtract the volume of irrigant from the total drainage
4. Ensure that urine and irrigant drain into two separate bags

Client Case Scenario 43: Doug Mullens is admitted to hospital with calcium-based urinary calculi. **Items 489 to 491 refer to this client case scenario.**

489. Mr. Mullens, who is about to have surgery to remove his urinary calculi, needs education about a:
1. Cystometry
2. Cystolithiasis
3. Cryoextraction
4. Cystolithectomy

490. Which background knowledge helps the nurse understand the reasons for a strict 200-mg calcium diet for 3 days with daily urinary calcium tests for Mr. Mullens?
    1. Excessive calcium intake has little influence on renal stone formation
    2. The thyroid hormone controls the serum levels of calcium and phosphorus
    3. If calcium excretion is still elevated on the test diet, dietary influences can be ruled out
    4. If calcium excretion is lowered on the test diet, hyperparathyroidism can be identified as the cause of the calculi

491. The diet ordered for Mr. Mullens is to contain 400 mg of calcium, a low calcium level. The foods permitted on this diet would include:
    1. Chocolate pudding
    2. Roast beef with baked potato
    3. Salmon loaf with cheese sauce
    4. Vanilla ice cream with chocolate syrup and nuts

492. The pathology report states that a client's urinary calculus is composed of uric acid. The nurse should instruct the client to avoid:
    1. Milk and fruit
    2. Eggs and cheese
    3. Organ meats and extracts
    4. Red meats and vegetables

493. The diet of choice for a client with renal calculi of calcium oxalate composition would be:
    1. Low in purines, alkaline ash
    2. Low in methionine, acid ash
    3. Low in calcium and oxalate, acid ash
    4. Low in calcium and oxalate, alkaline ash

494. The purpose of peritoneal dialysis is to:
    1. Reestablish kidney function
    2. Clean the peritoneal membrane
    3. Provide fluid for intracellular spaces
    4. Remove toxins and metabolic wastes

Client Case Scenario 44: Kerri Jenner has acute renal failure. **Items 495 to 498 refer to this client case scenario.**

495. The nurse understands that metabolic acidosis develops in renal failure as a result of:
    1. Inability of renal tubules to secrete hydrogen ions and conserve bicarbonate
    2. Depression of respiratory rate by metabolic wastes causing carbon dioxide retention
    3. Impaired glomerular filtration causing retention of sodium and metabolic waste products

    4. Inability of renal tubules to reabsorb water to achieve dilution of the acid contents of the blood

496. Mr. Jenner is to receive a very low-protein diet. This diet is based on the principle that:
    1. A high-protein intake ensures an adequate daily supply of all amino acids to compensate for losses
    2. Essential and nonessential amino acids are necessary in the diet to supply materials for tissue protein synthesis
    3. Urea nitrogen cannot be used to synthesize amino acids in the body, so all the nitrogen for amino acid synthesis must come from the dietary protein
    4. If the diet is low in protein and supplies only essential amino acids, the reduced amount of metabolic waste products will decrease stress on the kidneys

497. Mr. Jenner complains of tingling of the fingers and toes and muscle twitching. This is caused by:
    1. Acidosis
    2. Calcium depletion
    3. Potassium retention
    4. Sodium chloride depletion

498. Mr. Jenner becomes confused and irritable. The nurse realizes that this behavior may be caused by:
    1. Hyperkalemia
    2. Hypernatremia
    3. An elevated BUN
    4. Limited fluid intake

Client Case Scenario 45: Lily Norris has chronic renal failure and is hospitalized to receive hemodialysis. **Items 499 to 503 refer to this client case scenario.**

499. The main indication for hemodialysis for Mrs. Norris is:
    1. Ascites
    2. Acidosis
    3. Increase in blood pressure
    4. High and rising potassium levels

500. The kidney dialysis machine primarily makes use of the physical principle of:
    1. Osmosis
    2. Dialysis
    3. Filtration
    4. Diffusion

501. To gain access to a vein and an artery, an external shunt is used for Mrs. Norris' hemodialysis. The most serious problem with an external shunt is:

1. Septicemia
2. Clot formation
3. Exsanguination
4. Sclerosis of vessels

502. When caring for Mrs. Norris who has had an arteriovenous shunt inserted for her hemodialysis, the nurse should:
1. Cover the entire cannula with an elastic bandage
2. Use strict aseptic technique when giving shunt care
3. Notify the physician if a bruit is heard in the cannula
4. Take the blood pressure every 4 hours from the arm that contains the shunt

503. The nurse working in the hemodialysis unit runs a high risk of developing:
1. Infectious hepatitis
2. Hemolytic hepatitis
3. Type A viral hepatitis
4. Type B viral hepatitis

Gastrointestinal

504. Energy stored as ATP, ADP, and other high-energy compounds is formed chiefly by:
1. Peptidation
2. Respiration
3. Hydrolysis of fats
4. Oxidation of glucose

505. A black client describes abdominal discomfort following ingestion of milk. The nurse recognizes that this may be the result of a genetic deficiency of the enzyme:
1. Lactase
2. Maltase
3. Sucrase
4. Amylase

506. One of the main functions of bile is to:
1. Split protein
2. Emulsify fats
3. Help synthesize vitamins
4. Produce an acid condition

507. The nurse is instructing a group about food preparation. They are told to avoid using products in damaged cans because they might contain the anaerobic spore-forming rod:
1. *Escherichia coli*
2. *Clostridium tetani*
3. *Salmonella typhosa*
4. *Clostridium botulinum*

508. When teaching an athletic teenage client about nutritional intake, the nurse should explain that the carbohydrate food that would provide the quickest source of energy is a:
1. Glass of milk
2. Slice of bread
3. Chocolate candy bar
4. Glass of orange juice

509. The end products of protein digestion, amino acids, are absorbed from the small intestine by:
1. Simple diffusion because of their small size
2. Filtration according to the osmotic pressure direction
3. Active transport with the aid of vitamin B_6 (pyridoxine)
4. Osmosis caused by their greater concentration in the intestinal lumen

510. A complete protein, a food protein of high biologic value, is one that contains:
1. All 22 of the amino acids in sufficient quantity to meet human requirements
2. All 8 of the essential amino acids in correct proportion to meet human needs
3. The 8 essential amino acids in any proportion because the body can always fill in the difference needed
4. Most of the 22 amino acids from which the body will make additional amounts of the 8 essential amino acids needed

511. The statement that is true about the sources of vitamin K is:
1. Vitamin K is found in a wide variety of foods, so there is no danger of deficiency
2. Almost all vitamin K sufficient for metabolic needs is produced by intestinal bacteria
3. Vitamin K is rarely found in dietary food sources, so a natural deficiency can easily occur
4. Usually vitamin K can easily be absorbed without assistance, so all that is consumed is absorbed

512. Vitamin C is related to tissue integrity and hemorrhagic disease. It controls such disorders by:
    1. Preventing tissue hemorrhage by providing essential blood-clotting materials
    2. Preserving the structural integrity of tissue by protecting the lipid matrix of cell walls from peroxidation
    3. Facilitating adequate absorption of calcium and phosphorus for bone formation to prevent bleeding in the joints
    4. Strengthening capillary walls and structural tissue by depositing cementing material to build collagen from ground substance and thus prevent tissue hemorrhage

513. The main function of adipose tissue in fat metabolism is synthesizing and:
    1. Releasing glucose for energy
    2. Regulating cholesterol production
    3. Using lipoproteins for fat transport
    4. Storing triglycerides for energy reserves

514. Many vitamins and minerals regulate the chemical changes of cell metabolism by acting in a coenzyme role. This means that the vitamin or mineral:
    1. Forms a new compound by a series of complex changes
    2. Is not a part of the enzyme controlling a particular reaction
    3. May be a necessary catalyst present for the reaction to proceed
    4. Prevents unnecessary reactions by neutralizing the controlling enzyme

515. Because fat is insoluble in water, it cannot travel freely in the blood. Therefore the main type of compound formed to serve as a vehicle of transport is:
    1. Lipoprotein
    2. Triglyceride
    3. Phospholipid
    4. Plasma protein

516. Twenty-two amino acids are involved in total body metabolism building and rebuilding various tissues. Of these, 8 are essential amino acids. This means that:
    1. These 8 amino acids can be made by the body because they are essential to life
    2. These 8 amino acids are essential in body processes and the remaining 14 are not
    3. The body cannot synthesize these 8 amino acids and thus they must be obtained from the diet

    4. After synthesizing these 8 amino acids, the body uses them in key processes essential for growth

517. The food group lowest in natural sodium is:
    1. Milk
    2. Meat
    3. Fruits
    4. Vegetables

518. The terms saturated and unsaturated, when used in reference to fats, relate to degree of:
    1. Color
    2. Taste
    3. Density
    4. Digestibility

519. When the transport fat compounds accumulate to abnormal levels in the blood, the diet may be modified as one effort to control them. The foods most affected by such diet therapy would be:
    1. Fruits
    2. Grains
    3. Animal fats
    4. Vegetable oils

520. The breakdown of triglyceride molecules can be expected to produce:
    1. Fatty acids
    2. Amino acids
    3. Urea nitrogen
    4. Simple sugars

521. Megadoses of vitamin A are taken by a client. The nurse should question this practice because:
    1. The vitamin is highly toxic even in small amounts
    2. The liver has a great storage capacity for the vitamin, even to toxic amounts
    3. The vitamin cannot be stored, and the excess amount would saturate the general body tissues
    4. Although the body's requirement for the vitamin is very large, the cells can synthesize more as needed

522. Most of the work of changing raw fuel forms of carbohydrates to the refined usable fuel glucose is accomplished by enzymes located in the:
    1. Mouth
    2. Small intestine
    3. Large intestine
    4. Stomach mucosa

523. Vitamin A is a fat-soluble vitamin produced by humans and other animals from its precursor

carotene-provitamin A. One of the main sources of this vitamin is:
1. Oranges
2. Skim milk
3. Tomatoes
4. Leafy greens

524. A client is to have gastric gavage. When the gavage tube is inserted the nurse should place the client in the:
1. Supine position
2. Mid-Fowler's position
3. Low-Fowler's position
4. High-Fowler's position

525. A client expresses aversion to meals and eats only small amounts. The nurse should provide:
1. Nourishment between meals
2. Small portions more frequently
3. Only foods the client likes in small portions
4. Supplementary vitamins to stimulate appetite

526. The term used to most accurately describe a client's lack of interest in food is:
1. Apathy
2. Anoxia
3. Anorexia
4. Dysphagia

Client Case Scenario 46: Mr. Blanchard has been experiencing lower abdominal discomfort intermittently for the past 2 months. He is admitted to hospital for GI tests. **Items 527 to 534 refer to this client case scenario.**

527. A flat plate radiograph of the abdomen is ordered for Mr. Blanchard. The nurse recognizes that he should receive:
1. No special preparation
2. A low soapsuds enema
3. Nothing by mouth for 8 hours
4. A laxative the evening before the x-ray

528. Barium salts in the GI series serve to:
1. Fluoresce and thus illuminate the alimentary tract
2. Give off visible light and illuminate the alimentary tract
3. Dye the alimentary tract and thus provide for color contrast
4. Absorb x-rays and thus give contrast to the soft tissues of the alimentary tract

529. Specific nursing responsibility in preparing Mr. Blanchard for a sigmoidoscopy and barium enema includes:

1. Giving castor oil the afternoon before
2. Withholding food and fluid for 8 hours
3. Administering soapsuds enemas until clear
4. Ensuring Mr. Blanchard's understanding of what is to happen

530. During administration of the barium enema, Mr. Blanchard complains of intestinal cramps. The nurse should:
1. Give it at a slower rate
2. Discontinue the procedure
3. Stop until cramps are gone
4. Lower the height of the container

531. The maximum safe height at which the container of fluid can be held when administering an enema is:
1. 30 cm
2. 37 cm
3. 45 cm
4. 66 cm

532. The nurse explains to Mr. Blanchard that visualization of the GI tract after a barium enema is made possible by:
1. Barium physically coloring the intestinal wall
2. The high x-ray absorbing properties of barium
3. The high x-ray transmitting properties of barium
4. The chemical interaction between barium and the electrolytes

533. A sigmoidoscopy is performed as a diagnostic measure. For this examination, Mr. Blanchard should be placed in the position known as:
1. Sims'
2. Prone
3. Lithotomy
4. Knee-chest

534. As part of Mr. Blanchard's preparation for a sigmoidoscopy, the nurse should:
1. Administer an enema the morning of the examination
2. Provide a container for the collection of a stool specimen
3. Withhold all fluids and foods for 24 hours before the examination
4. Explain to Mr. Blanchard that a chalklike substance will have to be swallowed

Client Case Scenario 47: Gerry Banks is diagnosed with cancer of the tongue following the discovery of a mass on a routine dental check-up. **Items 535 and 536 refer to this client case scenario.**

535. When assessing Mr. Banks with cancer of the tongue, the specific adaptation the nurse should expect to find is:
1. Halitosis
2. Leukoplakia
3. Bleeding gums
4. Substernal pain

536. The nurse recognizes that Mr. Banks had an increased risk of developing cancer of the tongue because there was history of:
1. Nail biting
2. Poor dental habits
3. Frequent gum chewing
4. Heavy consumption of alcohol

537. Clients with fractured mandibles usually have them immobilized with wires. The life-threatening problem that can develop postoperatively is:
1. Infection
2. Vomiting
3. Osteomyelitis
4. Bronchospasm

538. The chief complaint in a client with Vincent's angina is:
1. Chest pain
2. Shortness of breath
3. Shoulder discomfort
4. Bleeding oral ulcerations

539. After undergoing surgery for removal of impacted molars, the client should be instructed to notify the physician if there is:
1. Foul odor to the breath
2. Pain and swelling after 1 week
3. Pain associated with swallowing
4. Tenderness in the mouth when chewing

540. A client with a hiatus hernia complains about having difficulty sleeping at night. Appropriate intervention would be:
1. Sleeping on two or three pillows
2. Eliminating carbohydrates from the diet
3. Suggesting a large glass of milk before retiring
4. Administering antacids such as sodium bicarbonate

541. To limit symptoms of gastroesophageal reflux (GERD), the nurse should advise the client to:

1. Avoid heavy lifting
2. Lie down after eating
3. Increase fluid intake with meals
4. Wear an abdominal binder or girdle

Client Case Scenario 48: Morry Steel is diagnosed with peptic ulcer disease. **Items 542 to 545 refer to this client case scenario.**

542. Most peptic ulcers occurring in the stomach are in the:
1. Pyloric portion
2. Cardiac portion
3. Esophageal junction
4. Body of the stomach

543. The basic goal underlying Mr. Steel's unique dietary management of peptic ulcer disease is to:
1. Provide optimal amounts of all important nutrients
2. Increase the amount of bulk and roughage in his diet
3. Eliminate chemical, mechanical, and thermal irritation
4. Promote psychologic support by offering him a wide variety of foods

544. Mr. Steel develops a GI bleed and is treated medically by infusing medication through an intravenous line. A drug commonly used for this purpose is:
1. Vasopressin (Pitressin)
2. Neostigmine (Prostigmin)
3. Propantheline (Pro-Banthine)
4. Phytomenadione (Mephyton)

545. Mr. Steel is scheduled for a pyloroplasty and vagotomy because of strictures caused by ulcers unresponsive to medical therapy. The nurse reinforces Mr. Steel's understanding by stating that the vagotomy serves to:
1. Increase the heart rate
2. Hasten gastric emptying
3. Eliminate pain sensations
4. Decrease secretions in the stomach

Client Case Scenario 49: Mrs. Bucci, an 80-year-old homemaker, is admitted because of cancer of the stomach. She undergoes a subtotal gastrectomy. **Items 546 to 552 refer to this client case scenario.**

546. After a subtotal gastrectomy is performed, Mrs. Bucci is returned to the unit with an IV solution infusing and a nasogastric tube in place. The nurse notes that there has been no nasogastric

drainage for $1/2$ hour. There is an order to irrigate the nasogastric tube prn. The nurse should insert:
1. 30 ml of normal saline and withdraw slowly
2. 20 ml of air and clamp off suction for 1 hour
3. 50 ml of saline and increase pressure of suction
4. 15 ml of distilled water and disconnect suction for 30 minutes

547. Two hours after the subtotal gastrectomy the nurse notes that the drainage from Mrs. Bucci's nasogastric tube is now bright red. The nurse should:
1. Notify the physician immediately
2. Clamp the nasogastric tube for one hour
3. Recognize that this is an expected finding
4. Irrigate the nasogastric tube with iced saline

548. One of the major problems after a subtotal gastrectomy is the prevention of pulmonary complications. The nurse can best achieve this by:
1. Administering PEEP every 4 hours
2. Maintaining a consistant oxygen flow rate
3. Ambulating to increase respiratory exchange
4. Promoting frequent turning, moving, and deep breathing to mobilize bronchial secretions

549. Several days following her surgery, Mrs. Bucci develops dumping syndrome. The nurse understands that dumping syndrome refers to:
1. Nausea due to a full stomach
2. Rapid passage of osmotic fluid into the jejunum
3. Reflux of intestinal contents into the esophagus
4. Buildup of feces and gas within the large intestine

550. The wisest dietary guidelines for Mrs. Bucci would be:
1. Increasing intake of dietary roughage
2. Avoiding oral feedings for a prolonged period
3. Gradually resuming small, easily digested feedings
4. Allowing the selection of personally preferred foods

551. The nurse designs a health teaching program specifically for Mrs. Bucci. This plan should include:
1. A warning to avoid all gas-forming foods
2. An explanation of the therapeutic effect of a high-roughage diet
3. Encouragement to resume previous eating habits as soon as possible

4. A thorough explanation of the dumping syndrome and how to limit or prevent it

552. The nurse should be aware that following her gastrectomy, Mrs. Bucci may develop pernicious anemia because:
1. Vitamin B_{12} is only absorbed in the stomach
2. The stomach parietal cells secrete the intrinsic factor
3. The hemopoietic factor is secreted in the stomach
4. Chief cells in the stomach secrete the extrinsic factor

553. A client with gastric ulcer disease asks the nurse the reason for antibiotic therapy that includes metronidazole (Flagyl). The nurse should explain that antibiotics are prescribed to:
1. Treat *Helicobacter pylori* infection
2. Reduce hydrochloric acid secretion
3. Augment the immune response
4. Potentiate the effect of antacids

554. The nurse would expect an antrectomy may be performed if a client has a diagnosis of:
1. Cataracts
2. Otosclerosis
3. Gastric ulcers
4. Trigeminal neuralgia

555. A client with gastric ulcers would probably describe the associated pain as:
1. An ache radiating to the left side
2. An intermittent colicky flank pain
3. A gnawing sensation relieved by food
4. A generalized abdominal pain intensified by moving

556. When caring for a client with a nasogastric tube attached to suction, the nurse should:
1. Irrigate the tube with physiologic saline
2. Use sterile technique when irrigating the tube
3. Withdraw the tube quickly when decompression is terminated
4. Allow the client to have small chips of ice or sips of water unless nauseated

557. A serious danger to which a client with intestinal obstruction is exposed because of intestinal suction is excessive loss of:
1. Protein enzymes
2. Energy carbohydrates
3. Vitamins and minerals
4. Water and electrolytes

558. During a percutaneous endoscopic gastrostomy (PEG) tube feeding, the observation that indicates that the client is unable to tolerate a continuation of the feeding would be:
1. A passage of flatus
2. Epigastric tenderness
3. A rise of formula in the tube
4. The rapid flow of the feeding

559. Three days after admission for a cerebral vascular accident, a client has a nasogastric tube inserted and is receiving intermittent feedings. To best evaluate if a prior feeding has been absorbed the nurse should:
1. Evaluate the intake in relation to the output
2. Aspirate for a residual volume and reinstill it
3. Instill air into the stomach while auscultating
4. Compare the client's body weight to the baseline data

560. Clients receiving full strength tube feedings most commonly develop diarrhea because of:
1. Increased fiber intake
2. Bacterial contamination
3. Inappropriate positioning
4. High osmolarity of the feedings

561. The nurse should administer a nasogastric tube feeding slowly to reduce the hazard of:
1. Distention
2. Flatulence
3. Indigestion
4. Regurgitation

562. A hormone that stimulates the flow of pancreatic enzymes is:
1. Enterocrinin
2. Pancreozymin
3. Enterogastrone
4. Cholecystokinin

563. The major digestive changes in fat are accomplished in the small intestine by a lipase from pancreas. This enzymatic activity:
1. Synthesizes new triglycerides from dietary fat consumed
2. Emulsifies the fat globules and reduces their surface tension
3. Easily breaks down all the dietary fat to fatty acids and glycerol
4. Splits off all the fatty acids in only about 25% of the total dietary fat consumed

564. Secretin and pancreozymin are hormones secreted by the:
1. Liver
2. Adrenals
3. Pancreas
4. Duodenum

565. Surgery may be needed to excise a pseudocyst of the pancreas. A pseudocyst of the pancreas:
1. Is generally a malignant growth
2. Is filled with pancreatic enzymes
3. Contains necrotic tissue and blood
4. Is a pouch of undigested food particles

566. The nurse understands that an acute attack of pancreatitis can be precipitated by heavy drinking because:
1. Alcohol promotes the formation of calculi in the cystic duct
2. The pancreas is stimulated to secrete more insulin than it can immediately produce
3. The alcohol alters the composition of enzymes so they are capable of damaging the pancreas
4. Alcohol increases enzyme secretion and pancreatic duct pressure and causes backflow of enzymes into the pancreas

567. Following pancreatic surgery, clients are at risk for developing respiratory tract infections because of the:
1. Length of time required for surgery
2. Proximity of the incision to the diaphragm
3. Lowered resistance caused by bile in the blood
4. Transfer of bacteria from the pancreas to the blood

568. Jaundiced clients are susceptible to postoperative hemorrhage because their blood does not clot normally due to the fact that:
1. Excess bile salts in the blood inhibit synthesis of prothrombin in the liver
2. Excess bile salts in the blood inhibit synthesis of vitamin K and prothrombin in the liver
3. Decreased bile salts in the blood inactivate prothrombinase and prevent formation of thrombin from prothrombin
4. Lack of bile in the intestine causes inadequate vitamin K absorption, which causes inadequate prothrombin synthesis by the liver

569. The nurse understands that for a client to utilize fat-soluble vitamins, the body must produce:
1. HCl
2. Bile
3. Lipase
4. Amylase

Client Case Scenario 50: Ali Brown, a 45-year-old obese woman, is admitted to emergency complaining of nausea, belching, gas, and right upper quadrant pain. She states that she has had attacks after eating fatty or fried foods. **Items 570 to 577 refer to this client case scenario.**

570. Before scheduling Mrs. Brown for endoscopic retrograde cholangiopancreatography (ERCP), the nurse should assess her:
    1. Urine output
    2. Bilirubin level
    3. Serum glucose
    4. Blood pressure

571. Mrs. Brown has an interference in bile utilization caused by cholecystitis and cholelithiasis. The nurse understands that the ejection of bile into the alimentary tract is controlled by the hormone:
    1. Gastrin
    2. Secretin
    3. Enterocrinin
    4. Cholecystokinin

572. Mrs. Brown experiences discomfort after ingesting fatty foods because:
    1. Fatty foods are hard to digest
    2. Bile flow into the intestine is obstructed
    3. The liver is manufacturing inadequate bile
    4. There is inadequate closure of the ampulla of Vater

573. The nurse assesses Mrs. Brown for the development of obstructive jaundice, which would be evidenced by:
    1. Inadequate absorption of fat-soluble vitamin K
    2. Light amber urine, dark brown stools, yellow skin
    3. Dark-colored urine, clay-colored stools, itchy skin
    4. Straw-colored urine, putty-colored stools, yellow sclerae

574. Mrs. Brown is scheduled for a cholecystectomy. The physician orders vitamin K because it is used in the formation of:
    1. Bilirubin
    2. Prothrombin
    3. Thromboplastin
    4. Cholecystokinin

575. The nurse in the postanesthesia unit notices that Mrs. Brown has serosanguinous fluid on the abdominal dressing. The nurse should:
    1. Change the dressing
    2. Reinforce the dressing
    3. Apply an abdominal binder
    4. Remove the tape and apply new tape

576. Following Mrs. Brown's abdominal cholecystectomy, the nurse should assess for signs of respiratory complications because the:
    1. Incision is close to the diaphragm
    2. Length of time required for the surgery is prolonged
    3. Client's resistance is lowered because of bile in the blood
    4. Bloodstream is invaded by microorganisms from the biliary tract

577. After her cholecystectomy, Mrs. Brown's diet will probably be:
    1. High in fat and carbohydrate to meet energy demands
    2. High in protein and calories to promote wound healing
    3. Low in fat to avoid painful contractions in the area of the wound
    4. Low in protein and carbohydrate to avoid excess calories and help the client lose weight

Client Case Scenario 51: Myra Mack is admitted to hospital to recover from an acute episode of alcoholism. Her physician orders thiamine chloride and nicotinic acid. **Items 578 to 580 refer to this client case scenario.**

578. The most therapeutic diet for Mrs. Mack would be:
    1. High protein, low carbohydrate, low fat
    2. Low protein, high carbohydrate, high fat, soft
    3. High carbohydrate, low saturated fat, 1800 calories
    4. Protein to tolerance, moderate fat, high calorie, high vitamin, soft

579. The nurse should teach Mrs. Mack that the vitamins ordered are needed for the maintenance of:
    1. Elimination
    2. Efficient circulation
    3. The nervous system
    4. Prothrombin formation

580. Because the detoxification of alcohol damages tissues, a high-calorie diet fortified with vitamins should be encouraged to protect Mrs. Mack's:
    1. Liver
    2. Kidneys
    3. Adrenals
    4. Pancreas

Client Case Scenario 52: Mr. Simone is admitted with cirrhosis of the liver, malnutrition, ascites, and elevated BP. **Items 581 to 589 refer to this client case scenario.**

581. The nurse recognizes that the main role of the liver in relation to fat metabolism is:
    1. Producing phospholipids
    2. Storing fat for energy reserves
    3. Oxidizing fatty acids to produce energy
    4. Converting fat to lipoproteins for rapid transport out into the body

582. Mr. Simone has long-standing poor nutrition, including a protein deficiency. This deficiency leads to:
    1. Decreased bile in the blood
    2. Fat accumulation in the liver tissue
    3. Coagulation of blood in microcirculation
    4. Tissue anabolism and positive nitrogen balance

583. The most therapeutic diet for Mr. Simone would be:
    1. High protein, low carbohydrate, low fat
    2. Low protein, low carbohydrate, high fat, soft
    3. High carbohydrate, low saturated fat, 1200 calories
    4. Low sodium, protein to tolerance, moderate fat, high calorie, high vitamin, soft

584. In regard to Mr. Simone's ascites, the nurse should understand that the portal vein:
    1. Brings blood away from the liver
    2. Enters the superior vena cava from the cranium
    3. Brings venous blood from the intestinal wall to the liver
    4. Is located superficially on the anteromedial surface of the thigh

585. When assessing Mr. Simone's portal hypertension, the nurse should be alert for indications of:
    1. Liver abscess
    2. Intestinal obstruction
    3. Perforation of the duodenum
    4. Hemorrhage from esophageal varices

586. The nurse is aware that the symptoms of portal hypertension in Mr. Simone are chiefly the result of:
    1. Infection of the liver parenchyma
    2. Fatty degeneration of Kupffer cells
    3. Obstruction of the portal circulation
    4. Obstruction of the cystic and hepatic ducts

587. The nurse understands that the ascites Mr. Simone demonstrates is due in part to:
    1. The escape of lymph into the abdominal cavity directly from the inflamed liver sinusoid
    2. Increased plasma colloid osmotic pressure due to excessive liver growth and metabolism
    3. The decreased levels of ADH and aldosterone due to increasing metabolic activity in the liver
    4. Compression of the portal veins, with resultant increased back pressure in the portal venous system

588. The physician orders a paracentesis to relieve Mr. Simone's ascites. Before the procedure, the nurse should instruct Mr. Simone to:
    1. Empty his bladder
    2. Eat foods low in fat
    3. Remain NPO for 24 hours
    4. Assume the supine position

589. The nurse would expect Mr. Simone to exhibit varicose veins because of:
    1. Increased plasma hydrostatic pressure in veins of the extremities
    2. Toxic irritating products released into the blood from the diseased organs
    3. Ballooning of vein walls due to decreased venous pressure and incompetent valves
    4. Decreased plasma protein concentration resulting in the pooling of blood in the venous system

Client Case Scenario 53: Mel Ponton is admitted for esophageal varices related to hepatic cirrhosis. **Items 590 to 595 refer to this client case scenario.**

590. The basic pathophysiologic problem in cirrhosis of the liver causing esophageal varices is:
    1. Ascites and edema
    2. Portal hypertension
    3. Loss of regeneration
    4. Dilated veins and varicosities

591. Mr. Ponton's emergency medical treatment for bleeding esophageal varices that is unrelated to the control of hemorrhage is:
    1. Gastric lavage
    2. Gastric suctioning
    3. Balloon tamponade
    4. Aminocaproic acid (Amicar)

592. Intubation is indicated for Mr. Ponton. The type of tube most likely to be used would be a(an):
    1. Levin tube
    2. Salem sump

3. Miller-Abbott tube
4. Sengstaken-Blakemore tube

593. The nurse administers Neomycin to Mr. Ponton to prevent the formation of:
   1. Bile
   2. Urea
   3. Ammonia
   4. Hemoglobin

594. In an effort to prevent hepatic coma in Mr. Ponton, it may become necessary to:
   1. Give Fleet enemas
   2. Eliminate protein from the diet
   3. Prepare for emergency surgery
   4. Eliminate carbohydrate from the diet

595. The nurse should assess Mr. Ponton for indications of hepatic coma. One classic sign of hepatic coma is:
   1. Bile-colored stools
   2. Elevated cholesterol
   3. Flapping hand tremors
   4. Depressed muscle reflexes

596. The cooked food most likely to remain contaminated by the virus that causes hepatitis Type A is:
   1. Canned tuna
   2. Broiled shrimp
   3. Baked haddock
   4. Steamed lobster

597. Prophylaxis for hepatitis B includes:
   1. Screening of blood donors
   2. Sterilizing the water supply
   3. Avoiding shellfish in the diet
   4. Limiting hepatotoxic drug therapy

598. In the client with hepatitis B the earliest indication of parenchymal damage to the liver usually is:
   1. A rise in bilirubin
   2. An alteration in proteins
   3. A rise in alanine aminotransferase
   4. An elevation of alkaline phosphatase

599. When caring for a client with hepatitis A the nurse should take special precautions to:
   1. Prevent droplet spread of infection
   2. Use caution when bringing food to the client
   3. Use gloves when removing the client's bedpan
   4. Wear mask and gown before entering the room

600. The major cause of posttransfusion hepatitis is:
   1. Hepatitis Type A
   2. Hepatitis Type B
   3. Hepatitis Type C
   4. Hepatitis Type D

601. A client with hepatic cirrhosis begins to develop slurred speech, confusion, drowsiness, and a flapping tremor. With this evidence of impending hepatic coma, the diet would probably be changed to:
   1. 20 g protein, 2000 calories
   2. 70 g protein, 1200 calories
   3. 80 g protein, 2500 calories
   4. 100 g protein, 1500 calories

602. When assessing a client with liver insufficiency the nurse would expect:
   1. Anuria
   2. Fetor hepaticus
   3. Blepharospasm
   4. Globus hystericus

603. The nurse should assess a client with liver cirrhosis and hepatic coma for:
   1. Icterus
   2. Urticaria
   3. Uremic frost
   4. Hemangioma

604. The laboratory test that would indicate that the liver of a client with cirrhosis is compromised and Neomycin enemas might be helpful would be:
   1. Ammonia level
   2. White blood count
   3. Culture and sensitivity
   4. Alanine aminotransaminase level

Client Case Scenario 54: Gerald Olgen has been diagnosed with cancer of the liver. He is in a debilitated state and is admitted for palliative treatment. **Items 605 to 607 refer to this client case scenario.**

605. On admission the objective information that would be most helpful for future monitoring of Mr. Olgen's condition would be:
   1. Diet history
   2. Bowel sounds
   3. Present weight
   4. Pain description

606. The nurse would expect Mr. Olgen to complain of fatigue because a readily available form of energy, although limited in amount, is stored in the liver by conversion of glucose to:
1. Glycerol
2. Glycogen
3. Tissue fat
4. Amino acids

607. The nurse would expect Mr. Olgen to have difficulty digesting fatty foods because the liver is involved in the production of:
1. Bile
2. Lipase
3. Amylase
4. Cholesterol

Client Case Scenario 55: Mrs. Ergotano is admitted with anorexia, weight loss, abdominal distention, and abnormal stools. A diagnosis of malabsorption syndrome is made. **Items 608 to 612 refer to this client case scenario.**

608. To meet Mrs. Ergotano's needs the nurse should:
1. Allow her to eat food preferences
2. Institute IV therapy to improve hydration
3. Maintain NPO status, because food precipitates diarrhea
4. Encourage consumption of meats at mealtime and high protein snacks

609. A striking clinical improvement should be noted in Mrs. Ergotano after administration of:
1. Folic acid
2. Vitamin B_{12}
3. Corticotropin
4. A gluten-free diet

610. When planning dietary teaching for Mrs. Ergotano the nurse should include the need to avoid:
1. Rice or corn
2. Milk or cheese
3. Fruit or fruit juices
4. Wheat, rye, or oats

611. A typical food combination that can be served to Mrs. Ergotano would be:
1. Roast beef, baked potato, carrots, tea
2. Cheese omelet, noodles, green beans, coffee
3. Creamed turkey on toast, rice, green peas, milk
4. Baked chicken, mashed potatoes with gravy, zucchini, Postum

612. Mrs. Ergotano is to have an enema. The rectal catheter should be inserted:

1. 5 cm
2. 10 cm
3. 15 cm
4. 20 cm

Client Case Scenario 56: Jenny Worth, 18 years old, is admitted with acute onset of right lower quadrant pain. Appendicitis is suspected. **Items 613 to 618 refer to this client case scenario.**

613. To determine the etiology of the pain, Miss Worth should be assessed for:
1. Urinary retention
2. Gastric hyperacidity
3. Rebound tenderness
4. Increased lower bowel motility

614. Miss Worth's condition is associated with:
1. Poor dietary habits
2. Infection of the bowel
3. Hypertension and resultant edema
4. Compromised circulation to the appendix

615. Miss Worth has an appendectomy and develops peritonitis. The nurse should assess her for an elevated temperature and:
1. Hyperactivity
2. Extreme hunger
3. Urinary retention
4. Local muscular rigidity

616. The position that is indicated for Miss Worth is the:
1. Sims' position
2. Semi-Fowler's position
3. Trendelenburg position
4. Dorsal recumbent position

617. Four days after abdominal surgery Miss Worth has not passed any flatus and there are no bowel sounds. Paralytic ileus is suspected. In this condition there is an interference caused by:
1. Decreased blood supply
2. Impaired neural functioning
3. Perforation of the bowel wall
4. Obstruction of the bowel lumen

618. The physician orders a rectal tube for Miss Worth to help relieve her abdominal distention. To achieve maximum effectiveness, the nurse needs to leave the tube in situ:
1. 15 minutes
2. 30 minutes
3. 45 minutes
4. 60 minutes

619. A 93-year-old client is admitted with severe abdominal pain, anorexia, nausea, and vomiting for 24 hours. A markedly elevated temperature and WBCs are increased. The primary reason for performing surgery is most likely that:
    1. The client's symptoms on admission were life threatening
    2. Surgery is usually indicated for clients with the diagnosis of diverticulitis
    3. In some instances diverticulitis is difficult to differentiate from carcinoma except surgically
    4. The client's age indicated immediate correction of the potentially fatal condition was needed

620. The most important method of preventing amebic dysentery is:
    1. Tick control
    2. Killing biting gnats
    3. Proper sewage disposal
    4. Proper pasteurization of milk

621. When teaching a client about intussusception, the nurse explains that it is:
    1. Kinking of the bowel onto itself
    2. A band of connective tissue compressing the bowel
    3. Telescoping of a proximal loop of bowel into a distal loop
    4. A protrusion of an organ or part of an organ through the wall that contains it

Client Case Scenario 57: Jake Weinberg is admitted to hospital with diverticulitis. An ileostomy is performed. **Items 622 to 624 refer to this client case scenario.**

622. When caring for Mr. Weinberg the nurse would:
    1. Encourage him to eat foods high in residue
    2. Explain that the drainage can be controlled with daily irrigations
    3. Expect the stoma to start draining on the third postoperative day
    4. Anticipate that emotional stress can increase intestinal peristalsis

623. Mr. Weinberg may suffer from anemia because:
    1. Folic acid is absorbed only in the terminal ileum
    2. The hemopoietic factor is absorbed only in the terminal ileum
    3. Iron absorption is dependent on simultaneous bile salt absorption in the terminal ileum
    4. The trace elements copper, cobalt, and nickel, required for hemoglobin synthesis, occur only in the ileum

624. The sport that should be avoided by Mr. Weinberg is:
    1. Skiing
    2. Football
    3. Swimming
    4. Track events

Client Case Scenario 58: Martin Fink enters hospital with diarrhea, anorexia, weight loss, and abdominal cramps. A tentative diagnosis of colitis has been made. **Items 625 to 633 refer to this client case scenario.**

625. When eliciting a health history from Mr. Fink the nurse bases the interview on the knowledge that colitis is commonly associated with:
    1. Chemical stress
    2. Endocrine stress
    3. Physiologic stress
    4. Psychologic stress

626. Vitamins are administered parenterally for Mr. Fink because:
    1. More rapid action results
    2. They are ineffective orally
    3. They decrease colon irritability
    4. Intestinal absorption may be inadequate

627. Mr. Fink receives an enema and should be placed in the:
    1. Sims' position
    2. Back-lying position
    3. Knee-chest position
    4. Mid-Fowler's position

628. To decrease GI irritability, the nurse should teach Mr. Fink to minimize use of:
    1. Table salt and rice products
    2. Sugar products and proteins
    3. Milk products and cola drinks
    4. Triglycerides and amino acids

629. The symptoms that the nurse should expect when assessing Mr. Fink are:
    1. Leukocytosis, anorexia, weight loss
    2. Anemia, hemoptysis, weight loss, abdominal cramps
    3. Diarrhea, anorexia, weight loss, abdominal cramps, anemia
    4. Fever, anemia, nausea and vomiting, leukopenia, diarrhea

630. The physician orders daily stool examinations for Mr. Fink in order to determine:
1. Ova and parasites
2. Culture and sensitivity
3. Fat and undigested food
4. Occult blood and organisms

631. The most serious complication associated with chronic inflammation of the bowel is:
1. Ileus
2. Bleeding
3. Perforation
4. Obstruction

632. The physician orders a low-residue diet for Mr. Fink. The nurse would know that the dietary teaching is understood when Mr. Fink states, "I can eat:
1. Baked fish, macaroni with cheese, strained carrots, fruit gelatin, and milk."
2. Cream soup and crackers, omelet, mashed potatoes, roll, orange juice, and coffee."
3. Stewed chicken, baked potato with butter, strained peas, white bread, plain cake, and milk."
4. Lean roast beef, buttered white rice with egg slices, white bread with butter and jelly, and tea with sugar."

633. Mr. Fink may need to make the decision to have a colectomy if advised by the physician. A significant factor in this decision may have been the knowledge that:
1. Surgical treatment cures ulcerative colitis
2. It would be temporary until the colon heals
3. Ulcerative colitis can progress to Crohn's disease
4. Without surgery he would be unable to eat table foods

Client Case Scenario 59: Jack Gray is admitted to hospital with extensive carcinoma of the descending portion of the colon with metastasis to the lymph nodes. **Items 634 to 644 refer to this client case scenario.**

634. The operative procedure that would probably be performed for Mr. Gray is a(an):
1. Ileostomy
2. Colectomy
3. Colostomy
4. Cecostomy

635. The nurse administers neomycin sulfate to Mr. Gray prior to surgery to:
1. Destroy intestinal bacteria
2. Increase the production of vitamin K
3. Decrease the incidence of any secondary infection
4. Decrease the possibility of postoperative urinary tract infection

636. Neomycin is especially useful prior to colon surgery because it:
1. Will not affect the kidneys
2. Acts systemically without delay
3. Is poorly absorbed from the GI tract
4. Is effective against many organisms

637. Following his surgery, the nurse should protect Mr. Gray's skin surrounding the stoma by using:
1. Alcohol
2. Mineral oil
3. Skin barriers
4. Tincture of benzoin

638. The primary step toward long-range goals in Mr. Gray's rehabilitation involves his:
1. Mastery of techniques of ostomy care
2. Readiness to accept an altered body function
3. Awareness of available community resources
4. Knowledge of the necessary dietary modifications

639. When teaching Mr. Gray to care for a new stoma, the nurse should advise him that irrigations be done at the same time every day. The time selected should:
1. Be approximately 1 hour before breakfast
2. Provide ample uninterrupted bathroom use at home
3. Approximate Mr. Gray's usual daily time for elimination
4. Be about halfway between the two largest meals of the day

640. If, during the ostomy irrigation, Mr. Gray complains of abdominal cramps, the nurse should:
1. Discontinue the irrigation
2. Lower the container of fluid
3. Advance the catheter about 2.5 cm
4. Clamp the catheter for a few minutes

641. When performing the colostomy irrigation, the nurse inserts the catheter into the stoma:
1. 5 cm
2. 10 cm
3. 15 cm
4. 20 cm

642. The nurse should indicate to Mr. Gray that the distance of the container above the stoma should be no more than:

1. 15 cm
2. 25 cm
3. 30 cm
4. 45 cm

643. When teaching Mr. Gray what might be expected on discharge, the nurse should discuss the:
    1. Need for special clothing
    2. Importance of limiting activity
    3. Periodic dilation of the stoma
    4. Bland, low-residue diet regimen

644. Mr. Gray should follow a diet that is:
    1. Rich in protein
    2. Low in fiber content
    3. High in carbohydrate
    4. As close to normal as possible

645. The solution of choice used to maintain patency of an intestinal (Cantor) tube is:
    1. Sterile water
    2. Isotonic saline
    3. Hypotonic saline
    4. Hypertonic glucose

646. A client has a transverse colostomy. When inserting a catheter for irrigation, the nurse should:
    1. Use an oil-base lubricant
    2. Instruct the client to bear down
    3. Apply gentle but continuous force
    4. Direct it toward the client's right side

647. A client has surgery for an incarcerated hernia. The physician returns the incarcerated tissue to the abdominal cavity and uses a mesh to reinforce the muscle wall, thereby preventing a future recurrence. This procedure is referred to as a:
    1. Herniotomy
    2. Herniectomy
    3. Hernioplasty
    4. Herniorrhaphy

648. A client with a cerebral vascular accident becomes incontinent of feces. When establishing a bowel training program, the nurse must remember that the most important factor is the:
    1. Use of medication to induce elimination
    2. Plan to schedule a definite time for attempted evacuations
    3. Client's previous habits in the area of diet and use of laxatives
    4. Timing of elimination to take advantage of the gastrocolic reflex

Client Case Scenario 60: Eric Robert, a 34-year-old professor, enters the hospital for a hemorrhoidectomy. **Items 649 to 654 refer to this client case scenario.**

649. When Mr. Robert is admitted for a hemorrhoidectomy, the nurse should observe the area for the presence of:
    1. Pruritus
    2. Flatulence
    3. Anal stenosis
    4. Rectal bleeding

650. Mr. Robert asks what caused this problem to occur. The nurse explains that it generally results from:
    1. Constipation
    2. Hypertension
    3. Eating spicy foods
    4. Poor bowel control

651. Before ligation of hemorrhoids, the nurse should expect the physician will suggest that Mr. Robert eat a:
    1. Bland diet
    2. Clear liquid diet
    3. High-protein diet
    4. Low-residue diet

652. Postoperative care for Mr. Robert should include:
    1. Occlusive dressings to the area
    2. Encouraging showers when needed
    3. Administration of laxatives and stool softeners
    4. Administration of enemas to promote defecation

653. While helping Mr. Robert reestablish a regular pattern of defecation, the nurse should base the teaching on the principle that:
    1. Inactivity produces muscle atonia
    2. The gastrocolic reflex initiates peristalsis
    3. Increased fluid promotes ease of evacuation
    4. Increased potassium is needed for normal neuromuscular irritability

654. When teaching Mr. Robert to include more bulk in the diet, the nurse recognizes that the action of bulk to promote defecation is a consequence of the:
    1. Irritating effect of fiber on the bowel wall
    2. Action of the multiflora of the large intestine
    3. Tendency of smooth muscle to contract when stretched
    4. Direct chemical stimulation of the colonic musculature

Client Case Scenario 61: Joann Jerry, an elderly client in an extended care facility, is suspected of being impacted. **Items 655 to 657 refer to this client case scenario.**

655. The nurse suspects Mrs. Jerry has become impacted when she states:
    1. "I have a lot of gas pains."
    2. "I don't have much of an appetite."
    3. "I feel like I have to go and just can't."
    4. "I haven't had a bowel movement for 2 days."

656. The assessment by the nurse that indicates the probable presence of a fecal impaction in Mrs. Jerry would be:
    1. Tympanites
    2. Fecal liquid seepage
    3. Bright red blood in the stool
    4. Decreased number of bowel movements

657. With the knowledge that Mrs. Jerry is accustomed to taking enemas periodically to avoid constipation, the nurse should:
    1. Arrange to have enemas ordered
    2. Have the physician order a daily laxative
    3. Offer her a large glass of prune juice and warm water each morning
    4. Realize that enemas will be necessary because the normal conditioned reflex has been lost

Neuromuscular

658. The nurse understands that hemiplegia involves:
    1. Paresis of both lower extremities
    2. Paralysis of one side of the body
    3. Paralysis of both lower extremities
    4. Paresis of upper and lower extremities

659. An overexercised muscle that has an insufficient oxygen supply may become sore from a buildup of:
    1. Acetone
    2. Lactic acid
    3. Butyric acid
    4. Acetoacetic acid

660. Stimulation of the vagus nerve results in:
    1. Tachycardia
    2. Slowing of the heart
    3. Dilation of the bronchioles
    4. Coronary artery vasodilation

661. A feeling of pleasantness or unpleasantness, varying in degree from mild to intense, occurs when sensory impulses reach the:
    1. Thalamus
    2. Basal ganglia
    3. Hypothalamus
    4. Cerebral cortex

662. An arterial anastomosis present at the base of the brain that is important in maintaining the integrity of the cerebral neurons is the:
    1. Volar arch
    2. Circle of Willis
    3. Brachial plexus
    4. Brachiocephalic sinus

663. The medulla has centers for:
    1. Control of sexual development
    2. Voluntary movement, taste, skin sensations
    3. Control of breathing, heartbeat, blood vessel diameter
    4. Fat metabolism, temperature regulation, water balance

664. A client with a spinal cord injury asks the nurse when walking will be possible. The nurse's reply is based on the knowledge that destroyed nerve fibers in the brain or spinal cord do not regenerate because they lack:
    1. Nuclei
    2. Nissl bodies
    3. A neurilemma
    4. A myelin sheath

665. The fact that a client cannot close the right eye can be explained by nonconduction of:
    1. The 2nd cranial nerve
    2. The 3rd cranial nerve
    3. The 4th cranial nerve
    4. The 7th cranial nerve

666. A client has a dilated right pupil. The nurse understands that this adaptation is related to:
    1. The 2nd cranial nerve
    2. The 3rd cranial nerve
    3. The 4th cranial nerve
    4. The 7th cranial nerve

667. A client's mouth is drawn over to the left. This suggests injury to the:
    1. Left facial nerve
    2. Right facial nerve
    3. Left abducent nerve
    4. Right trigeminal nerve

668. Tendon reflexes, for example, the knee-jerk on the right side of a client's body, are found to be exaggerated. Therefore the nurse is aware that impulses are still being conducted by the:
    1. Basal ganglia
    2. Pyramidal tracts
    3. Upper motoneurons
    4. Anterior horn neurons

669. A physician performs a lumbar puncture. To do this procedure a needle must be inserted into the:
1. Pia mater
2. Foramen ovale
3. Aqueduct of Sylvius
4. Subarachnoid space

670. Coordination of skeletal muscles and equilibrium are controlled by the:
1. Thalamus
2. Cerebellum
3. Hypothalamus
4. Medulla oblongata

671. Reflex control of respiration occurs in the:
1. Cerebellum
2. Hypothalamus
3. Cerebral cortex
4. Medulla and pons

672. The nurse should be aware that a common misconception about the autonomic nervous system is that:
1. Both sympathetic and parasympathetic impulses continually affect most visceral effectors
2. The autonomic nervous system is regulated by impulses from the hypothalamus and other parts of the brain
3. Sympathetic impulses stimulate while parasympathetic impulses inhibit the functioning of any visceral effector
4. Visceral effectors (e.g., cardiac muscle, smooth muscle, glandular epithelial tissue) receive impulses only via autonomic neurons

673. The relay center for sensory impulses is the:
1. Thalamus
2. Cerebellum
3. Hypothalamus
4. Medulla oblongata

674. Internal organs, such as the bladder and the esophagus, are most directly under the control of the:
1. Spinal cord
2. Central nervous system
3. Peripheral nervous system
4. Autonomic nervous system

675. Neural impulses travel in one direction because:
1. Polarization occurs laterally
2. Axons secrete acetylcholine
3. Sodium pump does not work in reverse
4. Cholinesterase acts along the entire axon

676. The terminals of axons supplying skeletal muscle release:
1. ATP
2. Epinephrine
3. Acetylcholine
4. Cholinesterase

677. An indication of parasympathetic dominance in a client under stress would be:
1. Constipation
2. Goose pimples
3. Excess epinephrine secretion
4. Increased hydrochloric acid secretion

678. Following a cerebrovascular accident a client remains unresponsive to sensory stimulation. The lobe of the cerebral cortex that registers general sensations such as heat, cold, pain, and touch is the:
1. Frontal lobe
2. Parietal lobe
3. Occipital lobe
4. Temporal lobe

679. The stage of sleep associated with psychologic rest is:
1. Stage 1
2. Stage 4
3. REM sleep
4. Non-REM sleep

680. Cold applications for short periods of time produce:
1. Local anesthesia
2. Peripheral vasodilation
3. Depression of vital signs
4. Decreased viscosity of blood

681. When caring for an anxious, fearful client an indication of sympathetic nervous system control identifiable by the nurse would be:
1. Dry skin
2. Skin pallor
3. Pulse rate of 60
4. Constriction of pupils

682. When transporting a client on a stretcher the nurse makes certain that the client's arms do not hang down over the edge. By taking this precaution the nurse prevents injury to the:
1. Solar plexus
2. Celiac plexus
3. Basilar plexus
4. Brachial plexus

683. A homeless person is brought to the emergency room after prolonged exposure to cold weather. The nurse should assess the client for hypothermia, which would be manifested by:
1. Stupor
2. Erythema
3. Increased anxiety
4. Rapid respirations

684. The nurse assists the physician in performing a lumbar puncture. When pressure is placed on the jugular vein during a lumbar puncture, there is normally a rise in the spinal fluid pressure. This is referred to as:
1. Homans' sign
2. Romberg's sign
3. Chvostek's sign
4. Queckenstedt's sign

685. To prevent toxoplasmosis, the nurse should instruct clients to avoid:
1. Contact with cat feces
2. Working with heavy metals
3. Ingestion of fresh water fish
4. Excessive radiation exposure

686. It is most important for the nurse to observe a client with the diagnosis of tetanus for:
1. Muscular rigidity
2. Respiratory tract spasms
3. Restlessness and irritability
4. Spastic voluntary muscle contractions

687. A characteristic manifestation of rabies includes:
1. Diarrhea
2. Memory loss
3. Urinary stasis
4. Pharyngeal spasm

688. The nurse is aware that bacteria that produce meningitis may enter the central nervous system via the:
1. Genitourinary tract
2. Gastrointestinal tract
3. Cranial apertures or sinuses
4. Integumentary system via the pores

689. Impulses initiated by stimulation of pain receptors are conducted by the:
1. Reticulospinal tracts
2. Posterior white columns
3. Lateral spinothalamic tracts
4. Ventral spinothalamic tracts

690. Electric stimulation by the use of a peripheral nerve implant or dorsal column stimulator is used in intractable pain. The nurse should explain to the client that after surgery:
1. Tub baths should not be taken
2. Analgesics will no longer be necessary
3. The transmitter must be worn externally
4. The device may interfere with the television remote control

691. A procedure done to relieve intractable pain in the upper torso is a:
1. Rhizotomy
2. Rhinotomy
3. Cordotomy
4. Chondrectomy

692. Following abdominal surgery a client complains of pain. The first action by the nurse should be to:
1. Reposition the client
2. Monitor the vital signs
3. Administer the ordered analgesic
4. Determine the characteristics of the pain

693. The part of the ear that contains the receptors for hearing is the:
1. Utricle
2. Cochlea
3. Middle ear
4. Tympanic cavity

694. The ear bones that transmit vibrations to the oval window of the cochlea are found in the:
1. Inner ear
2. Outer ear
3. Middle ear
4. Eustachian tube

695. Nerve deafness would most likely result from an injury or infection that damaged the:
1. Vagus nerve
2. Cochlear nerve
3. Vestibular nerve
4. Trigeminal nerve

696. A labyrinthectomy can be performed to treat Ménière's syndrome. This procedure results in:
1. Anosmia
2. Absence of pain
3. Reduction of cerumen
4. Permanent deafness

697. Otosclerosis is a common cause of conductive hearing loss. With such a partial hearing loss:
1. Stapedectomy is the procedure of choice
2. Hearing aids usually restore some hearing
3. The client is usually unable to hear base tones

4. Air conduction is more effective than bone conduction

698. A client who complains of tinnitus is describing a symptom that is:
1. Objective
2. Functional
3. Prodromal
4. Subjective

699. Physiologically the middle ear (containing the three ossicles) serves primarily to:
1. Maintain balance
2. Translate sound waves into nerve impulses
3. Amplify the energy of sound waves entering the ear
4. Communicate with the throat via the eustachian tube

700. The vision cycle in the eye requires vitamin A. Here the vitamin functions as:
1. An integral part of the retina's pigment called melanin
2. A part of the rods and cones that controls color blindness
3. The material in the cornea that prevents cataract formation
4. A necessary component of rhodopsin (visual purple), which controls light-dark adaptations

701. The nurse is aware that the optic chiasm:
1. Forms a cavity in which the eyeball is fixed
2. Receives nerve impulses from the optic tracts
3. Is a crossing of some optic nerves in the cranial cavity
4. Is the space posterior to the lens with the consistency of jelly

702. When the ciliary muscles contract they:
1. Close the eyelids
2. Focus the lens on near objects
3. Focus the lens on distant objects
4. Bring about convergence of both eyes

Client Case Scenario 62: Lena Fergus has primary closed-angle glaucoma. **Items 703 to 706 refer to this client case scenario.**

703. When caring for Mrs. Fergus, the nurse should understand that the goal of therapy is:
1. Controlling intraocular pressure
2. Resting the eye to reduce pressure
3. Dilating the pupil to allow for an increase in the visual field
4. Preventing secondary infections that can add to the visual problem

704. Drugs instilled in Mrs. Fergus' eye are administered by the method known as:
1. Topical
2. Injection
3. Intraocular
4. Insufflation

705. The nurse should recognize that further teaching is needed when Mrs. Fergus states, "It would be dangerous for me to:
1. Use any sedatives."
2. Become constipated."
3. Use atropine in any form."
4. Release my emotions by crying."

706. Mrs. Fergus should be advised to:
1. Take laxatives daily
2. Use eyewashes on a regular basis
3. Keep an extra supply of eye medication on hand
4. Have corrective lens prescriptions checked every 3 months

Client Case Scenario 63: Sim Lee is diagnosed with open-angle glaucoma. **Items 707 and 708 refer to this client case scenario.**

707. The first symptom Mrs. Lee is most likely to exhibit is:
1. Constant blurred vision
2. Sudden attacks of acute pain
3. Impairment of peripheral vision
4. A sudden, complete loss of vision

708. The nurse explains to Mrs. Lee that the chief aim of treatment is:
1. Controlling intraocular pressure
2. Promoting the healing process by resting her eye
3. Dilating the pupil to allow for an increase in her visual field
4. Preventing secondary infections that may add to her visual problem

Client Case Scenario 64: Christopher Styles is brought to the ophthalmologist's office by his wife. He has minimal vision in his left eye and tells the nurse "I'm sure it's a cataract; my brother just had cataract surgery." **Items 709 to 712 refer to this client case scenario.**

709. A cataract is:
1. An opacity of the lens
2. A thin film over the cornea
3. A crystallinization of the pupil
4. An increase in the density of the conjunctiva

710. After Mr. Styles has cataract surgery, the nurse should:
    1. Teach him coughing and deep breathing techniques
    2. Encourage eye exercises to strengthen the ocular musculature
    3. Keep Mr. Styles in the supine position with the head immobilized
    4. Advise Mr. Styles to refrain from vigorous brushing of his teeth and hair

711. After examination, the physician informs Mr. Styles that he has a detached retina. When he asks about the condition, the nurse should explain that retinal detachment is a:
    1. Consequence of optic-retinal atrophy
    2. Degeneration of the choroid and optic chiasm
    3. Division between the photoreceptor and neural layers of the retina
    4. Separation between the sensory portion of the retina and the pigment layer

712. The goal of surgery for Mr. Styles is to:
    1. Promote growth of new retinal cells
    2. Adhere the sclera to the choroid layer
    3. Graft a healthy piece of retina in place
    4. Create a scar that aids in healing retinal holes

Client Case Scenario 65: Bart Miller is admitted to emergency with delirium tremens due to alcohol withdrawal. **Items 713 and 714 refer to this client case scenario.**

713. The nurse should assign Mr. Miller to a:
    1. One-bed room next to the bathroom
    2. One-bed room next to the nurses' station
    3. Two-bed room next to the nurses' station
    4. Two-bed room at the quiet end of the unit

714. The nurse understands that chlordiazepoxide HCl (Librium) is given to Mr. Miller to combat his:
    1. Emotional problems
    2. Detoxification from alcohol
    3. Motor and sensory impairments
    4. Fluid and electrolyte imbalances

715. The preferred treatment for malignant melanoma of the eye is:
    1. Radiation
    2. Enucleation
    3. Cryosurgery
    4. Chemotherapy

716. The most frequently occurring type of brain tumor is a:
    1. Glioma
    2. Meningioma
    3. Neurofibroma
    4. Pituitary adenoma

717. A client is to have a parotidectomy to remove a cancerous lesion. A postoperative complication that may be distressing to the client is:
    1. A tracheostomy
    2. Frey's syndrome
    3. Facial nerve dysfunction
    4. An increase in salivation

Client Case Scenario 66: Brian Brown, who has a history of seizures, is admitted with partial occlusion of the left carotid artery. Items 718 to 721 refer to this client case scenario.

718. Mr. Brown has been taking phenytoin (Dilantin) for 10 years. When planning care for Mr. Brown, it is most important that the nurse:
    1. Obtain a history of his seizure incidence
    2. Place an airway, suction, and restraints at his bedside
    3. Ask him to remove any dentures and eyeglasses
    4. Observe him for increased restlessness and agitation

719. The primary responsibility of a nurse if Mr. Brown has a generalized motor seizure is:
    1. Determining if an aura was experienced
    2. Inserting a plastic airway between his teeth
    3. Clearing the immediate environment for safety
    4. Administering the prescribed prn anticonvulsant

720. Mr. Brown is scheduled for an arteriogram at 1000 and is to have nothing by mouth before the test. Because he is scheduled to receive phenytoin (Dilantin) at 0900, the nurse should:
    1. Omit the 0900 dose of the drug
    2. Give the same dosage of the drug rectally
    3. Ask the physician if the drug can be given IV
    4. Administer the drug with 30 ml of water at 0900

721. Mr. Brown questions the nurse regarding his medication after discharge. The nurse should explain that this medication:
    1. Will prevent the occurrence of seizures
    2. Will probably have to be continued for life
    3. Needs to be taken only in periods of emotional stress
    4. Can usually be stopped after a year's absence of seizures

Client Case Scenario 67: Bruce Short suffered head injuries in a motor vehicle accident. **Items 722 to 731 refer to this client case scenario.**

722. Injury to the brain is particularly likely to cause death if it involves the:
    1. Pons
    2. Medulla
    3. Midbrain
    4. Thalamus

723. When Mr. Short is unconscious, the nurse should expect him to be unable to:
    1. Hear voices
    2. Control elimination
    3. Move spontaneously
    4. React to painful stimuli

724. Soon after being admitted to the hospital, Mr. Short's temperature rises to 39° C. The nurse recognizes that this suggests injury of the:
    1. Pallidum
    2. Thalamus
    3. Temporal lobe
    4. Hypothalamus

725. When caring for Mr. Short, the nurse should assess for:
    1. Decreased carotid pulses
    2. Bleeding from the oral cavity
    3. Altered level of consciousness
    4. Absence of deep tendon reflexes

726. Mr. Short regains consciousness and has no paralysis of the extremities. This suggests non-involvement of the:
    1. Parietal lobe
    2. Basal ganglia
    3. Precentral gyrus
    4. Postcentral gyrus

727. Mr. Short is extremely confused. The nurse provides new information slowly and in small amounts because:
    1. Confusion or delirium can be a defense against further stress
    2. Destruction of brain cells has occurred, interrupting mental activity
    3. Teaching is based on information progressing from the simple to the complex
    4. A minimum of information should be given, since he is unaware of surroundings

728. Mr. Short complains of hearing ringing noises. The nurse recognizes that this assessment suggests injury of the:

    1. Frontal lobe
    2. Occipital lobe
    3. Sixth cranial nerve (abducent)
    4. Eighth cranial nerve (vestibulocochlear)

729. Mr. Short has a possible skull fracture. The nurse should:
    1. Observe him for signs of brain injury
    2. Check for hemorrhaging from the oral cavity
    3. Elevate the foot of the bed if he develops symptoms of shock
    4. Observe for symptoms of decreased intracranial pressure and temperature

730. Mr. Short has expressive aphasia. As a part of the long-range planning, the nurse should:
    1. Provide positive feedback when he uses a word correctly
    2. Wait for him to verbally state needs regardless of how long it may take
    3. Suggest that he get help at home because the disability is permanent
    4. Help the family to accept the fact that Mr. Short cannot participate in verbal communication

731. Of the following combinations of symptoms the most indicative of increased intracranial pressure for Mr. Short is:
    1. Weak rapid pulse, normal blood pressure, intermittent fever, lethargy
    2. Rapid weak pulse, fall in blood pressure, low temperature, restlessness
    3. Slow bounding pulse, rising blood pressure, elevated temperature, stupor
    4. Slow bounding pulse, fall in blood pressure, temperature below 36° C, stupor

Client Case Scenario 68: Mrs. Henry has had a stroke. **Items 732 and 733 refer to this client case scenario.**

732. Dexamethasone may be administered to Mrs. Henry to:
    1. Improve renal blood flow
    2. Maintain circulatory volume
    3. Reduce intracranial pressure
    4. Prevent the development of thrombi

733. Mrs. Henry has now been receiving dexamethasone (Decadron) for 3 weeks to control cerebral edema. The planned effect of the drug is to:
    1. Suppress production of antibodies
    2. Increase fluid removal from the tissues
    3. Increase elasticity of the ventricle walls
    4. Reduce CSF secretion by the choroid plexus

Client Case Scenario 69: Heidi Byrne is suffering from trigeminal neuralgia (tic douloureux). **Items 734 to 739 refer to this client case scenario.**

734. When planning nursing care for Mrs. Byrne, the nurse should specifically:
    1. Apply iced compresses to her affected area
    2. Be alert to prevent dehydration or starvation
    3. Initiate exercises of the jaw and facial muscles
    4. Emphasize the importance of brushing her teeth

735. The nurse would expect Mrs. Byrne to exhibit:
    1. Multiple petechiae
    2. Unilateral muscle weakness
    3. Excruciating facial and head pain
    4. Uncontrollable tremors of the eyelid

736. The nurse would also expect Mrs. Byrne to demonstrate:
    1. Prolonged periods of sleep due to anxiety
    2. Hyperactivity due to medications received
    3. Exhaustion and fatigue due to extreme pain
    4. Excessive talkativeness due to apprehension

737. To prevent precipitating a painful attack in Mrs. Byrne the nurse should:
    1. Avoid walking swiftly past Mrs. Byrne
    2. Keep Mrs. Byrne in the prone position
    3. Discontinue oral hygiene temporarily
    4. Massage both sides of her face frequently

738. To limit triggering further pain for Mrs. Byrne, the nurse should instruct her to:
    1. Drink iced liquids
    2. Avoid oral hygiene
    3. Apply warm compresses
    4. Chew on the unaffected side

739. When developing a teaching plan for Mrs. Byrne, the nurse should include an explanation that the medication used to treat this disorder is:
    1. Ascorbic acid
    2. Morphine sulfate
    3. Allopurinol (Purinol)
    4. Carbamazepine (Tegretol)

740. The nurse should expect a client with an exacerbation of multiple sclerosis to experience:
    1. Double vision
    2. Resting tremors
    3. Flaccid paralysis
    4. Mental retardation

Client Case Scenario 70: Patricia Zeno is a client with a history of myasthenia gravis. **Items 741 to 748 refer to this client case scenario.**

741. Clients with myasthenia gravis, Guillain-Barré syndrome, or amyotrophic lateral sclerosis experience:
    1. Progressive deterioration until death
    2. Increased risk of respiratory complications
    3. Deficiencies of essential neurotransmitters
    4. Involuntary twitching of small muscle groups

742. Myasthenia gravis most frequently affects:
    1. Males ages 15 to 35 years
    2. Children ages 5 to15 years
    3. Females ages 10 to 30 years
    4. Both sexes ages 20 to 40 years

743. Mrs. Zeno asks the nurse why the disease has occurred. The nurse bases the reply on the knowledge that there is:
    1. A genetic defect in the production of acetylcholine
    2. A reduced amount of neurotransmitter acetylcholine
    3. A decreased number of functioning acetylcholine receptor sites
    4. An inhibition of the enzyme AChE leaving the end plates folded

744. Respiratory complications are common for Mrs. Zeno because of:
    1. Narrowed airways
    2. Impaired immunity
    3. Ineffective coughing
    4. Viscosity of secretions

745. To provide safe care for Mrs. Zeno, it is most important for the nurse to check the bedside for the presence of:
    1. A tracheostomy set
    2. An intravenous setup
    3. A hypothermia blanket
    4. A syringe and edrophonium HCl (Tensilon)

746. Mrs. Zeno has been receiving neostigmine (Prostigmin). This drug acts by:
    1. Stimulating the cerebral cortex
    2. Blocking cholinesterase action
    3. Replacing deficient neurotransmitters
    4. Accelerating transmission along neural sheaths

747. Mrs. Zeno continues to become weaker despite treatment with neostigmine. Edrophonium HCl (Tensilon) is ordered:

1. For its synergistic effect
2. To rule out cholinergic crisis
3. To confirm the diagnosis of myasthenia
4. Because of the client's resistance to neostigmine

748. The prognosis for Mrs. Zeno is most likely to be:
    1. Excellent with proper treatment
    2. Slowly progressive without remissions
    3. Chronic, with exacerbations and remissions
    4. Poor, with death occurring in a few months

Client Case Scenario 71: Lee Purcell is a 72-year-old gentleman with Parkinson's disease. **Items 749 to 751 refer to this client case scenario.**

749. Parkinson's disease is caused by:
    1. Disintegration of the myelin sheath
    2. Degeneration of the corpora quadrigemini
    3. Reduced acetylcholine receptors at synapses
    4. Degeneration of neurons of the basal ganglia

750. The nurse would expect Mr. Purcell to exhibit:
    1. A flattened affect
    2. Tonic-clonic seizures
    3. Decreased intelligence
    4. Changes in pain tolerance

751. Levodopa appears to be useful in treating Mr. Purcell because it can:
    1. Improve myelination of neurons
    2. Increase acetylcholine production
    3. Replace the dopamine in the brain cells
    4. Cause regeneration of injured thalamic cells

Client Care Scenario 72: Gunther Fritz, a 32-year-old car salesman, suffered a spinal cord injury in a motor vehicle accident, resulting in paraplegia. **Items 752 to 758 refer to this client case scenario.**

752. A nurse finds Mr. Fritz under the wreckage of his car. He is conscious, breathing satisfactorily, and lying on his back complaining of pain in the back and an inability to move the legs. The nurse should first:
    1. Leave Mr. Fritz lying on his back with instructions not to move and then go seek additional help
    2. Gently raise Mr. Fritz to a sitting position to see if the pain either diminishes or increases in intensity
    3. Roll Mr. Fritz onto his abdomen, place a pad under his head, and cover him with any material available
    4. Gently lift Mr. Fritz onto a flat piece of lumber and, using any available transportation, rush him to the closest medical institution

753. Once admitted to hospital, the physician indicates that Mr. Fritz is a paraplegic. The family asks the nurse what this means. The nurse explains that:
    1. Upper extremities are paralyzed
    2. Lower extremities are paralyzed
    3. One side of the body is paralyzed
    4. Both lower and upper extremities are paralyzed

754. The nurse recognizes that one major early problem for Mr. Fritz will be:
    1. Bladder control
    2. Client education
    3. Quadriceps setting
    4. Use of aids for ambulation

755. The nurse should expect Mr. Fritz to have some spasticity of the lower extremities. To prevent the development of contractures, careful consideration must be given to:
    1. Active exercise
    2. Deep massage
    3. Use of a tilt board
    4. Proper positioning

756. Nursing care should include turning Mr. Fritz every 2 hours primarily to:
    1. Prevent pressure ulcers
    2. Keep Mr. Fritz comfortable
    3. Improve circulation in the lower extremities
    4. Prevent flexion contractures of all his extremities

757. Mr. Fritz should be encouraged to drink fluids primarily to prevent:
    1. Dehydration
    2. Constipation
    3. Urinary tract infections
    4. Fluid and electrolyte imbalance

758. Rehabilitation plans for Mr. Fritz:
    1. Should be left up to Mr. Fritz and his family
    2. Should be considered and planned for early in his care
    3. Are not necessary, because he will return to former activities
    4. Are not necessary, because he will probably not be able to work again

Client Case Scenario 73: Jo Maxwell has a cervical injury after falling from a scaffold. He is placed on a Stryker frame. **Items 759 to 761 refer to this client case scenario.**

759. Mr. Maxwell is placed on a Stryker frame because it:
    1. Promotes body functions
    2. Helps prevent deformities
    3. Allows vertical turning of Mr. Maxwell
    4. Allows horizontal turning of Mr. Maxwell

760. Before releasing the pivot pins and turning Mr. Maxwell's Stryker frame, it is most important for the nurse to:
    1. Observe Mr. Maxwell for signs of hypotension
    2. Secure all bolts and straps to ensure Mr. Maxwell's safety
    3. Tell Mr. Maxwell to hold on to the bottom part of the frame
    4. Get another nurse, since this procedure requires two people

761. When Mr. Maxwell complains of a severe headache and nasal congestion, the nurse should assess for:
    1. Suprapubic distention
    2. Increased spinal reflexes
    3. Adventitious breath sounds
    4. A sharp drop in blood pressure

Client Case Scenario 74: Harman Walker has quadriplegia following a motorcycle accident. **Items 762 to 764 refer to this client case scenario.**

762. When caring for Mr. Walker on a CircOlectric bed, the nurse understands that the benefit of this bed is that:
    1. A receptacle for elimination is easily accessible
    2. Just two people must be present when turning Mr. Walker
    3. Mr. Walker is rotated from side to side to prevent decubiti
    4. Postural hypotension after prolonged bed rest can be prevented

763. Mr. Walker is also placed on a tilt table daily. Each day the angle of the head of the table is gradually increased. The nurse explains to Mr. Walker that the tilt table is used to:
    1. Facilitate turning
    2. Prevent pressure sores
    3. Promote hyperextension of the spine
    4. Prevent loss of calcium from the bones

764. The majority of clients like Mr. Walker are taught to use wheelchairs because:
    1. It prepares them for bracing and crutch walking
    2. It assists them in overcoming orthostatic hypotension
    3. They usually are not and never will be functional walkers
    4. They have the strength in the upper extremities for self-propulsion

Client Case Scenario 75: Colleen O'Reilly, 62 years of age, has been admitted to hospital after having had a cerebral vascular accident involving the right cerebral cortex and cranial nerves resulting in left hemiplegia and hemiparesis. **Items 765 to 779 refer to this client case scenario.**

765. Mrs. O'Reilly is comatose on admission. The nurse would expect her to:
    1. Exhibit incontinence
    2. Be responsive to painful stimuli
    3. Have twitching or picking motions
    4. Respond with some purposeful motions

766. One of the primary nursing objectives for Mrs. O'Reilly is maintenance of her airway. To achieve this objective the nurse should initially place Mrs. O'Reilly in the:
    1. Prone position
    2. Lateral position
    3. Supine position
    4. Trendelenburg position

767. Mrs. O'Reilly has dysphagia and may experience difficulty in:
    1. Writing
    2. Focusing
    3. Swallowing
    4. Understanding

768. Mrs. O'Reilly has dysarthria and initial nursing care requires provision for:
    1. Liquid formula diet
    2. Routine hygienic needs
    3. Prevention of aspiration
    4. Effective communication

769. The blood pressure should not be obtained using Mrs. O'Reilly's affected arm because circulatory impairment may:
    1. Produce inaccurate readings
    2. Hinder restoration of function
    3. Precipitate the formation of a thrombus
    4. Cause excessive pressure on the brachial artery

770. Mrs. O'Reilly is confined to bed rest. Forty-eight hours following the CVA the nurse should institute:
    1. Active exercises of all extremities
    2. Passive range-of-motion exercises
    3. Light weight-lifting exercises of the right side
    4. Exercises that would actively capitalize on returning muscle function

771. The nurse can best prevent footdrop for Mrs. O'Reilly by the use of:
    1. Splints
    2. Blocks
    3. Cradles
    4. Sandbags

772. Mrs. O'Reilly's position should be changed every:
    1. Hour
    2. 2 hours
    3. 3 hours
    4. 4 hours

773. Urinary retention and overflow may become a problem for Mrs. O'Reilly and is evidenced by:
    1. Frequent voidings
    2. Oliguria and edema
    3. Continual incontinence
    4. Decreased urine production

774. Mrs. O'Reilly is transferred to a rehabilitation unit. A basic concept about rehabilitation is:
    1. Rehabilitation needs are best met by the client's family and community resources
    2. Rehabilitation is a specialty area with unique methods for meeting the client's needs
    3. Rehabilitation needs, immediate or potential, are exhibited by all clients with a health problem
    4. Rehabilitation is unnecessary for clients returning to their usual activities following hospitalization

775. Mrs. O'Reilly demonstrates paralysis of the left:
    1. Lower extremity and lower jaw
    2. Arm, left leg, and left side of the face
    3. Arm, left leg, and right side of the face
    4. Upper extremity and left side of the face

776. The nurse contributes to Mrs. O'Reilly's rehabilitation by:
    1. Beginning active exercises
    2. Making a referral to the physical therapist
    3. Positioning Mrs. O'Reilly to prevent deformity
    4. Not moving her affected arm and leg unless necessary

777. The nurse plans to facilitate Mrs. O'Reilly's independence by:
    1. Establishing long-range goals for the client
    2. Reinforcing success in tasks accomplished
    3. Pointing out errors and helping to correct them
    4. Demonstrating ways the client can regain independence

778. Mrs. O'Reilly begins using a cane specifically to:
    1. Maintain balance and improve stability
    2. Relieve pressure on weight-bearing joints
    3. Prevent further injury to weakened muscles
    4. Aid in controlling involuntary muscle movements

779. For optimum nutrition the nurse may find that Mrs. O'Reilly needs assistance with eating. To accomplish this goal, the nurse should:
    1. Request that her food be pureed
    2. Feed Mrs. O'Reilly to conserve the client's energy
    3. Have a family member assist Mrs. O'Reilly with each meal
    4. Encourage Mrs. O'Reilly to participate in the feeding process

Client Case Scenario 76: Lucia Grott is diagnosed as having expressive aphasia. **Items 780 and 781 refer to this client case scenario.**

780. The nurse anticipates that Miss Grott will have difficulty with:
    1. Speaking and/or writing
    2. Following specific instructions
    3. Understanding speech and/or writing
    4. Recognizing words for familiar objects

781. As part of the planning of long-term care for Miss Grott, the nurse should:
    1. Help Miss Grott accept this disability as permanent
    2. Begin helping Miss Grott associate words with physical objects
    3. Wait for Miss Grott to verbalize needs regardless of how long it may take
    4. Help family members accept the fact that they cannot verbally communicate with Miss Grott

Client Case Scenario 77: Philip Wilson has a herniated lumbar disc, and a microdiscectomy and a laminectomy are performed. **Items 782 to 786 refer to this client case scenario.**

782. The most common manifestation of a herniation of a lumbar disc is:
    1. Loss of control of elimination
    2. Pain radiating to the hip and leg
    3. Paralysis of both lower extremities
    4. Overgrowth of tissue on the lower back

783. Prior to surgery, Mr. Wilson would experience a sudden increase in pain when:
    1. Coughing or sneezing
    2. Sitting on cold surfaces
    3. Standing for extended periods
    4. Lying supine with the knees flexed

784. After microdiscectomy the nurse should assess Mr. Wilson for:
    1. Cerebral edema
    2. Spasms of the bladder
    3. Sensory loss in the legs
    4. Pain referred to the flanks

785. Postoperatively, the nurse should:
    1. Encourage Mr. Wilson to cough frequently
    2. Logroll Mr. Wilson by utilizing the draw sheet
    3. Assess Mr. Wilson for indications of peritonitis
    4. Instruct Mr. Wilson to bend the knees when turning

786. In contrast to caring for Mr. Wilson with a lumbar laminectomy, when caring for a client with a cervical laminectomy the nurse:
    1. Should maintain the client's head in a flexed position
    2. Has the added responsibility of removing oral secretions
    3. Must keep the client's head at a 45-degree angle from the spine
    4. Should provide range-of-motion exercise early during the postoperative period

Skeletal

Client Case Scenario 78: Henry King has suffered with gout for the last 6 years. He takes Allopurinol regularly on the advise of his physician. **Items 787 and 788 refer to this client case scenario.**

787. The objective of Mr. King's Allopurinol therapy is to:
    1. Increase joint mobility
    2. Decrease synovial swelling
    3. Decrease uric acid production
    4. Prevent crystallization of uric acid

788. One drug that may be an alternative for Mr. King and that has long been known to be of value in the prevention and treatment of acute attacks of gout is:
    1. Colchicine
    2. Hydrocortisone
    3. Ibuprofen (Motrin)
    4. Probenecid (Benemid)

789. Two days after the initial injury a sprain accompanied by edema is treated with the application of compresses. The appropriate temperature range for the compresses would be:
    1. 18.3° C to 26.1° C
    2. 26.6° C to 33.3° C
    3. 34.0° C to 36.1° C
    4. 36.6° C to 40.5° C

790. The synovial fluid of the joints minimizes:
    1. Efficiency
    2. Work output
    3. Friction in the joints
    4. Velocity of movements

791. The type of membrane that lines the knee joint is:
    1. Serous
    2. Mucous
    3. Synovial
    4. Epithelial

792. Compact bone is stronger than cancellous bone because of its greater:
    1. Size
    2. Weight
    3. Volume
    4. Density

793. A client with systemic lupus erythematosus questions the nurse as to the source of this disease. The nurse is aware that this is a disease of:
    1. Joints
    2. Bones
    3. Connective tissue
    4. Purine metabolism

Client Case Scenario 79: Mrs. Martin, age 68 years, is admitted with severe back pain. She has a history of osteoporosis. Items 794 to 797 refer to this client case scenario.

794. The risk of osteoporosis is increased for Mrs. Martin when she:

1. Receives long-term steroid therapy
2. Has a history of hypoparathyroidism
3. Engages in strenuous physical activity
4. Consumes excessive amounts of estrogen

795. Mrs. Martin's osteoporosis may be caused by:
    1. Estrogen therapy
    2. Hypoparathyroidism
    3. Prolonged immobility
    4. Excess calcium intake

796. Mrs. Martin is vulnerable to:
    1. Fatigue fractures
    2. Pathologic fractures
    3. Greenstick fractures
    4. Compound fractures

797. The nurse should encourage Mrs. Martin to increase her intake of:
    1. Red meat
    2. Soft drinks
    3. Turnip greens
    4. Enriched grains

Client Case Scenario 80: Barbara Bond, 35 years of age, has undergone a midthigh amputation following injury in a motor vehicle accident. **Items 798 to 804 refer to this client case scenario.**

798. Rehabilitation for Mrs. Bond should begin:
    1. Before the surgery
    2. During the convalescent phase
    3. On discharge from the hospital
    4. When it is time for a prosthesis

799. In preparing Mrs. Bond for ambulation with crutches, the nurse should recognize that Mrs. Bond needs further teaching when she states, "I must practice:
    1. Sitting down and standing up."
    2. Ambulating several hours a day."
    3. Standing and maintaining balance."
    4. Doing active exercises for muscle strengthening."

800. To promote early and efficient ambulation for Mrs. Bond, the nurse should:
    1. Keep her backrest elevated
    2. Place pillows under her stump
    3. Encourage Mrs. Bond to lie supine
    4. Turn Mrs. Bond to the prone position periodically

801. When Mrs. Bond is allowed up, the nurse should teach her to:
    1. Keep her hip in extension and adduction
    2. Keep her hip raised with the stump elevated
    3. Walk with crutches until her stump is completely healed
    4. Lift her shoulder and hip on her affected side when taking a step

802. Before ambulation is started and to make walking with crutches easier, the nurse should teach Mrs. Bond:
    1. Use of the trapeze to strengthen her biceps muscles
    2. The importance of keeping her affected limb in extension and abduction to prevent contractures
    3. Isometric exercises of her hamstring muscles while sitting in a chair until her circulatory status is stable
    4. Exercises with or without weights to strengthen her triceps, finger flexors, wrist extensors, and elbow extensors

803. The crutch gait the nurse should teach Mrs. Bond when wearing a prosthesis is the:
    1. Four-point gait
    2. Three-point gait
    3. Tripod crutch gait
    4. Swing-through crutch gait

804. To control edema of the stump a week after Mrs. Bond's amputation, the nurse should:
    1. Administer the prescribed diuretic
    2. Restrict Mrs. Bond's oral fluid intake
    3. Keep her stump elevated on a pillow
    4. Rewrap the elastic bandage as necessary

Client Case Scenario 81: Les Sork has a long leg cast applied after fracturing his leg in a downhill skiing accident. **Items 805 to 807 refer to this client case scenario.**

805. Because of Mr. Sork's long leg cast, the nurse should observe for signs that indicate compromised circulation such as:
    1. Foul odor
    2. Swelling of the toes
    3. Drainage on the cast
    4. Increased temperature

806. To prepare Mr. Sork for crutch walking, the nurse should encourage him to:
    1. Use the trapeze to strengthen the biceps muscles
    2. Keep the affected limb in extension and abduction
    3. Sit up straight in a chair to develop the back muscles
    4. Do exercises in bed to strengthen the upper extremities

807. The principle that the nurse should use when teaching Mr. Sork the four-point gait is:
    1. Elbows should be maintained in rigid extension
    2. Most of weight should be supported by the axillae
    3. Mr. Sork must be able to bear weight on both of his legs
    4. The affected extremity should be kept about 15 cm off the ground

808. When a client has paraplegia, the least effective method of preventing contractures of the joints of the lower extremities would be:
    1. Changing bed position q2h
    2. Maintaining proper bed positions
    3. Providing the client with active exercise instructions
    4. Passively moving the extremities through ROM several times daily

809. Formation of urinary calculi is a complication that may be encountered by the client with paraplegia. A factor that contributes to this condition is:
    1. High fluid intake
    2. Inadequate kidney function
    3. Increased intake of calcium
    4. Increased loss of calcium from the skeletal system

810. A client is placed into a whirlpool tub for range-of-motion exercises. Rehabilitating exercises carried out under water use:
    1. Water vapor
    2. Water pressure
    3. Water temperature
    4. Water's buoyant force

811. The nurse understands the joints most likely to be involved in a client with osteoarthritis are the:
    1. Hips and knees
    2. Ankles and metatarsals
    3. Fingers and metacarpals
    4. Cervical spine and shoulders

812. When preparing a teaching plan for a client with hypertrophic arthritis it would be inappropriate for the nurse to include a discussion of:
    1. Heberden's nodes
    2. Degenerative arthritis
    3. Nonankylosing arthritis
    4. Marie-Strümpell disease

813. To prevent deformities of the knee joints in a client with an exacerbation of arthritis, the nurse should:
    1. Discourage use of the knee joint
    2. Keep the client on a regimen of bed rest
    3. Encourage motion of the joint within limits of pain
    4. Immobilize the joint with pillows for a period of several weeks

814. A client with arthritis reports receiving the following dietary suggestions over the years. The recommendation for a daily diet that the nurse should reinforce is the use of:
    1. Wheat germ and yeast
    2. Yogurt and blackstrap molasses
    3. Multiple vitamin supplements in large doses
    4. A variety of meats, fruits, vegetables, milk, cereal grains

Client Case Scenario 82: Hariet Olin, a 38-year-old school teacher with rheumatoid arthritis, is admitted to hospital with severe pain and swelling of the joints of both hands. **Items 815 to 823 refer to this client case scenario.**

815. The primary consideration when caring for Mrs. Olin is:
    1. Surgery
    2. Comfort
    3. Education
    4. Motivation

816. The laboratory test that the nurse should refer to in reference to Mrs. Olin's diagnosis is:
    1. Pancreatic lipase
    2. Bence Jones protein
    3. Antinuclear antibody
    4. Alkaline phosphatase

817. A regimen of rest, exercise, and physical therapy is ordered for Mrs. Olin. This regimen will:
    1. Prevent arthritic pain
    2. Halt the inflammatory process
    3. Help prevent the crippling effects of the disease
    4. Provide for the return of joint motion after prolonged loss

818. Mrs. Olin asks the nurse why the physician is going to inject hydrocortisone into her affected joints. The nurse explains that the most important reason for doing this is to:
    1. Relieve pain
    2. Reduce inflammation
    3. Provide psychotherapy
    4. Prevent ankylosis of the joint

819. When planning nursing care for Mrs. Olin, the nurse should take into consideration the fact that:
1. Inflammation of the synovial membrane will rarely occur
2. Bony ankylosis of the joint is irreversible and causes immobility
3. Complete immobility is desired during the acute phase of inflammation
4. If redness and swelling of a joint occur, they signify irreversible damage

820. The nurse should know that Mrs. Olin will most often have pain and limited movement of the joints:
1. When her room is cool
2. After assistive exercise
3. In the morning on awakening
4. When the latex fixation test is positive

821. The diet the nurse would expect the physician to order for Mrs. Olin would be:
1. Salt free and low in fiber
2. High calorie with low cholesterol
3. High protein with minimal calcium
4. Regular diet with vitamins and minerals

822. The medication the nurse would expect to be prescribed to relieve Mrs. Olin's pain is:
1. Xanax 0.5 mg, tid
2. Aspirin, 0.6 g, q4h
3. Codeine, 30 mg, q4h
4. Meperidine, 30 mg, q4h prn

823. Range-of-motion exercises for Mrs. Olin should be:
1. Passively performed by the nurse
2. Avoided if any discomfort is present
3. Preceded by heat or cold application
4. Gradually increased for aerobic benefits

Client Case Scenario 83: Maggie Lund, age 72 years, has degenerative arthritis and is admitted to hospital for a total left hip replacement. **Items 824 to 830 refer to this client case scenario.**

824. Mrs. Lund's surgery may be done:
1. In a "laminar airflow room"
2. Using three separate stages
3. Early in the disease process
4. With Mrs. Lund in lithotomy position

825. Following surgery, the nurse should avoid placing Mrs. Lund:
1. In a supine position
2. On the affected side
3. On the unaffected side
4. In a low semi-Fowler's position

826. To prevent Mrs. Lund from experiencing circulatory complications, the nurse should make sure that she is:
1. Turned from side to side q3h
2. Exercising the ankles and other uninvolved joints
3. Ambulated as soon as the effects of anesthesia are gone
4. Permitted to be up in a chair as soon as the effects of anesthesia are gone

827. When Mrs. Lund is in the right side-lying position, the nurse ensures that she has a firm pillow placed between the thighs and that the entire length of the upper leg is supported. The most important reason for this is to prevent:
1. Strain on the operative site
2. Thrombus formation in the leg
3. Flexion contractures of the hip joint
4. Skin surfaces from rubbing together

828. When caring for Mrs. Lund who is currently immobilized, the nurse should remember to use principles of body mechanics by:
1. Bending at the waist to provide the power for lifting
3. Placing the feet apart to increase the stability of the body
2. Keeping the body straight when lifting to reduce pressure on the abdomen
4. Relaxing the abdominal muscles and using the extremities to prevent strain

829. When Mrs. Lund is ambulated from the bed to a chair, the nurse encourages her to stand on the unaffected leg before sitting in a chair (no weight-bearing on the involved limb). This is important because:
1. This will help maintain strength in the unaffected limb
2. There is increased circulation in the lower extremities
3. This is the quickest method of getting Mrs. Lund to and from the bed
4. This reduces the amount of help necessary to move Mrs. Lund from the bed to the chair

830. When ready to walk with crutches after hip surgery, Mrs. Lund will probably be taught:
1. Swing-through gait
2. Two-point crutch walking
3. Four-point crutch walking
4. Three-point crutch walking

Client Case Scenario 84: Mario Ray, a 67-year-old retired plumber, falls and is unable to get up. His daughter calls an ambulance and he is brought to the emergency room, where it is found that he has a fracture of the neck of the left femur. Mr. Ray is admitted to the orthopedic unit, put in Buck's extension, and prepared for surgery the next day. **Items 831 to 833 refer to this client case scenario.**

831. On examination of Mr. Ray, the nurse would expect to find:
   1. Adduction with internal rotation
   2. Abduction with external rotation
   3. Shortening of the affected extremity with external rotation
   4. Lengthening of the affected extremity with internal rotation

832 The nurse should explain to Mr. Ray that the chief reason for applying skin traction such as Buck's traction prior to surgery is to:
   1. Relieve muscle spasm and pain
   2. Prevent contractures from developing
   3. Keep him from turning and moving in bed
   4. Maintain the limb in a position of external rotation

833. The nurse should know that, following a fracture of the neck of the femur, the desirable position for Mr. Ray's limb is:
   1. Internal rotation with extension of the knee
   2. Internal rotation with flexion of the knee and hip
   3. External rotation with flexion of the knee and hip
   4. External rotation with extension of the knee and hip

834. Contractures that develop most frequently after fracture of the hip are:
   1. Internal rotation with abduction
   2. External rotation with abduction
   3. Flexion and adduction of the hip with flexion of the knee
   4. Hyperextension of the knee joint with foot-drop deformity

835. Aseptic necrosis can occur following a fracture of the head of the femur. The nurse should be aware that this is caused by:
   1. Infection at the site of the wound
   2. Weight-bearing before fracture is healed
   3. Immobilization after reduction of the fracture
   4. Loss of blood supply to the head of the femur

836. Intramedullary nailing is used in the treatment of:
   1. Slipped epiphysis of the femur
   2. Fracture of the shaft of the femur
   3. Fracture of the neck of the femur
   4. Intertrochanteric fracture of the femur

837. When teaching crutch walking to a client following an internal fixation of a hip fracture, the nurse should instruct the client to place weight on:
   1. The upper arms
   2. The axillary region
   3. Palms of the hands
   4. Both lower extremities

838. In any disaster concerning a number of people, the function that contributes most to saving of lives is sorting, or triage. When determining priority of needs, the people who need immediate care are those with:
   1. Closed fractures of major bones
   2. Partial thickness burns of 10% of the body
   3. Significant penetrating or perforating abdominal wounds
   4. Severe lacerations involving open fractures of major bones

Drug-related Responses

839. Radium is stored in lead containers because:
   1. Radium is a heavy substance
   2. The lead functions as a barrier
   3. Heat is produced as radium disintegrates
   4. Lead prevents disintegration of the radium

840. A client is receiving an antihypertensive drug intravenously for control of severe hypertension. The client's blood pressure is unstable and is at 160/94 before the infusion. Fifteen minutes after the infusion is started the blood pressure rises to 180/100. The response to the drug would be described as a(n):
   1. Allergic response
   2. Synergistic response
   3. Paradoxical response
   4. Individual hypersusceptibility

841. Before giving a client digoxin, the nurse should obtain the:
   1. Apical heart rate
   2. Radial pulse in both arms
   3. Radial pulse on the left side
   4. Difference between apical and radial pulses

Client Case Scenario 85: Mrs. Ivor is placed on nitroglycerine SL. Items 842 and 843 refer to this client case scenario.

842. Evaluation of the effectiveness of Mrs. Ivor's nitroglycerine SL is based on:
1. Relief of anginal pain
2. Improved cardiac output
3. A decrease in blood pressure
4. Dilation of superficial blood vessels

843. The nurse should teach Mrs. Ivor to suspect that nitroglycerin SL tablets have lost their potency when:
1. The tablets are three or more months old
2. Pain is unrelieved but facial flushing is increased
3. Onset of relief is delayed, but the duration of relief is unchanged
4. Pain occurs even after taking the tablet prophylactically to prevent its onset

844. When teaching a client receiving prazosin (Minipress) for hypertension why orthostatic hypotension occurs, the nurse knows that this antihypertensive causes vasodilation by:
1. Depleting acetylcholine
2. Stimulating histamine release
3. Blocking the response to norepinephrine
4. Decreasing adrenal release of epinephrine

845. A client receiving propranolol hydrochloride (Inderal) should be told to expect:
1. Dizziness with strenuous activity
2. Acceleration of the heart rate after eating a heavy meal
3. Flushing sensations for a few minutes after taking the drug
4. Pounding of the heart for a few minutes after taking the drug

846. A client with a history of arthritis has an acute episode of right ventricular heart failure and is receiving furosemide (Lasix). The physician lowers the client's usual dosage of aspirin. The nurse's explanation for the lower dose is based on the knowledge that:
1. Aspirin accelerates metabolism of furosemide and decreases the diuretic effect
2. Aspirin in large doses after an acute stress episode increases the bleeding potential
3. Competition for renal excretion sites by the drugs causes increased serum levels of aspirin
4. Use of furosemide and aspirin concomitantly increases formation of uric acid crystals in the nephron

847. A client asks the nurse why the physician has prescribed captopril (Capoten). The nurse explains it is an effective:

1. Diuretic
2. Hypnotic
3. Tranquilizer
4. Antihypertensive

848. The physician prescribes quinidine sulfate (Quinicardine) and digoxin (Lanoxin) for a client with atrial fibrillation. The nurse should understand that the goal of the drug therapy plan is to:
1. Suppress irritability of atrial and ventricular myocardial tissue
2. Slow SA node firing rate and decrease irritability of the atrial myocardial tissue
3. Decrease atrial irritability and slow transmission of impulses through the AV node
4. Stimulate SA node control of conduction and shorten the refractory period of atrial tissue

849. In addition to a decreased apical rate, the nurse should teach a client to withhold the prescribed digoxin if the client experiences:
1. Singultus
2. Chest pain
3. Blurred vision
4. Decreased urinary output

850. A client is to be discharged on a diuretic and digitalis. The nurse reviewing the client's diet would be especially careful to look for adequate sources of potassium because:
1. Potassium is a necessary ion for normal body function
2. Potassium is a cofactor for several important enzymes
3. Under conditions of hypokalemia, digitalis exerts toxic effects on the heart
4. Under conditions of hyperglycemia, digitalis exerts toxic effects on the heart

851. A client complains of fatigue and dyspnea and appears jaundiced. The nurse questions the client about medications taken routinely. In light of the symptoms, the nurse should be most concerned about:
1. Multivitamin with iron daily
2. Methyldopa (Aldomet) 250 mg bid
3. Chlordiazepoxide (Librium) 10 mg qid
4. Aspirin 600 mg just prior to admission

852. A client is receiving aminophylline intravenously to relieve severe asthma. The nurse should observe for:
   1. Hypotension
   2. Visual disturbances
   3. Decreased pulse rate
   4. Decreased urinary output

853. When teaching a client about nitroglycerine therapy, the nurse should include the importance of:
   1. Limiting the number of tablets to four per day
   2. Discontinuing the medication if a headache develops
   3. Making certain the medication is stored in a dark container
   4. Increasing the number of tablets if dizziness or hypertension occurs

854. When anticipating drug therapy for a client who is experiencing a cardiac arrest because of ventricular fibrillation, the nurse should initially prepare:
   1. Lidocaine HCl (Xylocaine) 50 mg IV bolus
   2. Dopamine HCl (Intropin) 400 mg in 500 ml D5W
   3. Epinephrine HCl (Adrenalin) 1 mg at 1:10,000 solution
   4. Sodium bicarbonate (NaHCO3) 1 mEq per kilogram of body weight

Client Case Scenario 86: Dolly Sherman is admitted with a diagnosis of partial occlusion of the left common carotid artery. She is admitted to hospital for stabilization of her Coumadin. **Items 855 to 857 refer to this client case scenario.**

855. Mrs. Sherman's prothrombin time (PT) has been somewhat unstable and the nurse interviews her to identify factors contributing to the problem. The nurse should assess Mrs. Sherman's:
   1. Use of analgesics
   2. Use of sleeping medications
   3. Intake of vitamin tablets or capsules
   4. Compliance with the plan for taking Coumadin

856. Mrs. Sherman is receiving IV heparin sodium and oral warfarin sodium (Coumadin) concurrently while in hospital. When Mrs. Sherman expresses concern about why both heparin and Coumadin are needed, the nurse's explanation is based on knowledge that the plan:
   1. Allows clot dissolution and prevents new clot formation

2. Permits the administration of smaller doses of each drug
   3. Immediately provides maximum protection against clot formation
   4. Provides anticoagulant intravenously until the oral drug reaches its peak effect

857. Mrs. Sherman is to be discharged while still receiving Coumadin. When discussing the adverse effects of Coumadin, the nurse should tell Mrs. Sherman to consult with the physician if:
   1. Blood appears in urine
   2. Swelling of the ankles increases
   3. The ability to concentrate diminishes
   4. Increased transient ischemic attacks occur

858. A female client with a history of a seizure disorder has been placed on Coumadin because of thrombophlebitis. After a weekly prothombin time the client telephones the clinic to find out if the anticoagulant dosage is to be changed. At the same time, the client mentions that she is out of the prescribed sleeping medication, but will get more at the time of her next appointment in three weeks. The nurse tells her to come for a refill immediately because:
   1. She may develop withdrawal symptoms
   2. Absence of sleep may precipitate seizures
   3. Discontinuance of the drug may affect the prothrombin level
   4. Control of seizures is dependent on the combined action of phenytoin (Dilantin) and the sleeping medication

859. The drug the nurse should expect the physician to order if symptoms of Coumadin overdose are observed would be:
   1. Heparin
   2. Vitamin K_1
   3. Protamine sufate
   4. Iron-dextran (Imferon)

860. The mercurial diuretics alter active transport systems in the kidney tubules, resulting in increased excretion of sodium and, secondarily, water. The principle explaining the secondary water loss (diuresis) is:
   1. Osmosis
   2. Diffusion
   3. Filtration
   4. Active transport

861. A client receiving hydrochlorothiazide (Hydro-Diuril) asks what this drug actually does. The nurse explains that the planned therapeutic effect of the drug is to:

1. Increase the glomerular filtration rate
2. Decrease the reabsorption of potassium
3. Increase the excretion of sodium and chloride
4. Decrease the amount of fluid reabsorption in Henle's loop

862. Vitamin B$_6$ is given with isoniazid (INH) because it:
    1. Improves the nutritional status of the client
    2. Enhances tuberculostatic effect of isoniazid
    3. Provides the vitamin when isoniazid is interfering with natural vitamin synthesis
    4. Accelerates destruction of remaining organisms after inhibition of their reproduction by isoniazid

863. A client with pulmonary tuberculosis is to receive streptomycin sulfate after discharge from the hospital. The physician plans to have the client come twice a week to the clinic for administration of the drug. The spaced dosage is planned to:
    1. Increase compliance with the therapy plan
    2. Lessen risk of adverse effects of the drug on neural tissue
    3. Minimize disruption of the rest hours required for recovery
    4. Lessen tissue trauma from injections while the client's resistance is low

864. The client is to receive isoproterenol (Isuprel) prn. The nurse administers this drug to:
    1. Produce sedation
    2. Relax bronchial spasm
    3. Decrease blood pressure
    4. Increase bronchial secretions

865. A client has been receiving Librium, 10 mg qid, for the past 5 days. The nurse should question giving the medication if the client exhibits:
    1. Hypotension
    2. Blurred vision
    3. Muscle twitching
    4. Extreme drowsiness

866. The nurse administers alprazolam (Xanax) as ordered to an anxious client who has severe hypertension because it:
    1. Induces sleep
    2. Promotes rest
    3. Reduces hostility
    4. Produces hypotension

867. Early symptoms of morphine overdose include:
    1. Slow pulse, slow respirations, sedation

2. Slow respirations, dilated pupils, restlessness
3. Profuse sweating, pinpoint pupils, and deep sleep
4. Slow respirations, constricted pupils, and deep sleep

868. When preparing a client's analgesic medication, the nurse should know that meperidine is commonly available for administration as:
    1. Narcan
    2. Darvon
    3. Doriden
    4. Demerol

869. The nurse should be aware that the medication most frequently used to relieve anxiety and apprehension in the client with pulmonary edema is:
    1. Chloral hydrate
    2. Morphine sulfate
    3. Hydroxyzine (Atarax)
    4. Sodium phenobarbital

870. After a client with a history of a seizure disorder has received IV heparin sodium for 3 days following open heart surgery, the drug is discontinued. The nurse continues to observe the client closely during the early days of treatment with Coumadin because:
    1. Phenytoin increases the clotting potential
    2. Coumadin affects the metabolism of phenytoin
    3. Coumadin action is greater in clients with seizure disorders
    4. Seizures increase the metabolic degradation rate of Coumadin

Client Case Scenario 87: Kristi Scully is admitted to emergency following a tonic-cloric seizure. She has a history of epilepsy. **Items 871 to 875 refer to this client case scenario.**

871. The physician prescribes phenobarbital sodium for Miss Scully. The nurse would know that she understood the teaching about the side effects of phenobarbital when Miss Scully states, "I should call the doctor if I develop:
    1. Loss of appetite or persistent fatigue."
    2. Anal itching or dizziness when I stand up."
    3. Diarrhea or a rash on the upper part of my body."
    4. Decreased tolerance to common foods or constipation."

872. The expected effect of phenytoin (Dilantin) is to:
    1. Produce an antispasmodic action on the muscles
    2. Prevent depression of the central nervous system
    3. Control nerve impulses originating in the motor cortex
    4. Alter the permeability of the cell membrane to potassium

873. Miss Scully is scheduled to receive phenytoin (Dilantin) 100 mg, orally at 1800 hours but is having difficulty swallowing capsules. The nurse should:
    1. Insert a rectal suppository containing 100 mg phenytoin
    2. Open the capsule and sprinkle the powder in a cup of water
    3. Administer 4 ml of phenytoin suspension containing 125 mg/5 ml
    4. Obtain a change in the prescribed administration route to allow IM administration

874. When caring for Miss Scully, the nurse plans health teaching and emphasizes meticulous oral hygiene because phenytoin (Dilantin):
    1. Causes hypertrophy of the gums
    2. Increases alkalinity of the oral secretions
    3. Irritates the gingiva and destroys tooth enamel
    4. Increases plaque and bacterial growth at the gum lines

875. Folic acid is also prescribed for Miss Scully because folic acid:
    1. Improves absorption of iron from foods
    2. Content of common foods is inadequate
    3. Prevents the neuropathy caused by phenytoin
    4. Absorption from foods is inhibited by phenytoin

876. Levodopa is prescribed for a client with Parkinson's disease. The nurse should know that this drug:
    1. Is poorly absorbed if given with meals
    2. Must be monitored by weekly laboratory tests
    3. Causes an initial euphoria followed by depression
    4. May cause a side effect of orthostatic hypotension

877. The effectiveness of carbamazepine (Tegretol) in the management of tic douloureux is determined by monitoring the client's:

1. Pain relief
2. Liver function
3. Cardiac output
4. Seizure activity

878. Edrophonium HCl (Tensilon) is used for the diagnosis of myasthenia gravis because this drug will cause a temporary increase in:
    1. Symptoms
    2. Consciousness
    3. Blood pressure
    4. Muscle strength

879. To assist the medical team in prescribing an effective antibiotic, the most valuable test is the:
    1. Serologic test
    2. Sensitivity test
    3. Susceptibility test
    4. Tissue culture test

880. After receiving streptomycin for 2 weeks as part of the medical regimen for tuberculosis, the client states, "I feel like I am walking like a drunken seaman." The nurse withholds the drug and promptly reports the problem to the physician because the signs may be a result of the drug's effect on the:
    1. Cerebellar tissue
    2. Peripheral motor end plates
    3. Internal capsule and pyramidal tracts
    4. Vestibular branch of the eighth cranial nerve

881. The nurse administers co-trimoxazole (Septra) as ordered to combat urinary tract infections. This drug belongs to the group of drugs known as:
    1. Antiseptics
    2. Analgesics
    3. Uricosurics
    4. Sulfonamides

882. A client who has been diagnosed as having Lyme disease is started on tetracycline therapy. When administering oral tetracycline, the nurse should:
    1. Administer medication with meals or a snack
    2. Provide orange or other citrus fruit juice with the medication
    3. Provide medication an hour before milk products are ingested
    4. Offer antacids 30 minutes after administration if GI side effects occur

883. A client has an urticarial response to tetracycline and ampicillin. Diphenhydramine hydrochloride (Benadryl) is administered to:

1. Destroy histamine in tissues and reverse the urticarial response
2. Inhibit release of vasoactive substances and dilate tissue capillaries
3. Compete with histamine for receptors and interfere with vasodilation
4. Metabolize histamine and inhibit release of substances causing intense itching

884. A client with tetanus is to continue taking ampicillin after discharge. The nurse should explain the need to:
    1. Take ampicillin with meals
    2. Notify the physician if diarrhea develops
    3. Store the ampicillin in a light-resistant container
    4. Continue the drug until a negative culture is obtained

885. A client will be taking sulfisoxazole (Sulfizole) at home. The nurse instructs the client to:
    1. Measure and record urine output
    2. Strain urine for crystals and stones
    3. Stop the drug if the urinary output increases
    4. Maintain the exact time schedule for drug taking

886. The physician orders 650 mg of quinine dihydrochloride to be given over an 8-hour period by IV drip in 1000 ml of normal saline to a client with malaria. The IV equipment is calibrated at 20 drops per milliliter. To deliver the correct dosage, the solution must be set to flow at the rate of:
    1. 10 drops/min
    2. 21 drops/min
    3. 34 drops/min
    4. 42 drops/min

887. Whenever quinine is used, the nurse should be alert to symptoms of severe cinchonism, which include:
    1. Deafness, vertigo, and severe nausea
    2. Pruritus, urticaria, and difficulty in breathing
    3. Leg cramps, fever, and swollen painful joints
    4. Tinnitus, decreased auditory acuity, and paresthesias

888. After several days of IV therapy for chloroquine-resistant malaria, the physician replaces the IV injection with quinine sulfate, 2 g per day in divided doses. The nurse should administer this medication after meals to:
    1. Delay its absorption
    2. Minimize gastric irritation

    3. Decrease stimulation of appetite
    4. Reduce its antidysrhythmic action

889. Prior to the discharge of a client with Addison's disease, the physician prescribes hydrocortisone 10 mg tid. The nurse expects hydrocortisone to:
    1. Control excessive loss of potassium salts
    2. Decrease cardiac dysrhythmias and dyspnea
    3. Prevent hypoglycemia and permit the client to respond to stress
    4. Increase amounts of angiotensin II to raise the client's blood pressure

890. The nurse administers desmopressin acetate (DDAVP) to a client with diabetes insipidus. To evaluate the effectiveness of the drug the nurse should monitor the client's:
    1. Pulse rate
    2. Serum glucose
    3. Arterial blood pH
    4. Intake and output

891. A client is receiving isophane insulin suspension (NPH) and regular insulin daily. The nurse should instruct the client to:
    1. Give the 2 insulins in the same syringe when the ratio is 1:1
    2. Mix the 2 insulins in any required dosage in the same syringe
    3. Give the 2 insulins separately unless the ratio of dosage is greater than 1:1
    4. Administer each insulin in a separate syringe using different sites for injection

892. While a client is receiving dexamethasone (Decadron) the nurse should test the client's blood for glucose every 4 hours because the drug:
    1. Has a glucose component
    2. Accelerates glucose metabolism
    3. Mobilizes liver stores of glycogen
    4. Lowers the renal threshold for glucose

893. The physician plans to reduce a client's dexamethasone (Decadron) dosage gradually and to continue a lower maintenance dosage. The nurse explains that the reason for the gradual dosage reduction is to allow:
    1. Production of antibodies by the immune system
    2. Return of cortisone production by the adrenal glands
    3. Building of glycogen and protein stores in liver and muscle
    4. Time to observe for return of increased intracranial pressure

894. A client with rheumatoid arthritis has been taking a steroid medication for the past year. A complication of the prolonged use of this medication is:
1. Leukopenia
2. Elevated C-reactive protein
3. Elevated sedimentation rate
4. Hypochromic, normocytic anemia

895. A client with rheumatoid arthritis is receiving Entrophen. The nurse should teach the client to report symptoms of salicylate intoxication, which include:
1. Polyuria
2. Confusion
3. Hypertension
4. Laryngeal spasm

896. Gold salts may be used to treat rheumatoid arthritis. A serious side effect of this drug is:
1. Kidney damage
2. Persistent nausea
3. Pulmonary emboli
4. Cardiac decompensation

897. The nurse should be aware that the drug of choice in rheumatoid arthritis is:
1. Imuran
2. Aspirin
3. Cortisone
4. Gold salts

898. A client with rheumatoid arthritis is receiving aurothioglucose, a gold compound. It is most important that the nurse monitor the client for:
1. Hypertension
2. Cutaneous lesions
3. Thrombocytopenia
4. Elevated blood glucose

899. During chemotherapy for cancer of the lung, the nurse expects the client to develop soreness of the mouth and anus because:
1. These tissues are poorly nourished because the client is anorectic
2. The entire GI tract is involved because of the direct irritating effects of chemotherapy
3. These tissues normally divide rapidly and are damaged by the chemotherapeutic agent
4. The side effects of the chemotherapeutic agents tend to concentrate in these body areas

900. A client is receiving a form of folic acid intramuscularly during intraarterial chemotherapy with methotrexate. The drug is being administered intramuscularly to:

1. Provide levels of folic acid required by blood-forming organs
2. Provide the metabolite required for destruction of cancer cells
3. Provide folic acid, which acts synergistically with antineoplastic drugs to destroy cancer cells
4. Increase production of phagocytic cells required to remove debris liberated by disintegrating cancer cells

901. The physician orders antibiotic therapy for a client receiving chemotherapy because these agents destroy rapidly growing cells in the:
1. Liver
2. Blood
3. Lymph nodes
4. Bone marrow

902. The nurse is aware that many of the chemotherapeutic agents used in the treatment of cancer cause:
1. Leukocytosis
2. Bone marrow depression
3. Decreased sedimentation rate
4. Increased hemoglobin and hematocrit

903. A client says, "I take 2.5 ml of baking soda in a glass of water when I get heartburn." The nurse suggests that the client use an antacid preparation that contains aluminum hydroxide and magnesium hydroxide such as Maalox. This response is based on the fact that antacids:
1. Contain little if any sodium
2. Are readily absorbed by the stomach mucosa
3. Have no direct effect on systemic acid-base balance
4. Cause few side effects such as diarrhea or constipation

904. The physician orders ranitidine (Zantac) for a client with peptic ulcer disease. The nurse should teach the client that Zantac is a drug whose main action is to:
1. Increase gastric motility
2. Neutralize gastric acidity
3. Increase histamine release
4. Inhibit gastric acid secretion

905. A client reports taking calcium carbonate (TUMS) frequently. The client should be advised that this practice may lead to:
1. Diarrhea
2. Water retention
3. Rebound hyperacidity
4. Bone demineralization

MEDICAL-SURGICAL
ANSWERS AND RATIONALES

Growth and Development

1. **3 Accidents are common during young adulthood. (IM; ED; GD)**
   1 Kidney dysfunction is not a problem specific to any one stage of growth.
   2 Cardiovascular disease is a common health problem in middle adulthood.
   4 Glaucoma is a common health problem in the older adult.

2. **2 Bones become more fragile with advancing age because of osteoporosis, often associated with lower circulating levels of estrogens or testosterone. (AN; PA; GD)**
   1 Carelessness is a characteristic applicable to certain individuals rather than to people within a developmental level.
   3 Although prolonged immobility is associated with bone demineralization, hip fractures also occur in active elderly individuals.
   4 Rheumatoid diseases certainly can affect the skeletal system but do not increase the incidence of hip fractures.

3. **1 As a result of the normal stresses on the body, the incidence of chronic illness increases in the elderly population. (AN; ED; GD)**
   2 Younger individuals have greater physiologic reserves and chronic illnesses are not common.
   3 Same as answer 2.
   4 Same as answer 2.

4. **3 Generally, female voices have a higher pitch than male voices and the elderly with presbycusis (hearing loss caused by the aging process) have more difficulty hearing these higher-pitched sounds. (DC; PA; GD)**
   1 Cerumen becomes drier and harder as a person ages.
   2 There is no greater incidence of tympanic tears caused by the aging process.
   4 The epithelium of the lining of the ear becomes thinner and drier.

5. **1 Cancer of the prostate occurs mainly in men over 60; screening via palpation and** by testing for prostatic specific antigen (PSA) should be performed at regular medical checkups. (DC; TC; GD)
   2 The largest percentage of HIV-positive individuals are in the 20 to 39-year-old age group, not the middle adult (45 to 65 years old) and late adult (over 65 years old) years.
   3 Same as answer 2.
   4 Triglyceride levels should be done at all regular physical examinations; in addition to older adults, there is evidence of plaque formation in young children, adolescents, and young adults.

Emotional Needs Related to Health Problems

6. **2 Nursing diagnosis defines an actual or potential health problem faced by the client. (AN; TC; EH)**
   1 This is the plan of care made prior to implementation; it follows the nursing diagnosis but is not part of it; it is a step in the nursing process.
   3 This is part of data collection prior to making the nursing diagnosis; it is the first step of the nursing process.
   4 Intervention follows the nursing diagnosis; it is part of the nursing process but not part of the nursing diagnosis.

7. **1 The primary nurse provides or oversees all aspects of care, including assessment, implementation, and evaluation of that care. (AN; TC; EH)**
   2 A clinician is an expert teacher or practitioner in the clinical area.
   3 The title given to a specially prepared nurse for one very specific clinical role.
   4 The nurse coordinator oversees all the staff and clients on a unit and coordinates care.

8. **4 When a plan does not effectively produce the desired outcome, the plan should be changed. (AN; TC; EH)**
   1 Time is not relevant in the revision of a care plan.
   2 Client response is the determinant, not the nursing diagnosis.
   3 Various methods may have the same outcome; effectiveness is most important.

9. **2 The nursing process is more than identifying a nursing problem. It is a step-by-step process that scientifically provides for client's nursing needs. (AN; TC; EH)**

1 This is incomplete; implementation of care is one aspect of the nursing process.

3 This is incomplete; goal establishment is one aspect of the nursing process.

4 This is incomplete; the nursing process goes beyond identification of a problem.

10. **3 The initial step in any process using problem solving is the collection of data. (DC; TC; EH)**

1 Goals are set after nursing needs are established.

2 Nursing needs can be determined only after assessment.

4 Evaluation is the last phase of the nursing process.

11. **1 Feedback permits the client to ask questions and express feelings and allows the nurse to verify client understanding. (EV; PS; EH)**

2 Medical assessment does not necessarily include nurse-client relationships.

3 Team conferences are subject to all members' evaluations of a client's status.

4 Nurse-client communication should be evaluated by the client's verbal and behavioral responses.

12. **2 Open-ended questions provide a milieu in which people can verbalize their problems rather than be placed in a situation of forced response. (IM; PS; EH)**

1 This can be threatening to the client, who may not have the answer to these questions.

3 False reassurance is detrimental to the nurse-client relationship and does not promote communication.

4 Direct questions do not open or promote communication.

13. **2 An individual is held legally responsible for actions committed against another individual or an individual's property. (AN; TC; EH)**

1 This is related to battery, which involves physical harm.

3 This is the definition of negligence.

4 This is the definition of a crime.

14. **3 False imprisonment and battery are wrongs committed by one person against another in a willful intentional way without just cause and/or excuse. (AN; TC; EH)**

1 Malpractice, which is professional negligence, is classified as an unintentional tort; assault, which is knowingly threatening another, is an intentional tort.

2 Malpractice and negligence are both unintentional torts.

4 Negligence, which is classified as an unintentional tort, involves exposure of another's person or property to unreasonable risk of injury by acts of commission or omission; invasion of privacy is an intentional tort.

15. **4 The reporting of possible child abuse is required by law, and the nurse's identity can remain confidential. (AN; TC; EH)**

1 The nurse is functioning in a professional capacity and therefore can be held accountable.

2 Although the Good Samaritan Act protects health professionals, the nurse would still be responsible for acting as any reasonably prudent nurse would in a similar situation.

3 Same as answer 2.

16. **1 Each province or territory is charged with the responsibility of protecting the health and welfare of its populace, which it does by regulating nursing practice. (AN; TC; EH)**

2 Although the members of the profession can also benefit from a clear description of their role, this is not the primary purpose of the law.

3 The employing agency does assume responsibility for its employees and therefore benefits from maintenance of standards, but this is not the purpose of the law.

4 Professional standards are established by the profession to assure quality care for the public.

17. **3 Informed consent means the client must comprehend the surgery, the alternatives, and the consequences. (EV; ED; EH)**

1 This explanation is not within nursing's domain.

2 Although this is true, it does not determine the client's ability to give informed consent.

4 Although this is true, initially the nurse should assess the client's knowledge in relation to the surgery.

18. **4 There is no evidence of incompetence. Because the client has not been certified as incompetent, the right of informed consent is retained. (IM; TC; EH)**

1 The client can sign the consent, and the client's signature requires only one witness.

2 Because there is no evidence of incompetence, the client should sign the consent.

3 Same as answer 2.

19. **3 The nurse was negligent in using a stretcher with worn straps. Such an oversight did not reflect the actions of a reasonably prudent nurse. (EV; TC; EH)**

1 The nurse is responsible for own actions and must ascertain the adequate functioning of equipment.

2 The hospital shares responsibility for safe, functioning equipment.

4 The nurse is responsible for determining the safety of hospital equipment.

20. **2 The client still had the right to make decisions regarding hours of sleep and time of medication. The concept of invasion of rights or intrusion applies. (EV; TC; EH)**

1 Although this statement may be true, it has no bearing on the legality of the situation.

3 Respondeat superior (let the master respond) indicates that employers may be liable for torts committed by employees within their employment. In this case the client has the right to make decisions about self-care.

4 Sleeping medications are to be given at the client's bedtimes, not at the convenience of the nursing staff.

21. **4 The parasympathetic nervous system (a branch of the autonomic nervous system) causes increased GI motility and secretions. The adrenal cortex releases glucocorticoids, which also stimulate the GI tract, increasing the acidity of the secretions. (AN; PS; EH)**

1 They do not affect involuntary muscles of the colon.

2 Same as answer 1.

3 The stress function of the pancreas is not directly related to the intestines but is related to glycogen release from the liver. The sympathetic nervous system decreases GI motility.

22. **4 Nurses must actively try to understand their own feelings and prejudices, because these will affect the ability to assess a client's behavior objectively. (DC; PS; EH)**

1 Understanding a client's emotional conflict can be accomplished only after dealing with one's own feelings.

2 The health team members should work together for the benefit of all clients, not just this client.

3 Information from significant others is beneficial, but only after nurses are able to deal with their own feelings.

23. **3 At this time the client is using this behavior as a defense. Quiet acceptance can be an effective interpersonal technique, since it is nonjudgmental. (EV; PS; EH)**

1 The nurse may be the target of a broad array of emotions; by focusing on only behaviors that affect the nurse, the full scope of the client's feelings are not considered.

2 During periods of overt hostility, perceptions are altered, making it difficult to evaluate the situation rationally.

4 Withdrawal signifies nonacceptance and rejection.

24. **2 Relaxation of muscles and facial expression are examples of nonverbal behavior; nonverbal behavior is a better index of feelings because it is less likely to be consciously controlled. (EV; PS; EH)**

1 Increased activity may be an expression of anger or hostility.

3 Clients may suppress verbal outbursts despite feelings and become withdrawn.

4 Refusing to talk may be a sign that the client is just not ready to discuss feelings.

25. **4 The response demonstrates that the nurse cares about the client and will have time for the client's special emotional needs. Such an approach allays anxiety and reduces emotional stress, which is beneficial in clients with cardiovascular disease. (IM; PS; EH)**

1 This indicates a lack of interest in the client, and interferes with developing an effective nurse-client relationship.

2 This statement does not respond to the client's need, and cuts off communication.

3 Same as answer 2.

MEDICAL-SURGICAL ANSWERS

26. **2 Clients adapting to illness frequently feel afraid and helpless and strike out at health team members as a way of maintaining control or denying their fear.** (DC; PS; EH)
   1 There is no evidence that the client denies the existence of a health problem.
   3 Although disorders such as cerebral vascular accidents and atherosclerosis, which are associated with hypertension, may lead to cerebral anoxia, there is insufficient evidence to support this conclusion in this situation.
   4 Capoten (an antihypertensive) is a renin-angiotensin antagonist that reduces blood pressure and does not cause behavior changes; Xanax reduces anxiety and may cause transient hypotension, not hypertension.

27. **1 An honest nurse-client relationship should be maintained so that trust can develop.** (IM; TC; EH)
   2 Although other health team members may need to be informed eventually, the initial action should concern only the nurse-client relationship.
   3 Same as answer 2.
   4 This does nothing to establish communication about feelings or motivation behind behavior.

28. **4 Seeking other opinions to disprove the inevitable is a form of denial employed by individuals having illnesses with a poor prognosis.** (DC; PS; EH)
   1 If the client is crying, the client is aware of the magnitude of the situation and is past the stage of denial.
   2 Criticism that is unjust is often characteristic of the stage of anger.
   3 This is common during the depression experienced as one moves toward acceptance.

29. **2 Bargaining is one of the stages of dying in which the client promises some type of desirable behavior to postpone the inevitability of death.** (AN; PS; EH)
   1 Frustration is a subjective experience, a feeling of being thwarted, but not one of the stages of dying.
   3 Classified as the fourth stage, depression represents the grief experienced as the individual recognizes the inescapability of fate.
   4 Rationalization is a defense mechanism in which attempts are made to justify or explain an unacceptable action or feeling.

30. **3 When an individual reaches the point of being able intellectually and psychologically to accept death, anxiety is reduced and the individual becomes detached from the environment.** (DC; PS; EH)
   1 Although detached, the client is still concerned and may use this time constructively.
   2 Although resigned to death, the individual is not euphoric.
   4 At the stage of acceptance, the client is no longer angry or depressed.

31. **4 Client is in acceptance; detachment is a coping mechanism often needed by the client, especially when facing a devastating illness, and should be accepted by the nurse.** (PL; PS; EH)
   1 Ignoring the behavior does not convey a willingness to listen and denies the client's feelings.
   2 Coping mechanisms are needed by the client as psychologic protection and must not be taken away until the client is able to replace one for another.
   3 The client is past the denial phase and is in acceptance.

32. **4 In the stage of acceptance the client frequently detaches the self from the environment and may become indifferent to family members. In addition, the family may take longer to accept the inevitable death than does the client.** (PL; PS; EH)
   1 Although the family may not understand the anger, dealing with the resultant behavior may serve as a diversion.
   2 Denial is often exhibited by both client and family at the same time.
   3 During this stage the family is often able to offer emotional support, and sometimes false reassurances, thus fulfilling one of their needs.

33. **4 The nurse's presence communicates concern and provides an opportunity for the client to initiate communication if needed. Silence is an effective interpersonal technique that permits the client to direct the content and extent of verbalizations without the nurse's imposing on the client's privacy.** (PL; PS; EH)
   1 Crying, which is so much a part of depression, usually ceases when the individual reaches acceptance.
   2 During acceptance the client may decide not to have visitors, preferring time for personal reflection.

3 Detached from the environment, the client may find the details of various hospital procedures lose significance.

34. **3 This promotes an exploration of the client's dilemma; this response encourages further communication. (IM; PS; EH)**
   1 Although this is true, this response is not supportive and abandons the client.
   2 It is inappropriate for the nurse to give advice; keeping feelings to self does not promote self-expression.
   4 It is inappropriate for the nurse to give advice; the nurse is directing the client to be judgmental.

35. **4 Although a hysterectomy may be performed, conservative management may include cervical conization and laser treatment that would not preclude future pregnancies; clients have a right to be informed by their physician of all treatment options. (IM; PS; EH)**
   1 This currently is not the issue for this client.
   2 This denies the validity of the client's feelings.
   3 Same as answer 2.

36. **2 This response reflects and verbalizes the client's feelings in a nonjudgmental way. (IM; PS; EH)**
   1 The husband did not indicate this; the client's perception is altered by her own feelings.
   3 This demonstrates a lack of acceptance of the client's feelings.
   4 Such feelings are common and need to be verbalized; surgery should not be postponed.

37. **4 Many people are ashamed or have a distorted body image when they know they have a long-term disorder. (EV; PS; EH)**
   1 Lapses of memory are not common in diabetes until advanced vascular changes occur in the brain.
   2 Diabetes is not a valid reason for not hiring an individual.
   3 This is a judgmental statement; the word "favorable" has individual interpretations.

38. **3 Open communication helps to decrease anxiety, ultimately lowering acid secretion. (IM; TC; EH)**
   1 Knowledge itself does not always reduce anxiety.
   2 Antibiotics, while controlling *Helicobacter pylori*, will have no direct effect on the client's anxiety.
   4 This is false reassurance.

39. **2 Surgery on the bowel has no direct anatomic or physiologic effect on sexual performance. However, psychologic factors could hamper this function, and the nurse should encourage verbalization. (IM; PS; EH)**
   1 There is no reason why sexual relationships must be curtailed.
   3 Although it may take several months to resume satisfying sexual relationships, the surgery has no direct physiologic effect.
   4 Although a partner should understand the nature of the surgery, the focus at this time should be on the client.

40. **2 Ulcerative colitis is linked to psychoemotional stress and generally is exacerbated when conflicts exist. (PL; PS; EH)**
   1 During an acute episode, a low-residue diet is prescribed to rest the colon.
   3 Endocrine activity is not the only causative factor.
   4 No physiologic change can be made surgically to alter the disease; an ileostomy may be done to rest the large intestine.

41. **1 Visits by family members can allay anxiety and consequently reduce emotional stress, an important risk factor in cardiovascular disease. (PL; PS; EH)**
   2 Family, community, or work problems conveyed by phone may cause anxiety; social communications with the family should be permitted.
   3 Television programs can cause anxiety or excitement, which would increase the metabolic rate and cardiac output.
   4 The client may be disturbed by current news. This would raise the metabolic rate, increasing oxygen demands on the heart.

42. **2 Open communication lines are always important in relieving anxiety and reducing stress, which might interfere with postoperative recovery. (IM; PS; EH)**
   1 This does not acknowledge the client's feelings and therefore does not deal with the source of the anxiety.
   3 Learning does not occur when anxiety levels are too high.
   4 Reassurances do not allow for open communication and invalidate the emotions experienced by the client.

43. **1 Nonjudgmentally identifying the client's feelings encourages further verbalization about those feelings and the diet. (IM; PS; EH)**
2 This response is inappropriate; there is no mention of specific foods.
3 The nurse should first acknowledge the client's feelings and then assess the client's level of knowledge before imparting such information.
4 This suggests that adherence to the prescribed medical regimen is unnecessary.

44. **2 The nurse should pick up all clues to client anxiety and allow for verbalization. This response recognizes the client's feelings. (IM; PS; EH)**
1 This response negates the client's feelings and presents a negative connotation about the procedure.
3 This response focuses on the task rather than on the client's feelings.
4 Same as answer 1.

45. **3 This recognizes that the client is upset and by indirect questioning helps facilitate communication. (IM; PS; EH)**
1 The client has not verbalized being upset and may be unaware of or unable to verbalize the actual cause of the emotions.
2 An assumption is being made about the basis for the behavior; this does not focus on the client's feelings.
4 False reassurance blocks communication.

46. **3 Although the client who has suffered a CVA may be emotionally labile, the major factors determining the reaction to illness are past experiences and coping mechanisms. (DC; PS; EH)**
1 Although care is important, basic coping mechanisms and personality are already established.
2 The site of the CVA may influence behavior and affect the client's emotional response to the disease, but to a lesser extent.
4 Emotional response does not depend on one's ability to understand the underlying physiologic causes of disease.

47. **2 To aid in motivation, the nurse should focus on the positive aspects of the client's progress. (IM; TC; EH)**
1 Short-term attainable goals provide positive reinforcement for the client; goal setting should be done by the client or shared with the nurse.

3 This negative reinforcement may result in discouragement.
4 Having individuals actually perform is more beneficial than telling or showing them what to do.

48. **2 The nurse's positive attitude encourages and motivates the client. (IM; TC; EH)**
1 As many objectives as necessary should be used.
3 This attitude on the part of the nurse may discourage the client's attempts to attain the highest goals possible.
4 Same as answer 3.

49. **2 Changes in self-image and family role can initiate a grieving process with a variety of emotional responses. (DC; PS; EH)**
1 This cannot be assumed from the situation described unless the client's feelings are elicited.
3 Same as answer 1.
4 The ability to cope successfully with an illness varies widely among individuals.

50. **4 To foster communication and cooperation, family members should be involved in planning and implementing care. (IM; PS; EH)**
1 This intervention does not focus on the client's feelings or needs.
2 The nurse remains responsible; the spouse may promote dependency in the client to satisfy a need to control.
3 Same as answer 1.

51. **3 Because of the profound effect of paralysis on body image, the nurse should provide the client with an environment that permits exploration of feelings without judgment, punishment, or rejection. (IM; PS; EH)**
1 Attempts to distract the client may be interpreted as denial of the client's feelings and will not resolve the underlying conflict.
2 This is an important part of nursing care but it is not specific to this client.
4 Same as answer 2.

52. **4 The first action should be to remove the victim from a source of further injury. (IM; TC; EH)**
1 Preventing further injury and reestablishing breathing are the priorities.
2 Breathing is the priority once further injury is avoided.
3 This wound would be treated after the victim is moved from danger and patency of the airway is verified.

53. **1 People in panic could initiate the panic reaction in those who appear to be in control. (IM; PS; EH)**
   2 Comatose individuals will not cause panic in others.
   3 Euphoric individuals would not adversely affect others.
   4 Depressed people will be calm and not affect others.

Fluid and Electrolytes

54. **3 Hypotonic solutions are less concentrated (contain less than 0.85 g of sodium chloride in each 100 ml) than body fluids. (AN; PA; FE)**
   1 Isotonic solutions are those which cause no change in the cellular volume or pressure, because their concentration is equivalent to that of body fluid.
   2 This relates to two compounds that possess the same molecular formula but that differ in their properties or in the position of atoms in the molecules; isomers.
   4 This contains more than 0.85 g of sodium chloride in each 100 ml.

55. **3 Increased respiration blows off carbon dioxide, which decreases hydrogen; the pH rises (less acidity). Decreased respiration results in carbon dioxide buildup, which increases hydrogen; the pH falls (more acidity). The kidneys either conserve or excrete bicarbonate, which helps to adjust the pH. (AN; PA; FE)**
   1 Interaction of these two does not maintain the pH.
   2 Although the circulatory system carries fluids and electrolytes to the kidneys, it does not interact with the urinary system to regulate plasma pH.
   4 Same as answer 1.

56. **1 Blood plasma and interstitial fluid are both part of the extracellular fluid and are of the same ionic composition. (AN; PA; FE)**
   2 The osmotic pressure is the same.
   3 The composition is the same.
   4 Ionic composition is the same; the main cation of both would be sodium.

57. **2 The excreted ammonia combines with hydrogen ions in the glomerular filtrate to form ammonium ions, which are excreted from the body. This mechanism helps rid the body of excess hydrogen, maintaining acid-base balance. (AN; PA; FE)**
   1 Osmotic pressure is not affected by excretion of ammonia.
   3 Ammonia is formed by the decomposition of bacteria in the urine; ammonia excretion is not related to the process and does not control bacterial levels.
   4 Ammonia excretion does not affect hemopoiesis.

58. **3 Because the plasma colloidal oncotic pressure (COP) is the major force drawing fluid from the interstitial spaces back into the capillaries, a drop in COP caused by albuminuria results in edema. (AN; PA; FE)**
   1 Hydrostatic tissue pressure is unaffected by alteration of protein levels; colloidal pressure is affected.
   2 Hydrostatic pressure is influenced by the volume of fluid and the diameter of the blood vessel, not by the presence of protein such as albumin.
   4 The osmotic pressure of tissues is not affected.

59. **2 The average adult human body is about 60% water. A newborn infant's body is about 80% water and reaches the 60% figure approximately 1 year after birth. (AN; PA; FE)**
   1 This is the percent for a newborn infant.
   3 The percent for the elderly may be as low as 40%.
   4 This represents complete dehydration of tissues.

60. **2 The osmoreceptors are located in the hypothalamus. Under conditions of dehydration they stimulate the neurohypophysis to release ADH into the blood. (AN; PA; FE)**
   1 Receptors for alterations in osmotic pressure are not located in the blood.
   3 The kidney tubules are the target organ for ADH; they reabsorb more water from the glomerular filtrate.
   4 This is the posterior lobe of the pituitary gland and is the source of antidiuretic hormone (ADH).

61. **4 The kidneys regulate fluid balance by adjusting the amount of fluid reabsorbed from the glomerular filtrate. (AN; PA; FE)**
   1 The liver does not play a major role in fluid balance.
   2 The heart is primarily a pump for the movement of blood.
   3 The role of the lungs is minimal.

62. **2 Interstitial fluid constitutes about 16% of body weight, which is 10 to 12 L in an adult male of 68 kg. (AN; PA; FE)**
1 Plasma is 4% of body weight (2.8 L).
3 This is part of the intracellular component.
4 This is derived from extracellular fluid and is calculated as part of the 20% of the total body weight.

63. **4 The concentration of potassium is greater inside the cell and is extremely important in establishing a membrane potential, a critical factor in the cell's ability to function. (AN; PA; FE)**
1 Sodium is the most abundant cation of the extracellular compartment.
2 Calcium is the most abundant electrolyte in the body; 99% is concentrated in the teeth and bones.
3 Chloride is an extracellular anion.

64. **2 Approximately 25 of the 40 L of body fluid are in the cells. (AN; PA; FE)**
1 Interstitial fluid makes up 16%.
3 Extracellular fluid makes up 20%.
4 Intravascular fluid makes up 4%.

65. **1 The fluid in a bottle hung over a person lying down possesses potential energy. When that fluid is allowed to drip into the person intravenously, its potential energy is then converted to kinetic energy (energy of motion). (AN; TC; FE)**
2 Energy is not being stored in this action; rather stored energy is converted to energy of motion.
3 No chemical reaction occurs when fluid drips into a vein.
4 No chemical reaction or formation of new substances occurs when fluid drips into a vein.

66. **1 A molar (1 M) solution contains 1 gram-molecular weight of solute per liter of solution. Molarity is not as informative as normality because the latter is based on the actual chemical-combining properties of the substance involved. (AN; PA; FE)**
2 A normal (1 N) solution is defined as containing 1 gram-equivalent weight of solute per liter of solution. In human body fluids the milliequivalent (1/1000 of the gram-equivalent) is a more convenient term for expressing concentration, because the gram-equivalent is rather large.
3 This deals with the osmotic pressure of two liquids; isotonic solutions have equal osmotic pressure.

4 A solution holding all the solute it can at a given temperature and pressure is a saturated solution.

67. **3 Arterial blood has a narrow pH range of 7.35 to 7.45. Venous blood is more acidic and closer to 7.35 than is arterial blood, which is normally closer to a pH of 7.45. (DC; TC; FE)**
1 This is very acidic and needs immediate treatment.
2 This is slightly acidic for both arterial and venous blood.
4 This is alkaline and needs treatment.

68. **1 Retention of carbon dioxide after exhausting the available bicarbonate ions as buffers will cause a lower pH (respiratory acidosis). (DC; PA; FE)**
2 Hyperventilation will cause respiratory alkalosis.
3 The loss of carbon dioxide reduces the body's level of carbonic acid, causing respiratory alkalosis.
4 Tissue necrosis results from localized tissue anoxia and will not cause the systemic response of respiratory acidosis; this is caused by excessive carbonic acid resulting from a respiratory insufficiency.

69. **2 The pH of blood is maintained within the narrow range of 7.35 to 7.45. When there is an increase in hydrogen ions, acidosis results and is reflected in a lower pH. (DC; PA; FE)**
1 This is too acidotic and may not be compatible with life.
3 This is within the normal range for pH.
4 This is slightly alkaline.

70. **3 Once treatment with insulin for diabetic ketoacidosis is begun, potassium ions reenter the cell, causing hypokalemia; therefore potassium, along with the replacement fluids, is generally supplied. (AN; TC; FE)**
1 Potassium would not correct this.
2 Flaccid paralysis would not occur in diabetic ketoacidosis; potassium replaces that which has reentered the cell after insulin therapy.
4 Knowing the relationship of insulin and potassium, the nurse should recognize that treatment with KCl is prophylactic, aborting any development of dysrhythmias.

71. **2 Sodium bicarbonate is a base and one of the major buffers in the body. (AN; PA; FE)**

1 Potassium is not a buffer; only a base can buffer an acid.

3 Carbon dioxide is carried in aqueous solution as carbonic acid (H_2CO_3); an acid does not buffer another acid.

4 Sodium chloride is not a buffer; it is a salt.

72. **2 Excessive loss of gastric fluid results in excessive loss of hydrochloric acid and can lead to alkalosis; the HCl is not available to neutralize the sodium bicarbonate ($NaHCO_3$) secreted into the duodenum by the pancreas. The intestinal tract absorbs the excess bicarbonate and alkalosis results. (DC; TC; FE)**

1 Loss of HCl will move the pH to a basic level.

3 Oxygen is not drawn from the blood by gastric lavage.

4 Gastric fluid does not regulate osmotic pressure in the blood; also, the volume of blood would be altered not by loss of gastric fluid but by severe dehydration.

73. **2 Prolonged use of sodium bicarbonate may cause systemic alkalosis as well as retention of sodium and water. (IM; TC; FE)**

1 This statement is inaccurate in describing the effects of sodium bicarbonate.

3 Same as answer 1.

4 Same as answer 1.

74. **4 Release of the adrenocortical steroids (cortisol) by the stress of surgery causes renal retention of sodium and excretion of potassium. (EV; TC; FE)**

1 Although sodium may be depleted by nasogastric suction, retention by the kidneys generally balances this loss.

2 This is not depleted by surgery or urinary excretion.

3 Same as answer 2.

75. **2 Potassium, the major intracellular cation, functions with sodium and calcium to regulate neuromuscular activity and contraction of muscle fibers, particularly heart muscle. In hypokalemia these symptoms develop. (DC; PA; FE)**

1 These symptoms do not indicate an electrolyte imbalance.

3 These symptoms would indicate hypocalcemia, which does not generally occur in colitis.

4 Nausea and vomiting might occur with prolonged potassium deficit; however, this is not an early sign; leg and abdominal cramps occur with potassium excess, not deficit.

76. **3 Dehydration is a danger because of fluid loss with GI suction. (EV; TC; FE)**

1 Based on the data provided, this symptom is not likely to occur.

2 Same as answer 1.

4 Same as answer 1.

77. **1 Because IV solutions enter the body's internal environment, all solutions and medications utilizing this route must be sterile to prevent the introduction of microbes. (IM; TC; FE)**

2 The medication can be mixed with the IV solution in many ways; sterility takes priority.

3 The amount and type of solution depend on the medication; sterility takes priority.

4 The needle does not have to be changed if sterility is maintained.

78. **1** $$\frac{\textbf{Amount to be infused} \times \textbf{Drop factor}}{\textbf{Time of infusion in minutes}}$$

(EV; TC; FE)

2 This is an incorrect calculation; it is too rapid; it would infuse in approximately 4 hours.

3 This is an incorrect calculation; it is too rapid; it would take between 2 and 3 hours to infuse.

4 This is an incorrect calculation; it would infuse too rapidly.

79. **4**

Intake (ml)		Output (ml)	
IV fluid	350	Voiding	
NG tube feeding	600	0830	150
		1300	220
Water	150	1515	235
Vitamin	30	Aspirated stomach contents	25
	1130		630

(EV; TC; FE)

1 This is a miscalculation; too little intake and too much output.

2 Same as answer 1.

3 This is a miscalculation; too little intake and output.

80. **4 Fluid and electrolyte disturbances occur because of fever, profuse diaphoresis, vomiting, and diarrhea. (DC; PA; FE)**

1 This symptom is not associated with complications of malaria.

2 Same as answer 1.

3 These symptoms are not associated with complications of malaria.

81. **3 ADH causes increased reabsorption of water by renal tubules, which dilutes sodium levels causing hyponatremia. (DC; TC; FE)**
   1 ADH will decrease urine volume.
   2 ADH causes fluid retention.
   4 ADH does not alter glucose metabolism.

82. **2 Potassium replacement is generally not indicated in the initial management of burns because hyperkalemia results from the liberation of potassium ions from the injured cells. (EV; TC; FE)**
   1 This will be given with colloidal Ringer's solution in various combinations depending on the client's needs.
   3 This will be given with colloidal and dextrose solutions in various combinations depending on the client's needs.
   4 This will be given with Ringer's and dextrose solutions in various combinations depending on the client's needs.

83. **4 After 24 hours there is increased risk of contamination of the solution and the container should be changed. (PL; TC; FE)**
   1 It is unnecessary to change the bag this often.
   2 Same as answer 1.
   3 Same as answer 1.

84. **1**

$$\frac{\text{Amount to be infused} \times \text{Drop factor}}{\text{Amount of time (in minutes)}}$$

$$\frac{2000 \times 10 = 20,000}{12 \times 60 = 720} = 27.77 \text{ drops/minute}$$

   (EV; TC; FE)
   2 This is an incorrect calculation and would result in excessive fluid administration.
   3 Same as answer 2.
   4 Same as answer 2.

85. **3 The liver manufactures albumin, the major plasma protein. A deficit of this protein will lower the osmotic (oncotic) pressure in the intravascular space, leading to a fluid shift. (AN; PA; FE)**
   1 The enlarged liver compresses the portal system, causing increased rather than decreased pressure.
   2 The kidneys are not the primary source of the pathologic condition. It is the liver's ability to manufacture albumin that maintains the colloid oncotic pressure.
   4 Potassium is not produced by the body, nor is its major function the maintenance of fluid balance.

86. **2 IV fluids do not provide proteins required for tissue growth, repair, and maintenance. Therefore tissue breakdown occurs to provide the essential amino acids. (EV; PA; FE)**
   1 The primary cause is lack of protein intake; each liter provides approximately 170 calories, which is insufficient to meet minimal energy requirements. Tissue breakdown will result.
   3 Weight loss is caused by insufficient intake of nutrients; vitamins will not prevent weight loss.
   4 An infusion of 5% dextrose in water may decrease the electrolyte concentration because of a fluid shift.

87. **2 When an IV infusion is infiltrated, it should be removed to prevent swelling of the tissues and pain. (EV; TC; FE)**
   1 Elevation does not change the position of the IV cannula; the infusion must be discontinued.
   3 This would add to the infiltration of fluid.
   4 Soaks may be applied, if ordered, after the IV is removed.

88. **2 Albumin acts to elevate the BP to normal levels when it is administered slowly and oral fluid intake is restricted. It causes fluid to move from the interstitial spaces into the circulatory system. Administration should not exceed 5 to 10 ml/minute. (IM; TC; FE)**
   1 Rapid administration could cause circulatory overload; high fluid intake would limit the shift of fluid from the interstitial to the intravascular compartment, interfering with the optimal effects of the drug.
   3 Rapid administration could cause circulatory overload; fluid is restricted, not withheld.
   4 Fluids are restricted to facilitate the optimal effects of the drug, which shifts fluids from the interstitial tissues to the intravascular compartment.

89. **4 Blood albumin, a protein, establishes the plasma colloid osmotic (oncotic) pressure because of its high molecular weight and size, which helps prevent cerebral edema postoperatively. (AN; PA; FE)**
   1 Blood clotting involves blood protein fractions other than albumin; for example, prothrombin and fibrinogen are within the alpha and beta globulin fractions.
   2 Red cell formation (erythropoiesis) occurs in red marrow and can be related to albumin only indirectly; albumin is the blood transport

protein for thyroxine, which stimulates metabolism in all cells, including those in red bone marrow.

3 Albumin does not activate WBCs; white blood cells are activated by antigens and substances released from damaged or diseased cells.

90. **1 Diuretic therapy that affects the loop of Henle generally involves the use of drugs that directly or indirectly increase urinary sodium, chloride, and potassium excretion. (EV; TC; FE)**

2 Sodium restriction does not necessarily accompany administration of furosemide (Lasix).

3 Dyspnea does not directly result in a depletion of electrolytes.

4 Unless otherwise ordered, oral intake is unaffected.

91. **3 Potassium is lost with the urine during diuresis. Hypokalemia, in turn, predisposes the client to digitalis toxicity. (EV; TC; DR)**

1 This electrolyte is not lost as a result of digitalis-induced diuresis.

2 Same as answer 1.

4 Same as answer 1.

92. **1 Hypokalemia causes a flattening of the T wave of the ECG because of its effect on muscle function. (DC; PA; FE)**

2 Hypokalemia causes a depression of the ST segment.

3 Hypokalemia causes a widening of the QRS complex.

4 Hypokalemia does not cause a deflection of the Q wave.

93. **1 Potassium follows insulin into the cells of the body, thereby raising the cellular potassium and preventing fatal dysrhythmias. (AN; PA; FE)**

2 Insulin does not cause excretion of these substances.

3 Potassium is not excreted as a result of this therapy; it shifts into the intracellular compartment.

4 The potassium level has no effect on pancreatic insulin production.

94. **3 Hypokalemia promotes mental confusion and apathy with poor muscle contractions and weakness; these effects are related to the diminished magnitude of the neuronal and muscle cell resting potentials. Abdominal distention results from flaccidity of the intestine and abdominal musculature. (EV; PA; FE)**

1 These are signs of sodium excess.

2 These are signs of hyperkalemia.

4 These are signs of diabetic ketoacidosis.

95. **3 To calculate the rate of fluid infusion:**

$$\frac{\text{Amount of fluid to be infused} \times \text{Drop factor}}{}$$

$$\frac{1000 \times 15}{8 \times 60} = \frac{15000}{480} = 31.25 = 31 \text{ drops/min}$$

(EV; TC; FE)

1 This is an incorrect calculation, resulting in an inadequate administration of fluid.

2 Same as answer 1.

4 This is an incorrect calculation, resulting in an excessive administration of fluid.

96. **1 These signs may indicate calcium depletion. (PL; TC; FE)**

2 Symptoms associated with hypomagnesemia include tremor, neuromuscular irritability, and confusion.

3 Symptoms associated with metabolic acidosis include deep rapid breathing, weakness, and disorientation.

4 Symptoms associated with hypokalemia include muscle weakness and malaise.

97. **2** $\dfrac{50 \text{ ml} \times 15 \text{ drops/min}}{20} = \dfrac{750}{20} = 37.5$

37.5 is rounded to 38. (EV; TC; FE)

1 This rate is too slow; it would take longer than 20 minutes to infuse.

3 This rate is too fast; it would infuse in less than 20 minutes.

4 Same as answer 3.

Cardiovascular

98. 3 **With anemia there is a greater return of blood to the heart from the peripheral vessels; the greater volume of blood returning to the heart stretches it and results in greater cardiac output. With polycythemia the heart must work harder to propel the more viscous blood through the circulatory system.** (DC; PA; CV)

1 Pressure is not involved; the terms anemia and polycythemia both refer to the number of cells present in a given volume (viscosity).

2 Temperature is not involved; the terms anemia and polycythemia both refer to the number of cells present in a given volume (viscosity).

4 Surface tension is not involved; the terms anemia and polycythemia both refer to the number of cells present in a given volume (viscosity).

99. 3 **The pulse increases to meet increased tissue demands for oxygen in the febrile state.** (DC; PA; CV)

1 Fever may not cause difficulty in breathing.

2 Pain is not related to fever.

4 Blood pressure is not necessarily elevated in fever.

100. 3 **Assessment of the pedal pulse should include the strength of the pulse (rated 0 to 4+). Symmetry, the correspondence of homologous parts on opposite sides of the body, indicates whether the pulses are equal.** (DC; TC; CV)

1 Contractility is not a characteristic of pulse but of the heart; rate is not measured with pedal pulses.

2 Color of skin is not a pulse characteristic; rhythm relates to radial and apical pulses, not pedal pulses.

4 Local temperature is not a characteristic of the pedal pulse; pulsations are not visible in pedal pulses.

101. 3 **Pulse pressure is obtained by subtracting the diastolic from the systolic readings after the blood pressure has been recorded.** (EV; TC; CV)

1 This is only a partial factor in determining pulse pressure; it is not the pulse pressure itself.

2 This is not pulse pressure; it is pulse deficit.

4 This is not pulse pressure.

102. 1 **Antibodies produced against group A beta-hemolytic streptococci sometimes interact with antigens in the heart's** valves, causing damage and symptoms of rheumatic heart disease; early recognition and treatment of streptococcal infections has limited the occurrence of rheumatic heart disease. (DC; PA; CV)

3 The most common causes of meningitis, an infection of the membranes surrounding the brain and spinal cord, include *Streptococcus pneumoniae*, *Neisseria meningitides*, and *Haemophilus influenzae*.

2 Hepatitis, an inflammation of the liver, is caused by the hepatitis A virus (HAV), not by bacteria.

4 Rheumatoid arthritis is thought to be an autoimmune disease; it is not caused by microorganisms such as beta-hemolytic streptococci.

103. 4 **A drop in blood pressure, rapid pulse, cold clammy skin, and oliguria are all signs of shock, which, if not treated promptly, can lead to death.** (EV; TC; CV)

1 This is an expected response; the client will push out the airway as the effects of anesthesia subside.

2 Snoring respirations are common because of the depressant effects of anesthesia.

3 Shallow respirations are common because of the depressant effects of anesthesia.

104. 1 **Paralysis of the sympathetic vasomotor nerves after administration of spinal anesthesia results in dilation of blood vessels, which causes a subsequent drop in blood pressure.** (AN; PA; CV)

2 These receptors are sensitive to oxygen and carbon dioxide tension; they are not related to postural hypotension and are not affected by spinal anesthesia.

3 The strength of cardiac contractions is not affected by spinal anesthesia and postural hypotension.

4 The cardiac accelerator center neurons in the medulla regulate heart rate; they are not related to postural hypotension and are not affected by spinal anesthesia.

105. 2 **Localized sensory changes may indicate nerve damage, impaired circulation, or thrombophlebitis. Activity should be limited, and the physician notified.** (IM; TC; CV)

1 Symptoms may indicate a serious problem, and the physician must be notified.

3 Rubbing or massaging the legs is contraindicated because of possible dislodging of a thrombus if present.

4 Bed rest is indicated to prevent the possibility of further damage or creation of an embolus.

106. **3 The sympathectomy causes dilation of the blood vessels in the lower extremities; the resulting shift in the fixed blood volume lowers systemic blood pressure. (EV; TC; CV)**
1 Fluid losses associated with surgery may gradually lower BP and are compensated by endocrine and renal mechanisms.
2 Although anesthesia depresses vital signs, generally there is not a sudden drop in BP postoperatively.
4 Epinephrine would increase BP by stimulating cardiac contractility.

107. **3 The pulmonary capillary beds are the first small vessels (capillary beds) that the embolus encounters once it is released from the calf veins. (EV; PA; CV)**
1 This would not occur because the embolus would enter the pulmonary system first.
2 Same as answer 1.
4 Dry gangrene occurs when the arterial rather than the venous circulation is compromised.

108. **3 An appendectomy is a relatively simple operation; the client is generally out of bed the same day. With an ambulatory client there is less risk of venous stasis, a condition that predisposes the individual to thrombus formation and emboli. (EV; PA; CV)**
1 Although generally ambulated the first day postoperatively, the client often is hampered by pain; pelvic surgery increases risk.
2 The client may or may not be out of bed the same day depending on the surgical approach; mobility may be hampered by a Foley catheter.
4 Vein ligation is performed for varicose veins; the diseased vein is removed, placing an additional burden on the deep venous system and possibly increasing the risk of thrombi.

109. **4 Thrombophlebitis is inflammation of a vein that occurs with the formation of a clot. Signs include pain (especially on dorsiflexion of the foot), redness, warmth, tenderness, and edema. (DC; TC; CV)**
1 Intermittent claudication (pain when walking resulting from tissue ischemia) may occur with peripheral vascular disease.
2 Pitting edema does not occur in thrombophlebitis.
3 Pain occurs on flexion of the foot (Homans' sign).

110. **4 The client who is on bedrest must do exercises such as dorsiflexion of the feet to prevent venous stasis and thrombus formation. (IM; TC; CV)**
1 Limiting fluid intake may lead to hemoconcentration and subsequent thrombus formation.
2 This improves pulmonary function rather than prevents venous stasis.
3 This actually promotes venous stasis by compressing the popliteal space.

111. **3 Support hose apply external pressure on the veins, preventing the retrograde pressure or flow that may occur in the standing or sitting positions; application before arising prevents the veins from having the opportunity to become engorged. (IM; TC; CV)**
1 If the feet are permitted to be dependent before the stockings are put on, venous pooling and edema may occur; application of elastic stockings at this time can cause tissue trauma.
2 Because they promote venous return, they do not need to be worn when the legs are elevated when sleeping.
4 Stockings must be removed so the legs can be washed and dried at least daily. They usually need not be worn while in bed with the feet elevated because gravity prevents venous pooling.

112. **1 The vessels branching from the circle of Willis provide excellent collateral circulation for the brain; partial blockage of one vessel is compensated by flow through other vessels. (AN; PA; CV)**
2 These take blood away from the brain.
3 This is not collateral circulation.
4 Same as answer 3.

113. **2 After removal of an arterial obstruction by endarterectomy, adequate circulation may be monitored by observation of skin color, pulses, and skin temperature. (EV; PA; CV)**
1 Appetite does not change as a result of vascular surgery.
3 Bowel habits would not be altered after surgery.
4 Turgor would be affected by changes in hydration.

MEDICAL-SURGICAL ANSWERS

114. **2** **Constriction of the peripheral blood vessels and the resulting increase in blood pressure impair circulation and limit the amount of oxygen being delivered to body cells, particularly in the extremities.** (PL; ED; CV)

1 Nicotine constricts all peripheral vessels, not just superficial ones; its primary action is to cause spasm; it will not dilate deep vessels.

3 Nicotine constricts rather than dilates peripheral vessels.

4 Same as answer 3.

115. **4** **Injured tissue cannot heal properly because of cellular deprivation of oxygen and nutrients; ulceration and gangrene may result; diminished sensation decreases awareness of injury.** (DC; PA; CV)

1 Emotional stress does not cause tissue injury; however, because of vasoconstriction, it may prolong healing.

2 Poor hygiene is only one stress that may cause tissue trauma; protein is not related to this disease.

3 Caffeine stimulates the cerebral cortex; it does not contribute to ulceration or deprivation of oxygen.

116. **3** **Buerger's disease (thromboangiitis obliterans) is characterized by vascular inflammation, usually in the lower extremities, leading to thrombus formation. As a result of impaired circulation, there is burning pain and intermittent claudication.** (DC; PA; CV)

1 These symptoms are not related to thromboangiitis obliterans.

2 Blanching is not related to thromboangiitis obliterans.

4 Fatigue and blanching of the skin are not related to thromboangiitis obliterans.

117. **4** **The Trendelenburg test evaluates the backflow of blood through defective valves. If, after raising the legs to empty the veins, the client stands and the veins fill from above the site of the suspected varicosity, the diagnosis is supported.** (DC; PA; CV)

1 This is not a simple test that the nurse can perform.

2 This test is used to determine injury of the pyramidal tract in adults; if present, it is obtained by firmly stroking the lateral aspect of the sole of the foot.

3 This is a test for position sense; the client loses balance when standing erect with feet together and eyes closed.

118. **2** **The legs should be elevated to promote venous return by gravity.** (IM; PA; CV)

1 This position increases pressure on the popliteal space, which may interfere with venous return from the legs.

3 Flexion of the knees and hips with the legs lower than the heart interferes with venous return.

4 Dorsiflexion of the feet places tension on the suture line and should be avoided; placing the legs lower than the level of the heart will not promote venous return.

119. **3** **Unexpressed rage or anger affects the sympathetic nervous system, precipitating the release of epinephrine and norepinephrine, constricting the blood vessels, and thus raising arterial blood pressure.** (DC; PE; CV)

1 Although the renin-angiotensin mechanism may contribute, kidney failure is not the primary cause of essential hypertension.

2 This may contribute but is not the primary cause.

4 Same as answer 2.

120. **3** **If there is a decrease in urinary output with increased conservation of body fluid, the blood pressure will be increased and vice versa.** (AN; PA; CV)

1 These cause a rapid response and have a short-term effect.

2 This may cause a short-term increase, but does not have a long-term effect.

4 Same as answer 1.

121. **3** **Many antihypertensive agents lower peripheral vascular resistance and may cause orthostatic hypotension. Therefore blood pressure should be monitored in both a supine and an upright position.** (AN; TC; CV)

1 Assessment prior to administration will not yield information related to effectiveness.

2 This is too short a time for determination of the drug's effect.

4 Change in position causes hypotension; when a position has been maintained for 5 minutes, the blood pressure has probably stabilized.

122. **4** **Sitting on the edge of the bed before getting up is recommended because it**

gives the body a chance to adjust to the effects of gravity on circulation in the upright position. (PL; PA; CV)

1 Support hose would not be worn continuously and would not prevent hypotension.

2 This would not prevent episodes of orthostatic hypotension.

3 Energetic tasks do not increase hypotension.

123. **2 An improper reading of the level of mercury will be obtained if the reader is not perpendicular to the column. An error of parallax results when an object is displaced by an observer's altered position. (PL; TC; CV)**

1 Too narrow a cuff can result in erroneously high readings; not an error of parallax.

3 Standing close to the manometer is not explicit; there may or may not be a resultant error of parallax depending on whether the examiner is perpendicular to the column of mercury.

4 Elevating the arm above the level of the heart will result in erroneously low readings; not an error of parallax.

124. **2 Clients and their families should be included in dietary teaching; families provide support that promotes compliance. (PL; ED; CV)**

1 The dietitian is a resource person who can give specific, practical information about diet and food preparation once the client has a basic understanding of the reasons for the diet.

3 Foods high in sodium will also have to be restricted; this teaching is inadequate.

4 The client should be included in own care; the client will ultimately assume the responsibility.

125. **2 Angina pectoris is pain in the chest that is caused by hypoxia of the cardiac muscle. (DC; PA; CV)**

1 Mitral insufficiency refers to an incompetent mitral valve; it could be only indirectly related to angina.

3 There is no cell death in angina.

4 A coronary thrombosis is an aggregation of platelets, clotting factors, and blood cellular elements that reduces the lumen of the artery; it may progress to a complete obstruction, resulting in a myocardial infarction.

126. **2 The two coronary arteries are the first branches of the aorta and carry blood with a high oxygen content to the myocardium. (AN; PA; CV)**

1 They carry blood with high oxygen content to the myocardium, not to the endocardium.

3 They carry blood with high oxygen content to the myocardium.

4 This is a function of the pulmonary veins.

127. **2 Ischemia causes tissue injury and the release of chemicals, such as bradykinin, that stimulate sensory nerves and produce pain. (AN; PA; CV)**

1 Arterial spasm, resulting in tissue hypoxia and pain, is associated with angina pectoris.

3 Arteries, not veins, are involved in the etiology of a myocardial infarction.

4 Tissue injury and pain occur in the myocardium.

128. **3 Anginal pain, which can be anticipated during certain activities, may be prevented by dilating the coronary arteries immediately before engaging in the activity. (IM; ED; CV)**

1 One tablet is generally administered at a time; doubling the dosage may produce severe hypotension and headache.

2 The sublingual form of nitroglycerin is absorbed directly through the mucous membranes and should not be swallowed.

4 When the pain is relieved, rest will generally prevent its recurrence by reducing oxygen consumption of the myocardium.

129. **4 Cholesterol is a sterol found in tissue; it is attributed in part to diets high in saturated fats. (IM; PA; CV)**

1 Cholesterol is also produced by the body.

2 Only animal foods furnish dietary cholesterol.

3 Cholesterol is needed for the synthesis of bile salts, adrenocortical and steroid sex hormones, and provitamin D.

130. **3 Whole milk is high in saturated fat. (IM; ED; CV)**

1 Most fish have a low fat content.

2 Corn oil is high in unsaturated fat.

4 Soft margarine is high in unsaturated fat.

131. **3 Vegetables and whole grains are low in fat and may reduce the risk of heart disease. (IM; ED; CV)**

1 Animal-derived products such as milk are high in saturated fats.

2 Meats are high in saturated fats.

4 Same as answer 2.

2. **3 Blood samples from the right atrium, right ventricle, and pulmonary artery would all be about the same with regard to oxygen concentration. Such blood contains slightly less oxygen than does systemic arterial blood. (AN; PA; CV)**

1 These contain slightly more carbon dioxide than does blood in the pulmonary vein, which has had some of its CO_2 expelled into the alveoli.

2 These contain less oxygen than does the pulmonary vein, which will carry oxygenated blood to the circulation.

4 It contains the same amount as do samples from the right atrium and right ventricle.

133. **4 The pulse should be assessed because the trauma at the insertion site may interfere with blood flow distal to the site. There is also danger of bleeding or occlusion. (IM; TC; CV)**

1 The client does not usually require additional rest after catheterization.

2 This would be determined on an individual basis; it is not routine.

3 It is not necessary to check the ECG every 30 minutes following the procedure.

134. **3 Myocardial infarction (MI) may cause increased irritability of tissue or interruption of normal transmission of impulses. Dysrhythmias occur in about 90% of clients after MI. (DC; TC; CV)**

1 Hypokalemia may result when clients are taking cardiac glycosides and diuretics; this is a complication associated with therapy, not a pathologic entity related to the MI itself.

2 Anaphylactic shock is caused by an allergic reaction, not by an MI.

4 Cardiac enlargement is a slow process and is not a complication that can be observed.

135. **2 The heart's apex is between the fifth and sixth ribs at the midclavicular line. It is closest to the chest wall here, so auscultation is easier. (PL; TC; CV)**

1 Although it may be possible to auscultate the heart in this area, it is usually easier to do so over the apex.

3 Same as answer 1.

4 Same as answer 1.

136. **1 LD, CK and AST (GOT) are enzymes released into the blood from cardiac muscle cells when the myocardium is damaged. (DC; PA; CV)**

2 Calcium level will not diagnose MI; there is no test called APPT; APTT assesses blood clotting time.

3 The sedimentation rate identifies the presence of inflammation or infection but is not specific; ALT identifies tissue destruction but it is more specific for liver injury.

4 The Paul-Bunnell test identifies heterophilic antibodies in infectious mononucleosis; it would not be specific for myocardial infarction.

137. **1 Until the client's condition has reached some degree of stability after myocardial infarction, routine activities such as changing sheets are avoided so the client's movements will be minimized and the cardiac work load reduced. (IM; TC; CV)**

2 Activity is contraindicated because it increases oxygen consumption and cardiac work load.

3 Changing all the linen causes unnecessary movement, which increases oxygen demands and makes the heart work harder.

4 Any activity is counterproductive to rest; rest must take precedence so the cardiac work load will be reduced.

138. **2 Adverse effects of digoxin include many types of dysrhythmias. An apical pulse rate less than 60 or above 120 contraindicates administration of the drug. Because the client will be taking the medication at home, it is necessary to teach the client how to take an accurate pulse and to contact the physician if the rate falls outside the parameters mentioned. (PL; TC; CV)**

1 The client will be assuming responsibility for drug administration at home; teaching is more of a priority than the nurse's assessments at this time.

3 Same as answer 1.

4 Same as answer 1.

139. **1 Desired anticoagulant effect is achieved when the activated partial thromboplastin time is 1.5 to 2 times normal. (EV; TC; CV)**

2 Although absence of bleeding suggests that the drug has not reached toxic levels, it does not indicate its effectiveness.

3 This does not affect viscosity.

4 Weakness and confusion are not related to anticoagulant therapy.

140. **2 The high vascularity of the nose, combined with its susceptibility to trauma (e.g., sneezing, nose blowing), makes it a frequent site of hemorrhage. (EV; TC; DR)**
    1 This symptom is usually not associated with anticoagulant therapy.
    3 Same as answer 1.
    4 Same as answer 1.

141. **3 Coumarin derivatives are ordered day by day, based on the prothrombin time of the client. This test gives an index of the individual's clotting ability. (PL; TC; CV)**
    1 Clotting time is the time required for blood to form a clot; it is not used for dosage calculation.
    2 Bleeding time is the time required for blood to cease flowing from a small wound; it is not used for coumarin dosage calculation.
    4 Sedimentation rate is a test used to determine the presence of inflammation or infection; it does not indicate clotting ability.

142. **1 Temperatures of 38° C or greater lead to an increased metabolism and cardiac workload. (AN; TC; CV)**
    2 An elevated temperature is not an early sign of developing cerebral edema, although the temperature may rise eventually because of medullary compression.
    3 Fever is unrelated to hemorrhage; in hemorrhage with shock, the temperature decreases.
    4 Although these symptoms are caused by an elevated temperature, it is not the reason for notifying the physician.

143. **4 Since the client is up more at home, edema usually increases. (IM; ED; CV)**
    1 Serosanguineous drainage will persist after discharge.
    2 These should not be expected and are, in fact, signs of postpericardotomy syndrome.
    3 These symptoms will persist longer, as it takes 6 to 12 weeks for the sternum to heal.

144. **2 Shock may have different etiologies (e.g., hypovolemic, cardiogenic, septic, anaphylactic) but always involves a drop in blood pressure and failure of the peripheral circulation because of sympathetic nervous system involvement. (AN; PA; CV)**
    1 Shock can be reversed by the administration of fluids, plasma expanders, and vasoconstrictors.
    3 It may be a reaction to tissue injury but has many different etiologies (e.g., hypovolemia, sepsis, anaphylaxis).

    4 Hypovolemia is only one cause; shock may also be septic, cardiogenic, or anaphylactic; it always involves a drop in blood pressure.

145. **1 Adrenalin is used to treat shock because the induced arterial constriction reduces blood pooling (vessels cannot hold as much blood) and increases venous return and cardiac output. (AN; PA; CV)**
    2 Digoxin slows and strengthens the heartbeat; it does not cause vasoconstriction.
    3 A sympathectomy interferes with autonomic vasoconstriction; it reduces venous return.
    4 Tourniquets constrict veins of the extremities and reduce venous return.

146. **4 This position is useful in treating shock since it promotes gravity-induced venous return. Warmth and fluids are also supportive to the person. (IM; TC; CV)**
    1 These are not methods used in the treatment of shock.
    2 This promotes venous pooling, which compounds shock.
    3 Same as answer 1.

147. **3 The CVP is a measure of the pressure within the right atrium. For an accurate reading the zero point must be level with the right atrium. This is at approximately the midaxillary line. (IM; TC; CV)**
    1 A normal CVP reading ranges from approximately 4 to 12 cm H_2O.
    2 A high reading indicates circulatory overload.
    4 The client must be supine only when the reading is taken.

148. **3 The CVP is to be recorded when the client is horizontal and the zero point of the manometer is at the midaxillary line (level of the right atrium). (IM; TC; CV)**
    1 This position alters the relationship of the midaxillary line and right atrium; inaccurate readings will be obtained.
    2 Same as answer 1.
    4 Same as answer 1.

149. **4 The catheter is placed in the pulmonary artery. Information regarding left ventricular function is obtained when the catheter balloon is inflated. (IM; ED; CV)**
    1 Information on stroke volume, the amount of blood ejected by the left ventricle with each contraction, will not be provided by a pulmonary catheter.
    2 Cardiac output is not usually measured via the pulmonary artery catheter used for continuous monitoring of the client.
    3 Although CVP can be obtained with the pulmonary catheter, it is not as specific as a pulmonary wedge pressure, which reflects pressure in the left side of the heart.

150. **2 The Nurse Practice Act states that nurses diagnose human responses to actual or potential health problems. The nurse used knowledge and intervened. (EV; PA; CV)**
    1 Because the client's symptoms reflected an immediate need for oxygen, postponement of treatment could result in further deterioration of the client's condition.
    3 Same as answer 1.
    4 Same as answer 1.

151. **2 An open flame or spark from static electricity (e.g., leather-soled shoes, wool, silk, nylon and Dacron blankets, ungrounded electric appliances) can initiate an explosion and fire in the presence of higher than normal oxygen levels. (IM; TC; CV)**
    1 Oxygen is not flammable; however, it increases the rate of combustion.
    3 Oxygen is not unstable.
    4 Oxygen does not increase apprehension; by reducing dyspnea and shortness of breath, it usually reduces apprehension.

152. **3 Oxygen via nasal cannula is the most comfortable and least intrusive, since the cannula extends minimally into the nose. (EV; PE; CV)**
    1 This method is oppressive, and clients complain of feeling "suffocated" when it is used.
    2 Same as answer 1.
    4 Same as answer 1.

153. **4 Adams-Stokes syndrome is a result of complete atrioventricular block. The ventricles take over the pacemaker function in the heart, but at a much slower rate than that of the SA node. As a result there is decreased cerebral circulation, causing syncope (DC; PA; CV)**
    1 These symptoms are unrelated to Adams-Stokes.
    2 These are symptoms of a cerebrovascular accident.
    3 Same as answer 1.

154. **3 Bradycardia refers to a heart rate of less than 60 per minute. It may be a physiologic adaptation to long-term exercise, cardiac disease, or digitalis toxicity. (AN; TC; CV)**
    1 This condition is described as a dysrhythmia; whereas bradycardia is also considered a dysrhythmia, the rhythm is usually regular.
    2 Tachycardia is the term used for rapid heart rates.
    4 This is called a bigeminal rhythm.

155. **3 Ventricular fibrillation is a death-producing dysrhythmia because the heart is not functioning as a pump. Immediate action is required or death will occur as a result of anoxia to the brain and other vital organs. (EV; TC; CV)**
    1 This is not a lethal dysrhythmia.
    2 Same as answer 1.
    4 This may require intervention and insertion of a pacemaker but is not lethal.

156. **1 Atropine blocks vagal stimulation of the SA node, resulting in an increased heart rate. (PL; PA; CV)**
    2 Digoxin (Lanoxin) slows the heart rate; hence it would not be indicated in this situation.
    3 Lidocaine hydrochloride (Xylocaine) decreases myocardial sensitivity and would not increase heart rate.
    4 Procainamide hydrochloride (Pronestyl) is an antidysrhythmic drug; it would not stimulate the heart rate.

157. **4 Bundle branch block interferes with the conduction of impulses from the AV node to the ventricle supplied by the affected bundle. Conduction through the ventricles is delayed, as evidenced by a widened QRS complex. (DC; PA; CV)**
    1 Changes in the T waves and/or ST segments usually occur as a result of cardiac damage.
    2 P waves, produced when the SA node fires to begin a cycle, are present in bundle branch block.
    3 Same as answer 1.

158. **3 Ventricular fibrillation will cause irreversible brain damage and then death**

within minutes because the heart is not pumping blood. Defibrillation or CPR until defibrillation is possible must be initiated immediately. (AN; TC; CV)

1 Although this condition requires prompt treatment, a client will live if treatment is withheld for several minutes.

2 Same as answer 1.

4 Same as answer 1.

159. **3 Cardioversion involves administration of precordial shock, which is synchronized with the R wave to interrupt the heart rate. It is used for atrial fibrillation, paroxysmal atrial tachycardia (PAT), and ventricular tachycardia when pharmaceutical preparations fail. The heart is stopped by the electric stimulation, and it is hoped that the SA node will take over as pacemaker. (AN; TC; CV)**

1 Because there are no R waves, the shock would not be delivered.

2 Same as answer 1.

4 Premature ventricular beats suggest an irritable myocardium and generally respond well to antidysrhythmic agents.

160. **2 Ventricular fibrillation is a death-producing dysrhythmia and, once identified, must be terminated immediately by precordial shock (defibrillation). This is usually a standing physician's order in a cardiac care unit. (PL; TC; CV)**

1 Oxygen is administered to correct hypoxia; it does not take priority over defibrillation.

3 CPR is instituted only when defibrillation fails to terminate the dysrhythmia.

4 Bicarbonate is administered to correct acidosis; it does not take priority over defibrillation.

161. **1 The height of the ventricular complexes must be sufficient to be picked up by the voltmeter, which will sound an alarm if the heart rate is outside the high and low parameters. (AN; TC; CV)**

2 The pulse generator (pacemaker) may be either an internal or an external device but is generally not part of the monitor.

3 The oscilloscope is the screen on which the electrical signals from the heart are displayed.

4 The synchronizer is used only during cardioversion to ensure that the electric shock is delivered during the QRS complex.

162. **3 Lidocaine hydrochloride (Xylocaine) decreases the irritability of the ventricles**

and is used in the treatment of ectopic beats originated by a ventricular focus. (IM; TC; CV)

1 Digoxin slows and strengthens ventricular contractions; it will not rapidly correct ectopic beats.

2 Furosemide (Lasix), a diuretic, does not affect ectopic foci.

4 Norepinephrine bitartrate (Levophed) is a sympathomimetic and is not the drug of choice for ventricular irritability

163. **2 The precordial shock during cardioversion must not be delivered on the T wave or ventricular fibrillation may ensue. By placing the synchronizer in the "on" position, the physician presets the machine so it will not deliver the shock on the T wave. (IM; TC; CV)**

1 The energy level may be set from 50 to 400 watt-seconds.

3 This will not ensure that the shock is not delivered on the T wave.

4 Same as answer 3.

164. **3 The pacemaker (PM) electrode is inserted via the venous system into the right ventricle, where PM-generated impulses can directly stimulate the ventricles. (IM; PA; CV)**

1 Stimulation of the SA node would be inadequate because of inability of the left bundle branch to transmit the impulse to the Purkinje fibers of the left ventricle.

2 The pacing catheter must directly stimulate the ventricles; the left atrium cannot transmit the impulse.

4 The pacing catheter must directly stimulate the ventricles; this site is too far from the ventricles.

165. **2 The SA node is the heart's natural pacemaker. An electronic pacemaker is used in some persons to supply an impulse that stimulates the heart to more efficient action. (AN; PA; CV)**

1 This is modified cardiac muscle, which receives impulses from the SA node and conducts them to the ventricular walls via the bundle of His and Purkinje fibers.

3 This is special cardiac muscle, which receives impulses from the AV node and conducts them to the ventricular walls.

4 Sympathetic fibers to the heart do not act as pacemakers to initiate and regulate the heartbeat.

166. **3 A demand pacemaker functions only when the heart rate falls below the set rate of the pacemaker. The client can detect pacemaker malfunctions by monitoring the pulse rate and noting a drop below the set rate. (PL; TC; CV)**
   1 The client need not alter previous sleeping habits.
   2 Normal activity may be resumed when healing has occurred.
   4 Demand pacemakers function only when the heart rate drops below a predetermined level.

167. **3 Functioning pacemakers initiate impulses when the client's pulse rate falls below the preset rate. (EV; TC; CV)**
   1 The client's heart beat may still be irregular.
   2 The client's heart rate may exceed the pacemaker.
   4 The pacemaker affects the rate, not the volume of the pulse.

168. **1 Asystole refers to the absence of atrial and ventricular contractions, which can cause death within minutes. (DC; TC; CV)**
   2 This might be bradycardia (less than 60 beats per minute) or heart block (a partial or complete interruption in transmission of impulses from the sinoatrial node to the ventricles).
   3 The heartbeat has ceased in asystole.
   4 This would be tachycardia if the heart rate was 100 to 150 beats per minute.

169. **2 Irreversible brain damage will occur if a client is anoxic for more than 4 minutes. (IM; TC; CV)**
   1 The age of the client does not affect the code.
   3 Although a variety of emergency medications must be available, their administration is ordered by the physician.
   4 Prior heart rate is of minimal importance. Rhythm is more significant.

170. **1 Help must be obtained immediately. (IM; TC; CV)**
   2 The nurse has already checked the carotid pulse; this action would waste valuable time.
   3 Prior to pulmonary resuscitation, tilt the head back, pinch the nose, and give two, rather than four, full lung inflations.
   4 This would not be done until the airway was open, two breaths were given, and reassessment indicated that there was no carotid pulse.

171. **4 The sternum must be depressed at least 3.7 to 5 cm to compress the heart ade-** quately between the sternum and vertebrae and to stimulate cardiac pumping action. (IM; TC, CV)
   1 This distance is ineffectual for an adult.
   2 Same as answer 1.
   3 Same as answer 1.

172. **4 This provides the best leverage for depressing the sternum. Thus, the heart is adequately compressed and blood is forced into the arteries. Grasping the fingers keeps them off the chest and concentrates the energy expended in the heel of the hand while minimizing the possibility of fracturing ribs. (IM; PA; CV)**
   1 Both hands must be utilized; pressure on the lower portion of the sternum may fracture the xiphoid process, which can injure vital underlying organs.
   2 Pressure spread over two hands may inadequately compress the heart and fracture the ribs.
   3 Application of pressure by the fingers is less effective; this provides inadequate cardiac compression.

173. **1 Congestive heart failure is the failure of the heart to pump adequately to meet the needs of the body, resulting in a backward buildup of pressure in the venous system. Adaptations by the body include edema, ascites, hepatomegaly, tachycardia, dyspnea, and fatigue. (DC; PA; CV)**
   2 These symptoms are generally not related to a specific disorder.
   3 These symptoms might indicate coronary insufficiency or infarction.
   4 This vague complaint is not specific to CHF; it might indicate a variety of pulmonary conditions.

174. **3 Measuring an area is an objective assessment and is not subject to individual interpretations. (DC; TC; CV)**
   1 Assessing for pitting is a subjective technique.
   2 Although assessing fluid balance by weighing a client is important, it does not determine the degree of edema in a specific extremity.
   4 Although monitoring the intake and output helps in assessing fluid balance, it does not determine the degree of edema in a specific extremity.

175. **4 In right ventricular heart failure, blood backs up in the systemic capillary beds; the increase in plasma hydrostatic pres-**

sure shifts fluid from the intravascular compartment to the interstitial spaces, causing edema. (AN; PA; CV)

1 This would occur with crushing injuries or if proteins were pathologically shifting from the intravascular compartment to the interstitial spaces.

2 Although a decrease in colloid osmotic (oncotic) pressure can cause edema, it results from lack of protein intake, not increased hydrostatic pressure associated with right ventricular heart failure.

3 Increased fluid pressures within the tissue would result in fluid shifts into the intravascular compartment.

176. **3 Failure of the right ventricle causes an increase in pressure in the systemic circulation. To equalize this pressure, fluid moves into the tissues, causing edema, and into the abdominal cavity, causing ascites. (AN; PA; CV)**

1 There is no loss of cellular constituents of blood in right ventricular heart failure.

2 Ascites is the accumulation of fluid in an extracellular space, not intracellular.

4 The opposite results when there is an increase in hydrostatic pressure.

177. **2 Elevation of an extremity promotes venous and lymphatic drainage by gravity. (PL; PA; CV)**

1 This is a dependent function of the nurse.

3 This is a dependent function of the nurse.

4 This procedure will have little effect on edema.

178. **4 With air conditioning, blood vessels in the skin remain partially constricted, preventing extensive blood flow through the skin. Such extensive skin blood flow would ordinarily occur in hot weather to promote radiation of heat from the body; however, the heart must then work to pump the blood through many extra miles of blood vessels in the skin. (AN; PA; CV)**

1 Body temperature is maintained.

2 There is decreased circulation to the skin in a cool environment versus a warm environment, which makes it beneficial to the person with cardiopulmonary problems.

3 Same as answer 2.

179. **1 Mitral stenosis impairs blood flow from the left atrium to the left ventricle. This backs up blood into the pulmonary veins and lungs. The result may be pulmonary edema. (DC; PA; CV)**

2 Pulmonic stenosis tends to cause a bulging of the intraventricular septum.

3 Severe arterial sclerosis of the coronary arteries narrows the arterial lumen, which can result in a decreased blood supply to the myocardium causing hypoxia and angina.

4 Tricuspid disease may cause jugular vein distension and hepatic congestion.

180. **4 Application of rotating tourniquets keeps blood in the extremities, decreasing venous return, which reduces pulmonary artery pressure and relieves pulmonary congestion. (PL; TC; CV)**

1 A wet phlebotomy is used only occasionally to reduce venous return to the heart; a dry phlebotomy (rotating tourniquets) is usually effective.

2 Extreme dyspnea and congestion necessitate a high-Fowler's position.

3 At times oxygen must be delivered under pressure to overcome the pressure of the edema fluid, but this is less common and is generally the responsibility of the inhalation or respiratory therapist.

181. **2 Six liters provide enough oxygen without adversely altering the client's blood gases, which would cause increased respiratory distress. (PL; TC; CV)**

1 This is insufficient.

3 Higher concentrations of oxygen may depress CO_2 and raise O_2 concentrations, interfering with the impetus to breathe.

4 Same as answer 3.

182. **1 Irritability and restlessness increase the metabolic rate (and the heart rate) and blood pressure. This complicates congestive heart failure. (AN; PA; CV)**

2 Restlessness does not directly influence respirations; an increase in cardiac workload would increase respirations.

3 Restlessness alone usually does not elevate the body temperature.

4 Restlessness does not affect oxygen supply.

MEDICAL-SURGICAL ANSWERS

183. **3 The orthopneic position allows maximum lung expansion because gravity reduces the pressure of the abdominal viscera on the diaphragm and lungs. (IM; PA; CV)**
    1. Elevation of the extremities should be avoided because it increases venous return, placing an increased workload on the heart.
    2. Excessive coughing and mucus production is characteristic of pulmonary edema and does not need to be encouraged.
    4. Positioning for postural drainage does not relieve acute dyspnea; furthermore, it increases venous return to the heart.

184. **1 The tourniquets must be rotated in a clockwise direction at 15-minute intervals so venous outflow in any one extremity is not occluded more than 45 minutes at a time. (PL; TC; CV)**
    2. Because tourniquets are applied to three of the four extremities, only one tourniquet is rotated at a time.
    3. Arterial blood flow cannot be totally occluded, or cell death will occur.
    4. One extremity is left without a tourniquet every 15 minutes.

185. **2 Application of rotating tourniquets keeps blood in the extremities, decreasing venous return to reduce pulmonary artery pressure and relieve pulmonary congestion. (AN; TC; CV)**
    1. The aim is to maintain adequate arterial flow to prevent tissue hypoxia.
    3. Capillary blood flow is not primarily affected.
    4. Visceral blood flow is not primarily affected.

186. **4 Right ventricular heart failure causes increased pressure in the systemic venous system, which leads to a fluid shift into the interstitial spaces. Because of gravity, the lower extremities are first affected in an ambulatory client. (DC; TC; CV)**
    1. Pulmonary disease would not result in varying degrees of edema.
    2. Pulmonary edema results in severe respiratory distress and peripheral edema.
    3. Myocardial infarction itself does not cause peripheral edema.

Blood and Immunity

187. **4 Immunization programs prevent the occurrence of disease and are considered primary interventions. (AN; PA; BI)**
    1. This is a tertiary intervention.

2. This is a secondary intervention.
3. Same as answer 1.

188. **3 Viscosity, a measure of a fluid's internal resistance to flow, is increased as the number of red cells suspended in plasma increases. (AN; PA; BI)**
    1. The number of cells does not affect the blood pH.
    2. The hematocrit would be higher.
    4. RBCs do not affect immunity.

189. **2 Plasma proteins do not easily pass through the capillary endothelium; however, the slight leakage through the capillary endothelium is important and results in edema if not corrected (one of the lymphatic system's functions is to return "leaked" plasma proteins to the blood). (AN; PA; BI)**
    1. Blood gases (oxygen and carbon dioxide) pass through capillary endothelium easily.
    3. Glucose and ions pass through the capillary endothelium easily.
    4. Amino acids and water pass through the capillary endothelium easily.

190. **2 The gamma globulin fraction in the plasma is the fraction that includes the antibodies. (AN; PA; BI)**
    1. Albumin helps regulate fluid shifts by maintaining the plasma oncotic pressure.
    3. Thrombin is involved in clotting.
    4. Hemoglobin carries oxygen.

191. **2 In active immunity, plasma cells provide antibodies in response to a specific antigen. (AN; PA; BI)**
    1. Eosinophils are involved in phagocytosis of antigen-antibody complexes.
    3. Erythrocytes (red blood cells) carry oxygen in the bloodstream.
    4. Lymphocytes are white blood cells that become plasma cells.

192. **4 Brief pressure is generally enough to prevent bleeding. (IM; TC; BI)**
    1. Complications are rare; no special positioning is required.
    2. Complications are rare; frequent monitoring is unnecessary.
    3. The site is cleansed prior to aspiration.

193. **3 The client has a weakened immune response; instructions regarding rest, nutrition, and avoiding unnecessary expo-**

sure to people with infections help reduce the risk of infection. (IM; ED; BI)

1. Although the onset of AIDS may be delayed, it represents the extreme of the continuum caused by HIV infection.
2. The client may experience social isolation as a result of society's fears and misconceptions; these are beyond the client's control.
4. Although Kaposi's sarcoma is related to HIV infection there are no specific measures to prevent its occurrence.

194. **2 Although blood is screened for the antibodies, there is a period between the time a potential donor is infected and the time when antibodies are detectable; there is still a risk but it is minimal. (IM; ED; BI)**

1. There is no current method of destroying the virus in a blood transfusion.
3. The screening test involves identification of the antibody, not the virus itself.
4. Although many people consider autotransfusion for elective procedures, a trauma victim does not have this option.

195. **1 Epidemiologic evidence has implicated breast milk in HIV transmission. (DC; TC; BI)**

2. These behaviors are not believed to transmit HIV.
3. This is unrelated to modes of transmission of HIV.
4. HIV transmission does not occur from casual contact.

196. **4 Vaseline breaks down the properties of condoms and would increase the risk of condom failure. (EV; ED; BI)**

1. Using Vaseline instead of a water-soluble lubricant shows a lack of knowledge about condom use, a form of safer sex.
2. Although the person is attempting to be responsible, there is a lack of knowledge and the behavior is unsafe.
3. Condom use shows the client has some understanding about the transmission of HIV.

197. **3 A person cannot contract HIV by eating from dishes previously used by an individual with AIDS; normal care is adequate (IM; ED; BI)**

1. This is unnecessary.
2. This is unnecessary; it may make the client feel different and create a feeling of isolation.
4. Same as answer 1.

198. **3 Painless enlargement of the cervical lymph nodes is often the first sign of Hodgkin's disease, a malignant lymphoma of unknown etiology. (DC; PA; BI)**

1. Axillary enlargement occurs after cervical.
2. Inguinal enlargement occurs later.
4. Mediastinal involvement follows after the disease progresses.

199. **2 For reasons unknown, Hodgkin's disease occurs most frequently between 15 and 30 years of age. (DC; PA; BI)**

1. It is less common in children.
3. It is uncommon in later years.
4. It is uncommon during middle years.

200. **2 Radiation exposure may lead to depression of the bone marrow, with subsequent insufficient WBCs to combat infection. (PL; ED; BI)**

1. There is no increase in the number of cells; therefore viscosity is not increased.
3. Red cell production is decreased by radiation.
4. Bone structure is not affected by treatment; pathologic fractures may occur in response to disease.

201. **3 Depression of the bone marrow interferes with hemopoiesis and results in anemia. (EV; PA; BI)**

1. There is a decrease in the number of cells and therefore a decrease in viscosity.
2. Pathologic fractures result from the disease, not the treatment.
4. Radiation causes increased susceptibility to infection as a result of the decreased number of white blood cells.

202. **1 Polycythemia vera results in pathologically high concentrations of erythrocytes in the blood; increased viscosity promotes the tendency toward thrombosis. (AN; PA; BI)**

2. The fragility of blood cells does not affect the viscosity of the blood.
3. Hypertension is usually related to narrowing or sclerosing of arteries, not to increased number of blood cells.
4. There is an increased number of RBCs in polycythemia; their immaturity is not related to the increased viscosity.

MEDICAL-SURGICAL ANSWERS

203. **1 An elevated plasma bilirubin level could indicate an increased rate of red cell destruction (bilirubin is a product of free hemoglobin metabolism); the individual may have a hemolytic anemia (e.g., sickle cell anemia, glucose 6-phosphate dehydrogenase deficiency).** (AN; PA; BI)
  2 This does not involve the destruction of red blood cells with subsequent liberation of bilirubin.
  3 A decreased amount of bile pigment would be liberated.
  4 Oxygen-carrying ability is reflected by hemoglobin.

204. **3 Iron is needed in the formation of hemoglobin.** (PL; TC; BI)
  1 Dextran is a plasma volume expander; it does not affect erythrocytes.
  2 The client's anemia is caused by gastrointestinal bleeding, not the process of RBC production.
  4 Vitamin B_{12} is a water-soluble vitamin that must be supplemented when an individual has pernicious anemia.

205. **1 Because of its great blood supply and general fragility, the spleen, when ruptured, must be removed to prevent possible hemorrhage, septicemia, or peritonitis.** (AN; TC; BI)
  2 This is not the reason for performing a splenectomy.
  3 This does not explain the reason for its removal.
  4 Although rupturing of the spleen may cause hemorrhage, septicemia, or peritonitis, it does not cause liver disease.

206. **3 Because the spleen has such vascularity, hemorrhage may occur and result in abdominal distention.** (DC; TC; BI)
  1 Although an elevated temperature is common, it is usually not the result of infection; the incidence of infection is not higher after a splenectomy, except in children and it would not occur in the immediate postoperative period.
  2 The incidence of obstruction is not higher than for other abdominal surgery.
  4 The incidence is not higher after splenectomy than after other abdominal surgery.

207. **3 Postoperative pain will cause splinting, shallow breathing, and underaeration of the lung's left lower lobe because of close proximity of the spleen to the diaphragm.** (PL; PA; BI)

  1 This would be true of any surgery and is not specific to a splenectomy.
  2 Same as answer 1.
  4 Same as answer 1.

208. **1 Malaria is caused by the protozoan *Plasmodium falciparum*, which is carried by mosquitoes.** (IM; TC; BI)
  2 Ingestion of untreated water will not enable protozoa to enter the blood stream.
  3 Ingestion of contaminated food will not facilitate the entry of protozoa into the blood stream.
  4 Exposure to crowds will not enable the protozoa to enter the blood stream.

209. **3 Parasites invade the erythrocytes, subsequently dividing and causing the cell to burst. The spleen enlarges from the sloughing of red blood cells.** (DC; PA; BI)
  1 WBCs (leukocytes) are not increased in number.
  2 RBCs (erythrocytes) are not increased in number.
  4 Malaria is an infestation, not an infection or inflammation.

210. **4 Maintaining adequate nutritional and fluid balance is essential to life and must be accomplished during periods when intestinal motility is not too excessive so that absorption can occur.** (PL; TC; BI)
  1 While shaking chills may occur, seizures do not generally occur.
  2 Peritoneal dialysis is not generally used in the treatment of malaria.
  3 Infection may occur only through direct serum contact or a bite from an infected *Anopheles* mosquito.

211. **3 Quinine sulfate is used in malaria when the plasmodia are resistant to the less toxic chloroquine. However, a new strain of *Plasmodium*, resistant to quinine, must be treated with a combination of quinine (quick acting), pyrimethamine, and sulfonamide (slow acting).** (IM; ED; BI)
  1 The aim of therapy is to eliminate the asexual erythrocytic parasite, which is responsible for the symptoms, not to control them.
  2 Reinfestation can occur with a different species or strain of *Plasmodium*.
  4 This would not occur if drug therapy is successful.

212. **2 *Plasmodium falciparum* in persons who have been treated with quinine causes**

hemoglobinuria, intravascular hemoly-sis, and renal failure as a result of destruction of red blood cells. (DC; PA; BI)

1 This symptom is unrelated to the development of blackwater fever.

3 Same as answer 1.

4 Same as answer 1.

213. **1 Platelets (thrombocytes) adhere to the intima of damaged vessels within sec-onds after injury, releasing substances that promote hemostasis. (AN; PA; BI)**

2 Leukocytes play no role in clotting; they pro-tect the body against microorganisms.

3 Erythrocytes are red blood cells; they carry oxygen and play no role in coagulation.

4 Red blood cells play no role in clotting; they carry oxygen to all body cells.

214. **3 Thromboplastin is a substance released by platelets that initiates the clotting process by converting prothrombin to thrombin. (AN; PA; BI)**

1 Bile does not contain thromboplastin.

2 Plasma does not produce thromboplastin.

4 RBCs do not produce thromboplastin.

215. **3 Fibrinogen is a soluble plasma protein that becomes the insoluble gel, fibrin, during the clotting process. (AN; PA; BI)**

1 Fibrin is the insoluble gel formed from fibrino-gen by the action of thrombin.

2 Thrombin is needed to convert fibrinogen to fibrin; it is also needed in platelet aggregation.

4 Prothrombin is the precursor of thrombin; it becomes fibrinogen.

216. **3 Calcium acts as a catalyst to convert pro-thrombin to thrombin. Thrombin acceler-ates the formation of insoluble fibrin from the soluble fibrinogen. (AN; PA; BI)**

1 Fluorine is a gas of the halogen group and is not involved in clotting; sodium fluoride helps harden tooth enamel.

2 Chloride is an extracellular anion that helps regulate osmotic pressure and combines with hydrogen to form hydrochloric acid; it is not involved with clotting.

4 Iron is essential for the synthesis of hemoglo-bin, which is not involved in clotting.

217. **4 Vitamin K, synthesized by the bacterial flora of the intestine, promotes the liver's synthesis of prothrombin, an important blood-clotting factor. (AN; PA; BI)**

1 Vitamin K does not promote platelet aggrega-tion.

2 Vitamin K does not affect calcium ionization.

3 Vitamin K does not promote fibrinogen for-mation.

218. **3 Hypersensitivity to a foreign substance can cause an anaphylactic reaction. Histamine is released, causing bronchial constriction, increased capillary perme-ability, and dilation of arterioles. This decreased peripheral resistance is associ-ated with hypotension and inadequate circulation to major organs. (AN; PA; BI)**

1 These are the problems that result from bronchial constriction and vascular collapse.

2 Arterioles dilate, capillary permeability increases, and eventually vascular collapse occurs.

4 Dilation of arterioles occurs.

219. **3 Hypersensitivity results from the produc-tion of antibodies in response to exposure to certain foreign substances (allergens). Prior exposure is necessary for the devel-opment of these antibodies. (AN; PA; BI)**

1 This is not a sensitivity reaction to penicillin; hay fever and asthma are atopic conditions caused by atopens.

2 It would be an active immunity.

4 Antibodies have been developed in a prior exposure to the allergen, in this case peni-cillin.

220. **4 Tetanus immune globulin provides anti-bodies against tetanus. This is used if the client has never received tetanus toxoid or antitoxin, which confer active immu-nity (the body makes its own antibodies in response to the antigen). (IM; PA; BI)**

1 DTP vaccine—diphtheria and tetanus toxoid combined with pertussis vaccine—produces active, not passive, immunity; in addition, DTP is not usually given to adults, Td is used.

2 Administration of this substance would pro-duce active immunity.

3 Same as answer 2.

221. **2 Tetanus antitoxin provides antibodies, which confer immediate passive immu-nity. (IM; PA; BI)**

1 Antitoxin does not stimulate production of antibodies.

3 It provides passive, not active, immunity.

4 Passive immunity, by definition, is not long lasting.

222. **2 Gamma globulin, an immune globulin, contains most of the antibodies circulating in the blood. When injected into an individual, it prevents a specific antigen from entering a host cell. (EV; TC; BI)**
    1 This does not stimulate antibody production.
    3 This does not affect antigen-antibody function.
    4 Same as answer 1.

223. **2 The client is unconscious. Although the spouse can consent, there is no legal power to refuse a treatment for the client unless previously authorized to do so by a power of attorney or a health care proxy; the court can make a decision for the client. (IM; TC; BI)**
    1 This alternative does not have a legal basis, and the nurse could be held liable.
    3 Although a nurse is legally licensed to teach, this will not meet the client's needs.
    4 Same as answer 1.

224. **1 Core rewarming with heated oxygen and administration of warmed po or IV fluids is the preferred method of treatment. (AN; PA; BI)**
    2 The victim would be too weak to ambulate; ambulation would expend energy.
    3 Oral temperatures are not the most accurate assessment of core temperature because of environmental influences.
    4 Warmed oral feedings are advised; gastric gavage would be unnecessary.

Respiratory

225. **4 Because atelectasis involves collapsing of the alveoli distal to the bronchioles, breath sounds would be diminished in the lower lobes. (DC; PA; RE)**
    1 A client would have rapid, shallow respirations to compensate for poor gas exchange.
    2 Atelectasis results in a loose, productive cough.
    3 Atelectasis results in an elevated temperature.

226. **3 The residual volume is the amount of air remaining in the lungs after maximum exhalation. (AN; PA; RE)**
    1 This is normally under the individual's control. The force exerted by the abdominal thrust surpasses that which the individual is voluntarily capable of exerting.
    2 Same as answer 1.
    4 Same as answer 1.

227. **3 After a submucosal resection (SMR), hemorrhage from the area is frequently detected by vomiting of blood that has been swallowed. (DC; TC; RE)**
    1 Crepitus would be caused by leakage of air into tissue spaces; it is not usually a complication of SMR.
    2 Headaches in the back of the head would not be a complication of a submucosal resection.
    4 The area under the tongue is not involved in this surgery.

228. **4 The respiratory center in the medulla responds primarily to increased carbon dioxide concentration in the blood. (AN; PA; RE)**
    1 Oxygen is normally not the primary stimulus to breathing; it functions as a primary stimulus in individuals who have chronic hypercapnia.
    2 This is not a stimulant; it is a by-product of muscular activity.
    3 These are not stimulants for respiration; they are involved in transmission of neural impulses.

229. **3 The lower the PO_2 and the higher the PCO_2, the more rapidly oxygen dissociates from the oxyhemoglobin molecule. (AN; PA; RE)**
    1 It must be associated with an increase in carbon dioxide pressure.
    2 It must be associated with a decrease in oxygen pressure.
    4 Oxygen dissociations would be decreased in this situation.

230. **3 Carbon monoxide (CO) binds with hemoglobin more avidly than does oxygen. The progressive results are dyspnea, asphyxia, and death. (AN; PA; RE)**
    1 Carbon monoxide does not block carbon dioxide transport; it binds with hemoglobin.
    2 Carbon monoxide inhibits oxygen transport, not vasodilation.
    4 Carbon monoxide does not form bubbles in the blood plasma; bubbles in tissues are caused by increased nitrogen, as in decompression sickness (bends).

231. **1 With an oxygen debt, a muscle would show primarily low levels of oxygen and low levels of ATP caused by the low levels of aerobic respiration and high levels of lactic acid formation. (DC; PA; RE)**

2 Low levels of calcium are present.

3 Low levels of glycogen are present.

4 High levels of lactic acid are present.

232. **3 Accumulated carbon dioxide (CO_2) will powerfully stimulate the breathing center of the brainstem, forcing resumption of respiration even if the person has fainted first. (AN; PA; RE)**

1 Increased carbon dioxide will stimulate breathing.

2 This is unrelated; it will occur with changes in pressure, as in decompression sickness.

4 Rising carbon dioxide, not oxygen, will stimulate breathing.

233. **1 An AmbuBag is a piece of equipment that can be compressed at regular intervals by hand for temporary ventilation of the client in respiratory arrest. (PL; TC; RE)**

2 Ventricular fibrillation requires immediate defibrillation.

3 The AmbuBag is used to ventilate a client, not to measure respiratory output.

4 Wound drainage systems, not an AmbuBag, may be used for gross incisional drainage.

234. **3 The phrenic nerves conduct motor impulses to the diaphragm; cutting one phrenic nerve will paralyze the portion of the diaphragm innervated by that nerve. (AN; PA; RE)**

1 Phrenic nerves take motor impulses to the diaphragm, not the lungs.

2 Phrenic nerves are motor, not sensory, nerves.

4 Paralysis of the diaphragm will result on the same side.

235. **4 This is the acid-fast causative organism of tuberculosis. (AN; PA; RE)**

1 This is not an acid-fast organism.

2 Same as answer 1.

3 Same as answer 1.

236. **2 Tidal volume (TV) is defined as the amount of air exhaled normally after a normal inspiration. (AN; PA; RE)**

1 This is the expiratory reserve volume (ERV).

3 This is the residual volume (RV).

4 The volume of air that can be forcibly inspired over and above a normal inspiration is the inspiratory reserve volume (IRV).

237. **1 The tidal volume is the amount of air inhaled and exhaled while breathing normally. (DC; PA; RE)**

2 This is air that can be forcibly expired after deep inspiration.

3 This is the maximum amount of air that can be expired after expiration of the tidal volume.

4 This is the maximum amount of air that can be inspired following the inspiration of the tidal volume.

238. **4 Thoracic pressure is reduced because thoracic volume is increased as the diaphragm descends. (AN; PA; RE)**

1 Contraction of the diaphragm causes inspiration.

2 Rising pressure in the alveoli and the intrapleural space or relaxation of the diaphragm expels air from the alveoli.

3 Same as answer 2.

239. **2 The orthopneic position is a sitting position that permits maximum lung expansion for gaseous exchange, because the abdominal organs do not provide pressure against the diaphragm and gravity facilitates the descent of the diaphragm. (IM; PA; RE)**

1 This position does not permit the diaphragm to descend by gravity, and pressure of the abdominal organs against the diaphragm limits its movement.

3 This position does not maximize lung expansion to the same degree as the orthopneic position.

4 Same as answer 3.

240. **3 Orthopneic position refers to sitting up and leaning slightly forward. This drops the diaphragm, allowing the lungs more room for expansion. (IM; PA; RE)**

1 Horizontal positions do not allow the gravitational effect on the diaphragm and thus do not maximize air exchange.

2 Same as answer 1.

4 The Trendelenburg position forces the diaphragm up, interfering with lung expansion.

241. **3 Hemoptysis is expectoration of blood-stained sputum derived from the lungs, bronchi, or trachea. (DC; PA; RE)**

1 Hematuria refers to blood in the urine.

2 Hematoma refers to a local accumulation of blood in the tissues.

4 Hematemesis refers to vomiting of blood.

242. **4 This may occur because of the high osmotic pressure of the aspirated ocean water. (DC; TC; RE)**
1 Hypoxia and acidosis may occur after a near drowning.
2 This is not a sequela of near drowning.
3 Hypovolemia occurs because fluid is drawn into the lungs by the hypertonic salt water.

243. **4 Streptococcal organisms are present on the skin, mucous membranes, and in the environment at all times. The most frequent portals of entry are the respiratory tract and breaks in the skin. (AN; PA; RE)**
1 All are caused by streptococci.
2 Vaccinations are not available for most of these conditions; there is an antitoxin for scarlet fever, but antibiotics are now used.
3 Bacteria are not classified as parasites.

244. **1 Furosemide (Lasix) acts on the loop of Henle by increasing the excretion of chloride and sodium. (AN; TC; RE)**
2 Although used in the treatment of edema and hypertension, this drug is not as potent as furosemide.
3 Same as answer 2.
4 This is a potassium-sparing diuretic; it is less potent than thiazide diuretics.

245. **3 Destruction of the alveolar walls leads to diminished surface area for gaseous exchange and an increased CO_2 level in the blood. (AN; PA; RE)**
1 Pleural effusion occurs when there is seepage of fluid into the intrapleural space; this does not occur with emphysema.
2 Infectious obstructions occur in conditions in which microorganisms invade lung tissue; emphysema is not an infectious disease.
4 Muscle paralysis may occur in diseases affecting the neurologic system; emphysema does not affect the neurologic system; therefore it is not a neurologic disease.

246. **3 Because the client's condition is described as terminal, the nursing priority should be directed toward providing comfort. (PL; TC; RE)**
1 Although these are important aspects of nursing care, provision of comfort retains priority in the care of a dying client.
2 Same as answer 1.
4 Same as answer 1.

247. **3 There are several modes for the administration of oxygen. Selection is based on the disease and the client's adaptation. Oxygen-induced hypoventilation is a particular concern for clients with COPD. (AN; TC; RE)**
1 Although consideration may be given to activity, selection is based on the pathologic condition and therapeutic needs.
2 Although anatomy may be one factor considered, selection depends on the therapeutic effect relative to the client's disease and needs.
4 Although these will be taken into consideration, the ultimate decision is based on the pathologic condition and therapeutic needs.

248. **4 Clients with COPD (chronic obstructive pulmonary disease) respond only to the chemical stimulus of low oxygen levels. Administration of high concentrations of oxygen will eliminate the stimulus to breathe, leading to decreased respirations and lethargy. (EV; TC; RE)**
1 Cyanosis is caused by excessive amounts of reduced oxyhemoglobin; because oxygen is being administered, cyanosis may be reduced.
2 Rising carbon dioxide levels cause lethargy rather than anxiety.
3 High concentrations of oxygen will eliminate the stimulus to breathe, so the respiratory rate would decrease.

249. **2 Loss of elasticity causes difficult exhalation, with subsequent air trapping. Clients who have emphysema are taught to use accessory abdominal muscles and to breathe out through pursed lips to help keep the air passages open until exhalation is complete. (AN; PA; RE)**
1 Expiration is difficult because of air trapping and poor elasticity.
3 There will be decreased vital capacity.
4 Diaphragmatic breathing is a learned mechanism that is beneficial.

250. **3 Coughing is needed to raise the secretions for expectoration. (IM; TC; RE)**
1 Oxygen will not mobilize the secretions.
2 A sitting position will allow secretions to remain in the lungs unless coughing is encouraged.
4 Rest should be encouraged only after coughing to bring up secretions mobilized by postural drainage.

251. **2 Because family members are old enough to understand the client's needs, they should be encouraged to participate in the care. (PL; TC; RE)**
 1 Self-care increases oxygen utilization, causing fatigue and dyspnea.
 3 This deprives the client of a support system.
 4 Overworking the client causes undue fatigue and dyspnea; frequent rest periods should be incorporated into the plan.

252. **3 The etiology of a spontaneous pneumothorax is commonly the rupture of blebs on the lung surface. Blebs are similar to blisters. (DC; PA; RE)**
 1 Pleural friction rub would result in pain on inspiration, not a pneumothorax.
 2 A tracheoesophageal fistula would cause aspiration of food and saliva, resulting in respiratory distress.
 4 The client had no history of trauma.

253. **3 As a person with a tear in the lung inhales, air moves through that opening into the intrapleural space. This creates a positive pressure and causes partial or complete collapse of the lung. (AN; PA; RE)**
 1 Mediastinal shift occurs toward the unaffected side.
 2 This is not an impending problem.
 4 There is loss of intrathoracic negative pressure.

254. **1 A pneumothorax results in decreased surface area for gaseous exchange. If the unaffected pleural regions cannot compensate, carbon dioxide builds up in the blood (hypercapnia). The client becomes drowsy and may lose consciousness. The body attempts to compensate by increasing the respiratory and pulse rates and by the renal retention of bicarbonate. (DC; TC; RE)**
 2 Hypokalemia causes extreme muscle weakness, abdominal distention, and changes in the ECG pattern.
 3 Carbon dioxide builds up in the blood, and the PO_2 is lowered because of the decreased surface area for gaseous exchange.
 4 Acidosis occurs with elevated PCO_2.

255. **2 Sudden chest pain occurs on the affected side; it may also involve the arm and shoulder. (DC; PA; RE)**
 1 Bloody vomitus is unrelated to pneumothorax.
 3 Decreased chest motion would occur because of failure to inflate the involved lung.

 4 The shift toward the unaffected side is caused by pressure from the pneumothorax.

256. **2 The ribs may penetrate the pleura and lung, allowing air to fill the pleural space and collapse the lung. (DC; PA; RE)**
 1 Scoliosis involves altered vertebral alignment, not the ribs.
 3 This does not occur.
 4 Same as answer 3.

257. **2 Pressure within the pleural cavity causes a shift of the heart and great vessels to the unaffected side. This not only decreases the capacity of the unaffected lung but also impedes the filling of the right side of the heart and leads to a decreased cardiac output. (AN; PA; RE)**
 1 Infection is not caused by a mediastinal shift.
 3 This complication might occur in severe chest trauma, not in mediastinal shift.
 4 The volume of the unaffected lung may decrease because of pressure from the shift.

258. **2 Fluctuations occur with normal inspiration and expiration until the lung is fully expanded. If these fluctuations do not occur, the chest tube may be clogged or kinked; coughing should be encouraged. (EV; TC; RE)**
 1 The binder does not prevent tension on the tube; it would be contraindicated, because it limits thoracic expansion.
 3 The tube should be clamped only if ordered or if an air leak is suspected.
 4 The client may not be agitated; morphine depresses respirations and is usually avoided.

259. **4 Chest x-ray films or radiographs reveal the degree to which the lung fills the pleural cavity and also the presence of any mediastinal shift. (EV; PA; RE)**
 1 This would be an indicator of expansion of both lungs, and would not be specific to expansion of the affected side.
 2 The chest tubes may have minimal drainage; this is not an indicator.
 3 These are not normal chest sounds and do not indicate the degree of lung expansion.

MEDICAL-SURGICAL ANSWERS

260. **1 Alupent is a selective beta-2 adrenergic antagonist that causes increased heart contraction (positive inotropic effect) and increased heart rate (positive chronotropic effect). If toxic levels are reached, side effects occur and the drug should be withheld until the physician is notified. (IM; TC; RE)**

2 This is false reassurance and a false statement; the drug will have to be withheld until the physician is notified.

3 Controlled breathing may be helpful in allaying a client's anxiety; however, the drug may be producing side effects and should be withheld.

4 Same as answer 2.

261. **2 As a result of the narrowed airways, exhalation is difficult, leaving air trapped in the lung. Distention of alveolar walls to accommodate this volume leads to emphysema. (DC; PA; RE)**

1 Atelectasis is the collapse of lung tissue.

3 Pneumothorax is the term that describes the collapse of a lung.

4 Pulmonary fibrosis is a condition in which fibrous connective tissue spreads over normal lung tissue.

262. **1 Hypersecretion of the mucous glands provides an excellent, warm, moist medium for microorganisms. (IM; ED; RE)**

2 Asthma is not a disease that is voluntarily controlled.

3 Coughing must be encouraged; it prevents retention of mucus, which is an excellent medium for microorganisms. Excessive secretions also limit gaseous exchange.

4 Anxiety is not willfully controlled.

263. **2 Turning the client to the side promotes drainage of secretions and prevents aspiration, especially when the gag reflex is not intact. This position also brings the tongue forward, preventing it from occluding the airway in the relaxed state. (IM; TC; RE)**

1 The risk of aspiration is increased when this position is assumed by a semialert client.

3 This increases the risk of aspiration; this position may flex the neck in an individual who is not alert, interfering with respirations.

4 This position is not generally used for a postoperative client because it interferes with breathing.

264. **2 Maintenance of a patent airway is always the priority, because airway obstruction impedes breathing and may result in death. (AN; TC; RE)**

1 This is important in the client's postoperative care; however, oxygenation is the priority.

3 Same as answer 1.

4 Same as answer 1.

265. **2 During radiation therapy with radium implants the client is placed in isolation so that exposure to radiation of family and staff will be decreased. (IM; TC; RE)**

1 This is unnecessary.

3 Excess exposure to radiation is hazardous to personnel.

4 Rubber gloves will not protect the nurse from radiation.

266. **2 Because of the location of the spleen, expansion of the thoracic cavity during inspiration causes pain at the operative site. (DC; PA; RE)**

1 Pain does not occur on expiration, for the lungs deflate and decrease pressure on the operative site.

3 Because limited activity decreases oxygen consumption, shortness of breath is not a common complaint.

4 This is not to be expected; accumulation of secretions can be avoided by coughing and deep breathing.

267. **3 With the head elevated, rather than horizontal or dependent, fluid will not collect in the interstitial spaces around the trachea. (PL; TC; RE)**

1 This may cause aspiration if the gag reflex has not returned.

2 Same as answer 1.

4 Same as answer 1.

268. **3 Cancerous lesions in the pleural space increase the osmotic pressure, causing a shift of fluid to that space. (AN; PA; RE)**

1 Excessive intake is normally balanced by increased urine output.

2 Inadequate chest expansion results from pleural effusion and is not the cause of it.

4 A bronchoscopy does not involve the pleural space.

269. **3 The phrenic nerve stimulates the diaphragm. After destruction of the nerve on the operative side, the diaphragm will**

move upward, decreasing the size of the empty space and helping to prevent mediastinal shift. (AN; PA; RE)

1 Would occur if both nerves were severed.
2 Because the phrenic nerve stimulates the diaphragm, its effect on postoperative pain would be negligible.
4 There is less excursion because the nerve has been severed.

270. **2 Inadequate dental hygiene may predispose a person to oral infections but would be only remotely involved in laryngeal neoplasms because of the anatomical relationship of the oral cavity and the larynx. (DC; PA; RE)**

1 Irritation by air pollutants may initiate a tissue change that can lead to malignancy.
3 Alcohol is an irritant that may initiate a tissue change that results in a malignant neoplasm.
4 Tissue alterations caused by repeated microbiologic stress may result in a malignant neoplasm.

271. **2 The inner cannula, if nondisposable, must be removed, cleaned with peroxide, and rinsed with saline to remove mucus accumulation and prevent occlusion. (IM; TC; RE)**

1 The obturator is used only for inserting the outer cannula.
3 The status of the cuff has no effect on tracheostomy care.
4 The outer cannula is left in place, its patency maintained through suctioning.

272. **2 During suctioning of a client, negative pressure (suction) should not be applied until the catheter is ready to be drawn out because, in addition to the removal of secretions, oxygen is being depleted. (IM; TC; RE)**

1 The asepsis of the catheter can be maintained during one suctioning session; a new sterile catheter should be used for each new session of suctioning.
3 A cough reflex may be absent or diminished in some clients; the catheter should be inserted approximately 12 cm (4 to 5 inches) or just past the end of the tracheostomy tube.
4 The inner cannula is not removed during suctioning; it may be removed during tracheostomy care.

273. **2 Immediately prior to administration, an assessment of vital signs is necessary to determine whether any contraindications to analgesia exist (e.g., hypotension, a respiratory rate of 12 or less). (EV; PA; RE)**

1 Pain prevents both psychologic and physiologic rest.
3 Before administration, the nurse must check the physician's orders, the time of the last administration, and the client's vital signs.
4 Prior to determining the time of the last dose, the nurse should obtain the client's vital signs; the client's status must be evaluated further.

274. **2 A chest tube drains the leaking chyle from the thoracic area; TPN provides nutrition, boosts immune defenses, and decreases thoracic duct flow; bed rest is recommended because lymphatic flow increases with activity. (PL; PA; RE)**

1 A gastrostomy tube will not drain fluid from the thoracic area; a high-fat diet is contraindicated but bed rest is recommended.
3 This has no relationship to the drainage of chyle from the thoracic area; a fat-poor diet and bed rest are recommended.
4 The nasogastric tube does not drain fluid from the thoracic area; a fat-poor diet and bed rest are recommended; a low-fat diet of medium chain triglycerides will reduce the production and flow of chyle.

275. **2 The respiratory membrane, consisting of the alveolar and capillary walls, is extremely thin. This thinness facilitates exchange of respiratory gases without the need for additional energy. (AN; PA; RE)**

1 Osmosis is diffusion of water through a selective membrane.
3 Filtration is a process to prevent passage of certain-sized particles.
4 This mechanism is utilized when energy is required to move matter against a concentration gradient.

276. **3 The absence of bacteria in the sputum indicates that the disease can no longer be spread by the airborne route. (EV; PA; RE)**

1 Once an individual has been infected, the test will always be positive.
2 Treatment is over an extended period; eventually the client may not have an active disease, but still remains infected.
4 This is not evidence that the disease will not be transmitted.

MEDICAL-SURGICAL ANSWERS

277. 2 Expectoration of blood is an indication that the lung itself was damaged during the procedure; a pneumothorax or hemothorax may occur. (EV; TC; RE)

1 Increased lung expansion should improve cerebral oxygenation and decrease confusion if present.

3 Increased breath sounds are anticipated as the lung is closer to the chest wall after the fluid in the pleural space is removed.

4 A decreased rate may indicate improved gaseous exchange and is not evidence that the client is in danger.

278. 2 Suctioning also removes oxygen, which can cause cardiac dysrhythmias; the nurse should try to prevent this by hyperoxygenating the client prior to and after suctioning. (IM; PA; RE)

1 To prevent trauma to the trachea, suction should only be applied while removing the catheter.

3 This kind of movement could cause tracheal damage.

4 Suction only as needed; excessive suctioning irritates the mucosa, which increases secretion production.

Endocrine

279. 1 Glucose catabolism is the main pathway for cellular energy production. (AN; PA; EN)

2 Glucose is not used directly for this process; ATP is the energy source.

3 Same as answer 2.

4 Same as answer 2.

280. 2 Ingested glucose not used immediately for energy needs is stored in the liver as glycogen and broken down when the blood glucose level falls (glycogenolysis). (AN; PA; EN)

1 Not all foods provide glucose; ingested glucose may meet immediate needs but must be converted to glycogen for storage; glycogen is converted to glucose as needed.

3 This is formation of glucose from protein or fat.

4 This is digestion.

281. 1 Insulin functions by facilitating the transport of glucose through the cell membrane and by increasing the deposits of glycogen in muscle. Both cellular glucose and muscle glycogen can be utilized for energy. (AN; PA; EN)

2 Thyroxine stimulates the rate of oxygen consumption and thus the rate at which carbohydrates are burned; it is not the main controlling hormone.

3 Adrenal steroids stimulate glyconeogenesis.

4 Growth hormone accelerates protein anabolism and stimulates growth.

282. 3 As a result of osmotic pressures created by increased serum glucose, the cells become dehydrated; the client must receive fluid and then insulin. (AN; PA; EN)

1 Oxygen therapy is not necessarily indicated.

2 Carbohydrates would increase the blood glucose, which is already high.

4 Although dietary instruction may be appropriate if the problem is related to dietary noncompliance, such instruction is inappropriate during the crisis.

283. 1 In starvation there are inadequate carbohydrates available for immediate energy, and stored fats are used in excessive amounts. (DC; PA; EN)

2 There is no fat in alcohol; no fat oxidation occurs.

3 This does not require the use of great amounts of fat; calcium is deposited to form callus.

4 This does not require the use of great amounts of fat.

284. 4 Oral hypoglycemics may be helpful when some functioning of the beta cells exists, as in Type II (NIDDM) diabetes. (PL; PA; EN)

1 Rapid-acting regular insulin is needed to reverse ketoacidosis.

2 Obesity as a symptom does not offer enough information to determine the status of beta-cell function.

3 Clients with Type I (IDDM) diabetes have no function of the beta cells.

285. 2 Ketones are given off when fat is broken down for energy. (AN; PA; EN)

1 Although rarely used, sodium bicarbonate may be administered to correct the acid-base imbalance resulting from ketoacidosis; acidosis is caused by excess acid, not excess base bicarbonate.

3 Diabetes does not interfere with removal of nitrogenous wastes.

4 Carbohydrate metabolism is hampered in the diabetic.

286. 2 Infection increases the body's metabolic rate, and insulin is not available for increased demands. (DC; PA; EN)

1 Although emotional stress will affect glucose levels, diabetic ketoacidosis will rarely result.

3 Increased insulin dose will lead to insulin shock if diet is not increased as well.

4 This would result in insulin shock (insulin coma).

287. 1 **IV fluids are given to combat dehydration in acidosis and to keep an IV line open for administration of medications. When the electrolyte levels have been evaluated, potassium may be added if needed. (IM; TC; EN)**

2 In acidosis potassium ions initially shift from intracellular to extracellular fluids, which results in hyperkalemia; as acidosis is corrected, hypokalemia may occur and then potassium may be administered.

3 This is an intermediate-acting insulin; rapid-acting insulin such as regular insulin is indicated in an emergency.

4 This is not indicated; abnormally high serum potassium levels will revert once dehydration is corrected.

288. 2 **Regular insulin is rapid acting and should be used when immediate action is desired. (IM; TC; EN)**

1 This is intermediate-acting insulin; it is not indicated for use in an emergency.

3 This is not a form of insulin; it is a simple protein.

4 This is a long-acting insulin that is not indicated in an emergency.

289. 3 **Kussmaul respirations occur in diabetic coma as the body attempts to correct a low pH caused by accumulation of ketones (ketoacidosis); HHNC affects people with Type II diabetes who still have some insulin production; the insulin prevents the breakdown of fats into ketones. (EV; PA; EN)**

1 Fluid loss is common to both because elevated blood glucose ultimately leads to polyuria.

2 Glycosuria is common to both conditions.

4 Hyperglycemia is common to both conditions.

290. 1 **Glucagon, produced by the alpha cells in the islets of Langerhans, is an insulin antagonist. It mobilizes glycogen storage in the liver, leading to an increased blood glucose level. (AN; PA; EN)**

2 This stimulates an increase in blood glucose, not glycogen.

3 Glucagon does not compete with insulin; it promotes the conversion of glycogen to glucose.

4 Glucagon is not a glucose substitute.

291. 1 **The ketones produced excessively in diabetes are acetoacetic acid, beta-hydroxybutyric acid, and acetone. The major ketone, acetoacetic acid, is an alphaketoacid that lowers the blood pH, resulting in acidosis. (DC; PA; EN)**

2 Glucose is not an acid; it does not change the pH.

3 Lactic acid is produced as a result of muscle contraction; it is not unique to diabetes.

4 This is a product of protein metabolism.

292. 1 **In the absence of insulin, which facilitates the transport of glucose into cells, the body breaks down proteins and fats to supply energy; ketones, a byproduct of fat metabolism, accumulate causing metabolic acidosis (pH below 7.35). (AN; PA; EN)**

2 The pH of food ingested has no effect on the development of acidosis.

3 The opposite is true.

4 Cholesterol level has no effect on the development of acidosis.

293. 4 **The urinary catheter and drainage bag should always remain a closed sterile system; urine should be drawn only from the catheter, not the collection bag. (IM; TC; EN)**

1 The system should remain closed so that there will be fewer microorganisms entering the urinary system.

2 This would not yield a fresh specimen indicating present acetone levels.

3 The system should remain closed so that there will be a decreased possibility of urinary system infection.

294. 4 **In the absence of insulin, glucose cannot enter the cell or be converted to glycogen, so it remains in the blood. Breakdown of fats as an energy source causes an accumulation of ketones, which results in acidosis. The lungs, in an attempt to compensate for lowered pH, will blow off CO_2 (Kussmaul respirations). (EV; PA; EN)**

1 Hyperglycemia and a low CO_2 combining power would be present.

2 Hyperglycemia and increased acidity would be present.

3 High acidity and a low CO_2 combining power would be present.

MEDICAL-SURGICAL ANSWERS

295. 4 **The bicarbonate-carbonic acid buffer system helps maintain the pH of the body fluids; in metabolic acidosis there is a decrease in bicarbonate due to an increase of metabolic acids.** (DC; PA; EN)
1 The pH is decreased.
2 The PO_2 is not decreased in diabetic acidosis.
3 The PCO_2 may be decreased by the body's attempt to eliminate CO_2 to compensate for a low pH.

296. 1 **Regular insulin is rapid acting (30 to 60 minutes) and is used to meet a client's immediate insulin needs.** (PL; TC; EN)
2 This is an intermediate-acting insulin, which has an onset of 1 to $2^1/2$ hours; in diabetic acidosis the individual needs rapid-acting insulin.
3 This is an intermediate-acting insulin, which has an onset of 1 to 2 hours; in diabetic acidosis the individual needs rapid-acting insulin.
4 This is a long-acting insulin, with an onset of 4 to 8 hours and a peak of 10 to 30 hours.

297. 1 **Because the brain requires a constant supply of glucose, hypoglycemia triggers the response of the sympathetic nervous system, which causes these symptoms.** (EV; TC; EN)
2 These symptoms are consistent with dehydration, which is often associated with hyperglycemic states.
3 These are associated with hyperglycemia; these symptoms are caused by the breakdown of fats as a result of inadequate insulin supply.
4 Hypoglycemia causes the compensatory mechanism of hunger. Because blood glucose is low, the renal threshold is not exceeded, and there is no glycosuria.

298. 3 **Glucagon, an insulin antagonist produced by the alpha cells in the islets of Langerhans, leads to the conversion of glycogen to glucose in the liver.** (IM; TC; EN)
1 It stimulates glycogenolysis, the conversion of glycogen to glucose.
2 It is an insulin antagonist.
4 It does not stimulate the storage of glucose but rather is released by the conversion of glycogen to glucose.

299. 1 **Liquids containing simple carbohydrates are most readily absorbed and thus increase blood sugar quickly.** (IM; TC; EN)
2 Although a solution of 50% dextrose may be given if the client is comatose, 5% dextrose does not supply sufficient carbohydrates.

3 This will not alter the current situation.
4 Complex carbohydrates and protein take longer to elevate blood glucose, so they should be administered after simple carbohydrates.

300. 1 **The Nurse Practice Act states that the nurse will do health teaching and administer nursing care supportive to life and well-being.** (EV; ED; EN)
2 The teaching was essential prior to discharge.
3 The client is responsible for self-care.
4 Health teaching is an independent function of the nurse.

301. 2 **Each client should be given an individually devised diet selecting commonly used foods from the Good Health Eating Guide; family members should be included in the diet teaching.** (PL; ED; EN)
1 Rigid diets are difficult to comply with; substitutions should be offered.
3 Nutritional requirements are different for each individual depending on many factors, such as activity level, degree of compliance, and physical status.
4 Seasonings do not affect the management of diabetes mellitus.

302. 2 **The client needs further teaching because these foods cannot be exchanged; they are not on the same exchange list.** (EV; ED; EN)
1 No further teaching is necessary because this is an equal exchange.
3 Same as answer 1.
4 Same as answer 1.

303. 1 **An understanding of the diet is imperative for compliance. A balance of carbohydrates, proteins, and fats usually apportioned over three main meals and two between-meal snacks needs to be tailored to the client's specific needs, with due regard for activity, diet, and therapy.** (IM; ED; EN)
2 Although restriction of calories and concentrated sweets is essential, a total dietary regimen must be followed to ensure adequate nutrition and control of the disease.
3 This is true; however, indigestion is not the basis for the client's problems.
4 Total caloric intake, rather than the distribution of meals, is the major factor in weight gain.

304. 2 **A combination of diet, exercise, and medication is necessary to control the disease; the interaction of these thera-**

pies is reflected by the serum glucose. (EV; TC; EN)

1 Weight loss may occur with inadequate insulin.

3 Acquisition of knowledge does not guarantee its application.

4 Insulin alone is not enough to control the disease.

305. **3 Glucagon is an insulin antagonist produced by the alpha cells in the islets of Langerhans. It causes the breakdown of glycogen and protein to glucose. (AN; PA; EN)**

1 Acidosis occurs when there is a high serum glucose level; therefore glucagon is not indicated.

2 Diabetes mellitus involves a decreased insulin production.

4 Glucagon is not indicated in idiosyncratic reactions to insulin.

306. **4 Insulin stimulates cellular uptake of glucose and also stimulates the membrane-bound pump for sodium and potassium ions, leading to the influx of potassium into cells. The resulting hypokalemia is offset by parenteral administration of potassium. (AN; PA; EN)**

1 Hypokalemia may be caused by the movement of potassium back into the cells as dehydration is reversed.

2 Hypokalemia may occur because the potassium moves back into the cells as dehydration is reversed.

3 Anabolic reactions are stimulated by insulin and glucose administration; potassium is drawn into the intracellular compartment, necessitating a replenishment of extracellular potassium.

307. **1 During treatment for acidosis the client may develop hypoglycemia; careful observation for this complication should be made by the nurse, even without an order. (EV; TC; EN)**

2 Withholding all glucose may cause insulin shock; monitoring glucose is indicated to prevent this.

3 The regulation of insulin depends on the physician's orders for coverage.

4 Whole milk and fruit juices contain large amounts of carbohydrates, which are contraindicated in this period immediately following ketoacidosis.

308. **2 Because the client has severe diabetes, it is essential that the blood glucose level be determined before meals to evaluate the success of control of diabetes and the possible need for insulin coverage. (EV; PA; EN)**

1 To prevent flexion contractures of the hip, the client should not sit in a chair for a prolonged time.

3 This could result in a hip flexion contracture.

4 Raising the head of the bed flexes the hips, which could result in hip flexion contractures.

309. **2 Because water is not being reabsorbed, urine is dilute, resulting in a low specific gravity. (DC; PA; EN)**

1 Diabetes insipidus is not a disorder of glucose metabolism; blood levels are not affected.

3 Loss of fluid may actually lower blood pressure.

4 As fluid is lost from the vascular compartment, serum osmolarity increases.

310. **4 Antidiuretic hormone (ADH), from the posterior pituitary, promotes water uptake by the kidney tubules; the result is decreased urinary output—an antidiuretic effect. (AN; PA; EN)**

1 The adrenal cortex does not produce ADH; the antidiuretic effect from the aldosterone that is secreted by the adrenal cortex is a secondary, osmotic effect of sodium reabsorption and not a direct antidiuretic effect (as is caused by ADH).

2 The adrenal medulla does not produce ADH.

3 The anterior pituitary does not produce ADH.

311. **1 The antidiuretic hormone aids the body in retaining fluid by causing the nephrons to reabsorb water. (AN; PA; EN)**

2 Reabsorption of glucose is not affected, only the reabsorption of water.

3 The glomeruli are not affected.

4 Same as answer 3.

312. **2 Endocrine gland secretions (hormones) are inactivated by the liver and other tissues fairly rapidly; continuous hormonal secretion by the endocrine glands is regulated by immediate feedback controls, and the body's metabolism is always close to being suitable to the body's immediate needs. (AN; PA; EN)**

1 This time interval does not represent secretory patterns of the endocrine glands.

3 Same as answer 1.

4 Same as answer 1.

313. 2 Somatotropin promotes growth by accelerating amino acid transport into cells. Oversecretion after full growth and epiphyseal closure results in acromegaly, with enlargement of bones and overlying soft tissue in the feet, hands, lower jaw, and cheeks. This growth hormone also increases blood glucose levels. (AN; PA; EN)

1 Oversecretion of testosterone would affect secondary sexual characteristics.

3 This causes hyperthyroidism; it is not produced by the hypophysis.

4 TSH would increase stimulation of the thyroid gland.

314. 2 The hypophysis (pituitary) does not directly regulate insulin release. This is controlled by serum glucose levels. Because somatotropin release will stop after the hypophysectomy, any elevation of blood glucose caused by somatotropin will also stop. (EV TC; EN)

1 This effect may be expected after a hypophysectomy because follicle-stimulating hormone and follicle-stimulating hormone releasing factor will no longer be present to stimulate spermatogenesis.

3 Thyroid-stimulating hormone will not be present; extrinsic thyroxine will have to be taken.

4 ACTH, which stimulates glucocorticoid secretion by the adrenal glands, is absent and cortisone will have to be administered.

315. 4 Because the pituitary gland is located in the brain, edema following surgery may result in increased intracranial pressure. (EV; TC; EN)

1 This may follow any surgery because of the effects of anesthesia and is not a specific occurrence following cranial surgery.

2 Although this may be the result of pressure on the medulla caused by increased intracranial pressure, it is not an initial sign of increased ICP.

3 Same as answer 1.

316. 3 Hyperplasia of the adrenal cortex leads to increased secretion of cortical hormones, which causes signs of Cushing's syndrome. (DC; PA; EN)

1 This malfunction of the pituitary would result in Simmond's disease (panhypopituitarism), which has symptoms similar to Addison's disease.

2 ACTH stimulates production of adrenal hormones. Inadequate ACTH would result in addisonian symptoms.

4 Cushing's syndrome results from excessive cortical hormones.

317. 3 Glucocorticoids (e.g., cortisone) and mineralocorticoids (e.g., aldosterone) are secreted by the adrenals. (AN; PA; EN)

1 The gonads secrete testosterone (primarily in males) and estrogen and progesterone (primarily in females).

2 The pancreas secretes insulin and glucagon.

4 The anterior pituitary (adenohypophysis) regulates secretions such as STH, FSH, LH, LTH, TSH, and ACTH; it also secretes prolactin and endorphins.

318. 4 Excess glucocorticoids cause hyperglycemia and signs of diabetes mellitus may develop. (AN; PA; EN)

1 Adrenocortical hormones cause sodium retention and subsequent weight gain.

2 ACTH affects the adrenal cortex, not the pancreas.

3 Although muscle wasting is associated with excessive corticoid production, this will not cause diabetes mellitus.

319. 2 Cushing's syndrome results from excess adrenocortical activity. Signs include slow wound healing, buffalo hump, hirsutism, weight gain, hypertension, acne, moon face, thin arms and legs, and behavioral changes. (DC; PA; EN)

1 Menorrhagia (excessive menstrual bleeding) and dehydration do not occur; menses may cease or be scanty because of virilization; water balance is maintained by mineralocorticoid production.

3 Pitting edema does not occur except when congestive heart failure is present and severe. There is no increase in frequency of colds since the ability to adapt to pathogens is not affected.

4 Menses may become irregular or scanty, and headaches are not caused by this syndrome.

320. 2 As a result of increased cortisol levels, clients experience increased blood glucose. (DC; PA; EN)

1 Increased mineralocorticoids will decrease urine output.

3 Sodium is retained by the kidneys but potassium is excreted.

4 The immune response is suppressed.

321. 4 Adrenal steroids help an individual adjust to stress. Unless received from external

sources, there would be no hormone available to cope with surgical stresses after an adrenalectomy. (AN; TC; EN)

1 Glucose stores (glycogen) will be utilized after surgery to adapt to surgery. Insulin is the hormone that facilitates conversion of glucose to glycogen.
2 The inflammatory effect of the adrenals would be obliterated after removal.
3 Steroids would result in fluid retention, not loss.

322. **4 Hydrocortisone succinate (Solu-Cortef) is a glucocorticoid. A client undergoing bilateral adrenalectomy must be given adrenocortical hormones so that adjustment to the sudden lack of these hormones that occurs with this surgery can take place. (PL; TC; EN)**

1 Because the adrenal glands are removed, ACTH will have no target gland on which to act.
2 Insulin is produced by the pancreas, and its function is not altered by this surgery.
3 Because the surgery involves the adrenals, not the pituitary gland, secretion of pituitary hormones will not be affected.

323. **1 After an adrenalectomy, adrenal insufficiency causes hypotension because of fluid and electrolyte alterations. (EV; TC; EN)**

2 Hypoglycemia may be a problem stemming from the loss of glucocorticoids.
3 Hyponatremia may occur because of the lack of mineralocorticoid production.
4 Potassium ions may be retained because of the lack of mineralocorticoids.

324. **3 These agents are classified as antiinflammatory or immunosuppressive. Glucocorticoids interfere with the body's response to microorganisms but do not directly promote the spread of enteroviruses. (AN; PA; EN)**

1 Immunosuppressant action causes bone marrow depression, which decreases the number of WBCs.
2 They interfere with antibody production.
4 They interfere with the release of enzymes responsible for the inflammatory response.

325. **3 ACTH is released in response to decreased blood levels of cortisol. The ACTH then stimulates release of more adrenocortical hormone. (AN; PA; EN)**

1 Cortisol has antiinflammatory properties, which delay wound healing.
2 As a glucocorticoid it increases gluconeogenesis in the liver.
4 Cortisol assists the body in adapting to stress.

326. **2 The adrenal glands, stimulated by the sympathetic nervous system, secrete epinephrine during stressful situations. The ensuing alarm reaction involves rapid adjustment of the body to meet the emergency situation. (AN; PA; EN)**

1 There may be modification in secretion of thyroid hormones, but it is not directly related to meeting emergency situations.
3 There may be modification in secretion of pituitary hormones, but it is not directly related to meeting emergency situations.
4 There may be modification in secretion of pancreatic hormones, but it is not directly related to meeting emergency situations.

327. **4 Mineralocorticoids such as aldosterone cause the kidneys to retain sodium ions. With sodium, water is also retained, elevating blood pressure. Absence of this hormone thus causes hypotension. (AN; PA; EN)**

1 Estrogen is a female sex hormone produced by the ovaries; it does not affect blood pressure.
2 Androgens are produced by the adrenal cortex; they have an effect similar to that of the male sex hormones; they do not affect blood pressure.
3 The major effect of glucocorticoids such as hydrocortisone is on glucose, not on sodium and water metabolism; absence of this hormone would not cause significant hypotension.

328. **4 Because of diminished glucocorticoid production, there is a decreased inflammatory effect. (IM; TC; EN)**

1 Glucocorticoids are involved with metabolism; however, this does not directly affect susceptibility to infection.
2 The respiratory system is not affected.
3 There is hyponatremia and hyperkalemia in this disorder; however, these do not alter the defense against infection.

329. **3 Glucocorticoids help maintain blood sugar and liver and muscle glycogen content. A deficiency of glucocorticoids causes hypoglycemia, resulting in breakdown of protein and fats as energy sources. (AN; PA; EN)**
   1 These three symptoms are not related to fluid balance.
   2 Emaciation results from diminished protein and fat stores and hypoglycemia, not from an alteration in electrolytes.
   4 Masculinization does not occur in this disease.

330. **2 Exertion, either physical or emotional, places additional stress on the adrenal glands, which may precipitate an addisonian crisis. (IM; TC; EN)**
   1 Low levels of adrenocortical hormones will cause fatigue, and exercise may result in crisis because of increased metabolic demands.
   3 Diversional activities are important to all clients, not just those with Addison's disease.
   4 Because of the limits imposed by the adrenal disease, the amount of exercise that the client may desire may not be consistent with the amount tolerated.

331. **3 Lack of mineralocorticoids causes hyponatremia, hypovolemia, and hyperkalemia. Dietary modification, as well as administration of cortical hormones, is aimed at correcting these electrolyte imbalances. (PL; TC; EN)**
   1 There is no disturbance in the eosinophil count.
   2 Lymphoid tissue does not change in this disease.
   4 Although glucocorticoids are involved in metabolic activities, including carbohydrate metabolism, the primary aim of therapy is to restore electrolyte imbalance. Lack of electrolyte balance is life threatening.

332. **4 Lack of mineralocorticoids (aldosterone) leads to loss of sodium ions in the urine and subsequent hyponatremia. (IM; ED; EN)**
   1 Potassium intake is not encouraged; hyperkalemia is a problem because of insufficient mineralocorticoids.
   2 This disease is caused by idiopathic atrophy of the adrenal cortex; tissue repair of the gland is not possible.
   3 Vitamins are not directly energy producing.

333. **4 Fludrocortisone acetate (Florinef) has a strong effect on sodium retention by the**

kidneys, which leads to fluid retention (weight gain and edema). **(IM; ED; EN)**
   1 Mood swings frequently occur with fludrocortisone therapy; this is not an indication of a problem.
   2 Fluid retention and hence decreased urination may occur.
   3 Fatigue may occur with adrenal insufficiency and is not related to cortisone therapy.

334. **1 The thyroid gland produces thyroxine (T_4) and triiodothyronine (T_3), which help regulate oxidation in all body cells. (AN; PA; EN)**
   2 The primary regulator is the thyroid; the adrenals influence metabolism of carbohydrates in times of stress.
   3 The pituitary gland is involved in secondary regulation because it secretes TSH, which stimulates thyroid production of thyroxine and triiodothyronine.
   4 The pancreas regulates glucose metabolism by secretion of insulin.

335. **1 Myxedema is the severest form of hypothyroidism. Decreased thyroid gland activity means reduced production of thyroid hormones. (AN; PA; EN)**
   2 This results from excess growth hormone in adults once the epiphyses are closed.
   3 This results from an excess, not a deficiency, of thyroid hormones.
   4 This results from excess glucocorticoids.

336. **3 Decreased production of thyroid hormones lowers metabolism, which leads to decreased heat production and cold intolerance. (DC; PA; EN)**
   1 Lethargy, rather than irritability, is expected.
   2 Decreased metabolism requires less oxygen, so the pulse rate is generally slower.
   4 The skin is dry and coarse, not moist.

337. **3 An individual treated for a thyroid problem by intake of radioactive iodine (^{131}I) becomes mildly radioactive, particularly in the region of the thyroid gland, which preferentially absorbs the iodine. Such clients should be treated with routine safety precautions. (EV; TC; EN)**
   1 Because radioactive iodine is internalized, the client becomes the source of radioactivity.
   2 The amount of radioactive iodine used is not enough to cause high radioactivity.
   4 Same as answer 1.

338. **2 Because of the individual's increased metabolic rate, a high-calorie diet is needed to meet the energy demands of the body and prevent weight loss. (PL; TC; EN)**
 1 Modification of the consistency is unnecessary.
 3 Sodium is not restricted because clients with hyperthyroidism perspire heavily and lose sodium.
 4 GI motility is increased and does not require the additional stimulus of increased roughage.

339. **2 Lugol's solution adds iodine to the body fluids, exerting negative feedback on the thyroid tissue and decreasing its metabolism and vascularity. (PL; TC; EN)**
 1 This drug interferes with production of thyroid hormone but causes increased vascularity and size of the thyroid.
 3 This is a topical antiseptic.
 4 This is a synthetic thyroid hormone; its use is contraindicated because there is already an excessive production of thyroid hormone.

340. **3 The possibility of respiratory complications caused by edema of the glottis or injury to the recurrent laryngeal nerve could require a tracheostomy. (PL; TC; EN)**
 1 Sandbags are not necessary because the client can move the head when the neck is supported.
 2 Hemostats are not kept at the bedside; if hemorrhage occurs it will most likely be internal and a vessel could not be clamped.
 4 Nasogastric suction would usually not be necessary; clients would rarely have a nasogastric tube.

341. **4 Thyroid surgery sometimes results in accidental removal of the parathyroid glands. A resultant hypocalcemia may lead to contraction of the glottis, causing airway obstruction; edema also causes obstruction. (IM; TC; EN)**
 1 The airway takes priority.
 2 Speaking is important to determine the status of the glottis.
 3 The client should be maintained in a semi-Fowler's position to maximize respiratory excursion.

342. **1 If the laryngeal nerves are injured bilaterally during surgery, the vocal cords will tighten, interfering with speech. If one cord is affected, hoarseness develops. This can be evaluated simply by having the client speak every hour. (EV TC; EN)**

 2 This ability is not influenced by laryngeal nerve damage.
 3 Same as answer 2.
 4 Same as answer 2.

343. **2 Parathyroid removal eliminates the body's source of parathyroid hormone, which increases blood calcium. The resulting low body fluid calcium affects muscles, including the diaphragm, resulting in dyspnea, asphyxia, and death. (EV; PA; EN)**
 1 Loss of the thyroid gland would upset thyroid hormone balance and might cause myxedema.
 3 The parathyroids are not involved in regulating plasma volume; the pituitary and adrenal glands are.
 4 The parathyroids do not regulate the adrenal glands.

344. **3 Thyroid trauma, thyroid surgery, or psychologic stress in a client with hyperthyroidism may lead to the release of abnormally high levels of thyroid hormones. This intensifies all symptoms of hyperthyroidism—thyroid storm (increased pulse, elevated temperature, restlessness, vomiting, and often death). (AN; PA; EN)**
 1 Iodine would bind with thyroxine, decreasing the potential storm.
 2 Tetany occurs from this inadvertent surgical excision.
 4 Anesthesia would depress metabolism, not increase it.

345. **2 A decreased TSH assay together with an elevated T_3 (triiodothyronine) level may indicate hyperthyroidism. (IM; ED; EN)**
 1 X-ray results would not indicate thyroid disease, and elevation of T_4 (thyroxine) might indicate hyperthyroidism. However, this could be a false reading because of the presence of thyroid-binding globulin (TBG) and is inadequate for diagnosis when used alone.
 3 PO_2 is not specific to thyroid disease, and the thyroglobulin level is most useful to monitor for recurrence of thyroid carcinoma or response to therapy.
 4 The results with the sequential multichannel autoanalyzer (SMA 12) are not specific to thyroid disease; the protein-bound iodine test is not definitive because it is influenced by the intake of exogenous iodine.

346. **4 Parathormone increases blood calcium by accelerating calcium absorption from the intestine and kidneys and releasing calcium from bone. Vitamin D promotes calcium absorption from the intestine.** (AN; PA; EN)

1 Phosphorus and ACTH do not interact to regulate calcium levels. Phosphorus is a component of bone; ACTH, produced by the anterior pituitary, stimulates the adrenal cortex to secrete the corticosteroid hormones.

2 Vitamin A and thyroid hormone do not interact to regulate calcium levels. Vitamin A is essential for the normal function of epithelial cells and visual purple; calcitonin, from the thyroid gland, lowers serum calcium.

3 Ascorbic acid (vitamin C) and growth hormone do not interact to regulate calcium levels. Vitamin C promotes collagen production and the formation of bone matrix; growth hormone, produced by the anterior pituitary, controls the rate of skeletal growth.

347. **1 Calcitonin, a thyroid gland hormone, prevents the reabsorption of calcium by bone. It also inhibits the release of calcium from bone. The net result is lowered serum calcium levels.** (AN; PA; EN)

2 Aldosterone regulates fluid and electrolyte balance by promoting the retention of sodium and water and the excretion of potassium.

3 Calcitonin lowers serum calcium levels; the other thyroid hormones (thyroxine and triiodothyronine) control the body's metabolic rate.

4 Parathyroid hormone promotes the intestinal absorption of calcium and mobilizes calcium from the bones to increase blood calcium levels.

348. **4 Hyperparathyroidism causes calcium release from the bones, leaving them porous and weak.** (DC; TC; EN)

1 Tetany is the result of low calcium; in this condition serum calcium is high.

2 Seizures are caused by increased neural activity, a condition not related to this disease.

3 Graves' disease is the result of increased thyroid, not parathyroid, activity.

349. **2 Fluids help prevent the formation of renal calculi associated with high serum calcium.** (PL; TC; EN)

1 Additional calcium intake could raise already high levels of serum calcium.

3 Seizures are associated with low, not high, serum calcium.

4 Rest is contraindicated because bone destruction is accelerated.

350. **2 Parathormone hormone increases osteoclastic activity, resulting in breakdown of bone substance and release of calcium into the blood.** (AN; TC; EN)

1 It increases blood calcium and will thereby prevent tetany.

3 Although blood calcium does increase, blood phosphate also increases.

4 The hormone calcitonin, released by the thyroid gland, increases the incorporation of calcium into the bones.

Integumentary

351. **2 Unwashed hands are considered contaminated and are used to turn on sink faucets. The use of foot pedals or a paper towel barrier prevents recontamination of washed hands.** (AN; PA; IT)

1 They are not considered contaminated for this reason; areas cannot be sterile.

3 It has nothing to do with the number of people; it is related to being touched by contaminated hands.

4 Although bacterial growth is facilitated in moist environments, this is not why sinks are considered contaminated.

352. **4 Soap helps by reducing the surface tension of water, but friction is necessary for the removal of microorganisms.** (IM; TC; IT)

1 Although this aspect of hand washing is important, without friction it has minimal value.

2 Although soap reduces surface tension, without friction it has minimal value.

3 Although water flushes some microorganisms from the skin, without friction it has minimal value.

353. **4 The absorption of fluids by gauze results from the adhesion of water to the gauze threads. The surface tension of water causes contraction of the fiber, pulling fluid up the threads.** (EV; TC; IT)

1 This is separation of substances in solution utilizing their differing rates of diffusion through a membrane.

2 This is movement of molecules from high to low concentration.

3 This refers to movement of water through a semipermeable membrane.

354. **3** **Intact skin is the first line of defense against entry of microorganisms. A surgical incision is a portal of entry, so a technique that requires the absence of all microorganisms (surgical asepsis) is essential. (AN; TC; IT)**
    1 Wound asepsis is incorrect terminology.
    2 Medical asepsis utilizes clean technique to minimize the spread of microorganisms; when there is a break in the skin, such technique is insufficient.
    4 Concurrent disinfection refers to measures initiated to control the spread of infection while an infection is present; concurrent asepsis is incorrect terminology.

355. **3** **Vitamin C (ascorbic acid) plays a major role in wound healing. It is necessary for the maintenance and formation of strong collagen, the major protein of most connective tissues.(PL; PA; IT)**
    1 Vitamin A is important for the healing process; however, vitamin C cements the ground substance of supportive tissue.
    2 Vitamin K plays a major role in blood coagulation.
    4 Vitamin B_{12} is needed for red blood cell synthesis and a healthy nervous system.

356. **4** **Because pressure is force developed per unit of area over which the force is applied, as the area decreases the pressure increases. The tip of a needle or the point of a knife has an extremely small area, and consequently a very high pressure can be developed for a given force. (AN; TC; IT)**
    1 The length and shape of the needle have no relevance to the ease of penetration; the small point in relation to energy developed at the point of insertion is the prime factor.
    2 Although some energy is required to insert the needle, the amount is very little because the area at the tip of the needle is so small.
    3 Although a factor, texture relationship is not the primary reason for ease of insertion; the small point in relation to energy developed at the point of insertion is the prime factor.

357. **4** **The temperature range for tepid applications is somewhat below body temperature. (IM; TC; IT)**
    1 This temperature is too cool to be considered tepid.
    2 Same as answer 1.
    3 Same as answer 1.

358. **4** **Conduction is the conveyance of energy such as heat, cold, or sound by direct contact. (AN; PA; IT)**
    1 Direct contact is not necessary to convey heat by radiation.
    2 This refers to retention of heat, not its transfer.
    3 This is the transfer of heat by air circulation (e.g., by fans or open windows).

359. **4** **Cholesterol is an absolutely essential structural and functional component of most cellular membranes. That it is associated with atherosclerotic plaques does not detract from its essential functions in membrane structure and steroid hormone metabolism. (AN; PA; IT)**
    1 Cholesterol is not necessary for blood clotting; calcium and vitamin K are.
    2 Cholesterol is not essential for bone formation; calcium, phosphorus, and calciferol are.
    3 Cholesterol is not involved in muscle contraction; potassium, sodium, and calcium are.

360. **3** **Oxygen perfusion is impaired during prolonged edema, leading to tissue ischemia. (AN; PA; IT)**
    1 This is not a complication resulting from long-term edema.
    2 Same as answer 1.
    4 Same as answer 1.

361. **3** **In gangrene the release of iron from hemoglobin as erythrocytes disintegrate in necrotic tissue results in ferrous sulfide formation, causing darkening of the tissues. (AN; PA; IT)**
    1 Heme constitutes the pigment portion of the hemoglobin molecule, which gives blood its red color; it does not cause the darkening of tissue associated with gangrene.
    2 Ferric chloride is used as a reagent; it is also used topically as an antiseptic and as an astringent; it is not related to gangrene.
    4 Proteins are not insoluble.

MEDICAL-SURGICAL ANSWERS

362. **4** *Clostridium welchii* **(perfringens) is a spore-forming bacterium that produces a toxin that decays muscle, releasing a gas; it is one of the major causative agents for gas gangrene. (DC; PA; IT)**
   1 This disease is caused by *Bacillis anthracis*, not Clostridium.
   2 *Clostridium tetani* enters the body via puncture of the skin and affects the nervous system; gas gangrene does not occur with this organism.
   3 *Clostridium botulinum* contaminates food that is then ingested, causing botulism.

363. **3 Psoriasis is characterized by dry, scaly lesions that occur most frequently on the elbows, knees, scalp, and torso. (DC; PA; IT)**
   1 Pruritis, if present at all, is generally mild.
   2 Petechiae are not characteristic.
   4 Macules are erythematous flat spots on the skin as in measles; no scales are present.

364. **2 Steroids are applied locally and usually covered with plastic (or Saran Wrap) at night to reverse the inflammatory process. (IM; TC; IT)**
   1 Solar rays are used in the treatment of psoriasis.
   3 Potassium permanganate is an antiseptic astringent used on infected, draining, or vesicular lesions.
   4 The plaques are not necrotic and therefore do not require debriding.

365. **1 Scabies is caused by the itch mite** *(Acarus scabiei)*, **the female of which burrows under the skin to deposit eggs. It is intensely pruritic and is transmitted by direct contact or, in a limited way, by soiled sheets or undergarments.(DC; PA; IT)**
   2 Scabies is an acute infection.
   3 It is caused by the itch mite, a parasite.
   4 It is an infectious disease and is unrelated to allergies.

366. **3 Pemphigus is primarily a serious disease characterized by large vesicles called bullae. Although potentially fatal, it can be relatively controlled by steroid therapy. (IM; PA; IT)**
   1 Pemphigus is a disease of the skin.
   2 Same as answer 1.
   4 Same as answer 1.

367. **1 The connective tissue degeneration of SLE leads to involvement of the basal** cell layer, producing a butterfly rash over the bridge of the nose and in the malar region. (DC; PA; IT)
   2 This occurs in scleroderma and may advance until the client has the appearance of a living mummy.
   3 This occurs in muscular dystrophy, which is characterized by muscle wasting and weakness.
   4 This occurs in polyarteritis nodosa, a collagen disease affecting the arteries and nervous system.

368. **1 Scleroderma is an immunologic disorder characterized by inflammatory, fibrotic, and degenerative changes. (AN; PA; IT)**
   2 This is not involved in development of scleroderma.
   3 Same as answer 2.
   4 Same as answer 2.

369. **4 A partial-thickness burn over 30% of the body is considered critical. Shock, infection, electrolyte imbalance, and respiratory distress are life-threatening complications that can occur. (DC; PA; IT)**
   1 Burns involving less than 30% of the body surface of older children and adults under 50 years of age are generally less severe; the condition would be rated accordingly.
   2 Same as answer 1.
   3 Same as answer 1.

370. **2 The leukocyte count would not be affected in the first few hours. (AN; TC; IT)**
   1 Pain is present in partial-thickness burns because the sensory nerves are not damaged.
   3 Replacement of fluids and electrolytes is essential in all burned clients.
   4 Inhalation of hot air can cause laryngeal edema and would be a concern.

371. **4 The circulating air bed disperses body weight over a larger surface, which reduces pressure against the capillary beds allowing for tissue perfusion. (PL; TC; IT)**
   1 These beds are used for clients who are immobile; they do not increase mobility.
   2 This bed will have no effect on the development of contractures.
   3 This bed will have no effect on the development of orthostatic hypotension.

372. **3 An increased hematocrit level indicates hemoconcentration secondary to fluid loss. (DC; PA; IT)**

1 This may be used to indicate dehydration from burns, but interpretation can be complicated by other conditions accompanying burns that also cause elevation of the BUN.

2 The pH levels reflect acid-base balance.

4 The sedimentation rate is not used as an indicator of fluid loss; it indicates the presence of an inflammatory process.

373. **4 As the amount of tissue involved increases, there is greater extravasation of fluid into the tissues. Thus the relationship of fluid loss to body surface is directly proportional. Several formulas are used to estimate fluid loss based on percent of body surface burned. (AN; PA; IT)**

1 This is incorrect; the relationship is proportional.

2 Same as answer 1.

3 Same as answer 1.

374. **1 The fluid level in the manometer fluctuates with respiration because the changes in thoracic pressure affect the pressure in the right atrium. (DC; PA; IT)**

2 To approximate the level of the right atrium, the "O" level should be even with the midaxillary line.

3 Although the CVP line is not used routinely for blood samples, blood can be easily aspirated.

4 The positive pressure of a ventilator alters the central venous pressure readings, so the ventilator must be removed when CVP is taken.

375. **2 An autograft is one taken from an uninjured area of the same person's body. (AN; PA; IT)**

1 An allograft is skin taken from the same species.

3 A homograft is skin taken from the same species.

4 A heterograft or xenograft is skin taken from a different species.

376. **4 A heterograft or xenograft involves the grafting of tissues from a different species. (AN; PA; IT)**

1 This type of graft does not exist.

2 An allograft is skin taken from the same species.

3 A homograft is skin taken from the same species.

377. **1 *Clostridium tetani* can develop in partial- and full-thickness burns that contain dead tissue. (PL; PA; IT)**

2 Although gamma globulin provides passive immunity against certain infectious agents, it is not specifically indicated in the treatment of burns.

3 Isuprel is an adrenergic drug used in the treatment of bronchospasm and heart block.

4 This drug is indicated for hypoprothrombinemia caused by the deficiency of vitamin K; it is not related to burns.

378. **4 Application of a solution of sodium bicarbonate (a mild alkali) after a thorough flushing with water is the best way to treat acid-splashed skin, because the alkali will neutralize residual acid on the skin. (IM; ED; IT)**

1 Sodium sulfate is a neutral salt, which would serve no immediate first-aid benefit.

2 Sodium chloride is a neutral salt, which would serve no immediate first-aid benefit.

3 Although sodium hydroxide is an alkali and would neutralize acid, it is too strong and can also cause burns.

379. **1 This first-aid treatment will chemically neutralize residual alkali still on the skin. It will not reverse the chemical burns already caused by the alkali but will minimize additional chemical change. (IM; TC; IT)**

2 A weak base will not neutralize alkaline substances.

3 This is a neutral substance; it will not neutralize a base.

4 This would not affect the pH.

380. **2 A nurse may independently treat human responses to actual or potential health problems. (EV; TC; IT)**

1 Activity parameters must be prescribed by the physician.

3 Providing supportive care is an independent, not dependent, function of the nurse.

4 Surgical wound debridement is performed by the physician.

381. **3 Lymphadenopathy occurs in clients with malignancies that have metastasized. (DC; PA; IT)**

1 Skin is generally dry and itchy.

2 Nikolsky's sign occurs in clients with pemphigus.

4 Erythema of the palms is not a symptom of melanoma.

MEDICAL-SURGICAL ANSWERS

382. **1 A sarcoma is defined as a malignant tumor whose cells resemble those of the supportive (connective) tissues of the body.** (AN; PA; IT)
2 Carcinoma refers to a malignant neoplasm of epithelial tissue.
3 Although collagen is the substance used to form the connective tissue, the term collagenoma is incorrect.
4 Osteoblastomas are benign tumors of the bone.

383. **4 Basal cell carcinoma, the most common type of skin cancer, is most closely linked to solar ultraviolet radiation.** (DC; PA; IT)
1 Although skin type is a genetically determined risk factor, it cannot be altered and it is influenced by solar ultraviolet radiation.
2 Diet is not a risk factor.
3 Smoking is not a risk factor.

384. **1 Radiation in controlled doses is therapeutic. When uncontrolled or in excessive amounts, it is carcinogenic.** (IM; ED; IT)
2 Therapeutic doses are helpful in whatever areas are being treated.
3 Physical status does not affect the outcome of radiation therapy.
4 The nutritional status of the cells does not influence radiation's effect.

385. **3 Infection is caused by viral contact with the dermal layer of skin; cleansing the wound with soap and water helps remove superficial contaminants.** (IM; TC; IT)
1 Antivenins are not effective against microbiological stresses.
2 A pressure dressing will not prevent infection.
4 Application of a tourniquet may impair circulation and will not prevent infection.

386. **4 If the area is not kept both clean and dry, drainage from the colostomy can quickly cause a breakdown of the skin around the stoma. This, in combination with a warm moist surface, also predisposes the individual to infection.** (PL; TC; IT)
1 Although oral fluids are withheld until peristalsis returns, it is essential that parenteral fluids be administered to replace the losses incurred by surgery.
2 Same as answer 1.
3 The client is often unable to accept the altered body image and must be given time to adjust before participating actively in dressing changes.

Reproductive and Genitourinary
Reproductive

387. **3 A sharp rise in luteinizing hormone production triggers the rupture of the follicle and ovulation.** (AN; PA; RG)
1 Estrogen stimulates the thickening of the endometrium.
2 Progesterone prepares the endometrium for the implantation of the fertilized ovum.
4 FSH stimulates the development of the graafian follicle.

388. **4 The function of progesterone is to relax the uterus and maintain a succulent endometrium to foster implantation of the fertilized ovum.** (AN; PA; RG)
1 Ovulation is stimulated by increases in the levels of luteinizing hormone (LH) and estrogen.
2 Menstruation is controlled by regulating factors from the hypothalamus and pituitary (FSH-RH, FSH, LH-RH, LH); these hormones stimulate the production of ovarian follicles, ovulation, estrogen, and progesterone by the ovarian cells.
3 Capillary fragility is often associated with deficiency of vitamin C (ascorbic acid); progesterone is not responsible.

389. **4 Estrogen is found in the follicular fluid of the ovaries and aids in the growth of the endometrium.** (AN; PA; RG)
1 The luteinizing hormone promotes the development of ovarian follicles as well as stimulating ovulation and the production of estrogen and progesterone by the ovarian cells.
2 The luteinizing hormone promotes the development of ovarian follicles as well as stimulating ovulation and the production of estrogen and progesterone; progesterone prepares the endometrium for implantation and the breasts for lactation.
3 These hormones prepare the breasts for milk secretion (lactation).

390. **1 A generous supply of blood is carried by the uterine arteries (branches of the internal iliac arteries). The vaginal and ovarian arteries also supply the uterus with blood by anastomosing with the uterine vessels.** (AN; PA; RG)
2 The aorta does not supply the uterus directly.
3 The hypogastric or internal iliac arteries supply the pelvic wall and viscera.
4 The hypogastric arteries (internal iliac) supply the pelvic wall and gluteal area, and the exter-

nal branches (called uterine arteries) supply the uterus and genitalia; the aorta does not supply the uterus directly.

391. **4 The gonadotropins, follicle-stimulating hormone and luteinizing hormone, are concerned with ovarian changes that produce ovulation. Estrogen is increased because of secretion from the developing follicle. Progesterone is higher because of secretion from the corpus luteum. The hormones work in concert to stimulate the menstrual cycle. (AN; PA; RG)**
   1 The gonadotropins must work in concert with estrogen and progesterone for the cycle to be completed.
   2 These must work in concert with FSH and LH; otherwise there is no cycle.
   3 Progesterone is also required for the menstrual cycle to be completed.

392. **3 The time between ovulation and the next menstruation is relatively constant. Within a 30-day cycle the first 15 days are preovulatory, ovulation occurs on day 16, and the next 14 days are postovulatory. Ovulation therefore occurs on January 17. (DC; PA; RG)**
   1 This is within the first 15 days and is the pre-ovulatory phase.
   2 Same as answer 1.
   4 This is within the last 14 days of the cycle and is postovulatory.

393. **4 Bleeding between periods is abnormal. Bleeding other than during the menstrual period is known as metrorrhagia. (AN; PA; RG)**
   1 Bleeding may not be limited to ovulation.
   2 The amount varies from spotting to frank bleeding; it is not occult.
   3 Menorrhagia is the term used to describe excessive bleeding during menstruation.

394. **1 Primitive sex cells, called spermatogonia, are present in newborn males. At puberty these cells mature and form spermatozoa (spermatogenesis). (AN; PA; RG)**
   2 Spermatogenesis does not occur until puberty.
   3 Spermatogonia or primitive sex cells are found at this time.
   4 Only immature cells are found during this period.

395. **3 Sperm cells are very fragile and can be destroyed by heat, resulting in sterility. (AN; PA; RG)**
   1 Sperm do not move through the urine; they are found in semen.
   2 Sperm are motile, achieving this by motion of their flagella; they move from the epididymis to the vas deferens to the ejaculatory ducts to the urethra.
   4 During this period the testes are not suspended.

396. **2 Candidiasis (*Candida* infection) arises in certain individuals when local resistance is decreased through prolonged antibiotic therapy or with certain diseases (e.g., diabetes) and debilitating conditions (e.g., drug addiction). (EV; PA; DR)**
   1 *Coxiella burnetii*, a rickettsia, is not part of the normal flora; it is spread by contact with infected animals, drinking contaminated milk, or the bite of a vector tick.
   3 *Streptococcus* organisms would be responsive to antibiotic therapy and are not considered part of the normal flora.
   4 The varicella-zoster virus is not part of the normal flora.

397. **1 *Neisseria gonorrhoeae* is a gram-negative diplococcus commonly infecting the urogenital tract of both males and females. (DC; PA; RG)**
   2 Meningococci are associated with infections of the brain and spinal cord.
   3 Pneumococci are associated with infections of the respiratory tract.
   4 This is the spirochete that causes syphilis.

398. **3 Condylomata acuminata are variably sized cauliflower-like warts occurring principally on the genitals or the anogenital skin or mucosa of both females and males; they are generally associated with poor hygiene. (AN; PA; RG)**
   1 Scabies is an infestation of the skin by *Sarcoptes scabiei* (itch mite).
   2 Herpes zoster is an acute vesicular skin infection caused by the varicella-zoster virus (VZV).
   4 Condylomata acuminata are warts occurring on the genitals or the anogenital skin or mucosa of both females and males; the epididymis is part of the male reproductive system and is an internal structure.

MEDICAL-SURGICAL ANSWERS

399. 1 Massive doses of penicillin may limit CNS damage if treatment is started before neural deterioration from syphilis occurs. (PL; TC; RG)

2 Tranquilizers are used to modify behavior, not to treat general paresis.

3 Paresis is not a behavior and is therefore not suitably treated with behavior modification.

4 Electroconvulsive therapy is used in the treatment of certain psychiatric disorders.

400. 3 Gonorrhea is caused by a gram-negative diplococcus, *Neisseria gonorrhoeae*. (AN; PA; RG)

1 This is a lactobacillus found in the vagina; it does not cause gonorrhea.

2 This is the spirochete that causes syphilis.

4 Staphylococci are constantly present on the skin and in the upper respiratory tract; they commonly cause suppurating infection.

401. 3 In males the inflammatory process associated with the infection may lead to destruction of the epididymis. In females the gonorrheal infection causes destruction of the tubal mucosa and eventually tuboovarian abscesses. (IM; ED; RG)

1 Gonorrhea has become more difficult to treat because many gonococci have become penicillin resistant.

2 Gonorrhea is a common sexually transmitted disease.

4 *Neisseria gonorrhoeae* will invade internal structures, particularly the epididymis in males and the fallopian tubes in females.

402. 2 Penicillin inhibits the synthesis of bacterial cell walls. It is effective against *Neisseria gonorrhoeae*, a gram-negative diplococcus. (PL; TC; RG)

1 Colistin sulfate is effective against most gram-negative enteric pathogens such as *Escherichia coli*.

3 Actinomycin is an antineoplastic agent.

4 Chloramphenicol is a broad-spectrum antimicrobial agent; however, it can cause bone marrow depression, so its use is limited to severe infections that do not respond to less toxic drugs.

403. 3 *Trichomonas vaginalis* is a protozoan that favors an alkaline environment. (AN; PA; RG)

1 A yeast is a unicellular, usually oval, nucleated fungus; it does not cause trichomonal infections.

2 A fungus is a simple parasitic plant; it does not cause trichomonal infections.

4 A spirochete is a motile spiral-shaped bacterium; it does not cause trichomonal infections.

404. 1 Because *Trichomonas vaginalis* favors an alkaline environment, vinegar, an acid, is utilized to decrease the pH of the vagina. (PL; TC; RG)

2 Tap water will not alter the pH.

3 Normal saline will not alter the pH.

4 An increase in pH would create an environment conducive to the growth of microorganisms.

405. 4 Metronidazole (Flagyl) is a potent amebicide. It is extremely effective in eradicating the protozoan *Trichomonas vaginalis*. (PL; TC; RG)

1 Penicillin is administered for its effect on bacterial, not protozoal, infections.

2 Gentian violet is a local antiinfective that is applied topically and may cause discoloration of the skin; it is particularly effective against *Candida albicans*.

3 Nystatin is an antifungal used for infections caused by *Candida albicans*.

406. 4 Dorsal recumbency takes advantage of the anatomic position of the vaginal tract and prevents undue retention or too rapid return of the douche. (IM; TC; RG)

1 This promotes retention of the douche.

2 This promotes rapid return of the douche before the therapeutic effect is achieved.

3 Same as answer 1.

407. 3 This is the anatomic direction of the vaginal tract in the back-lying position. (IM; ED; RG)

1 The vaginal tract may be injured when the douche nozzle is not directed with consideration of normal anatomy.

2 Same as answer 1.

4 Same as answer 1.

408. 4 Some spermatozoa will remain viable in the vas deferens for a variable time after vasectomy. (IM; ED; RG)

1 Although it is considered a permanent form of sterilization, there has been some success reversing the procedure.

2 The procedure does not affect sexual functioning.

3 Precautions must be taken to prevent fertilization until absence of sperm in the semen has been verified.

409. **2 When the testes are twisted, a decrease in their blood supply occurs. This can result in gangrene. (AN; TC; RG)**
1 Pain can be alleviated through the use of medication.
3 Although edema occurs, the testes do not rupture.
4 Sperm are continually produced, so their destruction is not the concern.

410. **2 Persistent pain of any kind is usually a symptom, and the client should seek medical attention (IM; ED; RG)**
1 Although diversion is a method to alter pain perception, the presence of pain requires investigation of possible causes.
3 Although a nutritious diet is beneficial, iron does not prevent the pain of dysmenorrhea.
4 Voluntary relaxation of the abdominal muscles does not cause cessation of uterine contractions.

411. **3 Gonorrhea frequently is an ascending infection and affects the fallopian tubes. (DC; PA; RG)**
1 Syphilis, if untreated, may spread to the nervous system via the blood; it does not usually cause ascending infection of the fallopian tubes.
2 Abortion should not cause inflammation of the fallopian tubes.
4 This is not an infection, it is an aberrant growth; it would not cause inflammation of the fallopian tubes.

412. **2 The Fowler's position facilitates localization of the infection by pooling pelvic drainage. (IM; TC; RG)**
1 This position does not make use of gravity to promote drainage of exudate.
3 This position does not make use of gravity to promote pelvic drainage.
4 Same as answer 3.

413. **2 Mild hypocalcemia sometimes occurs during menstruation. An increase in dietary calcium just before and during menstruation may eliminate or relieve the occasional abdominal cramps resulting from this temporary disorder. (DC; PA; RG)**
1 Hypokalemia (lowered potassium levels) is evidenced by malaise and muscle weakness.
3 Hyperglycemia (elevated blood glucose levels) is evidenced by polyuria, polydipsia, polyphagia, weight loss, and urine that is positive for sugar and acetone.

4 Hypernatremia (elevated sodium levels) is evidenced by agitation, tissue turgor, and oliguria.

414. **1 Laparoscopy involves direct visualization of the uterus via fiberoptics. The procedure is carried out through a transabdominal stab wound. (DC; TC; RG)**
2 This test yields data on hormone levels and it is usually done prior to delivery.
3 This procedure involves blowing air through the fallopian tubes to test for patency.
4 This test would give information on tissue abnormalities.

415. **3 Ulcerations may occur when the vagina and uterus are inverted. (DC; PA; RG)**
1 Exudate would not be present with procidentia.
2 Development of ulcerations, not edema, is usually the problem.
4 The vagina would be everted, and therefore discharge would not be present.

416. **2 Moist compresses may be indicated to prevent ulcerations. (IM; TC; RG)**
1 Ambulation would encourage the development of ulcerations.
3 This would be ineffective; gravity alone does not correct the procidentia.
4 The tissue should be protected, and manipulation, which causes irritation, should be avoided.

417. **2 Changes in the pH of the vaginal tract cause cellular alteration and destruction. (DC; PA; RG)**
1 The direct effects of labor and delivery will not cause cervical erosion; erosion involves continuous inflammation or ulceration.
3 Same as answer 1.
4 Same as answer 1.

418. **2 Douches with acidic solutions such as vinegar and water bring back the normal pH of the vaginal tract. (AN; TC; RG)**
1 Comfort may be enhanced by correcting the pathologic disorder, but it is not the main goal of the treatment.
3 Although this may be a secondary benefit, a vinegar and water solution would not be required.
4 The use of vinegar will only indirectly affect bacterial growth because it acidifies the environment.

419. **2 Erosion of the cervix frequently occurs at the squamocolumnar junction, the most common site for carcinoma of the cervix. (PL; TC; RG)**

1 This may be present as erosion develops into carcinoma; however, spotting may be the earliest sign and will be eliminated when the cancer is treated; treatment of the erosion is done to prevent the cancer from progressing.
3 Even though a cervical erosion is treated, another may occur and repeat treatment may be necessary.
4 Infection may occur in the cancerous area accompanied by profuse, malodorous discharge; treatment of the erosion is done to prevent cancer, not the secondary infection.

420. **4 Polyps are usually benign but should undergo biopsy because epidermoid cancer occasionally arises from cervical polyps. (DC; TC; RG)**

1 Bleeding may occur whether they are malignant or not.
2 This is untrue; polyps are rarely the precursors of uterine cancer.
3 This is untrue; polyps are usually benign.

421. **2 This recognizes the client's feeling of anxiety as valid. (IM; PS; RG)**

1 This does not recognize the client's concerns and may inhibit the expression of feelings.
3 This is false reassurance. Although a condyloma is a benign wart, the papilloma virus that causes it can bring about neoplastic changes in the cervical tissue, which if not interrupted leads to cervical carcinoma.
4 This is not true and does not recognize the client's concerns.

422. **4 Any abnormal sign of vaginal bleeding may indicate cervical cancer and must be checked by a physician. (DC; PA; RG)**

1 There are few nerve endings; discomfort is a late sign.
2 Discharge becomes foul smelling only after there is necrosis and infection; it is not an early sign.
3 If pressure occurs, it is not an early symptom because the cancer must be extensive to cause pressure.

423. **4 The endocervical surface is frequently altered by metaplasia or covered by a variant of squamous epithelium. It is thus called the transitional zone. This** area is often distorted by eversion and laceration, especially in pregnancy. Therefore it is a frequent site for carcinoma. Erosion in this area most frequently leads to squamous cell carcinoma, accounting for 95% of cervical cancer. **(DC; PA; RG)**

1 Extension to lymph nodes is a later stage.
2 Adenocarcinoma, accounting for only 5% of cervical cancers, may be found in the endocervical glands.
3 The cervix is the lower portion of the uterus; the juncture of the uterine body with the cervical canal is called the internal os; erosion most frequently occurs distal to this point, between the external and internal ossa, closer to the external.

424. **1 When the cancerous cells are completely confined within the epithelium of the cervix without stromal invasion, it is stage 0 and called carcinoma in situ or preinvasive carcinoma. (AN; PA; RG)**

2 This is Stage I A; there is minimal stromal invasion.
3 This is Stage II B and involves the area around the broad ligaments but not the pelvic wall; there is extension to the corpus of the uterus.
4 This is Stage I; lymph node metastasis occurs about 10% of the time.

425. **4 Pain and elevated temperature may indicate toxic effects. Excessive sloughing of tissue can cause hemorrhage or infection. (EV; TC; RG)**

1 These are expected side effects of internal radiotherapy.
2 These are associated with need to maintain position, not with radium itself.
3 These are expected side effects of internal radiotherapy.

426. **3 Normal activity must be limited so that the implant will not become dislodged. (IM; TC; RG)**

1 While the client is receiving therapy, alpha, beta, and gamma rays will be emitted. Therefore the nurse should employ the principles of time and distance when providing care. The extent of exposure to the client must be monitored and kept within safe limits depending on the type and amount of rays emitted.
2 This is not necessary; adherence to principles of time and distance will protect the nurse from excessive exposure.

4 This is not necessary; however, all bed linens must be examined carefully for dislodged radium prior to sending to the laundry.

427. **1 Time, distance, and shielding are the important factors in determining the amount of radiation the visitor receives. Restriction of each visitor to a 10-minute stay minimizes the risk of exposure. Many institutions will not allow visitors while an implant is in place. (IM; TC; RG)**
2 The urine is not radioactive, so no precautions are indicated.
3 Lead aprons are effective shields against x-rays but not against rays emitted by internal sources of radiation.
4 Radium implants will not affect the location of IM injections.

428. **4 Radium, a radioactive isotope, is used to destroy or delay the growth of malignant cells; packing maintains the insert in its correct placement to maximize the effect on cancerous tissue and minimize the effect on normal tissue. (AN; TC; RG)**
1 The packing must be readjusted or replaced to protect normal tissue from damage from the radium implant.
2 This is not true.
3 There should be no active bleeding with radium implants although there may be cellular sloughing.

429. **2 Radium must be handled with long-handled forceps because distance helps limit exposure. (IM; TC; RG)**
1 A nurse is not responsible for cleaning radium implants.
3 Foil-lined rubber gloves do not provide adequate shielding from the gamma rays emitted by radium.
4 The amount and duration of exposure are important in assessing the effect on the client; however, this will not affect safety during removal.

430. **3 Prior to discharge it is important for the nurse to instruct the client to follow through with medical care at specified intervals. (PL; ED; RG)**
1 Fluids are not reduced unless other cardiac or renal pathology is present.
2 A low-residue diet is indicated to avoid pressure from a distended colon only when the implant is in place; the radium implant is removed before discharge.

4 If diet is adequate, multivitamins are unnecessary.

431. **3 Doxorubicin hydrochloride (Adriamycin) is a chemotherapeutic agent classified as an antibiotic. It achieves its therapeutic effect by inhibiting the synthesis of RNA. This blocks protein synthesis and cell division. (AN; TC; RG)**
1 This is not a physiologic action of Adriamycin.
2 Same as answer 1.
4 Same as answer 1.

432. **4 A hysterectomy involves only removal of the uterus. The ovaries, which secrete estrogen and progesterone, are not removed. Therefore menopause will not be precipitated but will occur naturally. (IM; ED; RG)**
1 If the ovaries were being removed, older women might have less severe symptoms than younger women; however, in this instance there would be no symptoms.
2 The nurse should serve as a resource person; the comment does not answer the question.
3 This is incorrect; it fails to point out the difference between myth and reality.

433. **4 The prescribing of medications is the legal responsibility of the physician. In addition, the use of hormones is controversial and depends on the physician's beliefs and the client's needs. (IM; ED; RG)**
1 This is an evasive response; the client is left without direction.
2 Hormones may be used to prevent the development of severe symptoms.
3 This is an evasive response; it does not answer the client's question.

434. **3 Estrogen receptor protein-positive tumors have a more dramatic response to hormonal therapies that reduce estrogen. (IM; ED; RG)**
1 This does not influence breast reconstruction.
2 Estrogen contributes to tumor growth; supplements are not indicated.
4 This is unrelated to metastasis.

435. **2 A definitive diagnosis of the cellular changes associated with benign prostatic hypertrophy is made by biopsy with subsequent microscopic evaluation. (DC; TC; RG)**
  1 Palpation of the prostate gland is not a definitive diagnosis; it only reveals size and configuration.
  3 This test would not yield a definitive diagnosis because malignant cells might not be present in the fluid.
  4 This would give information as to the activity of phosphorus in the body; however, no definitive diagnosis could be made.

436. **2 The serum acid phosphatase is elevated when the cancer extends beyond the prostate, whereas the serum alkaline phosphatase is elevated in bony metastasis. (EV; TC; RG)**
  1 Elevated creatinine levels may be caused by impaired renal function as a result of blockage by an enlarged prostate but do not indicate that metastasis has occurred.
  3 Elevated BUN levels may be caused by impaired renal function as a result of blockage by an enlarged prostate but do not indicate that metastasis has occurred.
  4 Nonprotein nitrogen refers to waste products from metabolism of protein and includes urea, creatinine, uric acid, and ammonia.

437. **2 The phenolsulfonphthalein and urea clearance tests evaluate the kidneys' ability to excrete a particular substance from the blood. The urine concentration or specific gravity is an indicator of the kidneys' ability to concentrate urine. (DC; PA; RG)**
  1 These tests are not generally ordered (as grouped) to determine kidney disease.
  3 Same as answer 1.
  4 Same as answer 1.

438. **3 Inability to empty the bladder, as a result of pressure exerted by the enlarging prostate on the urethra, causes a backup of urine into the ureters and finally the kidneys (hydronephrosis). (DC; PA; RG)**
  1 BPH develops over the client's life span; it is not congenital.
  2 It is uncommon for BPH to become malignant.
  4 This level is elevated in prostatic carcinoma.

439. **3 The exudate from herpes virus type 2 is highly contagious; gown and gloves provide a barrier, a concept related to medical asepsis. (IM; TC; RG)**
  1 The organism is not in respiratory tract secretions; the organism is present in the exudate from active lesions.
  2 This is unnecessary.
  4 This is not an airborne infectious disease.

440. **4 Although the usual incubation period of syphilis is about 3 weeks, clinical symptoms may appear as early as 9 days or as long as 3 months after exposure. (IM; PA; RG)**
  1 The normal incubation period is 21 days.
  2 Same as answer 1.
  3 Same as answer 1.

441. **1 The tertiary stage is noncontagious; tertiary lesions contain only small numbers of treponemes; fatal cases involve the aorta, CNS, or eye. (AN; PA; RG)**
  2 The primary stage lasts 8 to 12 weeks; the chancre is teeming with spirochetes, and the individual is contagious.
  3 The incubation stage lasts 2 to 6 weeks; spirochetes proliferate at entry site, and the individual is contagious.
  4 The duration of the secondary stage is variable (about 5 years); skin and mucosal lesions contain spirochetes, and the individual is highly contagious.

442. **3 Although the treatment of choice is penicillin, clients who are allergic must be given other antimicrobial agents to avoid an anaphylactic reaction. (DC; TC; RG)**
  1 The portal of entry does not influence treatment.
  2 The chancre is present only in the primary stage; it does not alter treatment.
  4 Although contacts should be identified and notified, treatment should not be delayed.

443. **1 Gonorrhea is a highly contagious disease transmitted through sexual intercourse. The incubation period varies, but symptoms usually occur 2 to 10 days after contact. Early effective treatment prevents complications. (DC; TC; RG)**
  2 The parents may be unaware that their child has gonorrhea.
  3 Contracting venereal disease is not necessarily indicative of promiscuity.
  4 Most birth control measures do not protect against the transmission of sexually transmitted disease.

444. **1 Penicillin is specific for *Neisseria gonorrhoeae* and eradicates the microorganism; other treatment regimens are available for resistant strains. (IM; ED; RG)**
2 If the disease progresses before diagnosis is made, complications such as sterility, valve damage, or joint degeneration may occur.
3 Transmission is not controlled; the organism is eliminated.
4 If tubal structures, valves, or joints degenerate, the pathologic changes will not be reversed by antibiotic therapy.

Genitourinary

445. **3 Specimens can be analyzed for specific information that is objective. (DC; PA; RG)**
1 The client's verbal history of the illness is subjective data.
2 Direct observations without precise measurements are subjective.
4 Feelings are experienced by an individual and cannot be uniformly measured.

446. **1 A strange environment, as well as the anxiety associated with private body functions like elimination, interferes with the client's ability to relax the urinary sphincter to void. (IM; TC; RG)**
2 This method might be helpful in some situations; however, it does not take into account the common anxiety of voiding in a strange environment.
3 Same as answer 2.
4 Same as answer 2.

447. **1 Depending on the purpose of the collection, a preservative to prevent breakdown of the specimen may be necessary. (IM; TC; RG)**
2 This is not necessary.
3 The last specimen should be collected as close as possible to the end of the 24-hour period and added to the urine collected.
4 This is not necessary, nor is the measurement of each voiding during the 24-hour collection, unless the client is on intake and output.

448. **2 The kidneys are ultimately responsible for maintaining fluid and electrolyte balance by excretion or retention based on the body's needs. (AN; PA; RG)**
1 Aldosterone will cause retention of sodium ions by the nephrons and subsequent fluid retention.
3 The lungs eliminate water and carbon dioxide only if excess carbonic acid is present; their role in fluid and electrolyte balance is less extensive than the kidneys'.
4 Antidiuretic hormone has a direct effect on the nephrons, resulting in water retention.

449. **2 Because the plasma colloid oncotic pressure (COP) opposes glomerular filtration, a decrease in blood proteins will increase the glomerular filtration rate (GFR). (AN; PA; RG)**
1 Glomeruli are clusters of capillaries, not arteries.
3 Volume is determined by the amount of water reabsorbed in the tubules.
4 This does not affect the glomerular filtration rate.

450. **2 Osmosis is the diffusion of water through a selectively permeable membrane. Such membranes include cellular membranes and capillary walls. Osmosis occurs in the kidney tubules and in all capillary beds. (AN; PA; RG)**
1 Dialysis is the diffusion of small molecules, other than water, down their concentration gradients through a selectively permeable membrane.
3 Diffusion is the process by which particulate matter in a fluid moves from an area of greater concentration to an area of lesser concentration.
4 Active transport is the movement of molecules against a concentration gradient and requires energy input; osmosis and diffusion are passive processes.

451. **2 Refrigeration retards the growth of bacteria and may preserve the specimen for several hours. (IM; TC; RG)**
1 Growth of bacteria will alter the pH and the glucose and protein levels in the urine; it must be refrigerated to retard growth.
3 Same as answer 1.
4 This represents an unnecessary waste of time, effort, and money.

452. **2 The prostate gland is a tubuloalveolar gland shaped like a ring, with the urethra passing through its center. (AN; PA; RG)**
1 The epididymis lies along the top and sides of the testes.
3 The seminal vesicles are on the posterior surface of the bladder.
4 This gland lies below the prostate.

453. 2 The Foley catheter is always positioned so that the level of the bladder with the catheter inserted is higher than the level of the drainage container; gravity causes urine flow. (AN; PA; RG)

1 This refers to a property of matter.

3 This refers to the movement of water across a semipermeable membrane; it is not responsible for the flow of urine through a catheter.

4 This refers to the passage of molecules from an area of higher concentration to one of lower concentration.

454. 4 Cleansing the urinary meatus and adjacent skin removes accumulated bacteria, limiting the possible introduction of microbes into the urinary tract. (PL; TC; RG)

1 Although cleansing the perineal area is helpful, it is actually the organisms closest to the meatus that gain entry to the urinary tract first.

2 Although encouraging fluids helps prevent urinary stasis and subsequent infection, the most common source of infection is microorganisms from around the meatus.

3 Irrigations require opening the closed drainage system and allowing the entry of microorganisms; this increases the risk of infection.

455. 3 Catheter patency ensures drainage and prevents bladder distention and other complications. Therefore patency of a catheter should be established prior to notifying the physician. (IM; TC; RG)

1 Assessment is necessary prior to consultation with the physician.

2 Patency of the catheter should be assessed first. Milking the tubing may be necessary if the catheter is clogged. Milking a catheter is usually required when the drainage is viscous rather than clear.

4 Irrigation is avoided if possible because of the associated risk of infection.

456. 3 An indwelling catheter dilates the urinary sphincters, keeps the bladder empty, and short-circuits the normal reflex mechanism based on bladder distention. When the catheter is removed, the body must adapt to functioning once again. (AN; PA; RG)

1 Although this could cause difficulty in voiding, there are no data presented to draw this conclusion.

2 This would not cause this problem.

4 Same as answer 1.

457. 2 Cystitis is an inflammation of the bladder that causes frequency, urgency, pain on micturition, and hematuria. (DC; PA; RG)

1 Pyelitis is an inflammation of the pelvis of the kidney, causing flank pain, chills, fever, and weakness.

3 Nephrosis is a kidney condition in which there is proteinuria, hypoalbuminemia, and edema.

4 Pyelonephritis is a diffuse pyogenic infection of the pelvis and parenchyma of the kidney that causes flank pain, chills, fever, and weakness.

458. 3 Ammonium chloride causes metabolic acidosis. As a result the kidneys secrete the excess hydrogen ions, increasing the acidity of the urine. An acid urine is essential for the antibacterial action of methenamine mandelate (Mandelamine). (AN; TC; RG)

1 Ammonium chloride is an acidifier and thus does not promote healing.

2 By acidifying the urine this drug enhances the antibacterial action of methenamine mandelate; it does not decrease bladder irritation.

4 Combining these drugs will have no effect on uric crystal stone formation.

459. 4 Because the female urethra is closer to the anus than in the male, it is at greater risk of becoming contaminated. (AN; PA; RG)

1 Urinary pH is within the same range in both males and females.

2 Hormonal secretions have no effect on the development of bladder infections.

3 The position of the bladder is the same in males and females.

460. 1 Cloudy urine usually indicates purulent drainage associated with infection. (DC; PA; RG)

2 Viscosity is a subjective characteristic that would not be measurable.

3 Specific gravity yields information related to fluid balance.

4 Sugar and acetone are not affected by urinary tract infections.

461. 3 An enlarged prostate constricts the urethra, interfering with urine flow causing retention. When the bladder fills and approaches capacity, small amounts can be voided but the bladder never empties completely. (AN; PA; RG)

1 Edema does not cause the client to void frequently in small amounts because of decreased production of urine.

2 Dysuria is painful or difficult urination that is not part of the client's symptoms.

4 The urge to void is caused by stimulation of the stretch receptors as the bladder fills with urine; in suppression little or no urine is produced.

462. **3 Bethanechol chloride (Urecholine) improves the muscle tone of an atonic bladder, facilitating micturition. (AN; TC; RG)**

1 Carbachol is a miotic used in the treatment of glaucoma.

2 Neosporin is an antibiotic; it does not aid in increasing bladder muscle tone.

4 Pilocarpine hydrochloride is a miotic, used in the treatment of glaucoma.

463. **2 This is considered a routine procedure to meet basic physiologic needs and is covered by a consent signed at the time of admission. (EV; TC; RG)**

1 The catheter is inserted to aid the health team in assessing the client.

3 This treatment does not require special consent.

4 Same as answer 3.

464. **3 The total amount of irrigation solution instilled into the bladder is eliminated with urine and therefore must be subtracted from the total output to determine the volume of urine excreted. (IM; TC; RG)**

1 An accurate specific gravity cannot be obtained when irrigating solutions are being instilled into the bladder.

2 Hourly outputs are indicated only if there is concern about renal failure or oliguria.

4 Twenty-four hour urine tests would not be accurate if the client was receiving continuous irrigations.

465. **3 Hepatitis Type B is transmitted by blood or blood products. The hemodialysis and routine transfusions needed for a client in renal failure constitute a great risk of exposure. (EV; TC; RG)**

1 Peritonitis is a danger in peritoneal dialysis.

2 Renal calculi are not a complication of hemodialysis; they often occur in clients confined to prolonged bed rest because of demineralized bones.

4 Dialysis does not involve the bladder and would not contribute to the development of a bladder infection.

466. **3 The length of the urethra is shorter in females than in males; therefore microorganisms have a shorter distance to travel to reach the bladder. The proximity of the meatus to the anus in females also increases this incidence. (DC; PA; RG)**

1 Fluid intake may be adequate in both males and females and would not account for the difference.

2 Hygienic practices can be poor in males or females; however, the anatomic length of the urethra in females predisposes them to infection.

4 Mucous membranes are continuous in both males and females and would not make a difference.

467. **4 The causative organism should be isolated prior to institution of antibiotic therapy. (PL; TC; RG)**

1 This test will not determine the infective organisms causing the problem.

2 The bowel is not affected by the diagnosis; enemas are not required.

3 Catheterization is not a routine procedure for urethritis.

468. **4 Changes in the amount of blood in the urine may indicate progressive increases in kidney damage. (DC; PA; RG)**

1 This is unrelated to hematuria.

2 This is unrelated to hematuria; it is associated with breakdown of adipose tissue.

3 Same as answer 1.

469. **3 Relaxation of the pelvic musculature causes the uterus to drop, with a subsequent relaxation of the vaginal walls, most often as a result of childbirth. A rectocele is protrusion of the rectal wall into the vagina, whereas a cystocele is protrusion of the bladder into the vaginal wall. (AN; PA; RG)**

1 This does not cause either a rectocele or a cystocele.

2 Same as answer 1.

4 Same as answer 1.

470. **3 As the uterus drops, the vaginal wall relaxes. When the bladder herniates into the vagina (cystocele) and the rectal wall herniates into the vagina (rectocele), the individual feels pressure or pain in the lower back and/or pelvis. When there is an increase in intraabdominal pressure in the presence of a cystocele, incontinence results. (DC; PA; RG)**

1 These do not indicate cystocele and rectocele; they are common with infection.

2 These do not indicate cystocele and rectocele.

4 Same as answer 2.

471. **1** **The effects of anesthesia and the inflammatory process may impede voiding, leading to urinary retention; an indwelling catheter empties the bladder continuously, preventing retention.** (AN; TC; RG)

2 Distention causes discomfort; this is avoided by preventing retention.

3 Because the bladder is continually empty when an indwelling catheter is in place, it loses tone. This is an expected but undesirable effect.

4 Distention places pressure on the suture line; this is avoided by preventing retention.

472. **1** **Dysuria, nocturia, and urgency are all signs of an irritable bladder.** (EV; PA; RG)

2 This is not an indication of bladder irritability.

3 Same as answer 2.

4 Same as answer 2.

473. **3** **The occurrence of bladder tumors is related to smoking, radiation, and schistosomiasis.** (DC; PA; RG)

1 Jogging is unrelated to the development of tumors.

2 Ingestion of cola has not been linked to bladder tumors.

4 Vibrations may result in musculoskeletal or kidney problems; they are unrelated to bladder tumors.

474. **4** **Preoperative cleansing of the bowel is mandated prior to surgical resection and formation of a urinary conduit.** (PL; TC; RG)

1 Fluids should not be restricted until after midnight of the operative day.

2 Muscle-tightening exercises have no effect on this procedure.

3 The stoma of an ileal conduit is not irrigated.

475. **3** **The ureters are implanted in a segment of the ileum, and urine drains continually because there is no sphincter.** (EV; PA; RG)

1 Ileal conduits are not neurologically innervated; therefore no peristalsis exists.

2 No feces are present in an ileal conduit.

4 Nutrients are not normally absorbed from urine.

476. **1** **Because of the anatomic position of the incision, drainage would flow by gravity and accumulate under the client lying in the supine position.** (EV; TC; RG)

2 Nail beds would indicate peripheral perfusion, not early hemorrhage.

3 Respiratory hemorrhage is not common after kidney surgery.

4 Blood pressure decreases in hemorrhage, and pulse increases.

477. **4** **Dressings retain an undetermined amount of drainage, which would lead to an inaccurate reading.** (IM; TC; RG)

1 Weighing dressings is the most accurate method of estimating postoperative drainage. The nurse must subtract the dry weight of the dressings to determine fluid loss.

2 Counting of saturated pads allows for some degree of objectivity in the assessment, but it is not the most accurate.

3 Measuring drainage that has seeped through is not as accurate as weighing; however, it does allow for more objective measurement.

478. **4** **A suprapubic prostatectomy involves an abdominal incision to gain access to the prostate through the bladder. Postoperatively the client has a suprapubic cystotomy tube to instill a GU irrigant to dilute the urine and limit clot formation as well as a Foley catheter under tension to limit bleeding and drain urine.** (PL; PA; RG)

1 The ureters are not involved in this surgery.

2 The kidneys are not involved in this surgery.

3 An incision is made in the lower abdomen; a ureteral catheter is not used.

479. **3** **Because of the vascularity of the involved tissue, hemorrhage and shock constitute the immediate postoperative danger after a prostatectomy.** (DC; TC; RG)

1 Bladder spasms may occur but are not potentially life threatening; observing for hemorrhage is the priority.

2 Impotence is a relatively rare complication.

4 A Foley catheter is used; leakage of urine may occur for a few days after the Foley catheter is removed due to sphincter trauma.

480. **1** **The bladder is a sterile body cavity. Any time a solution or catheter is introduced into the urinary meatus, strict surgical asepsis is required.** (IM; TC; RG)

2 Excessive pressure can traumatize the lining of the urinary tract.

3 The solution is generally administered at room temperature.

4 This would only be done if the fluid did not return by gravity; the negative pressure exerted during aspiration may cause trauma.

481. **2 The catheter must be reinserted by the physician to ensure bladder emptying, maintain pressure at the operative site, and prevent hemorrhage. (IM; TC; RG)**
1 Because of the danger of further trauma to the urethra and surgical site, the surgeon should insert the catheter.
3 Irrigations require a physician's order.
4 In addition to urinary drainage, the balloon of the urethral catheter exerts pressure against the prostate to help control bleeding and should be reinserted.

482. **2 Following this type of surgery pain is associated with bearing down; to prevent constipation the client should be instructed to increase fluid, fiber, and activity. (IM; ED; RG)**
1 The client is past childbearing age.
3 The anterior colporrhaphy is expected to reduce incontinence.
4 The colporrhaphy involves only the vaginal wall, the rectum should not be involved.

483. **3 A balloon tube is inserted into the renal pelvis to drain urine, necessitating an incision into the kidney (nephrostomy). (PL; TC; RG)**
1 Ileostomy is the surgical implantation of the ileum into the abdominal wall; it is not related to urinary disease.
2 Cecostomy is the surgical creation of a temporary opening into the cecum to relieve obstruction; this is not done for urinary problems.
4 Ureterostomy is the surgical implantation of the ureter in the abdominal wall; it would be performed if the bladder were involved.

484. **2 Although other solutions may be ordered, irrigations of the bladder usually employ normal saline (0.9% NaCl), which is a solution of approximately the tonicity of normal body fluids. (PL; TC; RG)**
1 This is a hypotonic solution, which may be absorbed by body tissues.
3 Same as answer 1.
4 Genitourinary irrigants usually contain an antimicrobial agent such as neosporin; indiscriminate use of such agents leads to the emergence of resistant strains of microorganisms.

485. **3 Frequency and a sense of urgency occur because of the irritation caused by the stone. (DC; PA; RG)**

1 Irritability may occur because of discomfort; twitching does not occur.
2 Pyuria may occur when infection is present; skin problems do not occur.
4 Pain radiates from the flank to the groin area.

486. **1 Urine is strained to determine whether any calculi or calcium gravel has been passed. (IM; TC; RG)**
2 Fluids should be encouraged to promote dilute urine and facilitate passage of the calculi.
3 Blood pressure assessment is of no particular importance to the client with kidney stones.
4 Administration of analgesics is based on time and need.

487. **1 Calcium and phosphorus are components of these stones and should therefore be avoided. Also an acid environment is not favorable to their development. (PL; TC; RG)**
2 Diets high in calcium must be avoided.
3 This diet is indicated for clients with gout.
4 Same as answer 2.

488. **3 Continuous bladder irrigation requires a three-way indwelling catheter so that the irrigant infuses through one port and both urine and irrigant drain out together through another port; the third port allows for inflation of the balloon that keeps the catheter in the bladder. (IM; TC; RG)**
1 The bedside drainage bag contains both irrigant and urine.
2 The purpose of CBI is to prevent obstruction of the catheter; stopping the irrigation would increase the risk of obstruction.
4 Both urine and irrigant mix in the bladder and drain from the same port.

489. **4 Cystolithectomy refers to the removal of bladder stones. (PL; ED; RG)**
1 Cystometry is the process of measuring the bladder's pressure and capacity.
2 Cystolithiasis denotes the presence of stones in the bladder.
3 Cryoextraction refers to the use of subfreezing temperatures in the removal of tissue; generally used in cataract extraction.

490. 3 This is a low calcium intake and continued high excretion levels would then have to be from other than a dietary source; recurrent infections and inadequate fluids contribute most to formation of calculi; most stones are calcium or oxalate in nature. (AN; TC; RG)

1 Calcium intake through the diet may affect the blood calcium levels.

2 Parathyroid hormone controls the serum calcium levels.

4 This is not conclusive evidence that parathyroidism is the cause.

491. 2 Roast beef and a baked potato have only moderate amounts of calcium compared with the other choices. (PL; TC; RG)

1 Pudding is made with milk and is high in calcium.

3 Cheese is high in calcium.

4 Ice cream is made with milk and is high in calcium.

492. 3 Uric acid stones are controlled by a low-purine diet. Foods high in purine, such as organ meats and extracts, should be avoided. (IM; ED; RG)

1 Calcium stones are controlled by a low-calcium, low-phosphate diet; milk, fruits, and vegetables need not be avoided with uric acid stones.

2 Cystine, not uric acid, stones are controlled by a low-methionine diet, which excludes meat, milk, eggs, and cheese from the diet.

4 Only organ meats must be avoided; vegetables do not need to be controlled.

493. 3 Calcium oxalate renal stones can be prevented by adhering to a diet low in calcium and oxalate and high in acid ash. (PL; TC; RG)

1 Purines are catabolized to uric acid and must be avoided in gout.

2 Methionine is an essential amino acid and must be included in the diet.

4 The diet should be high in acid, not alkaline, ash to control production of these stones.

494. 4 Peritoneal dialysis uses the peritoneum as a selectively permeable membrane for diffusion of toxins and wastes from the blood into the dialyzing solution. (AN; PA; RG)

1 Peritoneal dialysis acts as a substitute for kidney function; it does not reestablish kidney function.

2 The dialysate does not clean the peritoneal membrane; the semipermeable membrane allows toxins and wastes to pass into the dialysate within the abdominal cavity.

3 Fluid in the abdominal cavity does not enter the intracellular compartment.

495. 1 Bicarbonate buffering is limited, hydrogen ions accumulate, and acidosis results (AN; PA; RG)

2 The rate of respirations increases in metabolic acidosis to compensate for a low pH.

3 The retention of sodium ions is related to fluid retention and edema rather than to acidosis.

4 The fluid balance does not significantly alter the pH.

496. 4 The amount of protein permitted in the diet (usually below 50 g) depends on the extent of kidney function; excess protein causes a rise in urea, which should be avoided; adequate calories are also provided to prevent tissue catabolism that also results in an increase in metabolic waste products. (AN; TC; RG)

1 The diet used in managing renal failure is low in protein because the kidneys are unable to eliminate the waste products from the body.

2 The body is able to synthesize the nonessential amino acids.

3 Urea is a waste product of protein metabolism; the body is able to synthesize the nonessential amino acids.

497. 2 In renal failure, as the glomerular filtration rate decreases, phosphorus is retained. As hyperphosphatemia occurs, calcium is excreted. Calcium depletion (hypocalcemia) causes tetany. (DC; PA; RG)

1 The symptoms described are not characteristic of this condition.

3 Same as answer 1.

4 Same as answer 1.

498. 3 An elevated blood urea nitrogen, indicating uremia, is toxic to the central nervous system and causes mental cloudiness, confusion, and loss of consciousness. (DC; PA; RG)

1 Hyperkalemia is associated with muscle weakness, irritability, nausea, and diarrhea.

2 Hypernatremia is associated with firm tissue turgor, oliguria, and agitation.

4 If decreased fluid intake results in dehydration, it can cause fatigue, dry skin and mucous membranes, and rapid pulse and respiratory rates.

499. 4 Protein breakdown liberates cellular potassium ions, leading to hyperkalemia, which can cause cardiac dysrhythmia and standstill. The failure of the kidneys to maintain a balance of potassium is one of the main indications for dialysis. (PL; TC; RG)

1 Ascites occurs in liver disease and is not an indication for dialysis.

2 Dialysis is not the usual treatment for acidosis. This usually responds to administration of alkaline drugs.

3 Dialysis is not a treatment for hypertension; this is usually controlled by antihypertensive medication and diet.

500. 2 Hemodialysis exposes the blood to a solution that contains normal concentrations of nutrients and low concentrations of waste products; the blood and dialyzing solution are separated by a selectively permeable membrane. The movement of small molecules (wastes) from the blood to the dialyzing solution is an example of dialysis. (AN; PA; RG)

1 Osmosis is the movement of fluid through a selectively permeable membrane.

3 This would use hydrostatic pressure to pass water and solute through a permeable membrane.

4 This would be movement of solute particles in the direction of a pressure gradient from an area of greater concentration to an area of lesser concentration.

501. 3 Because an external shunt provides circulatory access to a major artery and vein, special safety precautions must be taken to prevent disconnection of the cannulas. Disconnection can cause unimpeded excessive blood loss and death. Clamps should be carried at all times by the client in case this emergency should arise. (EV; TC; RG)

1 Although a potential complication, this does not pose the same immediate threat to life as does exsanguination.

2 Same as answer 1.

4 Same as answer 1.

502. 2 Insertion of an arteriovenous shunt represents a break in the first line of defense against infection, the skin. An infection of an arteriovenous shunt can be avoided by strict aseptic (sterile) technique. (IM; TC; RG)

1 An elastic bandage would interfere with examination of the site.

3 A bruit is normally auscultated by virtue of the increased arterial pressure in the area.

4 To prevent damage to the shunt, blood pressure should not be measured in the affected arm.

503. 4 Hepatitis B is caused by a DNA virus and is transmitted by contact with infected blood. (AN; TC; RG)

1 Infectious or type A viral hepatitis is spread by contaminated food or water.

2 This is a fictitious disease.

3 Same as answer 1.

Gastrointestinal

504. 4 The aerobic oxidation of glucose occurring in the mitochondrion produces 38 moles of ATP for every mole of glucose oxidized. (AN; PA; GI)

1 This is the formation of peptide bonds.

2 This activity involves gaseous exchange.

3 The digestion, not hydrolysis, of fats is involved.

505. 1 Milk and milk products are not tolerated well because they contain lactose, a sugar that is converted to galactose by lactase. Lactose intolerance is common in those of African-American heritage (DC; PA; GI)

2 This enzyme assists in the digestion of maltose, which is not a milk sugar.

3 This enzyme assists in the digestion of sucrose, which is not a milk sugar.

4 This enzyme assists in the digestion of starch, which is not a milk sugar.

506. 2 The salts in bile act as detergents to break large fat droplets into smaller ones (emulsification), providing a larger surface area for the enzymatic action of fat-splitting enzymes (lipases). (AN; PA; GI)

1 Bile does not act on proteins.

3 Bile does not help synthesize vitamins; it emulsifies fat and thus assists in absorption of fat soluble vitamins.

4 Bile does not have an acid pH.

507. 4 This is the organism that causes botulism. (AN; ED; GI)

1 This is a normal inhabitant of the intestines; it is not anaerobic.

2 This is an anaerobic organism that causes tetanus.

3 *Salmonella*, a gram-negative rod, is not anaerobic.

508. **4 Orange juice has a higher proportion of simple sugars, which are readily available for conversion to energy. (PL; TC; GI)**
1 Milk contains fat and protein, which require a longer digesting time, and lactose, which is a disaccharide.
2 Bread contains carbohydrates, which require a longer time to digest because they must be converted to simple sugars.
3 Candy bars do not contain the high proportion of simple sugars found in orange juice; they also contain fat, which takes longer to digest.

509. **2 Amino acids are absorbed into the blood in the intestinal capillaries with the aid of vitamin B$_6$ via the energy-dependent system, active transport. (AN; PA; GI)**
1 Proteins are fairly large molecules; they do not passively diffuse.
3 This refers to movement across a semipermeable membrane; it does not apply to proteins.
4 Same as answer 3.

510. **2 Complete proteins contain sufficient amounts of all essential amino acids and are of animal origin. (AN; PA; GI)**
1 Not all 22 but rather the 8 essential and 2 semiessential (arginine and histidine) amino acids are needed during growth.
3 Sufficient amounts of all 8 essential amino acids must be present plus 2 semiessential (arginine and histidine), which are essential only during periods of growth.
4 The body cannot make the essential amino acids; they must be present in foods ingested.

511. **2 Vitamin K is synthesized by intestinal bacteria but is also found in liver, egg yolks, cheese, tomatoes, and green leafy vegetables. (AN; PA; GI)**
1 Vitamin K is found in a small variety of foods.
3 It is found in enough foods so that a natural deficiency usually does not occur.
4 Vitamin K is not easily absorbed; it is fat soluble and requires bile salts for its absorption.

512. **4 Vitamin C is an intercellular cement substance. (AN; PA; GI)**
1 This is the function of vitamin K.
2 This is the function of vitamin A.
3 This is the function of vitamin D.

513. **4 A triglyceride is composed of three fatty acids and a glycerol molecule. When energy is required, the fatty acids are mobilized from adipose tissue for fuel. (AN; PA; GI)**
1 This is not the function of adipose tissue; its main function is storage.
2 This is not a function of adipose tissue; cholesterol is produced in the liver.
3 This is not the function of adipose tissue in fat metabolism.

514. **3 A coenzyme is a nonprotein substance that, in the presence of a suitable enzyme, serves as a catalyst in chemical changes. (AN; PA; GI)**
1 A series of complex changes is not involved in formation of the enzyme controlling a particular reaction.
2 A coenzyme is a nonprotein that combines with an apoenzyme to form a complete enzyme.
4 The coenzyme does not neutralize the enzyme.

515. **1 Lipoproteins are simple proteins combined with lipid to facilitate circulation of fat in the blood. (AN; PA; GI)**
2 A triglyceride is insoluble in water.
3 A phospholipid is insoluble in water.
4 Plasma proteins do not contain fat.

516. **3 These amino acids are needed to maintain life and are not produced by the body. (AN; PA; GI)**
1 The essential amino acids cannot be made by the body.
2 All amino acids are needed for metabolism; however, arginine and histidine are necessary for growth, but not during adulthood.
4 The body does not synthesize these amino acids; they must be ingested in the diet.

517. **3 Fruits contain less natural sodium than do other foods. (AN; PA; GI)**
1 Milk is higher in natural sodium than is fruit.
2 Meat is higher in natural sodium than is fruit.
4 Vegetables are higher in natural sodium than is fruit.

518. **3 Saturated fats found in animal tissue are more dense than unsaturated fats, which are found in vegetable oils. (AN; PA; GI)**
1 This characteristic of food has no bearing on fat content.
2 Same as answer 1.
4 The denseness of fat has nothing to do with digestibility.

519. **3 Animal fats are high in dense saturated fats. (PL; TC; GI)**
   1 Fruits do not contain saturated fats.
   2 Grains do not contain saturated fats.
   4 Vegetable oils contain unsaturated fats.

520. **1 Because triglycerides are made up of fatty acids bonded (esterified) to glycerol, their breakdown releases fatty acids as well as glycerol. (AN; PA; GI)**
   2 Triglycerides do not contain amino acids.
   3 Triglycerides do not contain urea nitrogen.
   4 Triglycerides do not contain simple sugars.

521. **2 Vitamin A is a fat-soluble vitamin that accumulates in the body and is not significantly excreted even if extremely large amounts are ingested. After prolonged ingestion of extremely large doses, toxic effects (irritability, increased intracranial pressure, fatigue, night sweats, severe headache) can occur. (IM; TC; GI)**
   1 Vitamin A is toxic only after prolonged large dosages.
   3 Vitamin A can be stored in the liver.
   4 Vitamin A cannot be synthesized by the body.

522. **2 Pancreatic amylase (which enters the small intestine at the sphincter of Oddi) and sucrase, lactase, and maltase (which are released by epithelial cells covering the villi in the small intestine) are responsible for carbohydrate digestion. (AN; PA; GI)**
   1 Because ptyalin is present in saliva, some starch digestion occurs in the mouth.
   3 Digestion of carbohydrates is completed prior to their arrival in the large intestine, which is concerned primarily with fluid reabsorption.
   4 Limited carbohydrate digestion occurs in the stomach; pepsin begins the digestion of proteins.

523. **4 Deep green and yellow vegetables contain large quantities of the pigments alpha-, beta-, and gamma-carotene; beta-carotene is the major chemical precursor of vitamin A in human nutrition. (AN; PA; GI)**
   1 Oranges are considered a good source of both vitamin C and potassium.
   2 Levels of vitamin A are higher in whole milk than in skim milk.
   3 Tomatoes are a good source of vitamin C.

524. **4 The high-Fowler's position promotes optimal entry into the esophagus aided by gravity. (IM; TC; GI)**
   1 This position does not take full advantage of the effect of gravity.
   2 Same as answer 1.
   3 Same as answer 1.

525. **2 Small meals are not as psychologically overwhelming and do not upset the stomach as easily. They are therefore better tolerated. (PL; TC; GI)**
   1 If no attempts are made to decrease portions at regular mealtimes, aversion will usually persist.
   3 This does not ensure adequate nutrition; if the portion size is decreased, frequency must be increased.
   4 Administration of vitamins is a dependent nursing function.

526. **3 Anorexia refers to loss of appetite. (DC; PA; GI)**
   1 Apathy refers to lack of concern or emotion.
   2 Anoxia refers to lack of oxygen.
   4 Dysphagia refers to difficulty in swallowing.

527. **1 A flat plate film of the abdomen visualizes abdominal organs as they are. (PL; TC; GI)**
   2 No bowel preparation is indicated.
   3 The client may eat and drink as tolerated.
   4 Same as answer 2.

528. **4 Barium salts used in a GI series coat the inner lining of the GI tract and then absorb x-rays passing through. They thus outline the surface features of the tract on a photographic plate. (IM; PA; GI)**
   1 Barium does not fluoresce.
   2 Barium has no light-emitting properties.
   3 Barium has no properties of a dye.

529. **4 To promote understanding and allay anxiety, all diagnostic tests should be explained to the client. (IM; TC; GI)**
   1 Preparations for tests may vary depending on the client's condition.
   2 Same as answer 1.
   3 Same as answer 1.

530. 3 Administration of additional fluid when a client complains of abdominal cramps adds to discomfort because of additional pressure. By clamping the tubing a few minutes the nurse allows the cramps generally to subside and the enema can be continued. (EV; TC; GI)

1 Slowing the rate decreases pressure but does not reduce it entirely.

2 Cramps are not a reason to discontinue the enema entirely; temporary clamping of the tubing usually relieves the cramps and the procedure can be continued.

4 This will reduce the flow of the solution, which will decrease pressure but not reduce it entirely.

531. 3 If the height of the enema fluid container above the anus is increased, the force and rate of flow also increase. If the container is raised excessively, damage to the mucosa may result and the procedure will be much more difficult for the client to tolerate. (IM; TC; GI)

1 The enema container can be held up to 45 cm above the anus and still be considered within safe limits.

2 Same as answer 1.

4 This would be too high and could cause mucosal injury.

532. 2 Because the soft tissues of the GI tract lack sufficient quantities of x-ray–absorbing atoms (as are naturally present in the dense calcium salts of bone), an x-ray–absorbing coating of barium is used for radiologic studies. (AN; PA; GI)

1 Barium does not color the intestinal wall.

3 Barium absorbs x-rays.

4 Barium does not interact with electrolytes.

533. 4 This position maximally exposes the rectal area and facilitates entry of the sigmoidoscope. It is preferred. (IM; TC; GI)

1 The Sims' position does not expose the rectal area to the same extent as the knee-chest position does but can still be used for a sigmoidoscopy if the client is unable to maintain the knee-chest position.

2 Although prone refers to a face-down position, the rectal area is not exposed.

3 The lithotomy position is appropriate for gynecologic examinations.

534. 1 To permit adequate visualization of the mucosa during the sigmoidoscopy, the bowel must be cleansed with a nonirritating enema before examination. (IM; TC; GI)

2 Stool should be eliminated from the colon by an enema before the examination.

3 Because only the lower bowel is being visualized, keeping the client npo is unnecessary and debilitating; clear liquids and a laxative may be given the day before to limit fecal residue.

4 The client does not drink such a substance in preparation for a sigmoidoscopy.

535. 2 Leukoplakia are white thickened patches that tend to fissure and to become maligant; ulcerations in the mouth or on the tongue may indicate cancer. (DC; PA; GI)

1 Halitosis would not be an early sign or specific to cancer of the mouth.

3 Bleeding gums occur in gingival diseases.

4 Pain associated with cancer of the tongue would not radiate to the substernal area.

536. 4 Heavy alcohol ingestion predisposes an individual to the development of oral cancer. (DC; PA; GI)

1 Nail biting has no effect on the development of oral cancer.

2 Dental hygiene does not affect the development of oral cancer.

3 Gum chewing is not a contributing factor to development of oral cancer.

537. 2 Vomiting may result in aspiration of vomitus, because it cannot be expelled; this could cause pneumonia or asphyxia. (EV; TC; GI)

1 This is not a life-threatening problem.

3 Same as answer 1.

4 Same as answer 1.

538. 4 Vincent's angina (trenchmouth) is an infection of the mouth resulting in bleeding gums, pain on swallowing and talking, and fever. (DC; PA; GI)

1 This symptom is related to angina pectoris, resulting from insufficient oxygenation of myocardial tissue, not Vincent's angina.

2 Same as answer 1.

3 Same as answer 1.

539. 2 Pain and swelling should subside prior to 1 week postoperative. Continued pain may indicate infection. (EV; TC; GI)

1 The breath may have an odor because of dried blood in the oral cavity; this is to be expected during the postoperative period.

3 Painful swallowing may occur because of generalized trauma resulting from surgery and is to be expected.

4 Tenderness is expected during the postoperative period.

540. **1 Sleeping on pillows raises the upper torso and prevents reflux of the gastric contents through the hernia. (IM; ED; GI)**

2 This would have no effect on the mechanical problem of the stomach's entering the thoracic cavity.

3 Increasing the content of the stomach before lying down would aggravate the symptoms associated with a hiatal hernia.

4 The effect of antacids is not long lasting enough to promote a full night's sleep; sodium bicarbonate is not the antacid of choice.

541. **1 Heavy lifting increases intraabdominal pressure, allowing gastric contents to move up through the lower esophageal sphincter (regurgitation) causing heartburn (pyrosis). (IM; ED; GI)**

2 This encourages regurgitation and should be avoided.

3 Increasing fluids with meals increases gastric volume, causing distention and reflux.

4 Constrictive garments such as belts, binders, and girdles increase intraabdominal pressure and could lead to reflux.

542. **1 Almost all peptic ulcers in the stomach develop along the lesser curvature of the antral (pyloric) region. About 85% of all peptic ulcers occur within the first 2 cm of the duodenum. These regions are most exposed to acid conditions. (DC; PA; GI)**

2 This is less exposed to gastric secretions.

3 This is less exposed to gastric secretions; however, erosion may occur after repeated episodes of gastric reflux.

4 Same as answer 2.

543. **3 Irritation of the mucosa may cause increased bleeding or perforation and therefore should be avoided. (AN; TC; GI)**

1 All clients' diets should be nutritionally balanced; this is not specific to this client's problem.

2 Bulk and roughage may irritate the mucosa and should be decreased.

4 Psychologic support is not the primary goal; efforts should be made to include foods that are psychologically beneficial, but not at the expense of foods that are nonirritating to the mucosa.

544. **1 Pitressin is a vasoconstrictor that is used with great success in controlling GI bleeding. (PL; TC; GI)**

2 Neostigmine inhibits cholinesterase, permitting acetylcholine to function; it is used primarily for myasthenia gravis.

3 Pro-Banthine is a gastrointestinal anticholinergic; it decreases motility but has no effect on bleeding.

4 Mephyton is vitamin K; it promotes formation of prothrombin in the liver; although this action would be helpful, it would take too long to be of value in an emergency situation.

545. **4 The vagus nerve stimulates the stomach to secrete hydrochloric acid. When it is severed, this neural pathway is interrupted and there will be a decrease in stomach secretions. (IM; ED; GI)**

1 The portion of the vagus nerve that was severed innervated the stomach, not the heart; therefore the heart rate would not be affected.

2 The vagus nerve controls hydrochloric acid secretion, not gastric emptying; emptying is determined by the nature of foods being digested.

3 The vagus nerve is not a sensory nerve.

546. **1 Physiologic normal saline is used in gastric irrigation to prevent electrolyte imbalance. Because of the fresh gastric sutures, slow and gentle irrigation should be performed. Most surgeons, however, prefer gastric instillations. (IM; TC; GI)**

2 The purpose of irrigation is to maintain the patency of the tube for gastric decompression; with disconnection from suction a buildup of secretions and air can occur or the tube can become blocked by viscous drainage.

3 Increasing the pressure may cause damage to the suture line.

4 Same as answer 2.

547. **3 Nasogastric drainage is expected to be bright red at first and gradually darken within the first 24 hours after surgery. (DC; TC; GI)**

1 Bloody drainage is expected this soon after surgery and the physician does not need to be notified.

2 Nasogastric suction must be working and the tube must remain patent to prevent stress on the suture line.

4 The nasogastric tube is only irrigated if the physician orders it because of the danger of injury to the suture line; generally saline at room temperature would be ordered.

548. **4 To promote drainage of different lung regions, clients should turn every 2 hours. Deep breathing inflates the alveoli and promotes fluid drainage. (IM; TC; GI)**
1 Administration of PEEP is a dependent function of the nurse and is associated with a ventilator, not postoperative care.
2 Oxygen administration is a dependent function and is not generally required unless there is an underlying cardiac or respiratory disease.
3 During physical effort, individuals with abdominal incisions often revert to shallow breathing.

549. **2 When high-osmotic fluid passes rapidly into the small intestine, it causes hypovolemia. This results in a sympathetic response with tachycardia, diaphoresis, and dizziness. The symptoms are also attributed to a sudden rise and subsequent fall in blood sugar. (AN; PA; GI)**
1 The stomach is not full; its contents rapidly empty into the jejunum.
3 This could occur with intestinal obstruction; dumping syndrome is associated with increased motility originating in the jejunum. Reflux would need reverse peristalsis.
4 This is usually associated with paralytic ileus; dumping syndrome leads to increased intestinal motility.

550. **3 Small frequent feedings are tolerated best after a subtotal gastrectomy. (PL; TC; GI)**
1 Roughage may be irritating to the GI tract after surgery.
2 As soon as edema subsides, the individual is generally given small amounts of fluid and then the diet is gradually progressed.
4 Recuperation from gastric surgery may take up to 3 months; allowing only food preferences does not ensure inclusion of nutrients necessary for recovery.

551. **4 Symptoms of dumping syndrome occur to some degree in about 50% of all individuals who have undergone a gastrectomy. They include weakness, faintness, heart palpitations, and diaphoresis. It is therefore important to explain to the client that such symptoms can be minimized by resting after meals in the semi-Fowler's position, eating small meals, and omitting concentrated and highly refined carbohydrates. (PL; ED; GI)**
1 Gas-forming foods affect the intestines, not the stomach.

2 Modification of roughage is part of the management of intestinal rather than gastric disorders.
3 Eating habits must be modified to prevent rapid emptying of the stomach.

552. **2 Pernicious anemia is caused by a lack of vitamin B_{12}. Intrinsic factor, produced by the parietal cells of the gastric mucosa, is necessary for B_{12} absorption. (EV; PA; GI)**
1 B_{12} is absorbed in the ileum.
3 The intrinsic factor is secreted by the stomach; the hemopoietic factor is the combination of B_{12} and intrinsic factor.
4 Chief cells secrete the enzymes of the gastric juice.

553. **1 Approximately $^2/_3$ of clients with peptic ulcer disease have been found to have *Helicobacter pylori* infecting the mucosa and interfering with its protective function. (IM; ED; GI)**
2 Antibiotics do not affect acid secretion.
3 Antibiotics do not affect immunity.
4 Antibiotics do not increase the effect of antacids.

554. **3 The antrum is responsible for gastrin production, which stimulates hydrochloric acid secretion; its removal reduces HCl secretion and thus reduces irritation of the gastric mucosa. (DC; TC; GI)**
1 Removal by means of a laser beam, cryotechnique, or surgery is used when cataracts occur.
2 A stapedectomy, mobilization of the stapes, or a prosthetic implant would be used with otosclerosis.
4 A resection of the fifth cranial nerve would be done in trigeminal neuralgia.

555. **3 The act of eating allows the hydrochloric acid in the stomach to work on and be neutralized by food rather than irritate the gastric mucosa. (DC; PA; GI)**
1 This symptom is not specific to gastric ulcers.
2 This may indicate renal colic.
4 This is a generalized symptom not specific to gastric ulcers.

556. **1 To ensure continued suction, the patency of the tube should be maintained. Physiologic saline is used to prevent fluid and electrolyte disturbances during irrigation. (PL; TC; GI)**
2 The stomach is not considered a sterile body cavity, so medical asepsis is indicated.
3 Care must be taken to avoid traumatizing the mucosa.

4 Ice chips and water represent fluid intake, which must be approved by the physician; being hypotonic in nature, such intake may lower the serum electrolytes.

557. **4 Fluid and electrolytes are lost through intestinal decompression; on a daily basis about one-fifth of the total body water is secreted into and almost completely reabsorbed by the GI tract. (EV; TC; GI)**
   1 Because the client is kept npo, there would be no stimulus to cause enzymes to be secreted into the GI tract.
   2 IV dextrose supplies some carbohydrates as a source of energy; it would not be drawn from storage by intestinal decompression.
   3 Because the client is being kept npo, vitamins and minerals are not entering the GI tract and therefore are not lost.

558. **3 A rise in the level of formula within the tube indicates a full stomach. (EV; PA; GI)**
   1 Passage of flatus reflects intestinal motility, which does not pose a potential problem.
   2 Epigastric tenderness is not necessarily caused by a full stomach.
   4 A rapid inflow is the result of holding the container too high or using a feeding tube with too large a lumen.

559. **2 The presence of 50 ml or more of undigested formula may indicate impaired absorption; the volume of the next feeding may need to be reduced or the feeding postponed to reduce the risk of aspiration. (EV; TC; GI)**
   1 This evaluates fluid balance and is best performed over a 24-hour period.
   3 This is a method for evaluating placement.
   4 Although weighing the client regularly is important to evaluating overall nutritional progress, it cannot provide information about absorption of a particular feeding.

560. **4 The increased osmolarity (concentration) of many formulas draws fluid into the intestinal tract causing diarrhea; such feedings may need to be diluted initially until the client develops tolerance. (AN; TC; GI)**
   1 Formulas frequently have reduced fiber content, causing problems with constipation.
   2 Bacterial contamination is not a factor if feedings are administered as recommended by the manufacturer.
   3 Inappropriate positioning may increase the risk of aspiration, but does not increase diarrhea.

561. **4 Because the cardiac sphincter of the stomach is slightly opened to admit the nasogastric tube, rapid feeding could result in regurgitation. (IM; TC; GI)**
   1 Distention can be diminished by avoiding the instillation of air with the feeding.
   2 The speed of feeding does not cause flatulence, but the administration of air may.
   3 Indigestion is not hazardous to the client.

562. **2 This is the unique function of pancreozymin, which is secreted by the duodenal mucosa. It particularly affects the production of amylase. (AN; PA; GI)**
   1 Enterocrinin increases intestinal juice secretion.
   3 Enterogastrone lessens gastric secretion and motility.
   4 Cholecystokinin stimulates the flow of bile from the gallbladder.

563. **4 Lipase is a pancreatic enzyme that aids in the digestion of fat. (AN; PA; GI)**
   1 Lipase does not synthesize triglycerides.
   2 This is the function of bile.
   3 Lipase does not break down all dietary fat.

564. **4 The duodenum secretes several digestion-related hormones, including secretin, which elicits bicarbonate secretion from the pancreas, and pancreozymin, which elicits enzyme secretion from the pancreas. It also brings about gallbladder contraction and secretion of bile; in this function it is known as cholecystokinin. (AN; PA; GI)**
   1 The liver produces bile, which aids in the digestion of fat, but does not produce any hormones.
   2 The adrenals produce glucocorticoids, mineralocorticoids, and epinephrine.
   3 The pancreas produces the hormone insulin.

565. **3 A pseudocyst of the pancreas is an abnormally dilated space that contains blood, necrotic tissue, and enzymes and is surrounded by connective tissue. (AN; PA; GI)**
   1 This is an incorrect definition of a pseudocyst.
   2 Same as answer 1.
   4 Same as answer 1.

MEDICAL-SURGICAL ANSWERS

566. **4 Alcohol stimulates pancreatic enzyme secretion and an increase in pressure in the pancreatic duct. The backflow of enzymes into the pancreatic interstitial spaces results in partial digestion and inflammation of the pancreatic tissue. (AN; PA; GI)**
1 Although blockage of the bile duct with calculi may precipitate pancreatitis, this is not associated with alcohol.
2 Alcohol does not deplete insulin stores; the demand for insulin is unrelated to pancreatitis.
3 Although the volume of secretions increases, the composition remains unchanged.

567. **2 An incision close to the diaphragm (as in surgery of the pancreas) causes a great deal of pain when the client coughs and deep breathes. These clients tend to take shallow breaths, leading to inadequate expansion of the lungs, the accumulation of secretions, and infection. (AN; PA; GI)**
1 This is unrelated to the development of respiratory infections.
3 The elevation of serum bilirubin in the blood does not affect the immune mechanisms.
4 There is no evidence that an infection of the pancreas was present.

568. **4 Vitamin K is a fat-soluble vitamin and needs bile salts for its absorption from the upper segment of the small intestine. It is a catalyst in the carboxylation of glutamine to prothrombin. (AN; PA; GI)**
1 Bile salts do not inhibit the synthesis of prothrombin.
2 The liver does not synthesize vitamin K; the intestine does.
3 Bile salts do not affect prothrombinase (thromboplastin).

569. **2 Bile, a natural antioxidant, helps stabilize the vitamins and prevents destruction by oxygen. In addition, it is a transport vehicle for fat through the intestinal wall. (AN; PA; GI)**
1 This is stomach acid.
3 This is the digestive enzyme for lipids.
4 This is the digestive enzyme for starch.

570. **2 ERCP involves the insertion of a cannula into the pancreatic and common bile ducts during an endoscopy. The test is not performed if the client's bilirubin is greater than 3 to 5 mg/dl because cannulization may cause edema, which would increase obstruction of bile flow. (DC; PA; GI)**
1 This is not directly related to this test.
3 Same as answer 1.
4 Same as answer 1.

571. **4 Cholecystokinin is a widely distributed hormone whose functions include stimulation of gallbladder contraction and the release of pancreatic enzymes. It also functions as a neurotransmitter in the CNS. (AN; PA; GI)**
1 Gastrin stimulates the secretion of gastric juice.
2 Secretin promotes the production of bile by the liver and the secretion of pancreatic juice.
3 Enterocrinin stimulates the secretion of intestinal juice (succus entericus).

572. **2 When bile does not mix with foods in the intestine, emulsification of fats cannot occur and fat digestion is retarded. Stomach motility is also reduced, because increased stomach peristalsis depends on fat digestion in the small intestine. The bile trapped in the gallbladder acts as an irritant. (AN; PA; GI)**
1 Once emulsified by bile, fatty foods are readily broken down by digestive enzymes.
3 The production of bile is unaffected.
4 Obstruction would cause discomfort. Bile and pancreatic secretions enter the duodenum through the ampulla of Vater. With obstruction, edema and spasm occur, blocking the flow of enzymes and causing pain.

573. **3 These symptoms result from failure of bile to enter the intestines, with subsequent backup into the biliary system and diffusion into the blood. The bilirubin is carried to all body regions, including the skin (itching) and kidneys (excretion of bile-colored urine). The absence of bilirubin in the intestine results in clay-colored stools. (DC; PA; GI)**
1 Signs refer to objective findings of an examiner; the signs of inadequate absorption of vitamin K include ecchymosis, hematuria, and other bleeding.
2 The urine would be dark, reflecting increased serum bilirubin levels, and the stools would not be brown because the bile pigments would not be present in the GI tract.

4 If bile levels in the bloodstream are high, there would be bile in the urine, causing it to have a dark color.

574. **2 Vitamin K is necessary in the formation of prothrombin to prevent bleeding. It is a fat-soluble vitamin and is not absorbed from the GI tract in the absence of bile.** (AN; TC; GI)

1 Bilirubin is the bile pigment formed by the breakdown of erythrocytes.
3 Thromboplastin converts prothrombin to thrombin during the normal coagulation process.
4 Cholecystokinin is the hormone that stimulates pancreatic secretion and contraction of the gallbladder.

575. **2 The nurse should anticipate drainage and reinforce the surgical dressing as needed.** (IM; TC; GI)

1 Changing a dressing at this time unnecessarily increases the risk of infection.
3 An abdominal binder is rarely ordered and it would interfere with assessment of the dressing at this time.
4 Montgomery straps are utilized when frequent dressing changes are anticipated; they are not appropriate at this time.

576. **1 The location of the incision results in pain on inspiration or coughing. The subsequent reluctance to cough and deep breathe facilitates respiratory complications from retained secretions.** (DC; PA; GI)

2 This surgery does not take a prolonged period of time.
3 Bile does not impair inflammatory or immune responses.
4 A cholecystectomy is usually performed to treat cholelithiasis or cholecystitis; there is generally an inflammatory, not an infectious, process.

577. **2 Protein and calories provide energy, both of which are necessary for tissue building.** (PL; TC; GI)

1 A high-fat diet is contraindicated because fat requires bile to be absorbed; spasms in the biliary system may result in pain.
3 The obstruction has been corrected and painful contractions should not occur; dietary fat intake depends on individual tolerance.
4 This is inadequate for tissue repair.

578. **4 Protein helps correct severe malnutrition; moderate fat limits the need for bile; a high-calorie, high-vitamin diet prevents tissue breakdown.** (DC; PA; GI)

1 A diet high in protein, carbohydrates, and calories is needed to improve nutritional status.
2 A high-protein diet is essential in repairing tissues and restoring nutritional status.
3 This diet does not offer enough fat or calories.

579. **3 Thiamine and nicotinic acid help convert glucose for energy and therefore nerve activity.** (AN; PA; GI)

1 These vitamins do not affect elimination.
2 These vitamins are not related to circulatory activity.
4 Vitamin K, not thiamine and niacin, is essential for the manufacture of prothrombin in the liver.

580. **1 The liver detoxifies alcohol and is the organ most often damaged in chronic alcoholism. The high-calorie diet prevents tissue breakdown, which produces additional amino acids and nitrogen.** (AN; PA; GI)

2 These organs are not involved in detoxification of alcohol.
3 Same as answer 2.
4 This organ is not involved in detoxification of alcohol.

581. **4 In the liver a simple protein combines with a lipid to form a lipoprotein. Lipoproteins circulate freely in the blood and can be utilized easily and quickly in various metabolic processes.** (AN; PA; GI)

1 The liver does not produce phospholipids.
2 Fat is stored in adipose tissue.
3 The liver does not oxidize fat.

582. **2 Lipoproteins, a combination of a fat and a simple protein, have not been formed because of poor protein intake. Therefore fat accumulates in the liver.** (AN; PA; GI)

1 Elevations of bile in the blood occur because hepatic ducts are obstructed by the enlarged liver.
3 Individuals with cirrhosis of the liver are likely to have bleeding tendencies (rather than clotting) because of the decreased synthesis of prothrombin.
4 Deficiency of protein results in the breakdown of tissue (catabolism) and a negative nitrogen balance.

583. **4 Low sodium controls fluid retention, blood pressure, and consequently edema; low protein controls ammonia formation in proportion to the liver's ability to detoxify ammonia in forming urea; moderate fat and high calories and vitamins help repair a long-standing nutritional deficit. (PL; PA; GI)**
1 High-protein diets are contraindicated because of the liver's inability to detoxify ammonia.
2 Because protein is required for tissue regeneration, restriction is based on the liver's ability to detoxify ammonia; a high-fat diet is avoided because of the related cardiovascular risks and the related demand for bile.
3 Regeneration of tissue requires a high-calorie diet; 1200 calories is too low.

584. **3 The hepatic portal vein carries blood from the capillary beds of the viscera (small and large intestinal walls, stomach, spleen, pancreas, gallbladder) to the sinusoids of the liver. The hepatic veins drain the liver sinusoids into the inferior vena cava. (AN; PA; GI)**
1 The portal vein takes blood to the liver; the hepatic veins drain the liver sinusoids into the inferior vena cava.
2 Enters the superior vena cava from the capillary beds of the viscera.
4 Same as answer 2.

585. **4 The elevated pressure within the portal circulatory system causes elevated pressure in areas of portal systemic collateral circulation (most important, in the distal esophagus and proximal stomach). Hemorrhage is a possible complication. (DC; TC; GI)**
1 Liver abscesses may occur as a complication of intestinal infections; they are not related to portal hypertension.
2 This is not related to portal hypertension; it may be caused by manipulation of the bowel during surgery, peritonitis, neurologic disorders, or organic obstruction.
3 Perforation of the duodenum is usually caused by peptic ulcers; it is not a direct result of portal hypertension or cirrhosis.

586. **3 With obstruction of the portal vein there is an increase in pressure in the abdominal veins, which empty into the portal system. These veins develop collaterals to circumvent the obstruction. The collaterals are usually in the paraumbilical, hemorrhoidal, and esophageal areas. (AN; PA; GI)**

1 Although viral hepatitis may predispose to the development of cirrhosis, which in turn causes portal hypertension, most often it does not.
2 Kupffer cells are part of the reticuloendothelial system, which helps prevent infection and does not primarily affect venous pressure.
4 Obstruction of these ducts blocks the flow of bile, causing obstructive jaundice.

587. **4 In cirrhosis of the liver, fibrous scarring within the liver parenchyma, most often from alcohol toxicity, compresses the portal veins and causes a backup of blood and increased pressure within the portal system. Fluid seeps into the abdominal cavity (ascites), mainly from the surface of the liver. (AN; PA; GI)**
1 Lymph does not escape from the liver sinusoids.
2 Plasma osmotic (oncotic) pressure is decreased because of decreased albumin production.
3 Secretion of ADH and aldosterone increases as renal blood flow decreases.

588. **1 The bladder must be empty to decrease the chance of puncturing it during the paracentesis. (IM; TC; GI)**
2 This is not necessary.
3 Same as answer 2.
4 This is usually performed in the Fowler's position to assist the flow of fluid by gravity.

589. **1 The increased plasma hydrostatic pressure in the extremities resulting from heart failure or liver cirrhosis, possibly combined with a genetic weakness in the vein walls, may lead to varicose veins. (DC; PA; GI)**
2 Toxins are not responsible for varicose veins.
3 Distention of venous walls occurs as a result of increased rather than decreased pressure.
4 Decreased plasma protein causes fluid to move out of the vascular compartment into the interstitial spaces.

590. **2 Cirrhosis of the liver results in the development of extensive scar tissue within the liver structure; such scar tissue contracts around hepatic blood vessels, impeding blood flow and raising the pressure in the hepatic portal system. The physiologic response to slowly developing portal circulatory obstruction is the growth of collateral vessels linking portal veins with esophageal veins; as destruction progresses, the col-**

laterals become so large that they bulge into the esophageal lumen and are called esophageal varices. (DC; PA; GI)

1 Ascites and edema are the result of the pathophysiologic process in the liver, not the cause; the fluid is present in the interstitial spaces and abdominal cavity as a result of portal hypertension and decreased plasma protein.

3 The liver regenerates; but in the case of cirrhosis, scar tissue is formed.

4 The varicosities are the result of increased portal pressure.

591. **2 Gastric suctioning provides an estimate of the extent of bleeding but does not control it.** (AN; TC; GI)

1 Room temperature normal saline is instilled via a nasogastric tube to control hemorrhage; this promotes blood vessel constriction and prevents clot formation.

3 Balloon tamponade (Sengstaken-Blakemore tube) may be used to apply pressure against the bleeding varices.

4 Aminocaproic acid inhibits the fibrinolysis that may accompany hepatic cirrhosis.

592. **4 This tube has an esophageal balloon that on inflation exerts pressure, which retards hemorrhage.** (PL; TC; GI)

1 This is used for gastric decompression, gavage, or lavage; it has one lumen.

2 This is used for gastric decompression; it has two lumens, one for decompression and one for an air vent.

3 This is used for intestinal decompression.

593. **3 Neomycin destroys intestinal flora, which breaks down protein and in the process gives off ammonia. Ammonia at this time is poorly detoxified by the liver and can build up to toxic levels.** (IM; TC; GI)

1 Bile levels may be elevated because of biliary obstruction by the enlarged liver but are unaffected by Neomycin.

2 Urea is a by-product of protein metabolism formed in the liver as it detoxifies ammonia. The production of urea is hampered by severe liver damage and is unaffected by Neomycin.

4 Hemoglobin levels may be lowered as a result of cirrhosis and bleeding but are not increased by administration of Neomycin.

594. **2 Because protein breakdown gives off ammonia, which cannot be detoxified by the liver, protein should be eliminated from the diet.** (IM; TC; GI)

1 A Fleet enema would not affect ammonia levels, which are associated with hepatic coma; a Neomycin enema would limit intestinal bacteria, which breaks down protein, giving off ammonia.

3 No surgical intervention would affect ammonia levels associated with hepatic coma.

4 Carbohydrates are unrelated to protein breakdown and rising ammonia levels; eliminating carbohydrates would have no effect.

595. **3 An accumulation of nitrogenous wastes in hepatic coma affects the nervous system. Flapping tremors and generalized twitching occur in the second stage of this disease.** (DC; PA; GI)

1 The stool is often clay colored because of biliary obstruction by a cirrhotic liver.

2 Elevated cholesterol levels are not necessarily present.

4 As encephalopathy progresses to coma, all reflexes are absent.

596. **4 The temperature during steaming is never high enough or sustained long enough to kill organisms.** (IM; ED; GI)

1 Processing destroys the organisms.

2 Because of the extremely high temperature, broiling sufficiently destroys the virus.

3 Baking would destroy the organisms.

597. **1 Contacting hepatitis B through blood transfusions can be prevented by screening donors and testing the blood.** (PL; TC; GI)

2 This does not prevent transmission of hepatitis B.

3 Same as answer 2.

4 Same as answer 2.

598. **3 This is an enzyme, also known as glutamic-pyruvic transaminase, that is released early in the course of liver damage.** (DC; PA; GI)

1 This is not an early sign of liver damage.

2 Same as answer 1.

4 Same as answer 1.

599. 3 The virus is present in the stool of clients with hepatitis Type A, so special handling is required. The virus may also be present in the urine and in the nasotracheal secretions. (PL; TC; GI)

1 Hepatitis Type A is not usually transmitted via the air.
2 Bringing food to a client requires no precautions; however, disposable utensils should be used because the client's nasotracheal secretions contain the virus.
4 Same as answer 1.

600. 3 Hepatitis C, formerly called non-A, non-B hepatitis, is caused by an RNA virus that is transmitted parenterally. The incubation period is 5 to 10 weeks. (AN; PA; GI)

1. Hepatitis A, also known as infectious hepatitis, is caused by an RNA virus that is transmitted via the fecal-oral route. The incubation period is 2 to 6 weeks.
2 Hepatitis B is transmitted parenterally, sexually, and by direct contact with infected body secretions. The incubation period is 1 to 6 months.
4 Hepatitis D is a complication of hepatitis B.

601. 1 Because the liver is unable to detoxify ammonia to urea, protein intake should be further restricted when coma is inevitable. (PL; PA; GI)

2 This relatively high intake of protein will increase blood ammonia levels.
3 Same as answer 2.
4 Same as answer 2.

602. 2 The client's breath has a sweet odor because the liver is not metabolizing the amino acid methionine. (DC; PA; GI)

1 Anuria is characteristic of renal failure.
3 This refers to spasm of the eyelid associated with anxiety or cranial nerve pathology; it is unrelated to liver disease.
4 A sensation of a lump in the throat is associated with acute anxiety; it is unrelated to liver disease.

603. 1 Bile deposits will impart a yellowish tinge (jaundice or icterus) to the skin, often first observed in the sclerae. (DC; PA; GI)

2 Urticaria (or hives) is generally characteristic of an allergic response.
3 Uremic frost is characteristic of renal failure.
4 Hemangioma is a benign lesion composed of blood vessels.

604. 1 Increased ammonia levels indicate that the liver is unable to detoxify protein by-products. Neomycin reduces the amount of ammonia-forming bacteria in the intestines. (DC; PA; GI)

2 White blood cells may indicate infection; however, this would have no relationship to the need for Neomycin enemas.
3 Culture and sensitivity testing would identify the presence of a microorganism and the medication that would be effective in its eradication; it would not be indicated in cirrhosis.
4 Alanine aminotransferase (ALT), also called serum glutamic-pyruvic transaminase (SGPT), is a test to assess for liver disease but has no relationship to the need for Neomycin enemas.

605. 3 Weight is valuable objective information that can be helpful in determining the development or extent of ascites. (DC; TC; GI)

1 Diet history will not help in monitoring a client's condition.
2 Bowel sounds are objective data but do not help monitor the liver.
4 Pain is subjective.

606. 2 The liver stores carbohydrates as glycogen, which is a polymer of glucose. (DC; PA; GI)

1 Glycerol is a by-product of lipids and combines with three fatty acids to form triglyceride molecules.
3 Fat is not stored in the liver.
4 These are not a ready form of energy; combinations of amino acids form protein.

607. 1 Fatty acids are insoluble and must combine with bile to form water-soluble substances. (AN; PA; GI)

2 Lipase is a pancreatic enzyme.
3 Amylase, which digests starch, is found in saliva and pancreatic juice.
4 This is a component of bile. It is produced in the liver and stored in the gallbladder, but it is not the component of bile that emulsifies fats.

608. 4 The diet should be high in protein and calories, low in fat, and gluten free for individuals with malabsorption syndrome. Protein is needed for tissue rebuilding. (IM; TC; GI)

1 The client may prefer foods high in gluten, which would potentiate malabsorption.
2 IV therapy is a dependent function and does not provide all the necessary nutrients.

3 Diarrhea is caused by malabsorption, which accounts for the poor nutritional status; once the diarrhea is corrected, it is essential to compensate by providing a nutritious diet.

609. 4 Gluten, a cereal protein, appears to be responsible for morphologic changes of the intestinal mucosa in individuals with nontropical sprue (adult celiac disease). (EV; TC; GI)
1 Folic acid, along with antimicrobial agents, is used to treat tropical sprue; it causes dramatic improvement.
2 Vitamin B_{12} may be administered if macrocytic anemia or achlorhydria develops; however, it does not correct the major pathosis.
3 The use of corticosteroids may be advantageous with either form of sprue; however, this does not produce the same effect as specific treatments already described.

610. 4 Gluten is found in rye, wheat, and oat products. (PL; ED; GI)
1 Gluten is not found in these foods; they do not have to be avoided.
2 Same as answer 1.
3 Same as answer 1.

611. 1 These foods are low in gluten. (IM; TC; GI)
2 Flours used in the production of noodles are high in gluten.
3 Flours used in the production of bread are high in gluten.
4 Postum is a cereal drink high in gluten.

612. 3 A rectal catheter should be inserted approximately 15 cm to pass the rectal sphincters and reach where the gas accumulates. (IM; TC; GI)
1 An insertion to 5 centimeters will not allow the tube to pass the sphincters.
2 Although this may just pass the internal sphincter it will not reach the accumulated gas.
4 Deep insertion may damage the intestinal mucosa.

613. 3 Rebound tenderness is a classic subjective sign of appendicitis. (DC; PA; GI)
1 Urinary retention does not cause acute lower right quadrant pain.
2 Hyperacidity causes epigastric, not lower right quadrant, pain.
4 There is generally decreased bowel motility distal to an inflamed appendix.

614. 4 When circulation to the appendix is interfered with by a fecalith or foreign body, inflammation occurs. (AN; PA; GI)
1 Diet patterns do not predispose the individual to the development of appendicitis.
2 Bowel infections are rare and do not predispose the individual to the development of appendicitis.
3 Hypertension may cause generalized edema; local edema would not occur.

615. 4 Muscular rigidity over the affected area is a classic sign of peritonitis. (DC; TC; GI)
1 Malaise, rather than hyperactivity, is often associated with peritonitis.
2 Nausea is a common occurrence with peritonitis.
3 Urinary retention may occur following surgery, as a complication of anesthesia.

616. 2 The semi-Fowler's position aids in drainage and prevents spread of infection throughout the abdominal cavity. (IM; TC; GI)
1 The Sims' position is generally used for administration of enemas or rectal examination; it would not be helpful in draining the area.
3 The Trendelenburg position would contribute to the spread of infection throughout the abdominal cavity.
4 The dorsal recumbent position would not allow for localization of drainage.

617. 2 Paralytic ileus occurs when neurologic impulses are diminished, as from anesthesia, infection, or surgery. (EV; PA; GI)
1 Interference in blood supply would result in necrosis of the bowel.
3 Perforation of the bowel would result in pain and peritonitis.
4 Obstruction of the bowel lumen would initially cause increased peristalsis and bowel sounds.

618. 2 A rectal tube promotes maximum benefits in 30 minutes. This allows adequate time for gas to escape. (IM; TC; GI)
1 Fifteen minutes is not adequate time to permit removal of flatus.
3 After 30 minutes there would be minimal release of flatus.
4 Same as answer 3.

619. **1 The client's status requires immediate intervention; to delay treatment may prove dangerous because symptoms indicate possible perforation. (AN; TC; GI)**
  2 Diverticulitis can in most cases be treated by diet, rest, and antibiotic therapy.
  3 This is not true with the diagnostic techniques presently available.
  4 Age is not the factor; the symptoms indicate possible peritonitis.

620. **3 *Entamoeba histolytica*, the organism that causes amebic dysentery, is transmitted through excreta. (PL; PA; GI)**
  1 This is not a tick-borne disease.
  2 This organism is not transmitted by gnats.
  4 This organism is not transmitted via milk.

621. **3 Intussusception is the telescoping or prolapse of a segment of the bowel within the lumen of an immediately connecting part. (IM; ED; GI)**
  1 Volvulus is a twisting of the bowel onto itself.
  2 Adhesions are bands of scar tissue that can compress the bowel.
  4 Herniation is the term that describes protrusion of an organ through the wall that contains it.

622. **4 Emotional stress of any kind can stimulate peristalsis and thereby increase the volume of drainage. (PL; PA; GI)**
  1 The client should be encouraged to eat a diet as normal as possible.
  2 Ileostomy drainage is liquefied and continuous, so irrigations are not indicated.
  3 The stoma will start to drain within the first 24 hours after surgery.

623. **2 Vitamin B$_{12}$ (extrinsic factor) combines with intrinsic factor, a substance secreted by the parietal cells of the gastric mucosa, forming hemopoietic factor. Hemopoietic factor is only absorbed in the ileum, from which it travels to bone marrow and stimulates erythropoiesis. (EV; PA; GI)**
  1 Folic acid is not absorbed in the terminal ileum.
  3 Iron absorption does not occur in the ileum.
  4 Trace elements are not absorbed in the ileum.

624. **2 Trauma to the abdominal wall and to the stoma should be avoided, so contact sports are contraindicated. (PL; TC; GI)**
  1 Trauma to the abdominal wall is a minimal risk in this sport.

  3 Same as answer 1.
  4 Same as answer 1.

625. **4 Personality and psychologic stresses cause pathologic changes that influence the development of ulcerative colitis. (DC; PA; GI)**
  1 Although this may be another causative factor, psychologic stress is more commonly associated with this disease.
  2 Same as answer 1.
  3 Same as answer 1.

626. **4 Because the mucosa of the intestinal tract is damaged, its ability to absorb vitamins taken orally is greatly impaired. (IM; PA; GI)**
  1 Although this is true, the risks associated with IV administration will outweigh the benefits unless other factors are considered.
  2 Vitamins are effective orally unless there is disease involving the GI tract that hampers absorption.
  3 IV vitamins do not decrease colonic irritability.

627. **1 To take advantage of the anatomic position of the sigmoid colon and the effect of gravity, the client should be placed in a left Sims' position for the enema. (IM; TC; GI)**
  2 This position does not facilitate the flow of fluid into the sigmoid colon by gravity.
  3 Same as answer 2.
  4 Same as answer 2.

628. **3 Milk and the caffeine in cola are chemically irritating to the intestinal mucosa. They also promote secretion of gastric juice. (IM; ED; GI)**
  1 Salt helps retain water and rice produces bulk, both of which promote motility.
  2 This is too general; except for those that contain lactose sugars, products containing sugar generally are not irritating to the mucosa; protein also is not irritating.
  4 These are absorbed slowly and are not irritating.

629. **3 Glucocorticoids and acetylcholine tend to increase peristalsis, causing cramping and diarrhea with subsequent weight loss. As ulceration occurs, loss of blood leads to anemia. (DC; PA; GI)**
  1 Leukocytosis or increased leukocytes in the blood is not common in this disease.

2 Hemoptysis (coughing up blood from the respiratory tract) is not a related symptom.

4 Fever may or may not be a symptom and leukopenia (deficiency in number of leukocytes) does not occur.

630. **4 Occult blood in the stool could indicate active bleeding; the stool should also be examined for microorganisms to detect early infections that could easily become systemic by spread through the damaged intestinal mucosa. (AN; PA; GI)**

1 There is no indication that parasites are present; the situation does not warrant this examination.

2 This situation does not warrant culturing.

3 This situation does not warrant these examinations.

631. **3 As a result of chronic irritation, the colon becomes thin and may perforate. (DC; TC; GI)**

1 Paralytic ileus may be a complication of surgical interventions involving the intestines or of perforation.

2 Bleeding may vary from a small amount to hemorrhage; this is not the most serious complication.

4 Obstruction rarely occurs, but if it does it is not the most serious complication.

632. **4 This is a low-residue diet and is necessary in the acute phase of ulcerative colitis to prevent irritation of the colon. (EV; ED; GI)**

1 Milk contains lactose, which is irritating to the colon and contraindicated in colitis.

2 The juice in this diet contains cellulose, which is not absorbed and irritates the colon; cream soup contains lactose, which is irritating to the colon.

3 Same as answer 1.

633. **1 When the diseased bowel is removed, the client's symptoms cease. (AN; TC; GI)**

2 Surgical removal of a body part is not temporary, but permanent.

3 Ulcerative colitis is unrelated to Crohn's disease; clients with ulcerative colitis have an increased risk for colorectal cancer.

4 This is not a true statement.

634. **3 The location of the tumor will usually indicate whether a colostomy, creation of an opening proximal to the tumor between the colon and the skin surface, is needed. (AN; TC; GI)**

1 An ileostomy is the creation of an opening between the ileum and the skin surface; it would not be done.

2 A colectomy is the surgical removal of a portion of the colon, with creation of an anastomosis; it is generally used in less extensive carcinoma.

4 A cecostomy is the creation of an opening between the cecum and the skin surface; it is usually a temporary procedure.

635. **1 Neomycin sulfate is poorly absorbed from the GI tract and is therefore used for sterilization of the intestines prior to bowel surgery. (IM; TC; GI)**

2 Because intestinal bacteria are destroyed, there is a decreased production of vitamin K.

3 Oral administration of Neomycin primarily affects intestinal bacteria.

4 Because it is poorly absorbed from the GI tract, Neomycin sulfate does not affect urinary tract infections.

636. **3 Because Neomycin is poorly absorbed from the GI tract, most remains in the intestines and exerts its antibiotic effect on the intestinal mucosa. In preparation for GI surgery the level of microbial organisms will be reduced. (AN; TC; GI)**

1 Neomycin is nephrotoxic.

2 Because it is poorly absorbed from the GI tract, the systemic effect is minimal.

4 Neomycin is mainly effective in suppression of intestinal bacteria.

637. **3 A skin barrier such as Stomahesive provides a protective coating that provides a barrier to gastrointestinal enzymes and protects against allergic reactions to the tape on the appliance. (IM; TC; GI)**

1 Alcohol tends to dry out the skin and mucous membranes, leading to irritation and breakdown.

2 Mineral oil is not an effective skin protectant and could interfere with adherence of any appliance.

4 This contains alcohol, which is drying and leads to skin irritation.

638. **2 The client must be ready to accept changes in body image and function; this acceptance will facilitate mastery of the techniques of colostomy care, special diets, and optimal use of community resources. (AN; PS; GI)**
    1 Specific knowledge can be imparted only when an individual is ready to learn; it requires acceptance of a new body image.
    3 Same as answer 1.
    4 Same as answer 1.

639. **2 Ample time in the bathroom must be ensured for the actual irrigation process and fecal returns, which may not be immediate. (PL; ED; GI)**
    1 The availability of adequate time takes precedence; this would not use the gastrocolic reflex that would occur after eating
    3 This is important, but the availability of adequate time takes precedence.
    4 Same as answer 1.

640. **4 The rapid rate of enema administration or ostomy irrigation often causes cramping. Additional fluid leads to more discomfort. Cramping will generally subside if the enema tubing is clamped for a few minutes; the procedure can then be continued. (IM; TC; GI)**
    1 Discontinuing the irrigation could lead to ineffective evacuation of the colon.
    2 Lowering the container will decrease the rate of flow, but fluid will continue to enter the colon if the container remains above the stoma.
    3 Indiscriminate advancing of the catheter can injure the mucosa and does not affect cramping.

641. **2 This is far enough to direct the flow of solution into the bowel. (IM; TC; GI)**
    1 This is inadequate; fluid may leak back around the catheter.
    3 An insertion of 15 cm may cause trauma to the mucosa.
    4 An insertion of 20 cm may cause trauma to the mucosa.

642. **4 A colostomy irrigation is much like a tap water enema. The solution must be held high enough to allow it to flow into the bowel but not so high that it flows rapidly, or it can cause cramping or mucosal injury. (IM; ED; GI)**

1 This does not represent maximum height permitted and may not ensure flow of solution into the bowel.
2 Same as answer 1.
3 Same as answer 1.

643. **3 The stoma of a colostomy must be dilated with a lubricated, gloved finger to prevent strictures and subsequent obstruction. (IM; ED; GI)**
    1 Clothing need not be special but should be nonconstricting.
    2 Once healing has occurred, activity is not limited.
    4 Diet should be as close to normal for the individual as possible; gas-forming foods should be avoided.

644. **4 Although foods that produce gas are generally avoided, the diet of an individual with a colostomy should be as close to normal as possible for optimal physiologic and psychologic adaptation. (PL; PA; GI)**
    1 A high-protein diet is important until healing occurs; but a balanced diet generally meets nutritional needs for protein.
    2 There is no need to limit fiber; it provides bulk necessary for unconstipated stools.
    3 Because absorption of nutrients is unaffected, there is no need to increase carbohydrate intake.

645. **2 Isotonic saline most closely resembles normal body fluids; it will not cause an imbalance by pulling extra fluids and electrolytes out of the circulation. (IM; TC; GI)**
    1 Hypotonic solutions would allow absorption of fluid into the circulation, resulting in dilution of electrolytes and possible circulatory overload.
    3 Same as answer 1.
    4 Hypertonic solutions would draw fluids out of the circulation into the GI tract; glucose provides a medium for bacterial growth.

646. **4 A transverse colostomy is an opening created in the transverse colon. The rectal tube should be pointed to the proximal intestine to evacuate the bowels. (IM; TC; GI)**
    1 A water-soluble lubricant is generally used to facilitate insertion.
    2 There are no sphincters so bearing down is unnecessary.
    3 Continual force may traumatize the mucosa; lack of nerve endings diminishes sensation.

647. **3 Hernioplasty involves not only the reduction of a hernia but also an attempt to change or strengthen the structure to prevent recurrence. (AN; PA; GI)**
1 Analysis of the word shows that it means an opening cut into the hernia; it does not refer to repair of a hernia.
2 There is no such word; hernias are not cut out. They are reduced and the area reinforced to prevent recurrence.
4 Herniorrhaphy is surgical repair of a hernia.

648. **2 Bowel training is a program for the development of a conditioned reflex that controls regular emptying of the bowel. The key to success in a conditioning program is adherence to a strict time for evacuation based on the client's individual schedule. (PL; TC; GI)**
1 The indiscriminate use of laxatives can result in dependency.
3 Although this should be considered, the cerebrovascular accident affects the responses of the client by altering motility, peristalsis, and sphincter control despite adherence to previous habits.
4 The passage of food into the stomach does stimulate peristalsis but is only one factor that should be considered when planning a specific time for evacuation.

649. **4 Rectal bleeding is a common problem when hemorrhoids are present. (DC; TC; GI)**
1 Pruritus is not a symptom that can be observed.
2 Flatulence is unrelated to hemorrhoids.
3 Anal stenosis is not a complication of hemorrhoids.

650. **1 Constipation and prolonged standing may cause this problem. (IM; ED; GI)**
2 Hypertension does not contribute to the development of hemorrhoids.
3 Spicy foods may irritate hemorrhoids but do not cause them.
4 Bowel control is unrelated to the development of hemorrhoids.

651. **4 A low-residue diet limits stool formation. (PL; PA; GI)**
1 Bland diets are usually employed in the management of upper, not lower, GI disturbances.
2 Although a clear diet is low in residue, it does not meet normal nutritional needs.
3 A high-protein diet is indicated postoperatively to promote healing.

652. **3 The client must be advised to avoid straining and constipation; stool softeners are widely used. (IM; TC; GI)**
1 Light dressings of witch hazel may be used to promote drainage and healing.
2 Baths are advised to promote healing and cleaning of the area.
4 Enemas may be ordered several days after surgery if the client has not had a bowel movement.

653. **2 Because stomach distention after eating results in contractions of the colon (gastrocolic reflex) promoting defecation, establishing some regularity of meals that includes adequate bulk or fiber will help establish routine patterns of defecation. (IM; ED; GI)**
1 Although increased fluid intake and activity facilitate elimination, in general they do not help establish a pattern.
3 Same as answer 1.
4 Increased potassium is not needed for normal elimination.

654. **3 Fiber absorbs water, swells, and consequently stretches the bowel wall, promoting peristalsis, mass movements, and defecation. Smooth muscle tends to contract when stretched because of the reflex activity of stretch receptors. (IM; ED; GI)**
1 Bulk caused by fiber does not irritate the bowel wall.
2 Bacterial action is not involved in the process by which bulk stimulates defecation.
4 There is no chemical stimulation.

655. **3 Because of the presence of feces in the colon, a client with a fecal impaction has the urge to defecate but is unable to. (DC; TC; GI)**
1 Flatulence may occur as a result of immobility, not just obstruction.
2 Anorexia may occur with an impaction but may also be caused by other conditions.
4 The frequency of bowel movements varies for individuals; it may be normal for this individual not to have a BM for several days.

MEDICAL-SURGICAL ANSWERS

656. 2 When the bowel is impacted with hardened feces, there is often seepage of liquid feces around the obstruction and thus uncontrolled diarrhea. (DC; PA; GI)

1 The bowel may become distended if completely obstructed, but this is a late symptom if it occurs at all.
3 This is indicative of lower GI bleeding.
4 There are often frequent liquid bowel movements in the presence of an impaction.

657. 3 Prune juice and warm water can be administered prophylactically by the nurse to promote defecation. Prune juice irritates the bowel mucosa, stimulating peristalsis. Increased fiber in the diet may also improve intestinal motility. (IM; TC; GI)

1 The routine use of enemas should be avoided because they promote dependency and can result in electrolyte imbalance.
2 The routine use of laxatives promotes dependency.
4 Same as answer 1.

Neuromuscular

658. 2 Hemiplegia is paralysis of one side of the body. (AN; PA; NM)

1 Paresis is a weakness or partial paralysis.
3 Paraplegia is the paralysis of both lower extremities and the lower trunk.
4 This is quadriplegia.

659. 2 The ache in muscles that have been vigorously worked without adequate oxygen supply is caused in part by the buildup of lactic acid. During rest the lactic acid is oxidized completely to carbon dioxide and water, providing ATP for further muscular contraction. (AN; PA; NM)

1 Acetone is not a product of muscle contraction; it is a ketone body and a by-product of acetoacetic acid metabolism.
3 Butyric acid is not a product of muscle contraction; it is a fatty acid occurring in feces, urine, and perspiration.
4 Acetoacetic acid is not a product of muscle contraction; it is a ketone body resulting from incomplete oxidation of fatty acids. It is also produced by the metabolism of lipids and pyruvates.

660. 2 Vagal stimulation slows the heart. The vagus is the principal nerve of the parasympathetic portion of the autonomic nervous system, and its axon terminals release acetylcholine. The response of the viscera to acetylcholine varies, but in general the organ is in a relaxed state. (DC; PA; NM)

1 This is an action of the sympathetic nervous system (accelerator nerve) caused by the release of norepinephrine.
3 Stimulation of the sympathetic nervous system dilates bronchioles in the lungs; the vagus nerve constricts them.
4 There are no parasympathetic fibers to the coronary blood vessels; sympathetic impulses dilate these vessels.

661. 1 The thalamus associates sensory impulses with feelings of pleasantness and unpleasantness; therefore it is partly responsible for emotions. The cortical limbic system is also involved in expression of emotions. (AN; PA; NM)

2 This is located in the cerebrum and controls all conscious functions.
3 This controls body temperature and serves as a neural pathway.
4 This is the outer layer of the cerebrum and controls mental functions.

662. 2 The arteries communicating (anastomosing) at the base of the brain are referred to as the circle of Willis. (AN; PA; NM)

1 This is an anastomosis of blood vessels that is located in the palm of the hand.
3 This is a nerve communication network in the region of the neck and axilla.
4 This is a single large branch of the aorta.

663. 3 The medulla, part of the brainstem just above the foramen magnum, is concerned with vital functions. (AN; PA; NM)

1 Sexual development is controlled by the hypothalamus (through releasing hormones) and the pituitary at puberty.
2 Voluntary movements are mediated through the somatomotor area of the frontal cerebral lobe. The opercular-insular area of the parietal cerebral lobe is concerned with taste sensations.
4 Temperature and water balance are controlled by the hypothalamus; fat metabolism is unrelated to the medulla.

664. 3 The Schwann cells that comprise the neurilemma of peripheral nerve fibers (dendrites and axons) are capable of supporting nerve fiber regeneration. (AN; PA; NM)

1 These are not involved in regeneration.

2 Same as answer 1.

4 The myelin sheath, produced peripherally by the Schwann cells and centrally by the oligodendrocytes, is not involved directly in the regenerative process.

665. **4 Lesions affecting the seventh cranial (facial) nerve cause paralysis of the eyelids. (DC; PA; NM)**

1 The optic nerve is concerned with vision; lesions result in visual field defects and loss of visual acuity.

2 The oculomotor nerve is concerned with pupillary constriction and eye movements; lesions result in ptosis, strabismus, and diplopia.

3 The trochlear nerve is concerned with eye movements; lesions result in diplopia, strabismus, and head tilt to the affected side.

666. **2 The third cranial (oculomotor) nerve contains autonomic fibers that innervate the smooth muscle responsible for constriction of the pupils. (DC; PA; NM)**

1 The optic nerve is concerned with vision; lesions result in visual field defects and loss of visual acuity.

3 The trochlear nerve is concerned with eye movements; lesions result in diplopia, strabismus, and head tilt to the affected side.

4 The facial nerve is concerned with facial expressions; lesions result in loss of taste and paralysis of the facial muscles and the eyelids (lids remain open).

667. **1 The facial nerve (seventh cranial) has motor and sensory functions. The motor function is concerned with facial movement, including smiling and pursing the lips. Nonconduction of the 7th nerve will cause drooping on the side of the problem. (DC; PA; NM)**

2 Nonconduction of the facial nerve on the right side would cause that side of the face to droop.

3 Nonconduction of the left abducent nerve would prevent abduction of the left eye.

4 Nonconduction of the trigeminal nerve would cause problems in mastication.

668. **4 Anterior horn neurons are also known as lower motoneurons. Their cell bodies are located in the anterior gray columns and are part of the reflex arc. (EV; PA; NM)**

1 Basal ganglia are islands of gray matter in each cerebral hemisphere; they are not part of the reflex arc.

2 Pyramidal tracts are motor nerve pathways from the brain that pass down the spinal cord to motor cells in the anterior horn; they are not part of the reflex arc.

3 Upper motoneurons are neurons in the cerebral cortex that conduct impulses to the spinal cord or the motor nuclei of the cerebral nerves.

669. **4 This is the space between the arachnoid and the pia mater. It is filled with cerebrospinal fluid. (IM; TC; NM)**

1 This is the innermost of the three meninges covering the brain and spinal cord.

2 This is an opening in the atrial septum in the fetal heart.

3 This is the cerebral aqueduct, between the third and fourth ventricles, in the midbrain.

670. **2 The cerebellum coordinates muscular activity and promotes balance. The other brain regions govern motor, sensory, and higher integrative functions. (AN; PA; NM)**

1 This controls conscious recognition of pain, temperature, and crude touch and pressure.

3 This is involved in temperature regulation; it controls and integrates the autonomic nervous system; it is the intermediary between the nervous and endocrine systems; it is associated with feelings of rage and aggression.

4 This controls the heartbeat, blood pressure, and reflexes such as vomiting and coughing.

671. **4 One of the centers for reflex control of respiration is in the medulla. Another important reflex respiratory center is in the pons. The other brain regions—cerebral cortex, hypothalamus, and cerebellum—may influence respiration but not so directly as the centers in the medulla and pons. (AN; PA; NM)**

1 This is the center for coordination and equilibrium.

2 This controls and integrates the higher autonomic functions; it influences respiration but not so directly as the centers in the medulla and pons.

3 This is the center of control for all conscious functions.

MEDICAL-SURGICAL **ANSWERS**

672. **3 Although sympathetic impulses usually control most visceral effectors in times of stress, parasympathetic fibers likewise stimulate increased gastric contractions and increased peristalsis. Sympathetic fibers also inhibit organs such as the bladder and cause relaxation of this organ. (AN; PA; NM)**
1 This statement is accurate.
2 Same as answer 1.
4 Same as answer 1.

673. **1 The thalamus receives sensory impulses from the spinothalamic tract and relays them to the cerebral cortex. (AN; PA; NM)**
2 The cerebellum is involved in motor activity and coordination.
3 The hypothalamus relays messages between the cortex and autonomic centers.
4 The medulla contains the vital respiratory, cardiac, and vasomotor centers.

674. **4 The autonomic nervous system functions to regulate visceral effectors and maintain internal equilibrium. (AN; PA; NM)**
1 The spinal cord transmits impulses from the periphery to the brain and from the brain to the periphery; it also integrates reflexes.
2 The CNS is concerned with overall control; it consists of the brain and spinal cord.
3 The peripheral nervous system conveys information from peripheral receptors to the central nervous system and information from the CNS to muscles and glands.

675. **2 Only axon terminals secrete acetylcholine, so nerve impulse propagation occurs in one direction only: from axon terminal to dendrite or cell body of the next neuron, or from axon terminal to effector organ (muscle or gland). (AN; PA; NM)**
1 Polarization refers to the resting potential of the neuron when one side of the membrane is negatively and the other side positively charged.
3 This refers to the active movement of sodium ions into the cell and back across the membrane to the opposite side, which promotes transmission of this impulse but does not affect the direction of the impulse.
4 Cholinesterase acts only at the synapse, inactivating acetylcholine at the myoneural junction.

676. **3 Axon terminals release acetylcholine at the myoneural junctions. As acetyl-**
choline contacts the sarcolemma, it stimulates the muscle fiber to contract. (AN; PA; NM)
1 ATP is not produced by axons; it is a nucleotide that gives off energy when it loses a phosphate radical.
2 Epinephrine is produced by the adrenal medulla and released by axons of the autonomic nervous system.
4 Cholinesterase is released by muscle cells to inactivate acetylcholine.

677. **4 Parasympathetic nerves increase peristalsis and secretion of gastric hydrochloric acid. (DC; PA; NM)**
1 The parasympathetic nervous system increases intestinal motility, which would result in diarrhea.
2 Goosebumps (piloerection), caused by contraction of the musculi arrectores pilorum, are under sympathetic control; vasoconstriction is also under sympathetic control.
3 Epinephrine is a sympathomimetic.

678. **2 Sensory impulses from temperature, touch, and pain travel via the spinothalamic pathway to the thalamus and then to the postcentral gyrus of the parietal lobe, the somatosensory area. (AN; PA; NM)**
1 This is the area of abstract thinking and muscular movements.
3 This is the area where nerve impulses are translated into sight.
4 This is the area where nerve impulses are translated into sound.

679. **3 REM (rapid eye movement) sleep is necessary for psychologic coping. The nurse should be aware that some medications affect this sleep stage and thereby alter emotional health. (AN; PA; NM)**
1 The individual is just drifting off to sleep; alpha brain waves are present.
2 The individual is in a deep sleep and is difficult to arouse; delta brain waves predominate; stages 1 and 4 are associated with physiologic rest.
4 The individual is in a light sleep and can be readily wakened; delta waves are interspersed with alpha waves; stages 1, 2, 3, and 4 are called non-REM sleep.

680. **1 Cold reduces the sensitivity of receptors for pain in the skin. In addition, local blood vessels constrict, limiting the amount of interstitial fluid and its related pressure and discomfort. (EV; TC; NM)**

2 Local blood vessels constrict.

3 Local cold applications do not depress vital signs.

4 Local cold applications increase blood viscosity.

681. **2 The sympathetic nervous system constricts the smooth muscle of blood vessels in the skin when a person is under stress. (DC; PA; NM)**

1 The sympathetic system stimulates rather than inhibits secretion by the sweat glands.

3 The parasympathetic system (vagus nerve) slows the pulse, and the sympathetic increases it.

4 This is not under sympathetic control; the parasympathetic system constricts the pupils.

682. **4 The brachial plexus is a maze of nerves extending from the axilla to the neck in the shoulder area; trauma to the arm may also injure this plexus. (AN; TC; NM)**

1 The solar plexus, also known as the celiac plexus, is where the splanchnic nerves terminate; it is unrelated to the arms.

2 The celiac plexus (solar plexus) is where the splanchnic nerves terminate; it is unrelated to the arms.

3 The basilar plexus is a venous plexus over the basilar part of the occipital bone; it is unrelated to the arms.

683. **1 This may occur after hypothermia because of slowed cerebral metabolic processes. (DC; TC; NM)**

2 Pallor, not erythema, would be present as a result of peripheral vasoconstriction.

3 Drowsiness occurs; the client is unable to focus on anxiety-producing aspects of the situation.

4 Respirations would be lowered.

684. **4 If there is no obstruction, pressure on the jugular vein causes increased intracranial pressure. This, in turn, causes an increase in spinal fluid pressure. (DC; PA; NM)**

1 Homans' sign is calf pain elicited by dorsiflexion of the foot if thrombophlebitis is present.

2 Romberg's sign is failure to maintain balance when the eyes are closed; indicates cerebellar pathology.

3 Chvostek's sign is twitching elicited by tapping the angle of the jaw if hypocalcemia is present.

685. **1 *Toxoplasma gondii*, a protozoan, can be transmitted by exposure to infected cat feces or ingestion of undercooked contaminated meat. (IM; PA; NM)**

2 Toxoplasmosis is not related to heavy metals.

3 *Toxoplasma gondii* is a parasite of warm-blooded animals; fish are not considered the source of contamination.

4 Toxoplasmosis is not related to radiation.

686. **2 Toxins from the bacillus invade nervous tissue; respiratory spasms may result in respiratory failure. (DC; PA; NM)**

1 Muscular rigidity can occur; however, this generalized condition is not life threatening.

3 These subjective symptoms are not life threatening.

4 Voluntary muscles may contract because of toxins from the bacillus; however, this is not life threatening.

687. **4 Painful pharyngeal spasms when swallowing or even looking at water are responsible for the use of the term hydrophobia to refer to rabies. (DC; PA; NM)**

1 The central nervous system is affected; diarrhea is not a concern.

2 Memory is not affected by this disease.

3 Urinary stasis is not a potential problem; catheterization can be employed.

688. **3 Infections of cranial structures can cause meningitis because bacteria travel by direct anatomical route to the meninges and cerebral spinal fluid (CSF). (AN; PA; NM)**

1 This part of the body does not come into contact with CSF.

2 Same as answer 1.

4 Same as answer 1.

689. **3 Pain and temperature sensations enter the posterior horns of the spinal cord, cross to the contralateral side, and travel upward via the spinothalamic tracts to the thalamus. There they synapse with other sensory neurons for transmission to the cortex. (AN; PA; NM)**

1 These are descending motor tracts. The lateral tracts facilitate impulse transmission to the skeletal muscles; the medial tracts inhibit transmission to the skeletal muscles.

2 The location of the fasciculus gracilis, which is involved with pressure sensation.

4 These are ascending tracts. They conduct impulses of crude touch, pain, and temperature.

MEDICAL-SURGICAL   ANSWERS

690. 3 Electrodes are attached to sensory nerves or over the dorsal column; a transmitter is worn externally and, by electric stimulation, may be used to interfere with the transmission of painful stimuli as needed. (IM; ED; NM)

1 Clients may bathe when the transmitter is disconnected.
2 The client may need analgesics in conjunction with the transmitter.
4 The device should not interfere with a remote control apparatus.

691. 1 A rhizotomy is the resection of posterior nerve roots to eliminate nerve impulses associated with severe pain from the thoracic area (as in lung cancer). (IM; TC; NM)

2 A rhinotomy is an incision into the nose.
3 A cordotomy is the surgical interruption of pain-conducting pathways in the spinal cord.
4 A chondrectomy is the surgical excision of a cartilage.

692. 4 The exact nature of the pain must be determined to distinguish whether this is pain caused by the surgery or is from some other cause. (DC; PA; NM)

1 This should be done later but the first action would be to determine the nature of the pain.
2. Same as answer 1.
3. Prescribed analgesics would be given after determining the exact nature of the pain.

693. 2 The dendrites of the cochlear nerve terminate on the hair cells of the organ of Corti in the cochlea. (AN; PA; NM)

1 The utricle is a membranous sac that communicates with the semicircular canals of the ear.
3 The middle ear contains bones (malleus, incus, stapes).
4 This is the part of the middle ear that contains the auditory ossicles; it is the area between the tympanic membrane and the bony labyrinth.

694. 3 The bones in the middle ear transmit and amplify air pressure waves from the tympanic membrane to the oval window of the cochlea, which is in the inner ear. The tympanic membrane separates the outer from the middle ear. (AN; PA; NM)

1 The organ of Corti, cochlea, and semicircular canals are found in the inner ear.
2 The outer ear consists of the pinna and outer ear canal.
4 This connects the middle ear and nasopharynx; it helps maintain the balance of air pressure.

695. 2 Because the organ of hearing is the organ of Corti, located in the cochlea, nerve deafness would most likely accompany damage to the cochlear nerve. (DC; PA; NM)

1 The vagus nerve would affect voice production.
3 The vestibular nerve would affect balance.
4 The trigeminal nerve would affect chewing movements.

696. 4 The labyrinth is the inner ear and consists of the vestibule, cochlea, semicircular canals, utricle, saccule, cochlear duct, and membranous semicircular canals. A labyrinthectomy is performed to alleviate the symptom of vertigo but results in deafness, because the organ of Corti and cochlear nerve are located in the inner ear. (EV; TC; NM)

1 Anosmia is loss of the sense of smell and would not be affected by surgery to the ear.
2 There is no pain associated with Ménière's syndrome.
3 Ménière's syndrome is not related to cerumen production.

697. 2 With a partial hearing loss the auditory ossicles have not yet become fixed; as long as vibrations occur a hearing aid may be beneficial. (AN; PA; NM)

1 When what is heard is useless or if there is total hearing loss then this procedure may be performed.
3 Although the base tones are particularly affected, all tones are affected.
4 With conduction hearing loss, bone conduction is more effective than air conduction.

698. 4 A subjective symptom such as ringing in the ears can be felt only by the client. (DC; PA; NM)

1 An objective symptom refers to signs that can be assessed through direct physical examination.
2 This term is not generally used to describe a symptom; a functional disease is one in which there is alteration in the ability to perform as intended without physiologic changes.
3 Prodromal refers to symptoms that are early indications of a developing disease; there is insufficient information to decide this from the situation described.

699. 3 The middle ear contains the three ossicles—malleus, incus, and stapes—which,

with the tympanic membrane and oval window, form an amplifying system. (AN; PA; NM)

1 The inner ear contains both the organ of hearing (the cochlea) and the organ of balance (the vestibule).

2 The pressure of sound waves is amplified in the middle ear and transmitted to the cochlea (inner ear), where it is detected by the organ of Corti and transmitted along the acoustic nerve.

4 Normally the eustachian tube, which connects the middle ear and nasopharynx, is closed and flat to prevent organisms from entering the middle ear; however, it allows air into the middle ear and thus equalizes pressure on both sides of the eardrum.

700. **4 Vitamin A is used in the formation of retinene, a component of the light-sensitive rhodopsin molecule. (AN; PA; NM)**

1 Melanin is a pigment of the skin.

2 Vitamin A does not influence color vision, which is centered in the cones.

3 The cornea is a transparent part of the anterior portion of the sclera; a cataract is an opacity of the normally transparent crystalline lens. Vitamin A does not prevent cataracts.

701. **3 The optic chiasm is the point of crossover of some optic nerve fibers in the cranial cavity at the base of the brain. The optic tracts conduct nerve impulses from the optic chiasm to other brain regions. (AN; PA; NM)**

1 The orbit is the cavity in which the eyeball is fixed.

2 Optic tracts conduct nerve impulses from the optic chiasm.

4 This is the vitreous body.

702. **2 The contraction permits the lens to return to its normal bulge, decreasing focal length and allowing focus on near objects. (AN; PA; NM)**

1 The ciliary muscles are intrinsic (within the eyeball); the third cranial nerve (oculomotor), an extrinsic nerve, controls movements of the eyelid.

3 In this case the ciliary muscles would relax.

4 The rectus and oblique muscles of the eye are involved in convergence.

703. **1 Glaucoma is a disease in which there is increased intraocular pressure resulting from narrowing of the aqueous outflow channel (canal of Schlemm). This can**

lead to blindness, caused by compression of the nutritive blood vessels supplying the rods and cones. (AN; PA; NM)

2 Intraocular pressure is not affected by activity of the eye.

3 Pupil dilation increases intraocular pressure because it narrows the canal of Schlemm.

4 Although secondary infections are not desirable, the priority is to maintain vision.

704. **1 Eye medications are applied directly to the eye. (IM; TC; NM)**

2 This route is not used for ocular medications.

3 Intraocular drugs are given by an ophthalmologist for severe infections.

4 Same as answer 2.

705. **1 Sedatives have no effect on the intraocular pressure. (EV; ED; NM)**

2 Additional teaching is not necessary; this should be avoided as it would raise the intraocular pressure.

3 Same as answer 2.

4 Same as answer 2.

706. **3 Because continued use of eyedrops is indicated, an extra supply should always be available. (IM; ED; NM)**

1 Although it is important to avoid constipation because straining may increase intraocular pressure, laxatives should not be taken on a routine basis.

2 Eyewashes (collyria) have no effect on the disease.

4 Corrective lenses do not need to be checked this frequently.

707. **3 Open-angle glaucoma has an insidious onset, with increased intraocular pressure causing pressure on the retina and blood vessels in the eye. Peripheral vision is decreased as the visual field progressively diminishes. (DC; PA; NM)**

1 This may occur with untreated acute angle closure glaucoma.

2 Pain occurs in acute angle closure, not open-angle glaucoma.

4 Occlusions of the central retinal artery would cause a sudden loss of vision.

MEDICAL-SURGICAL ANSWERS

708. **1 In glaucoma the intraocular pressure is elevated and must be returned to normal. (IM; ED; NM)**
2 Resting has no effect on this condition, for it will not decrease the pressure.
3 Dilation of the pupils may further increase the pressure by obstructing the canal of Schlemm; increased pressure reduces the visual field and leads to blindness.
4 Glaucoma does not lead to secondary infections.

709. **1 A cataract is a clouding of the crystalline lens or its capsule. (DC; PA; NM)**
2 This is not included in the pathophysiology related to cataracts.
3 Same as answer 2.
4 Same as answer 2.

710. **4 Activities such as rigorous brushing of hair and teeth cause increased intraocular pressure and may lead to hemorrhage in the anterior chamber. (IM; TC; NM)**
1 Coughing and deep breathing can increase intraocular pressure.
2 Weakening of the eye musculature is not related to cataracts.
3 This is unnecessary; cataract removal is usually done in the ambulatory surgery unit. Once stabilized, the client is generally discharged.

711. **4 Retinal detachment is a separation between the sensory retina and the retinal pigment epithelium. These layers are not attached by any special structures and can separate as a result of various pathologic processes. (AN; PA; NM)**
1 This statement does not explain the disease process involved.
2 Same as answer 1.
3 Same as answer 1.

712. **4 Scar formation seals the hole and promotes attachment of the two retinal surfaces. (AN; TC; NM)**
1 The retina is part of the nervous system; it does not regenerate or grow new cells.
2 The sclera is not involved; the retina adjoins and is nourished by the choroid.
3 This is not the treatment used; treatment includes the formation of a scar by the use of lasers or surgical "buckling."

713. **2 Proximity to the nurses' station is vital. The client must be observed frequently, because behavior is unpredictable. (IM; TC; NM)**
1 The client may be unable to ambulate safely to the bathroom; this choice does not indicate proximity of the room to the nurses' station.
3 Sharing a room with another client would disturb the other client.
4 Sharing a room with another client would disturb the other client; a room far from the nurses' station would prevent close observation.

714. **3 Librium is an antianxiety agent ordered to reduce the response to psychomotor stimuli. (AN; TC; NM)**
1 Emotional problems are masked, not resolved, by antianxiety agents.
2 Detoxification is a slow process that still occurs but the symptoms are modified.
4 Fluid and electrolyte balance is unaffected by this drug.

715. **2 Malignant melanoma of the eye is an intraocular tumor that metastasizes rapidly; therefore enucleation (removal of the eye) is the treatment of choice. (IM; TC; NM)**
1 This is only palliative at best.
3 Same as answer 1.
4 Same as answer 1.

716. **1 Gliomas account for about 45% of all brain tumors. (DC; PA; NM)**
2 Meningioma, which occurs in the meninges of the brain, accounts for about 20% of all brain tumors.
3 Neurofibroma is a tumor of nerve tissue but is more common in the peripheral nervous system.
4 An adenoma is a tumor involving glandular tissue; it may occur in the pituitary gland.

717. **3 The facial nerve may be damaged during surgery. Drooping of the area results from loss of muscle tone. (DC; PA; NM)**
1 A tracheostomy may not be performed; it is not a complication but rather a preventive measure.
2 This is also called auriculotemporal syndrome; it may follow infection and suppuration of the parotid gland; it is not a surgical complication.
4 The parotid is a salivary gland; its removal would decrease salivation.

718. **1 Phenytoin (Dilantin) is an anticonvulsant most effective in controlling tonic-clonic seizures. Data collection before planning nursing care for a client with a**

seizure disorder should always include a history of seizure incidence (type and frequency). (PL; TC; NM)

2 Although protection is important, restraints and airway insertion during a seizure often cause injury as a result of violent muscle contractions.

3 Although these may be removed during a seizure, the client's normal routines should be respected.

4 Increased restlessness may be evidence of the prodromal phase in some individuals, but symptoms vary so widely that the history of the client should be obtained.

719. **3 A seizure is generally self-limiting; the nurse's responsibilities include protecting the client from injury and assessing the characteristics of the seizure. (IM; TC; NM)**

1 During a seizure the client loses consciousness and would be unable to discuss any aura experienced.

2 Nothing should be forced into the client's mouth when the teeth are clenched during a seizure; this could damage the teeth or cause an airway occlusion if improperly placed.

4 Anticonvulsants are given on a regular basis, not prn, to achieve therapeutic levels; diazepam (Valium) may be given IV in an emergency to control status epilepticus.

720. **3 To achieve the anticonvulsant effect, therapeutic blood levels of phenytoin must be maintained. If the client is not able to take the prescribed oral preparation, the physician should be questioned about alternate routes of administration. (IM; TC; NM)**

1 Omission would result in lowered blood levels, possibly below the necessary therapeutic level to prevent a seizure.

2 The route of administration cannot be altered without physician approval.

4 The client is being kept npo.

721. **2 Seizure disorders are usually associated with marked changes in the electrical activity of the cerebral cortex, requiring prolonged or lifelong therapy. (IM; ED; NM)**

1 Seizures may occur despite drug therapy; the dosage may need to be adjusted.

3 A therapeutic blood level must be maintained through consistent administration of the drug.

4 Absence of seizures would probably result from medication effectiveness rather than from correction of the pathophysiologic condition.

722. **2 The medulla contains the vital respiratory, cardiac, and vasomotor centers. (AN; PA; NM)**

1 The pons conducts impulses; it contains reflex centers for cranial nerves V, VI, VII, VIII (trigeminal, abducent, facial, vestibulocochlear).

3 The midbrain deals with sensory input from the eyes and ears.

4 The thalamus relays sensory impulses to the cerebral cortex.

723. **2 An unconscious individual loses voluntary control of the sphincters surrounding the urethra and anus. (DC; PA; NM)**

1 This cannot be assumed; hearing is often the last sense to be lost.

3 Motion (although often purposeless) is possible in coma.

4 Unconscious clients may react to various degrees of pain.

724. **4 The hypothalamus connects with the autonomic area for vasoconstriction, vasodilation, and perspiration and with the somatic centers for shivering; therefore it is an important area for regulating body temperature. (AN; PA; NM)**

1 The pallidum is part of the basal ganglia; it is also called the globus pallidus. Together with the putamen, it comprises the lenticular nucleus; it is concerned with muscle tone, which is required for specific body movements.

2 The thalamus receives all sensory stimuli, except taste, for transmission to the cerebral cortex; it is also involved with emotions and instinctive activities.

3 The temporal lobe is concerned with auditory stimuli; it may also be involved with the sense of smell.

725. **3 An altered level of consciousness, as determined by the Glasgow Coma Scale, precedes other changes, such as vital sign alterations. (DC; TC; NM)**

1 Carotid circulation is not altered.

2 This would not occur in this situation.

4 Spinal reflexes generally remain intact.

MEDICAL-SURGICAL ANSWERS

726. **3 The precentral gyrus is the most posterior convolution of the frontal lobe and the primary motor area. Other gyri also contain motor neurons.** (AN; PA; NM)
   1 The parietal lobes translate nerve impulses into sensations such as taste, touch, and temperature.
   2 The basal ganglia are islands of gray matter within the cerebral hemispheres; one activity with which they are concerned is muscle tone.
   4 The postcentral gyrus is the primary sensory area of the cerebral cortex; it is unrelated to motor activity.

727. **1 Because their mental status prevents total awareness of reality, confused or delirious clients may protect themselves by assimilating small amounts of information at a time.** (AN; ED; NM)
   2 Confusion or delirium is not synonymous with brain destruction.
   3 Although this statement is true, teaching principles must be altered when dealing with a confused client who cannot handle the complex.
   4 A client may be aware of surroundings, but perception may be inaccurate.

728. **4 The eighth cranial nerve has two parts—the vestibular nerve and the cochlear nerve. Sensations of hearing are conducted by the cochlear nerve.** (DC; PA; NM)
   1 The frontal lobe is concerned with thinking, skeletal muscle tone, and biorhythms.
   2 The occipital lobe is concerned with sight, particularly shape and color.
   3 Cranial nerve VI (abducent) is concerned with abduction of the eye.

729. **1 Head injuries can cause trauma to the brain; and the client should be observed for signs of increased intracranial pressure (e.g., headache, dizziness, visual disturbances).** (PL; TC; NM)
   2 This is not indicated in this situation.
   3 Elevating the lower extremities should be avoided because it will increase intracranial pressure.
   4 The intracranial pressure may increase after trauma because of bleeding and edema.

730. **1 It is important to help the client who has expressive aphasia regain maximum communicative abilities early during the hospital stay; this action provides reinforcement.** (PL; PS; NM)

   2 This approach may increase client frustration and anxiety.
   3 Although expectations should be realistic, improvements are possible and should be encouraged.
   4 Some abilities do return, and therefore the client should be encouraged to participate.

731. **3 Increased intracranial pressure places tension on the brain stem, causing signs such as increased systolic blood pressure, slow bounding pulse, elevated temperature, and changes in the respiratory pattern.** (DC; PA; NM)
   1 These combinations of symptoms are not found when vital brain centers are subjected to increased pressure.
   2 Same as answer 1.
   4 Same as answer 1.

732. **3 As an antiinflammatory agent, dexamethasone (Decadron) helps prevent cerebral edema, which generally peaks between day 3 and 5 after a cerebral vascular accident (CVA); this medication may also be used following a ruptured cerebral aneurysm.** (AN; PA; NM)
   1 This drug is not given for this purpose.
   2 This is not the reason for giving this drug; although blood volume may increase because dexamethasone causes sodium retention, this is not beneficial to a client after a CVA.
   4 Same as answer 1.

733. **2 Decadron is a corticosteroid that acts on the cell membrane to prevent the normal inflammatory responses as well as stabilize the blood-brain barrier.** (EV; TC; NM)
   1 This is not an effect of corticosteroid therapy.
   3 Same as answer 1.
   4 Same as answer 1.

734. **2 The pain may prevent the client from ingesting anything by mouth.** (PL; TC; NM)
   1 Hot or cold foods or compresses should be avoided because they may trigger a painful attack.
   3 Exercises may precipitate an attack.
   4 This would initiate an acute attack of trigeminal neuralgia; often clients must limit oral hygiene to rinsing the mouth.

735. **3 Tic douloureux, also referred to as trigeminal neuralgia, is an inflammation of the fifth cranial (trigeminal) nerve, which innervates the midline of the face and head.** (DC; PA; NM)

1 Petechiae are minute subcutaneous hemorrhages; they are not present in this disorder.
2 Pain, not weakness, occurs in this disease.
4 The oculomotor (or third, not the fifth) cranial nerve innervates the eyelid.

736. **3 Severe constant pain, emotional stress, muscle tensing, and diminished nutritional intake can lead to exhaustion and fatigue. (DC; PA; NM)**
1 Because clients are apprehensive and have pain, prolonged periods of sleep usually do not occur.
2 Pain medications do not normally cause hyperactivity.
4 The client may be very quiet for fear of precipitating an attack.

737. **1 The nurse should avoid walking swiftly past the client because drafts or even slight air currents can initiate pain. (PL; TC; NM)**
2 The client may assume any position of comfort, but pressure on the face while in the prone position may trigger an attack.
3 Although the procedure for oral hygiene may be altered, it is necessary to prevent infection.
4 Massaging may trigger an attack and should be avoided.

738. **4 The client may be able to avoid stimulating the involved trigeminal nerve and thus prevent pain by chewing on the unaffected side. (PL; ED; NM)**
1 Food that is too hot or too cold can precipitate pain.
2 Although oral hygiene may initiate pain, it cannot be avoided. It can be modified to include rinsing the mouth or using a soft swab instead of tooth brushing.
3 Warm compresses may precipitate pain.

739. **4 Carbamazepine (Tegretol) is a nonnarcotic analgesic, anticonvulsive drug used to control pain in trigeminal neuralgia and to abort future attacks. It sometimes eliminates the need for surgery. (PL; TC; NM)**
1 Ascorbic acid is vitamin C. This vitamin is found in high concentrations in the adrenal gland and is utilized when the body is subject to stress as occurs with pain.
2 Morphine is a narcotic analgesic that will relieve severe pain but will not prevent its recurrence; prolonged frequent use is contraindicated because of possible addiction.
3 Allopurinal is used in the treatment of gout.

740. **1 Diplopia and nystagmus are experienced by clients with multiple sclerosis as a result of demyelination. (DC; PA; NM)**
2 Clients experience intention tremors, not resting tremors; resting tremors occur with Parkinson's disease.
3 Clients experience spastic paralysis as upper motoneurons are involved.
4 Although emotional affect and speech are affected, intelligence remains intact.

741. **2 As a result of muscle weakness, the vital capacity is reduced leading to increased risks of respiratory complications; impaired swallowing can also lead to aspiration. (DC; TC; NM)**
1 Although ALS is progressive, clients with myasthenia gravis may be stable with treatment and clients with Guillain-Barré syndrome may experience a complete recovery.
3 None of these diseases are caused by a lack of neurotransmitters.
4 Twitching is not expected with myasthenia gravis or Guillain-Barré syndrome.

742. **4 Myasthenia gravis is a degenerative disease that occurs equally in both sexes during adulthood. (AN; PA; NM)**
1 Myasthenia gravis occurs equally in both sexes.
2 Myasthenia gravis is not a disease that is common in childhood.
3 Same as answer 1.

743. **3 One of the pathologic changes is electron-microscopic evidence of fewer AChR sites; also, antibodies cause destruction and blockade at the acetylcholine receptor sites. (IM; PA; NM)**
1 There is no genetic defect in the production of acetylcholine; rather than a genetic cause, it is believed that myasthenia gravis has an autoimmune etiology.
2 Although the defect is at the neuromuscular junction, it is not a decrease in acetylcholine, but in the receptor sites.
4 This enzyme is inhibited by anticholinesterase drugs used to treat myasthenia gravis, leaving more acetylcholine available to the damaged or decreased acetylcholine receptors.

744. 3 Weakened muscles result in ineffective coughing; secretions are retained and provide a medium for bacterial growth. (AN; PA; NM)

1 Airways are not narrowed.

2 Immune mechanisms are not directly impaired.

4 Viscosity of secretions depends on fluid intake and humidity.

745. 1 A tracheostomy set may be necessary to establish an emergency airway in case of respiratory crisis. (PL; TC; NM)

2 An IV may or may not be started; it is not as critical as airway obstruction.

3 This is not indicated; the client is not febrile.

4 The effects of Tensilon are brief; it is used primarily for diagnostic purposes.

746. 2 Neostigmine, an anticholinesterase, inhibits the breakdown of acetylcholine, thus prolonging neurotransmission. (AN; TC; NM)

1 Neostigmine's action is at the myoneural junction, not the cerebral cortex.

3 Neostigmine prevents neurotransmitter breakdown but is not a neurotransmitter.

4 Neostigmine's action is at the myoneural junction, not the sheath.

747. 2 Tensilon improves muscle strength in myasthenic crisis; weakness persists if symptoms are caused by cholinergic crisis, which can result from toxic levels of neostigmine. (EV; TC; NM)

1 Tensilon is not used for synergistic effects; the duration of effect is brief.

3 The diagnosis has already been established and treatment initiated.

4 This is the same type of drug as neostigmine; no resistance is indicated.

748. 3 Myasthenia gravis is a chronic degenerative disorder with exacerbations that are precipitated by emotional stress, ingestion of alcohol, and physical stress such as infection. (AN; PA; NM)

1 The prognosis is not excellent; there is no cure.

2 The disease is characterized by exacerbations and remissions.

4 The disease is chronic; death does not occur within a short period but usually after the muscles of respiration are affected.

749. 4 Parkinson's disease involves destruction of the neurons of the substantia nigra, caudate nucleus, and globus pallidus of the basal ganglia. The cause of this destruction is unknown. (AN; PA; NM)

1 This pathologic condition is associated with multiple sclerosis.

2 This condition would result in auditory and visual problems; it is not associated with Parkinson's disease.

3 This condition is believed to be associated with myasthenia gravis.

750. 1 Destruction of the neurons of the basal ganglia results in decreased muscle tone. The masklike appearance and monotonous speech patterns can be interpreted as flat. (DC; PA; NM)

2 These are not associated with Parkinson's disease.

3 This is not associated with Parkinson's disease.

4 Same as answer 3.

751. 3 Levodopa is the precursor of dopamine. It is converted to dopamine in the brain cells, where it is stored until needed by axon terminals; it functions as a neurotransmitter. (AN; TC; NM)

1 This is not an action of L-dopa.

2 Same as answer 1.

4 This is not an action of L-dopa; neurons do not regenerate.

752. 1 To avoid additional spinal cord damage, the victim must be moved only with great care. Moving a person whose spinal cord has been injured could cause irreversible paralysis. (IM; TC; NM)

2 A back injury is suspected; therefore the person should not be moved.

3 A back injury precludes changing the person's position.

4 A flat board would be indicated; however, one rescuer could not move the person alone.

753. 2 Both legs and generally the lower part of the body are paralyzed in paraplegia. (IM; PA; NM)

1 There is no term to describe this condition; all parts below an injury are affected.

3 This is hemiplegia.

4 This is quadriplegia.

754. 1 Because of the location of the micturition reflex center (in the sacral region of the spinal cord), bladder function may be

impaired with lower spinal cord injuries. (DC; PA; NM)

2 Plans for education are usually postponed until the client has had a chance to deal with feelings; high anxiety interferes with learning.

3 These exercises require motor control, which the client does not have.

4 Because there is no voluntary control over the lower extremities, mobility is usually accomplished through the use of a wheelchair rather than ambulation.

755. **4 Correct positioning prevents the client from assuming incorrect positions, which could result in contracture formation. (PL; TC; NM)**

1 Because the client is paralyzed, active exercises are not possible.

2 Deep massage may dislodge thrombi that have formed as a result of venous stasis.

3 The tilt board is used primarily to prevent orthostatic hypotension or bone demineralization.

756. **1 Pressure ulcers easily develop when a particular position is maintained; the body weight, directed continuously in one region, restricts circulation and results in tissue necrosis. (AN; TC; NM)**

2 Clients often state that they are comfortable and wish to remain in one position.

3 Because turning is usually done laterally, the circulation to the lower extremities is not dramatically affected.

4 Proper positioning with supportive devices and ROM are more effective measures to prevent contractures.

757. **3 Clients with early spinal cord damage experience an atonic bladder, which is characterized by the absence of muscle tone, an enlarged capacity, no feeling of discomfort with distention, and overflow with a large residual. This leads to urinary stasis and infection. High fluid intake limits urinary stasis and infection by diluting the urine and increasing urinary output. (IM; PA; NM)**

1 Dehydration is not a major problem after spinal cord injury.

2 Constipation may occur because of the lack of neural stimulation, not decreased fluids.

4 A fluid and electrolyte imbalance is not a major problem after spinal cord injury.

758. **2 To promote optimism and facilitate smooth functioning, all rehabilitation should begin on admission to the hospital. (PL; TC; NM)**

1 Although the client and family should be included in planning, they are often unaware of the options available in the health care system; the nurse should be available to provide the necessary information and support.

3 Because paralysis is permanent alterations in normal life-style are required.

4 Because the paralysis is permanent rehabilitation plans should be made.

759. **4 The Stryker frame provides for horizontal changes of position to prone or supine while maintaining proper body alignment. (AN; TC; NM)**

1 Although the frame itself does not directly promote body functions or prevent deformities, it does enable the nurse to turn the client, which helps prevent complications of immobility.

2 This frame does not prevent deformities; it only provides for horizontal turning.

3 Vertical turning is not possible with a Stryker frame.

760. **2 The main nursing principles when turning a client on the Stryker frame are the maintenance of alignment and safety. Securing all bolts and straps ensures that the client is snug yet comfortably wedged between the frames. (IM; TC; NM)**

1 Because the client is being turned horizontally, hypotension is not a major problem.

3 After a cervical injury clients are often unable to use their arms.

4 The procedure does not require two nurses unless such a protocol is established by the institution.

761. **1 These are symptoms of autonomic dysreflexia, which is not commonly precipitated by a distended bladder. (DC; TC; NM)**

2 These are not associated with autonomic dysreflexia.

3 Same as answer 2.

4 Blood pressure rises suddenly with autonomic dysreflexia.

MEDICAL-SURGICAL ANSWERS

762. **4** **The CircOlectric bed turns clients from a horizontal supine position vertically to a horizontal prone position. It can also remain stationary in a vertical position. The change of position alters the body pressures periodically while the client is confined to the bed. (AN; PA; NM)**

1 Although in some mattresses a pad can be removed so that a bedpan may be inserted, a receptacle itself would be impractical, because the entire bed turns.

2 It is possible for one nurse to turn a client in a CircOlectric bed.

3 Lateral turning is not possible with a CircOlectric bed.

763. **4** **During prolonged inactivity bone reabsorption proceeds faster than bone formation, and lack of therapeutic weight bearing on bone results in demineralization. A tilt table provides gradual progressive weight bearing, which counters these effects. (IM; ED; NM)**

1 Lateral turning is possible and necessary if a client is immobile, but a tilt table does not make this possible.

2 The tilt table is used for scheduled periods in physical therapy; the nursing care required to prevent pressure ulcers must be consistently performed frequently throughout all shifts.

3 The tilt table does not cause hyperextension of the spine; the spine remains in functional body alignment.

764. **3** **Clients with quadriplegia do not have and never will have the muscle innervation, strength, or balance needed for ambulation. (AN; TC; NM)**

1 Bracing and crutch walking require muscle strength and coordination that an individual with quadriplegia does not have.

2 Orthostatic hypotension can be prevented by any upright positioning and does not necessarily require a wheelchair.

4 Quadriplegia refers to paralysis of all four extremities.

765. **1** **A comatose client loses voluntary control of elimination. (DC; PA; NM)**

2 Because there are different levels of coma, the individual may respond to intense stimuli such as pain.

3 Twitching motions may be evidence of abnormal cerebral electrical activity; such seizure-like activity is often present in comatose individuals.

4 Because cerebral functioning is depressed, purposeful or voluntary movement is absent.

766. **2** **Absence of a gag reflex is common after a CVA. To prevent aspiration, the client is positioned on the side to allow gravity to drain mucus in the nasopharyngeal area away from the trachea. (IM; TC; NM)**

1 Chest expansion is hindered in the prone position.

3 This position allows the tongue to occlude the airway and encourages the aspiration of secretions if the gag reflex is not intact.

4 This position interferes with respiration and leads to increased intracranial pressure.

767. **3** **Dysphagia is difficulty in swallowing. (DC; PA; NM)**

1 Writing is unrelated to dysphagia.

2 Focusing with the eyes is unrelated to dysphagia.

4 Understanding information is unrelated to dysphagia.

768. **4** **Clients with dysarthria have difficulty communicating verbally, and alternate means may be indicated. (PL; TC; NM)**

1 This is an important aspect of care but not related to dysarthria.

2 Same as answer 1.

3 Same as answer 1.

769. **1** **The paralyzed side has decreased muscle tone, which may lower blood pressure readings; tissue damage may also occur. (IM; TC; NM)**

2 The return of function to the affected extremity is not influenced by taking blood pressure; if it occurs, it is because of resolution of inflammation or resorption of blood in the area of the infarct.

3 Taking blood pressure does not precipitate the formation of thrombi.

4 There is no difference when pressure is exerted on the brachial artery in either arm.

770. **2** **Passive ROM exercises prevent the development of deformities and yet do not require any energy expenditure by the client who is confined to bed. Instituting ROM exercises is an independent nursing function. (PL; TC; NM)**

1 Bed rest is prescribed to decrease oxygen demands; active exercises markedly increase oxygen consumption.

3 Same as answer 1.

4 Same as answer 1.

771. **1 Various types of splints or boots are available to keep the foot in a position of dorsiflexion. (IM; TC; NM)**

2 Blocks elevate the frame of the bed and have no effect on position of the feet.

3 Cradles keep linen off of the client's abdomen and legs but do nothing to position the feet.

4 Sandbags help prevent lateral movement of an extremity or the head.

772. **1 Change of position every hour helps prevent the respiratory, urinary, and cutaneous complications of immobility. (PL; TC; NM)**

2 Too protracted a period in one position increases the potential for respiratory, urinary, and neuromuscular impairment; prolonged physical pressure increases the possibility of skin breakdown.

3 Same as answer 2.

4 Same as answer 2.

773. **1 Atony permits the bladder to fill without being able to empty. As pressure builds within the bladder, the urge to void occurs and just enough urine is eliminated to relieve the pressure and the urge to void. The cycle is repeated as pressure again builds. Thus small amounts are voided without emptying the bladder. (DC; TC; NM)**

2 These might be signs of renal failure.

3 Continual incontinence would not occur if urine were retained.

4 The total amount of urine produced and voided would be unchanged.

774. **3 All nursing intervention aims to assist an individual in maximizing capabilities and coping with modifications in life-style. (AN; PA; NM)**

1 All resources, including the private physician and acute care facilities, that can be beneficial to client rehabilitation should be utilized.

2 Rehabilitation is a commonality in all areas of nursing practice.

4 Rehabilitation is necessary to help clients return to a previous level of functioning after both illness and surgery.

775. **3 Cerebral damage on one side of the cortex causes alterations on the opposite side, because three fourths of the fibers originating in the cortex decussate (cross over) in the medulla before extending down the spinal cord. When there is cranial nerve damage, the same side of the body is affected, because the cranial nerves do not decussate but leave the cranial cavity by way of the small foramina in the skull. (DC; PA; NM)**

1 Hemiplegia refers to paralysis of one side of the body and affects both extremities; the right side of the face, not just the jaw, would be involved.

2 Facial muscles on the same side as the cerebral lesion are paralyzed because they are innervated by the cranial nerves, which originate above the points where the spinal nerves decussate.

4 Same as answer 1.

776. **3 To prevent deformity after a CVA, the client should be repositioned frequently and passive ROM exercises should be instituted. (IM; TC; NM)**

1 Active exercises require a physician's order; active exercises are impossible with paralyzed limbs.

2 The nurse must directly assist the client; periodic visits by the physical therapist are insufficient.

4 This would increase deformities and atrophy.

777. **2 Success is a basic motivation for learning. People receive satisfaction when a goal is reached. The more frequent the success, the greater is their satisfaction, which in turn motivates them to continue striving toward realistic goals. (PL; TC; NM)**

1 Progress toward long-range goals is often not readily apparent and may tend to discourage a client.

3 Constructive criticism is an important aspect in client teaching; but if not tempered with praise, it is discouraging.

4 An important part of teaching; but this will not necessarily motivate the client to attempt them.

778. **1 Left-sided paresis creates instability. Using a cane provides a wider base of support and, therefore, greater stability. (AN; TC; NM)**

2 Inflammation of these joints is not mentioned; therefore this is unnecessary.

3 Activity should not injure but strengthen weakened muscles.

4 The use of a cane would not prevent involuntary movements if they were present.

MEDICAL-SURGICAL ANSWERS

779. **4 As part of the rehabilitative process after a CVA, clients must be encouraged to participate in their own care to the extent to which they are able and to extend their abilities by establishing short-term goals.** (IM; TC; NM)

1 A client with a CVA may or may not have dysphagia; altering the consistency of food without the need to do so may make it less palatable.

2 Making the client feel helpless discourages independence.

3 This is unrealistic; family members may not be available because of other responsibilities.

780. **1 Damage to Broca's area, located in the posterior frontal region of the dominant hemisphere, causes problems in the motor aspect of speech.** (AN; PA; NM)

2 This would be associated with receptive aphasia, not expressive aphasia; receptive aphasia is associated with disease of Wernicke's area of the brain.

3 Although difficulty in writing may be associated with expressive aphasia, understanding speech would be associated with receptive aphasia.

4 Same as answer 2.

781. **2 Clients with expressive aphasia must be encouraged to associate words with objects so that communication is regained.** (PL; TC; NM)

1 Speech can usually be improved through therapy.

3 To avoid frustration, the client's needs should be anticipated.

4 Despite difficulty speaking, individuals with expressive aphasia can understand what is said to them.

782. **2 Because of pressure on the sciatic nerve, pain radiating to the hip and leg is common.** (DC; PA; NM)

1 This is not associated with a ruptured nucleus pulposus.

3 Although weakness (paresis) may occur, paralysis is not common.

4 Same as answer 1.

783. **1 These actions, as well as lifting and straining, cause an increase in the intraspinal pressure, resulting in pain.** (DC; PA; NM)

2 This does not affect the intraspinal pressure.

3 Although pain may increase as a result of

compression of the vertebrae, the increase is gradual, not sudden.

4 Flexing the knees and hips relieves pressure and pain.

784. **3 Inflammation from the trauma of surgery could lead to injury of the nerve root, with consequent motor or sensory dysfunction.** (EV; TC; NM)

1 Cerebral edema does not occur.

2 Urinary retention rather than spasticity may occur if pressure on the nerve root occurs as a result of edema or bleeding.

4 Pain is usually experienced at the operative site and in the legs as a result of edema around the cord.

785. **2 Logrolling maintains the alignment of the vertebral column.** (2: IM; TC; NM)

1 Coughing will increase the pressure of the cerebrospinal fluid surrounding the spinal cord and intensify the pain; incentive spirometry and turning should be used to prevent respiratory complications.

3 Peritonitis is not a danger because the abdominal cavity is not opened.

4 Extreme flexion of the knees is avoided postoperatively because it alters intervertebral pressure.

786. **2 Sore throat and oral secretions are additional problems of the client after cervical laminectomy.** (PL; TC; NM)

1 To prevent strain on the operative site, flexion of the head is avoided.

3 The head of the bed may be only slightly elevated after a cervical laminectomy.

4 Limited range of motion occurs after both operations.

Skeletal

787. **3 Allopurinol interferes with the final steps in uric acid formation by inhibiting the production of xanthinoxidase.** (AN; PA; SK)

1 This drug prevents the formation of uric acid.

2 Allopurinol has no effect on swelling of the synovial membranes.

4 Same as answer 1.

788. **1 Colchicine decreases the formation of lactic acid, which may promote the deposition of uric acid in the joints. It also decreases the inflammatory response.** (AN; PA; SK)

2 Hydrocortisone is an antiinflammatory; it is not used to treat gout.

3 Ibuprofen is a nonsteroid antiinflammatory agent; it does not prevent the formation of uric acid.

4 Benemid acts to inhibit the reabsorption of urate in the kidneys and, therefore, decreases uric acid in the blood; it is not useful in the treatment of acute gout but rather of chronic gout.

789. **4 Warm compresses (at or slightly above body temperature) dilate blood vessels, increasing blood flow to the area and decreasing edema. (IM; TC; SK)**

1 This temperature is too cool to increase blood flow to the area.

2 Same as answer 1.

3 Same as answer 1.

790. **3 Synovial fluid minimizes friction at joints by providing lubrication for the moving parts. (AN; PA; SK)**

1 Synovial fluid increases the efficiency of joint movements.

2 Synovial fluid increases work output.

4 Synovial fluid increases the speed of movements.

791. **3 Synovial joints, like the knee, shoulder, or articulations between the middle ear bones, are lined with synovial membrane. (AN; PA; SK)**

1 Serous membrane does not line joints but rather areas such as the thoracic and abdominal cavities.

2 Mucous membrane lines passages that open to the exterior of the body such as the mouth and the genitourinary tract.

4 Epithelium covers the internal and external organs of the body, including the skin.

792. **4 The greater density of compact bone makes it stronger than cancellous bone. Compact bone forms from cancellous bone by the addition of concentric rings of bone substance to the marrow spaces of cancellous bone; the large marrow spaces are reduced to haversian canals. (AN; PA; SK)**

1 Overall size does not determine strength.

2 Weight alone is not a factor.

3 Volume is not related to strength.

793. **3 Systemic lupus erythematosus is a chronic, autoimmune, systemic disease with inflammatory and degenerative changes in the body's connective tissue. (AN; PA; SK)**

1 It is connective tissue throughout the organs of the body that is affected, not joints.

2 Bones are not the focus of this disease.

4 Purine metabolism is affected in gout.

794. **1 Increased levels of steroids will accelerate bone demineralization. (DC; PA; SK)**

2 Hyperparathyroidism, not hypoparathyroidism, accelerates bone demineralization.

3 Weight bearing that occurs with strenuous activity promotes bone integrity by preventing bone demineralization.

4 Estrogen promotes deposition of calcium into bone.

795. **3 Prolonged immobility results in bone demineralization because there is decreased bone production by osteoblasts and increased resorption by osteoclasts. (DC; PA; SK)**

1 Estrogen helps prevent bone demineralization.

2 Hypoparathyroidism decreases mobilization of calcium from the bones and thus serum calcium is lowered.

4 Decreased calcium intake or absorption may precipitate osteoporosis.

796. **2 Pathologic fractures occur as a result of minimal injury to an already weakened bone; osteoporosis causes this weakening. (AN; PA; SK)**

1 Fatigue fractures occur when muscles are so fatigued that they no longer act as shock absorbers to protect the bone, a condition not related to osteoporosis.

3 Greenstick fractures occur in soft bones, usually just in children.

4 Compound fractures refer to the protrusion of the bone fragments through the skin. This is not related to osteoporosis.

797. **3 Turnip greens are high in calcium, but not in phosphorus. (IM; ED; GI)**

1 High levels of nitrogen from protein breakdown may increase calcium resorption from bone to serve as a buffer of the nitrogen.

2 Soft drinks that are high in phosphorus may interfere with calcium absorption from the GI tract.

4 Enriched grains that are high in phosphorus may interfere with calcium absorption from the GI tract.

798. **1 Rehabilitation should begin on admission; this includes preoperative discussion of the nature of the operation and rehabilitation techniques. (PL; TC; SK)**
  2 This is too late; valuable rehabilitation time has been wasted.
  3 Same as answer 2.
  4 Same as answer 2.

799. **2 Practicing ambulation without proper preparation of ambulation techniques and strengthening the involved muscle groups would not be helpful in the rehabilitation process and could exhaust the client. (EV; ED; SK)**
  1 Because different muscle groups are utilized, the client must be instructed even about what seem to be simple maneuvers; transfer from a sitting to a standing position must be accomplished before ambulation.
  3 Prior to ambulation the individual must be able to maintain balance.
  4 The muscles used for crutch walking are different from those used in normal ambulation; therefore they must be strengthened by active exercises prior to ambulation.

800. **3 Flexion contracture of the hip can be prevented by routinely placing the client in a prone position to extend the hip. (IM; TC; SK)**
  1 This can cause flexion of the hip, which will result in a hip contracture and affect balance.
  2 Same as answer 1.
  3 Lying in the supine position does not allow for full extension of the hip.

801. **1 This position offsets the development of hip deformities resulting from contractures. It also maintains the correct center of gravity when the client is upright. (IM; ED; SK)**
  2 This promotes flexion contracture of the hip.
  3 A prosthesis may be applied early in the postoperative period but requires a rigid dressing (cast) to prevent edema; ambulation can be facilitated by the use of a walker, crutches, parallel bars, or cane.
  4 This may alter the center of gravity and cause a loss of balance.

802. **4 Preparing muscles that will do the work in crutch walking is imperative. (IM; ED; SK)**
  1 The biceps are not the major muscles required for crutch walking.

  2 Contractures of the limb will not have a great influence on the ability to use crutches.
  3 Strengthening the hamstring muscles will not assist in the use of crutches.

803. **1 A four-point gait provides for weight bearing on all four extremities and maximum support during ambulation. (IM; ED; SK)**
  2 A three-point gait is used when one extremity cannot bear weight.
  3 Same as answer 2.
  4 A swing-through gait does not simulate ambulation; it is used when the individual can bear weight but lacks the muscular control needed for ambulation without an assistive device.

804. **4 Elastic bandages compress the stump, preventing edema and promoting stump shrinkage and molding; the bandage must be rewrapped when it loosens. (PL; TC; SK)**
  1 This would have a systemic effect on fluid balance; edema of the stump is a localized response to inflammation.
  2 Same as answer 1.
  3 Prolonged immobilization of the residual extremity in one position can lead to a flexion contracture of the hip.

805. **2 Constriction of circulation decreases venous return and increases pressure within the vessels. Fluid then moves into the interstitial spaces, causing edema. (EV; PA; SK)**
  1 This would indicate infection.
  3 Same as answer 1.
  4 Same as answer 1.

806. **4 In crutch walking the client uses the triceps, trapezius, and latissimus muscles. A client who has been in bed may need to implement an exercise program to strengthen these shoulder and upper arm muscles before initiating crutch walking. (IM; PA; SK)**
  1 This activity does not strengthen muscles used in crutch walking.
  2 Keeping the leg in abduction alters the center of gravity, which impedes ambulation.
  3 Back muscles are not used in crutch walking.

807. **3 In the four-point gait the client brings the left crutch forward first, followed by the right foot; then the right crutch is brought forward, followed by the left**

foot. Thus both legs must be able to bear some weight. (IM; ED; SK)

1 Although the arms are extended to allow the hands to bear weight, the elbows are not maintained in this position.

2 Pressure on the axillae may damage nerves in the area.

4 Both extremities must be able to bear weight.

808. **3 The paraplegic client is unable to exercise the lower extremities actively.** (IM; TC; SK)

1 Changing a position involves moving the extremities. Contractures develop as a result of prolonged immobility.

2 The use of pillows, splints, and other supportive devices helps maintain alignment and prevent the shortening of muscle fibers associated with contractures.

4 Passive ROM helps maintain joint mobility and muscle tone.

809. **4 Calcium that has left the bones as a response to prolonged inactivity enters the blood and may precipitate in the kidneys, forming calculi.** (AN; PA; SK)

1 Increased fluid intake is helpful in avoiding this condition by preventing urinary stasis.

2 Calculi may develop despite adequate kidney function; kidney function may be impaired by the presence of calculi and the high incidence of urinary tract infections associated with urinary stasis or repeated catheterizations.

3 Calcium intake is usually limited to prevent the increasing risk of calculi.

810. **4 Rehabilitating exercises carried out underwater minimize strain on the body. The buoyant force of the water makes the limbs easier to move.** (AN; PA; SK)

1 Vapors are produced above water as a result of evaporation; they do not facilitate exercise.

2 Exercises are carried out near the surface of the water where the water pressure would have little effect.

3 Water temperature would not assist movement.

811. **1 Osteoarthritis affects the hips and knees first because they are the weight-bearing joints and undergo the most stress.** (DC; PA; SK)

2 Although these are weight-bearing joints, normal motion is not as great as in the hips and knees; thus there is less degeneration.

3 Although the distal interphalangeal joints are frequently affected, the remaining interphalangeal joints and metacarpals are not.

4 These are not weight-bearing joints.

812. **4 Marie-Strümpell disease is synonymous with rheumatoid spondylitis, which involves fixation of joints (usually vertebral).** (PL; ED; SK)

1 Heberden nodules are the bony or cartilaginous enlargements of the distal interphalangeal joints that are associated with degenerative arthritis.

2 As the cartilage of the joints degenerates, there are hypertrophic changes of the bone edges, which eventually replace the articular cartilage.

3 Ankylosis occurs in rheumatoid arthritis, not in hypertrophic or degenerative arthritis.

813. **3 Exercise of involved joints is important to maintain optimal mobility and prevent buildup of calcium deposits.** (IM; TC; SK)

1 Immobilization causes loss of joint mobility and contractures.

2 Same as answer 1.

4 Same as answer 1.

814. **4 There is no special diet for arthritis. A balanced diet, consisting of foods from all levels of the food pyramid, is essential in maintaining good nutrition.** (IM; ED; SK)

1 Limiting the diet to particular foods does not provide all essential nutrients.

2 Same as answer 1.

3 If nutritional intake is adequate, multivitamins are unnecessary.

815. **2 Because pain is an all-encompassing and often demoralizing experience, the client should be kept as pain free as possible.** (PL; TC; SK)

1 Pain can usually be managed medically; surgery is used to correct deformity and facilitate movement.

3 Concentration on learning something is difficult when a client is in severe pain.

4 Motivation is difficult when a client is in severe pain.

MEDICAL-SURGICAL ANSWERS

816. **3 An antinuclear antibody test (ANA) may be positive in clients with autoimmune disorders such as rheumatoid arthritis and systemic lupus erythematosus. (IM; PA; SK)**
1 Pancreatic lipase is an enzyme that catalyzes the breakdown of lipids; this is a test used to diagnose pancreatic problems.
2 Bence Jones protein is a urine test helpful in diagnosing multiple myeloma.
4 Alkaline phosphatase is a blood test to determine phosphorus activity; it is generally used in diagnosing liver and biliary tract disorders and identifying periods of active bone growth or metastasis of cancer to bone.

817. **3 ROM exercises must be instituted to maintain mobility of joints. However, overuse may prevent resolution of the inflammation. (AN; TC; SK)**
1 Pain may persist but cannot be allowed to legitimize inactivity.
2 Activity will not prevent the inflammatory process; it may aggravate it.
4 Severely damaged joints may require prosthetic replacement.

818. **2 Steroids have an antiinflammatory effect that can reduce arthritic pannus formation. (AN; TC; SK)**
1 Pain relief results from the antiinflammatory actions of steroids.
3 Injection of a drug is not physiotherapy.
4 Ankylosis refers to fusion of joints. It is only indirectly influenced by steroids, which exert their major effect on the inflammatory process.

819. **2 Ossification of cartilage, particularly of the spine, causes fixation of the involved joints. (PL; TC; SK)**
1 Inflammation and thickening of the synovial membrane are characteristic of arthritis.
3 Although rest is essential, complete immobility would result in a loss of joint motion.
4 Redness and swelling are symptoms of local inflammation; they do not indicate irreversible damage.

820. **3 Inactivity over an extended time increases stiffness and pain in joints. (PL; PA; SK)**
1 This is not a factor; cold packs may decrease joint discomfort.
2 Assistive exercises help maintain joint mobility.
4 The latex fixation test is positive when the rheumatoid factor is found in blood serum; this factor is present in many conditions, including rheumatoid arthritis, aging, narcotic addiction, and SLE.

821. **4 There are no dietary restrictions, but iron and vitamins should be encouraged to normalize any underlying nutritional deficiencies. (PL; TC; SK)**
1 These nutritional restrictions are not indicated.
2 A high-calorie diet would increase the client's weight; this is contraindicated because it would increase the strain on weight bearing joints.
3 A normal protein intake should fulfill nutritional needs; there is no need to restrict calcium.

822. **2 Because of its antiinflammatory effect, aspirin is useful in treating arthritis symptoms. (IM; TC; SK)**
1 Xanax is an antianxiety, not an antiinflammatory, agent.
3 Narcotics should be avoided because they promote drug dependency and do not affect the inflammatory process.
4 Same as answer 3.

823. **3 Heat and cold reduce inflammation and discomfort. (IM; TC; SK)**
1 This will depend on the client's tolerance.
2 Avoiding exercise will increase the destructive effects of immobility.
4 Exercises are necessary to prevent contractures and permanent joint damage; aerobic exercises may be too strenuous and accelerate joint destruction.

824. **1 Laminar air flow decreases the risk of bone infection, because potentially contaminated air continuously flows away from the sterile field, decreasing the concentration of airborne pathogens. (IM; TC; SK)**
2 The procedure is performed at one time.
3 Surgery is generally considered when destruction of the femoral head and acetabulum is extensive.
4 The lithotomy position is used for gynecologic procedures; the side-lying position is generally used for hip surgery.

825. **2 Pressure on the operative site may cause unnecessary pain and impair circulation necessary for healing. (PL; TC; SK)**
1 This is acceptable because no stress is placed on the operative site.
3 Supine or on the unaffected side is the position of choice; however, a wedge, thigh

spreader, or pillows must be used to maintain abduction of the affected thigh; adduction can result in displacement of the prosthesis.

4 Same as answer 3.

826. **2 Ankle movement, particularly dorsiflex-ion of the foot, allows muscle contrac-tion, which compresses veins, reducing venous stasis and risk of thrombus for-mation. (PL; TC; SK)**

1 The client must be turned at least every 2 hours to help prevent the complications of immobility; 3 hours is too long to keep a client in one position.

3 The client is generally not allowed out of bed until at least 1 day postoperative.

4 This is too soon and sitting is contraindicated because hip flexion can cause displacement of the prosthesis.

827. **1 This supports the site; the involved leg must be maintained in alignment, avoid-ing adduction. (PL; TC; SK)**

2 The pillow will not affect venous return, which relates to thrombus formation.

3 Adduction, not flexion, contractures are of most concern after surgery.

4 Although friction is decreased when skin does not interface with skin, this is not the reason for separating the thighs and lower limbs.

828. **2 Placing the feet apart creates a wider base of support and brings the center of gravi-ty closer to the ground. This improves sta-bility. (IM; TC; SK)**

1 Bending at the waist should be avoided because it strains the lower back muscles; the power for lifting should be supplied by the muscles of the thighs and buttocks.

3 Pressure on the abdomen is prevented by tightening the abdominal and gluteal muscles to form an internal girdle; keeping the body straight does not reduce strain on the abdom-inal musculature.

4 Relaxing the abdominal muscles with physical activity increases strain on the abdomen.

829. **1 Some weight bearing on the uninvolved leg helps maintain its muscle tone. (IM; TC; SK)**

2 When the legs are in a dependent position without moving, venous return is impaired.

3 Speed is not important when ambulating.

4 This is an unacceptable rationale for care.

830. **4 The three-point gait, which requires con-siderable arm strength, is used when a limb cannot bear weight. The affected leg and crutches are advanced together, and the strong leg swings through. (IM; ED; SK)**

1 This is used for individuals who cannot move their lower extremities; it does not simulate normal ambulation.

2 This requires weight bearing on both feet.

3 Same as answer 2.

831. **3 As a result of contracting and pulling of the muscles on the two portions of bone, there is a characteristic shorten-ing of the femur with external rotation of the extremity. (DC; PA; SK)**

1 Lateral motion of the leg does not occur; the leg externally rotates.

2 Lateral motion of the leg does not occur.

4 The extremity externally rotates as the mus-cles contract; shortening, not lengthening, occurs.

832. **1 Buck's traction is frequently used in the treatment of a fractured hip to align the bones (reduction of fracture). If such traction were not employed, the muscles would go into spasm, shifting the bone fragments and causing pain. (IM; ED; SK)**

2 Buck's traction is usually a temporary measure prior to surgery; contractures result from a shortening of the muscles by prolonged immobility.

3 Although the affected extremity must be properly aligned, turning and moving the client is still necessary.

4 External rotation is contraindicated and pre-vented by the use of sandbags or trochanter rolls.

MEDICAL-SURGICAL ANSWERS

833. **1 A fracture in the neck of the femur will cause shortening of the femur and external rotation. To correct this malalignment, the client's leg should be extended and maintained in slight internal rotation. (PL; TC; SK)**
2 To reduce the fracture, it is necessary to maintain the leg in extension, counteracting the contraction of the quadriceps, which may cause overriding of bone fragments.
3 To reduce the fracture, it is necessary to maintain the leg in extension, counteracting the contraction of the quadriceps, which may cause overriding of bone fragments. External rotation of the thigh as a result of muscle contraction tends to misalign the bone fragments; therefore slight internal rotation or normal alignment is preferred.
4 External rotation of the thigh as a result of muscle contraction tends to misalign the bone fragments; therefore slight internal rotation or normal alignment is preferred.

834. **3 This type of contracture frequently occurs when the client lies in bed with knees bent and thighs not abducted. (DC; PA; SK)**
1 This does not describe a contracture.
2 Same as answer 1.
4 Although footdrop is a problem for all clients confined to bed, hyperextension of the knee is not normally possible.

835. **4 After a fracture, if blood supply is cut off or impaired, necrosis of the bone may occur from lack of oxygen and nutrient perfusion. (AN; PA; SK)**
1 Aseptic indicates that infection is not present.
2 Early weight bearing at the fracture site might result in trauma to bone; circulation would not be impaired.
3 Immobilization does not cut off circulation to the bone; it may cause contractures.

836. **2 Intramedullary nails are used to maintain bone alignment and provide support along the femur's length. (AN; TC; SK)**
2 Because this orthopedic problem does not affect the shaft of a long bone, an intramedullary nailing device is not appropriate.
3 Same as answer 1.
4 Same as answer 1.

837. **3 To prevent nerve damage in the axillary area, the palms should bear all the weight. (IM; ED; SK)**
1 This is unsafe and next to impossible to perform.
2 Pressure in the axillary area causes nerve damage to the brachial plexus.
4 Weight bearing on the affected lower extremity is initially contraindicated.

838. **4 This group would succumb quickly to severe blood loss if dressings as indicated were not applied. (PL; TC; SK)**
1 These individuals could wait for treatment per the triage routine.
2 Same as answer 1.
3 Same as answer 1.

Drug-related Responses

839. **2 Radium atoms are unstable and spontaneously disintegrate. This disintegration produces potentially harmful radiation; lead is a barrier to these radiations. (AN; PA; DR)**
1 Radium is not a heavy substance but an unstable one.
3 Heat is not produced during spontaneous disintegration; radiation is.
4 Disintegration of radium occurs in the lead containers.

840. **3 A paradoxical response to a drug is directly opposite the desired therapeutic response (EV; PA; DR)**
1 An allergic response induces an allergen-antibody reaction.
2 This response involves drug combinations that enhance each other.
4 This is a response to a drug that is more pronounced than the response observed in most of the population.

841. **1 Because digoxin slows the heart, the apical pulse should be counted for 1 minute prior to administration. If the apical rate is below 60 (bradycardia), digoxin should be withheld because its administration could further depress the heart rate. If the heart rate is above 120, digoxin should be withheld because the client may be in digitalis toxicity. (DC; TC; DR)**
2 This is not as accurate as apical pulse; the client may also have an atrial dysrhythmia, which would not be detected with the radial rate alone.
3 Same as answer 2.
4 This is the pulse deficit, not an indicator of heart rate.

842. **1 Cardiac nitrates relax the smooth muscles of the coronary arteries so that they dilate and deliver more blood to relieve ischemic pain. (EV; PA; DR)**
    2 Although cardiac output may improve because of improved oxygenation of the myocardium, this is not a basis for evaluating the drug's effectiveness.
    3 Although dilation of blood vessels and subsequent drop in BP may occur, this is not the basis for evaluating the drug's effectiveness.
    4 Although superficial vessels dilate, lowering BP and creating a flushed appearance, this is not a basis for evaluating the drug's effectiveness.

843. **1 Nitroglycerin tablets are affected by light, heat, and moisture. A loss of potency can occur after 3 months, reducing the drug's effectiveness in relieving pain. A new supply should be obtained routinely. (IM; ED; DR)**
    2 This does not necessarily indicate a loss of potency.
    3 Same as answer 2.
    4 Same as answer 2.

844. **3 Prazosin blocks the response to norepinephrine bound to alpha-adrenergic receptors relaxing smooth muscle in peripheral vessels, increasing circulation and decreasing blood pressure. (AN; ED; DR)**
    1 This is not an action of prazosin.
    2 Same as answer 1.
    4 Prazosin does not affect adrenal release of epinephrine.

845. **1 Because propranolol (Inderal) competes with catecholamines at the beta-adrenergic receptor sites, the normal increase in heart rate and contractility in response to exercise does not occur. This, combined with the drug's hypotensive effect, may lead to dizziness. (3, EV; TC; DR)**
    2 This drug does not increase the heart rate, but may cause bradycardia.
    3 This is not a side effect of this drug.
    4 Same as answer 3.

846. **3 Because furosemide (Lasix) and aspirin compete for the same renal excretory sites, salicylate toxicity may occur even with lower dosages. (AN; PA; DR)**
    1 Aspirin does not affect the metabolism of Lasix.

    2 This response does not take into account the other drug that the client is receiving.
    4 Although furosemide has a hyperuricemic effect similar to that of the thiazide diuretics, it is not potentiated by aspirin.

847. **4 Captopril (Capoten) is an antihypertensive because it inhibits conversion of angiotensin I to angiotensin II. (IM; ED; DR)**
    1 Capoten is an antihypertensive, not a diuretic; diuretics produce fluid excretion.
    2 Capoten is an antihypertensive, not a hypnotic; hypnotics promote sleep.
    3 Capoten is an antihypertensive, not a tranquilizer; tranquilizers reduce muscle tension and anxiety.

848. **3 Atrial fibrillation is the rapid discharge of impulses from a focus other than the SA node. Because not all these impulses are transmitted through the AV node, the ventricular response varies. Quinidine inhibits discharge of electric impulses from such ectopic foci, whereas digoxin delays the conduction of impulses from the AV node, slowing down the rate of ventricular response to impulses from the atria. (AN; TC; DR)**
    1 This is true of quinidine but does not explain the action of digoxin.
    2 This is only partially true. Digoxin increases vagal activity to slow the heart rate, and quinidine inhibits ion exchange across the cellular membrane; thus excitability of the atrial and ventricular myocardium is decreased, intraventricular and AV nodal conduction is slowed, and the refractory period is prolonged.
    4 Digoxin increases vagal activity to slow the heart rate, and quinidine inhibits ion exchange across the cellular membrane; thus excitability of the atrial and ventricular myocardium is decreased, intraventricular and AV nodal conduction is slowed, and the refractory period is prolonged.

849. **3 In addition to GI disturbances, visual disturbances such as blurred vision may be evidence of digitalis toxicity. Heart rates over 120 may also indicate toxicity. (EV; TC; DR)**
    1 This is not a symptom of digitalis toxicity.
    2 Same as answer 1.
    4 Same as answer 1.

850. 3 Toxic levels of digitalis overstimulate the vagus nerve, leading to depressed conduction through the AV node (AV block of any degree) as well as SA node depression (sinus bradycardia). In addition, ectopic pacemakers are accelerated, leading to multiple premature beats. Such pathologic effects are enhanced by low serum potassium levels from diuretics, vomiting, and nasogastric drainage as well as by chronic arterial hypoxemia and impaired renal function. (AN; TC; DR)

1 This is true but not specific to the situation described.
2 Vitamins act as coenzymes.
4 This is an untrue statement.

851. 2 Methyldopa is associated with acquired hemolytic anemia and should be discontinued to prevent disease progression and complications. (EV; TC; DR)

1 This is not associated with red blood cell destruction.
3 Same as answer 1.
4 Same as answer 1.

852. 1 Aminophylline, a theophylline derivative, promotes diuresis and relaxes smooth muscles, resulting in hypotension. (EV; TC; DR)

2 These are not a side effect of the drug.
3 Side effects include sinus tachycardia.
4 Urine output is increased.

853. 3 Nitroglycerine is sensitive to light and moisture and must be stored in a dark airtight container. (IM; ED; DR)

1 This medication is usually taken prn. The daily number may be as high as 12 to 15 tablets; if more than three are necessary in a 15-minute period, the doctor should be notified.
2 This may be an expected side effect and the medication should not be discontinued.
4 These signs indicate the physician may need to be notified and the dosage may need to be decreased .

854 3 Epinephrine HCl is the drug of first choice in ventricular fibrillation because its alpha adrenergic effects improve susceptibility to defibrillation. (PL; TC; DR)

1 Lidocaine HCl is used after epinephrine has been used.
2 Dopamine HCl is not a first line drug of choice in the management of ventricular fibrillation.
4 Sodium bicarbonate use is based on blood gas confirmation of the presence of acidosis.

855. 4 Compliance with the prescribed regimen, which includes taking the drug and having prothrombin times performed by the laboratory, is necessary for safe and effective warfarin sodium (Coumadin) therapy. The dosage of Coumadin is adjusted according to the prothrombin time (PT); if the client fails to take the drug as prescribed, the tests are not reliable in monitoring the response to therapy. (EV; TC; DR)

1 Although some medications can affect the absorption or metabolism of Coumadin and also should be investigated, this is less likely to be a cause of fluctuations in laboratory values.
2 Same as answer 1.
3 Same as answer 1.

856. 4 Coumarin anticoagulants are administered orally and take 2 or 3 days to achieve the desired decrease in prothrombin level. Heparin, which must be administered parenterally, has immediate effects. (PL; TC; DR)

1 These drugs do not dissolve clots already present.
2 Because each drug affects a different part of the coagulation mechanism, dosages must be adjusted separately.
3 This does not account for the reason for the administration of both drugs, because coumarin derivatives will not exert an immediate therapeutic effect.

857. 1 Coumarin derivatives cause an increase in the prothrombin time, leading to an increased risk of bleeding. Any abnormal or excessive bleeding must be reported, because it may indicate toxic levels of the drug. (EV; ED; DR)

2 Edema is not caused by bleeding.
3 This would not be caused by Coumadin.
4 TIAs are not caused by bleeding, which is the primary concern in clients receiving anticoagulants.

858. 3 Barbiturates decrease the body's response to warfarin sodium (Coumadin). As a result there is less suppression of prothrombin; when inhibition caused by barbiturates disappears, hemorrhage can occur. (IM; ED; DR)

1 Serious withdrawal symptoms are unlikely in this situation; however, indiscriminate use of the drug should be avoided.
2 Insomnia may increase seizure incidence, but methods to promote sleep other than barbiturates should be considered.

4 Sleeping medications are not used to control seizures, although barbiturates such as phenobarbital may be prescribed for this purpose three or four times a day.

859. **2 The antagonist for Coumadin is vitamin K₁, which is involved in prothrombin formation. (PL; TC; DR)**
   1 Heparin is an anticoagulant.
   3 Protamine sulfate is the antidote for heparin overdose.
   4 Imferon is an iron supplement, not an antidote for coumarin.

860. **1 The presence of excess sodium (a solute) in the nephric tubules effectively decreases the water concentration of the glomerular filtrate and urine; water passively diffuses (osmosis) from the kidney tubule cells into the urine to equalize the water concentration. (AN; PA; DR)**
   2 Diffusion is not specific to fluid; osmosis is.
   3 Filtration refers to solutes; none are being passed.
   4 Active transport requires energy; water is passively diffused from the tubule cells to the urine.

861. **3 Hydrochlorothiazide (HydroDiuril) inhibits sodium reabsorption in the nephron, causing an increased excretion of sodium and chloride. (IM; ED; DR)**
   1 Osmotic diuretics affect the glomerular filtration rate.
   2 Most diuretics cause loss of potassium; however, potassium-sparing diuretics, such as spironolactone, decrease this loss.
   4 Loop diuretics (e.g., furosemide, ethacrynic acid) inhibit the reabsorption of sodium and chloride at the ascending loop of Henle.

862. **3 INH (isoniazid) often leads to pyridoxine (vitamin B₆) deficiency because it competes with the vitamin for the same enzyme. This is most often manifested by peripheral neuritis, which can be controlled by regular administration of vitamin B₆. (AN; PA; DR)**
   1 A vitamin does not, in and of itself, improve nutritional status.
   2 Pyridoxine does not enhance the effect of INH.
   4 Pyridoxine does not destroy organisms.

863. **2 Because of potential damage to the eighth cranial (vestibulocochlear) nerve, the dosage is regulated according to the**

combination of drugs prescribed and the severity of the illness. **(PL; TC; DR)**
   1 Dosage spacing does not increase compliance with the regimen.
   3 Although rest is important, this is not the rationale behind spacing doses.
   4 Injection sites may be rotated to decrease tissue trauma.

864. **2 Isoproterenol stimulates the beta receptors of the sympathetic nervous system, causing bronchodilation and increased rate and strength of cardiac contractions. (IM; PA; DR)**
   1 Barbiturates and hypnotics produce sedation.
   3 Antihypertensives and diuretics help decrease blood pressure.
   4 This is not the action of Isuprel. Expectorants mobilize respiratory secretions.

865. **4 Drowsiness is a side effect of Librium and indicates excessive depression of the central nervous system. (EV; TC; DR)**
   1 This is an expected response with therapeutic levels.
   2 This is not commonly attributed to chlordiazepoxide.
   3 Although tremors are listed as a possible adverse reaction, hyporeactivity is more common.

866. **2 Alprazolam (Xanax)) is an anxiolytic. It promotes muscle relaxation, reducing anxiety and facilitating rest. (EV; TC; DR)**
   1 Drowsiness is a side effect of Xanax, caused by its depression of central nervous system activity.
   3 One of the possible adverse reactions to Xanax is hostility.
   4 Transient hypotension is a side effect of Xanax.

867. **4 Used for its analgesic effects, morphine is a CNS depressant. Its major adverse effect is respiratory depression. It can also cause lethargy, pupillary constriction, depressed reflexes, and it could lead to coma and death. (EV; TC; DR)**
   1 These symptoms occur to some extent with therapeutic doses because of their effect on the CNS; however, they are not symptoms of an overdose.
   2 Overdose causes miosis rather than dilated pupils.
   3 Although diaphoresis may accompany hypotension, it is only indirectly related to the drug and is not profuse.

MEDICAL-SURGICAL ANSWERS

868. **4 Meperidine hydrochloride is the generic name for Demerol. (AN; TC; DR)**
1 Naloxone is the generic name for Narcan.
2 Propoxyphene hydrochloride is the generic name for Darvon.
3 Glutethimide is the generic name for Doriden.

869. **2 The exact mode of action of morphine sulfate is unknown. However, it has a rapid onset, lowers blood pressure, decreases pulmonary reflexes, and produces sedation. (AN; TC; DR)**
1 Chloral hydrate is a hypnotic but is not appropriate for the acute situation described.
3 Hydroxyzine hydrochloride is generally used to control anxiety associated with less acute situations and is available in oral form only.
4 Phenobarbital has a slower onset than morphine and does not affect respirations and blood pressure to the same extent as morphine.

870. **2 Warfarin sodium (Coumadin) has been shown to inhibit the metabolism of phenytoin (Dilantin), which results in an accumulation of this drug in the body. (AN; TC; DR)**
1 By potentiating the anticoagulant, phenytoin decreases clotting potential.
3 This is true only if the client is receiving phenytoin to control the seizure disorder.
4 They do not have a significant effect on the metabolism of Coumadin.

871. **1 Phenobarbital depresses the CNS, particularly the motor cortex, producing side effects such as lethargy, loss of appetite, depression, and vertigo. (EV; ED; DR)**
2 These are not side effects of phenobarbital.
3 Same as answer 2.
4 Same as answer 2.

872. **3 The primary site of action is the motor cortex, where seizure activity is limited by maintaining the sodium ion gradient of the neurons. (AN; TC; DR)**
1 This incorrectly describes the pharmacologic action of Dilantin.
2 Same as answer 1.
4 Same as answer 1.

873. **3 When an oral medication is available in a suspension form, the nurse should use it for clients who cannot swallow capsules. (IM; TC; DR)**
1 The route of administration cannot be altered without physician approval.

2 Because a palatable suspension is available, it is a better alternative than opening the capsule.
4 Intramuscular injections should be avoided because of related risks of tissue injury and infection.

874. **1 Gingival hyperplasia is an adverse effect of long-term phenytoin (Dilantin) therapy. The incidence can be decreased by maintaining therapeutic blood levels and meticulous oral hygiene. (PL; ED; DR)**
2 Alkalinity is not related to Dilantin or to the gingival hyperplasia caused by Dilantin. The incidence can be decreased by meticulous oral hygiene.
3 These are not a direct effect of Dilantin.
4 Plaque and bacterial growth at the gum line are unrelated to Dilantin or to the hyperplasia caused by it. The incidence can be decreased by meticulous oral hygiene.

875. **4 Phenytoin inhibits folic acid absorption and potentiates the effects of folic acid antagonists. Folic acid therapy is often helpful in correcting certain anemias that can result from administration of phenytoin. (Dosage must be carefully adjusted because folic acid diminishes the effects of phenytoin.) (AN; TC; DR)**
1 Although folic acid plays a role in the formation of heme in hemoglobin, its prescription in this case is related to Dilantin.
2 The description of this situation does not provide data to arrive at this conclusion.
3 Neurologic side effects include an elevation of the excitability threshold of neurons; neuropathy is not prevented by folic acid.

876. **4 Levodopa is the metabolic precursor of dopamine. It reduces sympathetic outflow by limiting vasoconstriction, which may result in orthostatic hypotension. (EV; TC; DR)**
1 Levodopa should be administered with food to minimize gastric irritation.
2 Although periodic tests to evaluate hepatic, renal, and cardiovascular therapy are required for prolonged therapy, whether these tests should be done on a weekly basis has not been established.
3 Levodopa may produce either symptom, but no established pattern of such responses exists.

877. **1 Carbamazepine (Tegretol) is administered to control pain by reducing the**

transmission of nerve impulses in clients with trigeminal neuralgia (EV; PA; DR)

2 Liver function is monitored to detect an adverse reaction to carbamazepine, not to determine therapeutic effectiveness.

3 This medication is not given to influence cardiac output.

4 Tegretol is not administered for its anticonvulsant properties to clients with tic douloureux because seizures are not present with this disorder.

878. **4 Tensilon, an anticholinesterase drug, causes temporary relief of symptoms of myasthenia gravis in clients who have the disease and is therefore an effective diagnostic aid. (EV; TC; DR)**

1 There is a decrease in symptoms.

2 Consciousness is not affected.

3 Hypotension may occur.

879. **2 A culture and testing of the antibiotic sensitivity of secretions or drainage identify the causative organism (culture) and the antibiotics to which the organism is particularly sensitive or resistant (sensitivity). (AN; PA; DR)**

1 This is a test for antibody content.

3 This is a test to determine whether a pathogen is virulent.

4 This is a test for viral activity.

880. **4 Streptomycin is ototoxic and may cause damage to the auditory and vestibular portions of the eighth cranial nerve. (EV; TC; DR)**

1 The drug does not adversely affect the cerebellum.

2 The motor end plates of the peripheral nervous system are not affected.

3 These cells and tracts of the nervous system are not affected.

881. **4 Septra blocks two consecutive steps in bacterial synthesis of essential nucleic acids and protein. (AN; TC; DR)**

1 Septra is an antibiotic, not an antiseptic.

2 Septra is an antibiotic, not an analgesic.

3 Septra is an antibiotic; it does not inhibit the reabsorption of uric acid.

882. **3 Any product containing aluminum, magnesium, or calcium ions should not be taken in the hours before or after an oral dose, because it decreases absorption by as much as 25% to 50%. (IM; TC; DR)**

1 Food interferes with absorption; it should be given 1 hour before or 2 hours after meals or snacks.

2 Citrus juice has no influence on this drug.

4 Antacids will interfere with absorption of this drug.

883. **3 Diphenhydramine hydrochloride (Benadryl), like other antihistamines, competes with histamine at receptor sites. This alleviates the effects of histamine, which include increased dilation and permeability of capillaries (the cause of urticaria). (IM; TC; DR)**

1 Benadryl does not destroy histamine; it competes with histamine at receptor sites.

2 Benadryl does not cause these responses; histamine dilates capillaries.

4 Benadryl does not metabolize histamines.

884. **2 Diarrhea is a possible side effect that can be related to a superinfection; it can lead to fluid and electrolyte imbalance. (IM; ED; DR)**

1 Ampicillin is best absorbed when taken on an empty stomach with water.

3 Although storage in a tight container is necessary, protection from light is not.

4 A culture is generally not repeated unless the client's condition warrants it.

885. **1 To prevent crystal formation, the client should have sufficient intake to produce 1000 to 1500 ml of fluid per day while taking this drug. (IM; TC; DR)**

2 Straining urine is not indicated when a client is taking a urinary antibiotic.

3 Urinary decrease is of concern, since it may indicate urinary failure. If fluids are encouraged, the client's output should increase.

4 The drug need not be taken at a strict time daily.

886. **4**

$$\frac{1000 \text{ ml} \times 20 \text{ drops per ml}}{8 \text{ hr} \times 60 \text{ min}} = \frac{20{,}000}{480}$$

$$= 42 \text{ drops/min}$$

(EV; TC; GI)

1 This rate would be too slow.

2 Same as answer 1.

3 Same as answer 1.

887. **1** Signs of cinchonism, such as tinnitus, headache, dizziness, deafness, and nausea, indicate that toxicity caused by an overdose of quinine has occurred. (EV; PA; DR)
2 These are not signs of cinchonism.
3 Same as answer 2.
4 Tinnitus and diminished hearing are caused by maximum levels of quinine; however paresthesias do not occur.

888. **2** Quinine administered orally can cause gastric irritation, resulting in nausea and vomiting. By administering such a medication immediately after meals the nurse minimizes its irritating effect. (IM; TC; DR)
1 Absorption of the drug is not significantly affected by administration after meals.
3 The appetite is not affected by this drug as long as gastric irritation is avoided.
4 Quinidine sulfate or gluconate, not quinine, is given for its antidysrhythmic effect.

889. **3** Hydrocortisone is a glucocorticoid that has antiinflammatory action and aids in metabolism of carbohydrate, fat, and protein, causing elevation of blood sugar. Thus it enables the body to adapt to stress. (EV; TC; DR)
1 Potassium salts are retained in Addison's disease.
2 Cardiac dysrhythmias are caused by electrolyte imbalances, and dyspnea is caused by hypovolemia and decreased O_2 supply; neither is affected by hydrocortisone.
4 Lack of angiotensin II is not the cause of hypotension in this disorder.

890. **4** DDAVP replaces the ADH, facilitating reabsorption of water and consequent return of normal urine output and thirst. (EV; TC; DR)
1 Although a correction of tachycardia is consistent with correction of dehydration, the client is not dehydrated if the fluid intake is adequate.
2 DDAVP does not alter serum glucose; diabetes mellitus, not diabetes insipidus, results in hyperglycemia.
3 The mechanisms that regulate pH are not affected.

891. **2** Different types of insulin are compatible and are administered in the same syringe. However, the regular insulin is generally drawn up first because it is fast acting, and the possibility that a slower-acting insulin will enter the multidose vial is eliminated. (IM; TC; DR)
1 The ratio does not affect compatibility.
3 Same as answer 1.
4 This is unnecessary; unnecessary injections increase the risk of infection as well as causing additional discomfort.

892. **3** Dexamethasone (Decadron) increases gluconeogenesis, which may cause hyperglycemia. (EV; TC; DR)
1 Decadron does not contain a glucose component.
2 Glucose metabolism is not accelerated by Decadron.
4 The renal threshold for glucose is not affected by Decadron.

893. **2** Any hormone normally produced by the body must be withdrawn slowly to allow the appropriate organ to adjust and resume production. (IM; ED; DR)
1 Although important, this is not the reason for gradual withdrawal of the drug.
3 Same as answer 1.
4 Same as answer 1.

894. **1** Prolonged use of steroids may cause leukopenia as a result of bone marrow depression. (DC; PA; DR)
2 CRP (C-reactive protein) is present in acute inflammatory diseases and necrosis; it is not associated with steroids.
3 The sedimentation rate is elevated when inflammation is present; it is not associated with steroids.
4 This is the name given anemias that are characterized by decreased concentration of hemoglobin in erythrocytes; it is not a sequela of the use of steroids.

895. **2** Salicylates can cause ototoxicity as well as central nervous system effects such as confusion. (EV; TC; DR)
1 This is not an effect of salicylate intoxication.
3 Same as answer 1.
4 Same as answer 1.

896. **1** Gold salts, bound to plasma proteins, are distributed irregularly throughout the body but the highest concentration occurs in the kidneys. The slow excretion of gold salts cannot keep up with their intake; they accumulate in the kidneys, causing damage. (EV; TC; DR)

2 This is not a side effect associated with gold salts, such as Myochrysine.

3 Same as answer 2.

4 Same as answer 2.

897. **2 The antiinflammatory action of acetyl-salicylic acid (ASA) is effective in reducing the discomfort and pain associated with rheumatoid arthritis. (AN; PA; DR)**

1 Azathioprine (Imuran) is used in refractory rheumatoid arthritis and would be added to the medication regimen if nonsteroidal antiinflammatories, gold salts, or cortisone do not provide relief.

3 Cortisone is employed when more conservative treatment fails; its use is avoided because of associated adverse effects (e.g., osteoporosis, gastric ulceration, psychosis, decreased resistance, hirsutism, hyperglycemia, edema, hypertension).

4 Gold salts are employed if more conservative treatment fails; they must be administered intramuscularly and are highly toxic.

898. **3 Adverse reactions include blood dyscrasias, such as eosinophilia, thrombocytopenia, aplastic anemia, and leukopenia, which can be life threatening. (EV; TC; DR)**

1 This is not an adverse reaction to a gold compound.

2 Although cutaneous lesions can occur, they are not life threatening as thrombocytopenia can be.

4 Same as answer 1.

899. **3 Many chemotherapeutic agents function by interfering with DNA replication associated with normal cellular reproduction (mitosis). The normal rapid mitosis of the stratified squamous epithelium of the mouth and anus result in their being powerfully affected by the drugs. (EV; PA; DR)**

1 The state of nourishment would be applicable to all cells; although anorexia is common, this client may not be anorexic.

2 This effect is not caused by direct irritation; most agents are administered parenterally.

4 Chemotherapeutic agents affect the cells that are most rapidly proliferating, which include not only the cells of the GI epithelium but also those of the bone marrow and hair follicles.

900. **1 Methotrexate is a folic acid antagonist that can cause depression of bone marrow. This serious toxic effect is sometimes prevented by administration of folic acid. Some physicians advocate its administration after a course of methotrexate therapy so as not to interfere with methotrexate activity. (AN; TC; DR)**

2 Folic acid is a metabolite and does not destroy cancer cells.

3 Same as answer 2.

4 Methotrexate does not increase the production of phagocytes.

901. **4 Prolonged chemotherapy may slow the production of leukocytes in bone marrow and lymph nodes, thus suppressing the activity of the immune system. Antibiotics may be required to help counter infections that the body can no longer handle easily. (AN; TC; DR)**

1 The liver does not produce leukocytes.

2 Although leukocytes are circulating in both blood and lymph, these cells are more mature and thus more resistant to the effects of chemotherapy.

3 Same as answer 2.

902. **2 Most chemotherapeutic agents interfere with mitosis. The bone marrow consists of rapidly dividing cells, and therefore its activity is depressed. (EV; TC; DR)**

1 Because of bone marrow depression, leukopenia rather than leukocytosis can occur.

3 The ESR generally increases in the presence of tissue inflammation or necrosis.

4 If bleeding occurs, the hemoglobin and hematocrit may be decreased because of the decreased number of thrombocytes.

903. **3 Sodium bicarbonate is absorbed and can alter the acid-base balance. Antacids are not readily absorbed, so they do not alter acid-base balance. (AN; ED; DR)**

1 This is false; aluminum hydroxide and/or magnesium hydroxide preparations contain sodium and should be used only with caution.

2 This is false; nonsystemic antacids are insoluble and not readily absorbed.

4 This is false; these are side effects of nonsystemic antacids.

904. **4 It decreases gastric secretion by inhibiting histamine at H$_2$ receptors. (IM; ED; DR)**
1 It does not affect gastric motility.
2 It does not affect the pH of gastric secretions already present.
3 It is an H2 histamine receptor antagonist.

905. **3 Calcium carbonate's antacid action lowers gastric pH, which in turn stimulates renewed secretion of acid by the gastric mucosa. (2, IM; ED; DR)**

1 This medication causes constipation, not diarrhea.
2 Calcium carbonate does not contain sodium as do some antacids; thus, it does not promote fluid retention.
4 This antacid provides a source of calcium that would help prevent bone demineralization.

Comprehensive
Test

COMPREHENSIVE TEST

The questions in the comprehensive test have been developed to reflect the current Nurse Registration/Licensure examination format and guidelines. In order for you to achieve maximum learning from this experience we have divided the comprehensive test into two sections. Parts A and B each contain 125 questions, which together total 250 questions, the approximate number of questions that you will be presented with on a typical version of the Nurse Registration/Licensure examination. Approximately half of the 250 questions are presented as independent items while the remaining questions are grouped into Client Case Scenarios, where questions relate to a particular client who requires nursing care. You should allow about 1 minute per question and complete Part A within 3½ hours and Part B within 3½ hours. Allow yourself a 1-hour break between Parts A and B. This will reflect the testing session of the Nurse Registration/Licensure examination.

There are two methods you can use when taking the Comprehensive Test. One method is to answer the questions in Part A and then review the answers and rationales before completing Part B. This method will reinforce your immediate learning. An alternative method is to complete both Part A and Part B before checking the answers and rationales. This method will also reinforce learning and will better reflect the actual situation you will experience when taking the Nurse Registration/Licensure examination.

To help you analyze your mistakes on the Comprehensive Test and to provide a database for making study plans, worksheets have been included. These sheets are designed to aid you in identifying and recording errors in the way you process information and to help you identify and record gaps in knowledge. Follow directions that appear at the beginning of the Answers and Rationales for Comprehensive Test Questions. Use a separate worksheet for each part of the test. As you review material in class notes or this review book, pay special attention to correcting your most common problems and identifying the topics you need to review. It might be helpful to set priorities; review the most difficult topics first so that you will have time to review them more than once. The worksheets can be used to focus your future study. The comprehensive test questions are classified by five categories: (1) phases of the nursing process, (2) cognitive or affective domain, (3) client need, (4) content area/category of concern, and (5) client age and gender. Full descriptions of these categories and their subclassifications are presented in Chapter 1 and at the beginning of the Answers and Rationales for the Comprehensive Test Questions.

ANSWERS AND RATIONALES FOR COMPREHENSIVE TEST QUESTIONS

To enhance your study and review:
- First, find the parentheses containing five pairs of letters following the correct answers.
- The first pair of letters is the abbreviation for the step in the nursing process and two additional categories tested by the question: (DC) data collection, (AN) analysis and interpretation of data, (PL) planning care, (IM) implementation, (EV) evaluation, (CC) collaboration and coordination, (PP) professional practice. The Appendix provides a detailed list of Canadian registered nurse competencies found within each step in the nursing process, as well as the two additional categories. The list has been divided into four groups, each weighted from competencies of high importance (Group A) to competencies of relatively low importance (Group D). Thus, those competencies from Group A have the greatest representation on the Comprehensive Test, wheras those from Group D have the least representation. The groups reflect Canadian registered nurse competencies relative to their importance, frequency, and level of difficulty.
- The second pair of letters is the abbreviation for the cognitive level tested by the question: (KC) knowledge and comprehension, (AP) application, (CT) critical thinking for the cognitive domain, and (AF) affective for the affective domain.
- The third pair of letters is the abbreviation for the area of client need tested by the question: (PA) physiologic and anatomic equilibrium; (TC) therapeutic care; (ED) education and health promotion; (PS) psychosocial and emotional equilibrium.
- The fourth pair of letters is the abbreviation for the specific area of content or, as we call it, the category of concern tested by the question. The categories of concern used in medical, surgical, and pediatric nursing include (BI) blood and immunity; (CV) cardiovascular; (DR) drug-related responses; (EH) emotional needs related to health problems; (EN) endocrine; (FE) fluid and electrolyte; (GI) gastrointestinal; (GD) growth and development; (IT) integumentary; (NM) neuromuscular; (RG) reproductive and genitourinary; (RE) respiratory; (SK) skeletal.

The categories of concern used in childbearing and women's health nursing include (DR) drug-related responses; (EC) emotional needs related to childbearing and women's health; (HC) healthy childbearing; (HN) high-risk neonate; (HP) high-risk maternal-fetal conditions affecting childbearing; (NN) normal neonate; (RC) reproductive choices; (RP) reproductive problems; (WH) women's health.

The categories of concern used in mental health/psychiatric nursing include (AX) anxiety, somatoform, and dissociative disorders; (CS) crisis situations; (DD) dementia, delirium, and other cognitive disorders; (EP) emotional problems related to physical health and childbearing; (BA) disorders first evident before adulthood; (MO) disorders of mood; (PR) disorders of personality; (DR) drug-related responses; (EA) eating disorders; (PD) personality development; (SD) schizophrenic disorders; (SA) substance abuse; (TR) therapeutic relationships.

- The fifth pair of letters is the abbreviation for client age and gender tested by the question: (CM) child/adolescent - male, (CF) child/adolescent - female, (AM) adult male, (AF) adult female, (OM) older male, (OF) older female.

USING YOUR ANALYSIS OF THE QUESTIONS TO DEVELOP A FOCUS FOR STUDY

The question analysis provides an opportunity for you to review the questions on the Comprehensive Test that you answered incorrectly. For each question on the Comprehensive Test this book tells you why the correct answer is correct and why each of the other options is incorrect. The rationale for the correct answer includes in parentheses the specific areas measured by the question; that is, the type of nursing behavior, the cognitive or affective domain, the client need, the content area/category of concern, and the client age and gender tested. The categories of concern identify the specific content area covered by the question; they provide the basis for developing your own personal focus of study.

Use the *Focus for Study Worksheets* that are included with the answers and rationales for each part of the Comprehensive Test as you look over the list of questions you missed. You will also need to refer to the questions on the Comprehensive Test. By identifying the topic of each question and its category of concern, you can identify those areas in which you missed the greatest number of questions.

The worksheet has seven columns across the top of the page. The first column contains a list of the categories of concern used in this book. The other six columns, entitled pathophysiology (basic science), pharmacology, nutrition, diagnostic studies, physical care, and emotional care, are empty.

To develop a meaningful focus of study, simply follow these directions.

1. In the Comprehensive Test, reread each question you missed.
2. In the Answers and Rationales section, read the correct answer and the rationale for that answer.
3. Read the answer you chose and the reason your answer was incorrect.
4. Identify the category of concern for the question by looking at the fourth set of two letters in the parentheses following the correct rationale.
5. Find these same two letters in the category of concern column on the worksheet.
6. Now your professional judgment comes into action. Look at the question you missed and decide if the subject matter being questioned best fits under the general heading of pathophysiology (basic science), pharmacology, nutrition, diagnostic studies, physical care, or emotional care.
7. Write the number of this question in the box that intersects both the category of concern column and the general heading row. Make your numbers small so that you can enter the numbers of all applicable questions in the appropriate box. Do this for every question you answered incorrectly.
8. After you complete this process, you will be able to identify the areas of knowledge where you missed the most questions. These gaps, requiring additional study, may be in a topic area, a category of concern, or both. You may want to go over those questions you missed along with answers and rationales again to be sure you understand why you answered incorrectly and to identify the specific information you need to study.

It is important that you take the time to carefully complete the worksheets. The resulting information will assist you in identifying your areas of both strength and weakness and help you to use your study time effectively.

The topics that the worksheets demonstrate need further study can be found in the index of most nursing textbooks or in the review section of this book. You can therefore use whatever text or resource material is available to you and with which you are already familiar.

If you practice the subject matter, the knowledge you gain will provide you with the ability to answer questions. Remember, if you know the material, you can handle any question.

COMPREHENSIVE TEST: PART A

Client Case Scenario 1: Mrs. Rowan is a 32-year-old client who is a primigravida. Her pregnancy has been progressing uneventfully. Mrs. Rowan is now at 24 weeks gestation. **Items 1 to 6 refer to this client case scenario.**

1. Mrs. Rowan comes into the clinic for her prenatal checkup. Her blood pressure is 150/86 and she has gained 2.27 kg in the last 2 weeks. The nurse should:
   1 Take her temperature and pulse
   2 Prepare her for a vaginal examination
   3 Give her another appointment in 2 weeks
   4 Test her urine for the presence of albumin

2. Preeclampsia is first suspected in Mrs. Rowan's pregnancy when she has:
   1 Fluctuation of the BP
   2 Excessive weight gain
   3 Presence of albuminuria
   4 Progressive ankle edema

3. Mrs. Rowan is diagnosed with pregnancy-induced hypertension. The nurse would know that dietary teaching is effective when Mrs. Rowan says, "I should follow a diet that includes:
   1 High sodium and calories and low protein."
   2 Low sodium and calories and high protein."
   3 Normal sodium with ample calories and protein."
   4 Moderate sodium, low calories, and ample protein."

4. Mrs. Rowan is hospitalized and is receiving magnesium sulfate ($MgSO_4$) by IV push. Before administering each dose, the nurse should assess her:
   1 Temperature and pulse rate
   2 Respirations and patellar reflex
   3 Blood pressure and apical pulse
   4 Urinary output relative to fluid intake

5. What would the nurse place at Mrs. Rowan's bedside in preparation for the possibility of magnesium sulfate toxicity?
   1 Nalline
   2 Oxygen
   3 Calcium gluconate
   4 Suction equipment

6. The nurse should monitor Mrs. Rowan's hematocrit levels, which may be elevated due to her pregnancy-induced hypertension. Which of the following may cause this elevation?

1 Vasodilation caused by an alteration in circulating fluid
2 Agglutination of red cells caused by membrane fragility
3 Hemoconcentration caused by a decrease in plasma volume
4 Hemodilution of pregnancy caused by increases in blood volume

---

Client Case Scenario 2: Jason is a 10-year-old client who has been diagnosed as having Type I or insulin-dependent diabetes mellitus (IDDM). **Items 7 to 10 refer to this client case scenario.**

7. Jason is placed in a two-bed room. Which of the following children would be the best roommate for him?
   1 A 12-year-old girl with colitis
   2 A 9-year-old boy with asthma
   3 A 10-year-old girl with a fractured femur
   4 A 10-year-old boy with rheumatoid arthritis

8. Which of the following statements best describes Jason's Type I, insulin-dependent diabetes mellitus?
   1 IDDM does not always require insulin
   2 IDDM does not involve vascular changes
   3 IDDM occurs more often in obese children
   4 IDDM begins more rapidly than adult-onset diabetes

9. The physician orders 20 units of Humulin R insulin for Jason. The vial reads: 1 ml=100 units of Humulin R insulin. An insulin syringe is not available. Which of the following amounts, measured in a regular syringe, should the nurse administer?
   1 0.2 ml
   2 0.3 ml
   3 0.4 ml
   4 0.6 ml

10. As part of the teaching plan for Jason, the nurse should indicate that his need for insulin will likely decrease during which of the following times?
    1 At puberty onset
    2 When an infection is present
    3 When there is an emotional stress
    4 When active exercise is performed

Client Case Scenario 3: Carlie, a 4-year-old, is admitted to hospital exhibiting withdrawal. Following examination, she is diagnosed with autistic disorder. **Items 11 to 14 refer to this client case scenario.**

11. Since Carlie withdraws into her own world, relationships are difficult to establish. The nurse may be able to reach Carlie by:
    1 Body contact, such as cuddling
    2 Providing a quiet, safe place for rocking
    3 Encouraging participation in group activities
    4 Imitating and participating in the child's activities

12. When assessing Carlie, the nurse would expect her to demonstrate:
    1 Sad, blank facial expressions
    2 Flapping of hands and rocking
    3 Lack of response to any stimulus
    4 Inappropriate smiling with flat emotions

13. What interventions by the health care team would facilitate Carlie's play therapy?
    1 Play music and dance with her
    2 Talk to her while holding hands
    3 Provide mechanical and inanimate objects for play
    4 Provide her with brightly colored toys and blocks that can be held

14. Given a choice, which of the following would Carlie usually enjoy playing with?
    1 Cuddly toy
    2 Large red block
    3 Small yellow block
    4 Playground merry-go-round

Client Case Scenario 4: Mr. Lister, age 71 years, has been recently diagnosed with primary open-angle glaucoma. **Items 15 to 17 refer to this client case scenario.**

15. Why is it imperative that the nurse assist Mr. Lister in accepting the need for treatment for his glaucoma?
    1 Total blindness is inevitable
    2 Lost vision cannot be restored
    3 Surgery will only temporarily help the problem
    4 There is usually restriction in the use of both eyes

16. Which of the following ocular symptoms should the nurse expect Mr. Lister to demonstrate?
    1 Attacks of acute pain
    2 Constant blurred vision
    3 Impairment of peripheral vision
    4 A complete loss of central vision

17. The nurse would know that discharge teaching for Mr. Lister was effective when he states, "I should:
    1 Restrict my fluid intake."
    2 Avoid bending exercises."
    3 Use mydriatrics regularly."
    4 Avoid bright lights or darkness."

Client Case Scenario 5: Mr. Vitrie, age 42 years, has undergone an above-the-knee amputation after falling from a scaffold at a construction site where he worked. **Items 18 to 21 refer to this client case scenario.**

18. To prevent a contracture of Mr. Vitrie's hip, the nurse should:
    1 Elevate the head of his bed
    2 Place pillows under his stump
    3 Encourage him to sit in a chair as much as possible
    4 Encourage him to lie in the prone position several times daily

19. To promote early and efficient ambulation following an above-the-knee amputation, Mr. Vitrie should be encouraged to keep his hip:
    1 In a flexed position
    2 In functional alignment
    3 Extended and abducted
    4 Slightly raised when moving the stump

20. Which of following is a factor that may contribute to Mr. Vitrie developing stump shrinkage?
    1 Postoperative edema
    2 Development of skin turgor
    3 Reduction of subcutaneous fat
    4 Loss of tissue and bone during operation

21. Following his amputation, the nurse can help Mr. Vitrie prepare his stump for a prosthesis by encouraging him to:
    1 Abduct the stump when ambulating
    2 Hang the stump off the bed frequently
    3 Soak the stump in warm water twice a day
    4 Periodically press the end of the stump against a pillow

Client Case Scenario 6: Mrs. Dowle has just delivered a healthy baby boy. **Items 22 to 24 refer to this client case scenario.**

22. Two hours after delivery, the nurse finds that Mrs. Dowle's fundus is firm, shifted to the right, and two fingers above the umbilicus. This would indicate:
    1 A full bladder
    2 A normal process

3 Impending bleeding
4 Retained secundinae

23. After delivery, when checking Mrs. Dowle's signs, the nurse should normally find:
1 A decided bradycardia with no change in respirations
2 A decided tachycardia with a decrease in respirations
3 An elevated basal temperature with a decrease in respirations
4 A slight lowering of basal temperature with an increase in respirations

24. When helping Mrs. Dowle develop her parenting role, the nurse should:
1 Do things for the baby in her presence
2 Demonstrate baby bathing and care before discharge
3 Provide enough time for her and the baby to be together
4 Find out what she knows about babies and proceed from there

Client Case Scenario 7: Sarah is a 2½-year-old girl who has been admitted to a pediatric hospital with laryngotracheobronchitis (croup). **Items 25 to 28 refer to this client case scenario.**

25. When assessing Sarah, which of the following presentations should the nurse expect to find?
1 Expiratory stridor, crackles
2 Laryngospasm, barking cough
3 Bronchospasm, whooping cough
4 Productive cough, inspiratory stridor

26. Two hours after Sarah is admitted, the nurse observes an increase in her respiratory and cardiac rates. She is restless, with substernal and intercostal retractions. Which of the following actions should the nurse place as first priority?
1 Remove secretions with suction apparatus
2 Increase the level of oxygen being delivered
3 Strike the child on the back to dislodge mucus
4 Inform the physician of the child's respiratory status

27. An emergency tracheotomy is performed on Sarah. Suctioning of the tracheostomy should be done routinely and will also be indicated if she demonstrates which of the following problems? Sarah:
1 Tells the nurse of difficulty in breathing
2 Becomes restless, diaphoretic, and cyanotic

3 Has severe substernal retractions and stridor
4 Becomes restless, pale, or the pulse increases

28. Sarah's croup resolves. When teaching Sarah's parents about handling further episodes of croup at home, the nurse indicates that actions are to be directed at which of the following goals?
1 Dilation of the bronchi
2 Interruption of the spasm
3 Reduction of the inflammation
4 Depression of the cough center

Client Case Scenario 8: Mr. Voth, 32 years of age, is admitted to a mental health clinic because his family is concerned about his increasingly manic and ritualistic behavior. He has been previously diagnosed with obsessive-compulsive disorder. **Items 29 to 31 refer to this client case scenario.**

29. Mr. Voth's personality with an obsessive-compulsive disorder is probably characterized by:
1 Marked emotional maturity
2 Elaborate delusional system
3 Rapid, frequent mood swings
4 Doubts, fears, and indecisiveness

30. For Mr. Voth, it is most important that the nurse:
1 Allow him sufficient time to carry out the ritual
2 Promote reality by showing that the ritual serves little purpose
3 Try to ascertain the meaning of the ritual by discussing it with him
4 Interrupt the ritual to demonstrate that the ritual does not control what happens

31. If interrupted in his performance of the ritual, Mr. Voth would most likely react with:
1 Anxiety
2 Hostility
3 Aggression
4 Withdrawal

Client Case Scenario 9: Mrs. Low, 51 years of age, has lived with bronchial asthma for the past 6 years. **Items 32 to 36 refer to this client case scenario.**

32. What is the most probable cause of Mrs. Low's difficulty breathing?
1 A too rapid expulsion of air
2 Spasms of the bronchi, which trap the air
3 Hyperventilation due to an anxiety reaction
4 An increase in the vital capacity of the lungs

33. Nursing management for Mrs. Low should be directed toward:
    1 Curing the condition permanently
    2 Raising mucus secretions from the chest
    3 Limiting pulmonary secretions by decreasing fluid intake
    4 Convincing her that the condition is emotionally based

34. The nurse administers aminophylline via an IV drip to Mrs. Low. The purpose of this therapy is to:
    1 Reduce respiratory bacteria
    2 Promote rest and relaxation
    3 Stimulate smooth muscle relaxation
    4 Diminish inflammatory cell responses

35. The physician orders daily sputum specimens to be collected from Mrs. Low. When is it most appropriate for the nurse to collect these specimens?
    1 After activity
    2 Before meals
    3 On awakening
    4 Before a respiratory treatment

36. Mrs. Low is found to be allergic to dust. Her teaching plan should include the fact that:
    1 Housework must be done by someone else
    2 Damp-dusting the house will help limit dust particles in the air
    3 The condition must be accepted because dust cannot be limited
    4 The house must be redecorated because the environment must be dust-free

Client Case Scenario 10: Mrs. Joyce, age 63 years, has been diagnosed with cancer of the colon. She is admitted to hospital 3 days prior to surgery for a permanent colostomy. **Items 37 to 42 refer to this client case scenario.**

37. Mrs. Joyce is cooperative during all procedures, responds pleasantly when approached by nurses and does not question staff about the procedures being carried out. What behavior is most likely being exhibited? Mrs. Joyce:
    1 Feels reassured by frequent contacts with the nurses
    2 Is totally denying the illness and the need for surgery
    3 Is not verbalizing feelings about what will happen
    4 Has been fully informed by the physician about what to expect

38. Following surgery for a colostomy, the most effective way for the health care team to help Mrs. Joyce accept her colostomy would be to:

    1 Begin to teach self-care of the colostomy immediately
    2 Provide literature containing factual data about ostomies
    3 Contact a member of Colostomies, Inc. to speak with her
    4 Point out the number of important people who have had colostomies

39. Mrs. Joyce's postoperative diet orders are "diet as tolerated." Which principles should guide the nurse in helping Mrs. Joyce make food choices?
    1 Many foods will cause all individuals with a colostomy the same discomfort
    2 More rigid dietary rules limiting food choices are needed to provide security
    3 A low-residue diet should be followed indefinitely to avoid overstimulating the intestine
    4 A return to a regular diet as soon as possible gives psychologic support and more rapid physical rehabilitation

40. During a colostomy irrigation, Mrs. Joyce complains of abdominal cramps. What should the nurse do?
    1 Clamp the tubing and allow her to rest
    2 Reassure her and continue the irrigation
    3 Pinch the tubing so that less fluid enters the colon
    4 Raise the irrigating can to complete the irrigation quickly

41. Mrs. Joyce's colostomy is located on the left side of her abdomen. What type of stool should the nurse expect?
    1 Liquid
    2 Moist, formed
    3 Mucus coated
    4 Pencil shaped

42. When discussing the regaining of bowel control with Mrs. Joyce, the nurse should emphasize the importance of:
    1 A high protein diet
    2 An irrigation routine
    3 Managing fluid intake
    4 A soft low-residue diet

Client Case Scenario 11: Baby Terrence, a full-term male child, is delivered by his mother who is Rh negative. **Items 43 to 45 refer to this client case scenario.**

43. At the time of delivery, baby Terrence's blood is typed to determine the ABO group and the presence of the Rh factor. The nurse is aware that:

1 The Rh factor is not genetically determined
2 Not all infants of Rh-positive fathers are Rh positive
3 The Rh factor of the fetus is determined by the father
4 During gestation, the Rh factor of the fetus may change

44. Baby Terrence is Rh positive and his mother is Rh negative. Baby Terrence is to receive an exchange transfusion. The nurse knows that he will receive Rh-negative blood because:
1 It is the same as the mother's blood
2 It is neutral and will not react with his blood
3 It eliminates the possibility of a transfusion reaction occurring
4 Its RBCs will not be destroyed by maternal anti-Rh antibodies

45. When the nurse brings Terrence to his mother, she comments about the milia on the baby's face. The nurse should:
1 Tell her that all babies have them and they clear up in 2 to 3 days
2 Explain that these are birthmarks that will disappear with a few months
3 Instruct her about proper hand washing, since the milia can be infectious
4 Instruct her to avoid squeezing them or attempting to wash them off

Client Case Scenario 12: Mr. Letski, age 58 years, has just arrived in the recovery room following a segmental resection of the right lower lobe of the lung. He has a chest tube drainage system in place. **Items 46 to 49 refer to this client case scenario.**

46. When caring for Mr. Letski's chest tube drainage system, what action by the nurse would be most appropriate?
1 Add 3 to 5 ml of sterile saline to the water seal chamber
2 Raise the drainage system to bed level to check its patency
3 Mark the time and the fluid level on the side of the drainage system
4 Secure the chest catheter to the wound dressing with a sterile safety pin

47. What is the purpose of the water in the water seal chamber of Mr. Letski's chest tube drainage system?
1 Prevent entrance of air into the pleural cavity
2 Foster removal of chest secretions by capillarity
3 Facilitate emptying bloody drainage from the chest

4 Decrease the danger of sudden change in pressure in the tube

48. Mr. Letski has excessive respiratory secretions. In addition to encouraging him to cough, what independent nursing care should also be included?
1 Postural drainage
2 Turning and positioning
3 Administration of an expectorant
4 Percussion and vibration techniques

49. Mr. Letski is on oxygen therapy. What preventative measure regarding untoward effects should be taken by the nurse?
1 Humidifying the gas before delivery
2 Padding elastic bands of his face mask
3 Placing him in the orthopneic position
4 Taking his apical pulse before starting therapy

50. Which of the following problems associated with juvenile rheumatoid arthritis indicates the major difference between this disorder and the polyarthritis of rheumatic fever?
1 Some residual joint deformity
2 Some permanent cardiac damage
3 A link with the *Streptococcus* organism
4 An exacerbation during the winter months

51. When caring for a client receiving prolonged aspirin therapy, the nurse should be alert for symptoms of:
1 Urinary calculi
2 Atrophy of the liver
3 Prolonged bleeding time
4 Premature erythrocyte destruction

52. For clients who are terminally ill, the most important factor relative to therapeutic nurse-client relationships is the nurse's:
1 Feelings about the situation
2 Knowledge of the grieving process
3 Recognition of the family's ability to cope
4 Previous experience with terminally ill clients

53. Which food combinations can be included on a low-residue diet?
1 Baked fish, macaroni with cheese, strained carrots, fruit gelatin, milk
2 Creamed soup and crackers, omelet, mashed potatoes, bran muffin, orange juice, coffee
3 Stewed chicken, baked potato with butter, strained peas, white bread, plain cake, and milk
4 Lean roast beef, buttered white rice with egg slices, white bread with butter and jelly, tea with sugar

54. A client who is recovering from an acute bout of colitis is placed on a high-protein diet. What is the primary purpose of this diet?
    1 Repair tissues
    2 Slow peristalsis
    3 Correct the anemia
    4 Improve muscle tone

55. A 36-year-old pregnant woman accompanied by her husband is admitted to labor and delivery, and fetal monitoring is instituted. What should the nurse realize when a fetus is being monitored?
    1 Internal monitoring will be used in the latter part of labor
    2 The machinery can be very frightening to the laboring couple
    3 The mother may need a mild sedative every 4 hours for comfort
    4 Older primigravidas have more complications than younger women

56. A client with a history of endometriosis delivers a healthy baby. She expresses concern that the symptoms associated with endometriosis will return now that her pregnancy is over. What is the nurse's best response?
    1 "Pregnancy usually cures the endometriosis."
    2 "Endometriosis will usually cause an early menopause."
    3 "A hysterectomy will be necessary if the symptoms recur."
    4 "Breastfeeding your baby will delay the return of symptoms."

57. A client is breastfeeding her infant and complains that her breasts are swollen and painful. When teaching her about breastfeeding, what could the nurse say when explaining how to prevent engorgement in the future?
    1 "Use a bottle for feeding when you are experiencing discomfort."
    2 "Limit nursing to 4 to 6 minutes on each breast, four times a day."
    3 "Nurse the baby frequently and for at least 10 minutes on each breast."
    4 "Feed the baby four times a day. This will prevent rapid filling of the breast."

58. Following a radical neck dissection, a client returns to the unit with an endotracheal tube in place. The nurse should:
    1 Irrigate the tube to maintain patency
    2 Have a tracheostomy set at the bedside
    3 Change the dressing to observe for covert bleeding
    4 Reposition the endotracheal tube when the gag reflex returns

59. Following surgery a client is extubated in the postanesthesia unit. What observation would indicate to the nurse that acute respiratory embarrassment is occurring?
    1 Restlessness and confusion
    2 Anxiety and constricted pupils
    3 Decreased pulse and respirations
    4 Cyanosis and clubbing of the fingers

60. At the end of the first trimester of pregnancy a client complains of feeling tired. The nurse recognizes that this is probably related to the normal cardiovascular changes which:
    1 Increase BP
    2 Increase hematocrit
    3 Increase blood volume
    4 Decrease cardiac output

61. At delivery a mother observes a nevus vasculosus on her newborn's midthigh and becomes extremely upset. How can the nurse best respond?
    1 "This is a superficial area that will fade in a few days."
    2 "The area will spread rapidly and then regress."
    3 "This mark will not grow or fade, but will be covered by clothes."
    4 "Surgical removal will be necessary as soon as the infant is older."

62. During a prenatal class, how can the nurse best explain to participants an advantage of breastfeeding?
    1 Breastfeeding inhibits ovulation in the mother
    2 Allergic responses are diminished in breastfed infants
    3 Breastfed infants adhere more easily to a 4-hour schedule
    4 Breast milk has a larger concentration of protein than does cow's milk

63. The nurse teaches a couple about care of their newborn who has been circumcised. What statement by the father would indicate his understanding of the teaching?
    1 We will leave the infant undiapered
    2 We should observe for fussy behavior
    3 We will apply petroleum jelly gauze to the penis
    4 We should notify the clinic if yellow exudate occurs

64. The physician prescribes an estrogen-progestin oral contraceptive for a client. The nurse would know that teaching was effective when the client verbalizes that she should observe for the side effects of
   1 Nausea, rash, and bleeding
   2 Lethargy, syncope, and tachycardia
   3 Hypertension, calf and breast tenderness
   4 Bradycardia, visual changes, and hypertension

65. Which nursing approach would be most therapeutic when a new mother refuses to look at her infant who has a severe birth defect?
   1 Explain the problem to the family and encourage them to help comfort her
   2 Gently tell her that she should stop blaming herself for the child's handicap
   3 Reinforce the physician's explanation of the handicap and allow time for her to discuss her fears
   4 Wait until she has sufficiently recovered from the stress of delivery before bringing her the baby again

66. Which of the following parent responses might indicate an understanding of the development of toddlers when dealing with a temper tantrum?
   1 The child is ignored and isolated until behavior improves
   2 Restriction of a favorite food or activity is used for discipline
   3 The child is allowed to choose between two reasonable alternatives
   4 The parent gives in to the child before the tantrum becomes extensive

67. Which of the following actions might the nurse suggest to a parent to assist with teaching a toddler self-control?
   1 Rewarding good behavior
   2 Setting limits and being consistent
   3 Punishing the child for misbehavior
   4 Allowing the child to learn by mistakes

68. Mathew is a 5-year-old boy who has been diagnosed with lead poisoning. The nurse should suspect lead-induced renal damage to the proximal tubules of Mathew's kidneys when his urinalysis contains which substance?
   1 Calcium
   2 Albumin
   3 Potassium
   4 Phosphate

69. Which of the following actions by the nurse could best help prevent a reoccurrence of lead poisoning?

1 Discussing with the child's parents ways to renovate their home to remove sources of lead
2 Educating the parents about the dangers of lead ingestion and the type of treatment required
3 Initiating referrals to appropriate social and public health agencies for the management of the problem
4 Helping the parents recognize factors in interpersonal interactions and in the home environment that predispose the child to ingesting lead

70. When a client has a tracheostomy tube and is on a ventilator, the tracheostomy tube must:
   1 Have an inner cannula
   2 Be changed every week
   3 Be cleansed once a day
   4 Have a low-pressure cuff

71. Which of the following complications should the nurse be aware of when a client has a history of COPD?
   1 Kidney function
   2 Cardiac function
   3 Joint inflammation
   4 Peripheral neuropathy

72. When is the least appropriate time for the nurse to schedule segmental postural drainage treatments?
   1 At bedtime
   2 After a meal
   3 Before a meal
   4 On awakening

73. Which of the following tests would be done immediately to confirm the diagnosis of meningitis in a child?
   1 Blood cultures
   2 Lumbar puncture
   3 Meningomyelogram
   4 Peripheral skin smears

74. According to Piaget's theory of cognitive development, which of the following characteristics should a 6-month-old infant demonstrate?
   1 Early traces of memory
   2 Beginning sense of time
   3 Repetitious use of reflexes
   4 Beginning of object permanence

75. A client returns to the unit fully awake following a bronchoscopy and biopsy. What is the nurse's most appropriate action?
   1 Provide ice chips to reduce swelling
   2 Advise the client to cough frequently
   3 Evaluate the presence of a gag reflex
   4 Advise the client to stay flat for 2 hours

76. What is the most effective way for the nurse to loosen secretions for a client with an endotracheal tube in place?
    1 Increasing oral fluid intake
    2 Providing chest physiotherapy
    3 Administering humidified oxygen
    4 Instilling a saturated solution of potassium iodide

77. What is the most beneficial position for the nurse to place the client during the immediate postoperative period following a right pneumonectomy?
    1 In the high-Fowler's position
    2 Flat in bed with the knees flexed slightly
    3 On the right side with the head slightly elevated
    4 In the left Sims' position with the bed elevated 45 degrees

Client Case Scenario 13: Mr. Faber, an 80-year-old man, is scheduled for extensive head and neck surgery. Although the physician has explained the surgery, Mr. Faber remains anxious. **Items 78 to 83 refer to this client case scenario.**

78. How could the nurse intervene in assisting Mr. Faber to feel less anxious?
    1 Attempt to discover what is bothering him
    2 Elaborate on what the physician has already told him
    3 Teach him to use the suction equipment preoperatively
    4 Plan for postoperative communication, since a tracheostomy is likely

79. What is the purpose of placing Mr. Faber in high-Fowler's position following surgery?
    1 Prevent strain on the incision
    2 Promote drainage of the wound
    3 Provide stimulation for Mr. Faber
    4 Prevent edema at the operative site

80. What action is most appropriate by the nurse when Mr. Faber complains that his neck dressing is too tight?
    1 Assess for signs of constriction
    2 Observe the dressing for bleeding
    3 Explain that the tight dressing is necessary
    4 Loosen the dressing to relieve the pressure

81. Mr. Faber has a tracheostomy and is receiving mechanical ventilation. What aspect must the nurse be sure to check when observing the cuff of the tracheostomy tube?
    1 Must be inflated during suctioning
    2 Must remain deflated for 10 minutes every hour

    3 Should create a tight seal between the trachea and the tube
    4 Should allow only a slight air leak at the height of inspiration

82. What action should the nurse take when performing Mr. Faber's tracheal suctioning?
    1 Preoxygenate him before suctioning
    2 Apply negative pressure as the catheter is being inserted
    3 Be sure the cuff of the tracheostomy is inflated during suctioning
    4 Instill acetylcysteine (Mucomyst) into the tracheostomy prior to suctioning to loosen secretions

83. What action by the nurse is appropriate when performing Mr. Faber's tracheostomy care?
    1 Place him in the semi-Fowler's position
    2 Monitor his temperature after the procedure
    3 Maintain sterile technique during the procedure
    4 Use Betadine to clean the inner cannula when it is removed

---

Client Case Scenario 14: Rebecca is a newborn that has been born with meningomyelocele. **Items 84 to 88 refer to this client case scenario.**

84. The nurse should suspect that Rebecca is likely to develop hydrocephalus in which of the following situations?
    1 When her lower limbs lack movement
    2 When her Apgar score was five at 1 minute
    3 When her meningomyelocele is in the lumbosacral area
    4 When her head circumference is 2 cm larger than her chest circumference

85. When assessing Rebecca for hydrocephalus, which of the following presentations are indicative of increased intracranial pressure?
    1 Depressed fontanel, bulging eyes, irritability
    2 High shrill cry, decreased skin turgor, elevated fontanels
    3 Dilated scalp veins, depressed and sunken eyeballs, decreased BP
    4 Bulging fontanel, "sunset" eyes, projectile vomiting not associated with feeding

86. Discharge planning for Rebecca's parents should include teaching them to observe for the most common complications of shunt insertion. Which of the following presentations should the parents be taught to watch out for?
    1 Violent involuntary muscle contractions
    2 Excessive fluid accumulation in the abdomen

3 Eyes with sclerae that are visible above the irises

4 Fever accompanied by decreased responsiveness

87. When teaching parents to pump the valve of a ventriculoperitoneal shunt, the nurse should include the fact that the primary purpose of this procedure is to:
1 Keep the tubing of the shunt patent
2 Increase absorption of cerebrospinal fluid
3 Drain excessive cerebrospinal fluid rapidly
4 Divert the cerebrospinal fluid from the ventricles

88. Rebecca's meningomyelocele is repaired. Her parents are informed that she will be incontinent of urine. The teaching plan should also include which of the following information?
1 An ileal conduit will be necessary once she is in school
2 An indwelling bladder catheter is used for bladder management
3 She will probably be a candidate for an intermittent straight catheterization program
4 She will probably need to wear diapers for her lifetime, as bladder training will not be possible

Client Case Scenario 15: Mrs. Kim, a 22-year-old primigravida at term, is brought to hospital by her husband. They have attended preparation for childbirth classes and plan to be together during labour. On admission, Mrs. Kim states she has been constipated. She is having contractions 3 to 5 minutes apart, she has bloody show, and her membranes are intact. On vaginal examination, Mrs. Kim's cervix is fully effaced and 4 cm dilated. **Items 89 to 93 refer to this client case scenario.**

89. The nurse explains that constipation frequently occurs during pregnancy because of:
1 Changes in the metabolic rate
2 Pressure of the growing uterus on the anus
3 The slowing of peristalsis in the gastrointestinal tract
4 Increased intake of milk as recommended during pregnancy

90. When monitoring Mrs. Kim's labor, the nurse notices a gush of fluid from her vagina. After checking the fetal heart, the nurse should:
1 Place Mrs. Kim on her side and obtain her BP
2 Keep Mrs. Kim flat in bed and elevate her legs
3 Notify the physician immediately about the gush of fluid from the vagina
4 Place Mrs. Kim in a modified lithotomy position and inspect her perineum

91. Mrs. Kim's contractions decrease to 2 per 10 minutes. An oxytocin augmentation is commenced. What is the nurse's responsibility when monitoring Mrs. Kim's labor?
1 Flush the IV tubing if the flow slows
2 Monitor fetal heart tones every 2 hours
3 Shut off the infusion in the presence of hypertonic contractions
4 Obtain a physician's order to slow the IV in the presence of hypertonic contractions

92. When should the nurse be aware that the transitional phase of labor has probably begun?
1 Mrs. Kim complains of pain in the back
2 Mrs. Kim assumes the lithotomy position
3 Mrs. Kim perspires and has a flushed face
4 Mrs. Kim states that her pains have lessened

93. Shortly following delivery Mrs. Kim says she feels that she is bleeding. While checking the fundus, the nurse notes a steady trickling of blood from the vagina. What should the nurse's first action be?
1 Call the physician immediately
2 Check the client's BP and pulse
3 Hold the fundus firmly and gently massage it
4 Take no action, since this is a common occurrence

94. A 40-year-old woman in her twenty-second week of pregnancy is admitted with heavy bleeding and severe abdominal cramping. The client says to the nurse, "We wanted this baby so badly." The nurse's most therapeutic response would be:
1 "It must be difficult to lose something that was important to you both."
2 "A D & C will give you a new start. I bet you'll become pregnant again soon."
3 "You must be disappointed, but don't feel guilty. These things sometimes happen."
4 "It's not your fault. This is nature's way of dealing with babies that may have problems."

95. After experiencing a spontaneous abortion, a client states to the nurse, "We've always wanted this baby. How come this happened to us?" The nurse should be aware that the client is exhibiting which of the usual initial reactions to a loss?
1 Shock and denial
2 Despair and anger
3 Apathy and sadness
4 Dissociation and rationalization

96. Which of the following statements should the nurse use to explain an infant's cephalohematoma to a parent?
    1 The swelling results from tissue edema
    2 The soft sac will bulge when the infant cries
    3 It will resolve spontaneously in 3 to 6 weeks
    4 This condition is unusual with vaginal delivery

97. Nursing care of a newborn with a cephalohematoma should include which of the following primary objectives?
    1 Supporting the parents
    2 Recording neurologic signs
    3 Protecting the infant's head
    4 Applying ice packs to the hematoma

98. The physician tells a mother that her newborn has multiple visible birth defects. The mother seems quite composed and asks to see her baby. What would be the nurse's best response?
    1 Bring the baby to her immediately
    2 Tell her exactly what the baby looks like before bringing the baby to her
    3 Encourage her to express and explore her feelings, bring the baby to her, and stay with her during this time
    4 Show her some pictures, give her some literature, and discuss the treatment with her before bringing the baby to her

99. When caring for clients with atherosclerosis, the nurse should understand that atherosclerosis is:
    1 Development of atheromas within the myocardium
    2 A mobilization of free fatty acid from adipose tissue
    3 Development of fatty deposits within the intima of the arteries
    4 A loss of elasticity in and thickening and hardening of the arteries

100. What should the nurse's initial approach to creating a therapeutic environment for any client include?
    1 Providing for the client's safety
    2 Accepting the client's individuality
    3 Promoting the client's independence
    4 Explaining everything that is being done for the client

101. The nurse consults with a colleague regarding the need to put side rails up on the bed of a 73-year-old client who was admitted with a fractured hip. What is the purpose of this decision?
    1 As a safety measure because of the client's age

    2 Because all clients over 65 years of age should use side rails
    3 To be used as handholds and to facilitate the client's mobility in bed
    4 Because elderly people are often disoriented for several days after anesthesia

102. An elderly client is apprehensive about being hospitalized. The nurse realizes that one of the stresses of hospitalization is the strangeness of the environment and activity. How might this stress be limited?
    1 Using the client's first name
    2 Visiting with the client frequently
    3 Explaining what behavior is expected
    4 Listening to what the client has to say

103. The nurse consults with the dietitian regarding sodium intake for a client in congestive heart failure. Which of the following foods should be excluded?
    1 Fruits
    2 Grains
    3 Vegetables
    4 Processed foods

104. How should the nurse explain to the client that sodium restriction is an effective therapeutic tool in the treatment of congestive heart failure?
    1 Allows excess tissue fluid to be excreted
    2 Helps to control food intake and thus weight
    3 Aids the weakened heart muscle to contract and improves cardiac output
    4 Helps to prevent the potassium accumulation that occurs when sodium intake is higher

105. When a client has gluteal edema, why should the nurse avoid use of the gluteus maximus muscle for administration of intramuscular medications?
    1 Deposition of an injected drug causes pain
    2 Blood supply is insufficient for drug absorption
    3 Fluid leaks from the site for long periods after injection
    4 Tissue fluid dilutes the drug before it enters the circulation

106. The nurse would know that the client needed further teaching about preventing thrombi when the client states, "I should:
    1 Massage my legs."
    2 Increase my fluid intake."
    3 Perform range-of-motion exercises."
    4 Wear elastic stockings when out of bed."

107. What should the nurse remember while assisting a client with a repaired fractured hip to transfer between the bed and the wheelchair?
    1 During a weight-bearing transfer the client's knees should be slightly bent
    2 The appropriate proximity and visual relationship of wheelchair to bed must be maintained
    3 Transfers to and from the wheelchair will be easier if the bed is higher than the wheelchair
    4 The transfer can be accomplished by pivoting while bearing weight on both upper extremities and not on the legs

108. How should the nurse stand when assisting a client to ambulate following repair of a fractured right hip?
    1 Behind the client
    2 In front of the client
    3 On the client's left side
    4 On the client's right side

109. A surgical client has a portable wound-drainage system in place. What is an important nursing intervention to promote drainage?
    1 Irrigating the drainage tube with saline
    2 Applying warm compresses to the involved site
    3 Maintaining compression of the drainage system
    4 Keeping the involved area in a dependent position

110. Which statement should the nurse make in assisting a mother of a newborn with a cleft palate to feed her baby?
    1 "Since he tires easily, it is best to have him lying in bed while he is being fed."
    2 "He should be held in a horizontal position and fed slowly to avoid aspiration."
    3 "Give him brief rest periods and frequent burpings during feedings to expel swallowed air."
    4 "Try using a soft nipple with an enlarged opening so that he can get the milk through a chewing motion."

111. What is the nurse's first responsibility when caring for a client with a spinal cord injury during the initial postinjury period?
    1 Prevent urinary tract infections
    2 Prevent contractures and atrophy
    3 Avoid flexion or hyperextension of the spine
    4 Prepare the client for vocational rehabilitation

112. Two weeks after sustaining a spinal cord injury a client begins vomiting thick coffee-ground material and appears restless and apprehensive. What is the most important action by the nurse?
    1 Change the client's diet to bland
    2 Prepare for insertion of a nasogastric tube
    3 Check laboratory reports for hemoglobin level
    4 Collect a stool specimen and check for occult blood

113. A client who has sustained multiple serious injuries from a motor vehicle accident is diagnosed as having a stress ulcer. When caring for this client, what should the nurse immediately report?
    1 Nausea, weakness, and headache
    2 Dyspepsia, distention, and diarrhea
    3 Complaints of thirst and warm, flushed skin
    4 Tachycardia, diaphoresis, and cold extremities

114. A college athlete sustained a severance of the spinal cord while practicing on the trampoline. The physician explained to him that he is a paraplegic. Three weeks later the client says he must get out of the hospital to practice for an upcoming tournament. The nurse and doctor understand that the client is:
    1 Exhibiting denial
    2 Verbalizing a fantasy
    3 No longer able to adapt
    4 Extremely motivated to get well

115. The father of a child who is dying of cancer asks the nurse if he should tell his 7-year-old son that his sister is dying. What is the nurse's best response?
    1 "A child of his age cannot comprehend the real meaning of death, so don't tell him until the last moment."
    2 "Your son probably fears separation most and wants to know that you will care for him, rather than what will happen to his sister."
    3 "Why don't you talk this over with your doctor, who probably knows best what is happening in terms of your daughter's prognosis."
    4 "Your son probably doesn't understand death as we do but fears it just the same. He should be told the truth to let him prepare for his sister's possible death."

116. What is the best description of a somatoform disorder?
    1 A psychosomatic reaction to stress
    2 A conscious defense against anxiety
    3 A psychologic defense against stress
    4 An unconscious means to control conflict

117. Conversion disorder is the term used to describe the phenomenon wherein anxiety associated with stress or conflict has been repressed and converted into specific physical manifestations. What is one of the characteristics of the client's reaction to the physical symptom?
    1 Anger
    2 Anxiety
    3 Agitation
    4 Indifference

118. A client is scheduled for an occupational therapy group. While listening to instructions for the group project, the client experiences the feeling of weakness and is unable to move the right arm. After an assessment by the team, what would the nurse's best response be?
    1 "Exactly when did the weakness begin?"
    2 "Would you like to leave the group for a while?"
    3 "Is this similar to what you usually experience?"
    4 "What emotion were you feeling before you felt the weakness?"

119. How can the occurrence of a pattern of behavior that uses physical symptoms in response to stress be reduced by the nurse?
    1 Provide client teaching regarding medical care
    2 Teach the family how to decrease stress at home
    3 Assist the client in developing new coping mechanisms
    4 Decrease anxiety by limiting discussion of problems with the client

120. During a group therapy session some members accuse a client of intellectualizing to avoid discussing feelings. The client asks if the nurse agrees with the others. What would the nurse's best response be?
    1 "It seems that way to me, too."
    2 "You seem to need my opinion."
    3 "I'd rather not give my personal opinion."
    4 "What is your perception of my behavior?"

121. A 12-month-old child is admitted with delayed development, weight below the third percentile, and a diagnosis of failure to thrive. Which of the following infant behaviors might also support the possibility of parental neglect?
    1 Uncomforted by touch, withdrawn
    2 Cuddly; responsive to touch, and wants to be held
    3 A poor eater, sleeps soundly, and is easily satisfied

4 Responsive to adults, rarely cries, but shows little interest in the environment

122. Which of the following health care team actions should be encouraged by the nurse to best meet the needs of a neglected child?
    1 Plan to have staff members pick up and play with the child whenever they can
    2 Be as consistent a caregiver as possible, with stimulation that is moderate and purposeful
    3 Provide a vigorous schedule of stimulation geared to the child's present level of development
    4 Schedule care that allows the child stimulation and physical contact by several staff members

123. The nurse observes that an infant has head control and can roll over, but cannot sit up without support or transfer an object from one hand to another. At what age would the nurse assess this child's development?
    1 2 to 3 months
    2 3 to 4 months
    3 4 to 6 months
    4 6 to 8 months

124. Which of the following toys would be inappropriate for a 5-month-old infant?
    1 Brightly colored mobiles
    2 Snap toys, large snap beads
    3 Small rattles that the infant can hold
    4 Soft, stuffed animals that the infant can hold

125. A client is admitted to the recovery room after an abdominal hysterectomy. Which observation by the nurse should be reported to the physician immediately?
    1 An apical pulse of 90
    2 A decreased urinary output
    3 Serosanguinous drainage on the perineal pad
    4 Increased drainage from the nasogastric tube

COMPREHENSIVE TEST: PART B

Client Case Scenario 16: Zak is a 3 1/2-year-old boy who has been hospitalized for nephrotic syndrome. **Items 126 to 129 refer to this client case scenario.**

126. The physician prescribes steroid therapy for Zak. The nurse understands that the goal of this treatment is which of the following actions?
    1 Reduce BP
    2 Cause diuresis

3 Prevent infection

4 Provide hemopoiesis

127. Zak is placed on a low-sodium diet. Which of the following lunches planned by the nurse and dietician would best meet Zak's needs?
1 Macaroni and cheese, fresh pears, V-8 juice
2 Chicken, navy beans, fresh peaches, lemonade
3 Cheeseburger on a bun, fresh green beans, iced tea
4 Bacon and tomato sandwich, canned chicken noodle soup, low-sodium milk

128. Zak has significant edema and has been placed on bedrest. Which of the following diversions would be most appropriate, considering his developmental level and activity restriction?
1 Television viewing time
2 Squeaky stuffed animals
3 Little cars and a shoebox garage
4 Simple three- or four-piece wooden puzzles

129. Zak has been toilet trained for more than a year, but he has been wetting himself since hospitalization. His mother expresses concern over the behavior. Which of the following responses by the nurse would be the most therapeutic?
1 "He is wetting the bed to get attention. Reprimand him when he does this."
2 "The incontinence is due to his renal disease. It will improve as he gets better."
3 "This is a normal response to hospitalization. Ignore his regressive behavior and be supportive of him."
4 "He is using this regressive behavior to help him cope with hospitalization; just place him in diapers and say nothing."

Client Case Scenario 17: Mrs. King is a multipara and is admitted to the antenatal assessment unit with a history of decreased fetal movement at 36 weeks gestation. **Items 130 to 132 refer to this client case scenario.**

130. Mrs. King is scheduled for a oxytocin challenge test (OCT). The nurse caring for her understands that the OCT is used in evaluating the:
1 Fetal heart rate (FHR)
2 Uteroplacental function
3 Contractibility of the pregnant uterus prior to delivery
4 High-risk mother's ability to tolerate a vaginal delivery

131. When teaching Mrs. King about the OCT, what should the nurse emphasize is important to do?

1 Empty her bladder before the test
2 Take diazepam (Valium) 5 mg po 1/2 hour before the test
3 Be prepared to be in the hospital for 12 hours following the test
4 Eat nothing for 2 hours before the test and 6 hours after the test

132. Before the OCT, what should the nurse explain to Mrs. King?
1 The FHR will be monitored for 30 minutes prior to actual testing
2 A double-voided urine specimen will be collected prior to the test
3 At least six contractions must be observed before the test is discontinued
4 She will be placed in a right lateral position, which must be maintained throughout testing

Client Case Scenario 18: Mr. Sati, 78 years old, is hospitalized with a diagnosis of possible cancer of the pancreas. **Items 133 to 138 refer to this client case scenario.**

133. How should the nurse best respond when Mr. Sati asks if he has something serious, like cancer?
1 "What makes you think you have cancer?"
2 "I don't know if you do, but let's talk about it."
3 "Why don't you discuss this with your doctor?"
4 "Don't worry, we won't know until all the test results are back."

134. A complete blood count, urinalysis, and x-ray examination of the chest are ordered for Mr. Sati prior to surgery. How should the nurse respond when he asks why these tests are done?
1 "I don't know; the doctor ordered them."
2 "Don't worry, these tests are strictly routine."
3 "They are done to identify other health risks."
4 "They determine whether it's safe to proceed with surgery."

135. Mr. Sati is scheduled for an abdominal resection. What is the first priority of the health care team?
1 Alleviating Mr. Sati's anxiety
2 Recording accurate vital signs
3 Maintaining proper nutritional status
4 Teaching and answering all his questions

136. What is the most significant influence on Mr. Sati's perception of pain?
1 Age and sex
2 Overall physical status
3 Intelligence and economic status
4 Previous experience and cultural values

137. A progressive ambulation schedule is to be instituted for Mr. Sati the morning after surgery. He has been receiving antihypertensive medication and morphine sulfate for pain. When getting Mr. Sati out of bed, the nurse should first have him sit on the edge of the bed with his feet dangling. This action is taken because the nurse expects his adaptation may be:
    1 Abdominal pain
    2 Initial hypertension
    3 Respiratory distress
    4 Postural hypotension

138. On the second day after surgery, Mr. Sati complains of pain in the right calf. How should the nurse respond?
    1 Apply warm soaks
    2 Notify the physician
    3 Chart the symptoms
    4 Elevate the extremity

Client Case Scenario 19: Mr. Isaac, a 31-year-old man, has been diagnosed with myasthenia gravis. **Items 139 to 143 refer to this client case scenario.**

139. Because of the involvement of the ocular muscles, which early symptom of myasthenia gravis should the nurse assess Mr. Isaac for?
    1 Tearing
    2 Blurring
    3 Diplopia
    4 Nystagmus

140. A test that might be performed on Mr. Isaac to help confirm the diagnosis of myasthenia gravis involves the use of the drug:
    1 Prednisolone
    2 Disodium EDTA
    3 Phenytoin (Dilantin)
    4 Edrophonium (Tensilon)

141. Mr. Isaac is receiving neostigmine bromide (Prostigmin) for control of myasthenia gravis. In the middle of the night the nurse finds him weak, unable to move, and barely breathing. What signs would identify the problems as being related to neostigmine bromide?
    1 Distention of the bladder
    2 High-pitched, gurgling bowel sounds
    3 Fine tremor of the fingers and eyelids
    4 Rapid pulse with occasional ectopic beats

142. Mr. Isaac's family asks the nurse whether he will be an invalid. Recognizing the individuality of response to myasthenia gravis, what is the nurse's best response?

1 "Deformities will occur, but people with myasthenia will not become invalids."
2 "With continuous medication the progression of the disease can be controlled."
3 "The progression is slow, so people with myasthenia will spend their younger life with few problems."
4 "There will be periods when bed rest will be necessary and times when fairly normal activity will be possible."

143. Which diversional activity would best meet the nursing objectives for Mr. Isaac during periods of remission?
    1 Swimming with the family
    2 Watching television shows
    3 Short hikes with the family
    4 Teaching woodworking classes

Client Case Scenario 20: Mr. Gill, age 86 years, has been diagnosed with Alzheimer's disease. **Items 144 to 148 refer to this client case scenario.**

144. Which characteristics could the nurse expect when observing Mr. Gill?
    1 Transient ischemic attacks
    2 Remissions and exacerbations
    3 Rapid deterioration of mental functioning because of arteriosclerosis
    4 Slowly progressive deficits in intellect, which may not be noted for a long time

145. Mr. Gill frequently switches from being pleasant and happy to being hostile and sad without apparent external cause. How can the nurse best care for Mr. Gill?
    1 Try to point out reality to him
    2 Avoid Mr. Gill when he is angry and sad
    3 Encourage him to talk about his feelings
    4 Attempt to give nursing care when he is in a pleasant mood

146. What type of environment should be provided by the health care team for Mr. Gill?
    1 Familiar
    2 Variable
    3 Challenging
    4 Nonstimulating

147. Mr. Gill will need assistance in maintaining contact with society for as long as possible. Which therapy might help him achieve this goal?
    1 Psychodrama
    2 Recreation therapy
    3 Remotivation therapy
    4 Occupational therapy

148. What is the nurse's prime objective for Mr. Gill, when he is experiencing dementia and delirium?
    1 Diminished psychologic faculties
    2 Interaction with the environment
    3 Participation in educational activities
    4 Face-to-face contact with other clients

Client Case Scenario 21: Chris is a 7-year-old who is diagnosed with acute lymphocytic leukemia. **Items 149 to 152 refer to this client case scenario.**

149. Which of the following describes the pathophysiologic change underlying the symptoms of leukemia?
    1 Excessive destruction of blood cells in the liver and spleen
    2 Progressive replacement of bone marrow with fibrous tissue
    3 Proliferation and release of immature white blood cells into the circulating blood
    4 Destruction of red blood cells and platelets by an overproduction of white blood cells

150. Chris is placed on chemotherapy. Which of the following nursing actions describes a major objective for Chris while he is on his chemotherapy protocol?
    1 Check his vital signs every 2 hours
    2 Prevent his engaging in physical activity
    3 Have him avoid contact with infected persons
    4 Reduce unnecessary stimuli in his environment

151. Chris is placed on vincristine. Which of the following diets would be most appropriate considering the side effects of vincristine?
    1 Low in fat with regular fluids
    2 High in both roughage and fluids
    3 High in iron with decreased fluids
    4 Low in residue with increased fluids

152. The physician is planning to irradiate Chris' spine and skull. Which of the following explanations describes the rationale behind this treatment?
    1 Radiation will retard growth of cells in bone marrow of the cranium
    2 Radiation will decrease cerebral edema and prevent increased intracranial pressure
    3 Leukemia cells invade the nervous system more slowly, but the usual drugs are ineffective in the brain
    4 Neoplastic drug therapy without radiation is effective in most cases, but this is a precautionary treatment

Client Case Scenario 22: Mrs. Kelly is a 27-year-old gravida 1 para 0 with a childhood history of rheumatic fever resulting in a mild rheumatic heart disease. **Items 153 and 154 refer to this client case scenario.**

153. During her seventh week of pregnancy, Mrs. Kelly complains of some dependent edema in her ankles. How should the nurse advise her?
    1 Limit her fluid intake during the day
    2 Stop using salt for the next 3 months
    3 Elevate her legs more frequently during the day
    4 Call her physician immediately for a mild diuretic

154. Nutritional management is most important for Mrs. Kelly because of her cardiac problems. The nurse should advise her to eat a balanced diet with
    1 Moderate fats
    2 Limited protein
    3 Increased sodium
    4 Controlled calories

Client Case Scenario 23: Mrs. Finney, a 32-year-old, is admitted to hospital with a diagnosis of Addison's disease. **Items 155 to 160 refer to this client case scenario.**

155. Which of the following should the nurse reinforce when providing teaching to Mrs. Finney?
    1 A special low-salt diet
    2 Restriction of physical activity
    3 Hormone replacement therapy
    4 Frequent visits to the physician

156. When teaching about a diet appropriate for Mrs. Finney, which of the following should the nurse stress?
    1 Add a little extra salt to food
    2 Limit intake to 1200 calories
    3 Restrict the daily intake of fluids
    4 Omit protein foods at each meal

157. Mrs. Finney is receiving cortisone therapy. Which of the following should the nurse advise Mrs. Finney to report that could indicate adrenal crisis in the event that she neglects to take her medication?
    1 Dysphagia
    2 Hypertension
    3 Muscle spasms
    4 A high body temperature

158. Clients on prolonged cortisone therapy may exhibit adaptations caused by its glucocorticoid and mineralocorticoid actions. Which of the following side effects should the nurse teach Mrs. Finney and her family to observe for?
    1 Hypoglycemia and anuria
    2 Hypotension and fluid loss
    3 Anorexia and hyperkalemia
    4 Weight gain and moon face

159. Mrs. Finney expresses concern about the fact that she is developing signs of masculinity. What should the nurse tell her?
    1 That this is due to therapy
    2 It is a further sign of the illness
    3 Not to worry, because it will disappear with therapy
    4 That this is not important, so long as she gets better

160. When observing Mrs. Finney for cortisone overdose, which of the following should the nurse be particularly alert for?
    1 Hypoglycemia
    2 Severe anorexia
    3 Anaphylactic shock
    4 Behavioral changes

Client Case Scenario 24: Mr. Lee, a 66-year-old, is admitted to hospital in a depressed state. His family states that he has been agitated and has difficulty sleeping. **Items 161 to 166 refer to this client case scenario.**

161. Mr. Lee frequently tells the nurse, "Soon I will be dead." The nurse repeatedly tells him this is not true and urges Mr. Lee to forget about it and to go into the TV room and talk with the other clients. Mr. Lee becomes more agitated and ultimately has to be sedated. How might the nurse have altered this situation?
    1 Mr. Lee's delusions should be accepted without rebuff or argument
    2 He should be given tranquilizers before incidents such as this develop
    3 Mr. Lee's sleeplessness and agitation should have been treated as symptoms
    4 He needs to be encouraged and often gently pushed into relating to other clients

162. What should the nurse keep in mind when caring for Mr. Lee?
    1 Clients with simple depressions rarely attempt suicide
    2 Opportunities to attempt suicide are practically absent on a closed psychiatric unit
    3 Depressed clients are potentially suicidal during the entire course of their illness

    4 Once the severe depression begins to lift, the danger of suicide is no longer a problem

163. Mr. Lee appears preoccupied and remains seated when it is time for the clients to go to eat. What is the nurse's best response?
    1 Take Mr. Lee by the hand and lead him to the dining room
    2 Overlook Mr. Lee not eating and leave snacks in his room
    3 Tell Mr. Lee that now is the time to eat, since no food will be served later
    4 Ask Mr. Lee whether a tray in the room would be preferable to going to the dining room

164. Mr. Lee is eating very little at this time. The nursing care plan should be directed toward assisting him with meals. Besides encouraging nourishment, this nursing action also:
    1 Proves to him that food can be tolerated
    2 Provides him with some special attention
    3 Gets him into the dining room with the rest of the clients
    4 Shows that the staff considers him to be a worthwhile individual

165. Mr. Lee is taking lithium carbonate. Which of the following should the nursing staff carefully monitor?
    1 Serum levels
    2 Daily weights
    3 Leukocyte counts
    4 Psychomotor activity

166. Mr. Lee is going home for a 3-day weekend pass. In regards to his taking lithium carbonate, how should the nurse advise him?
    1 Have a snack with milk before going to bed
    2 Avoid participation in controversial discussions
    3 Adjust the lithium dosage if mood changes are noted
    4 Continue to maintain a normal sodium intake while at home

---

Client Case Scenario 25: Mrs. Morse, aged 82 years, is admitted to hospital with burns to her forearms and legs, after experiencing a fire in her apartment. **Items 167 to 171 refer to this client case scenario.**

167. Fluid shifts are a great danger to Mrs. Morse, who has partial- and full-thickness burns. What should the nurse initially expect to observe?
    1 A rise in blood volume
    2 Decreased capillary permeability
    3 A loss of sodium and an increase in blood potassium

4 Increased fluid shifts and irreversible shock after 2 hours

168. IV replacement is important for Mrs. Morse. What would the nurse expect Mrs. Morse's intake and output to be in the first 24 hours?
   1 Intake, 8000 ml; output, 480 ml
   2 Intake, 3000 ml; output, 2400 ml
   3 Intake, 6000 ml; output, 1200 ml
   4 Intake, 12000 ml; output, 4500 ml

169. The rate of fluid replacement for Mrs. Morse during the immediate hypovolemic stage is considered satisfactory if the urinary output is approximately:
   1 Half the intake
   2 Equal to the intake
   3 One-third the intake
   4 One-tenth the intake

170. Mrs. Morse is permitted food and fluids. Which diet should the nurse promote in order to enhance Mrs. Morse's nutritional status?
   1 Encourage an increased intake of sodium
   2 Limit caloric intake to decrease the work of the body
   3 Reduce protein intake to avoid overtaxing the kidneys
   4 Encourage drinking a variety of fluids containing vitamin C

171. Which of the following is an important nursing consideration when caring for Mrs. Morse?
   1 Death may still occur from septicemia
   2 The danger of physical complications is past
   3 Because of Mrs. Morse's need for rest, diversional therapy must be delayed
   4 Mirrors should be removed to decrease the client's anxiety about appearance

172. When caring for a client following a total left pneumonectomy, the nurse should palpate the client's trachea at least once a day because:
   1 The position may indicate mediastinal shift
   2 Nodular lesions may demonstrate metastasis
   3 Tracheal edema may lead to an obstructed airway
   4 The cuff of the endotracheal tube may be overinflated

173. A client in her fourth month of pregnancy calls the nurse and indicates that her husband just told her he has genital herpes. When teaching about sexual activity, which of the following should the nurse include?

   1 It will be necessary to refrain from all sexual contact during pregnancy
   2 The use of condoms by her husband during sexual activity will be required
   3 Sexual abstinence should be practiced during the last 6 weeks of pregnancy
   4 Meticulous cleaning of the hands and vaginal area after intercourse is essential

174. Early in the ninth month of pregnancy, a client experiences painless vaginal bleeding and is admitted to the hospital. What should her nursing care plan include?
   1 Administering vitamin K to promote clotting
   2 Performing a rectal examination to determine cervical dilation
   3 Administering an enema to prevent contamination during delivery
   4 Placing her in a semi-Fowler's position to increase cervical pressure

175. What is the most important weak or absent reflex for the nurse to report in the initial evaluation of a newborn?
   1 Gag
   2 Moro
   3 Babinski
   4 Tonic neck

176. During a developmental appraisal, which of the following observations of a 6-month-old infant should concern the nurse?
   1 Head lag
   2 Inability to sit unsupported
   3 Presence of the Babinski reflex
   4 Absence of Moro, tonic neck, and grasp reflexes

177. Proper positioning of an infant with hydrocephalus is essential to prevent breakdown of the scalp. Which of the following positions would be most appropriate in preventing skin breakdown?
   1 Supine and Trendelenburg
   2 Positioned on either side and flat
   3 Prone, with the legs elevated about 30-degrees
   4 Prone or supine, with the head elevated about 45-degrees

178. In the immediate postoperative period following a gastrectomy, the client's nasogastric tube is draining a light-red liquid. How long could the nurse expect this drainage?
   1 1 to 2 hours
   2 3 to 4 hours
   3 10 to 12 hours
   4 24 to 48 hours

179. Parenteral preparations of potassium are administered slowly and cautiously to prevent:
    1 Acidosis
    2 Cardiac arrest
    3 Psychoticlike reactions
    4 Edema of the extremities

180. The nurse obtains a health history from a client with peptic ulcer disease. Which statement by the client might indicate a possible contributing factor?
    1 "My blood type is A."
    2 "I smoke two packs of cigarettes a day."
    3 "I have been overweight most of my life."
    4 "My blood pressure has been high lately."

181. Which diet should the nurse encourage to assist a client when managing the dumping syndrome?
    1 Low-residue, bland diet
    2 Fluid intake below 500 ml
    3 Small frequent feeding schedule
    4 Low-protein, high-carbohydrate diet

182. A preterm infant is delivered. Which criteria should the nurse use in assessing gestational age of the infant?
    1 Breast bud size
    2 Fingernail length
    3 The presence of reflex stability
    4 The presence of simian creases

183. An infant has a noncommunicating hydrocephalus, and a ventriculoperitoneal shunt is performed. Which of the following is a nursing priority for the infant's postoperative care?
    1 Elevate the infant's head and chest
    2 Position the infant flat for about 48 hours
    3 Administer sedatives and analgesics to promote rest
    4 Encourage the parents to pick their child up to prevent crying

184. Which type of interview is most productive when the nurse first talks to a client in a clinic?
    1 Directive
    2 Exploratory
    3 Problem solving
    4 Information giving

185. A mother and father are in the waiting room for their first clinic appointment for their newborn. Accompanying them is their 18-month-old toddler. The infant is due for a bottlefeeding and the toddler is playing on the floor. At this time the nurse's best action would be to ask the father if he would mind:
    1 Giving the baby a bottle
    2 Taking the toddler for a walk
    3 Participating in the discussion
    4 Leaving the nurse and the mother alone

186. A client is admitted with a diagnosis of chronic adrenal insufficiency. Because of this condition, which room would be the least advisable for the client?
    1 With an elderly client who has a CVA
    2 With a middle-aged client who has pneumonia
    3 Next to a 17-year-old client with a fractured leg
    4 A private room that is away from the nurse's station

187. A client with adrenal insufficiency complains of weakness and dizziness on arising from bed in the morning. Which of the following is the most probable cause?
    1 A lack of potassium
    2 Postural hypertension
    3 A hypoglycemic reaction
    4 Increased extracellular fluid volume

188. Following an abdominal hysterectomy a client develops abdominal distention. Which nursing measures would most likely provide immediate relief?
    1 Ambulation and carbonated drinks
    2 Restriction of oral intake and frequent change of position
    3 Nasogastric intubation and administration of cholinergic agents
    4 Insertion of a rectal tube and application of heat to the abdomen

189. A client is receiving a H2 antagonist medication. The nurse explains that this drug is given prophylactically during the first few weeks after extensive burns to prevent:
    1 Colitis
    2 Gastritis
    3 Curling's ulcer
    4 Metabolic acidosis

190. A client is admitted with the diagnosis of possible placenta previa. What should the nursing care for this client involve?
    1 Inspecting for hemorrhage
    2 Withholding food and fluids
    3 Avoiding all extraneous stimuli
    4 Encouraging ambulation with supervision

191. What should the nurse be prepared for when a vaginal examination is to be performed on a client with possible placenta previa?
    1 Forceps delivery
    2 Induction of labor
    3 Cesarean delivery
    4 X-ray examination

192. The father of a 15-month-old child says to the nurse that he "does not believe in immunizations." Which of the following statements would be the nurse's best response?
    1 "You feel they may be harmful?"
    2 "Scientific evidence proves you wrong."
    3 "How can you risk the life of your child?"
    4 "Have you discussed this with a doctor?"

193. Which of the following immunizations are generally administered at about 12 months?
    1 Measles, mumps, rubella
    2 Diptheria, pertussis, tetanus, polio
    3 Pertussis, polio, tetanus, hemophilus
    4 Measles, mumps, rubella, hemophilus

194. Which of the following cells might be present in the urine of a child with a low platelet count?
    1 Casts
    2 Leukocytes
    3 Erythrocytes
    4 Lymphocytes

195. A newborn weighing 2840 g should have a daily intake of:
    1 888 ml of fluid and 500 calories
    2 740 ml of fluid and 450 calories
    3 592 ml of fluid and 400 calories
    4 532.8 ml of fluid and 375 calories

196. A client has a diagnosis of acute cholecystitis with biliary colic. In addition to pain in the right upper quadrant, what would the nurse expect the client to have?
    1 Melena and diarrhea
    2 Vomiting of coffee-ground emesis
    3 An intolerance to foods high in lipids
    4 Gnawing pain when the stomach is empty

197. On admission of a client to the labor and delivery unit the nurse asks the client about her marital status. The client refuses to answer and becomes very agitated, telling the nurse to leave. What is the nurse's most appropriate response?
    1 Insist on the information to complete the client's history
    2 Refer the client to a social service organization for assistance
    3 Question the family about the marital status of the client
    4 Restrict questions to those that are relevant to this situation

198. Following abdominal surgery, a client is transferred to the recovery room with a nasogastric tube in place. Which of the following nursing interventions would be most appropriate?
    1 Administer an antiemetic
    2 Elevate the head of the bed
    3 Check the patency of the tube
    4 Encourage the client to breathe deeply

199. Following a cholecystectomy the client should be assessed for signs of bleeding or hemorrhage. These observations are made because:
    1 Prostaglandins are released at the surgical site
    2 Diaphragmatic excursion places pressure on the suture line
    3 The inflammatory process interferes with platelet formation
    4 Blood clotting may be hindered by lack of vitamin K absorption

200. A client with a history of congestive heart failure admits to the nurse that a salt-restricted diet has not been followed and increased ankle edema, orthopnea, and dyspnea on exertion are now being experienced. In consultation with the health care team, what other signs of fluid retention should be monitored?
    1 Dizziness on rising
    2 Rhinitis and headache
    3 A weak and thready pulse
    4 A decreased hemoglobin and hematocrit

Client Case Scenario 26: Joanne is a 4-year-old with severe anemia. She is seen by the nurse in the clinic. **Items 201 to 204 refer to this client case scenario.**

201. In addition to weakness and fatigue, which of the following problems should the nurse expect Joanne to exhibit?
    1 Cold, clammy skin
    2 Increased pulse rate
    3 Elevated blood pressure
    4 Cyanosis of the nail beds

202. Which of the following problems associated with anemia best explains why Joanne becomes dizzy during periods of physical activity?
    1 An inflammation of the inner ear
    2 Insufficient cerebral oxygenation
    3 A sudden drop in blood pressure
    4 Decreased levels of serum glucose

203. Joanne is to receive a liquid iron preparation. Which of the following directions would be appropriate for the nurse to teach Joanne's mother?
    1 Administer this at least an hour before meals
    2 Explain that loose stools are common with iron
    3 Have Joanne take the diluted iron preparation through a straw
    4 Avoid giving Joanne orange or other citric juices with the iron preparation

204. Joanne is to have a blood transfusion. Which of the following problems is most likely associated with blood transfusion?
    1 Serum hepatitis
    2 Allergic response
    3 Pulmonary edema
    4 Hemolytic reaction

Client Case Scenario 27: Mrs. Rocky, a 78-year-old, is admitted to hospital for treatment of varicose veins. **Items 205 to 208 refer to this client case scenario.**

205. What is the most probable cause of Mrs. Rocky's varicose veins?
    1 Defective valves within the veins
    2 The formation of thrombophlebitis
    3 Atherosclerotic plaques along the veins
    4 External compression of the muscles of the legs

206. Which of the following indicators should the nurse expect Mrs. Rocky to exhibit?
    1 A positive Homans' sign
    2 Cramping sensations in the calf muscle
    3 Continuous edema of the affected extremity
    4 Coolness and pallor of the affected extremity

207. The evening prior to surgery, which care should the nurse provide to Mrs. Rocky?
    1 Apply a binder for support
    2 Ambulate Mrs. Rocky in the room
    3 Perform ROM exercises to her legs
    4 Assist Mrs. Rocky out of bed to a chair

208. Mrs. Rocky will have sclerotherapy on the veins that the doctor chose not to treat surgically. Which of the following factors should be considered?
    1 She is to avoid ambulation for 3 to 5 days
    2 The saphenous vein has no sign of aneurysms
    3 Mrs. Rocky understands the need to lose weight
    4 The valves at the saphenofemoral junction are competent

Client Case Scenario 28: Mrs. Story, age 37, is 39 weeks pregnant and diabetic. She is admitted to hospital to await delivery. **Items 209 to 211 refer to this client case scenario.**

209. Which of the following explanations by the nurse would best explain Mrs. Story's need for hospitalization?
    1 Complete rest prior to the work of delivery is essential
    2 Fetal development is complete and should be monitored
    3 Fetal death may occur after the thirty-sixth week of gestation
    4 Insulin needs to be administered intravenously before labor begins

210. What is the best response by the nurse when Mrs. Story asks why she can not continue to take the oral hypoglycemic pills she used prior to her pregnancy at this time?
    1 They may produce deformities in the fetus
    2 The effect of exogenous insulin on the fetus is uncertain
    3 During the latter part of pregnancy, diabetes can usually be controlled by diet alone
    4 The fetal pancreas compensates for the mother's inability to secrete adequate insulin

211. Mrs. Story delivers a male child. Which of the following problems should the nursery nurse be alert for?
    1 Poor sucking reflex
    2 Extreme restlessness
    3 Excessive birth weight
    4 Pallor of the skin and mucosa

Client Case Scenario 29: Mr. Bentley, age 19 years, is diagnosed with bipolar disorder. On admission to hospital, the nursing history reveals he has had recent periods of hyperactivity and combativeness. **Items 212 to 216 refer to this client case scenario.**

212. What is the legal implication for the health care providers who find Mr. Bentley beating another client?
    1 Mr. Bentley, who is known to have been combative, should have been sedated with tranquilizers
    2 Because of a history of hyperactivity and combativeness, Mr. Bentley should never be left unsupervised
    3 The admitting office should not have put Mr. Bentley, with a history of combativeness, in a two-bed room

4 Knowing that Mr. Bentley was frequently combative, close observation by the nursing staff was indicated

213. How should the nurse respond when Mr. Bentley becomes embarrassingly vulgar?
1 Restrict his contact with staff until this symptom passes
2 Tactfully tease Mr. Bentley about the use of such vulgarity
3 Discreetly refuse to talk to Mr. Bentley when he is speaking in this manner
4 Ask Mr. Bentley to limit the use of vulgarity while continuing the conversation

214. Which activities should the nurse encourage Mr. Bentley to get involved in?
1 Carving figures out of wood
2 Lacing tooled leather wallets
3 Stenciling designs on copper sheeting
4 Sanding and varnishing wooden bookends

215. Mr. Bentley becomes loud, noisy, and disruptive in the TV room, and the nurse asks him to be quiet or he will require isolation and safety measures. What are the legal implications of this situation?
1 The information given Mr. Bentley is actually a threat
2 Isolation is justified for Mr. Bentley's own protection
3 His behavior is to be expected and should be ignored
4 Mr. Bentley, who is hyperactive and disruptive, cannot be expected to understand instructions

216. Mr. Bentley demands to be allowed to go downtown to shop. Given that he does not have privileges at the present time, which of the following is the nurse's best response?
1 "You cannot leave the unit."
2 "You'll have to ask your doctor."
3 "Not right now. I don't have a staff member to go with you."
4 "I'm sorry, you can't go. Let's look through this new catalog."

Client Case Scenario 30: Andy is an infant who is born with trisomy 21, Down syndrome. **Items 217 to 221 refer to this client case scenario.**

217. Which of the following initial newborn assessment findings might indicate to the nurse that Andy has Down syndrome?
1 A rounded occiput

2 Asymmetric gluteal folds
3 A transverse palmar (simian) crease
4 Hypertonicity of the skeletal muscles

218. Which of the following problems are associated with Down syndrome?
1 Difficulty in hearing
2 High incidence of circulatory problems
3 Proneness to respiratory tract infections
4 A developmental lag after 1 or 2 years of age

219. The physician suspects that Andy has a congenital heart defect. Andy tires easily with feeding and has difficulty breathing. In which of the following positions should the nurse place Andy?
1 Supine with the knees flexed
2 Orthopneic with pillows for support
3 Prone with the head supported by pillows
4 Side-lying with the head and chest elevated

220. At 5 weeks of age, Andy has a cardiac catheterization. After the procedure, the leg used for the catheter site becomes mottled. Which nursing action would initially be the most appropriate?
1 Elevate the leg
2 Cover him with a blanket
3 Check the pulse in the extremity
4 Notify the physician of the situation

221. Which of the following objectives, associated with care for infants born with a genetic disability, should guide the nurse in caring for Andy?
1 Teaching him to nipple-feed
2 Helping the parents learn about their child
3 Frequent handling and rocking to keep him from crying
4 Preventing aspiration of formula by frequently bubbling him

Client Case Scenario 31: A nurse discovers Mrs. Alfonso, age 66 years, lying on the floor. **Items 222 to 226 refer to this client case scenario.**

222. What is the most appropriate response by the nurse?
1 Call for assistance
2 Establish an airway
3 Check the carotid pulse
4 Obtain the blood pressure

223. As the nurse is currently alone, what is the ratio of ventilations to cardiac compressions when performing cardiopulmonary resuscitation?
1 1:5
2 1:10
3 2:15
4 4:15

224. The emergency response team arrives and prepares for cardiac monitoring. What is the nurse's most appropriate action when preparing the skin area for placement of electrodes?
1 Scrub the area with povidone iodine solution
2 Use a scrubbing motion while cleansing the skin
3 Apply electrode paste only if the skin becomes excoriated
4 Moisten the area with normal saline before applying the electrodes

225. Mrs. Alfonso's cardiac monitor shows ventricular fibrillation. The nurse from CCU should prepare for which of the following?
1 Elective cardioversion
2 Immediate defibrillation
3 An IM injection of digoxin (Lanoxin)
4 An IV line for emergency medications

226. What should the nurse prepare to administer when it is suspected that Mrs. Alfonso is developing metabolic acidosis?
1 Regular insulin
2 Calcium gluconate
3 Potassium chloride
4 Sodium bicarbonate

Client Case Scenario 32: Mr. Wells, aged 88 years, is admitted to hospital with prostatic hypertrophy. He tells the nurse on morning rounds that he has not voided since last night. **Items 227 to 230 refer to this client case scenario.**

227. After assessing Mr. Wells and determining his bladder is distended, what is the most appropriate action by the nurse?
1 Encourage use of a urinal
2 Force fluids to induce voiding
3 Assist him into a warm shower
4 Apply pressure over the pubic area

228. Mr. Wells undergoes a suprapubic prostatectomy. What is the most appropriate action by the nurse to prevent secondary bladder infection?
1 Observe for signs of uremia
2 Attach the catheter to suction
3 Clamp off the connecting tubing
4 Change the dressings frequently

229. Mr. Wells complains of pain in the operative site. What is the most appropriate initial response by the nurse?
1 Administer the prescribed analgesic
2 Encourage intake of fluids to dilute urine

3 Inspect the drainage tubing for occlusion
4 Measure and record the vital signs before administering an analgesic

230. Which of the following is a most appropriate action in respect to Mr. Wells' postoperative care?
1 Have Mr. Wells stand to void
2 Aspirate the catheter with a bulb syringe
3 Discourage straining for a bowel movement
4 Notify the physician if Mr. Wells does not void in 12 hours

231. Which of the following is an initial nursing action after the birth of a preterm baby with an Apgar score of 8?
1 Apply an identification band
2 Check clamp and dress the umbilical cord
3 Assist the physician with resuscitative measures
4 Quickly dry the baby and place in a controlled, warm environment

232. What should the nurse expect of a baby about 1 hour after birth?
1 Crying and cranky
2 Hyperresponsive to stimuli
3 Relaxed and sleeping quietly
4 Intensely alert with eyes wide open

233. When changing a newborn, the nurse notices a brick-red stain on the diaper. The nurse should recognize this to be which of the following?
1 To be expected in female babies
2 A symptom of low iron excretion
3 A normal but uncommon occurrence
4 Due to medication given to the mother

234. Three days after birth, a newborn is slightly jaundiced. The nurse will know that this is due primarily to which of the following?
1 Immature liver function
2 An inability to synthesize bile
3 The mother's high hemoglobin level
4 High hemoglobin and low hematocrit levels

235. Why is it important for the nurse to apply eye patches to the newborn's eyes during phototherapy?
1 To be sure the eyes are closed
2 To prevent injury to conjunctiva and retina
3 To reduce overstimulation from bright lights
4 To limit excessive rapid eye movements and anxiety

236. What is the purpose of a **T** tube insertion following a cholecystectomy?
    1 Drain bile from the cystic duct
    2 Keep the common bile duct patent
    3 Prevent abscess formation at the surgical site
    4 Provide a port for contrast dye in a cholangiogram

237. What observations by the nurse would be considered normal when caring for a client 8 hours following the surgical creation of a colostomy?
    1 The presence of hyperactive bowel sounds
    2 The absence of drainage from the colostomy
    3 A dusky-colored, edematous-appearing stoma
    4 Bright bloody drainage from the nasogastric tube

238. Which of the following should the nurse teach the patient to limit to control uremia associated with renal failure?
    1 Fluid
    2 Protein
    3 Sodium
    4 Potassium

239. Which action by the nurse is most appropriate when caring for a client receiving peritoneal dialysis?
    1 Position the client from side to side if fluid is not draining properly
    2 Notify the physician if there is a deficit of 200 ml in the drainage fluid
    3 Maintain the client in a flat, supine position during the entire procedure
    4 Remove the cannula at the end of the procedure and apply a dry, sterile dressing

240. When discussing weight loss with an obese individual with Ménière's disease, it would be most therapeutic if the nurse suggests that the client:
    1 Limit intake to 900 calories a day
    2 Enroll in an exercise class at the local high school
    3 Get involved in diversionary activities when there is an urge to eat
    4 Keep a diary of all foods eaten each day, making certain to list everything

241. A new grandfather tells the nurse that he is anxious about feeling like a grandfather. What is the nursing priority in planning to meet the grandfather's needs?
    1 Encourage him to participate in a parenting class
    2 Provide time for him to be alone with and get to know the baby
    3 Provide a demonstration on diapering, feeding, and bathing the baby
    4 Provide the opportunity to ask questions after viewing a film about a new baby

242. A client is waiting for a renal transplant. When teaching about the transplant, what should the nurse tell the client?
    1 "Your urine production will be delayed after surgery."
    2 "The symptoms of rejection include fever, hypotension, and edema."
    3 "You will require immunosuppressive drugs daily for the rest of your life."
    4 "You will be unable to follow a full program of work and recreation, including sports."

243. A female client who has been abusing her son is undergoing treatment to control her behavior. Which statement by the client indicates the development of some insight into her behavior as a parent?
    1 "I promise that I won't get so angry when my son causes trouble again."
    2 "Once my son gets straightened out, I'll be better able to control my behavior."
    3 "I think the root of the problem is when my husband comes home after drinking."
    4 "If I feel angry at my son again, I'm going to go into the bedroom and punch a pillow."

244. A client is admitted to an alcohol-detoxification unit. After a team conference, which of the following is found to be a priority during the client's initial interview?
    1 An explanation of the unit's routines
    2 An explanation of the client's role on the unit
    3 A description of acceptable behavior on the unit
    4 A complete list of the unit's rules and regulations

245. A female client with a diagnosis of alcohol abuse appears disheveled and disorganized. Which plan would best gain the client's involvement in personal hygienic care?
    1 Assisting her in bathing and dressing by giving her clear, simple directions
    2 Drawing up a schedule with her and making certain that she adheres to it
    3 Bathing and dressing her each morning until she is willing to do it for herself
    4 Giving her a schedule and requiring her to bathe and dress herself each morning

246. When a client who is receiving peritoneal dialysis complains of severe respiratory difficulty, what is the most immediate nursing action?
    1 Notify the physician
    2 Discontinue the treatment
    3 Change the client's position
    4 Drain fluid from the peritoneal cavity

247. Which of the following nursing actions would assist in attempting to meet the emotional needs of a 4-year-old child receiving daily injections?
    1 Provide the child with a doll and other equipment and observe what happens
    2 Allow the child to play with a large needle and syringe and encourage acting out
    3 Encourage the child to draw pictures about what is happening and the associated feelings
    4 Explain the procedures to the child in simple terms at least one hour before they are scheduled

248. What suggestion by the nurse would assist the parents of a child who is diagnosed as being moderately retarded?
    1 Offer simple, repetitive tasks
    2 Concentrate on teaching detailed tasks
    3 Offer challenging, competitive situations
    4 Provide complete directions at the beginning of the task to be carried out

249. As a result of a transfusion reaction, a client suffers kidney damage. When determining kidney damage, what is the most significant clinical response that the nurse should assess?
    1 Polyuria
    2 Hematuria
    3 Decreased urinary output
    4 Acute pain over kidney area

250. A 4-year-old child who has never been separated from the parents or siblings is admitted to the hospital. What action could the nurse encourage the parents to take to assist the child?
    1 Bring a favorite toy to the hospital for the child
    2 Allow the nurse to be the child's major caregiver
    3 Visit the child as often as the hospital's rules allow
    4 Stay with the child throughout the hospitalization

COMPREHENSIVE TEST

ANSWERS AND RATIONALES

COMPREHENSIVE TEST: PART A

1. **4 Albumin in the urine is a sign of pregnancy-induced hypertension, as are an elevated BP and a weight gain of more than 1 kg per week. (EV; CT; PA; HP; AF)**
   1 BP and weight are more relative; changes in the pulse rate and temperature are not associated with pregnancy-induced hypertension.
   2 These signs indicate pregnancy-induced hypertension; treatment of this does not require vaginal examination.
   3 The signs indicate that pregnancy-induced hypertension may be present; the client may be seen more frequently than every 2 weeks.

2. **2 Weight gain caused by fluid retention is the earliest objective sign of mild preeclampsia. (AN; KC; PA; HP; AF)**
   1 Continued elevations are significant; emotional upset, anxiety, and other factors may cause fluctuations or variations in blood pressure.
   3 This may occur; however, it usually becomes evident after weight gain and a progressive increase in BP.
   4 Edema progresses as the signs of preeclampsia worsen because of abnormal retention of fluid.

3. **3 The latest concept concerning pregnancy-induced hypertension is that this condition is a consequence of salt loss during pregnancy and poor protein intake. The recommendations therefore call for a diet containing normal sodium, high protein, and a sufficient number of calories. (EV; AP; ED; HP; AF)**
   1 Low protein is contraindicated for normal fetal growth; there is no indication for increasing sodium.
   2 Lowering the intake of calories and sodium is detrimental to both fetus and mother.
   4 There is an additional daily requirement of 500 calories during pregnancy.

4. **2 The cumulative effects of magnesium sulfate include depressed respirations and an absent or weak knee-jerk reflex. (DC; CT; PA; HP; AF)**
   1 Temperature and pulse are not affected by administration of $MgSO_4$.
   3 The BP is monitored after administration of $MgSO_4$; the apical pulse is not relevant.
   4 Urinary output is increased after administration of $MgSO_4$.

5. **3 The antagonist for magnesium sulfate is calcium gluconate, and it needs to be at the bedside. (PL; CT; PA; HP; AF)**
   1 This is a narcotic antagonist.
   2 This would be ineffective if the action of magnesium is not reversed.
   4 This is not related to the toxic effect of magnesium sulfate; it may be necessary if the client convulses.

6. **3 In severe pregnancy-induced hypertension, fluid is drawn from the plasma into the tissues and the blood becomes more concentrated. This is reflected in the elevated hematocrit level. (AN; KC; PA; HP; AF)**
   1 Vasodilation would not alter the ratio of cells to fluid volume.
   2 Agglutination of red blood cells does not occur.
   4 The hemodilution results in a reduced hematocrit, since there is more blood volume than there are cells.

7. **4 Ten-year-old boys prefer the company of the same gender and age group. Also, the client needs to avoid stressful situations that would tend to increase exacerbations. (EV; CT; PS; GD; CM)**
   1 Same-gender roommates are desirable for companionship and to maintain boy/girl separateness of this age group.
   2 An eight-year-old boy will be too young for Jason to enjoy.
   3 Same-gender roommates are desirable for companionship and to maintain privacy needs.

8. **4 One of the characteristic differences between Type I and Type II diabetes mellitus is the rapid onset of the disease in Type I. Diabetes mellitus is often first diagnosed during acute ketoacidosis.** (AN; KC; PA; EN; CM)
1 Juveniles with diabetes are insulin dependent.
2 Vascular changes are complications associated with Type I diabetes mellitus.
3 Although adult-onset diabetes (Type II or NIDDM) often occurs in obese individuals, diabetes mellitus occurs in children of thin or normal build.

9. **1 100 units : 1 ml = 20 units : × ml**

$$100 \times = 20$$
$$\times = \frac{20}{100} = \frac{1}{5} = 0.2 \text{ ml}$$

(EV; AP; TC; DR; CM)
2 This dose is too large.
3 Same as answer 2.
4 Same as answer 2.

10. **4 Exercise reduces the body's need for insulin. Increased muscle activity accelerates the transport of glucose into the muscle cells, thus producing an insulin-like effect.** (PL; CT; ED; EN; CM)
1 With increased growth and associated dietary intake, the need for insulin increases.
2 An infectious process, if severe enough, may require increased insulin.
3 An emotional upset is a stress that increases the need for insulin.

11. **4 One begins by trying to enter the world where the child's attention is currently focused; this is a way of making human contact, since the child's usual contacts are inanimate objects.** (IM; AP; PS; BA; CF)
1 Autistic children generally cannot tolerate cuddling and will become rigid when anyone attempts to do so.
2 This would have no effect on the nurse's ability to reach the child; rather it would reinforce the withdrawal.
3 The autistic child is unable to participate in group activities.

12. **2 Isolated, unrelated activities predominate. The child's behavior reflects withdrawal or feelings of destructive rage.** (DC; KC; PS; BA; CF)
1 The facial expression is blank; sadness would be a response to the external world, from which the child has withdrawn.

3 The autistic child seems to overrespond to stimuli in the environment.
4 The autistic child rarely if ever smiles.

13. **3 Self-isolation and disinterest in interpersonal relationships lead the autistic child to find security in nonthreatening, impersonal objects.** (IM; AP; PS; BA; CF)
1 This would be too threatening to an autistic child.
2 Touching the child might prove to be too threatening.
4 These children do not respond to bright-colored toys and blocks as other children do unless there is movement involved.

14. **4 The rhythmic movement of the merry-go-round provides soothing and nonthreatening comfort to the autistic child, who cannot reach out to the environment.** (IM; AP; PS; BA; CF)
1 The autistic child rejects cuddling and anything that feels cuddly.
2 The child would prefer a mechanical object over a colored block.
3 Same as answer 2.

15. **2 Retinal damage caused by the increased intraocular pressure of glaucoma is permanent and is progressive if the disease is not controlled.** (PL; KC; PA; NM; OM)
1 Blindness may be prevented if treatment is early.
3 Surgery can open up drainage and permanently reduce pressure.
4 One eye may be affected, and there is no restriction in the use of the eyes.

16. **3 In glaucoma there is a loss of peripheral vision long before the central vision is affected. The client may also complain of seeing halos around light.** (DC; KC; PA; NM; OM)
1 Primary closed-angle glaucoma causes pain.
2 Blurred vision may be due to a refractive error; peripheral vision is affected in glaucoma.
4 This occurs when there is damage to the central retina; peripheral vision is affected in glaucoma.

17. **2 Exercise should not include bending and the Valsalva maneuver, which might increase intraocular pressure.** (EV; AP; ED; NM; OM)
1 Fluids may be taken as desired because they have no effect on intraocular pressure.

3 Mydriatics are contraindicated in glaucoma because they dilate the pupil, which increases intraocular pressure.

4 Lighting conditions have no effect on intraocular pressure.

18. 4 **The prone position stretches the flexor muscles, thus preventing hip flexion contractures.** (IM; AP; PA; NM; AM)

1 Elevating the head of the bed would cause hip flexion, which could result in a hip flexion contracture.

2 Elevating the stump would cause hip flexion, which could result in a hip flexion contracture.

3 Sitting flexes the hips, which could result in a hip flexion contracture.

19. 2 **Muscles that originate at the vertebrae or pelvic girdle and insert on the femur act to abduct, adduct, flex, extend, and rotate the femur. Normal body alignment should be maintained because it facilitates the safe and efficient use of muscle groups for balance and stability.** (IM; AP; PA; NM; AM)

1 This position does not approximate normal body alignment; hip flexion will alter the center of gravity and promote the development of a hip flexion contracture.

3 This position does not approximate normal body alignment; abduction of the stump will alter the center of gravity.

4 This interferes with the development of a normal gait; muscles that originate at the vertebrae and pelvic girdle should be used to move the stump.

20. 3 **Subcutaneous fat is reduced by the pressure of the initial constrictive bandage and the socket of the prosthesis.** (AN; KC; PA; NM; AM)

1 Edema is limited and contributes minimally to the size of the postoperative stump.

2 Restoration of skin turgor does not affect stump size.

4 Tissue and bone excised remain constant; after surgery there is no additional loss.

21. 4 **The client is usually instructed to push forcefully yet gently over the bone to toughen the limb for weight bearing. This process is begun by pushing the stump against increasingly harder surfaces.** (IM; AP; PA; NM; AM)

1 Abduction of the stump does not maintain normal alignment and should be avoided; it does not prepare the stump end for a prosthesis.

2 Dangling the stump does not help prepare it for a prosthesis and may impede venous return, which would prolong healing.

3 This would macerate the stump and hinder the use of a prosthesis.

22. 1 **A distended bladder usually displaces the fundus upward and toward the right.** (EV; KC; PA; HC; AF)

2 The normal position of the fundus is at the level of the umbilicus, or below, in the midline, rather than shifted to the right.

3 The fundus is firm; therefore bleeding at this time is not a problem.

4 If parts of the placenta and/or membranes were retained, bleeding would be present.

23. 1 **In the immediate postpartum period a slower-than-normal pulse rate can be anticipated as a result of a combination of factors, such as horizontal position, emotional relief and satisfaction, and enforced rest after labor and delivery.** (AN; AP; PA; HC; AF)

2 Bradycardia is more likely; respirations generally are unchanged.

3 The temperature may rise slightly, but respirations usually are unchanged.

4 Same as answer 3.

24. 3 **Parenting can begin only when the baby and mother get to know each other. To promote normal development, the nurse should provide time for parent-child interaction.** (PP; AP; ED; HC; AF)

1 This may make the mother feel incompetent and retard her mothering.

2 Time must be provided for the mother with the baby to return demonstrations and ask questions.

4 This is ineffective; knowledge does not ensure good mothering. Time with the infant is more important.

25. 2 **A predominant clinical sign of croup is reactive spasms of the laryngeal muscles, which produces partial respiratory obstruction. The cough is tight, with a barking metallic sound.** (DC; KC; PA; RE; CF)

1 Children with croup experience inspiratory rather than expiratory stridor.

3 Children with croup experience spasm of the larynx rather than the bronchi; whooping cough (pertussis) is a separate communicable disease.

4 The cough of croup is tight and nonproductive.

26. **4 The physician may have to be notified. A tracheostomy may be necessary to maintain an open airway. (IM; AP; TC; RE; CF)**
    1 The symptoms are not indicative of increased secretions; suctioning can precipitate sudden laryngospasm.
    2 Notification of the physician would be done immediately. In addition, increasing the level of oxygen will not be of significant assistance to a child whose airway is obstructing.
    3 This is ineffective for laryngeal spasms.

27. **4 These are some of the first signs of hypoxia; the airway must be kept patent to promote oxygenation. (IM; AP; PA; RE; CF)**
    1 The child will not be able to communicate verbally after a tracheotomy.
    2 These are late signs of hypoxia; suctioning should have been done well before this time.
    3 These are late signs of respiratory difficulty; suctioning and other measures should have been done well before this time.

28. **2 Spasm must be interrupted or hypoxia will occur. (AN; AP; ED; RE; CF)**
    1 The problem in croup is laryngeal spasm, not constriction of bronchi.
    3 This is not the priority; the spasm must be interrupted immediately.
    4 Same as answer 3.

29. **4 These disorders are characterized by anxiety and minor distortions of reality. The anxiety results in an inability to reach a decision, because all alternatives are threatening. (DC; KC; PS; PR; AM)**
    1 Just the opposite is true; part of emotional maturity is the ability to relate to people, and these people have difficulties in this area.
    2 This would be indicative of severe emotional illness, not an anxiety disorder.
    3 This would be indicative of a mood disorder.

30. **1 Rituals are a means for the individual to control anxiety. If not permitted to carry out the ritual, the client will probably experience unbearable anxiety. (IM; AP; PS; PR; AM)**
    2 The client understands this already but is unable to stop the activity.
    3 These clients have no idea what the ritual means; only that they must continue with it.
    4 This would have the effect of increasing anxiety in the client, possibly to panic levels.

31. **1 Since the compulsive ritual is used to control anxiety, any attempt to prevent the action would greatly increase the anxiety. (EV; KC; PS; PR; AM)**
    2 Underlying hostility is considered to be part of the disorder itself; not a reaction to an interruption of the ritual.
    3 This would be possible only if the anxiety reached panic levels and caused the person overtly to express anger.
    4 This is not a pattern of behavior associated with this disorder

32. **2 Asthma involves spasms of the bronchi and bronchioles as well as an increased mucus production. This decreases the size of the lumina, interfering with inhalation and exhalation. (AN; KC; PA; RE; AF)**
    1 This is not a mechanism involved in asthma, in which there is interference with both inhalation and exhalation.
    3 The client cannot hyperventilate because of mucosal edema, bronchoconstriction, and secretions, all of which cause airway obstruction. Emotional stress is only one of many precipitating factors such as allergens, temperature changes, odors, and chemicals.
    4 There will be a decrease in the vital capacity.

33. **2 In addition to dilation of bronchi, treatment is aimed at expectoration of mucus. Mucus interferes with gas exchange in the lungs. (PL; AP; PA; RE; AF)**
    1 This is an unrealistic goal; asthma is a chronic illness.
    3 Increased fluid intake helps liquefy secretions.
    4 Asthma has a psychogenic factor but this does not imply emotions are the only etiology; there is an interaction between the psyche and the soma.

34. **3 Aminophylline relaxes the smooth muscles, causing bronchodilation and thereby relieving respiratory distress and promoting rest. (EV; KC; PA; RE; AF)**
    1 Aminophylline is not an antibiotic.
    2 Aminophylline is not a skeletal muscle relaxant.
    4 This is the effect of corticosteroids.

35. **3 During sleep, mucus secretions in the respiratory tract move more slowly toward the throat. On awakening, increased ciliary motion raises such secretions more vigorously; this facilitates expectoration and the collection of sputum specimens. (PL; AP; PA; RE; AF)**

1 Although activity mobilizes secretions, there may not be any secretions present at the time of activity; sputum is most plentiful upon arising.

2 Sputum may leave an unpleasant taste in the mouth, which could interfere with appetite.

4 Sputum would more likely be collected after a respiratory treatment, because this mobilizes secretions due to positive pressure.

36. **2 Although dust cannot be avoided completely, use of a damp cloth helps eliminate the amount of airborne particles that might be inhaled. (PL; AP; ED; RE; AF)**

1 This is unrealistic.

3 This is untrue; there are ways to limit the amount of airborne particles.

4 Redecorating will not eliminate dust; it is a part of our environment.

37. **3 A diagnosis of cancer and a colostomy both drastically alter a person's self-image and body image. People react differently to this stress, often finding it difficult to express their concerns verbally; however, their actions may demonstrate an awareness of the situation. (EV; CT; PS; EP; OF)**

1 There is not enough information to determine this.

2 Same as answer 1.

4 Same as answer 1.

38. **3 Clients who have radical changes in their body image as a result of surgery are usually best able to relate to someone who has faced the same stress and successfully adapted. (PP; CT; PS; EP; OF)**

1 Clients cannot learn to do colostomy care until they psychologically accept the presence of the colostomy.

2 This would provide information but do little to aid acceptance.

4 This would do little to aid acceptance.

39. **4 A diet as close as possible to normal after a colostomy is recommended for the stated reason that individuals will discover their own food intolerances and should eat accordingly. (PL; KC; ED; GI; OF)**

1 Each person is an individual and reacts differently to foods.

2 Rigid dietary regulations usually increase anxiety; return to normally tolerated foods provides security.

3 A low-residue diet is not necessary; once healing occurs, a diet with adequate residue promotes peristalsis and colostomy functioning.

40. **1 Rapid instillation of fluid into the colon may cause abdominal cramps. By clamping the tubing, the nurse allows the cramps to subside so the irrigation can be continued. (EV; AP; TC; GI; OF)**

2 Emotional support will not interrupt the physical adaptation of abdominal cramps; the irrigation must be temporarily interrupted.

3 Although this may reduce the force of the fluid, it will not eliminate the flow of fluid completely; the irrigation should be temporarily interrupted.

4 This is contraindicated; this will increase the force of flow, which will increase the abdominal cramps.

41. **2 A colostomy located on the left side of the abdomen most likely would involve the descending colon. Since most but not all of the fluid would be absorbed, the stool would be moist and formed. (DC; KC; PA; GI; OF)**

1 This would be associated with a colostomy involving the ascending colon.

3 Stools are not usually covered with mucus; they may be moist but not mucoid.

4 This would be associated with conditions that narrow the intestinal lumen; this is not usually associated with a colostomy.

42. **2 Colostomy irrigations done daily at the same time help establish normal patterns of bowel evacuation. (IM; AP; ED; GI; OF)**

1 Initially after surgery, protein promotes healing; protein intake has no relationship to bowel control.

3 Although fluid is important to prevent hard stools, it will not help the client regain bowel control; a daily regimen is the priority.

4 A soft, low-residue diet is not necessary; it should be as close to normal as possible.

43. **2 A heterozygous father who is Rh positive coupled with a heterozygous Rh-positive or Rh-negative mother may produce an Rh-negative infant. (AN; KC; PA; HN; CM)**

1 The Rh factor is a genetically determined trait; it cannot be altered by time.

3 Rh factor is a genetically determined trait; it is influenced by both parents.

4 Same as answer 1.

44. **4 Giving Rh-positive cells would lead to further hemolysis; Rh-negative cells are not attacked by maternal antibodies. (PL; CT; PA; HN; CM)**
    1 This would be irrelevant because the blood cells usually do not come from the mother.
    2 This is not really neutral; it is only a temporary safeguard from further hemolysis.
    3 A reaction to other antigens in the cross-matched blood could still occur.

45. **4 These are tiny plugged sebaceous glands, and attempts to remove them will further irritate them; they will disappear by themselves. (IM; KC; ED; NN; CM)**
    1 This is not true because many infants do not have them; the mother may look for validation of this statement in other babies.
    2 These are not birthmarks; they result from maternal hormonal influences and are temporary.
    3 The white material is not pus and is not infectious.

46. **3 The fluid level and time must be marked so the amount of drainage in the chest tube drainage system can be evaluated. (IM; AP; TC; RE; AM)**
    1 The amount of sterile water used to create a water seal depends on the drainage system used and is usually more than 3 to 5 ml; once the water seal is created, the nurse usually does not add water.
    2 The drainage system must be kept below chest level to promote drainage of the pleural space so the lung can expand.
    4 The catheter is secured by skin sutures, not to the dressing itself.

47. **1 Atmospheric pressure is greater than the pressure inside the pleural space. If a chest tube were not attached to a drainage system closed by a water seal, air would enter the pleural space and collapse the lung (pneumothorax). (DC; AP; TC; RE; AM)**
    2 Capillarity is the tendency of cohesive liquid molecules to rise in a tube; this is not the purpose of water in a chest tube drainage system.
    3 This is the purpose of the drainage collection chamber and suction working together, not the water seal chamber.
    4 The concern is not primarily for pressure within the tube itself but to prevent atmospheric pressure from collapsing the lung.

48. **2 Turning and positioning prevent pooling of secretions in the lung and maximize lung expansion. (IM; AP; PA; RE; AM)**
    1 This is a dependent nursing function.
    3 Same as answer 1.
    4 Same as answer 1.

49. **1 Oxygen can dry the mucous membranes of the respiratory tract. Drying of mucous membranes can predispose to infection. (IM; KC; PA; RE; AM)**
    2 Padding is required because of irritation by some equipment; not related to the untoward effects of oxygen therapy.
    3 The orthopneic position promotes lung expansion and is often used in conjunction with oxygen therapy; not an untoward effect.
    4 Although vital signs should be assessed so the effect of treatment can be evaluated, an apical pulse is not necessary.

50. **1 Polyarthritis of rheumatic fever is transitory and does not cause deformity. Rheumatoid arthritis is chronic and causes changes in joints. (AN; KC; PA; SK; CF)**
    2 Cardiac damage is often associated with rheumatic fever.
    3 The etiology of rheumatic fever is related to a previous occurrence of strep throat; rheumatoid arthritis is unrelated.
    4 Juvenile rheumatoid arthritis involves chronic inflammation of the joints; exacerbations are most often related to stress.

51. **3 Aspirin interferes with platelet aggregation, thereby lengthening bleeding time. (EV; KC; TC; DR; AM)**
    1 Urate excretion is enhanced by high doses of aspirin.
    2 Aspirin is readily broken down in the GI tract and liver.
    4 Aspirin inhibits platelet aggregation; it does not destroy erythrocytes.

52. **1 To be truly effective in the relationship with the client, the nurse must know and understand personal feelings about terminal illness and death. (PP; KC; PS; CS; OF)**
    2 When dealing with terminal illness, knowledge alone is not enough to assure an effective nurse-client relationship.
    3 Although the family is an important part of the client's support system, the client's feelings are more important to the relationship.
    4 Previous experiences could be positive or negative and would not guarantee an effective nurse-client relationship.

53. **4 This grouping of foods does not contain high-residue fruits, vegetables, or whole grains, which are irritating to the intestinal mucosa, cause bulk, and increase peristalsis.** (PL; CT; PA; GI; AM)
    1 This choice includes vegetables and grain, which leave increased residue.
    2 This choice includes whole-grain foods, which leave increased residue.
    3 Same as answer 1.

54. **1 The affected areas of the intestine are in need of repair. Protein is required in the building and repairing of tissues.** (PL; KC; ED; GI; AF)
    2 Increased protein will not significantly affect peristalsis.
    3 Anemia may result from chronic bleeding; it usually is corrected, however, with increased iron and normal intake of protein.
    4 Protein is given to promote healing; once tissues are repaired, muscle tone may improve.

55. **2 Nurses can become very blasé about the equipment used in labor and forget that it may be frightening for the layperson.** (EV; CT; PS; EC; AF)
    1 Internal monitoring is only used if adequate readouts cannot be obtained on an external monitor.
    3 Sedation is never given on a routine basis to the client in labor.
    4 This is not universally true; older primigravidas may have totally uncomplicated labors.

56. **4 Lactation delays ovarian function after delivery. It will also therefore delay the symptoms of endometriosis.** (IM; AP; PA; WH; AF)
    1 Pregnancy temporarily suppresses ovarian function; the aberrant endometrial tissue is still present.
    2 Endometriosis may lead to sterility; it does not cause menopause.
    3 Conservative medical therapy will be used first; a hysterectomy is only a last resort.

57. **3 Frequent nursing reduces the possibility of engorgement. A 10-minute period provides for complete emptying of the breast.** (PL; AF; ED; HC; AF)
    1 A relief bottle will prevent emptying of the breast; this will increase pain and swelling.
    2 This does not provide for complete emptying of the breasts.
    4 This will not decrease engorgement.

58. **2 If a tracheostomy is not performed with radical neck surgery, tracheal edema may cause obstruction of the airway after the endotracheal tube is removed.** (PL; AP; TC; RE; AM)
    1 An endotracheal tube is not irrigated to maintain patency, as is a nasogastric tube; the endotracheal tube is in the trachea, leading to the lungs.
    3 Initially postoperative dressings should be removed by the surgeon.
    4 It is not necessary to reposition the endotracheal tube if the gag reflex returns; when the client is able to breathe independently, the anesthesiologist will remove the tube.

59. **1 Inadequate oxygenation of the brain may produce restlessness or behavioral changes. The pulse and respiration rates increase as a compensatory mechanism for hypoxia.** (EV; KC; PA; RE; AM)
    2 The pupils dilate with cerebral hypoxia.
    3 The pulse and respiration rates increase with hypoxia.
    4 Clubbing of the fingers, the result of increased vascularization, is an adaptation to prolonged hypoxia.

60. **3 The nurse should expect to see an increase in blood volume by as much as 40% above prepregnant levels. During pregnancy, fluid in all body compartments increases.** (AN; CT; PA; HC; AF)
    1 The BP remains essentially unchanged throughout pregnancy.
    2 The hematocrit decreases as a result of the hemodilution of pregnancy.
    4 An increase in cardiac output is seen as early as the end of the first trimester, because of increased blood volume.

61. **2 This is the usual pattern that a nevus vasculosus follows.** (IM; KC; ED; EC; AF)
    1 This is false; a nevus vasculosus involves the dermal and subdermal layers.
    3 This is false; a nevus vasculosus grows and fades. Saying it will be covered by clothes gives little reassurance.
    4 Surgical removal is not recommended.

62. **2 The antibody system is not functioning in neonates. Antibodies are transferred from the mother in breast milk. (IM; KC; ED; HC; AF)**
    1 Lactating mothers rarely ovulate for the first 9 weeks postpartum; however, they may anytime after that.
    3 Because of the higher carbohydrate content of breast milk, infants wake more easily; carbohydrate is digested more rapidly.
    4 Breast milk has 1.1 g protein/100 ml; cow's milk has 3.5 g/100 ml; whole cow's milk is unsuitable for infants.

63. **3 Petroleum gauze helps control bleeding and prevent adherence of the diaper. (EV; AF; ED; NN; CM)**
    1 This is not practical with a male infant.
    2 Fussy behavior is normal for a few hours after the procedure.
    4 Yellow exudate is normal; it is not part of an infectious process.

64. **3 The woman must watch closely for symptoms associated with side effects of these medications. Estrogen-progestin contraceptives have been associated with thrombophlebitis (calf pain) and breast malignancy (breast tenderness from estrogen-supported tumors), as well as cardiovascular changes (hypertension). (EV; AP; ED; RC; AF)**
    1 Nausea and rash are not associated with using estrogen-progestin contraceptives; however, breakthrough bleeding is a major side effect.
    2 Lethargy, syncope, and tachycardia are not side effects of oral contraceptives.
    4 Bradycardia and visual changes are not side effects; hypertension is a major side effect.

65. **3 This approach allows for ventilation of feelings and clarifies explanations that probably were not heard or understood because of anxiety. (PP; AF; PS; CS; AF)**
    1 This excludes the client from facing the problem, thereby increasing her feelings of loss of control.
    2 This closes off communication by not allowing free expression of grief.
    4 This supports avoidance of the reality of the situation; it does not help the problem.

66. **3 The parent's action allows the child to make a decision providing for developmental autonomy. (EV; AF; ED; GD; CM)**

1 Although tantrums as attention-getting devices largely must be ignored, ignoring the child will produce feelings of isolation and insecurity.
2 Boredom, hunger, and insecurity can lead to additional frustration and anger.
4 This could lead to the development of more manipulative tactics, since the action brought a degree of success initially.

67. **2 Children learn socially acceptable behavior when consistent, reasonable limits that provide guidelines are established. (IM; AP; ED; GD; CF)**
    1 Rewards should not always be necessary for good behavior; they will become expected.
    3 Authorities vary on their attitudes about punishment; punishment should not become the major means of teaching children to control their behavior.
    4 This is not always safe or reasonable for very young children.

68. **2 Albumin is not normally excreted in the urine. When found, it indicates renal disease. (EV; CT; PA; RG; CM)**
    1 Excess calcium is normally excreted.
    3 Potassium is normally excreted by the kidneys to maintain electrolyte balance.
    4 Excess phosphate is normally excreted.

69. **1 Active sharing of responsibility will prove most helpful. It will assure that lead sources are removed. (IM; AP; ED; NM; CF)**
    2 This will not resolve etiologic factors or accomplish prevention.
    3 This is a good idea, but does not guarantee action; concrete action should be taken first.
    4 This omits the need to remove lead from the environment; therefore, it will not assure prevention.

70. **4 A low-pressure cuff prevents constriction of the capillary bed, preventing tracheal necrosis. (PL; CT; TC; RE; AM)**
    1 The tracheostomy tube can be a single lumen tube or have both an inner and outer cannula.
    2 A tracheostomy tube, whether it is a single lumen tube or has both an inner and outer cannula, does not have to be changed weekly; it is usually changed every 2 to 3 weeks as necessary.
    3 The tracheostomy should be cleaned every 8 hours and whenever necessary.

71. **2 As a result of COPD, there is increased pressure in the pulmonary circulation. The right side of the heart hypertrophies**

**(called cor pulmonale), and right ventric-
ular heart failure may ensue.** (AN; KC; PA;
RE; AM)

1 This system is not as closely related to the pulmonary system as the cardiac system is; kidney problems do not usually occur.

3 The skeletal system is not truly related to the
pulmonary system; joint inflammation does
not occur.

4 Peripheral nerves are not as closely related to
the pulmonary system as the cardiac system is;
peripheral neuropathy does not occur.

72. **2 Productive coughing induced by postural
drainage can cause nausea and vomiting.**
(PL; KC; PA; RE; AM)

1 Since coughing must be encouraged after
treatment, sleep is postponed; but as breathing
is facilitated, sleep may then be more restful.

3 Approximately 1 hour before meals is a preferred time for postural drainage; the resulting
cough and mucus production will be less likely to affect dietary intake.

4 Upon awakening, mucus secretions are plentiful and tenacious; postural drainage at this
time would be most beneficial.

73. **2 A culture of CSF obtained would reveal
the presence of a causative organism (e.g.,
the pneumococcus, tubercle bacillus,
meningococcus, or streptococcus).** (AN; KC;
PA; NM; CF)

1 This is not a definitive test, although advisable;
occasionally it will prove positive when a CSF
culture is negative.

3 This is used to detect the presence of abnormalities by the injection of a contrast medium
into the subarachnoid space; it does not identify the organism.

4 This would demonstrate the presence of bacteria on the skin, not identify organisms in the
cerebrospinal fluid.

74. **4 The concept of object permanence begins
to develop around 6 months of age.** (DC;
KC; ED; GD; CM)

1 This occurs between 13 and 24 months.

2 Same as answer 1.

3 This occurs during the first several months of
life.

75. **3 After administration of a local anesthetic
during a bronchoscopy, fluids and food
should be withheld until the gag reflex
returns.** (EV; AP; TC; RE; AM)

1 Ice chips must not be given until the gag reflex
returns.

2 Coughing should not be encouraged; it might
initiate bleeding from the site of the biopsy.

4 To allow drainage and minimize the possibility of aspiration, the client should be kept in a
semi-Fowler's position.

76. **3 Because the client has an endotracheal
tube in place, secretions can be loosened
by the administration of humidified oxygen and by frequent turning.** (PL; CT; PA;
RE; AM)

1 A client with an endotracheal tube in place is
not permitted fluids by mouth.

2 This would be too vigorous for a client who
needs an endotracheal tube.

4 Potassium is never instilled into the lungs.

77. **3 To maintain normal expansion of the
remaining lung after a pneumonectomy,
the client should be positioned on the
operative side or the back.** (IM; AP; PA; RE;
AM)

1 A high-Fowler's position may cause the client
to slip down in the bed, diminishing thoracic
excursion.

2 Keeping the client flat will decrease lung
expansion; gatching a bed may cause peripheral circulatory complications.

4 The client should not be placed on the unaffected side; this will impede lung expansion.

78. **1 Various aspects of hospitalization and
diagnosis could cause the client anxiety.
The nurse should determine what dis-
turbs the client most.** (PP; AP; PS; EP; OM)

2 An anxious client will not be receptive to
learning.

3 This may cause the client unnecessary anxiety.

4 A tracheostomy may not be performed, depending on the extent of the surgery and edema.

79. **4 This position minimizes the discomfort
associated with venous engorgement. It
also promotes venous drainage by gravity, minimizing edema.** (IM; AP; PA; RE; OM)

1 This position would neither increase nor
decrease strain on the suture line.

2 Drainage from the wound would not be
affected.

3 Providing stimulation would not be a priority;
this position would not affect the degree of
stimulation.

80. **1 If the dressing is too tight, impaired cerebral circulation may result. (EV; AP; PA; CV; OM)**
    2 Bleeding would not cause the client to complain of tightness.
    3 This is untrue; impaired cerebral circulation may result from a tight dressing.
    4 The dressing may be loosened or removed only if indicated by the physician.

81. **4 The cuff should be inflated to the minimum occlusive volume, which allows the desired volume to be achieved but does not press against the trachea, constricting circulation. This can be judged by using a stethoscope to listen for a slight air leak at the back of the throat. (IM; AP; TC; RE; OM)**
    1 The cuff may be deflated during suctioning to prevent tracheal necrosis; secretions just above the cuff drop by gravity and can also be removed by suctioning.
    2 High-volume, low-pressure cuffs do not require routine deflation except to evaluate if the cuff is overinflated.
    3 The seal should be minimally occlusive; a tight seal could result in tracheal necrosis.

82. **1 Administration of 100% oxygen for a few minutes prior to suctioning reduces the risk of hypoxia, the major complication of suctioning. (IM; AP; TC; RE; OM)**
    2 Negative pressure is applied as the catheter is withdrawn.
    3 Tracheostomy tubes have cuffs; tracheostomy cuffs are indicated when a client is on mechanical ventilation.
    4 When ordered, this drug is usually given by inhalation, not instillation; 3 to 5 ml of normal saline can be instilled into the tracheostomy tube to loosen secretions.

83. **3 The tracheostomy site is a portal of entry for microorganisms. Sterile technique must be used; the most advantageous system is a closed tracheal suctioning catheter system. (IM; AP; TC; RE; OM)**
    1 The high-Fowler's position promotes maximum aeration of the lungs.
    2 Body temperature is not related to the suctioning procedure.
    4 The cannula, if it is not disposable, is generally cleaned with peroxide and saline.

84. **3 Hydrocephalus complicates approximately 90% of lumbosacral meningomyeloceles. (DC; KC; PA; NM; CF)**
    1 Paraplegia is not an indicator for the development of hydrocephalus.
    2 Hydrocephalic infants may or may not have a low Apgar score.
    4 This is normal for a newborn.

85. **4 Increased intracranial pressure results in pressure exerted against the cranium. This is especially evident in areas with less confinement, such as the fontanel (which bulges), the orbits (which are pushed forward so the eyelids are pulled taut and upper lids are above the irises [sunset eyes]), and the brain (vomiting center stimulated regardless of activity of eating). (DC; KC; PA; NM; CF)**
    1 The fontanel will show signs of increased fluid volume in the skull and therefore bulge.
    2 A high, shrill cry and decreased skin turgor are not signs associated with increased intracranial pressure.
    3 The eyeballs will show signs of increased fluid volume in the skull and be pushed forward, pulling the lids taut; systolic pressure is elevated and diastolic is the same or lower, creating a widening pulse pressure.

86. **4 These are associated with infection, the greatest postoperative hazard for children with shunts for hydrocephalus. (PL; CT; ED; NM; CF)**
    1 This may occur as a result of an infected shunt; however, it is not the most common complication.
    2 The peritoneum absorbs cerebrospinal fluid adequately; ascites is not a problem.
    3 These occur with progressively increasing intracranial pressure, usually before shunt insertion; it is considered a sign, not a symptom, of infection.

87. **1 Periodic pumping of the valve ensures the patency of the tubing and allows the fluid to move through. (IM; CT; ED; NM; CF)**
    2 Pumping the shunt does not affect the absorption of cerebrospinal fluid.
    3 Bleeding results if cerebrospinal fluid is drained too rapidly.
    4 This is the purpose of the shunt itself; pumping the valve only keeps the tubing patent.

88. **3 Most children with spinal cord damage from communicating hydrocephalus can be managed successfully with this approach.** (PL; AP; ED; NM; CF)
    1 Most children with spinal cord damage from this defect can be managed successfully with intermittent straight catheterization. An ileal conduit is not usually
    2 This is an inaccurate statement, and the least desirable approach because of recurrent urinary tract infections.
    4 This is a devastating and inaccurate statement to make to any young infant's parents.

89. **3 The growing uterus exerts pressure on the mesentery, slowing peristalsis; more water is reabsorbed from the colon and constipation results.** (AN; KC; ED; HC; AF)
    1 The metabolism increases but does not affect the bowel.
    2 The growing uterus tends to exert pressure on the bladder; it is way above the anus.
    4 Milk is not constipating.

90. **4 Rupture of the membranes and the gush of fluid can carry the umbilical cord downward. Immediate placement in the lithotomy position and inspection may lead to identification of prolapse and prevention of fetal distress.** (EV; CT; TC; HC; AF)
    1 These are routine intrapartal nursing measures.
    2 The supine position may decrease blood flow and cause hypoxia in the fetus as well as hypotension in the mother.
    3 The gush of fluid is due to rupture of membranes; unless it is meconium stained or followed by the cord, this is normal and needs no medical intervention.

91. **3 Hypertonic contractions of the uterus, if allowed to continue, can lead to fetal distress and uterine rupture; therefore the infusion should be discontinued so the hypertonic contractions cease.** (EV; AP; PA; DR; AF)
    1 The IV should be carefully monitored with an automatic pump to ensure a regulated and continuous flow.
    2 Fetal heart tones should be monitored more frequently (q 15 min) if a fetal monitor is not used.
    4 The resulting delay could lead to uterine rupture; the nurse should discontinue the infusion of oxytocin.

92. **3 As cervical dilation nears completion, labor is intensified with an increase in pain and energy expenditure.** (AN; KC; PA; HC; AF)
    1 Back pain usually indicates a posterior-lying position of the infant.
    2 The client is usually very restless and thrashes about, assuming no particular position.
    4 Pain is increased, since contractions are more frequent and intense, and they last longer.

93. **3 A relaxed uterus is the most frequent cause of bleeding in the early postpartum period. The uterus can be returned to a state of firmness by intermittent gentle fundal massage.** (EV; CT; PA; HC; AF)
    1 Immediate action is directed toward the client's safety; the physician is called if uterine massage does not control bleeding.
    2 Assessment of the uterus and massage take priority; then the vital signs are checked.
    4 Steady bleeding is neither common nor normal and must be attended to immediately.

94. **1 This response acknowledges the loss and the grieving process. It also encourages ventilation through acceptance.** (PP; AF; PS; CS; AF)
    2 This response does not recognize the loss; cuts off communication.
    3 Guilt feelings were never expressed by the client; this response may reflect the nurse's feelings.
    4 This minimizes the loss and may reflect the nurse's feelings. It also plants thoughts of a less-than-perfect fetus.

95. **1 Initial disbelief and denial help protect the ego from the pain of reality in a stressful situation.** (EV; AF; PS; CS; AF)
    2 This may result from guilt or feelings of inadequacy because of the loss, but occurs later.
    3 Once the initial shock is over, these are the usual results as the self realizes the loss.
    4 There is no evidence of either dissociation or rationalization.

96. **3 Cephalohematoma is a collection of blood between the skull bone and its periosteum as the result of trauma. It resolves spontaneously in 3 to 6 weeks. (IM; KC; ED; CV; CF)**
    1 Caput succedaneum is the result of tissue swelling; cephalohematoma is the result of bleeding over the skull.
    2 A cephalohematoma is a hard, indurated area that remains immobile even when the infant cries.
    4 This is trauma caused by pressure of the head against the birth canal, which occurs in vaginal delivery.

97. **1 Parents need support and reassurance that their child has no permanent damage. (AN; KC; PS; EH; CF)**
    2 Cephalohematomas do not cause impaired neurologic functioning.
    3 No special protection of the head is required; routine safety measures are adequate.
    4 Cephalohematomas resolve spontaneously; no ice is applied.

98. **3 Allowing the client time to talk about her feelings and staying with her when she sees the baby for the first time provides support, acceptance, and understanding. (PP; CT; PS; CS; AF)**
    1 This does not give the nurse a chance to assess the mother's feelings.
    2 This does not give the nurse a chance to assess the mother's feelings; anomalies are difficult to describe accurately in words.
    4 Showing pictures may not be helpful, and discussing treatment is premature.

99. **3 Atherosclerosis begins with the accumulation of fatty deposits (plaques) within the inner lining (intima) of the arteries, leading to a narrowing of the lumen. Later the plaques enlarge, cause greater occlusion, and harden by deposition of calcium (atheroarteriosclerosis), eventually increasing the work of the heart. (AN; KC; PA; CV; AM)**
    1 Atheromas develop within the intima of arteries, not in the cardiac muscle.
    2 Although atheromas or plaques are deposited from circulating fat, mobilization from adipose storage is not a prerequisite.
    4 This is arteriosclerosis.

100. **2 Each person is unique. The nurse should avoid making the client feel dehumanized. (PL; AP; PS; TR; AM)**
    1 Although safety is a priority, it is not the initial need.
    3 This would be a later nursing action.
    4 It is important that the client understand what is happening; however, individuality must be considered first.

101. **3 Devices such as side rails can help clients increase their mobility by facilitating movement in bed. Side rails are immovable objects and provide a handhold for leverage when changing positions. (CC; AP; TC; SK; AM)**
    1 The need to use side rails for safety must be evaluated for each individual based on the mental and physical status and hospital regulations.
    2 Same as answer 1.
    4 Same as answer 1.

102. **3 Explaining procedures and routines decreases the client's anxiety about the unknown. (IM; AP; PS; TR; AM)**
    1 The nurse should not confuse the role of professional with that of being a friend; the client should be called by the appropriate title (Mr., Miss, Ms., Mrs., etc.) unless the client requests otherwise.
    2 The nurse should not confuse the role of professional with that of being a friend; "visiting" has a social connotation.
    4 Although therapeutic, this does not change the fact that the hospital environment is strange to the client.

103. **4 Processed foods generally have sodium added to enhance the taste and help preserve the food. (CC; AP; ED; CV; OF)**
    1 Most fruits have a low sodium content.
    2 Although grain products contain sodium, the content is much less than that in processed food.
    3 Most vegetables have a low sodium content; however, carrots and celery should be avoided.

104. **1 A lowered concentration of extracellular sodium brings about a decrease in the release of ADH. This leads to increased excretion of urine. (AN; KC; ED; CV; OM)**
    2 The sodium restriction does not control the volume of food intake; weight is controlled by a low-calorie diet and by prevention of fluid retention.

3 The resulting elimination of excess fluid reduces the workload of the heart but does not improve contractility.

4 Potassium is inefficiently retained by the body; an adequate intake of potassium is needed.

105. 2 Fluid in the interstitial spaces impairs circulation, leading to poor absorption of drugs as well as predisposing to skin breakdown. (AN; KC; TC; IT; AM)

1 The pain caused by injection is influenced by the type and volume of the drug, not the site.

3 Interstitial fluid may leak from edematous tissue, but this is not the rationale for altering sites.

4 The dilution of the drug does not significantly affect absorption.

106. 1 This would be unsafe if a thrombus were developing because it could dislodge, causing a fatal embolus. (EV; AP; ED; CF; AF)

2 Fluids decrease blood viscosity, reducing the risk of thrombus formation.

3 This prevents venous stasis and promotes muscle tone; it propels venous blood toward the heart, facilitated by venous one-way valves.

4 These physically compress the veins, which prevents venous stasis, lowering the risk of thrombus formation.

107. 2 The wheelchair should be angled close to the bed so the client will have to make only a simple pivot on the stronger leg. When the wheelchair is within the client's visual field, the client will be aware of the distance and direction that the body must navigate to transfer safely and avoid falling (IM; AP; TC; SK; OM)

1 If the knees are flexed, the client may be unable to support his or her weight on the unaffected leg.

3 Moving a client back to bed in this situation would encompass moving against gravity.

4 The large muscles of the legs rather than the arms should be used to prevent muscle strain.

108. 3 When ambulating a client, the nurse walks on the client's stronger or unaffected side. This provides a wide base of support and therefore increases stability during the phase of ambulation that calls for weight bearing on the affected side as the unaffected limb moves forward. (IM; AP; TC; SK; OM)

1 This tends to change the center of gravity from directly above the feet and may cause instability.

2 Same as answer 1.

4 The nurse should stand on the client's stronger or unaffected side.

109. 3 Self-contained suction devices (such as Hemovac or Jackson Pratt) for wound drainage must be compressed for the suction to work. (PL; KC; TC; IT; AF)

1 Drainage tubes are generally not irrigated by nurses.

2 Application of heat is a dependent function and may increase inflammatory edema after surgery.

4 A dependent position impairs venous return and increases edema.

110. 3 The congenital defect prevents the infant from creating a tight seal with the lips to promote sucking. As a result the infant swallows large amounts of air when feeding. The mother should be taught to provide frequent rest periods and to bubble the infant often to expel the excess air in the stomach. (IM; AP; ED; GI; AF)

1 Infants with cleft lip and palate should be held upright during feedings.

2 Same as answer 1.

4 Newborn infants cannot chew.

111. 3 The priority of care at this time is to protect the spine from strain to prevent additional damage to the traumatized area while it heals. (IM; AP; PA; NM; AM)

1 Infection usually results from prolonged immobility; although important, it is not the immediate priority.

2 Although an important aspect of care, it is not the priority item in the immediate postinjury period.

4 Survival and safety take priority; vocational rehabilitation will assume greater importance after the client's condition stabilizes.

112. 2 The client should have a nasogastric tube inserted to prevent aspiration and keep the stomach decompressed. (IM; CT; TC; GI; AM)

1 Diet change requires a physician's order; clients who are vomiting may have food withheld.

3 This information is important; however, prevention of aspiration takes priority.

4 This would be indicated at the next bowel movement; however, maintenance of vital functions is most important.

113. **4 These signs are a result of sympathetic nervous system stimulation and could be indicative of hemorrhage from perforation and require immediate surgical intervention. (IM; CT; PA; GI; AM)**

1 These complaints should be noted; however, they are not indicative of potential priority problems.
2 These complaints should be noted, but they do not indicate an emergency situation that would threaten life.
3 These complaints should be noted because they may indicate early signs of diabetes mellitus; however, the nurse's primary observation should be for symptoms of perforation and shock.

114. **1 Denial is a pattern of defense often demonstrated in the self-protective stage of adaptation to illness. Thoughts and feelings are so painful and provoke such anxiety that the client rejects the existence of the paraplegia. (CC; CT; PS; CS; AM)**

2 From the information available, it cannot be assumed that the client is fantasizing; a fantasy is the transformation of undesirable experiences into imagined events to fulfill an unconscious wish or need.
3 Denial is a method of psychologic adaptation.
4 Motivation must have realistic goals in mind; the client is in denial.

115. **4 Children at early school age are not yet able to comprehend death's universality and inevitability, but fear it, often personifying death as a bogeyman or death angel. They need an opportunity to prepare for this. (PP; AF; PS; CS; AM)**

1 A child this age needs to know the seriousness of the illness and that recovery may not be possible.
2 Children of this age interpret death as separation and punishment; they fear this in addition to death itself.
3 This response only avoids the question.

116. **4 The individual cannot resolve the conflict consciously because of emotional pressure pulling in both directions. As anxiety increases, the unconscious seeks a solution. The conversion selected usually resolves the initial conflict by making action impossible, thus removing the need to select one or the other choice. (AN; KC; PS; AX; OF)**

1 There are no physical changes involved with this unconscious resolution of a conflict.
2 The conversion of anxiety to physical symptoms operates on an unconscious level.
3 A conversion reaction is a psychologic response to stress, not a defense against it.

117. **4 The development of the symptom is the unconscious method of reducing the anxiety. Because the symptom is meeting this need, it does not create anxiety itself but is passively accepted. (AN; KC; PS; PR; OF)**

1 There is no anger; symptoms are passively accepted.
2 There is no anxiety; the conflict is resolved by the physical symptom.
3 There is no agitation; symptoms are passively accepted.

118. **4 This response focuses the client on the relationship between emotion and physical symptoms in a nonthreatening, accepting manner. (CC; CT; PS; PR; OF)**

1 The nurse knows when the weakness began so it is redundant to ask.
2 This would provide a secondary gain; it implies sympathy and the client avoids an undesired activity.
3 This does not help pinpoint what the person was feeling when the weakness happened.

119. **3 Until the client learns new ways of dealing with anxiety, this pattern of behavior will continue. Learning new ways to operate will break the pattern. (PP; CT; PS; PR; OF)**

1 This would reinforce the sick role.
2 There is a certain amount of stress in everyday family situations, and the client, not the family, must learn new coping mechanisms.
4 This would be unrealistic; the client must learn to cope with problems.

120. **2 This helps the client identify behavior and feelings in a nonthreatening manner. (PP; AF; PS; TR; OF)**

1 This would be ganging up on the client.
3 This evasion and refusal to answer would have the psychologic effect of removing the nurse from the group.
4 The nurse's behavior is not the issue; the situation should be turned back to the client's behavior.

121. **1 These children have difficulty reaching out to the environment and tend to be withdrawn. They frequently get little response from the parents and do not learn how to respond to others.** (DC; KC; PS; EH; CF)

2 The child with failure to thrive is usually non-responsive or only poorly responsive to human contact.

3 These children show little satisfaction and are very difficult to comfort.

4 These children do not respond readily to human contact.

122. **2 A consistent caregiver enhances the formation of a trusting and mutually satisfying relationship between the child and the nurse.** (CC; AP; PS; EH; CF)

1 Overstimulation should be avoided.

3 Stimulation should proceed gradually and be geared to the present level of development.

4 A consistent caregiver enhances the development of trust.

123. **3 Head control and rolling over are achieved at 4 and 5 months, respectively. Transferring objects from one hand to another and sitting unsupported are achieved at 7 and 8 months.** (DC; KC; ED; GD; CM)

1 The ability to roll over is achieved by approximately 5 months of age.

2 Same as answer 1.

4 Transferring objects from hand to hand is usually achieved in approximately 7 months.

124. **2 Fine motor coordination is inadequately developed to manipulate snap toys.** (PL; KC; ED; GD; CM)

1 These are appropriate to stimulate visual attention.

3 The voluntary grasp will allow the child to hold the toy and the rattling sound will stimulate the auditory system.

4 These stimulate the sense of touch, and, since voluntary grasp appears at about 3 to 4 months, they would be handled satisfactorily.

125. **2 Accidental ligation of a ureter is a serious complication of a total abdominal hysterectomy. A decrease in urine output should be reported immediately to the surgeon.** (EV; CT; TC; WH; AF)

1 An apical rate of 90 falls within normal limits but should be evaluated in relation to the client's previous vital signs.

3 Serosanguineous vaginal drainage is to be expected.

4 A nasogastric tube is not routinely inserted.

COMPREHENSIVE TEST: PART B

126. **2 Although the exact mechanism is unknown, steroids produce diuresis in almost all children with nephrotic syndrome.** (IM; KC; PA; DR; CM)

1 Hypertension is not a common finding with nephrotic syndrome.

3 Steroids will not prevent infection and will in fact mask the symptoms of infection and delay treatment.

4 Steroids have no effect on the production of blood cells.

127. **2 Fresh vegetables and meat are lower in sodium compared to canned foods and cured meats.** (CC; AP; ED; FE; CM)

1 Cheese and canned juices have high sodium content and should be avoided.

3 Cheese is a high-sodium food; the bun would not be allowed unless it was low-sodium.

4 Bacon, bread, and canned soup all have high sodium content and should be avoided.

128. **3 This allows an active 3½-year-old to move within restrictions and encourages use of the imagination.** (IM; CT; ED; GD; CM)

1 Unless carefully selected, many shows are inappropriate and uninteresting for a 3½-year-old.

2 Although a 3½-year-old may still cling to a security toy, it would not allow for expenditure of energy.

4 This may provide the child with rest, but this activity is too simple for this age child and will not promote development.

129. **3 Regression frequently occurs during and after hospitalization; guilt about his regression should be avoided, but this behavior should not be encouraged.** (IM; AF; ED; EH; CM)

1 Although punishment is a form of attention, it will not help the child overcome the problem causing the behavior.

2 Nephrotic syndrome is not associated with neurogenic control of the bladder.

4 This will shame the child; accepting the child's regressive behavior but not encouraging it is the best response.

130. 2 **A positive OCT indicates uteroplacental insufficiency, which usually heralds potential fetal distress during delivery. Prompt intervention is indicated to deliver a healthy fetus.** (EV; KC; ED; HP; AF)

1 This is only part of the evaluation; the occurrence of decelerations and accelerations is also evaluated.

3 The small dose of oxytocin is too small to test completely the ability of the uterus to contract.

4 The OCT is unrelated to the mother; it is concerned only with the ability of the fetus to tolerate labor.

131. 1 **The OCT will take 1 to 2 hours, during which time the client is confined to bed. Movement on and off a bedpan should be avoided.** (IM; AP; ED; HP; AF)

2 Valium could interfere with the results of the OCT, since the baby would be sedated.

3 The client may go home 1 hour after the test.

4 No food restrictions are indicated for this test.

132. 1 **This is done to measure baseline FHR variability and to observe any FHR alteration without oxytocin-induced stress.** (IM; AP; ED; HP; AF)

2 There is no indication for this; the test is concerned only with observing the FHR.

3 This is incorrect; the test involves monitoring the fetal heart during three uterine contractions within a 10-minute period.

4 The semi-Fowler's position with a left-sided tilt is the position of choice.

133. 2 **The nurse should demonstrate to the client a recognition of the verbalized concern and a willingness to listen.** (PP; AF; PS; TR; OM)

1 The client did not state this as the diagnosis; this response puts the client on the defensive.

3 Avoiding the question indicates that the nurse is unwilling to listen.

4 This could increase anxiety and would not reduce worry; furthermore, it cuts off communication and denies feelings.

134. 3 **Certain diagnostic tests (e.g., CBC, urinalysis, chest x-ray examination) are done preoperatively to rule out the existence of health problems that could increase the risks involved with surgery.** (PP; AF; ED; RE; OM)

1 Lack of knowledge without a statement of plans to obtain the information suggests incompetence on the part of the nurse.

2 Feelings would not be dispelled by this response; it also blocks further communication.

4 This is false information; surgery poses a risk despite test results.

135. 1 **Anxiety experienced by a preoperative client can be a disruptive force affecting the client's ability to adapt psychologically and physiologically. For other nursing measures to be effective, it must be alleviated.** (CC; AP; PS; EH; OM)

2 Vital signs must be recorded, for they will serve as a baseline in postoperative assessment; however, reduction of anxiety is the first priority.

3 Diet is limited prior to surgery so residue in the intestines will be decreased.

4 Learning is hampered by high anxiety levels.

136. 4 **Interpretation of pain sensations is highly individual and is based on past experiences, which include cultural values.** (AN; AP; PS; PD; OM)

1 Age and sex affect pain perception only indirectly because they generally account for past experience to some degree.

2 Overall physical condition may affect one's ability to cope with stress; but unless the nervous system were involved, it would not greatly affect perception.

3 Intelligence is a factor in understanding pain, so it can be better tolerated, but it does not affect the perception of intensity; economic status has no effect on pain perception.

137. 4 **Following the administration of certain antihypertensives or narcotics, the client's neurocirculatory reflexes may have some difficulty adjusting to the force of gravity when assuming an upright position. Postural or orthostatic hypotension occurs, and there is a temporarily decreased blood supply to the brain.** (PL; AP; TC; DR; OM)

1 Abdominal pain will not be prevented by the intervention described.

2 Hypertension does not occur.

3 Respiratory distress is an adverse effect of morphine but is not prevented by the intervention described.

138 2 **Pain in the calf may be a sign of thrombophlebitis, a possible postoperative complication. If the thrombus becomes dislodged, it may lead to pulmonary embolism. Any client with this complaint should immediately be confined to bed, and the physician notified.** (AN; CT; TC; CV; OM)

1 Application of heat is a dependent nursing function.

3 Charting does not take precedence over notifying the physician of a potentially serious complication.

4 The leg should not be elevated above heart level without a physician's order; gravity may dislodge the thrombus, creating an embolism.

139. **3 In myasthenia gravis the sensitivity of the end plates at the postsynaptic junction to acetylcholine is reduced, interfering with muscle contraction. Inadequate contraction of the ocular muscles results in double vision (diplopia). (DC; AP; PA; NM; AM)**

1 This is not a symptom of myasthenia gravis.

2 Same as answer 1.

4 Nystagmus is a common symptom of multiple sclerosis.

140. **4 Tensilon is an anticholinesterase compound that drastically increases muscle strength when administered to an individual with myasthenia gravis. (IM; KC; PA; DR; AM)**

1 Prednisolone is a steroid; it is not used to diagnose this disease.

2 Disodium EDTA is a calcium-chelating agent that is not used in the treatment of myasthenia gravis.

3 Dilantin is an anticonvulsant; it is not used to test for myasthenia.

141. **2 Neostigmine bromide (Prostigmin) is an anticholinergic that increases the peristaltic activity of the intestines. The result is hyperactive bowel sounds. (EV; AP; PA; DR; AM)**

1 Bladder distention is not associated with neostigmine.

3 These are not side effects associated with neostigmine.

4 Bradycardia and hypotension may occur with neostigmine.

142. **4 The response should be kept as optimistic as possible while still being realistic. (PP; AF; ED; NM; AM)**

1 This is false reassurance; the client's status will depend on individual response.

2 Medication does not affect progression of the disease; it only treats the symptoms.

3 The individual response varies; this gives false reassurance.

143. **1 Swimming would help keep the muscles supple, without requiring fine motor activity. (AN; AP; ED; NM; AM)**

2 Sedentary activities are not helpful in maintaining muscle tone.

3 This might prove too rigorous for the client.

4 Woodworking requires fine motor activity and would be difficult for the client.

144. **4 Alzheimer's disease is an insidious atrophy of the brain resulting in a gradually diminished intellect. (DC; KC; PA; DD; OM)**

1 TIAs may precede a cerebral vascular accident; this is unrelated to Alzheimer's disease.

2 Alzheimer's is a progressive, deteriorating disease.

3 Alzheimer's is a slow, chronic deterioration of the brain; the role of arteriosclerosis is unclear.

145. **4 Since these clients do experience a lability of mood, it is best to attempt to establish a relationship and give care when they are feeling receptive. (PP; CT; PS; DD; OM)**

1 Clients with this disorder have limited contact with reality.

2 This rejects the client when the client needs the nurse most.

3 This may be of limited help; the client may be unable to do it.

146. **1 Sameness provides security and safety and reduces stress for the client. (CC; AP; PS; DD; OM)**

2 Clients with this disorder do not do well in a constantly changing environment.

3 A challenging environment would increase anxiety and frustration.

4 A nonstimulating environment would add to the client's diminishing intellect.

147. **3 Clients with long-term psychiatric problems who have limited contact with reality can usually still become involved with a remotivation therapy group. The demands of this type of group are limited and self-confining. (AN; KC; PS; DD; OM)**

1 This is suitable for working through emotional problems; these clients are unable to follow the dramatization of emotions.

2 The objective of such therapy is to develop social skills; these goals are inappropriate for clients with this disorder.

4 The objective of this therapy is to perform the activities of daily living.

148. 2 Clients are encouraged to interact with their environment by focusing their attention on some common "emotionally safe" article or activity that most clients can recognize and talk about. (PL; KC; PS; DD; OM)

1 This is more appropriate for clients who have a schizophrenic disorder than for those with dementia, delirium, or other cognitive disorder.
3 The focus is on interpersonal skills and becoming competent or maintaining competence in the activities of daily living.
4 They do have face-to-face contact with other clients, but that is not the objective of the group.

149. 3 Acute leukemia is an excessive, uncontrolled production of immature white blood cells that compete for nutrients and eventually crowd the bone marrow, preventing formation of other blood cells. (AN; KC; PA; BI; CM)

1 The liver and spleen are invaded by leukemic cells.
2 Proliferating cells depress bone marrow production of the formed elements of blood.
4 RBCs and platelets are crowded out by proliferation of leukemic cells.

150. 3 Infection from lowered resistance is a constant threat from the disease and from the immunosuppressant drugs, both of which affect white blood cells. (IM; CT; TC; DR; CM)

1 Although vital signs need to be checked to assess for changes in pulse or BP, unless there is other clinical evidence of bleeding, q2H readings are not needed.
2 The client needs to maintain the physical activity that can be tolerated.
4 Clients need stimuli appropriate for their developmental level except when acutely ill from drug therapy.

151. 2 Constipation from adynamic ileus can be prevented with high-fiber foods and liberal fluids. These will keep the stool bulky and soft, promoting evacuation. (IM; AP; PA; DR; CM)

1 Roughage and fluids are recommended to help minimize the constipation associated with vincristine.
3 Constipation is a common side effect of protein. A diet high in iron may increase constipation. In addition, there is no indication for iron.
4 Vincristine causes constipation; roughage and fluids are needed.

152. 3 The protective blood-brain barrier initially screens leukemic cells from the CNS. However, in advanced stages leukemic infiltration occurs. The chemotherapeutic agents, also screened out by the blood-brain barrier, are ineffective. (IM; KC; ED; NM; CM)

1 Radiation destroys leukemic cells.
2 Radiation does not decrease cerebral edema.
4 Irradiation of the cranium is needed because chemotherapy does not pass the blood-brain barrier.

153. 3 The dependent edema in the ankles is normal. It results from the increased pressure of the uterus on venous return. Elevating the legs encourages venous return. (IM; CT; ED; HC; AF)

1 This can be harmful; increased circulating blood volume during pregnancy must be maintained.
2 This is contraindicated; salt is necessary to retain fluid for the increased circulating blood volume during pregnancy.
4 Diuretics are not used during pregnancy; they may decrease the circulating blood volume.

154. 4 This is recommended to keep weight gain (up to 11 Kg) in balance and to control blood pressure. (PL; KC; ED; HP; AF)

1 Fats should be limited because they could cause an accumulation of unwanted adipose tissue.
2 Decreasing protein intake is not advised for clients with cardiac problems.
3 Increasing sodium intake is not advised for clients with cardiac problems.

155. 3 Clients with Addison's disease must take glucocorticoids regularly to enable them to adapt physiologically to stress and prevent an Addisonian crisis, a medical emergency similar to shock. (PL; CT; ED; EN; AF)

1 Sodium should be taken as desired because hyponatremia frequently occurs from diminished mineralocorticoid secretion.
2 Activity is permitted as tolerated.
4 Frequent visits are not indicated after control is established.

156. 1 Because of diminished mineralocorticoid secretion, clients with Addison's disease are prone to development of hyponatremia. Therefore the addition of salt to the diet is advised. (IM; AP; ED; EN; AF)

2 Caloric intake is determined on an individual basis; diet is not necessarily restricted to 1200 calories.

3 Fluids are not restricted in Addison's disease.

4 Protein is not omitted from the diet; ingestion of essential amino acids is necessary for normal metabolism.

157. **4 When there are not enough circulating glucocorticoids and mineralocorticoids to sustain normal functioning of the body, the following symptoms occur: hypotension, fever, pallor, tachycardia, and cyanosis, an Addisonian crisis. (EV; AP; ED; EN; AF)**

1 This does not occur in an Addisonian crisis.

2 Hypotension, not hypertension, is a sign of an Addisonian crisis.

3 Muscle spasms do not occur in an Addisonian crisis; the client usually progresses into a coma.

158. **4 Prolonged steroid therapy may produce Cushing's syndrome. Signs include slow wound healing, buffalo hump, hirsutism, weight gain, hypertension, acne, moon face, thin arms and legs, and behavioral disturbances. (IM; AP; ED; EN; AF)**

1 Cortisone therapy has a glucocorticoid action, which increases blood glucose levels.

2 Hypertension and fluid retention occur.

3 Hyperkalemia occurs with Addison's disease, not Cushing's syndrome.

159. **1 Some cortisol derivatives possess 17-ketosteroid (androgenic) properties, which result in masculinization. (PP; AP; ED; DR; AF)**

2 Masculinization is not part of the disease; it results from the androgens present in cortisol.

3 Saying not to worry denies the client's concerns; masculinization results from the therapy and will not go away.

4 This response denies the client's feelings.

160. **4 Development of mood swings and psychosis is possible from an overdose of glucocorticoids as a result of fluid and electrolyte alterations. (EV; KC; PA; DR; AF)**

1 This is not a sign of glucocorticoid overdose.

2 Same as answer 1.

3 Same as answer 1.

161. **1 Clients use delusions as a defense and cannot be argued out of them. The nurse's response did not demonstrate acceptance and only added to the client's anxiety and agitation. (PP; AP; PS; MO; OM)**

2 This would only serve to mask the problem rather than planning more suitable intervention.

3 There is nothing to indicate that treatment had not been started toward relieving these symptoms.

4 The client should have a one-to-one relationship with staff before attempting to relate to other clients on the unit.

162. **3 Feelings of hopelessness, helplessness, and isolation dominate the emotional state of the depressed client. The ability to attempt to act out suicide ideation frequently does not occur until psychomotor depression begins to lift. (AN; KC; PS; MO; OM)**

1 This is not true; these clients frequently attempt suicide.

2 A person intent on self-destruction will find a way on any type of unit.

4 This is when the danger is greatest; there is more energy at this time to follow through on a plan.

163. **1 Preoccupied clients are usually not aware of external events. The client has not refused to eat but has simply not responded to external stimuli. Taking the client by the hand to the dining room simply puts the client where the food is. (IM; AP; PS; MO; OM)**

2 The client may be too preoccupied to eat anything; part of the intervention should be directed toward meeting client's nutritional needs.

3 The client probably would not care and probably would not respond.

4 This would allow a withdrawal pattern of behavior to continue.

164. **4 Spending time with clients communicates to them that the staff members feel they are worthy of their attention and that someone cares. (IM; KC; PS; MO; OM)**

1 There is nothing to indicate that the client has a delusion regarding food.

2 Special attention is not the purpose; the goal is to increase the client's self-esteem, self-concept, and self-worth.

3 The goal is eventually to have the client relate to the other clients, not to get away from them.

COMPREHENSIVE TEST ANSWERS

165. 1 **The therapeutic level of lithium carbonate is very close to the toxic level. Therefore it is vital that blood levels of the drug be monitored twice a week during the acute phase and bimonthly once the client is on a maintenance dosage.** (EV; AP; PA; DR; OM)
    2 Lithium does not affect fluid retention; monitoring daily weights is not necessary.
    3 Lithium does not affect the leukocyte levels; monitoring the leukocyte count is unnecessary.
    4 Psychomotor activity should be normal once the maintenance dosage is achieved; careful monitoring of psychomotor activity is not a major priority.

166. 4 **Lithium decreases sodium reabsorption by the renal tubules. If sodium intake is decreased, sodium depletion can occur. In addition, lithium retention is increased when sodium intake is decreased; a low-sodium intake can lead to lithium toxicity.** (IM; AP; ED; DR; OM)
    1 This would not have any effect on the lithium therapy.
    2 If the client is well enough to go home for 3 days, participation in controversial discussions is not contraindicated.
    3 Clients should never adjust the dosage of prescribed medication without the physician's approval.

167. 3 **Because of tissue destruction, sodium ions are lost in the interstitial fluid, whereas potassium ions are liberated from the injured cells. The result is hyponatremia and hyperkalemia.** (AN; KC; PA; IT; OF)
    1 Blood volume decreases, and hypovolemic shock may occur.
    2 Capillary permeability is increased in burns.
    4 Fluid shifts may cause shock, but it is reversible with therapy.

168. 3 **Because of fluid loss via the burned area and sodium reabsorption by the kidneys, which pulls fluid, urinary output is diminished. However, output of 30 ml per hour or less is considered a sign of shock.** (IM; AP; PA; FE; OF)
    1 This amount would cause overload; output is less than 30 ml per hour.
    2 This amount of fluid replacement would be inadequate, and fluid loss excessive in the newly burned client; very little fluid is left to replace losses during the first few days.

    4 This intake is excessive, as is the output; these would not be expected in the newly burned client.

169. 3 **Since a great deal of intravascular fluid is lost during the first 48 hours through evaporation and in the exudate and edema, urinary output is not expected to equal the intake but increases from that of the first day. An output of less than 30 ml per hour is an indication of shock.** (EV; KC; PA; FE; OF)
    1 If half the intake is excreted, insufficient fluid is left to replace losses.
    2 This would not allow for replacement of fluid loss due to burns.
    4 This would probably indicate inadequate kidney perfusion, shock, or kidney damage.

170. 4 **Vitamin C is essential for wound healing. It provides a component of intercellular ground substance that develops into collagen and is necessary to build supportive tissue.** (IM; AP; PA; IT; OF)
    1 To prevent excess fluid retention, which would increase the cardiovascular workload, sodium intake should be regulated.
    2 Decreasing calories could increase the work of the body; this would promote catabolism of body tissue.
    3 To help in repairing damaged tissue, protein intake should be increased.

171. 1 **The skin is the first line of defense against infection. When much of it is destroyed, the individual is vulnerable to infection.** (PL; KC; PA; IT; OF)
    2 Complications such as infection and contractures may still occur during the acute phase and as the client is healing.
    3 Diversional therapy as tolerated may be helpful physically and emotionally.
    4 Removing mirrors can increase anxiety about body image and appearance and lead the client to conclude that the situation is even worse than it is.

172. 1 **After a pneumonectomy the mediastinum may shift toward the remaining lung, or the remaining lung could shift toward the empty space, dependent on the pressure within the empty space. Either of these shifts would cause the trachea to move from its normal midline position. (The trachea is palpated above the suprasternal notch.)** (EV; AP; PA; RE; OF)

2 Metastatic lesions would not appear rapidly.

3 Tracheal edema cannot be assessed through palpation; edema is not a concern when the endotracheal tube is in place.

4 The cuff of the endotracheal tube cannot be assessed through palpation of the trachea.

173. **3 Abstinence 4 to 6 weeks prior to delivery is the best way to avoid contracting the virus and having an outbreak prior to delivery. (IM; KC; ED; WH; AF)**

1 Abstinence is necessary only when disease symptoms are present in the partner and during the last 4 to 6 weeks.

2 Since the herpes virus is smaller than the pores of a condom, this kind of protection has limited effectiveness.

4 Washing is not enough to prevent contraction of this virus; contact has already been made.

174. **4 Placing the expectant mother in a semi-Fowler's position forces the heavy uterus to put temporary pressure on the blood vessels at the site of the separating placenta. This controls bleeding to some extent. (PL; CT; TC; HP; AF)**

1 There is no indication that the clotting mechanism is disturbed.

2 This is contraindicated when placenta previa is suspected; it may further dislodge the placenta.

3 This is contraindicated in any client admitted with vaginal bleeding.

175. **1 Absent or diminished gag reflex could be life threatening. The infant might aspirate mucus or formula. (AN; AP; TC; NN; CF)**

2 This is important but it may be delayed because the mother has been anesthetized; the gag reflex is of primary importance.

3 Same as answer 2.

4 Same as answer 2.

176. **1 Head lag in an infant 6 months old is abnormal and is frequently a sign of cerebral damage. (DC; CT; ED; NM; CM)**

2 The ability to sit unsupported is achieved at 7 to 8 months.

3 The Babinski reflex is normally present until 2 years of age.

4 The tonic reflex and grasp reflex usually disappear at 2 and 3 months, respectively.

177. **4 The infant can be positioned on the back or abdomen to allow for a routine change of head position. The head is elevated to decrease the intracranial pressure by gravity. (IM; AP; TC; NM; CF)**

1 Trendelenburg positioning would be contraindicated, because it might aggravate the ICP.

2 The head is elevated to minimize the increased pressure through gravity.

3 The head is elevated to decrease the intracranial pressure by gravity.

178. **3 The trauma of surgery normally results in some seeping or oozing of blood into the remaining gastric area, which is being immediately suctioned out of the body via the nasogastric tube. (EV; AP; TC; GI; AM)**

1 The trauma of surgery will result in some blood loss, which will continue until coagulation takes place; this is too short a time for this to occur.

2 Same as answer 1.

4 If light-red liquid is still draining 24 to 48 hours after surgery, it is abnormal; the physician should be notified.

179. **2 Too rapid administration can result in hyperkalemia, which can cause a long refractory period in the cardiac cycle and result in cardiac dysrhythmias and arrest. (IM; AP; TC; FE; AF)**

1 This statement is too general; there is no indication of whether it is respiratory acidosis or metabolic acidosis. Metabolic acidosis can cause hyperkalemia.

3 This reaction does not occur in hyperkalemia.

4 Hyperkalemia usually causes nausea, vomiting, and diarrhea, which may result in dehydration; in this instance fluid would shift from interstitial spaces to the intravascular compartment. With edema the fluid shift is in the opposite direction.

180. **2 Smoking increases the acidity of gastrointestinal secretions, which damages the mucosal barrier. (DC; AP; PA; GI; AM)**

1 While blood type O is more frequently associated with duodenal ulcer, type A has no significance.

3 This is unrelated to peptic ulcer disease.

4 This is not directly related to peptic ulcer disease.

181. **3 Small feedings reduce the amount of bulk passing into the jejunum and therefore reduce the fluid shifting into the jejunum.** (IM; AP; PA; GI; OM)
    1 Although a diet high in roughage may be avoided, a low-residue, bland diet is not necessary.
    2 Total fluid intake does not have to be restricted; however, fluids should not be taken immediately before, during, or after a meal because they promote rapid stomach emptying.
    4 Concentrated sweets pass rapidly out of the stomach and increase fluid shifts; consequently the diet should be low in carbohydrates. Protein is needed to promote tissue repair.

182. **1 The size of the breast bud is an indication of gestational age. Small, underdeveloped nipples reflect prematurity.** (DC; KC; ED; HN; CF)
    2 This is not related to gestational age.
    3 This is not a good indication of gestational age; reflexes may be impaired in full-term infants also.
    4 This is not present in normal newborns; it is a clinical manifestation of Down syndrome.

183. **2 A flat position helps prevent problems associated with too rapid reduction of intracranial fluid.** (IM; CT; TC; NM; CM)
    1 Elevation of the infant's head and chest will enhance the flow of CSF by gravity. During the immediate postoperative period, this can cause problems with too rapid reduction of CSF.
    3 Sedatives and analgesics are avoided. They can mask signs of impending loss of consciousness.
    4 Initially, positioning flat is important to prevent serious complications.

184. **2 The first step in the problem-solving process would be exploration so family needs could be identified.** (IM; KC; PS; TR; OM)
    1 Without exploring family needs first, the nurse would not know what direction the family needed.
    3 Without exploring family needs first, the nurse would not know the problems that needed solving.
    4 Without exploring family needs first, the nurse would not know what information was needed.

185. **3 Inclusion in the interview will avoid a feeling of ostracism for the father and will foster his cooperation.** (PP; CT; PS; TR; AM)
    1 Observing one parent feed the baby does not provide the nurse an opportunity to assess family interaction.

    2 Removing the father from the situation decreases his participation.
    4 The father is part of the family, and his feelings will affect the mother as well.

186. **2 Exposure to infection, cold, or overexertion of a client with chronic adrenocortical insufficiency (Addison's disease) can cause circulatory collapse.** (PL; CT; TC; EN; AM)
    1 This would be an appropriate room assignment.
    3 Same as answer 1.
    4 Same as answer 1.

187. **3 Deficiency of the glucocorticoids causes hypoglycemia in the client with Addison's disease. Signs of hypoglycemia include nervousness; weakness; dizziness; cool, moist skin; hunger; and tremors.** (AN; KC; PA; EN; AM)
    1 Hypokalemia is evidenced by nausea, vomiting, muscle weakness, and dysrhythmias.
    2 Weakness with dizziness on arising is called postural hypotension, not hypertension.
    4 This would be evidenced by edema, increased BP, and crackles.

188. **4 Abdominal distention, caused by retention of flatus, is a frequent postoperative problem. A rectal tube will usually accomplish expulsion of flatus in 20 to 30 minutes. Application of heat, in addition to its vasodilating effect, will relax tensed muscles.** (IM; AP; PA; WH; OF)
    1 Carbonated drinks increase flatulence.
    2 Although position changes may promote peristalsis, restriction of oral intake will not.
    3 Distention usually occurs as a result of flatus in the intestines and would not be alleviated by gastric decompression.

189. **3 Curling's ulcer (an ulcer of the upper GI tract) is related to the excessive secretion of stress-related hormones, which increases hydrochloric acid production. H2 antagonists decrease acid secretion.** (IM; KC; ED; DR; AM)
    1 This is not a complication of burns.
    2 Same as answer 1.
    4 This is not a complication of burns unless hypermetabolism or renal failure exists; it is not treated with H2 antagonists.

190. **1 To prevent further maternal and fetal complications, clients must be continuously observed for blood loss by the mon-**

itoring of external bleeding and the counting and weighing of pads. (IM; AP; TC; HP; AF)

2 This would be necessary only if bleeding were continuous and profuse; a cesarean delivery might be necessary.

3 This is unnecessary; there is no indication that the client is preeclamptic or that cerebral irritation is present.

4 To minimize further placental separation, the client would be kept on complete bed rest.

191. **3 A vaginal examination might precipitate severe bleeding, which would be life threatening to the mother and infant and necessitate an immediate cesarean delivery. (PL; AP; TC; HP; AF)**

1 This might lead to further placental separation and severe bleeding before the fetus could be delivered.

2 The vaginal examination might precipitate severe bleeding; there would be no time for induction of labor.

4 This would not be a priority after a vaginal examination, which can precipitate severe bleeding; an x-ray examination would not reveal placental separation, only fetal size and position.

192. **1 This allows the father to express his feelings and is nonjudgmental. (PP; AF; PS; BI; AM)**

2 Direct contradiction often causes defensive reactions and decreases future cooperation.

3 This value-laden statement will place the father on the defensive.

4 The father, as the parent, has a right to make his own decisions; this question will place him on the defensive.

193. **1 MMR is generally given at about 12 months. (IM; KC; ED; BI; CF)**

2 DPTP is given with hemophilus at 2, 4, 6, and 18 months

3 Same as 2.

4 Hemophilus is not given at 12 months.

194. **3 Low platelet count predisposes to bleeding, which may be evident in the urine. Red blood cells are seen microscopically in the sediment. (EV; KC; PA; BI; CM)**

1 Casts are seen in the urine in some kidney disorders.

2 White blood cells occur in the urine when there is a urinary tract infection.

4 Lymphocytes are not normally found in the urine.

195. **4 An infant should receive 60 calories and 88.8 ml of fluid per 454 g daily. (IM; CT; ED NN; CM)**

1 This is too much fluid and too many calories for an infant weighing 2840 g.

2 Same as answer 1.

3 Same as answer 1.

196. **3 An interference with bile flow into the intestine will lead to increasing inability to tolerate fatty foods. The unemulsified fat remains in the intestine for prolonged periods, and the result is inhibition of stomach emptying with possible gas formation. (DC; KC; PA; GI; AF)**

1 Melena is tarry stools associated with upper GI bleeding; diarrhea would be associated with increased intestinal motility.

2 Coffee-ground emesis is usually indicative of gastric bleeding; it is not associated with cholecystitis.

4 Gnawing pain when the stomach is empty is associated with peptic ulcers.

197. **4 Any other action would be an invasion of privacy. The marital status has no bearing on the needs of the client at this time. (PP; AF; PS; TR; AF)**

1 The client's marital status has no bearing on the course of labor.

2 There is no indication at this time that the client requires this referral.

3 This action would be an invasion of privacy.

198. **3 A nasogastric tube attached to suction removes gastric secretions and prevents vomiting. However, if it becomes clogged, secretions may accumulate, leading to distention, nausea, and vomiting. (IM; CT; TC; GI; AM)**

1 An antiemetic should be administered if nausea persists after the patency of the nasogastric tube is established.

2 To promote drainage of vomitus and prevent aspiration, the client should be initially turned on the side.

4 Deep breathing will not prevent vomiting if the nasogastric tube is not patent.

199. **4** **Bleeding disorders are common when bile does not flow through the intestine. Vitamin K, a fat-soluble vitamin requiring bile salts for its absorption, is needed by the liver to synthesize prothrombin.** (AN; CT; PA; GI; OM)

1 Prostaglandins regulate platelet aggregation and control inflammation and vascular permeability.

2 Diaphragmatic excursion itself does not put pressure on the suture line; deep breathing does result in pain.

3 This is untrue; platelets aggregate at the site of injury.

200. **4** **An increase in the extracellular fluid volume can cause a relative decrease in the hemoglobin and hematocrit by dilution of the blood.** (CC; CT; PA; FE; OF)

1 This occurs when the pooling of blood in the peripheral vessels causes hypotension; it rarely occurs with hypervolemia.

2 Headache might accompany overhydration, but rhinitis would not.

3 An increased fluid volume in the intravascular compartment (overhydration) will cause the pulse to feel full and bounding.

201. **2** **Inadequate oxygenation increases demands on the heart. This leads to tachycardia as the body tries to compensate.** (DC; AP; PA; BI; CF)

1 Anemia is usually caused by iron deficiency rather than by blood loss that could cause cold, clammy skin.

3 This is not generally an adaptation associated with decreased hemoglobin.

4 This results from excess carboxyhemoglobin; pallor is more common with anemia.

202. **2** **Decreased oxygen-carrying capacity of the blood may lead to hypoxia during exercise, when oxygen demand is greater.** (AN; KC; PA; BI; CF)

1 Although this may be a cause of dizziness, it is not directly related to anemia.

3 Same as answer 1.

4 Same as answer 1.

203. **3** **Liquid iron preparations may stain tooth enamel, so they should be diluted and administered through a straw.** (IM; AP; PA; DR; CF)

1 To avoid gastric irritation, iron should be given with food.

2 Constipation, rather than loose stools, often results from the administration of iron.

4 To improve absorption, iron may be given with orange juice.

204. **3** **The added cardiac workload of individuals with anemia receiving transfusions increases the risk of heart failure, leading to pulmonary edema.** (EV; CT; PA; RE; CF)

1 This is untrue. This problem occurs with frequent transfusions; it is not increased by anemia.

2 Same as answer 2.

4 Same as answer 2.

205. **1** **Varicose veins are dilated veins that occur as a result of incompetent valves. Varicosities may be due to numerous factors, including heredity, prolonged standing (which puts strain on the valves), and abdominal pressure on the large veins of the lower abdomen.** (AN; KC; PA; CV; OF)

2 Thrombophlebitis is usually a sequela of varicose veins.

3 Atherosclerotic plaques usually occur in arteries, not veins.

4 This is unrelated; this is the rationale for elastic stockings; their action limits venous pooling.

206. **2** **Because of the dilation in the veins and concomitant decrease in arterial flow, the client may experience heaviness or muscle cramps in the legs. Edema, if present, can be relieved by elevating the legs.** (DC; KC; PA; CV; OF)

1 Homans' sign is present in deep vein thrombosis.

3 Edema may be decreased when the extremity is elevated.

4 These signs may indicate early arterial occlusion.

207. **2** **Muscle contraction of the legs promotes venous return and prevents thrombus formation.** (IM; AP; TC; CV; OF)

1 Binders are not used.

3 Active exercises are more beneficial after vein ligation.

4 Sitting in a chair is generally avoided; it flexes the hip and keeps the legs dependent, which diminishes venous return.

208. **4** **Since the superficial vein (saphenous) will be obliterated, it is first necessary to**

determine whether the deep veins will be capable of supporting the return circulation. (PL; AP; PA; CV; OF)

1 Bed rest would promote stasis and thrombus formation.

2 This is insignificant; this vein is generally obliterated with sclerotherapy.

3 Weight loss is desired; however, it is not a prerequisite for surgery.

209. **3 Fetal death may occur in diabetic mothers after 36 weeks of gestation; it can result from acidosis and placental dysfunction; cesarean delivery or induction may be used as necessary. (IM; KC; ED; HP; AF)**

1 Exercise and ambulation are needed to promote adequate circulation and prevent thromboembolism.

2 Fetal growth continues as long as placental functioning is still intact.

4 This is not a routine procedure; insulin is administered according to need.

210. **1 The effects of oral hypoglycemics are not well known; such agents may be teratogenic. (IM; KC; ED; HP; AF)**

2 Oral hypoglycemics are not exogenous insulin.

3 There is often a need for larger amounts of insulin in the latter part of pregnancy.

4 The fetal pancreas does not compensate for the mother's diabetes but it does hypertrophy because of increased insulin secretion to cover increased circulating glucose.

211. **1 Feeding difficulties are due to hypoglycemic effects on the fetal CNS. (DC; CT; ED; HN; CM)**

2 This may be related to hypoxia, not lowered blood sugar.

3 Excessive birth weight is common but does not indicate hypoglycemia.

4 This may be related to prematurity; it is generally not related to hypoglycemia.

212. **4 The nurse, knowing the client was combative, was negligent in not providing close supervision; a reasonable, prudent nurse would have closely observed the client to protect against self-imposed injury as well as to protect others. (PP; AP; PS; MO; AM)**

1 It would be unrealistic to keep a client sedated at all times.

2 This is true of all clients, not only those who are combative.

3 The admitting office may have had no knowledge of the situation; therefore it was the nurse's responsibility.

213. **4 This sets appropriate limits for the client who cannot set self-limits; it rejects the behavior but accepts the client. (PP; CT; PS; MO; AM)**

1 This does not show acceptance of the client, nor does it help the client control behavior.

2 This may have the effect of reinforcing the behavior rather than decreasing it.

3 This does not deal with the problem directly. The nurse's response can confuse the client, because the client may not be aware of why the nurse is refusing to talk.

214. **4 Activities that release tension and use up energy can decrease anxiety. (PL; AP; PS; MO; AM)**

1 This activity requires too much concentration, and the client may use the tools in a self-injurious manner in the process.

2 This activity requires sitting still for prolonged periods and a dexterity that the client would probably find impossible at this time.

3 This activity requires too much concentration.

215. **1 A threat is a type of assault that is an intentional tort. (PP; AP; PS; MO; AM)**

2 Restraints would be cruel, illegal, and unnecessary for this client.

3 The client's behavior may be expected but should be dealt with directly. Behavior should never be ignored.

4 This generalization draws a conclusion that may not be true.

216. **4 Clients who are hyperactive are easily diverted. It is best to use this characteristic behavior rather than precipitate a confrontation. (PP; AP; PS; MO; AM)**

1 This response shows no consideration of how the client may feel.

2 This response shifts responsibility to the physician; the nurse should know that a shopping trip is unrealistic at this time.

3 This response does not deal with reality and only postpones having to deal directly with the problem.

217. **3 A simian crease is a common clinical manifestation. It is readily observable when present. (DC; KC; ED; NM; CM)**
1 Many children who do not have Down syndrome also have rounded occiputs.
2 This is not a characteristic of children with Down syndrome, but of children with congenital hip dislocation.
4 Children with Down syndrome usually manifest hypotonicity of skeletal muscles.

218. **3 Infants with Down syndrome have decreased muscle tone, which compromises respiratory expansion as well as the adequate drainage of mucus. These factors contribute to increased susceptibility to upper respiratory tract infections. (AN; AP; PA; RE; CH)**
1 Impaired hearing is not an expected problem in Down syndrome.
2 Cardiac, not circulatory, problems are common in children with Down syndrome.
4 Slowed development is usually apparent before this time.

219. **4 With the head and chest elevated, gravity promotes respiratory excursion; alternating side-lying positions allows for pulmonary drainage and expansion. (IM; AP; PA; RE; CM)**
1 This would permit the abdominal viscera to impinge on the diaphragm, impeding lung expansion.
2 It is difficult to maintain a 5-week-old infant in this position. In addition this position would not promote rest.
3 This position would make it difficult for the lungs to expand, causing difficulty in breathing.

220. **3 Some mottling is expected because of the circulatory disruption and arterial spasm. Further assessment (e.g., palpation of the pedal pulse) is done to rule out total occlusion. (IM; AP; PA; CV; CM)**
1 Elevation of the leg would be contraindicated as it might reduce arterial flow to the extremity and support bleeding from the puncture site.
2 Mottling would be generalized if due to the external temperature; a blanket would interfere with observation.
4 Other observations should be made before the physician is notified.

221. **2 Parents' responses to their children may greatly influence decisions regarding future care. Learning about their child**

and the child's problem can help lessen guilt feelings. **(PL; AP; ED; GD; CM)**
1 This is essential for all babies.
3 Same as answer 1.
4 Same as answer 1.

222. **1 The first step of cardiopulmonary resuscitation, after determining unresponsiveness, is calling for immediate assistance. (PP; AP; TC; CV; OF)**
2 Establishing an airway, assessing for breathlessness, and initiating rescue breathing would be done after calling for immediate assistance.
3 This would done after calling for immediate assistance.
4 Same as answer 3.

223. **3 CPR by one person is less efficient than that performed by two because of the two activities required. The 2:15 ratio is the most efficient way to provide minimally adequate tissue perfusion. (IM; KC; PA; CV; OF)**
1 This ratio would be used when two people were administering CPR.
2 Ineffective; would result in the circulation of unoxygenated blood.
4 Ineffective; blood would not be circulated while four breaths were being administered, and thus hypoxia would result.

224. **2 The area must be scrubbed to remove oils and debris, which may interfere with the conduction of electrical impulses. (IM; AP; PA; CV; OF)**
1 The use of an antimicrobial agent is unnecessary because there will be no break in the skin.
3 Electrode paste facilitates conduction of electrical impulses and is used regardless of excoriation.
4 Moisture will prevent adherence of the electrodes and thus interfere with impulse conduction.

225. **2 When ventricular fibrillation is verified, the first intervention is defibrillation. It is the only measure that will terminate this lethal dysrhythmia. (IM; CT; PA; CV; OF)**
1 Elective cardioversion delivers a shock during the R wave; since there is no R wave in ventricular fibrillation, the dysrhythmia would continue and death would result.
3 Digitalis preparations are not used in the treatment of ventricular dysrhythmias.
4 If not already in place, an IV line should be inserted as soon as the client is defibrillated.

226. **4 In the absence of oxygen, the body derives its energy anaerobically. This results in a buildup of lactic acid. Sodium bicarbonate, an alkaline drug, will help neutralize the acid, raising the pH. (PL; AP; PA; FE; OF)**
   1 Insulin is used in the treatment of diabetes mellitus; it lowers blood sugar by facilitating the transport of glucose across cell membranes.
   2 Calcium gluconate is used primarily in the treatment of hypocalcemia.
   3 Although potassium is essential for cardiac function, it will not correct acidosis.

227. **3 Warm water will often relax the urinary sphincter, enabling a client to void. (IM; AP; PA; RG; OM)**
   1 The client has already indicated an inability to void.
   2 Since the bladder is already distended, increased fluid intake will only increase pressure and may result in hydronephrosis.
   4 Pressure over a distended bladder induces pain, which causes muscular contraction of the urinary sphincters.

228. **4 After a suprapubic prostatectomy there is generally leakage of urine around the suprapubic tube. This leakage creates an environment in which bacteria can flourish if the dressing is not changed frequently. (IM; KC; PA; RG; OM)**
   1 Uremia is caused by inadequate kidney function; it is not directly related to bladder infection.
   2 Negative pressure on the bladder may traumatize the delicate tissue; urine should flow by gravity.
   3 Clamping off the tube causes urinary stasis, which increases the risk of infection.

229. **3 Pain after a suprapubic prostatectomy may denote retention of urine as a result of blocked drainage tubes or infection, or it may be a normal response to surgery. The possibility of any complication must first be investigated. (IM; AP; TC; RG; OM)**
   1 Analgesics can be administered after the cause of pain has been investigated.
   2 Encouraging fluids without a patent drainage tube will increase pressure and discomfort; assessment should occur before implementation.
   4 The need to measure vital signs is dependent upon the analgesic ordered; assessing the cause of pain takes priority.

230. **3 Straining applies pressure to the operative site. (IM; CT; TC; RC; OM)**
   1 A retention catheter is routinely put in place.
   2 To prevent trauma, negative pressure should not be exerted on the bladder.
   4 Same as answer 1.

231. **4 Cold stress produces hypoxia and acidemia. Because of physiologic factors, such as lack of brown fat, the preterm infant is more vulnerable to cool temperatures. (IM; AP; TC; HN; CM)**
   1 These are not a priority; keeping the baby warm is more important.
   2 Same as answer 1.
   3 This would only be necessary if the infant had an Apgar of 0 to 3.

232. **4 This is the first period of reactivity. The newborn is alert and awake. (AN; AP; ED; NN; CF)**
   1 This is untrue; after the initial cry, the baby will settle down and become quiet and alert.
   2 This occurs after the first sleep.
   3 First sleep usually occurs more than 1 hour after delivery.

233. **3 The brick-red color is caused by albumin and urates that are concentrated because of dehydration, which is normal in the first 10 days. (AN; CT; ED; NN; CF)**
   1 This is unrelated to the sex of the infant; it is not hormonally based.
   2 Iron is eliminated via the gastrointestinal tract.
   4 No medication used in delivery would cause this discoloration.

234. **1 Jaundice occurs because of the normal physiologic breakdown of fetal red blood cells and the immaturity of the infant's liver. (DC; KC; ED; NN; CM)**
   2 Conjugation and excretion, not synthesis of bile, are compromised because of the immature liver.
   3 This is unrelated to the infant's hemoglobin level; the mother and baby have separate circulations.
   4 Babies usually have high hemoglobin and high hematocrit levels.

235. **2 Eye patches are applied to prevent drying of the conjunctiva, injury to the retina, and alterations in biorhythms.** (IM; AP; TC; NN; CF)
   1 The baby will automatically close the eyes in response to bright lights and application of a patch.
   3 The baby should be exposed to bright lights periodically so normal rhythms will become established.
   4 These movements are automatic during sleep phases and will not be affected by eye patches.

236. **2 Exploration of the common bile duct may cause edema; a T tube prevents the edema from obstructing the duct.** (AN; AP; TC; GI; AF)
   1 The cystic duct is ligated when the gallbladder is removed.
   3 The T tube will not prevent the formation of an abscess.
   4 A T tube can be used to inject dye for a cholangiogram, but it is not inserted for that purpose.

237. **2 A colostomy does not function for 2 to 4 days postoperatively because of the lack of peristalsis.** (EV; AP; TC; GI; OM)
   1 Bowel sounds will be absent until peristaltic activity returns.
   3 This would indicate an interference with circulation to the stoma; the stoma should be cherry red.
   4 This would indicate gastric bleeding, which is abnormal.

238. **2 The waste products of protein metabolism are the main cause of uremia. The degree of protein restriction is determined by the severity of the disease.** (IM; AP; ED; RG; OF)
   1 Fluid restriction may be necessary to prevent edema, congestive heart failure, or hypertension; fluid does not directly influence uremia.
   3 Sodium is often restricted to control fluid retention, not uremia.
   4 Potassium is restricted to prevent hyperkalemia, not uremia.

239. **1 If fluid is not draining properly, the client should be positioned from side to side or with the head raised; or manual pressure should be applied to the lower abdomen to facilitate drainage by the use of external pressure and gravity.** (IM; AP; TC; RG; OF)
   2 This deficit is not enough to require notifying the physician.

3 The client's position may be changed prn; a supine position does not facilitate drainage by the use of gravity.
   4 The physician removes the cannula.

240. **4 Keeping a record of what one eats helps limit unconscious and nervous eating by making the individual aware of intake.** (IM; AP; ED; GI; OM)
   1 Limiting calories to 900 per day is a severe restriction and requires a physician's order.
   2 Exercise causes rapid head movements, which may precipitate a Ménière's attack.
   3 This is not always practical and is difficult to implement; assessment of dietary habits is the priority.

241. **2 This provides the opportunity for paternal-infant bonding. Handling the infant may reduce some of the grandfather's anxiety.** (IM; AP; PS; EC; OM)
   1 Although helpful, this does not meet the need for paternal-infant bonding.
   3 This does not recognize the grandfather's anxiety; also, he may not be ready to absorb this information.
   4 This is a simplistic approach to the grandfather's emotional needs and does not deal with the real situation.

242. **3 Immunosuppressive agents are administered to reduce the immune system's tendency to reject the transplanted organ.** (IM; AP; ED; RG; OF)
   1 Urine production occurs almost immediately.
   2 Although fever and edema would occur, hypotension would not; an increased BP would usually be due to fluid retention.
   4 This is untrue; recreation and exercise are encouraged. Only contact sports should be avoided.

243. **4 This response demonstrates some insight; the client assumes the responsibility for her behavior and devises a preliminary plan of action.** (EV; CT; PS; TR; OF)
   1 This response does not show insight; it places blame on the son and promises behavior that is probably beyond her ability.
   2 This response does not show insight but instead places responsibility for her abuse on the son's behavior.
   3 Same as answer 2.

244. 1 **This would provide some security because the client would know what to expect at different periods during the day.** (PP; AP; PS; SA; OF)
    2 This would be inappropriate and would probably increase the client's anxiety. There is no one prototype of a client's role.
    3 This would be inappropriate and would increase the client's anxiety and serve little purpose. Necessary limits should be individually set, not set by regulation.
    4 This would be inappropriate and would be somewhat overwhelming. Many of the regulations would not even apply to the client.

245. 1 **This action provides the disorganized client with the necessary structure to encourage participation and support self-image.** (PP; AP; PS; SA; OF)
    2 This would increase the client's anxiety and foster withdrawal. It would also decrease the client's level of functioning.
    3 This would increase dependency and add to the client's self-doubt.
    4 Same as answer 1.

246. 4 **When respiratory embarrassment occurs, possibly from pressure of the dialysate on the diaphragm, fluid should be removed and the client's vital signs and status observed.** (PP; AP; TC; RC; OF)
    1 The physician should be notified after immediate action is taken.
    2 Treatment is discontinued only if ordered.
    3 This may be indicated after the solution is drained and the diaphragmatic pressure decreased.

247. 1 **The 4-year-old can express feelings better through play than with words.** (PP; AP; PS; EH; CF)
    2 A needle is dangerous; even a play syringe would focus the child's attention on one aspect of treatment, without eliciting broader feelings.
    3 This may help the nurse understand emotional problems; however, it is not as helpful as play therapy in meeting the child's emotional needs.
    4 Understanding explanations requires abstract thinking; 4-year-olds think in a concrete manner.

248. 1 **For a child who is moderately retarded, simple repetitive tasks provide all the challenge needed.** (IM; AP; PS; BA; CF)
    2 This would be asking too much of a moderately retarded child.
    3 Same as answer 2.
    4 Moderately retarded children will not be able to follow many instructions given at a single time.

249. 3 **The cessation of renal function is usually evidenced by a decrease in output to less than 400 ml/24 hours.** (DC; AP; PA; RG; OF)
    1 Although this symptom is related to the renal system, its presence does not indicate kidney damage.
    2 Same as answer 1.
    4 Same as answer 1.

250. 3 **The 4-year-old child has developed trust but still needs frequent support from the parents.** (IM; AP; PS; EH; CF)
    1 The parents may bring a toy, but their presence to provide support and reinforce trust is more important.
    2 The parents should participate in their child's care as much as possible, so there will be no interference with the trust relationship and to provide support.
    4 This is appropriate for an infant who is just developing trust in the parents; hospitalization at 4 years of age should not interfere with this important aspect of personality development.

Focus for Study Worksheet			
Category of concern		**Pathophysiology (basic science)**	**Pharmacology**
Medical-Surgical and Pediatric Nursing	**BI** Blood and Immunity		
	CV Cardiovascular		
	DR Drug-related Responses		
	EH Emotional Needs Related to Health Problems		
	EN Endocrine		
	FE Fluid and Electrolyte		
	GI Gastrointestinal		
	GD Growth and Development		
	IT Integumentary		
	NM Neuromuscular		
	RG Reproductive and Genitourinary		
	RE Respiratory		
	SK Skeletal		
Childbearing and Women's Health Nursing	**DR** Drug-related Responses		
	EC Emotional Needs Related to Childbearing & Women's Health		
	HC Healthy Childbearing		
	HN High-risk Neonate		
	HP High-risk Maternal-Fetal Conditions Affecting Childbearing		
	NN Normal Neonate		
	RC Reproductive Choices		
	RP Reproductive Problems		
	WH Women's Health		
Psychiatric/Mental Health Nursing	**AX** Anxiety, Somatoform, and Dissociative Disorders		
	CS Crisis Situations		
	DD Dementia, Delirium, and Other Cognitive Disorders		
	EP Emotional Problems Related to Physical Health and Childbearing		
	BA Disorders First Evident Before Adulthood		
	MO Disorders of Mood		
	PR Disorders of Personality		
	DR Drug-related Responses		
	EA Eating Disorders		
	PD Personality Development		
	SD Schizophrenic Disorders		
	SA Substance Abuse		
	TR Therapeutic Relationships		

Focus for Study Worksheet—cont'd			
Nutrition	Diagnostic studies	Physical care	Emotional care

The RN Exam List of Competencies (By Group)

Group A: **71 Competencies**
50% to 65% of the RN Exam

Group B: **68 Competencies**
20% to 35% of the RN Exam

Group C: **50 Competencies**
5% to 15% of the RN Exam

Group D: **49 Competencies**
1% to 10% of the RN Exam

GROUP A

DATA COLLECTION

The nurse. . .
- establishes a professional relationship with the client during the initial nursing history (e.g., identifies self by name and role; answers client's questions; provides information concerning the physicial environment, expected routines, and services offered by the facility; interprets the nursing role with respect to availability, approachability, responsibility, and limitations).
- uses appropriate sources for data collection: the client.
- uses appropriate sources for data collection: knowledge from nursing, in related fields and disciplines.
- selects data collection techniques pertinent to the client and the situation (e.g., observation; auscultation; palpation; percussion; inspection; selected screening tests; interview; consultation; measuring; and monitoring).
- conducts an interview with the client using the principles of communication (e.g., listens actively; structures the interview in such a way as to obtain the necessary data).
- collects client-related biophysiological data, through observation and interview, for initial and ongoing nursing assessments (e.g., vital signs; circulatory and respiratory status; lifestyle factors such as sleep and exercise; sensory deficits in hearing, vision, and extremities; level of consciousness).
- collects client-related psychosocial data, through observation and interview, for initial and ongoing nursing assessments (e.g., cultural values, beliefs and customs related to health situation; developmental tasks; spiritual beliefs; family history; perception of present health situation).
- modifies the assessment phase to suit the client's health situation.
- records the data collected.

ANALYSIS AND INTERPRETATION OF DATA

The nurse. . .
- analyzes data by determining a relationship among the various data collected (e.g., determines a relationship among the client's color, blood gas report, and verbalization of dyspnea).
- interprets data based on scientific knowledge and norms (e.g., takes the analyzed data and determines that the client's color, blood gas report, and statement of dyspnea are not normal and that a problem exists with the respiratory system).

- interprets data taking into account the plan of care etablished by the health care team.
- formulates nursing diagnoses that identify actual or potential health problems.

PLANNING CARE

The nurse. . .
- facilitates the client's participation in the planning of care (e.g., fosters an environment that allows for questioning, exchange of information, and a creative approach to care).
- plans nursing interventions that are compatible with the client's existing resources.
- develops the plan of care by: prioritizing client needs.
- develops the plan of care by: establishing expected outcomes for the client.
- develops the plan of care by: identifying nursing interventions.
- develops the plan of care by: prioritizing nursing interventions.
- documents the plan of care.

IMPLEMENTATION

The nurse
- implements nursing interventions using agency policies and protocols, principles of safety, and appropriate resources (e.g., providing support to the client during procedures).
- helps the client to understand the interventions and their relationship to expected outcomes (e.g., possible risk, discomforts, inconveniences, costs).
- modifies interventions to suit the client's situation by: selecting interventions that are consistent with the priority of the health situation.
- modifies interventions to suit the client's situation by: selecting interventions that are consistent with the client's identified concerns and priorities.
- modifies interventions to suit the client's situation by: considering the client's tolerance when sequencing interventions.
- modifies interventions to suit the client's situation by: providing immediate interventions for urgent health situations.
- documents interventions by: using a concise and organized manner.
- documents interventions by: recording them as soon as possible, without compromising client safety.
- documents interventions by: identifying those that are pertinent to the client's situation.
- provides nursing interventions that assist the client to meet altered food and fluid needs by maintaining established peripheral intravenous therapy.

- promotes comfort and pain management by: medicating.
- gives the medication while applying the following principles: demonstrating knowledge of medications.
- gives the medication while applying the following principles: calculating dosage correctly.
- gives the medication while applying the following principles: determining dosage is safe.
- gives the medication while applying the following principles: preparing drug appropriately.
- gives the medication while applying the following principles: administering medication on time.
- gives the medication while applying the following principles: observing for desired effects.
- gives the medication while applying the following principles: observing for side effects.
- gives the medication while applying the following principles: observing for interactions.
- gives the medication while applying the following principles: justifying the administration of a p.r.n. medication.
- gives the medication while applying the following principles: assessing client's perception of the response to medication.
- promotes a safe environment by: correcting factors that are detrimental to the psychological safety of the client.
- uses principles of a helping relationship when providing nursing care by: demonstrating a helping attitude (e.g., empathy, warmth, respect).
- uses principles of a helping relationship when providing nursing care by: using therapeutic communication techniques (e.g., reflection, clarification, summarizing).
- uses principles of a helping relationship when providing nursing care by: identifying communication barriers.
- promotes acceptance of sexuality by: demonstrating nonjudgemental behavior.
- prepares the client for laboratory investigation, diagnostic examinations, and treatments using agency policies and procedures, principles of safety, and appropriate resources (e.g., explaining laboratory tests, diagnostic examinations, and treatments to the client; explaining normal or therapeutic values to the client; obtaining specimens from the client).
- intervenes in response to changes observed in the client's condition by: immediately intervening.
- intervenes in response to changes observed in the client's condition by: intervening according to protocol.
- acknowledges mourning by family members of a deceased client (e.g., offers privacy for them to talk and grieve; explains the compulsory procedures they must go through; ensures that all family members are in a condition to leave the hospital).
- plans for discharge by: anticipating client's health care needs on return to the community.
- plans for discharge by: verifying that the client is able to meet health care needs on discharge (e.g., medication administration, dietary alterations, selfcare activities, resource utilization).

EVALUATION

The nurse observes changes in the client's condition, on an ongoing basis.

COLLABORATION AND COORDINATION

The nurse acts as a health care team member by: establishing and maintaining effective communication with the health care team.

PROFESSIONAL PRACTICE

The nurse. . .
- practices within the provisions governing practice: nurses act and standards of practice.
- practices within the provisions governing practice: code of ethics
- practices within the provisions governing practice: regulations/bylaws respecting nursing acts.
- acts as a client advocate within the health care team by: assisting the client to gain access to quality health care in such a way as to maintain the client's health, safety, and integrity.
- acts as a client advocate within the health care team by: facilitating, ensuring, and monitoring the quality of care received by the client.
- acts as a client advocate within the health care team by: challenging questionable orders and decisions by medical and professional staff.
- acts as a client advocate within the health care team by: protecting individual rights to confidentiality, privacy, beliefs, values.
- acts as a client advocate within the health care team by: reporting incidents of unsafe nursing practice to the appropriate authority.
- acts as a client advocate within the health care team by: reporting unsafe practices of other members of the health team to the appropriate persons.
- assesses self in terms of: performance as a care provider.
- assesses self in terms of: knowledge/experience required to improve practice and promote professional growth.
- exercises judgement when performing agency procedures and job requirements.

- is accountable for own actions.
- assumes responsibility for nursing care, even when assigned to others.
- evaluates own workload, and identifies an unrealistic workload for self.
- having identified an unrealistic workload, asks for assistance if necessary.
- demonstrates behavior consistent with the professional role by accepting constructive feedback from colleagues.

GROUP B

DATA COLLECTION

The nurse uses appropriate sources for data collection: previous and current health records/nursing care plans.

ANALYSIS AND INTERPRETATION OF DATA

The nurse validates the interpretation of the data with other members of the health care team as required.

PLANNING CARE

N/A.

IMPLEMENTATION

The nurse. . .
- promotes ventilation and respiration by: performing cardiopulmonary resuscitation.
- promotes ventilation and respiration by: performing oral or nasal suctioning.
- promotes ventilation and respiration by: administering oxygen.
- promotes ventilation and respiration by: assisting client with deep breathing and coughing.
- promotes ventilation and respiration by: proper positioning.
- promotes circulation by: controlling bleeding.
- promotes circulation by: assisting the client with active and passive exercises.
- provides nursing interventions that assist the client to meet altered food and fluid needs by: promoting adequate oral fluid intake.
- provides nursing interventions that assist the client to meet altered food and fluid needs by: discontinuing intravenous therapy.
- provides nursing interventions that assist the client to meet altered food and fluid needs by: administering/maintaining blood transfusion.
- provides nursing interventions that assist the

client to meet altered food and fluid needs by: recording intake.
- promotes elimination by: caring for drainage tubes and collection devices.
- promotes elimination by: performing bladder catheterization.
- promotes elimination by: measuring output.
- promotes comfort and pain management by: positioning.
- gives the medication while applying the following principles: checking the chart for the original order.
- gives the medication while applying the following principles: identifying correct medication.
- gives the medication while applying the following principles: identifying client.
- gives the medication while applying the following principles: using appropriate administration technique.
- gives the medication while applying the following principles: recording medication appropriately.
- gives the medication while applying the following principles: documenting client's response to medication.
- promotes balance between rest/sleep and activity by: encouraging exercise and ambulation.
- promotes body alignment by: proper positioning.
- promotes hygiene by: assisting client to bathe or bathing client.
- promotes hygiene by: assisting with other aspects of personal hygiene (e.g., mouth care, foot care, perineal care).
- promotes tissue integrity by: providing skin care (e.g., washing, drying, positioning).
- promotes tissue integrity by: providing wound care (e.g., cleansing, dressing).
- prevents infection by: implementing established protocol for reporting.
- prevents infection by: practicing surgical asepsis.
- prevents infection by: practicing isolation techniques.
- prevents infection by: using universal precautions.
- promotes sensory stimulation by: talking with the client during nursing care.
- promotes a safe environment by: monitoring factors that are detrimental to the physical safety of the client (e.g., wet floors, inadequate lighting).
- promotes a safe environment by: monitoring factors that are detrimental to the psychological safety of the client (e.g., lack of privacy; sensory overload; too heavy or too limited schedules).
- promotes a safe environment by: correcting factors that are detrimental to the physical safety of the client.
- promotes a safe environment by: ensuring mechanical equipment/safety.

- promotes a safe environment by: supervising the activities of clients who are at risk.
- promotes a safe environment by: recognizing risks for incidents and accidents.
- promotes a safe environment by: utilizing safety measures to protect self from injury.
- promotes a safe environment by: taking the necessary precautions to prevent accidents, according to the client's condition (e.g., bed rails; accessibility of the call bell; being present when a client is agitated, when the client is transferred to the examination table, or is brought to the operating room; for transfers).
- uses principles of a helping relationship when providing nursing care by: using other means to communicate when barriers exist (e.g., interpreter, touch, gestures).
- uses principles of a helping relationship when providing nursing care by: using appropriate means to communicate with an unconscious client (e.g., talks to client, uses sensory stimulation that is familiar to client).
- uses teaching/learning principles to facilitate client/family learning by: using terminology appropriate for the client/family.

EVALUATION

The nurse. . .
- ensures that the client has received the planned care (e.g., verification with the client, with the staff, in the written documents).
- informs appropriate health team members of significant changes in the client's condition.
- revises the plan of care as indicated.
- evaluates nursing care by: verifying the client's progress toward the expected outcomes.

COLLABORATION AND COORDINATION

The nurse. . .
- informs nursing staff of pertinent information related to nursing care (e.g., changes made in the care plan, changes in the client's behavior).
- requests that the nursing staff report any noticeable changes in the client's condition.

PROFESSIONAL PRACTICE

The nurse. . .
- discovering that, when a client refuses a prescribed treatment, tries to find out the reason for the refusal.
- discovering that a client refuses a prescribed treatment, after discussing it with the client, refers the problem to the professional concerned if treatment is essential.
- discovering that a client refuses a prescribed treatment, records the refusal in the chart.
- asks help and guidance when unable to perform competently.
- questions the appropriate person when agency policies, procedures, and job requirements are considered inappropriate.
- refrains from practicing beyond competence.
- uses means to update competence (e.g., reading; courses; study days; conferences; fieldwork experience).
- demonstrates use of new nursing knowledge in practice.
- demonstrates an attitude of inquiry to enhance nursing practice.
- demonstrates respect for nursing colleagues.
- demonstrates a commitment to the profession of nursing.
- demonstrates behavior consistent with the professional role by: being receptive to change.
- demonstrates behavior consistent with the professional role by: being open to new ideas.
- demonstrates behavior consistent with the professional role by: being honest/sincere.
- demonstrates behavior consistent with the professional role by: practicing confidentiality.
- demonstrates behavior consistent with the professional role by: maintaining clients' privacy.
- demonstrates a caring attitude as the foundation for nursing practice.

GROUP C

DATA COLLECTION

The nurse. . .
- uses appropriate sources for data collection: family members/significant persons.
- uses scientific principles related to the data collection techniques used.
- validates the data with the client/family.

ANALYSIS AND INTERPRETATION OF DATA

The nurse. . .
- validates her interpretation of the data with the client/family.
- formulates nursing diagnoses that identify areas for health promotion.
- validates the nursing diagnoses with the client/family.
- validates the nursing diagnoses with the nursing team.

PLANNING CARE

The nurse. . .

- discusses with the client* the health care outcomes in regard to the health problem or nursing diagnoses.
- develops the plan of care by: establishing target dates.
- develops the plan of care by: identifying required resources.
- consults with members of the health care team in planning care.
- provides the rationale for the plan of care.

IMPLEMENTATION

The nurse. . .

- encourages the client/family to participate in the implementation of care (e.g., administration of insulin, intermittent catheterization).
- provides nursing interventions that assist the client to meet altered food and fluid needs by: maintaining total parenteral nutrition infusion.
- provides nursing interventions that assist the client to meet altered food and fluid needs by: maintaining established central venous intravenous therapy.
- promotes the client's positive self-concept by: facilitating client's integration of changes in body image.
- promotes the client's positive self-concept by: promoting use of effective coping techniques to deal with expected and unexpected life events (e.g., loss).
- promotes the client's positive self-concept by: supporting cultural and spiritual preferences.
- uses teaching/learning principles to facilitate client/family learning by: assessing learning needs.
- uses teaching/learning principles to facilitate client/family learning by: assessing readiness to learn.
- uses teaching/learning principles to facilitate client/family learning by: identifying strategies to facilitate change.
- uses teaching/learning principles to facilitate client/family learning by: validating learning objectives with client/family.
- uses teaching/learning principles to facilitate client/family learning by: implementing a teaching plan.
- uses teaching/learning principles to facilitate client/family learning by: using a variety of opportunities for teaching.

- uses teaching/learning principles to facilitate client/family learning by: creating an environment conducive to learning.
- uses teaching/learning principles to facilitate client/family learning by: using existing resources to support teaching.
- uses teaching/learning principles to facilitate client/family learning by: building on previous experience/education.
- uses teaching/learning principles to facilitate client/family learning by: evaluating the effectiveness of the teaching plan.
- identifies a rapidly changing health situation (e.g., clarifying the problem with the client; determining what the client can do in such a situation; verifying what the client expects of the nurse/support system; suggesting possible solutions; offering the client the necessary support in order to succesfully deal with the situation).
- intervenes in response to changes observed in the client's condition by: maintaining an efficient manner.
- applies the basic principles of rehabilitation (e.g., the beginning is initiated early; the process is gradual; the client's tolerance is respected; the client's improvements are pointed out even if they are minimal).
- plans for discharge by: initiating strategies to maintain continuity of care on discharge (e.g., teaching, referral, family consultation).
- plans for discharge by: validating the client's needs for return to the community.
- plans for discharge by: assisting the client in accessing community resources.

EVALUATION

The nurse evaluates nursing care by: validating the client's perception of their progress toward the expected outcomes.

COLLABORATION AND COORDINATION

The nurse. . .

- assigns health care activities to allied nursing personnel consistent with levels of expertise, education, job description, and client needs.
- provides rationale for the assignment of nursing activities based on client needs, nursing staff competence, nursing staff duties.
- coordinates the care plan to be implemented by other members of the nursing staff.
- acts as a health care team member by: presenting the client's perspective.

---

*Significant persons might be included in these discussions depending on the client's wish.

- acts as a health care team member by: coordinating with the client and other professionals the activities provided for in the therapeutic plan in order to ensure continuity.
- demonstrates leadership skills within the nursing team (e.g., team leader).
- recognizes the components of effective group structure and functioning.
- demonstrates team building skills that promote collegial relationships within the health care team.

PROFESSIONAL PRACTICE

The nurse. . .
- acts as a client advocate within the health care team by: ensuring appropriate and timely responses by health team members.
- discovering that a client refuses a prescribed treatment, accepts the client's decision.
- utilizes responsible practices that contribute to cost-effective use of health care resources.
- identifies and responds to professional, legal, and ethical issues that arise.
- promotes change, utilizing knowledge of formal and informal power structure and appropriate channels of communication.
- participates in planning changes that lead to improvement in the work setting.
- provides constructive feedback to colleagues.

GROUP D

DATA COLLECTION

The nurse. . .
- uses appropriate sources for data collection: other professionals/facilities/agencies.
- collects client-related environmental data, through observation and interview, for initial and ongoing nursing assessments (e.g., housing; work environment; urban or rural community).
- validates the data with other members of the health care team.

ANALYSIS AND INTERPRETATION OF DATA

N/A.

PLANNING CARE

The nurse describes steps in planning nursing care.

IMPLEMENTATION

The nurse. . .
- promotes ventilation and respiration by: using oropharyngeal airway and resuscitation bag.
- provides nursing interventions that assist the client to meet altered food and fluid needs by: assisting with menu/meal planning.
- provides nursing interventions that assist the client to meet altered food and fluid needs by: assisting with oral feeding.
- provides nursing interventions that assist the client to meet altered food and fluid needs by: inserting and removing nasogastric tubes.
- provides nursing interventions that assist the client to meet altered food and fluid needs by: performing gastric feeding via gastrostomy/nasogastric tube.
- provides nursing interventions that assist the client to meet altered food and fluid needs by: maintaining heparin/saline lock.
- promotes elimination by: using and teaching routines and dietary control.
- promotes elimination by: providing ostomy care.
- promotes elimination by: administering enemas and suppositories.
- promotes elimination by: disimpacting.
- promotes elimination by: irrigating bladder.
- promotes comfort and pain management by: applying heat and cold.
- promotes comfort and pain management by: using touch, massage, and stress reduction techniques.
- promotes comfort and pain management by: ensuring proper maintenance of orthesis and prosthesis.
- promotes balance between rest/sleep and activity by: pacing routines and activities.
- promotes balance between rest/sleep and activity by: facilitating diversional activity.
- promotes balance between rest/sleep and activity by: assisting the client with mobilizing devices.
- promotes balance between rest/sleep and activity by: using and teaching relaxation techniques.
- promotes body alignment by: caring for the client with external immobilizing devices.
- promotes sensory stimulation by: preventing overload of sensory stimulation (e.g., mechanical noise, lights).
- promotes sensory stimulation by: facilitating the presence of a significant person.
- promotes sensory stimulation by: touching the client when talking with them.
- promotes sensory stimulation by: using humor.
- promotes acceptance of sexuality by: teaching about safe sexual practices.

- promotes acceptance of sexuality by: promoting healthy sexuality.
- promotes acceptance of sexuality by: teaching about family planning.
- promotes the client's positive self-concept by: validating client's strengths.
- promotes social interaction of clients by: encouraging social participation.
- promotes social interaction of clients by: creating opportunities for social interaction.
- uses teaching/learning principles to facilitate client/family learning by: providing opportunities for client/family to practice new knowledge.
- with the client's consent, instructs family how they may participate in client care (e.g., hygiene, walking, stoma care, baby feeding).
- intervenes in response to changes observed in the client's condition by: intervening according to a standing order.
- justifies the choice of persons she notifies in an emergency situation (e.g., family, priest).

EVALUATION

The nurse evaluates nursing care by: determining the client's/family's satisfaction.

COLLABORATION AND COORDINATION

The nurse. . .
- describes the functions of the other categories of nursing staff.

- acts as a health care team member by: clarifying the nurses' role and responsibilities to other team members.
- acts as a health care team member by: contributing to the identification of health issue(s)/problems from the nursing perspective.
- acts as a health care team member by: sharing knowledge and expertise with others.
- acts as a health care team member by: referring problems to appropriate team members/agencies as necessary (e.g., seeking support in care the nurse cannot totally conduct—spiritual, nutritional).
- acts as a health care team member by: supporting the contribution of each member of the health care team.

PROFESSIONAL PRACTICE

The nurse. . .
- describes the independent and interdependent functions related to the role of the nurse.
- states the professional goals of nursing practice.
- recognizes the importance of research as a basis for nursing practice.
- incorporates relevant research findings in nursing practice.
- understands the function of the health care delivery system: within the province of licensure.

Reprinted with permission from the Canadian Nurses Association.

BIBLIOGRAPHY

BIBLIOGRAPHY

General

Canadian Pharmaceutical Association: *Compendium of pharmaceuticals and specialties,* ed 13, Ottawa, Ontario, 1995, Canadian Pharmaceutical Association.

McHenry L et al: *Mosby's pharmacology in nursing,* ed 19, St. Louis, 1995, Mosby.

The Canadian Red Cross: *Basic life support,* St. Louis, 1994, Mosby Lifeline.

Colombo, JR (ed): *Canadian global almanac,* Toronto, 1994, Mac Millan Canada.

Nair C, Karim R, Nyers C: Health care and health status: A Canada–United States statistical comparison, *Health Reports* 4(2): 181, 1992.

Health and Welfare Canada: *Nutrition recommendations: The report of the Scientific Review Committee,* 1990, Ottawa: Minister of Supply and Sciences, vol 24; 2303

Statistics Canada: *Mortality: Summary list of causes 1992,* Ottawa: Statistics Canada (Catalogue No. 84-209 annual)

Components of Nursing Practice

Angus DE, Turbayne E: *Path to the future: A synopsis of health and health care issues* (File: 492-273), Ottawa, 1995, National Nursing Competency Project.

Baumgart AJ, Larsen J, editors: *Canadian nursing faces the future,* ed 2, St. Louis, 1996, Mosby.

Du Gas L, Knor E: *Nursing foundations: A Canadian perspective,* Scarborough, ON, 1995, Appleton & Lange.

Kerr JR, MacPhail J, editors: *Canadian nursing: Issues and perspectives,* ed 3, St. Louis, 1996, Mosby.

Joint statement on terminal illness, *Canadian Nurse* 80(6): 24, 1984.

Minister of Supplies and Services Canada: *The charter of rights and freedom: A guide for Canadians* (Cat. No. CP45-24/1982-1), Ottawa, 1982, Publications Canada.

Rachlis M, Kushner C: *Strong medicine: How to save Canada's health care system,* Toronto, 1994, Harper Collins.

Registered Nurses Association of British Columbia: *Standards for nursing practice in British Columbia,* Vancouver, BC, 1992, Registered Nurses Association of British Columbia.

Rozovsky L: *The Canadian patient's book of rights: A consumer's guide to Canadian health law* (rev. ed.), Toronto, 1994, Doubleday.

Childbearing and Women's Health

Ministry of Health: *Baby's best chance: Parents' handbook of pregnancy and baby care,* ed 4, Toronto, 1994, Macmillan Canada.

Bloon R, Cropley C. *Neonatal resuscitation,* 1994, American Academy of Pediatrics and the American Heart Association (Endorsed in full by the Canadian Pediatrics Association.)

Bobak IM, Lowdermilk DL, and Jensen MD: *Maternity nursing,* ed 4, St. Louis, 1994, Mosby.

Bobak IM and Jensen MD: *Maternity and gynecologic care,* ed 5, St. Louis, 1993, Mosby.

British Columbia Reproductive Care Program: *British Columbia reproductive care program guidelines for maternal and newborn care,* Vancouver, British Columbia, 1995.

Dickason EJ et al: *Maternal and infant nursing care,* ed 2, St. Louis, 1994, Mosby.

Edge V and Miller M: *Women's health care,* St. Louis, 1994, Mosby.

Gilbert ES and Harmon JS: *Manual of high-risk pregnancy and delivery,* St. Louis, 1993, Mosby.

Health and Welfare Canada: *Family centred maternity and newborn care: National guidelines,* ed 4, Ottawa, 1988, Gage Publishing.

Lawrence RA: *Breastfeeding: A guide for the medical profession,* ed 4, St. Louis, 1994, Mosby.

Phillips CR: *Family-centered maternity/newborn care,* ed 3, St. Louis, 1992, Mosby.

Tucker SM: *Pocket guide to fetal monitoring,* ed 2, St. Louis, 1992, Mosby.

Weiner SM: *Clinical manual of maternity and gynecologic nursing,* St. Louis, 1989, Mosby.

Worthington-Roberts BS and Williams SR: *Nutrition in pregnancy and lactation,* ed 5, St. Louis, 1993, Mosby.

Psychiatric Mental Health Nursing

Aguilera DC: *Crisis intervention: Theory and methodology,* ed 7, St. Louis, 1994, Mosby.

Fawcett C: *Family psychiatric nursing,* St. Louis, 1993, Mosby.

Haber J et al: *Comprehensive psychiatric nursing,* ed 4, St. Louis, 1992, Mosby.

Keltner NL, Schwecke LH, and Bostrom CE: *Psychiatric nursing,* ed 2, St. Louis, 1994, Mosby.

Pasquali EA, Arnold HM, and DeBasio N: *Mental-health nursing: a holistic approach,* ed 3, St. Louis, 1989, Mosby.

Rawlins RP, Williams SR, and Beck CK: *Mental health-psychiatric nursing,* ed 3, St. Louis, 1993, Mosby.

Stuart GW and Sundeen SJ: *Principles and practice of psychiatric nursing,* ed 5, St. Louis, 1994, Mosby.

Sundeen SJ et al: *Nurse-client interaction: Implementing the nursing approach,* ed 5, St. Louis, 1994, Mosby.

Taylor CM: *Essentials of psychiatric nursing,* ed 14, St. Louis, 1994, Mosby.

Pediatric Nursing

Betz CL and Poster E: *Mosby's pediatric nursing reference,* ed 2, St. Louis, 1992, Mosby.

Betz CL et al: *Family-centered nursing care of children,* ed 2, Philadelphia, 1994, WB Saunders.

Engel J: *Pocket guide to pediatric assessment,* ed 2, St. Louis, 1993, Mosby.

Hazinski MF: *Nursing care of the critically ill child,* ed 2, St. Louis, 1992, Mosby.

Keller L and Weir A: *The outline series: Pediatric nursing,* St. Louis, 1994, Mosby.

Merenstein GB and Gardner SL: *Handbook of neonatal intensive care*, ed 3, St. Louis, 1993, Mosby.

Pipes PL and Trahms CM: *Nutrition in infancy and childhood*, ed 5, St. Louis, 1993, Mosby.

Wong DL: *Whaley & Wong's nursing care of infants and children*, ed 5, St. Louis, 1994, Mosby.

Wong DL: *Whaley & Wong's essentials of pediatric nursing*, ed 4, St. Louis, 1993, Mosby.

Wong DL and Whaley LF: *Clinical manual of pediatric nursing*, ed 3, St. Louis, 1990, Mosby.

Medical-Surgical Nursing

Berne RM and Levy MN, eds: *Physiology*, ed 3, St. Louis, 1993, Mosby.

Berne RM and Levy MN: *Cardiovascular physiology*, ed 6, St. Louis, 1992, Mosby.

Bowers AC and Thompson JM: *Clinical manual of health assessment*, ed 4, St. Louis, 1992, Mosby.

Brooks Tighe SM: *Instrumentation for the operating room: a photographic manual*, ed 4, St. Louis, 1994, Mosby.

Canobbio MM: *Cardiovascular disorders*, St. Louis, 1990, Mosby.

Christensen PJ and Kenney JW: *Nursing process: application of conceptual models*, ed 4, St. Louis, 1994, Mosby.

Clark JB, Queener SF, and Karb VB: *Pharmacological basis of nursing practice*, ed 4, St. Louis, 1993, Mosby.

Conover MB: *Understanding electrocardiography*, ed 6, St. Louis, 1992, Mosby.

Daily EK and Schroeder JS: *Techniques in bedside hemodynamic monitoring*, ed 5, St. Louis, 1994, Mosby.

Ebersole P and Hess P: *Toward healthy aging: human needs and nursing response*, ed 4, St. Louis, 1994, Mosby.

Gahart BL: *Intravenous medications*, ed 11, St. Louis, 1994, Mosby.

Gordon M: *Manual of nursing diagnosis*, 1995-1996, St. Louis, 1995, Mosby.

Groer MW and Shekleton ME: *Basic pathophysiology: a holistic approach*, ed 3, St. Louis, 1989, Mosby.

Kim MJ, McFarland GK, and McLane AM: *Pocket guide to nursing diagnosis*, ed 6, St. Louis, 1995, Mosby.

Kinney MK et al: *Comprehensive cardiac care*, ed 8, St. Louis, 1995, Mosby.

Lee G: *Quick emergency care reference*, St. Louis, 1992, Mosby.

Long BC, Phipps WJ, and Cassmeyer VL: *Medical-surgical nursing: a nursing process approach*, ed 3, St. Louis, 1993, Mosby.

Malasanos L et al: *Health assessment*, ed 4, St. Louis, 1990, Mosby.

Marriott HJL and Conover MB: *Advanced concepts in arrhythmias*, ed 2, St. Louis, 1989, Mosby.

McKenry LM and Salerno E: *Mosby's pharmacology in nursing*, ed 19, St. Louis, 1994, Mosby.

Meeker MH and Rothrock JC: *Alexander's care of the patient in surgery*, ed 10, St. Louis, 1994, Mosby.

Ogilvie RI et al: Report of the Canadian Hypertension Society Consensus Conference: 3. Pharmacologic treatment of essential hypertension, *Canadian Medical Association Journal* 149(5): 575–584, 1993.

Pagana KD and Pagana TJ: *Mosby's diagnostic and laboratory test reference*, ed 2, St. Louis, 1994, Mosby.

Perry AG and Potter PA: *Clinical nursing skills and techniques*, ed 3, St. Louis, 1994, Mosby.

Phipps WJ et al: *Medical-surgical nursing: concepts and clinical practice*, ed 5, St. Louis, 1994, Mosby.

Potter PA and Perry AG: *Fundamentals of nursing: concepts, process, and practice*, ed 3, St. Louis, 1993, Mosby.

Redman BK: *The process of patient education*, ed 7, St. Louis, 1993, Mosby.

Reeves RA et al: Report of the Canadian Hypertension Society Consensus Conference: 4. Hypertension in the elderly, *Canadian Medical Association Journal* 149(6):815–820, 1993.

Saxton DF and Ercolano-O'Neill N: *Basic math and meds for nurses: a programmed approach for calculations of drugs and solutions*, St. Louis, 1992, G. W. Manning & Associates.

Seidel HM et al: *Mosby's guide to physical examination*, ed 3, St. Louis, 1994, Mosby.

Sheehy SB: *Emergency nursing: principles and practice*, ed 3, St. Louis, 1992, Mosby.

Skidmore-Roth L: *Mosby's 1995 nursing drug reference*, ed 8, St. Louis 1994, Mosby.

Sundeen SJ et al: *Nurse-client interaction: implementing the nursing process*, ed 5, St. Louis, 1994, Mosby.

Thibodeau GA and Patton K: *Anatomy and physiology*, ed 2, St. Louis, 1993, Mosby.

Thompson JM et al: *Mosby's clinical nursing*, ed 3, St. Louis, 1993, Mosby.

Thompson JM and Bowers AC: *Health assessment: an illustrated pocket guide*, ed 3, St. Louis, 1992, Mosby.

Tucker SM et al: *Patient care standards: nursing process, diagnosis, and outcome*, ed 5, St. Louis, 1992, Mosby.

Urden LD, Davie JK, and Thelan LA: *Essentials of critical care nursing*, St. Louis, 1992, Mosby.

Vinsant-Crawford MO and Spence MI: *Commonsense approach to coronary care: a program approach*, ed 6, St. Louis, 1994, Mosby.

Weldy NJ: *Body fluids and electrolytes*, ed 6, St. Louis, 1992, Mosby.

Wilkins RL, Sheldon, RL, and Krider SJ: *Clinical assessment in respiratory care*, ed 3, St. Louis, 1994, Mosby.

Williams SR: *Nutrition and diet therapy*, ed 7, St. Louis, 1993, Mosby.

INDEX